HUTCHISON'S
PAEDIATRICS

HUTCHISON'S PAEDIATRICS

Edited by

Krishna M Goel
MD, DCH, FRCP (Lond, Edin and Glas), Hon FRCPCH
Formerly Honorary Senior Lecturer of Child Health
University of Glasgow and Consultant Paediatrician
at the Royal Hospital for Sick Children
Yorkhill, Glasgow, Scotland, UK

Devendra K Gupta
MS, MCh, FAMS, FRCS (Hon), DSc (Honoris Causa)
Professor and Head
Department of Paediatric Surgery
All India Institute of Medical Sciences
Ansari Nagar, New Delhi, India

Foreword
Meharban Singh

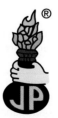

JAYPEE BROTHERS MEDICAL PUBLISHERS (P) LTD

New Delhi • Ahmedabad • Bengaluru • Chennai • Hyderabad
Kochi • Kolkata • Lucknow • Mumbai Nagpur • St Louis (USA)

Published by

Jitendar P Vij

Jaypee Brothers Medical Publishers (P) Ltd

Corporate Office

4838/24 Ansari Road, Daryaganj, **New Delhi** - 110002, India, Phone: +91-11-43574357

Registered Office

B-3 EMCA House, 23/23B Ansari Road, Daryaganj, **New Delhi** - 110 002, India

Phones: +91-11-23272143, +91-11-23272703, +91-11-23282021, +91-11-23245672

Rel: +91-11-32558559, Fax: +91-11-23276490, +91-11-23245683

e-mail: jaypee@jaypeebrothers.com, Website: www.jaypeebrothers.com

Branches

* 2/B, Akruti Society, Jodhpur Gam Road Satellite
  Ahmedabad 380 015, Phones: +91-79-26926233, Rel: +91-79-32988717
  Fax: +91-79-26927094, e-mail: ahmedabad@jaypeebrothers.com

* 202 Batavia Chambers, 8 Kumara Krupa Road, Kumara Park East
  Bengaluru 560 001, Phones: +91-80-22285971, +91-80-22382956, 91-80-22372664
  Rel: +91-80-32714073, Fax: +91-80-22281761, e-mail: bangalore@jaypeebrothers.com

* 282 IIIrd Floor, Khaleel Shirazi Estate, Fountain Plaza, Pantheon Road
  Chennai 600 008 Phones: +91-44-28193265, +91-44-28194897, Rel: +91-44-32972089
  Fax: +91-44-28193231, e-mail: chennai@jaypeebrothers.com

* 4-2-1067/1-3, 1st Floor, Balaji Building, Ramkote Cross Road
  Hyderabad 500 095, Phones: +91-40-66610020, +91-40-24758498, Rel: +91-40-32940929
  Fax:+91-40-24758499, e-mail: hyderabad@jaypeebrothers.com

* No. 41/3098, B and B1, Kuruvi Building, St. Vincent Road
  Kochi 682 018, Kerala, Phones: +91-484-4036109, +91-484-2395739, +91-484-2395740
  e-mail: kochi@jaypeebrothers.com

* 1-A Indian Mirror Street, Wellington Square
  Kolkata 700 013, Phones: +91-33-22651926, +91-33-22276404, +91-33-22276415
  Rel: +91-33-32901926, Fax: +91-33-22656075, e-mail: kolkata@jaypeebrothers.com

* Lekhraj Market III, B-2, Sector-4, Faizabad Road, Indira Nagar
  Lucknow 226 016, Phones: +91-522-3040553, +91-522-3040554, e-mail: lucknow@jaypeebrothers.com

* 106 Amit Industrial Estate, 61 Dr SS Rao Road, Near MGM Hospital, Parel
  Mumbai 400 012, Phones: +91-22-24124863, +91-22-24104532, Rel: +91-22-32926896
  Fax: +91-22-24160828, e-mail: mumbai@jaypeebrothers.com

* "KAMALPUSHPA" 38, Reshimbag, Opp. Mohota Science College, Umred Road
  Nagpur 440 009 (MS), Phone: Rel: +91-712-3245220, Fax: +91-712-2704275, e-mail: nagpur@jaypeebrothers.com

USA Office

1745, Pheasant Run Drive, Maryland Heights (Missouri), MO 63043, USA, Ph: 001-636-6279734

e-mail: jaypee@jaypeebrothers.com, anjulav@jaypeebrothers.com

Hutchison's Paediatrics

© 2009, Krishna M Goel, Devendra K Gupta

This book has been published in good faith that the material provided by contributors is original. Every effort is made to ensure accuracy of material, but the publisher, printer and editors will not be held responsible for any inadvertent error(s). In case of any dispute, all legal matters are to be settled under Delhi jurisdiction only.

First Edition : **2009**

ISBN 978-81-8448-586-8

Typeset at JPBMP typesetting unit

Printed at Replika Press Pvt. Ltd.

Contributors

Alison M Cairns
MSc, BDS, MFDS, FRCS (Edin), M Paed Dent (RCPSG)
Clinical Lecturer in Paediatric Dentistry
University of Glasgow, Dental Hospital and School
Glasgow, Scotland, UK

Anne Devenny
MBChB, MRCP (UK), FRCPCH
Paediatric Respiratory Consultant
Royal Hospital for Sick Children
Glasgow, Scotland, UK

Benjamin Joseph
MBBS, MS Orth, MCh Orth
Professor of Orthopaedics and
Head of Paediatric Orthopaedic Service
Kasturba Medical College, Manipal
Karnataka, India

Christina Halsey
BM, Bch, BA (Hons), MRCP, MRCPath
Leukaemia Research Fund Clinical Research Fellow
Royal Hospital for Sick Children
Glasgow, Scotland, UK

Craig McWilliam
MD, FRCP, FRCPath
Consultant Microbiologist
Royal Hospital for Sick Children
Glasgow, Scotland, UK

David James
MBChB, Dip Ed, DCH, DPM, FRCPsych, FRCP (Glas)
Retired Child Psychiatrist
Formerly at Department of Child and Family Psychiatry
Royal Hospital for Sick Children
Glasgow, Scotland, UK

Devendra K Gupta
MS, MCh, FAMS, FAMS (Hon), FRCS (Hon), DSc (Honoris Causa)
Professor and Head, Department of Pediatric Surgery
All India Institute of Medical Sciences
Ansari Nagar, New Delhi, India

Elizabeth A Chalmers
MBChB, MD, MRCP, FRCPath
Consultant Paediatric Haematologist
Royal Hospital for Sick Children
Glasgow, Scotland, UK

James Wallace
BSc, MR Pharma, FRCPCH (Hon)
Chief Pharmacist
Yorkhill Hospitals, Glasgow
Scotland, UK

Jugesh Chhatwal
MD, DCH
Professor and Head of Paediatrics
Christian Medical College, Ludhiana
Punjab, India

Kirsteen J Thompson
FRCS (Edin), Ophthalmologist
45, Station Road, Milngavie, Scotland, UK

Krishna M Goel
MD, DCH, FRCP (Lond, Edin and Glas), Hon FRCPCH
Formerly Honorary Senior Lecturer of Child Health
University of Glasgow and Consultant Paediatrician
Royal Hospital for Sick Children
Glasgow, Scotland, UK

Louis Low
MBChB, MRCP (UK), FRCP (Lond, Edin and Glas), FRCPCH
Professor of Paediatrics
The University of Hong Kong
Queen Mary Hospital, Pokfulam
Hong Kong

Margo Whiteford
BSc, FRCP
Consultant Clinical Geneticist
Ferguson-Smith Centre for Clinical Genetics
Yorkhill Hospital, Glasgow
Scotland, UK

Mary Mealyea
MBChB, Diploma in Dermatology
Associate Specialist in Paediatric Dermatology
Royal Hospital for Sick Children
Glasgow, Scotland, UK

Michael Morton
MPhil, MA, MBChB, FRCPsych, FRCPCH
Consultant Child and Adolescent Psychiatrist
Department of Child and Family Psychiatry
Royal Hospital for Sick Children
Glasgow, Scotland, UK

N Doraiswamy
MS, FRCS (Edin and Glas), FICS, FISS, FFAEM, FRCPCH
Consultant Surgeon (Retired)
Royal Hospital for Sick Children
Glasgow, Scotland, UK

Paul Galea
MD, DCH, FRCP (Glas), FRCPCH
Consultant Paediatrician
Royal Hospital for Sick Children, Glasgow, Scotland, UK

Peter Galloway
BSc, DCH, FRCP (Edin and Glas), FRCPath
Consultant Clinical Biochemist
Royal Hospital for Sick Children
Glasgow, Scotland, UK

Phyllis Kilbourn
International Director, Crisis Care Training International
International Office, PO Box 517
Fort Mill, South Carolina, USA

Prabhakar D Moses
MBBS, MD (Paed), MRCP (UK), FRCP (Edin), FCAMS
Professor and Head of Child Health Unit 111
Christian Medical College
Vellore, Tamil Nadu, India

Richard Welbury
BDS (Hons), MBBS, PhD, FDSRCS, FDSRCPS, FRCPCH
Professor of Paediatric Dentistry
University of Glasgow Dental Hospital and School
Glasgow, Scotland, UK

Robert Carachi
MD, PhD, FRCS (Glas, Eng), FEBPS
Professor of Surgical Paediatrics
University of Glasgow
Royal Hospital for Sick Children
Glasgow, Scotland, UK

Rosie Hague
MD, MRCP (UK), FRCPCH
Consultant Paediatric Id/Immunology
Yorkhill NHS Trust
Royal Hospital for Sick Children, Glasgow, Scotland, UK

Rosemary Sabatino
Trainer and Educator
Crisis Care Training International
International Office
PO Box 517, Fort Mill, South Carolina, USA

Sandra J Butler
BSc (Hons), MBChB, MRCPCH, FRCR
Consultant Paediatric Radiologist
Royal Hospital for Sick Children
Glasgow, Scotland, UK

Sanjay V Maroo
MBChB, M-Med, FRCR
Consultant Paediatric Radiologist
Royal Hospital for Sick Children
Glasgow, Scotland, UK

Sarada David
MS DO
Professor and Head
Department of Ophthalmology
Christian Medical College
Vellore, Tamil Nadu, India

Shilpa Sharma
MBBS, MS, MCh, DNB
Senior Research Associate
Department of Paediatric Surgery
All India Institute of Medical Sciences
Ansari Nagar, New Delhi, India

Syed Rehan Ali
MB, DCH, MRCPI
Consultant and Senior Instructor in Neonatal Medicine
Department of Paediatrics and Child Health
Aga Khan University Hospital
Karachi, Pakistan

Tahmeed Ahmed
MBBS, PhD
Head, Nutrition Programme Scientist, Clinical Sciences Division
International Centre for Diarrhoeal Diseases Research, B
Dhaka, Bangladesh

Trevor Richens
MBBS, BSc (Hons), MRCP (Lond)
Consultant Paediatric Cardiologist
Royal Hospital for Sick Children, Glasgow
Scotland, UK

Zulfiqar Ahmed Bhutta
MBBS, FRCP, FRCPCH, FCPS, PhD
The Husein Lalji Dewraj Professor and Chairman
Department of Pediatrics and Child Health
The Aga Khan University and Medical Center
Karachi, Pakistan

Foreword

Children constitute the foundation of the human race and the basic aim of paediatrics is to ensure that every child is assisted to achieve his/her optimal genetic potential for physical growth and mental development. There is increasing evidence that seeds of most adult diseases are sown in childhood, and effective health care of children is, therefore, crucial to ensure that every child is assisted to become a strong, healthy and productive adult. The art and understanding of health problems of children have undergone rapid advances with a dual challenge of delivery of primary or essential health care at their doorsteps, to the most intensive care in a tertiary care setting with various grades of care in-between.

The scope of paediatrics has now become broader, encompassing the vital period of adolescence. Above all, paediatrics is now being recognized as a separate independent discipline in undergraduate medical curriculum in most countries.

Hutchison's Paediatrics has been created by taking excerpts as rennet from "Children's Medicine and Surgery" edited by Cockburn, Carachi, Goel and Young, which have been amplified with outstanding contributions of core contents by eminent international paediatric experts under the authoritative patronage of legendary Hutchison.

Editors Krishna M Goel and Devendra K Gupta deserve our accolades for creating a comprehensive Textbook of Paediatrics covering practically all the medical and surgical conditions of children from birth through adolescence. The contributors have provided state-of-the-art information and their own personal experiences pertaining to the fields of their expertise. Each chapter has laid emphasis on anatomical and physiological background, etiopathogenesis, clinical spectrum, diagnosis and management in a lucid manner. The text is amply supported by illustrations, line diagrams, charts, tables and photographs. The format, composing and quality of production are commendable.

I have no doubt that *Hutchison's Paediatrics* would fulfill the felt needs of graduate and postgraduate students in paediatrics and paediatric surgery as well as paediatricians and family physicians because of cultural, ethnic, social, economic and ecological similarities.

Meharban Singh
MD, FAMS, FIAP, FIMSA, FAAP
Ex-President
National Neonatology Forum of India and
Indian Academy of Paediatrics

Former Professor and Head
Department of Paediatrics
All India Institute of Medical Sciences
New Delhi, India

Preface

The patterns of childhood disease throughout the world are changing with advancing knowledge, altering standards of living, life style and rising levels of medical care. The origins of physical and mental health and disease lie predominantly in the early development of the child. Most of the abnormalities affecting the health and behaviour of children are determined prenatally or in the first few years of life by genetic and environmental factors. The range of contributors indicates that they are all experts in their particular fields. The authors have summarised the current knowledge of causation and have indicated where health education and prevention might reduce the burden of childhood ill health. We seek in this book to provide practical advice about the diagnosis, investigation and management of the full spectrum of childhood disorders, both medical and surgical. We have tried to indicate and where appropriate to describe, techniques and laboratory investigations which are necessary for advanced diagnosis and up-to-date therapy. Attention is directed to the special problems which arise in the developing countries.

It is intended in a true apprenticeship fashion of pedagogy to provide a manageable, readable and practical account of clinical paediatrics for medical undergraduates, for postgraduates specialising in paediatrics and for general practitioners whose daily work is concerned with care of children in health and sickness. The authors had to be selective in deciding what to exclude in order to keep the book manageable and practical.

We would like to express our immense gratitude to our colleagues who have provided us with help and advice in writing this book. The willingness with which they gave us their time in spite of many other commitments leaves us permanently in their debt.

We are especially grateful to the parents and to the many children and their families who contributed to our knowledge and understanding of paediatrics and willingly gave permission to reproduce photographs of their children. Also a book such as this cannot be written without reproducing material reported in the medical literature. We acknowledge here with gratitude the permission granted free of charge by individual publishers to reproduce material for which they hold the copyright.

Our deepest thanks go to Professor Forrester Cockburn, Professor Dan Young and Professor Robert Carachi, who most kindly passed on to us their rights of the book entitled 'Children's Medicine and Surgery' from which some material has been used.

We particularly wish to thank the Hutchison family for allowing us to use the name of the late Professor James Holmes Hutchison, the author of 'Practical Paediatric Problems' to enable us to title this book *Hutchison's Paediatrics*. Even today Hutchison's name is highly respected in the paediatric world.

Finally, we would like to express our thanks to Jean Hyslop, Medical Artist, who created the line drawings and art work and helped to integrate the text with the illustrations.

Krishna M Goel
Devendra K Gupta

Contents

Chapter 1

Paediatric History and Examination

Krishna M Goel, Robert Carachi

THE HISTORY

Semeiology (The study of symptoms).

Disease

'A condition in which, as a result of anatomical change or physiological disturbance, there is departure from the normal state of health'. There is a lot of variation in normal people.

CLINICAL MANIFESTATIONS OF DISEASE

Symptoms

Something the patient feels or observes which is abnormal, e.g. pain, vomiting, loss of function. A good history will provide a clue to the diagnosis in 80% of patients.

Signs

Physical or functional abnormalities elicited by examination, e.g. tenderness on palpation, a swelling, a change in a reflex picked up on physical examination. Always inspect, palpate, percuss then auscultate.

The Patient

Why do patients go to the doctor?
• They are alarmed. They believe themselves to be ill and are afraid
• Relief of symptoms
• Cure
• Prognosis.

The Doctor

• Helps diagnose disease
• Symptoms + signs → differential diagnosis → Δ definitive diagnosis
• Acquired knowledge allows recognition + interpretation + reflection → therapy + prognosis.

How is Knowledge Acquired?

• Reading: 10% - 20% retention
• Taught by others: 10% retention, e.g. lectures, tutorials, computer programs
• Personal experience: 80% retention, e.g. bedside teaching

A Description of the Disease

1. Knowledge of the causation (aetiology).
2. Pathological, anatomy and functional changes which are present (morphology).
3. Assembly of all the relevant facts concerning the past and present history (symptoms).
4. Full clinical examination and findings (signs).
5. Simple laboratory tests such as an examination of the urine or blood and X-rays (investigations).

Prognosis

Depends on:
1. Nature of the disease.
2. Severity.
3. Stage of the disease.
   Statistical statements about prognosis can often be made, e.g. the average expectation of life in chronic diseases or the percentage mortality in the acute cases. These must be applied with great caution to individual patients. Patients expect this more and more with internet access. Often information has to be interpreted. They may be testing your knowledge and comparing it to other doctors or information obtained.

Syndrome

A group of symptoms and/or signs which commonly occur together, e.g. Down's syndrome, Wiedemann-Beckwith syndrome (*).

> **WARNING!**
> When discussing medical matters in a patient's hearing, certain words with disturbing associations should be avoided. This is so, even if they are not relevant to the particular individual.

* *Oxford Dysmorphology Database*

History and Documentation

History of Present Condition

a. General Description

The taking of an accurate history is the most difficult and the most important part of a consultation. It becomes progressively simpler as the physician's knowledge of disease and experience increases but it is never easy. As far as possible the patients' complaints list should be written (in order of relevance), unaltered by leading questions but phrased in medical terms. When the patient's own phraseology is used, the words should be written in inverted commas, e.g. "giddiness", "wind", "palpitation" and an attempt should be made to find out precisely what they mean to the patient.

1. *Onset* - The order of onset of symptoms is important. If there is doubt about the date of onset of the disease, the patient should be asked when he last felt quite well and why he first consulted his doctor.
2. *Therapy* - Notes on any treatment already received and of its effect, if any, must be made as it might alter disease states, e.g. appendicitis masked by drug treatment for a UTI.

b. Symptomatic Enquiry

After the patient has given a general description of his illness, the system mainly involved will usually but by no means always, be obvious. The patient should then be questioned about the main symptoms produced by diseases of this system. This should be followed by enquiries directed towards other systems. Remember different systems may produce similar symptoms.

This systematic enquiry runs from the 'head to the toes' (32 questions). However, relevant questions are grouped together under systems. Here are some examples.

Alimentary Tract Questions

- **Abdominal pain or discomfort (24):**
  Site, character, e.g. constant or colicky, radiation, relationships to food and bowel actions. Shift in site.
- **Nausea and vomiting (15):**
  Frequency and relationship to food, etc. (positive vomiting), amount of vomitus, contents, colour, blood (haematemesis), etc.

- **Flatulence (16, 26):**
  Eructation (belching) and passage of flatus.
- **Bowels (25):**
  Constipation (recent or long standing, severity); diarrhoea (frequency and looseness of motions); presence of blood and mucus in faeces; altered colour of faeces – black from altered blood (melaena); clay coloured in obstructive jaundice; bulky and fatty in steatorrhoea, piles. Tenesmus painful sensation and urgent need to defecate (Rectal Pathology).
- **Appetite and loss of weight (17):**
  Recent looseness of clothing. Types of food in diet, amounts eaten.
- **Difficulty in swallowing (18a):**
  Food hard or soft, fluids, level at which food 'sticks'. Pain, regurgitation. Progression from solid food to liquid.
- **Heartburn, acid eructations, "and belching".**
- **Jaundice (17):**
  Constant or fluctuating.
  N.B. Steatorrhoea: bulky pale foul smelling and greasy stools due to
  a. Depressed fat digestion (pancreatic lipase and bile)
  b. Depressed fat absorption (small intestine mostly jejunum)

Cardiovascular System Questions

- **Breathlessness (11):**
  On exertion (DOE) (degree) on at rest (DAR), time especially if wakes at night, position, relieving factors, gradual/sudden onset, change, duration (PND), precipitating factors, number of pillows used.
- **Pain in chest (19):**
  Site on exertion or at rest, character, radiation, duration, relief by drugs, etc. accompanying sensations, e.g. breathlessness, vomiting, cold sweats, pallor, frequency, other relieving factors.
- **Swelling of ankles (23):**
  Time of day.
- **Swelling of abdomen (27):**
  Tightness of trousers or skirt, bloatedness.
- **Palpitation (20):**
  - Patient conscious of irregularity or forcefulness of heart beat.
  - Dizziness and faints – hypertension pain.
- **Pain in the legs on exertion (22):**
  Intermittent claudication at rest or exertion, other vascular problems.
- **Coldness of feet (23):**
  Raynaund's phenomenon.

- **Dead fingers or toes (22):**
  Pain, sensation, ulceration, diabetes.

Respiratory System Questions

- **Cough (12):**
  Character, frequency, duration, causing pain, timing. Productive.
- **Sputum (13):**
  Quantity, colour (frothy, stringy, sticky odour), colour when most profuse (during the day and the year and the affect of posture (bronchiectasis) presence of blood haemoptysis. Is the blood red or brown? Is it pure blood or 'specks'? e.g. acute or chronic bronchitis.
- **Breathlessness (11):**
  On exertion or at rest. Expiratory difficulty, precipitating factors, cough, fog, emotion, change of environment, wheezing.
- **Pain in chest:**
  Location, character, affected by respiration, coughing. Position? ($\uparrow\downarrow$ pain). Weight loss.
- **Hoarseness (10):**
  With or without pain (involvement of recurrent laryngeal nerve. Other associated features eg neurological.
- **Throat (10):**
  Soreness, Tonsillitis, ulcers, infection.
- **Nasal discharge or obstruction (7):**
- **Bleeding from nose (8):**
  Epistaxis.
- **Sweating (14):**
  Day or night, associated symptoms, amounts.
- **Wheezing (12):**
  Asthma, chest infection, relieving factor, COPD
- **Smoking.**

Central Nervous System Questions

- **Loss of consciousness (1):**
  Sudden, warning, injuries, passage of urine, duration, after effects. Precipitating factor, witnesses?
- **Mental state (3):**
  Memory, independent opinion of relative or friend sought. Orientation.
- **Headache (2):**
  Character, site, duration, associated symptoms, e.g. vomiting, aura, timing.
- **Weakness or paralysis of limbs or any muscles (21):**
  Sudden, gradual or progressive onset, duration, visual disturbance.
- **Numbness or 'pins and needles' in limbs or elsewhere (22):**
  Paraesthesine, backpain, diabetes.

- **Giddiness or staggering (5):**
  True vertigo, clumsiness, staggering, ataxia.
- **Visual disturbance (4):**
  Seeing double (diplopia) dimness, zig zag figures (fortification spectra).
- **Deafness or tinnitus (6):**
  Discharge from ears, pain, hearing loss.
- **Speech disturbance (9):**
  Duration, onset, nature. Problems with reading or understanding.

Genito Urinary System Questions

- **Micturation (29):**
  Frequency during day and night, retention, dribbling, amount of urine passed. Pain or smarting (dysuria). Stress incontinence, urgency incontinence.
- **Urine (30):**
  Colour and amount – smell, blood, colour, frothy.
- **Lumbar pain (28):**
  Radiation. ROM, history of trauma, mechanical.
- **Swelling of face or limbs (23):**
  Presence on rising, drugs, improve with movement, pain.
- **Menstruation (31):**
  Age of onset (menarche) age of cessation (menopause). Regularity, duration, amount of loss, pain (dysmenorrhoea). Inter-menstrual discharge - character, blood or otherwise. Vaginal discharge, quantity, colour (normally clear), smell, irritation. Any hormone replacement therapy (HRT), child bearing age.
- **Periods:**
  Time of menopause
  Postmenopausal bleeding
  Last normal menstrual period LNMP
  Menstrual cycle No. of days/interval, e.g. 4/28
  Regular or irregular, e.g. 2 - 8/
  Interval longest or shortest, e.g. 21 - 49
  Increase or decrease in flow.

Locomotor System Questions

- **Swelling:**
  One joint or multiple joints.
  Pain – Back (22):
  When worse during day. Effect of exercise. Lifting.
- **Stiffness:**
  Effect of exercise.
- **Previous bone or joint injury:**
  N.B. Pain in joints. Where worse in morning or later during day/night. Whether it radiates from one joint to another.

Skin Questions

- **Occupation (32):**
  Exposure to irritants and drugs:
- **Rashes:**
  Type, situation, duration, any treatment, painful, itching, (psoriasis).

Past History

1. Diabetes
2. Hypertension
3. Rheumatic fever
4. Heart disease
5. C.F.
6. Spina bifida
7. Other illnesses

Illnesses, operations, injuries. Routine X-ray examinations. In female - obstetrical history (a) number of deliveries and abortions, e.g. 3 + 1, (b) type of delivery, e.g. NA, SO, forceps, (c) complication of puerperium or pregnancy.

Family History

Married, number and health of children, health of partners, any illnesses in parents, grand-parents, brothers, sisters, longevity or short lives, any illnesses similar to patients.

Drug History

- Social and personal history:
- Occupation:

INTRODUCTION

At all times the doctor must show genuine concern and interest when speaking with parents. The parents and the child must feel that the doctor has the time, interest and competence to help them. A physician who greets the child by name irrespective of age will convey an attitude of concern and interest. Parents tell us about the child's signs and symptoms although children contribute more as they grow older.

The doctor-patient relationship gradually develops during history-taking and physical examination. Considerable tact and discretion are required when taking the history especially in the presence of the child: questioning on sensitive subjects should best be reserved for a time when the parents can be interviewed alone. It may therefore be necessary to separate the parent and the child-patient when taking the history especially when the problems are related to behaviour, school difficulties and socioeconomic disturbances in the home environment.

Table 1.1: History-taking—The paediatric patient
• Presenting problem
• History of the presenting problem
• Previous history:
• Pregnancy and delivery
• Neonatal period and infancy
• Subsequent development
• Other disorders or diseases
• Dietary
• Immunisation
• Family history
• Parents
• Siblings
• Others
• Draw a family tree if indicated

The medical student having been instructed in the history-taking and physical examination of adults needs to appreciate the modifications necessary when dealing with the child-patient. A basic template for history-taking is useful and serves as a reminder of the ground to be covered (Table 1.1). Initially the medical student may be confused because of the need to obtain information from someone other than the patient, usually the mother. Useful information may be obtained by observing the infant and young child during the history-taking. The older child should be given an opportunity to talk, to present their symptoms and to tell how they interfere with school and play activities.

The simple act of offering a toy, picture book or pen-torch is often an effective step toward establishing rapport. Rigid adherence to routine is both unnecessary and counter productive. A lot may be learned of the family constellation and the parent-child relationship by simply observing the parent(s) and child during the history-taking and physical examination. Therefore watching, listening and talking are of paramount importance in paediatric practice and are invaluable in arriving at a working diagnosis.

Key Learning Point
Useful information may be obtained by observing the infant and young child during the history-taking.

History of Present Complaint

Even before language develops in the infant (Latin - without speech) parents can detect altered behaviour and observe abnormal physical signs. It is sensible to commence with the history of the presenting observations because that is what the parents have come to talk about. In the newborn infant the history from the attending nurse and medical staff is important.

Every endeavour should be made to ask appropriate questions and discuss relevant points in the history in order to identify the nature of the child's problems and come to a tentative diagnosis. Ask what the child is called at home and address the child with this name since otherwise he/she may be less forthcoming. Let the parents give the history in their own way and then ask specific questions. Ask, how severe are the symptoms; have the symptoms changed during the past days, weeks or months; has there been any change recently in the child's appetite, energy or activities; has the child been absent from school; has anyone who cares for the child been ill; has the child been thriving or losing weight; what change in behaviour has there been; has there been a change in appetite, in micturition or bowel habits. An articulate older child can describe feelings and symptoms more accurately, as the child's memory for the time and sequence of events may be more precise, than the parents.

Past Medical History

The past history is the documentation of significant events which have happened in the child's life and which may be of relevance in coming to a diagnosis. Therefore the doctor should try to obtain relevant information concerning the past from the family and any other sources that are available. It is useful if the events are recorded in the sequence of their occurrence. A careful history should contain details of pregnancy, delivery, neonatal period, early feeding, the child's achievement of developmental milestones and details of admissions to hospital, with date, place and reason for admission. A complete list of current medication including vitamins and other supplements should be obtained. An enquiry should be made of any drug or other sensitivity which should always be prominently recorded. Details of immunisation and all previous infectious diseases should be elicited.

Key Learning Point
Dietary history is of vital importance in paediatric history-taking especially if the child is not thriving or has vomiting, diarrhoea, constipation or anaemia.

Mother's Pregnancy, Labour, Delivery and the Neonatal Period

The younger the child, the more important is the information about the period of intrauterine life. The history of pregnancy includes obstetric complications during the pregnancy; history of illness, infection or injury and social habits, e.g. smoking of the mother are important. Drug or alcohol ingestion and poor diet during pregnancy may have an adverse effect on the fetus and

lead to problems. The estimated length of gestation and the birth weight of the baby should be recorded. Details of any intrapartum or perinatal problems should be recorded.

Dietary History

The duration of breastfeeding should be recorded or the type of artificial feed and any weaning problems. The dietary history can be of major importance in paediatric history-taking. If the patient is not thriving or has vomiting, diarrhoea, constipation or anaemia then the physician must obtain a detailed dietary history. The dietary history should not only include solid foods but also the consumption of liquid foods and any other supplements such as vitamins. In this way the quality of the diet and the quantity of nutrients can be assessed and compared to the recommended intake. Any discrepancy between the actual and recommended intake may have a possible bearing on the diagnosis.

Developmental History

Inquiries about the age at which major developmental milestones in infancy and early childhood were achieved are necessary when faced with an infant or child who is suspected of developmental delay. On the other hand the child who is doing well at school and whose physical and social activities are normal, less emphasis on the minutiae of development is needed. Some parents are vague about the time of developmental achievements unless, very recently acquired but many have clear recall of the important events such as smiling, sitting and walking independently. It can be helpful to enquire whether this child's development paralleled that of other children.

Family and Social History

The health and educational progress of a child is directly related to the home and the environment. Medical, financial and social stresses within the family sometimes have a direct or indirect bearing on the child's presenting problem. It is therefore essential to know about the housing conditions and some information of parental income and working hours, as well as the child's performance in school and adjustment to playmates.

The family history should be thoroughly evaluated. The age and health of the close relatives are important to record. Heights and weights of parents and siblings may be of help especially when dealing with children of short stature, obesity, failure to thrive, or the infant with an enlarged head. Consanguinity is common in some cultures and offspring of consanguinous marriages have an increased chance of receiving the same recessive gene from each parent and thus developing a genetically determined disease. Therefore it is important to draw a family tree and to identify children at high risk of genetic disease, and to make appropriate referrals.

Key Learning Point

A history of recent travel abroad, particularly in tropical areas, is important as the child may have a disorder uncommon in his/her own country but having been contracted in another country where disease may be endemic.

PHYSICAL EXAMINATION

The physical examination of the paediatric patient requires a careful and gentle approach. It should be carried out in an appropriate environment with a selection of books or toys around, which can be used to allay the apprehension and anxiety of the child. More can be learned by careful inspection than by any other single examination method. The baby should be examined in a warm environment in good light. Nappies must be removed to examine the baby fully. We look first at the baby as a whole noting especially the colour, posture and movements. Proceed to a more detailed examination starting at the head and working down to the feet "Top to Toe".

It is important to realise that the child may be apprehensive with a stranger, especially when faced with the unfamiliar surroundings of a surgery or hospital outpatient department. It is essential that the doctor be truthful with the child regarding what is going to be done. The child should never be made to face sudden unexpected manouevres and should be allowed to play with objects such as the stethoscope. It may be useful to let him or her examine a toy animal or doll to facilitate gaining confidence. Infants and young children are often best examined on the mother's lap where they feel more secure. The doctor should ensure that his hands and instruments used to examine the child are suitably warmed. It is not always mandatory to remove all the child's clothes, although it is often essential in the examination of the acutely ill child. Procedures which may produce discomfort such as examination of the throat, ears or rectal examination should be left until towards the end of the examination. The order of the examination may be varied to suit the particular child's needs. Awareness of the normal variations at different ages is important.

A thorough physical examination is a powerful therapeutic tool especially if the problem is one primarily of inappropriate parental anxiety. Understandably parents do not usually accept reassurance if the doctor has not examined the child properly. Examination of the infant or child is often preceded by recording the patient's height, weight and head circumference on the growth chart. This may have been done by a nurse before the doctor sees the family. These measurements are plotted on graphs or charts which indicate the percentiles or standard deviations at the various ages throughout childhood. If these measurements are outwith the 3rd to 97th centile for children of that sex and age further study is indicated. If previous records of height, weight or head circumference are available for comparison with the current measurements this may provide considerable help towards diagnosis and management. Inquiry of parental height, weight or head size may also be important, e.g. familial macrocephaly or constitutional short stature.

General Inspection

The general appearance of the child may suggest a particular syndrome. Does the child look like the rest of the family? The facies may be characteristic in Down's Syndrome and other chromosomal disorders or in mucopolysaccharidoses. Peculiar odours from an infant may provide a clue to diagnosis of aminoacidurias, such as Maple Syrup disease (maple syrup like odour), Phenylketonuria (mousy odour), or Trimethylaminuria (fishy odour). A more detailed examination should then be performed. The most valuable of the doctor's senses are his eyes as more can be learned by careful inspection and also on watching the patient's reactions than any other single procedure.

Colour

Should be pink with the exception of the periphery which may be slightly blue. Congenital heart disease is only suggested if the baby has central cyanosis. A pale baby may be anaemic or ill and requires careful investigation to find the cause. A blue baby may have either a cardiac anomaly or respiratory problems and rarely methhae-moglobinaemia.

Posture and Movements

A term baby lies supine for the first day or two and has vigorous, often asymmetric movements of all limbs. In contrast a sick baby adopts the frog position with legs abducted, externally rotated and is inactive. Older infants and children should be observed for abnormal movements, posture and gait.

Key Learning Points

- Always leave the most upsetting parts of the examination until the end such as inspection of the throat or taking the blood pressure.
- If epiglottitis is a possibility do not examine the throat because obstruction may be precipitated.

Skin

The skin is a major body organ which, because of the larger surface area in relationship to weight, of the young means that the skin is relatively more important in the immature. It forms a barrier against environmental attack and its structure and function reflects the general health of the child, i.e. in states of malnutrition and dehydration. The presence of any skin rash, its colour and whether there are present macules, papules, vesicles, bullae, petechiae or pustules should be recorded (see Box). The skin texture, elasticity, tone and subcutaneous thickness should be assessed by picking up the skin between the fingers. Pigmented naevi, strawberry naevi, haemangiomata or lymphangiomata may be present and may vary in size and number. They may be absent or small at birth and grow in subsequent days or weeks.

Dermatological Terminology	
Macule:	area of discolouration, any size, not raised-flat with skin
Papule:	small raised lesion (< 5mm)
Petechiae:	haemorrhage in skin, non-blanching (< 1mm)
Purpura:	haemorrhage in skin, non-blanching (2-10 mm in diameter)
Ecchymoses:	large bruise, non-blanching
Vesicle:	small blister, elevated, fluid-filled (< 5mm)
Bullae:	large blister: elevated, fluid-filled (> 5mm)
Weal:	elevation in skin, due to acute oedema in dermis, surrounding erythematous macule
Pustule:	elevated, pus-filled
Lichenification:	thickened skin, normal lines in skin more apparent

Head

The head should be inspected for size, shape and symmetry. Measurement of the head circumference [occipital frontal circumference (OFC)] with a non-elastic tape by placing it to encircle the head just above the eyebrows around maximum protuberance of the occipital bone should be performed and charted. In the infant the skull should be palpated to determine the size and tension in the fontanelles and assess the skull sutures (Figure 1.1). Premature fusion of sutures suggests craniostenosis. In the neonate the posterior fontanelle may be very small and subsequently closes by three months of age but the anterior fontanelle is larger, only closing at around 18 months. A tense and bulging fontanelle suggests raised intracranial pressure and a deeply sunken one suggests dehydration.

Large fontanelles, separation of sutures, delayed closure of the fontanelles may be associated with raised intracranial pressure or other systemic disorders such as hypothyroidism and rickets.

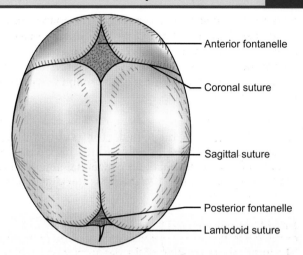

Fig. 1.1: Top of head – anterior fontanelle and cranial sutures

Ears

Position and configuration of the ears should be observed. Whilst abnormalities such as low setting of the ears is frequently associated with renal tract anomalies absence of an ear or non development of the auricle will require early referral to an otolaryngologist. It often requires the parent to hold the child on his or her lap and provide reassurance during the examination. Methods of doing this are illustrated in Figure 1.2. Parents are usually very competent in detecting hearing impairment. The exception to this is where the child is mentally retarded. All infants should be given a screening test for hearing at 6 months of age. Simple testing materials are required, e.g. a cup and spoon, high and low pitched rattles, devices to imitate bird or animal sounds, or even snapping of finger tips are

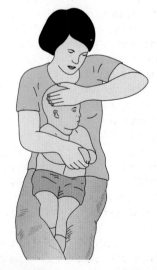

Fig. 1.2: Method of restraining a child for examination of the ear

usually effective if hearing is normal. The sounds should be made quietly at a distance of 2 - 3 feet out of view of the child. By 6 months of age a child should be able to localise sound. To pass the screening test the child should turn and look directly at the source of the sound.

Eyes

These should be inspected for subconjuctival haemorrhages which are usually of little importance, for cataracts, for papilloedema and congenital abnormalities such as colobomata (Figs 1.3 A and B). 'Rocking' the baby

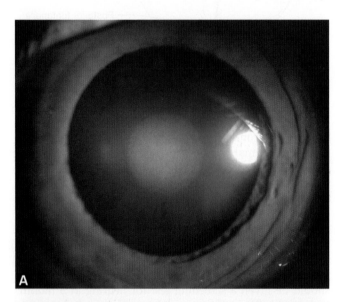

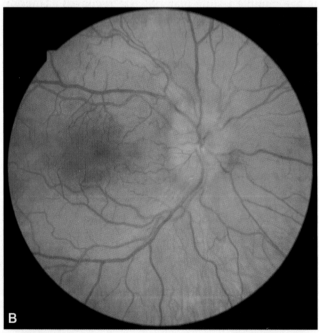

Figs 1.3A and B: A. Congenital cataract **B.** Papilloedema

from the supine to vertical position often results in the eyes opening so they can be inspected. Squint is a condition in which early diagnosis and treatment is important. There are two simple tests which can be carried out to determine whether or not a squint is present.

a. The position of the "corneal light reflection" should normally be in the centre of each pupil if the eyes are both aligned on a bright source of light, usually a pen torch. Should one eye be squinting then the reflection of the light from the cornea will not be centred in the pupil of that eye. It will be displaced outwards if the eye is convergent and inwards towards the nose if the eye is divergent. It may be displaced by such a large amount that it is seen over the iris or even over the sclera, where of course it may be rather more difficult to identify, but with such obvious squints the diagnosis is usually not in doubt.

b. In the "cover test" one chooses an object of interest for the child, e.g. a brightly coloured toy with moving components. When the child is looking at the object of interest the eye thought to be straight is covered with an opaque card and the uncovered eye is observed to see whether it moves to take up fixation on the object of interest. If the child has a convergent squint then the eye will move laterally to take up fixation, and this is the usual situation since convergent squints are four times more common than divergent squints. If the eye were divergent it would move medially.

The commonest cause for apparent blindness in young children is developmental delay. Assessment of whether a young baby can see is notoriously difficult, Fixation should develop in the first week of life but an early negative response is of no value as the absence of convincing evidence of fixation is not synonymous with blindness. The failure to develop a fixation reflex results in ocular nystagmus, but these roving eye movements do not appear until the age of 3 months.

A misleading response may be obtained when a bright light stimulus is applied to a child preferably in a dimly lit room. The normal response is a blinking or "screwing up" the eyes and occasionally by withdrawing the head. This is a subcortical reflex response and may be present in babies despite them having cortical blindness. The absence of this response increases the probability of blindness.

Face

Abnormalities of facial development are usually obvious and an example is the infant with cleft lip. Associated with this there may be a cleft palate but full visual examination of the palate including the uvula is necessary to ensure that the palate is intact and there is not a submucous cleft of the soft palate or a posterior cleft. Submucous and soft palate clefts cannot be felt on palpation.

Mouth

Inspection of the mouth should include visualisation of the palate, fauces and the dentition. A cleft lip is obvious but the palate must be visualised to exclude a cleft. The mouth is best opened by pressing down in the middle of the lower jaw. A baby is rarely born with teeth but if present these are almost always the lower central incisors. The soft palate should be inspected to exclude the possibility of a submucous cleft which could be suggested by a bifid uvula. Small fibromata are sometimes seen in the gums. They are white and seldom require treatment. These are normal. The lower jaw should be seen in profile as a receding chin (micrognathia) may be the cause of tongue swallowing or glossoptosis (Pierre Robin Syndrome) and it may be associated with a cleft palate.

Neck

Examination of the neck may reveal congenital goitre and midline cysts which may be thyroglossal or dermoid in origin. Lateral cysts which may be of branchial origin or sometimes there may be extensive swellings which may be cystic hygroma or lymphangiomata. In early infancy a sternomastoid tumour may be palpable in the mid region of the sternomastoid muscle. Associated with this there may be significant limitation of rotation and lateral flexion of the neck. Palpation along the clavicle will define any tenderness or swelling suggestive of recent or older fracture.

Chest

The shape, chest wall movement and the nature and rate of the breathing (30 to 40 per minute) as well as the presence of any indrawing of the sternum and rib cage should be noted. In a normal baby without respiratory or abdominal problems the abdomen moves freely during breathing and there is very little chest movement. Most of the movements of the breathing cycle are carried out by the movement of the diaphragm. The nipples and axilliary folds should be assessed to exclude conditions such as absent pectoral muscles.

Cardiovascular

Examination of the cardiovascular system of infants and children is carried out in a similar manner to that of adults. The examiner should always feel for femoral pulses and ascertain whether there is any radio-femoral or brachio-femoral delay as this would suggest the possibility of coarctation of the aorta. The most important factor in recording the blood pressure of children is to use a cuff of the correct size. The cuff should cover at least two thirds of the upper arm. If the cuff size is less than this a falsely high blood pressure reading may be obtained. In small infants relatively accurate systolic and diastolic pressures as well as mean arterial pressures can be obtained by use of the doppler method. The apex should be visible and palpable and the position noted. The precordial areas should be palpated for the presence of thrills. If the apex beat is not obvious look for it on the right side of the chest as there could be dextrocardia or a left-sided congenital diaphragmatic hernia with the heart pushed to the right or collapse of the right lung. All areas should be auscultated while the baby is quiet Systolic murmurs may be very harsh and can be confused with breath sounds.

Lungs

Small children frequently cry when the chest is percussed and when a cold stethoscope is applied. If the mother holds the child over her shoulder and soothes him it is often easier to perform a thorough chest examination. Light percussion can be more valuable than auscultation in some situations but the basic signs are similar to those found in an adult. Breath sounds are usually harsh, high pitched and rapid. Any adventitious sounds present are pathological. Percussion of the chest may be helpful to pick up the presence of a pleural effusion (stony dull), collapse, consolidation of a lung (dull) or a pneumothorax (hyper-resonant). These pathological states are usually associated with an increase in the respiratory rate, as well as clinical signs of respiratory distress.

Abdomen

In the infant the abdomen and umbilicus are inspected and attention should be paid to the presence of either a scaphoid abdomen which in a neonate may be one of the signs of diaphragmatic hernia or duodenal atresia or a distended abdomen which suggests intestinal obstruction especially if visible peristalsis can be seen. Peristalsis from left to right suggests a high intestinal obstruction whereas one from the right to the left would be more in keeping with low intestinal obstruction. Any asymmetry of the abdomen may indicate the presence of an underlying mass. Abdominal movement should be assessed and abdominal palpation should be performed with warm hands.

Palpation of the abdomen should include palpation for the liver, the edge of which is normally felt in the newborn baby, the spleen which can only be felt if it is pathological and the kidneys which can be felt in the first 24 hours with the fingers and thumb palpating in the renal angle and abdomen on each side. The lower abdomen should be palpated for the bladder and an enlargement can be confirmed by percussion from a resonant zone, progressing to a dull zone. In the baby with abdominal distension where there is suspicion of perforation and free gas in the abdomen, the loss of superficial liver dullness on percussion may be the only physical sign present early on. Areas of tenderness can be elicited by watching the baby's reaction to gentle palpation of the abdomen. There may be areas of erythema, cellulitis, oedema of the abdominal wall and on deeper palpation crepitus can occasionally be felt from pneumatosis intestinalis (intramural gas in the wall of the bowel).

Auscultation of the abdomen in the younger patients gives rather different signs than in the adult. The infant even in the presence of peritonitis may have some bowel sounds present. However, in the presence of ileus or peritonitis breath sounds become conducted down over the abdomen to the suprapubic area and in even more severe disorders the heart sounds similarly can be heard extending down over the abdomen to the suprapubic area.

Perineal examination is important in both sexes. Examination of the anus should never be omitted. Occasionally the anus is ectopic, e.g. placed more anteriorly than it should be, stenotic or even absent. The rectal examination is an invasive procedure and should be carried out in a comfortable warm environment, preferably with the child in the left lateral position and the mother holding the hand of the child at the top end of the bed.

The testes in boys born at term should be in the scrotum. The prepuce cannot be and should not be retracted. It is several months or years before the prepuce can be retracted and stretching is both harmful and unnecessary. In girls the labia should be separated and genitalia examined

The presence of a swelling in the scrotum or high in the groin may suggest torsion of a testis and requires urgent attention. The testis which cannot be palpated in the scrotum and cannot be manipulated into the sac, indicates the presence of an undescended testis which will need to be explored and corrected before the age of 2 years. A swelling in the scrotum which has a blueish hue to it suggests the presence of a hydrocele due to a patent processus vaginalis and one can get above such a swelling in most children. Palpation of the scrotum is initially for testes but if gonads are not present then palpation in the inguinal, femoral and perineal regions to determine presence of undescended or ectopic testes should be carried out.

Conditions such as hypospadias, epispadias, labial adhesions or imperforate hymen should be diagnosed on inspection.

Limbs

Upper and lower limbs are examined in detail. Hands and feet should be examined for signs and those experienced in dermatoglyphics may define a finger print pattern which is consistent in various syndromes. The presence of a simian palmar crease may suggest trisomy 21 (Down's Syndrome) and thumb clenching with neurological disease. The feet, ankles and knees should be examined for the range of movement in the joints and tone of the muscles. The femoral head may be outside the acetabulum at birth in true dislocation of the hip or it may be dislocated over the posterior lip of the acetabulum by manipulation, in which case the hip is described as unstable, dislocatable or lax. There are conditions in which the acetabulum is hypoplastic and shallow and the femoral head itself is distorted. Congenital dislocation of the hip is more common after breech deliveries in girls and in certain parts of the world. All newborn infants should be screened shortly after birth. The infant is placed supine with the legs towards the examiner and each hip is examined separately. The knee and hip of the baby are flexed to 90% and the hip fully abducted by placing the middle finger over the greater trochanter and the thumb on the inner side of the thigh opposite the position of the lesser trochanter. When the thigh is in the mid-abducted position, forward pressure is exerted behind the greater trochanter by the middle finger. The other hand holds the opposite femur and pelvis steady. A dislocated femoral head is felt to slip over the acetabular ridge and back into the acetabulum as a definite movement. This part of the test is called the Ortolani manouvre. The second part of the test is the Barlow procedure. With the infant still on his back and the legs and hands in the same position the hip is brought into the position of mid-abduction with the thumb exerting gentle pressure laterally and posteriorly; at the same time the palm exerts posterior and medial pressure. If a hip is dislocatable the femur can be felt to dislocate over the posterior lip of the acetabulum. There is need for caution in performing this test and no force should be employed. Caution is particularly required in infants born with neural tube defects and paralysis of the lower limbs.

The knees, ankles and feet should be examined. Dorsiflexion of the feet should allow the lateral border to come in contact with the peroneal compartment of the leg. Failure indicates a degree of talipes - equino-varus (TEV) which is of concern to the parents although with simple physiotherapy there are seldom longterm problems in the absence of underlying neurological abnormality.

Spine

With the baby held face-downwards fingers should be run along the spine excluding spinal defects such as spina bifida occulta and noting the presence of the common post-anal dimple, a tuft of hair, a pad of fat and haemangioma. A Mongolian blue spot is commonly seen over the sacrum in Asian babies. The presence of a posterior coccygeal dimple or a sacral pit is common in babies and is due to tethering of the skin to the coccyx.

When one stretches the skin and the base of the pit can be seen then nothing needs to be done about it. Very rarely there is communication with the spinal canal which could be the source of infection and cause meningitis.

Stool and Urine Examination

Examination of a stool which is preferably fresh is often informative. The colour, consistency and smell are noted as well as the presence of blood or mucus. Urine examination is also important in children since symptoms related to the urinary tract may be non-specific.

Neurological Examination

The neurological examination of the young infant and child is different from that routinely carried out in the adult. Muscle tone and strength are important parts of the examination. In infants muscle tone may be influenced by the child's state of relaxation. An agitated hungry infant may appear to be hypertonic but when examined in a cheerful post-prandial state the tone reverts to being normal. The examination of the neurological system cannot be complete without the evaluation of the child's development level relating to gross motor, fine motor and vision, hearing and speech and social skills. All older children should be observed for gait to detect abnormal co-ordination and balance

Older children may be tested for sense of touch and proprioception as in adults. Tests of sensation as well as motor power must be performed in the paediatric patient but are difficult to assess in the very young child. The normal newborn has a large number of primitive reflexes (Moro, asymmetric tonic neck, glabellar tap, sucking and rooting process). The *Moro-reflex* is a mass reflex which is present in the early weeks after birth. Its absence suggests cerebral damage. It consists of throwing out of the arms followed by bringing them together in an embracing movement. It can be demonstrated by making a loud noise near the child. The *sucking reflex* is present at birth in the normal baby as is the *swallowing reflex*. If the angle of the baby's mouth is touched by the finger or teat the baby will turn his head towards it and search for it. It is looking for its mother's nipple and is known as the *rooting or searching reflex*.

The grasp reflex is illustrated by gently stroking the back of the hand so that the fingers extend and on placing a finger on the palm of the baby it takes a firm grip. Similar reflexes are present in the toes. If the baby is held up under the arms so that his feet are touching a firm surface he will raise one leg and hesitatingly put it down in front of the other leg, taking giant strides forwards. This is the *primitive walking reflex*.

Tendon reflexes such as the biceps and knee jerks are easily obtainable but the ankle and triceps jerks are not readily elicited. Important as an indication of nervous system malfunction are muscle tone, posture, movement and the primitive reflexes of the newborn that have been described. Plantar reflex is usually extensor and is of little diagnostic importance in the first year. Delay in disappearance of the primitive reflexes suggests cerebral damage.

A GUIDE TO EXAMINATION OF A CHILD-PATIENT

Checklist of Bodily Systems

GENERAL EXAMINATION

- Is the child unwell, breathless or distressed?
- Level of consciousness
- Is the child cyanosed, pale or jaundiced (in carotinaemia the sclerae are not yellow)?
- ENT examination: child's ears, nose and throat
- Is the child dehydrated? - skin turgor, sunken eyes, sunken fontenelle
- Nutritional state
- Peripheral perfusion: capillary refill time-should occur within 2 secs
- Does the child have any dysmorphic features, i.e. an obvious syndrome?
- Check blood pressure, temperature and pulses, i.e. radial and femoral
- Hands: for clubbing (look at all fingers), peripheral cyanosis, absent nails (ectodermal dysplasia), pitted nails (psoriasis), splinter haemorrhages
- Height, weight and head circumference (OFC): plot these on a percentile chart
- Rash: generalised or localised, bruises, petechiae, purpura, birth marks (learn dermatological terminology - (see Box on Page 7)
- Abnormal pigmentation: café au lait spots, Mongolian blue spots
- Palpate for lymph nodes in the neck (from behind), axillae, groins any subcutaneous nodules
- Teeth: any dental caries, a torn lip frenulum (physical abuse)
- Genitalia: injuries to genitalia or anus – sexual abuse

Head

- Shape: normal, small (microcephaly, large (macro-ceohaly), plagiocephaly, brachycephaly, oxycephaly (turricephaly). Feel the sutures. Is there evidence of craniostenosis?
- Hair: alopecia, seborrhoea of the scalp
- Eyes: subconjunctival haemorrhage, ptosis, proptosis, squint, nystagmus, cataract, aniridia, optic fundi
- Mouth: thrush, fauces, tonsils, teeth, palate

- Ears: normal, low-set, shape, pre-auricular skin tags
- Anterior fontenelle: diamond shaped, open, closed, sunken, bulging, tense
- Head circumference: measure the child's OFC and plot it on a growth chart (if not done under general examination)

Neck

Short, webbed (Turner syndrome), torticollis
Thyroid: enlarged, bruit
Swellings:
1. Midline: thyroglossal cyst, goitre (Figs 1.4A and B)
2. Lateral: lymph nodes, branchial cyst, cystic hygroma, sternomastoid tumour

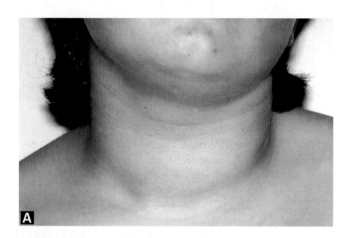

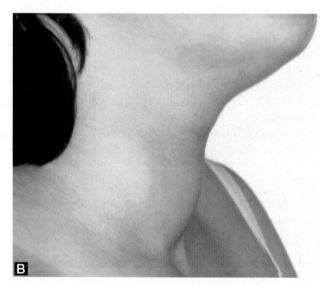

Fig. 1.4A and B: Goitre in Hashimotos thyroiditis –
A. AP neck and **B.** lateral view neck

RESPIRATORY SYSTEM

Inspection

- Use of accessory muscles of resp iration
- Intercostal recession, any stridor, audible wheeze
- Shape: normal, pectus carinatum (undue prominence of the sternum-pigeon chest,
- Pectus excavatum (funnel chest), Harrison's sulci, hyperinflation (increased A-P diameter)
- Count the respiratory rate
- Scars of past surgery (look at the front and the back of the chest)

Palpation

- Chest wall movement: Is it symmetrical?
- Feel the trachea: central or deviated
- Tactile vocal fremitus (over 5 years of age–ask the child to say 99)

Percussion

- Percuss all areas: normal, resonant, hyper-resonant, dull (collapse, consolidation), stony dull (pleural effusion)

Auscultation

- Air entry, vesicular (normal), absent breath sounds (pleural effusion), bronchial (consolidation)
- Added sounds: wheeze, inspiratory or expiratory, crackles (fine versus coarse), pleural friction rub
- Vocal resonance

CARDIOVASCULAR SYSTEM

Inspection

- Are there features of Down's (ASD, VSD), Turner's (coarctation of the aorta), or Marfan's (aortic incompetence)
- Cyanosis: peripheral, central
- Hands: clubbing, splinter haemorrhages (endocarditis)
- Oedema: praecordium, ankles, sacrum
- Praecordium for scars of past surgery

Palpation

- Pulses: radial/brachial/femoral - radio-femoral delay (synchrony of the two pulses), rate
- Character of pulse-collapsing, volume
- Heart rate-rhythm
- Apex beat: position (normal position in children 4th-5th left intercostal space in the mid-clavicular line), beware of dextrocardia
- Palpate for a parasternal heave and for precordial thrills

PERCUSSION OF THE HEART IS NOT NORMALLY UNDERTAKEN IN CHILDREN

Auscultation

- Listen to all four valve areas (apex, lower L sternal edge, upper L sternal edge, upper R sternal edge
- Quality of heart sounds
- Additional sounds, i.e. clicks, murmur (timing of the murmur)
- Blood pressure – use a cuff that covers at least 2/3rd of the upper arm or use Doppler

GASTROINTESTINAL SYSTEM

Inspection

- General distension
- Superficial veins-direction of flow, striae, umbilicus
- Masses, scars, visible peristalsis

Palpation and Percussion

- First lightly palpate the entire abdomen, keep looking at the child's face all the time
- Localised tenderness, rebound tenderness, rigidity
- Masses
- Ascites-percuss for the shifting dullness
- Spleen, liver, kidneys
- Hernial orifices
- Genitalia (testes), anus (site)

Auscultation

Bowel sounds: absence implies ileus

NERVOUS SYSTEM

- Level of consciousness
- Right or left handed
- Orientation, memory (past - present)
- Speech
- Posture

Cranial Nerve

1st	Smell-ability of each nostril to different smells
2nd	Visual acuity, visual fields, pupils (size, shape, reaction to light and consensual); Fundoscopy - papilloedema, optic atrophy, cataract
3rd	Palsy-unilateral ptosis, fixed dilated pupil, eye down and out
4th	Palsy-diplopia on looking down and away from the affected side
5th	Palsy-motor - jaw deviates to the side of lesion Sensory - corneal reflex lost
6th	Palsy - convergent squint
7th	Facial nerve lesions: weakness

Only the lower 2/3rd is affected in UMN lesions, but all of one side of the face in LMN lesions. Ask the child to screw-up eyes, raise eyebrows, blow out cheeks, show teeth

8th	Hearing, balance and posture
9th and 10th	Gag reflex - look at palatal movement
11th	Trapezii - shrug your shoulders
12th	Tongue movement - deviates to the side of lesion

Cerebellar Function

- Jerk nystagmus (worse on gaze away from midline)
- Truncal ataxia (if worse when eyes closed then lesion is of dorsal columns; not cerebellum)
- Intention tremor – Ask the child to pick up a small object and watch for tremor
- Past pointing – Ask the child to cover one eye with one hand and with the index finger of the other hand ask him to touch his nose and then touch your finger
- Gait – Ask the child to walk normally and then walk heel – toe look for ataxic gait

LOCOMOTOR SYSTEM

Arms

- Tone, muscle bulk, muscle power – oppose each movement
- Joints: hands – swollen/tender MCP/PIP joints, test joints for hypermobility
- Reflexes: biceps (C5,6) and triceps (C7,8) – compare both sides
- Hand: ask child to squeeze your fingers/spread fingers,
- Coordination: finger-nose touching
- Sensation: test light touch

Legs

- Tone, quadriceps/gastrocnemius bulk
- Power – oppose each movement
- Coordination – rub heel up and down shin ("heel - shin test")
- Joints: swollen, tender, patella tap test (effusion in knee)
- Reflexes: knee (L3,4) ankle (S1,2), plantar reflex – the plantar is normally up-going in infants until they begin to walk
- Feet: any deformity: are arches high or low?

Sensation

- Joint position sense
- Fine touch discrimination

Gait

Ask the child to walk normally across room

Gower's Sign

Ask the child to stand from supine. A child will normally sit up from lying and then stand. In Duchenne muscular dystrophy, the child will have to roll over onto their front and then climb up their legs.

DEVELOPMENTAL ASSESSMENT

This should be carried out under four headings: gross motor, fine motor and vision, hearing and speech and social behaviour. These milestones are based for a child who is aged 6 weeks to 5 years.

Birth to 6 weeks

Gross Motor

Marked head lag at birth on pulling to sit. By 6 weeks moderate head lag on pull to sit prone, brings chin momentarily off couch.

Fine Motor and Vision

Can see at birth. By 6 weeks, can fix and follow across to 90°.

Hearing and Speech

Can hear at birth. Startles and quietens to a soothing voice.

Social Behaviour

Stops crying when picked up. By 6 weeks, smiling to familiar noises and faces.

3 to 6 Months

Gross Motor

By 3 months, on ventral suspension brings head above level of back. Prone lifts head and upper chest off couch. By 6 months, sits with support or tripod sits. Beginning to weight bear. Rises to stand when supported.

Fine motor and Vision

By 3 months, holds hands loosely open and has hand regard. By 6 months, reaches for toys with palmar grasp. Transfers hand-to-hand and hand-to-mouth.

Hearing and Speech

Can laugh, gurgle and coo. Starts to babble around 6 months. Will turn when called.

Social Behaviour

Holds on to bottle or feeding cup when fed. Frolics when played with. Examines and plays with hands and places feet in mouth.

6 to 9 months

Gross Motor

By 6 months can roll from front to back. Sits unsupported with a straight back. Begins to pivot around on arms and legs into the crawling position.

Fine Motor and Vision

Small objects picked up between index finger and thumb in a pincer grasp. Transfers from hand to hand.

Hearing and Speech

By 9 months, shouts to gain attention. Vocalises non-specific syllables such as "dada" and "mama".

Social Behaviour

Turns when talked to. Resists when objects taken away. Tries to reach for objects out of reach. Likes to feed with fingers.

9 to 12 Months

Gross Motor

By 9-10 months most infants are crawling. 10% normal infants never crawl, but move around by rolling, padding or bottom shuffling. These children are often late walkers and may not walk alone until 2 years. By 9-12 months, begins to pull to standing and cruise.

Key Learning Point
Delayed walking could be due to the fact that the child is a bottom shuffler. There is a family history of bottom shuffling. It is autosomal dominant in inheritance. Rest of the developmental milestones are within the normal range.

Fine Motor and Vision

Will bang two cubes together. Looks for fallen objects.

Hearing and Speech

By 9-12 months, usually have 1 or 2 recognisable words in addition to "mama" and "dada".

Social Behaviour

Enjoys imitative games such as clapping hands and waving goodbye. Shy with strangers until the end of the first year.

12 - 18 Months

Gross Motor

By 12 months, can walk with hands held and begins to stand alone.

By 18 months, climbs onto chair and up stairs. Holds on to toys while walking.

Fine Motor and Vision

Pincer grip refined. Tiny objects can be picked up delicately. Points at objects with index finger. Can be persuaded to give objects to another on request. Builds a tower of two or three bricks.

Hearing and Speech

Vocabulary of several words. Comprehension is more advanced than speech at this age. Enjoys looking at pictures on a book and points and babbles while doing this.

Social Behaviour

By 12 months indicates wants, usually by pointing. Drinks from a cup and helps to feed themselves. Begins to help with dressing. Learns to throw. Enjoys simple games such as peek-a-boo.

2 Years

Gross Motor

Can walk, run, squat and climb stairs two feet per step.

Fine Motor and Vision

Builds tower of six or seven cubes. Spontaneous scribbling. Hand preference. Holds pencil with thumb and first two fingers. Imitates vertical lines.

Hearing and Speech

Uses 50 or more recognisable words and understands many more. Forms simple sentences. Carries out simple instructions.

Social Behaviour

Feeds with a spoon, drinks from a cup. Usually dry through day (variable). Demands mother's attention. Tantrums when frustrated. Instant gratification.

3 Years

Gross Motor

Climbs stairs one foot per step. Pedals a tricycle. Kicks a ball.

Fine Motor and Vision

Copies a circle, imitates a cross. Builds a tower of nine cubes. Threads beads.

Hearing and Speech

Speaks in sentences and may know a few colours. Recites nursery rhymes. Counts to 10.

Social Behaviour

Eats with fork and spoon. Dry through night. Likes to help in adult activities. Vivid imaginary play. Joins in play with others.

4 Years

Gross Motor

Walks up and down stairs one foot per step. May hop.

Fine Motor and Vision

Copies cross (also V T H O). Draws a man with head, legs and trunks. Picks up very small objects and threads beads. Knows four primary colours.

Hearing and Speech

Intelligible speech. Knows name, address and usually age.

Listens to and tells stories. Enjoys jokes.

Social Behaviour

May wash, dress, undress, but not yet manage laces. Understand taking turns, as well as sharing. Appreciates past, present and future time.

5 Years

Gross Motor

Catches a ball.

Fine Motor and Vision

Draws triangle and detailed man.

Hearing and Speech

Clear speech.

Social Behaviour

Comforts others, group play.

Primitive Reflexes

- Rooting reflex: appears–birth, disappears – 4 months
- Palmar/plantar reflex: appears–birth, disappears – 4months
- Stepping reflex: appears-birth, disappears – 4 months
- Moro reflex: appears–birth, disappears – 4 months
- Tonic neck reflex: appears–1 month, disappears – 6 months
- DELAY IN DISAPPEARANCE OF THE PRIMITIVE REFLEXES SUGGESTS CEREBRAL DAMAGE

Growth and Development

Louis Low

NORMAL GROWTH

Human growth is determined by an interaction of genetic and environmental factors. The Infancy-Childhood-Puberty (ICP) Growth Model breaks down the human linear growth curve into three additive and partly superimposed components (Fig. 2.1). There are different growth promotion systems for each component. The infancy phase describes the period of rapid growth in utero and in infancy and this phase of growth is predominantly nutritionally dependent. Maternal nutrition before and during pregnancy are important determinants of foetal growth and low pre-pregnancy weight increases the risk of intrauterine growth retardation (OR 2.55). An additional intake of 300 Kcal and 15 grams of protein per day are recommended for pregnant mothers above the recommended intake of non-pregnant women. Nutrient supply to the growing foetus is the dominant determinant in foetal growth, which is also dependent in placental function. Multiple approaches of nutritional intervention control of infection and improved antenatal care to pregnant women will be more effective than any single intervention. Nutritional deprivation during pregnancy can have an epigenetic effect on foetal growth extending over many generations. Cytokines are essential for implantation and insulin-like growth factor II (IGF-II) is important for placental growth. Apart from nutrition, hormones and growth factors have an important role in the control of foetal growth. Foetal insulin secretion is dependent on the placental nutrition supply and foetal hyperinsulinaemia stimulates cell proliferation and foetal fat accumulation from 28 weeks gestation onwards. Thyroid hormone, which affects cell differentiation and brain development, is also regulated by nutrition. Cortisol is essential for the prepartum maturation of different organs including the liver, lung, gut and pituitary gland. Although growth hormone (GH) is important in postnatal growth, it plays an insignificant role in foetal growth except for an effect on foetal fat content. Animal knockout studies and human observations have shown that IGFs are most important for metabolic, mitogenic and differentiative activities of the foetus. IGF-II is more important in early embryogenesis. In humans, foetal body weight is more closely correlated with the concentration of foetal serum IGF-1 than IGF-II.

In the childhood phase of growth, hormone like growth hormone, thyroid hormone and growth factors like insulin-like growth factors begin to exert their influence from the end of the first year of life. A delay in the onset of the childhood phase of growth will result in faltering of growth during this critical period. The growth faltering commonly observed between 6 to 18 months of life in children from developing countries are due to nutritional and socio-economic factors rather than ethnic differences. The importance of the growth hormone and IGF-1 axis and other hormones in the childhood phase of growth will be described in a subsequent section of this chapter. A short-lived growth acceleration between seven to eight years of age can be observed in two-thirds of healthy children followed by a fall in growth velocity before the onset of puberty. The pubertal phase of growth is controlled by

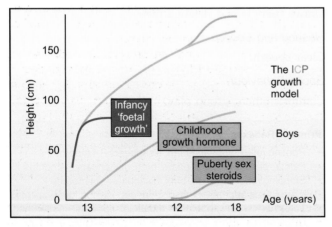

Fig. 2.1: Analysis of linear growth using a mathematical model
(J. Karlberg, et al. Acta Paediatrica Scand. 1987; 76: 478)

nutrition, health, GH-IGF-1 axis and pubertal secretion of adrenal androgens and sex steroids. The onset of the childhood component has been known to be positively associated with the magnitude of the foetal/infancy component. The height at onset of puberty is an important determinant of the final adult height. The onset of puberty component is negatively correlated with the height at onset of puberty.

The United Nations Children's Fund (UNICEF) has identified access to nutritionally adequate diet, health care for mothers and children, and environmental health factors as conditioning factors of child growth worldwide. The care required includes care of women in the reproductive age, breastfeeding and feeding practices, psychological care, food preparation, hygiene and home health practices. Low food intake and the burden of common childhood infectious diseases, diarrhoea, respiratory infections and infestations limit the full realization of the genetic potential in children from developing countries. As more and more women join the workforce, their duration of time spent in child care and income generation will determine whether child care is compromised. Quality child care will not be affordable or accessible to low-income working mothers. Environmental pollution (air, heavy metals and smoking) can affect the growth of children especially those living in developing countries undergoing rapid economic transition. The negative effects of active and passive smoking in mothers on foetal growth and growth in early life have been well characterised. Environmental exposure to lead in children has been linked to impaired physical growth, neuro-development and delayed puberty. Mercury poisoning from industrial pollution and teething powder and drugs are less common. There are claims of association of increased mercury exposure with neurodevelopment deficits. No significant association of prenatal and postnatal exposure to methylmercury from fish consumption with childhood neurodevelopment has been found in populations with high fish consumption. A negative association between environmental sulphur dioxide, total suspended particulates and exposure to herbicide and birth weight has been consistently reported in the literature. Impaired growth in infancy and childhood is associated with short adult stature and impaired cognitive development. The World Health Organization (WHO) Global Database on Child Growth and Malnutrition provides information on growth and nutrition worldwide (http://www.who.intnutgrowthdb) base on the National Center for Health statistic (NCHS)/WHO international growth reference. The prevalence of wasting in preschool children in Cambodia, Indonesia, Indian subcontinent, some island states in the Indian Ocean and some countries in Africa and Middle East has remained above 10%. According to WHO, 110 million stunted children live in Asia in 2005. With the improvement in socio-economic conditions and healthcare in most countries, there is a dramatic secular increase in mean stature of populations from Asia and other developing countries while the positive secular trends in growth have slowed or even plateaued in developed countries in Europe and North America.

Although malnutrition remains a problem in some parts of the world, there is now a worldwide obesity epidemic in both developing and developed countries. The reason for the increase in body weight in children in the community is multifactorial including genetic, cultural differences, dietary changes especially increase in intake of high fat energy dense foods, but most importantly the increasing sedentary life-style adopted by different sectors of the population. The decrease in daily physical activity is due to mechanization and computerization. Time spent watching television and playing or working on the computer is now regarded as a surrogate marker of inactivity in children. The health burden of excessive weight gain in childhood will be amplified in the years to come and urgent action by international organizations, governments and all national and region stake-holders is needed.

ASSESSMENT AND MONITORING OF GROWTH

A clinician should take the opportunity to assess the growth of each child at each clinical encounter. The head circumference should be measured as the biggest circumference between the frontal region and the occipital prominence using a non-stretchable measuring tape. The body weight should be measured with a calibrated electronic scale, without shoes or socks and the child wearing light clothing. In infants and young children, the supine length should be measured with an infant stadiometer (Fig. 2.2). Children older than 2 years of age should be measured standing using a wall-mounted stadiometer (Fig. 2.3) without shoes or socks, with the eyes and external auditory meatus held in the same plane and a slight upward pressure exerted on the jaw and occiput. The anthropometric measurements should be plotted accurately on the appropriate chart.

The monitor of growth in children and adolescents has been widely used by paediatricians as a marker of their general well-being. The normal pattern of growth in children is traditionally described in an up-to-date ethnic specific growth chart. Growth references are valuable tools for accessing the health of individuals and for health planner to assess the well-being of populations. In a survey involving 178 countries, growth monitoring in the first six years of life is an integral part of paediatric care in most countries worldwide. Two thirds of these countries use the NCHS/WHO growth reference while more developed countries use their own national growth reference. In developing countries, health care workers monitor growth to detect and intervene when children have growth

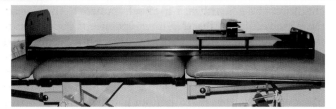

Fig. 2.2: Stadiometer for measurement of supine length

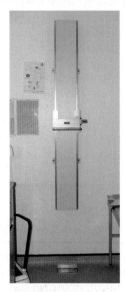

Fig. 2.3: Wall mounted stadiometer for height measurement

faltering. In developed countries, growth monitoring has been regarded as a useful tool for detecting unrecognized organic diseases, provision of reassurance to parents and for monitoring the health of children in the population. Understanding the ethnic differences in childhood and pubertal growth will help in our interpretation of results of surveillance of child growth based on the NCHS/WHO growth standard which has a number of limitations. A WHO Multicenter Growth Reference has been developed based on a longitudinal study of exclusively breastfed children from birth to twenty-four months and a cross-sectional study of children from 18 to 71 months from six countries (Brazil, Ghana, India, Norway, Oman and the United States). Babies in the Euro-Growth Study who were breastfed according to the World Health Organization (WHO) recommendations showed higher weight gain in the first 3 months of life and were lower in weight and length between 6 to 12 months as compared to the NCHS/WHO growth reference. No significant differences in growth from the NCHS reference in these children have been noted between 12 to 36 months. The finding is similar to that of the WHO Multicenter Growth Reference. The WHO Multicenter Growth reference has recently been completed (Acta Paediatr 2006; 95 (Suppl 450): 1-106) and will be the gold standard for assessing growth of children worldwide in the future.

Despite widespread acceptance of routine growth monitoring of children as the standard of care, a recent meta-analysis questioned the benefits of growth monitoring in childhood, as there have been very few trials that evaluated the impact of this practice on childhealth. Infants should be weighed at birth and at times of their immunization. Surveillance of children's weight beyond one year is only recommended in children whose growth causes clinical concern. Clinicians should pay more attention to growth parameter collected during clinical consultations. Length measurement should only be done in children under 2 years of age if there is a concern in their growth or weight gain.

In a normal population, less than 5% of the infants will drop their weight through two centile lines and less than 1% of infants will have a fall in weight across three centile lines in the first year of life. A baby would be regarded as failing to thrive if there is a fall in weight across more than two centile lines in infancy. In the United Kingdom, it has been recommended that primary care physicians should refer children for assessment if their heights falls below the 0.4th percentile (-2.67SD) and a single height measurement at school entry using this criteria has been found to be a sensitive marker for undiagnosed organic disease. The sensitivity of this recommended height screening test can be improved by making a correction for the height of the parents. Height measurements taken during other clinical encounters during childhood are further opportunities for referral using the 0.4th percentile as the cut-off for action. Clinicians have long placed a lot of emphasis on growth assessment using height velocity, which is calculated from the difference between two height measurements, thereby combining the imprecision of the two readings. Successive measurements of height over time in an individual are highly correlated whereas successive annual growth velocities are not. This suggests that growth velocity estimates are not reliable and does not have a useful role in routine growth monitoring. Despite its imprecision, a grossly abnormal growth velocity can still be regarded as an indicator of disease. Whether routine height screening every two to three years between five and twelve years of age will be cost effective in detecting silent disease without the capacity to cause harm within the paediatric population remains to be proven. However, routine monitoring of the height and weight in both developing and developed countries is likely to continue in the years to come.

In the monitoring of overweight and underweight, both the World Health Organization (WHO) and the International Obesity Task Force (IOTF) have suggested the use of different body mass index [BMI derived from weight (kg) /height² (in meters)] cut-offs for identifying these problems in the clinical and public health setting. The WHO has adopted the updated BMI reference based on the United States NHANES I data collected in 1971-1974 (http://www.cdc.gov/growth charts) while IOTF has adopted an International BMI reference derived from six population growth studies (Cole TJ et al. BMJ 2000; 320:1270) as the gold standard for international comparison. The WHO proposed a BMI below the 5th percentile, above 85th percentile and 95th percentile as cut-offs for underweight, overweight and obesity. The IOTF established BMI percentile cut-offs at different ages based on extrapolation of adult BMI cut-offs of $25kg/m^2$ and $30kg/m^2$ for overweight and obesity. In addition, national BMI references are now available in many developed countries. The cut-offs based on the United States reference data are related to some measures of morbidity but the newly developed IOTF BMI cut-off points for children still require validation with data on morbidity measures like blood pressure, serum lipids, insulin resistance and diabetes. In a meeting organised by WHO/International Association for the Study of Obesity (IASO)/IOTF in Hong Kong in 1999, the experts were of the opinion that a lower BMI cut-offs might need to be set for adult Asian populations because of their predisposition to deposit abdominal fat. The proposed revised BMI cut-off is $23kg/m^2$ and $25kg/m^2$ for overweight and obesity respectively (http://www.idi.org.au/obesity_report.htm)

The Growth Hormone—IGF-1 Axis

The pulsatile secretion of growth hormone from the pituitary gland is under the control of the stimulatory action of growth hormone releasing hormone (GHRH) and the suppressive effect of somatostatin. Multiple neurotransmitters and neuropeptides are involved in hypothalamic the release of these hormones. Growth hormone is essential for normal human growth in childhood and adolescence. The liver is the organ with the highest GH receptor concentrations and is the main source of GH binding protein (cleaved extracellular portion of the GH receptor) found in the circulation. After binding to its receptor and inducing dimerization, GH activates the JAK2/STAT pathway to bring about the stimulation of epiphyseal growth, osteoclast differentiation, lipolysis and amino acid uptake into muscles. The more important growth promotion action of GH is mediated by insulin-like growth factor-1 (IGF-1). Circulating IGF-1 comes predominantly from the liver and is associated with IGF binding protein 3 (IGFBP-3) and the acid labile submit (ALS) to form a ternary complex. The action of IGF-1 is modified by six binding proteins in the circulation. Although IGF-1 is important in foetal growth, serum concentration of IGF-1 is low in foetal life and in early infancy. A significant rise in IGF-1 and IGFBP-3 concentrations is observed in normal children from 10 months onwards. There is further progressive rise of serum IGF-1 to two to three times the adult serum concentrations

as the children progress through puberty. The serum IGF-1 level in childhood is also dependent on nutrients availability. It has now been shown that the local generation of IGF-1 in tissues in response to GH rather than the circulating IGF-1 is essential for normal growth; liver-specific IGF-1 knockout mice have low circulating IGF-1 levels and yet they have near normal growth. Short stature has been reported in humans with mutations in the genes of GHRH, GH, GH receptor, STAT5b, IGF-1, ALS and IGF-1 receptor.

PUBERTY

Puberty is defined as the maturational transition of an individual from the sexually immature state to adulthood with the capacity to reproduce. The hypothalamic-pituitary-gonadal axis is active in utero and at birth. After this period of activation, the axis undergoes a long period of relative quiescence from 3 to 6 months after birth until late childhood when pubertal development occurs. The onset of puberty is the result of decreasing sensitivity of the regulatory system of gonadotropin secretion (gonadostat) to the negative feedback of the small amounts of gonadal steroids secreted by the prepubertal gonads, as well as a decrease in the central neural inhibition of gonadotrophin releasing hormone (GnRH) release. Disruption of genes controlling the migration of GnRH neurons from the olfactory epithelium to the forebrain can result in delayed puberty. The initiation of puberty is associated with a decrease in trans-synaptic inhibition by GABAergic neurons and an activation of excitatory glutamatergic neurotransmission in the control of GnRH secretion. There is also evidence that glial to neuron signalling through growth factors is important in the neuro-endocrine control of puberty. The timing of puberty is also influenced by nutrition and metabolic cues. A direct relationship between a particular ratio of fat to lean body mass and onset of puberty has been described. Leptin plays a role in informing the brain of peripheral energy stores and body composition and may act as a permissive signal for the onset of puberty. Evidence for genetic regulation of the timing of puberty is suggested by the correlation of the age of onset of puberty in mother and their offspring's and also in twin studies. It has been suggested that 50-80% of the variance in pubertal onset may be genetically controlled.

With the onset of puberty, there is increasing pulsatile secretion of luteinising hormone (LH) and to a lesser extent follicle-stimulating hormone (FSH) mainly at night through gradual amplification of GnRH pulse frequency and amplitude. In pubertal boys and girls, sleep-entrained pulsatile GnRH secretion every 60 to 90 minutes progressing to become more regular throughout the day. In boys, the pulsatile gonadotropin secretion stimulates the testes to develop and the Leydig cells to produce testosterone. Testosterone production increases progressively and is responsible for the metabolic changes and the development of secondary sexual characteristics. Both LH and FSH are required for the development and maintenance of testicular function. In early puberty in girls, circulating FSH level increases disproportionately to the LH level in response to GnRH stimulation. Gonadotropin stimulation leads to a rapid rise in ovarian oestrogen production before menarche. When the concentration of oestradiol rises above 200pg/ml for a few days, the negative feedback on GnRH and gonadotropin release turns to positive feedback leading to the ovulatory LH surge. In humans, the ability of the hypothalamus to stimulate gonadotropin secretion in response to positive feedback effects of oestrogen does not occur until after menarche. In adult females, the GnRH pulse frequency starts at 90 minutes in early follicular phase, increases to one pulse every 60 minutes in mid-follicular phase and slows to one pulse every 4 to 6 hours in the lateral phase.

From the age of 6-8 years onwards, there is a progressive rise in adrenal androgens secretion up to 20 years of age. This process of maturation of the adrenal gland, referred to as adrenarche, is responsible for pubic and axillary hair development and this event occurs independent of the maturation of the hypothalamic-pituitary-gonadal axis although the timing of the two processes are usually related in normal puberty. Adrenarche is coincident with the mid-childhood adiposity rebound and there is evidence that nutritional status measured as a change in the body mass index (BMI) is an important physiological regulator of adrenarche.

The progressive changes in the secondary sexual characteristics have been described in a standardized format by Tanner (Figs 2.4 and 2.5). There is considerable variation in the age of onset and the tempo of progression of puberty among normal children. Over the last century, children have tended to be taller in stature and reach sexual maturity at an earlier age. In a recent population study from the United States, 5% and 15% of the white and African American girls had breast development before the age of 7 years. Since the mean age of menarche in these American girls have not changed significantly over time, puberty in American girls is associated with earlier onset of breast development but with a slower tempo of pubertal progression. An age of onset of puberty before the age of 9 years in boys and before 7 years in girls will be regarded as premature. Girls and boy without signs of puberty by the age of 13 years and 14 years should be monitored carefully and considered for evaluation of delayed puberty. The mean age of onset on menarche can vary from 11.2 years in African Americans to 13.7 years in China. Light-dark rhythm and climatic conditions have little effect on the age of menarche. Children adopted from developing countries have early puberty as a general feature.

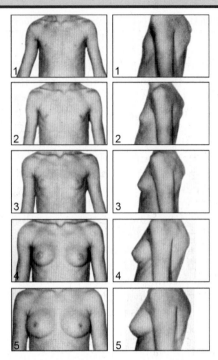

Fig. 2.4: Standards for breast development (From Tanner 1969) Reproduced by permission from Endocrine and Genetic Diseases of Childhood and Adolescence by Gardner, Lytt.I., 1975, WB Saunders Company

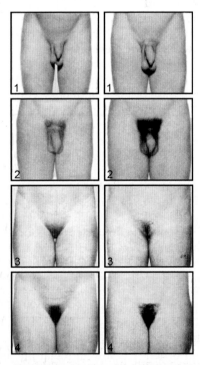

Fig. 2.5: Standards for pubic hair ratings in boys and girls (From Tanner 1969) Reproduced by permission from Endocrine and Genetic Diseases of Childhood and Adolescence by Gardner, Lytt.I. 1975, WB Saunders Company

CHILD DEVELOPMENT

Development in children is predominantly determined by genetic factors but a significant contribution comes from environmental factors (maternal nutrition during pregnancy, birth, socio-economic factors, nutrition and health after birth). Intellectual Development in childhood and adolescence is a complex and dynamic process with the interaction between genes and the environment continuously changing over time. Antenatal and postnatal depression, maternal malnutrition, maternal smoking during pregnancy, antenatal exposure to organic pollutants and adverse child care practice can disrupt the development of different psychomotor domains in infancy and childhood. Home environment, parent-child relationship, parenting style and discipline practices and school environment can have a major influence in the socioemotional and cognitive growth of an individual in childhood and adolescence. Traditionally, early childhood development can be described in stages in four functional skill areas: gross motor, fine motor, language and speech, social and emotional development. It is also important for paediatricians to be familiar with the development of the special senses, like hearing, vision, taste, smell, sensation and proprioception. Timing of achievement of major milestones in the various domains of development can vary enormously in normal children. Sound knowledge of development in childhood and adolescence allow us to recognise global or specific developmental delay beyond the normal acceptable age, disordered developmental sequence or developmental regression.

GROSS MOTOR DEVELOPMENT

Motor development progresses in a cephalocaudal direction with suppression of primitive reflexes and development of postural tone and secondary protective reflexes. The primitive reflexes including the Moro, grasp, stepping and asymmetric tonic neck reflexes must have disappeared by 3-6 months of age before head control (4 months) and independent sitting at 6-8 months can occur. Prior to walking, an infant can crawl on all four limbs, bottom shuffle, commando creep or roll along the ground. Shufflers, creepers and rollers tend to attain independent walking at a later age than infants who crawl on all fours. Thus early locomotor patterns can result in significant variation in the age of achieving independent walking. A delay in walking beyond 18 months of age is a warning sign in children who have crawling as the early locomotor pattern. An infant will stand holding on furniture by 9 months, cruise round furniture by 12 months and walk independently by 13-15 months. At 18 months, a child can climb onto a chair and walk up and down stairs two feet per step by 24 months of age. By 2½ years, a child should be able to stand on tip-toes, jump on both feet and kick a ball. A 3 year old child can walk backwards and can ride a tricycle. There is further development of gross motor skill and balance with age and most children can participate in a variety of activities like swimming, skating, gymnastics and ball games by 6-7 years of age.

FINE MOTOR DEVELOPMENT IN EARLY CHILDHOOD

The development of fine motor skills in childhood is condition upon the development of normal vision. Voluntary movements and fine motor manipulations require the co-ordinated development of nervous system and visuomotor co-ordination. Visual fixation can be demonstrated in babies by 4-6 weeks of life. The grasp reflex is usually inhibited by 3 months of age and babies can be seen to open their hands, clasp and unclasp their hands at the midline of the body. Between 3 to 5 months, babies will find their hands interesting and persistence of "hand regard" beyond 5 months is unusual. By 6 months, babies can reach and grasp an object (one inch cube) with the palm of their hands (palmar grasp). Putting objects to the mouth is a common activity at this age. Transfer of objects from one hand to the other can be seen at 6 months. By 9 months, babies can hold a cube in each hand and bring them together for comparison. Grasping of small objects with the thumb and index finger (pincer grasp) can be achieved between 9-12 months. Casting of objects is frequently observed towards the end of the first year of life but voluntary release of an object on command will only take place at 15 months. By 15 months, a child can hold a pen in his/her palm and scribble. The child can build a tower of 2-3 cubes between 15-18 months. At 2 years, a child's ability to manipulate small objects continues to improve (Fig. 2.6). Hand dominance can be

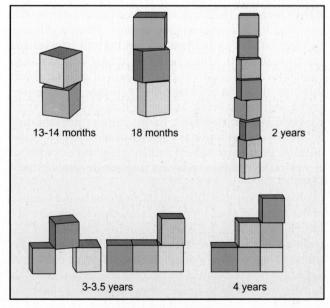

13-14 months   18 months   2 years

3-3.5 years   4 years

Fig. 2.6: Build cubes

observed at 2½ years and the child can scribble and draw a line or circle with a tripod pen grip. At 3 years, a child can build a tower of 8 to 9 cubes and copy building patterns using three to four cubes. The child can eat with a fork or spoon. By 4 years, a child can draw a man showing body parts and copy some alphabets. Between 5 to 6 years, a child can write well and eat properly with knife and fork.

LANGUAGE AND SPEECH DEVELOPMENT IN CHILDHOOD

Language can be defined as an arbitrary set of symbols, which when combined in a particular sequence, allows an individual to convey a specific message or conceptualization and transmit them to another individual. When the transmission of messages between individuals is performed verbally, then the action is referred to as speech. Language acquisition is a complex process integrating interaction between many factors. Genetic factors possibly play an important role early in the developmental process but neurological (cerebral palsy, neuromuscular disorders, hearing impairment, autism), cognitive (mental retardation, specific learning disabilities, specific developmental language impairment), environmental (psychosocial deprivation, bilingual or multi-lingual environments), cultural differences, maternal depression, large sibship) factors are important determinants of speech development. Impaired hearing is associated with impairment in language and speech development and the prevalence of severe hearing loss has been estimated to be between 1:900 to 1:2500 newborn infants. It has been shown that universal newborn hearing screening, using auditory brainstem response (ABR) or two-step screening (ABR – ABR) and otoacoustic emissions (OAE), enables the early identification of infants with moderate to severe hearing impairment. There is evidence that early diagnosis of impaired hearing and intervention can be associated with a better-improved language and communication skills by 2 to 5 years of age. Cochlear implant is an alternative to children with severe sensorineural hearing loss who do not benefit from conventional hearing-aids. Early cochlear implantation before 3 years of age has been associated with a better outcome in terms of speech and language development as compared to children receiving cochlear implants in later life.

A one-month-old baby will startle to sound but location of the source of sound presented at ear level is present at 6 months. At 3 months, they respond to the call of their names, smile, laugh or are comforted in response to the sound of the mother's voice. Babies can make consonant sounds at 3 months (e.g. ba, ka, da) and deaf infants are usually referred to as quiet babies at this stage. Babbling in strings will usually occur after 6 months of age. At 12 months, the baby understands some simple commands and uses increasing variety of intonation when babbling. At one year, an infant will understand simple commands like "blow a kiss" or "wave bye-bye". They will be able to say a few words with meaning and will have at least 6 recognizable words with meaning by 18 months. At 18 months, they can name body parts on request and start to use word combinations. By 2 years, children have a vocabulary of many words and can speak in simple sentences. A 9 month old child can look for an object after being hidden, demonstrating their grasp of the concept of object permanence. Before the development of expressive speech, infants of one year can indicate their desire by pointing or gesture. They demonstrate definition by use of common objects like cup, brush, comb and spoon. Symbolisation will occur at 18 months with the child imitating the mother's household chore or feeding a doll. Between 18 to 22 months, children can engage in constructive symbolic play with toys of miniature.

Both expressive and receptive language involves three important aspects, namely, phonology and articulation, semantics and syntax. The co-ordinated neuromuscular mechanisms, which produce the desire sequence of phonemes, constitute expressive phonology. The neurological process involved in the identification of the phonemes in a spoken message is referred to a receptive phonology. Semantics refers to the process involved in relating a spoken word to its meaning. In most cases, a thought cannot be expressed simply by a single word. In constructing a spoken message, syntax governs the particular order of words as they appear sequentially in speech. Syntax also governs the use of tense, plurality, grammar and the relationship between the different words. Syntactic process words in conjunction with the semantic process in deriving the meaning conveyed by a sequence of words. The use of two to three word combinations in young children involves the omission of function words, which are used in the more complex adult speech. The simple word combinations also reflect the reduced memory capacity of young children. By 3 years, a child can use plurals, pronouns and prepositions (e.g. under, behind, in front of) in their speech. Most young children are disfluent but child should be wholly intelligible and have few infantile substitutions or consonant substitutions at the age of 4 years. As children become older and with experience, they incorporate new rules and expand rules already acquired, in such a fashion that their speech becomes progressively a close approximation to the syntactic structure characteristic of adult speech. After the age of 6 years, children are able to engage in a long conversation with family members and their peers. They can perform simple tasks in command. At 7 years, children should be able to express their thoughts in speech and writing.

As the number of children raised in bilingual or multilingual families increases, paediatricians should have some knowledge of the normal patterns of bilingual language acquisition. A child may acquire two languages simultaneously with an initial undifferentiated simple language composed of elements from both languages. By 2 to 3 years of age, the child begins to be able to differentiate the two languages. The child can use the appropriate language when speaking to a particular person or in a particular environment (e.g. home or school). Normal children in bilingual families can also acquire the two languages in a sequential manner. In this situation, the first or dominant language is acquired first in the usual manner and then the children will develop an understanding of the second language drawing on the experience with the first language. There may be a period of selective mutism before the child can switch from one language to the other proficiently. Bilingualism may contribute to delay in language development but is not a cause of disorder of language or cognitive development. Parents should be consistent in setting the boundaries for where each language is spoken.

SOCIAL DEVELOPMENT

By 4 weeks of age, babies show social smile in response to the carer and enjoyment to cuddling, bathing and the voice of the mother. At 6 months, a baby is able to finger feed and is more wary of strangers. A child can drink from a cup with help and enjoy songs and nursery rhymes at 9 months of age. They also desire a comfort object (like a soft toy, cloth or blanket) and become anxious when they are separated from their carers (separation anxiety). Babies can play pat-a-cake or wave bye-bye and show affection to family members towards the end of the first year. At 18 months, they can feed themselves with a spoon and they can feed themselves properly using knife and fork at 4 years. The age of achievement of bladder and bowel control is variable but is usually towards the end of the second year of life but bedwetting at night can persist into mid or late childhood. Beyond two years of age, children are increasing mobile and are curious and interested in exploring their environment. They can help with dressing and bathing. They can manage to use the toilet independently by age three. At the age of 4 years, they can groom and dress themselves and brush their teeth. At age 18 months, children are contented to play by themselves at 2 years; they still play alone or alongside other children (parallel play). At 3 years, they start playing with other children and start making friends. They share toys and develop the concept of being helpful to others.

EMOTIONAL AND COGNITIVE DEVELOPMENT

Soon after birth, a baby demonstrates a keen interest in human faces and voices. They also become aware of other sensations like hunger and noxious stimuli and respond to unpleasant sensations by crying. Even at one month, a baby exhibits different dimensions of behaviour like activity, placidity, irritability, excitability and anger regulation that is commonly referred to as temperament. Infants with different temperament are at increased risk of behavioural problems in later life. The bonding of a baby with the parents depends on the baby's temperament and the personality, sensitivity and caring nature of the parents. At 6 months, a baby already becomes aware of the emotional state of the parents or carer through their actions and their voices. Secure attachment relationship between infant and mother, and to a certain extent, with fathers and caregivers will be established towards the end of the first year of life. Secure mother-infant bonding buffers a baby against the short-term influence of adverse psycho-social effects in childhood development. By one year, infants start to develop their own sense of identity. They have fluctuating moods, occasionally throw temper tantrums but will also show affection towards familiar people. In the next 2 to 3 years, young children become increasingly aware of other people's intension desires and emotions. They begin to show empathy (comfort a crying baby). They are inquisitive and constantly ask questions. They recognise primary colours (2½ to 3 years) and begin to grasp the concept of numbers and time. They play and communicate with other children. They have increased memory capacity and reasoning and problem solving skills. They can remember and give an account of past events. Children learn from observing and experiencing repeated stimuli and social situations, imitating and experimenting with speech and actions. They apply a set of concrete rules for exploring and interacting with the outside world. Their ability to appreciate logical arguments improves with age. They become aware of their body image and develop self-esteem. Their self-concept becomes differentiated and they begin to realize that they are not always competent in different developmental domains. During middle childhood, children further develop their fundamental skills of reading, writing, mathematics, long-term memory and recall. They will be able to comprehend complex instructions. Significant amount of learning will be acquired during the school hours. Adolescence is the period of transition from childhood to mature adulthood with physical maturation and acquisition of reproductive capability and socio-economic and independence from the family. With the increasing number of young people entering into tertiary education, this period of adolescent development has been lengthened in the developed world. Adolescents become increasingly competent in logical and scientific reasoning and these abilities are reflected in their ability to analyse and solve problems in mathematics and science and formulate arguments and opinions in different fields of study. They are able to think in abstract terms and develop an understanding of issues like responsibility, morality, peer relationships and sexuality.

DEVELOPMENT ASSESSMENT

A comprehensive child health assessment would not be complete without a proper developmental history, examination and assessment of emotion and mental well-being of the child. To obtain a developmental history, ask the parents open-ended questions and to elaborate on developmental concerns, if any, and provide examples of their concerns. A paediatrician should be able to identify "developmental red flags" (Table 2.1), developmental delay, disordered developmental sequence and developmental sequence and developmental regression. Observations and interactive assessment in different developmental domains (gross motor, fine motor, visuo-spatial co-ordination, language and speech, emotion and social behaviour, cognition, hearing and vision) should be carried out. After assessment, a profile of developmental abilities and difficulties should form the basis for the necessity of referral for multidisciplinary specialist assessments by developmental paediatrician, psychologist, speech, physio-and occupational therapists.

Intelligence tests have been used to assess the innate cognitive ability, and to indicate deficiencies of different domains of development in a child who is struggling and under achieving in school. The Wechsler Intelligence Scale for Children (WISC-III and IV) is one of the most widely used intelligence quotient (IQ) tests and has been translated into many languages and validated. Some Wechsler subtests do not require skills in English and may be used to address referrals of non-English speaking children for certain developmental problems. The tests provide four index scores reflecting verbal comprehension, perceptual reasoning, working memory and processing speed. An IQ test is the first step towards the assessment of specific learning disabilities and the provision of support and intervention for children with difficulties in schools. A high IQ score however, does not guarantee future success

Table 2.1: Developmental "Red Flags" in infancy and early childhood
1. No visual following by 8 weeks and poor eye contact
2. Unco-ordinated eye movements with head turning after 3 months
3. Persistent fisting (especially with thumbs adducted across the palms beyond 3 months
4. No head control by 6 months
5. Not sitting independently by 10 months
6. Unable to walk alone at 18 months
7. No pointing to show demand or interest by 14 months
8. No words with meaning by 18 months
9. Not joining two words by 30 months
10. Features of pervasive developmental disorders (compulsive and ritualistic activities, severe language delay, poorly developed social relationship, abnormal attachment to inanimate objects, inappropriate affect and tantrums, developmental delay).

in life. Children with an uneven developmental profile on IQ testing will require further specialist neuropsychological assessment using specialised test instruments for memory, visuo-spatial skills, language, attention, motor skills, social cognitive and planning and execution of tasks.

In recent years, there is increasing demand for paediatricians to develop skills in dealing with children with behavioural and emotional disorders. Measurements of behavioural and emotional well-being and adjustment in children and their family members can be achieved using the Child Behaviour Check List (CBCL) for parents, teachers and older children. Paediatricians should be aware of common presentations of such disorders and have some knowledge of neuropsychological test instruments for the assessment of childhood depression, anxiety, obsessive-compulsive, attention deficit hyper activity disorders, eating disorders and conduct disorders. These conditions will be discussed in greater details under the different chapters of this book.

Neonatal Paediatrics

Paul Galea, Syed Rehan Ali, Zulfiqar A Bhutta

3.1 Fetal and Neonatal Medicine

INTRODUCTION

Given a normal genetic endowment, a healthy well-nourished mother, a normal pregnancy and delivery, the provision of appropriate nutrition and a supportive home and community environment, a child will grow and develop normally. It is not possible to separate the reproductive health needs of women and the health of the newborn infant. Adverse genetic and environmental factors can compromise the health of an individual from the time of conception. Processes of cell division within the individual organs of the developing embryo, fetus, infant and child are dependent on adequate nutrition and freedom from environmental insult. The healthy child is one who shows no evidence of defective organ function and has normal growth and development.

Interventions aimed at lowering perinatal or neonatal mortality must address maternal health, the social position of women and the provisions for ensuring maternal health during pregnancy and delivery.

EMBRYONIC DEVELOPMENT

The ovum is fertilised by the sperm usually in the fallopian tube and is propelled along the tube to the uterus while undergoing repeated cell division. The resulting ball of cells (morula) develops a cavity (blastocoele) at which stage the ovum is known as a blastocyst. The multiplying cells of blastocyst form the inner cell mass whilst cells nearer to the surface develop into trophoblast. For a time the trophoblast and the inner cell mass remain connected by a stalk of cells known as the body stalk. The trophoblastic cells then begin to erode into the uterine endometrium eventually to form the placenta.

The Embryo

The ovum or blastocyst penetrates and eventually becomes completely embedded in the endometrium, which is then known as the decidua. Two cavities develop in the inner cell mass of the blastocyst. One is the amniotic sac and the other yolk sac. Between them is a cellular area called the embryonic plate because it is from this area that the embryo grows. In the embryonic plate area the cells become grouped into three primitive layers known as the ectoderm, the mesoderm and the endoderm. Subsequently the skin, certain mucus membranes and the central nervous system develop from the ectoderm; the blood, muscle, bones and certain organs from the mesoderm; and the lungs, alimentary mucosa, bladder, pancreas and parts of the liver from the endoderm. Amniotic fluid, which fills the amniotic sac, serves to protect and encourage the growth of the embryo, which derives its nutrient from the yolk sac pending the development of a rudimentary placenta. The yolk sac is connected by vitelline duct with the embryonic gut. The amniotic cavity gradually envelops the embryo and at the same time brings the yolk sac and the vitelline duct into contact with the body stalk to form the umbilical cord. Development of the cord is usually complete by the sixth week.

Placental Development

Buds of multiplying cells sprout out from the trophoblast where it comes into contact with the decidua and form the villi. These multiply in number to cover the entire ovum. Some of the villi become attached to the deep layer of the decidua (decidua basalis) and anchor the ovum to the decidua. Others penetrate decidual blood vessels around the third week after fertilisation. The villi develop to contain a central core of fetal mesoderm and embryonic vessels in which fetal blood circulates and two cellular layers: an inner-Langhan's layer or cytotrophoblast - and an outer- the syncytium or syncytiotrophoblast. Tropho-blast is responsible for the absorption of nutrients from maternal blood into the fetal circulation and for the return of waste products through the arterial vessels of the developing umbilical cord. By the end of the third month the placenta acquires a discoidal shape consisting of some 15 to 20 clumps (cotyledons) of chorionic villi anchored to the decidua basalis.

Twinning

In most instances twin pregnancy results from fertilisation of a single ovum (monozygote). There is one placenta, one chorion and two amniotic sacs. Exceptionally, however, two placentas may develop. Where in a twin pregnancy fertilisation of two ova has taken place (dizygote), there are two placentas, which may, however, fuse and have the appearance of a single placenta. Dizygotic twins may be born with separate placentas or with an apparently single placenta with two separate amniotic sacs (diamniotic) and two chorionic membranes (dichorionic). Monozygotic twins may be born with a) separate placentas and membranes, b) one placenta and dichorionic, diamniotic membranes, c) one placenta with monochorionic membranes. Monozygotic twins originate from the division of one fertilised egg and are identical. Splitting can occur at different stages of development. Early splitting (2 to 3 days) after conception will result in a different outcome from intermediate splitting (4 to 7 days) and late splitting (8-12 days), see Fig. 3.1.1. When the splitting is delayed beyond 13 days the twins may be fused (conjoined or "Siamese"). Twins of different sex must be dizygotic. In Europe, approximately 33% of monozygous twins are dichorial, 66% monochorial-diamniotic and 1% monochorionic-monoamniotic. Decisions as to whether twins are identical or not cannot always be made by examination of the placentas and membranes and it may require blood grouping and DNA finger printing analyses to make the final determination.

Key Learning Points
• It is difficult to determine twin zygosity from examination of the placenta and membranes. • Blood grouping and DNA analysis are required to make a definite diagnosis

Placental Function

The placenta transfers CO_2 from fetal tissues to the maternal circulation and obtains oxygen and other nutrients from the maternal blood in the intervillous spaces. Chorionic villi are capable of selective absorption of substances necessary for embryonic and fetal growth. In addition to the transfer of all nutrient materials necessary for the formation of the embryo and fetus the waste products of fetal metabolism such as urea and heat are transferred back across the placenta to maternal blood.

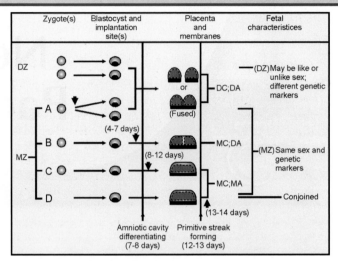

Fig. 3.1.1: Twins, zygosity and structure of the membranes

The placenta acts as a protective carrier preventing the passage of some, but by no means all, potentially harmful substances from the maternal circulation. Viruses such as those of rubella, cytomegalovirus, HIV and parvovirus can pass the barrier as can the spirochaete of syphilis, the bacillus of tuberculosis and the protozoon of toxoplasmosis.

Temporary passive immunity to many infections is acquired from the mother through placental transfer of IgG antibodies to infections previously experienced by the mother. Transfer of fetal antigens in a reverse direction can take place. Rhesus positive cells from a fetus may enter the circulation of the rhesus negative-mother and stimulate the formation of antibodies. Other substances, which can penetrate the placental barrier, include alcohol, nicotine and sedative, anaesthetic, antibiotic and other drugs.

The placenta functions as an endocrine organ for the production of oestrogens and other hormones. Maternal hormones can also transfer to the fetus to a varying degree.

Disturbance of normal placental growth and function can result in abnormalities of embryonic and fetal development. Abnormalities of placental structure and size, degenerative change and premature separation of the placental cotyledons can result in damage to the developing fetus.

Key Learning Points
• The placenta meets all the fetus's respiratory and nutritional needs during intrauterine life. • It is able to block the passage of several, but not all, organisms from mother to fetus. • The placenta prepares the fetus for extrauterine life by actively transporting trace metals and iron, and immunoglobulins, from mother to fetus.

The Embryo

Embryonic development takes place during the first 8 weeks after conception. Rudimentary eyes, ears, and the projecting buds representing the beginnings of limb formation are recognisable about 4 weeks after conception. At this stage the embryo consists of a large head and a rather tapering body and weighs approximately 1 to 1.3 grams and measures 9 to 12 millimetres in length. By the 8th week the hands and feet are recognisable; the external genitalia are developing and the head has assumed a recognisable shape. The name embryo has been used by custom until the end of the 8th week. Thereafter the embryo becomes a fetus. At 12 weeks the placenta is well developed, the umbilical cord begins to show normal spiral characteristics and fingers and toes are identifiable. By 12 weeks the fetus measures 9 cm in length and weighs about 30 grams. Centres of ossification are present in many bones. By 24 weeks of conception hair appears on the head and the deposition of subcutaneous fat begins. As subcutaneous fat is laid down in increasing amount the skin acquires a smooth texture and pink colour and the body develops a more rotund appearance. At 40 weeks the fetus measures approximately 51 cm in length and weighs about 3,200 grams with the male being slightly larger and heavier than the female. During fetal development various organ systems differentiate anatomically and progressively through a series of cells divisions, which are genetically determined in number and type. If intrauterine development of one or more organ systems does not progress normally this may result in fetal death or the delivery of an infant with anatomical and functional abnormalities.

The introduction of embryonic and fetal ultrasound by Ian Donald in Glasgow in 1957 brought about a revolution in our ability to assess fetal growth and development of individual organs. Gestational age, that is the age from conception, is generally calculated by reference to the date of the first day of the last menstrual cycle, which gives menstrual age. The mean interval between conception and delivery (gestational age) is around 265 days. More usually the duration of pregnancy, dated from the last menstrual period gives an average duration for a term pregnancy of 280 days. The first day of the last menstrual period is generally accepted as the date from which the gestational age is calculated to the nearest week. Since the introduction of ultrasonic techniques accurate assessments of fetal age can be obtained. Measurement of crown rump length in early pregnancy (12 weeks) gives a very accurate assessment of fetal maturity. In later pregnancy, measurements of trunk area in relation to skull area can give accurate assessment of fetal growth and development. Doppler ultrasound is used to assess fetal and placental blood flow and can give an early indication of placental failure or fetal circulatory anomalies. Measurement of fetal growth rate can be determined as can the presence of fetal anomalies some of which may be treated before delivery.

The introduction of ultrasound has allowed the development of techniques such as amniocentesis, chorionic villus biopsy and fetal blood and tissue sampling to be developed and to allow prenatal diagnosis of a wide range of inherited metabolic disorders and chromosomal defects. Fetal monitoring techniques using fetal electrocardiograms, heart rates and the determination of fetal pH by obstetricians has helped reduce the number of infants damaged by prenatal and intranatal disorders.

Birth

Adaptation from the fetal intrauterine state to the infant extrauterine state is not without its problems. The move from complete dependence on placenta and maternal tissues for life support to a dependence on the individual organs of the infant is complex. The infant systems principally involved in the initial stages are the respiratory, cardiovascular and nervous systems. Later, digestive, renal and hepatic, skin and musculoskeletal function become of more importance.

Key Learning Points
• The fetus is entirely dependent on the placenta for oxygenation but exists in a relatively hypoxic environment compared to the newborn baby who uses the lungs for oxygenation.
• Fetal haemoglobin and polycythaemia compensate for this relative hypoxia.
• Major adaptations in the cardiovascular and respiratory systems occur at birth, which allow the change from intra- to extrauterine life.

Respiration

Fetal breathing movements are necessary for normal lung development and can be affected by extrinsic factors such as maternal smoking. The fetal lung produces a fluid, which is normally swallowed although some may be expelled into the amniotic sac by fetal movement. Fetal blood gas exchange is dependent on a good blood flow on both the maternal and fetal sides of the placenta. Fetal tissues in utero are relatively hypoxaemic (20 - 30 mmHg/ 3-4 kPa is partly due to the large requirement of the placental tissues for oxygen and partly to the relative imbalance of fetal and maternal blood flow with uneven blood gas exchange in the cotyledons. There is, however, a large margin of safety in placental gas exchange to compensate for small rapid changes in maternal blood gas status. Larger changes in fetal blood gas status may be reflected in fetal tachycardia which is the first true sign of fetal distress and which may be sufficient to compensate for a temporary period of difficulty such as that which occurs during a uterine contraction. Progressive hypoxaemia of the fetus is manifest as bradycardia with associated fetal tissue acidaemia. The introduction of continuous recording of fetal heart rate in relation to the state of uterine contraction and the use of fetal scalp blood for measurement of hydrogen ion concentrations has allowed fairly exact measurement of fetal tissue hypoxia. Measurements of beat-to-beat variation in fetal heart rate give a sensitive indication of impending fetal hypoxaemia. The fetus is able to regulate blood distribution and in states of hypoxaemia can vasoconstrict the vessels supplying skin, limbs, lungs and abdominal organs to allow more oxygen to be made available to the heart and brain. Some of the metabolic acid (lactic acid) produced in the under-perfused tissue areas where anaerobic glycolysis is taking place, returns to the central circulation and is evident as a metabolic acidosis.

Key Learning Points

The major adaptations in the respiratory system at birth include:
- Clearing of lung liquid by thoracic compression during vaginal delivery and absorption into pulmonary lymphatics;
- Alveolar expansion aided by markedly reduced surface tension of fluid coating the alveolar as a result of surfactant action and
- A large drop in pulmonary vascular resistance allowing a major increase in pulmonary blood flow.

Initiation of Respiration

Normal vaginally delivered infants make their first respiratory movement within a few seconds of complete delivery. The time interval between the appearance of the nose and first breath is usually between 20 to 30 seconds. Within 90 seconds of complete delivery most infants have started rhymthic respirations. The strong initial respiratory efforts and the subsequent rhythmic activities of respiratory muscles are largely dependent upon brain stem respiratory centres which are influenced by several factors as listed in

Table 3.1.1 into starting and continuing respiration. Ventilation is regulated by the PCO_2 and hydrogen ion concentration [H^+] perfusing chemoreceptors in the medulla. Breathing is also stimulated by a decrease in PO_2 acting on chemoreceptors in the carotid bodies. This hypoxic drive may assume great importance if the medullary centres have been depressed by hypoxia or maternal anaesthesia or analgesia. In the healthy newborn infant at delivery the sensory stimuli and blood-gas alterations are sufficient to arouse in the brain motor impulses which produce the initial muscle movements in the diaphragm and intercostal muscles required to create the intermittent negative intrathoracic pressures which allow air to enter and leave the alveoli. Although a falling oxygen tension and increase in CO_2 tension at first stimulate the respiratory centres persistence of hypoxia and hypercarbia will depress these functions. An infant who has been chronically hypoxic during labour may have a non-responsive respiratory centre.

Fetal Circulation

A variable proportion of oxygenated fetal blood from the placenta travels from the umbilical vein where the PO_2 is 4.0 kPa (30 mmHg) directly to the inferior vena cava via the ductus venosus. Most inferior vena caval blood is directed through the foramen ovale into the left atrium where after mixture with pulmonary venous blood it enters the left ventricle and is pumped towards the head and upper limbs. A smaller flow of inferior vena caval blood enters the right atrium, mixes with poorly oxygenated blood returning from the superior vena cava and enters the right ventricle. From the right ventricle this blood mainly enters the ductus arteriosus, bypassing the lungs and entering the descending aorta. This relatively less oxygenated blood

Table 3.1.1: Factors which can initiate or influence the patterns of neonatal respirations	
Thermal	Chilling through loss of heat at about 2.5 kj/min
Pain	Skin, muscle and tendon receptors
Pressure	Gravity (departure from liquid environment), increased intrathoracic pressures during delivery, changes in intratracheal and intrathoracic pressure
Tactile	Trigeminal area particularly important
Receptors in lungs and pleura	Hering-Breuer reflex
Receptors in muscle, tendon and joints of limbs, spine and chest wall	Stimulated by alterations in posture during and after delivery
Auditory	
Visual	
Olfactory	
Cord clamping:	
Increased arterial pressure	Carotid baroreceptors
Decreased arterial PO_2	Aortic and carotid body receptors
Increased arterial PCO_2	Direct effect on respiratory center
Increased arterial [H^+]	

supplies the trunk, abdominal organs and lower limbs and also the lungs through the bronchial arteries. Blood from the abdominal aorta returns through the umbilical arteries to the placenta. This pattern of circulation is maintained through cardiac contractility and muscle tone in the fetal vessel walls. Pulmonary arterial pressure is higher than left ventricular and aortic pressure because of a higher resistance in the pulmonary arterioles than in the ductus arteriosus and aorta. Muscle tone in fetal blood vessels depends largely on the oxygen content of the blood perfusing them, mediated locally through prostaglandins and also on autonomic activity predominantly affecting the small vessels.

Key Learning Points
The lungs are superfluous to the fetus. In the fetal circulation the lungs are bypassed because the high pulmonary vascular resistance allows oxygenated placental blood returning to the right atrium to flow to the left atrium via the foramen ovale and the ductus arteriosus

Circulatory Changes at Birth

The vascular changes associated with gas exchange being transferred from placenta to lungs take place abruptly with cord clamping, cessation of umbilical arterial and venous flow and removal of the low resistance placental circuit. Pulmonary arterial blood flow increases dramatically when the infant lungs expand and are the result of a reduced pulmonary arteriolar resistance and functional closure of the ductus arteriosus, ductus venosus, foramen ovale and umbilical vessels. The foramen ovale and ductus venosus close mainly as a result of mechanical pressure changes. The constriction of the ductus arteriosus and dilation of the pulmonary arterioles is mediated through the increased oxygen content of blood perfusing these vessels and vasoactive substances. Inhibition of the dilator prostaglandins, PGE_2 and PGI_2, which maintain ductal patency during fetal life, contribute to ductal closure. Asphyxia of the infant during or after birth maintains a patent ductus arteriosus and increases the pulmonary vascular resistance thus maintaining the fetal situation and causing profound hypoxia (Fig. 3.1.2).

Key Learning Points
• At birth the lungs become essential to the fetus.
• The first few breaths cause lung expansion and air to flow to the alveoli.
• The drop in pulmonary vascular resistance allows a vast increase in pulmonary blood flow.
• The pressure gradient and blood flow across the foramen ovale are reversed leading to its closure.
• Improved blood oxygenation stimulates ductal closure.

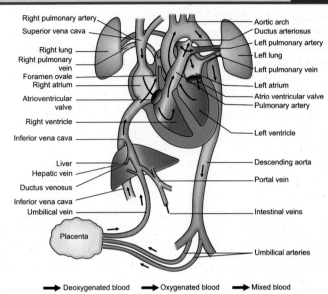

Fig. 3.1.2: Schematic representation of the fetal circulation

The First Breath

The lung fluid within the intra-alveolar spaces and tracheo-bronchial tree of the fetus is either expressed during the normal birth process or absorbed into pulmonary lymphatics. In the normal infant sensory stimuli initiate a first breath, which requires the creation of a negative intra thoracic pressure. This opens the terminal airways and expands the stiff (low-compliance) fluid filled lungs. Lung compliance (volume for unit pressure change) increases six fold aided by the presence of surfactant, which lowers the surface tension in the fluid film lining the alveolus. There is an accompanying reduction in the intrathoracic negative pressure. Infants born at term have an average tidal volume of 20 ml and a breathing frequency of about 30 breaths per minute creating a minute ventilation of about 600 ml per min. Preterm infants may have tidal volumes as low as 5 to 10 ml. During the first few days of life there may be minor degrees of right to left shunting through the foramen ovale and ductus arteriosus. Because of an inadequate ventilation/perfusion balance some blood is not fully oxygenated during passage through the lungs. This can be aggravated by an absence or deficiency of alveolar surfactant material produced by Type 2 alveolar lining cells or pneumonocytes. Prematurely born infants develop the respiratory distress syndrome when surfactant production is inadequate.

At term the fetal blood haemoglobin concentration is between 16 and 18 g/dl and is predominantly (60-80%) fetal haemoglobin (HbF). The PO_2 at which blood is 50% saturated with oxygen in the term fetus is only about 2.6 kPa (20 mmHg) but in the mother about 4.0 kPa (30 mmHg). This greater affinity of HbF for oxygen enables the fetal blood to take up oxygen readily from maternal blood. Although fetal red cells are avid for oxygen fetal tissues have a very low PO$_2$ (approximately 2.0 kPa) and the fetus is able to unload more of this oxygen to the fetal tissues.

Asphyxia

Asphyxia is defined as a combination of hypoxaemia, hypercapnoea and metabolic acidaemia. Fetal responses to asphyxia and haemorrhage during delivery are prompted by chemoreceptor and baroreceptor activity causing release of catecholamines. This catecholamine surge, which occurs during normal delivery, improves breathing by increasing lung surfactant, lung liquid absorption, lung compliance and bronchiolar dilatation. It mobilises energy from fat and glycogen reserves, stimulates gluconeogenesis by liver and increases blood flow to brain and heart.

Significant asphyxia causes an initial period of tachycardia followed by vagal bradycardia so that there is a combined autonomic response when hypoxaemia is severe, similar to those responses found in submerging mammals. In the "diving reflex" there is a sympathetic discharge with noradrenaline release causing a redistribution of blood flow to increase cardiac, cerebral and adrenal flow and to diminish flow to the skin of the trunk and limbs, skeletal muscle, liver, kidneys and intestine. There is also a vagally mediated bradycardia. During delivery fetal noradrenaline values exceed maternal and this ratio is markedly increased in asphyxial states. After birth in the acutely asphyxiated infant there is an initial period of rapid breathing (hyperpnoea) followed by a period of initial or primary apnoea and then regular gasping follows. This gasping ceases about 8 minutes after birth. The apnoeic period, which follows the last spontaneous gasp, is called secondary or terminal apnoea and death will ensue unless resuscitation is successfully instituted. Acute asphyxia of the fetus may occur with sudden complete placental separation or umbilical cord obstruction but the more common hypoxic insults are intermittent or subacute and are detected with fetal heart monitoring and blood sampling.

Case Study 1: A Baby with Intrapartum Asphyxia

A 26 year old primigravida was admitted in established labour at 39 weeks gestation. Initial assessment showed a fetal heart rate of 140 beats/min with good beat to beat variation. After 2 hours fetal tachycardia was noted with the rate increasing to 190 beats/min and then rapidly falling to <100/min. The mother complained of severe abdominal pain and her uterus felt tense. Abruptio placentae was diagnosed and she was delivered by emergency LSCS. The amniotic fluid was heavily blood stained. The baby was limp and pale and made no attempt at breathing or crying. Birthweight was 3200 gm.

Contd...

Contd...

The baby was transferred to the resuscitaire where facial oxygen was administered while heavily blood stained amniotic fluid was sucked out from the throat. There was no response to this stimulation. Apgar score at 1 minute was HR 30/min (1) Respiration absent (0) Colour very pale (0) response to stimuli (0) marked hypotonia (0) Total 1/10. The baby was intubated and more blood stained fluid sucked from the trachea. Cardiac massage was given at 100 beats /min and assisted ventilation started with 100% oxygen, 30 cm water pressure and one puff to every 7 chest compressions. An umbilical venous catheter was passed for venous access. Capillary blood gases at 2 minutes showed a pH of 6.95, pCO$_2$ 5.8, pO$_2$ 7.6, Base excess -16. A half correction of the acidosis with 8.4% sodium bicarbonate was given via the umbilical catheter.

The heart rate improved to 150/min followed by an improvement in colour and the start of irregular respiration. The baby grimaced occasionally and flexed her limbs. At 5 minutes she had an Apgar score of 7/10, heart rate >100/min (2) regular respiration (2) centrally pink but cyanosed peripherally (1) facial grimacing (1) slight hypotonia (1).

She was breathing regularly by 7 minutes and was extubated at 10 minutes. Resuscitation was stopped except for facial oxygen which was continued until 12 min when she was fully pink.

Assessment and Early Prognosis

When possible a time clock with a clearly visible second hand should be commenced at the time of infant's delivery. It is customary to aspirate the nasal and oral passages carefully immediately after delivery using a sterile, plastic tipped catheter. This removes amniotic and lung fluid from the oro-pharynx and stops the aspiration of blood, meconium and other debris into the upper airway. Excess fluid is normally dried from the infant's skin with a warm towel and the infant checked briefly for the presence of severe congenital anomalies such as spina bifida and microcephaly. The Apgar score is assessed at one minute and if the infant is apnoeic gentle sensory stimuli such as the blowing of cold air/oxygen over the infant's face through a facemask should be tried. If such stimuli fail to initiate breathing movements tracheal intubation should commence at 2 minutes. A heart rate of less than 80 per minute would be an indication for intubation and ventilation before 2 minutes of age. Virginia Apgar's clinical score based on heart rate, respiratory effort, muscle tone, responses to stimuli and skin colour has been found valuable in the assessment of the newborn (Table 3.1.2). The score is usually made at 1 minute after birth and repeated at 5 minutes. Apgar chose a time interval of 1 minute because at this time most infants in her large series had achieved their lowest scores. The five-minute score has been shown to have some correlation with subsequent brain damage whereas the one minute score gives some index of the need for active resuscitation, correlates well with biochemical assessment of acidosis and is inversely proportional to the neonatal death rate.

Table 3.1.2: Clinical evaluation of the newborn infant (Apgar scoring method). Sixty seconds after complete birth of the infant (disregarding the cord and placenta) the five objective signs are evaluated and each given a score of 0, 1 or 2. A score of 10 indicates an infant in the best possible condition

Apgar score SIGN	0	1	2
Heart rate	absent	<100 /min	>100/min
Respiratory effort	absent	weak cry,	good cry
Colour	blue, pale	body pink Blue extremities	pink
Muscle tone	limp	some flexion of extremities	active movements
Reflexes (stroking sole of foot)	no response	grimace	good cry

Ventilation

Lung inflation at a rate of 20 to 30 times per minute, maintaining inflation for approximately 1 second, at inflation pressures limited to 30 cm water should be instituted. Chest movement should be observed and the chest auscultated to ensure adequate air entry on both sides of the chest. If there is no entry, the tube is likely to be in the oesophagus and it should be withdrawn and the infant reintubated. Air entry to the right lung alone indicates that the endotracheal tube has entered the right main bronchus and air entry to the left lung usually improves if the endotracheal tube is withdrawn slowly whilst listening over the unventilated lung. Occasionally a pneumothorax or a diaphragmatic hernia can confuse the picture. Should the heart rate fail to increase in spite of adequate ventilation it is likely that the infant has a severe metabolic acidaemia and the injection of sodium bicarbonate 8.4% intravenously over 3 to 5 minutes, 10 ml to a normal term infant and 5 ml to a preterm infant should be given. If the heart rate remains less than 100 external cardiac massage at 100 to 120 beats per minute should be instituted. Seven cardiac compressions should be alternated with ventilation. If opiates have been given to the mother in the 6 hours prior to delivery and the infant fails to establish respiratory efforts, naloxone 0.01 mg per kg can be given by intravenous or intramuscular injection. Even when respiratory depression is thought to be due to maternal opiates the same indications for intubation and intermittent positive pressure ventilation (IPPV) should be used. The infant should be extubated as soon as regular respiration and good colour are achieved. When the infant is born without pulsation or heart sounds (Apgar 0-1) but a fetal heart is recorded up to 20 minutes before delivery, intubation, external cardiac massage, intravenous sodium bicarbonate and endotracheal adrenaline 1 ml of 1:10,000 IU should be given. If there is no heartbeat by 10 minutes of age or there is no respiratory effort by 30 minutes after institution of resuscitation these attempts should be abandoned. If intermittent but inadequate respiratory movements occur then it is reasonable to ventilate the infant for 24 hours, assess the neurological status and make a decision whether to withdraw or continue support. Resuscitation units with overhead heating, a time clock, an oxygen supply and a 30 cm water pressure valve should be available in all areas where at risk infants are to be delivered. It is most important to maintain the infant's temperature and prevent cooling during resuscitation. Much of the heat loss is from the head of the infant and this must be covered and the infant warmed with an appropriate heating unit. The majority of infants who require resuscitation can be extubated within 1 to 2 minutes and are probably not at significant risk and should be returned to their mothers for nursing supervision. Those requiring longer resuscitation may require admission to a special or intensive care nursery for subsequent observation for apnoea, convulsions and neurological status. Such infants require a check of their haemoglobin, blood glucose and blood gas determinations at intervals determined by the clinical status of the infant. If the term infant has no convulsions and is feeding normally within 48 hours the long-term prognosis is usually good.

Initial resuscitation may be carried out using a bag and facemask (Fig. 3.1.3). After the airway has been adequately cleared with gentle suction (-5 cm water) the mask is positioned to ensure an adequate face seal and the bag with a 30 cm H_2O leak-valve inflated at a rate of 20 to 30 per minute. A complication can be gaseous distension of the stomach. When prolonged bag and mask ventilation is necessary the insertion of a nasogastric tube may help.

BIRTH RELATED DISORDERS

Perinatal Health Services

Improved standards of care in the UK and other developed countries have resulted in a very marked reduction in

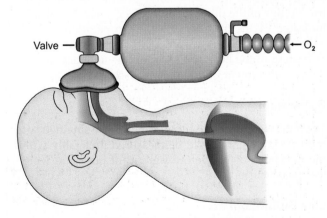

Fig. 3.1.3: Bag and mask ventilation

maternal mortality due to childbirth during the past century from over 500 maternal deaths per 100,000 deliveries at the beginning of the century in the UK to levels where maternal mortality rate is no longer a useful measure by which to assess the success of maternity services. The current maternal mortality rate in most developed countries is 1 per 10,000 births or less. Attention is now focused on infant morbidity and mortality. Many infant deaths in the first year of life are due to causes directly or closely related to factors occurring during fetal life or delivery.

Definitions

The following definitions are based on current World Health Organisation definitions. Those involved in collecting and disseminating perinatal statistics whether at national, regional, area, district, or local hospital level should adhere to standard definitions. It is appreciated that gestational age often cannot be determined by reference to the last menstrual period. None the less, whichever method of gestational age assessment is used the definitions of various gestational age categories are still appropriate. The definitions highlight the need for all live births and fetal deaths to be accurately weighed as soon as possible after birth.

Live Birth

"Live birth is the complete expulsion or extraction from its mother of a product of conception, irrespective of the duration of the pregnancy, which, after such separation, breathes or shows any other evidence of life, such as beating of the heart, pulsation of the umbilical cord, or definite movement of voluntary muscles, whether or not the umbilical cord has been cut or the placenta is attached; each product of such a birth is considered live born".

Fetal Death

Fetal death is death prior to the complete expulsion or extraction from its mother of a product of conception irrespective of the duration of the pregnancy. The death is indicated by the fact that after such separation the fetus does not breathe or show any other evidence of life, such as beating of the heart, pulsation of the umbilical cord, or definite movement of voluntary muscles.

Birthweight

The first weight of the fetus or newborn obtained after birth. This weight should be measured preferably within the first hour of life before significant postnatal weight loss has occurred.

Low Birthweight

Less than 2,500 g (up to, and including, 2499 g).

Gestational Age

The duration of gestation is measured from the first day of the last normal menstrual period. Gestational age is expressed in completed days or completed weeks (e.g. events occurring 280 to 286 days after the onset of the last normal menstrual period are considered to have occurred at 40 weeks of gestation). Measurements of fetal growth, as they represent continuous variables, are expressed in relation to a specific week of gestational age (e.g. the mean birthweight for 40 weeks is that obtained at 280 - 286 days of gestation on a weight-for-gestational age curve).

Preterm

Less than 37 completed weeks. (Up to and including the 258th day of gestation).

Term

From 37 to less than 42 completed weeks (259 days up to and including 293 days).

Post Term

42 completed weeks or more (294 completed days or more).

Perinatal Mortality Statistics

National perinatal statistics should include all fetuses and infants delivered weighing at least 500 g or, when birth weight is unavailable the corresponding gestational age (22 weeks) or body length (25 cm crown-heel), whether alive or dead. It is recognised that legal requirements in many countries may set different criteria for registration purposes, but it is hoped that countries will arrange the registration or reporting procedures in such a way that the events required for inclusion in the statistics can be identified easily. In the United Kingdom the "fetal death" component of perinatal mortality includes only those fetuses, which have completed 24 weeks (168 days) in the uterus. Fetuses below this age whether stillborn or live born are classified as abortions. There is much sense in defining perinatal mortality as "fetal deaths weighing 500 g or more plus deaths occurring less than 7 completed days after birth in babies weighing 500 g or more". The inclusion of extremely low birthweight babies within the definition of perinatal mortality underlines the need for all fetal deaths and live births to be accurately weighed. In this way perinatal mortality can be analysed within specific birthweight groups and when comparing perinatal mortality rates, allowances can be made for differences in birthweight distributions between populations.

Early Neonatal Death (included in Perinatal Mortality)

Death less than 7 completed days from birth.

Late Neonatal Death
(not included in Perinatal Mortality)

Death from 7 completed days to less than 28 days from birth.

Post-neonatal Death

Death from 28 completed days to less than 1 year from birth (i.e. up to and including 364 days).

Birth rate is the number of births, live and still, registered per 1000 of the population.

Stillbirth rate is the number of stillbirths registered per 1000 live and stillbirths.

Neonatal mortality rate is the number of deaths registered of infants dying under the age of 28 days per 1000 registered live births in the same year.

Perinatal mortality rate is the number of stillbirths and early neonatal deaths per 1000 live and stillbirths.

Infant mortality rate is the number of deaths registered of infants dying under 1 year of age per 1000 registered live births in the same year.

Post perinatal infant mortality rate is the number of deaths between the 8th day and end of the first year of life per 1000 live births.

Perinatal Mortality

In most countries where population growth has not out-stripped the economic growth there has been a steady fall in perinatal mortality. Since 1940 the perinatal mortality rate in Scotland has fallen from 65 per 1000 total births to less than 9 per 1000 in the year 2000. This change is largely due to improvement in living standards and in particular to higher standards of nutrition and hygiene. Improved antenatal care, a reduction in family size and improved perinatal care are other major factors in the improved outcome for all birthweight and gestational age categories during this time. There has also been a marked fall in the infant mortality rate partly due to a reduction in deaths during the first week of life. A reduction in the post neonatal mortality rate (deaths after the first 28 days) is largely attributed to a reduction in sudden unexplained infant deaths. The lower the birthweight and gestational age the higher the neonatal mortality rates.

Once it is possible to collect this type of information within national populations it becomes possible to identify preventable factors. By the study of such data for individual hospitals or individual urban and rural areas much can be learned of the success or failure of the methods of care and prevention. Many of the environmental factors such as maternal nutrition, hygiene, housing conditions, smoking, alcohol intake, maternal age and family size are known to influence stillbirth, neonatal and perinatal death rates and probably also the quality of survival. A reduction in preterm and low birthweight deliveries could significantly improve outcome. Prevention of congenital malformation is likely to have a major effect on the quality of survival of the larger infants. Measurements of the quality of life of those who survive are not easily obtained. Improvements in obstetric and neonatal practice have significantly reduced the number of term-asphyxiated infants and this has reduced the numbers of children with cerebral palsy in this mature group.

The collection of such data is essential, not only to audit outcome for the population but to detect potential harmful practices in perinatal care. One example of a harmful effect was the delayed feeding of preterm infants practised during the1950's, which led to impaired school performance and cerebral palsy in many of the children so treated. The association of retrolental fibroplasia with oxygen therapy is another example. Good record keeping is an absolute requisite for the accurate collection of basic information about an infant's pre and postnatal condition and this information can act as a basis of an ongoing life-long record of health for that individual.

The Parents

The most important factors determining the outcome for an individual infant are the parents. In the traditional family the birth or impending birth of a new infant is a major family and life event. Parents may seek advice before embarking on a pregnancy and this attitude to planned parenthood is in part related to improved education and increased knowledge of hereditary factors and an ability to examine the embryo and fetus in utero as well as to control fertility. Parents are mainly concerned about possible abnormal development of their child before birth. Apart from this concern parents are also anxious to make sure that they will be able to look after their new infant properly. Problems may arise because of inadequate housing, low income, ill health and family size. Many legal and ethical dilemmas are faced by society as they come to terms with technologies of *in vitro* fertilisation and prenatal screening and diagnostic tests for a variety of inherited metabolic and other abnormalities. Preparation for parenthood begins in childhood when children watch their own parents and relatives methods of child rearing. Educational programmes within schools should be encouraged to add instruction in parentcraft to lessons on home management and sex education and education authorities should ensure that teachers have appropriate knowledge and understanding of the importance of these matters. Of major importance is the need in many so-called developed countries to encourage young women to breast feed their infants. The role of the father in the support of the mother and child is crucial and the joint responsibilities of the two parents in the creation of a healthy child and healthy community cannot be over emphasised.

CONGENITAL ABNORMALITIES

Congenital means present at birth and malformations evident at birth represent only a small proportion of the seriously malformed products of gestation. Most cause embryonic and fetal death at an early stage of pregnancy and are generally unrecognised when they are aborted. The remaining abnormal fetuses, whether live-born or stillborn, have congenital abnormalities caused by a wide variety of genetic and environmental factors, some known and others as yet unrecognised. Potentially remedial developmental anomalies are present in more than 2 per 1000 live-born infants. Many abnormalities are now diagnosed antenatally by means of different modes of testing including alpha feto protein screening and fetal ultrasound. Prompt and effective management of these malformations is one of the most important aspects of neonatal surgery.

Aetiology

Of the many factors responsible for congenital malformations some are clearly defined. These include genetic and environmental factors including malnutrition, infections, drugs, smoking, alcohol, vascular incidents, the effects of chemotherapy, radiotherapy, ultrasound and second-generation malformations. There are clusters and trends in the incidence of congenital malformations, e.g. spina bifida in the West of Scotland as in many other countries has shown a decline in recent years. The interaction of genetic predisposition and environmental factors is well described. There are congenital malformations, which predispose to malignancy such as those skin abnormalities related to chromosome fragility syndromes, the Beckwith Wiedemann syndrome which is associated with Wilm's tumours.

When clinical examination of the newborn infant reveals a congenital malformation it is important to look for other abnormalities since there are sometimes more than one abnormality present. Where there are a series of abnormalities present then this may allow the identification of a syndrome. There are now a number of databases available for the categorisation of such malformation groupings. Many malformations are now detected prenataly but some may only become evident in later childhood or indeed in adult life.

Developmental Anomalies and the Parents

Parents whose child is born with a defect are always concerned to know the cause. Two common questions asked are "Is the defect due to any fault in the father or mother?" and "Will a second child be likely to have a similar or other defect?" Unfortunately a satisfactory answer is not always possible. It is, however, important that someone with understanding of the psychological impact of the birth of a deformed child on the family should interview the parents within the first few days after the birth. The doctor must give a simple and honest appraisal and attempt to dispel the shame or guilt felt by the parents. Facial deformities such as cleft lip and extensive facial haemangiomata are particularly distressing to parents.

Abnormal Development

As in 60% of the cases of congenital abnormality there is no identifiable cause and therefore no ability to take preventive action the paediatrician and paediatric surgeon continue to be faced with the management of such infants. Most of the abnormalities have resulted from a disturbance in the embryological development. In general terms these abnormalities arise because of:

*   Failure of development, e.g. amelia, microcephaly,
*   Failure to unite, e.g. cleft lip, spina bifida
*   Failure to divide, e.g. syndactyly, Siamese twins
*   Failure to canalize, e.g. intestinal atresias
*   Failure to migrate, e.g. malrotation of bowel, Hirschsprung Disease
*   Failure to atrophy, e.g. branchial clefts, thyroglossal cyst
*   Excess division, e.g. polydactyly, duplex renal systems

The medical and surgical management of such abnormalities are dealt with in the various organ chapters.

Perinatal Injuries

During the last two to three decades there has been a gratifying decline in the incidence of "mechanical" birth injuries. Trauma is at times an inevitable accompaniment of the mechanics of birth even when delivery is spontaneous and uncomplicated. The nature of the injury varies greatly and depending upon the site and severity may be of minor or major significance.

Antenatal Injury

During induction of labour superficial trauma generally of a minor degree can result from the rupturing of membranes, the application of scalp electrodes or the taking of fetal blood samples. Occasionally during Caesarean section fetal skin may be incised. Mechanical injury during delivery may be precipitated when there is disproportion between the size of the fetal head and the maternal pelvis, excessive uterine contractions (augmented labour), abnormal presentations, low birth weight and instrumental delivery.

Injury to Superficial Tissues

A caput succedaneum consists of oedematous swelling and bruising in the superficial tissues of the presenting part of the fetus. In vertex presentations the caput is not sharply defined and may extend across suture lines. If presentation is abnormal the caput will be formed elsewhere. There is pitting oedema of the affected tissues present at birth, which disappears within 48 hours. Abrasions are sometimes present in the skin overlying the caput and unless particular care is taken may allow entry of organisms leading to sepsis. Bruising and minor abrasions of the scalp not infrequently result from the application of a vacuum extractor.

Cephalhaematomata (Subperiosteal haematoma)

This is a swelling resulting from bleeding between the periosteum and underlying skull bone and is therefore restricted to the limits of that bone (usually parietal). The swelling is not usually present at birth but becomes evident on the second or third day and may increase in bulk and in extent for a few days. It is well-defined, may persist for a number of weeks or even months but invariably disappears completely. The swelling is at first fluctuant later becoming firmer as absorption of fluid takes place. A firm ring of calcification becomes palpable, sometimes extending to form a localised hard elevation around the site of the original swelling. Occasionally they may be bilateral. In general neither a caput succedaneum nor a cephalhaematoma need cause concern. It is important that infants with cephalhaematomata receive vitamin K.

Subaponeurotic Haemorrhage (Subgaleal haemorrhage) occasionally results from the application of a vacuum extractor. The swelling caused by this haemorrhage extends across the lines of the sutures and is a potentially dangerous complication. There can be excessive blood loss and vitamin K prophylaxis must be ensured.

Low Birthweight Infants (LBW)

Low birthweight infants (LBW) is a phrase used to describe all infants weighing less than 2500 g. These infants are at a major disadvantage when compared with those weighing more than 2500 g. Very low birthweight (VLBW) is a phrase used to describe infants weighing less than 1500 g. Mortality increases with reducing maturity and birth weight. Such infants require the facilities available in neonatal intensive care units and where these are available survival rates of 90% can be achieved for infants weighing between 1001 g to 1500 g. VLBW infants account for about 10% of the number of LBW infants but for about 60% of the perinatal deaths in LBW infants. Management of these infants poses an important challenge for those responsible for the care of the newly born infant.

Key Learning Points

Low birthweight is the result of either premature delivery or impaired intrauterine growth. Impaired intrauterine growth may be caused by poor placental function and nutrition (light-for-dates baby with small body and relatively large head) or by intrauterine infections or chromosomal abnormalities (small-for-dates baby with small head and small body).

Preterm Infants

A birth is preterm if it occurs up to and including the 258th day of gestation. Most preterm infants are of low birth weight and weigh less than 2500 g at birth. LBW may be caused by preterm delivery or poor fetal growth. Infants weighing less than the 10th percentile of the weight distribution for their gestational age are termed light for dates and infants over the 90th centile heavy for dates. Some infants who are born light for dates have a normal birth length but others have a combination of low birth weight and low birth length and are termed small for dates or small for gestational age. Frequently the chest and head circumference in these small infants are below the 10th centile. This growth failure may be detected prenatally. It is important to recognise infants who have failed to grow adequately in utero as they have different problems from those LBW infants who are adequately nourished but delivered preterm. The external signs and scoring system used are shown in Table 3.1.3 and Figure 3.1.4.

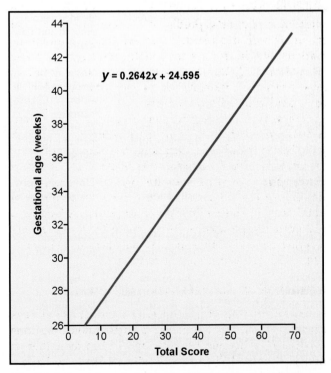

Fig. 3.1.4: Graph for calculation of gestational age from total score

Table 3.1.3: Scoring system for external criteria of maturation

Score* External sign	0	1	2	3	4
Oedema	Obvious oedema of hands and feet; pitting over tibia	No obvious oedema of hands and feet; pitting over tibia	No oedema		
Skin texture	Very thin gelatinous	Thin and smooth	Smooth; medium thickening Rash or superficial peeling	Slight thickening Superficial cracking and peeling especially of hands and feet	Thick and parchment like; superficial or deep cracking
Skin colour	Dark red	Uniformly pink	Pale pink; variable over body	Pale; only pink over ears, lips, palms, or soles	
Skin opacity (trunk)	Numerous veins and venules clearly seen, especially over abdomen	Veins and tributaries seen	A few large vessels clearly seen over abdomen	A few large vessels seen indistinctly over abdomen	No blood vessels seen
Lanugo (over back)	No lanugo	Abundant; long and thick over whole back	Hair thinning especially over lower back	Small amount of lanugo and bald areas	At least half of back devoid of lanugo
Plantar creases	No skin creases	Faint red marks over anterior half of sole	Definite red marks over > anterior ½; indentations over < anterior $\frac{1}{3}$	Indentations over > anterior $\frac{1}{3}$	Definite deep indentations over > anterior $\frac{1}{3}$
Nipple formation	Nipple barely visible; no areola	Nipple well defined; aerola smooth and flat, diameter < 0.75 cm	Areola stippled, edge not raised, diameter < 0.75 cm	Areola stippled, edge not raised, diameter > 0.75 cm	
Breast size	No breast tissue palpable	Breast tissue on one or both sides, < 0.5 cm diameter	Breast tissue both sides; one or both 0.5 - 1.0 cm	Breast tissue both sides; one or both > 1 cm	
Ear form	Pinna flat and shapeless, little or no incurving of edge	Incurving of part of edge of pinna	Partial incurving whole of upper pinna	Well defined incurving whole of upper pinna	
Ear firmness	Pinna soft, easily folded, no recoil	Pinna soft, easily folded, slow recoil	Cartilage to edge of pinna, but soft in places, ready recoil	Pinna firm, cartilage to edge; instant recoil	
Genitals Male	Neither testis in scrotum	At least one testis high in scrotum	At least one testis right down		
Female (with hips half abducted)	Labia majora widely separated, labia minora protruding	Labia majora almost cover labia minora	Labia majora completely cover labia minora		

*If score differs on two sides, take the mean.

From Dubowitz LMS, Dubowitz V, Goldberg C (1970). Clinical assessment of gestational age in the newborn infant. Journal of Pediatrics 77, 1-10; adapted from Farr V, Mitchell RG, Neligan GA, Parkin JM (1966). The definition of some external characteristics used in the assessment of gestational age in the newborn infant. Developmental Medicine 8, 507-11.

THE PRETERM INFANT

Preterm delivery is the major cause of low birthweight and is associated with a greatly increased risk of mortality and morbidity. The degree of risk increases progressively in the more preterm infant. Although improved methods of management have increased the chance of survival and its quality the risk of complications remains sufficiently high to justify every effort being taken to prevent preterm delivery (Table 3.1.4)

When mother goes into preterm delivery every effort should be made to admit her promptly to a maternity unit with tertiary intensive care for her newborn. The mother's uterus is the ideal transport incubator for transferring the infant to such a unit. The use of beta-agonists such as Ritodrine which act as uterine relaxants may delay delivery long enough to allow the institution of maternal Dexamethasone therapy to induce fetal lung maturation.

Clinical Features

The preterm infant's head and abdomen appear relatively large whilst the skin is soft in texture and pink in colour. A generalised lack of subcutaneous tissue results in prominence of the body skeleton with a thin, lined face, loose skin over the limbs and the frequent appearance of intestinal peristalsis visible through the abdominal wall. The infant sleeps more or less continuously, the cry is infrequent and feeble and respiratory movements may be rhythmic with periodic spells of apnoea. Muscular hypotonicity results in the characteristic posture in which the limbs are widely abducted, knees and ankles flexed, head lolling to one side. The ability to suck and to co-ordinate sucking and swallowing is poorly developed in the VLBW infant. Oedema may be present at birth or become marked during the first 24-48 hours. Severe oedema is an unfavourable omen and may be associated with maternal antepartum haemorrhage, pre-eclampsia or

Table 3.1.4: Factors carrying a high risk of preterm delivery	
Maternal	• Age below 20 years • Height: less than 155 cm • Poor socio-economic status • Heavy workload • Poor nutrition • Unmarried
Obstetric	• Primiparity • Pre-eclampsia • Antepartum haemorrhage • Smoking • Previous history of preterm delivery and chronic ill health
Fetal	• Multiple pregnancy • Congenital abnormalities • Slow intrauterine growth

diabetes mellitus. The heart rate in preterm infants averages 140 per min. The respiratory rate is 40-50 per min in the first 24 hours thereafter decreasing to 35-45. A continued rapid rate should arouse suspicion of the respiratory distress syndrome or pneumonia. Preterm infants have high surface area to body weight ratios and little reserve of subcutaneous or brown adipose tissue. During the first few days they lose water rapidly through their skin and these physical characteristics make it difficult for them to maintain their temperatures. Cold exposure greatly jeopardises their survival and particular attention must be paid to ensuring the correct ambient temperatures. Liver immaturity will predispose to "physiological" jaundice but early establishment of feeding and phototherapy have reduced the risk of neurological damage from hyper-bilirubinaemia.

The skin and mucous membrane surfaces are easily damaged in preterm infants and such breaches of these protective layers, together with a limited immunological competence predispose preterm infants to infections. They fail to show the signs found in older infants with sepsis and a very high degree of suspicion of infection must be maintained. Any infant suspected of having an infection requires culture of urine, blood and sometimes cerebrospinal fluid and the commencement of therapy with an appropriate broad-spectrum antibiotic.

A combination of septicaemia, hyperbilirubinaemia and hypoxia with metabolic acidaemia predisposes the infant to central nervous system damage. Intraventricular haemorrhage from the fragile poorly supported vessels in the germinal matrix of the brain results from a combination of hypoxia, hypotension and disordered cerebral blood flow. The commonest clinical signs of intraventricular haemorrhage are apnoeic episodes, convulsions or unexplained deterioration in clinical state. Mortality from intraventricular haemorrhage is high as is morbidity in the survivors because of obstructive hydrocephalus and periventricular leucomalacia.

As more and more immature infants survive it is important to maintain longer-term follow-up to assess the effectiveness of medical interventions in the management of these infants. Children born too soon do show impairment of performance at school age, which may not only be, related to the preterm delivery but also to early postnatal management particularly the provision of adequate nutrition.

Management

It is likely that most infants with birth weights of under 2 kg will be managed in hospital.

Maintenance of Body Temperature

Babies weighing < 2000gm need incubator care to maintain an adequate body temperature. The temperature within the incubator should be between 32 -35 degrees C and the humidity controlled above 50% to reduce skin evaporation and the resultant cooling. Room temperature should be kept at 27 -29 degrees C to reduce temperature fluctuations. Babies are dressed in bonnets, mittens and caps to conserve body heat but this may not be practicable in the very ill baby or VLBW babies who have to be nursed naked for observations to be made. In such cases covering the baby with a bubble plastic blanket or nursing in a perspex humidified headbox may help to reduce heat loss.

Nutrition and the Preterm Infant

In the normal term human infant there is a continuum of growth which, given a normal labour and delivery, together with satisfactory establishment of breastfeeding, proceeds uninterrupted during the change from the intrauterine to extrauterine existence. In the first few days, whilst breastfeeding is established, some infant nutrient reserves are mobilised to maintain cell division and growth in most major organs. For the infant born preterm it is almost impossible to prevent disruption of genetically predetermined programmes of cellular divisions, growth, maturation and activities. The more immature the infant at birth, the greater the difficulty of ensuring adequate nutrition and the more likely the infant is to suffer the consequences of impaired tissue growth, development and function. Nutritional deficits may result in disordered central nervous system function in childhood and in disordered cardiovascular and cerebrovascular function in later life. The infant born preterm has two major problems. The first is lack of nutritional reserve and the second is immaturity of organ function.

Nutritional Reserves

Virtually all of the fat, carbohydrate and protein in the preterm infant is structural whereas in the term infant there are reserves of glycogen, fat and other nutrients. After oxygen requirements have been met the next immediate need for survival in the preterm infant is an adequate water supply. It has been calculated that a VLBW infant might survive 3 to 4 days, a term infant 30 days and an adult 90 days if supplied with water alone. In starvation states a minimal energy expenditure of about 76 kcal per kg per 24 hours (0.32 MJ) is necessary to maintain life if new functional peptides and proteins such as hormones and enzymes are to be manufactured by the preterm infant. They can only be obtained by the destruction of structural proteins in organs such as muscle and liver if there is any failure to supply exogenous protein or amino acid. A relative excess of water particularly extracellular water, in the preterm infant confers no protection against dehydration since the obligatory daily turnover of water is equal to 15 to 20% of the total body water pool. Water-soluble

vitamins B and C transfer readily from mother to fetus so that at term fetal tissue concentrations of these vitamins exceed maternal. Fetal concentrations of the fat soluble vitamins A, D, E and K are not as high as adult values and because of their high rate of utilisation and low initial values preterm infants quickly run into deficit unless an early adequate intake is assured.

Immaturity of Organ Function

Lung immaturity results in many preterm infants requiring ventilatory assistance. Renal immaturity reduces water tolerance and can be aggravated by exogenous osmotic loads in the form of glucose, amino acids and electrolytes or endogenous from urea production. A preterm infant has virtually no response to a water load in the first 3 to 5 days of life. By one month of postnatal age the preterm infant can concentrate urine to approximately 400 mosmol/kg and by 3 months of postnatal age this can reach 750 mosmol/kg. Both kidneys and lungs are important in the maintenance of acid-base balance. Lung immaturity may cause hypercarbia with respiratory acidosis and hypoxia with metabolic acidosis both of which interfere with cell membrane and tissue function. Renal threshold for bicarbonate is lower in the preterm newborn who relies on the reclamation of bicarbonate at the proximal tubules as the ability to excrete hydrogen ions in combination with ammonia as ammonium ions is limited. The principal urinary buffer is the phosphate buffer disodium, monohydrogen phosphate (Na_2, HPO_4) and unless phosphate intake is adequate the preterm infant has a limited capacity to excrete titratable acid. Renal mechanisms largely under the influence of ADH and aldosterone are mainly responsible for electrolyte balance and extracellular fluid volume control. In preterm infants presented with large or imbalanced quantities of electrolyte, either parenterally or from tissue breakdown, or with kidneys poorly perfused or poorly oxygenated, gross distortion of fluid and electrolyte occur readily. Maintenance of good renal perfusion and oxygenation is a key factor in promoting anabolism. Hyper oxygenation will decrease renal blood flow as much as hypoxia and aggravate a catabolic state. Preterm birth creates stress, which imposes increased demands on endocrine function at a time when particular endocrine responses may be absent, poor or even inappropriate of functions of the gastrointestinal tract, the liver and exocrine pancreas make the maintenance of the anabolic state difficult. Structural development of the fetal gut is well in advance of functional capacity and there is a progressively changing pattern of enzyme differentiation during fetal life. With preterm delivery the later developing enzymes responsible for amino acid metabolism and gluconeogenesis may not yet be "switched on". Preterm infants are at particular risk of damaging hypoglycaemia as a result of the combination of a limited reserve of glycogen and reduced ability to synthesise glucose. An infant born preterm is an unphysiological creature who is unable to root, suck and swallow in a co-ordinated fashion because of central nervous system immaturity. Immaturity of other organs, which subserve normal gastrointestinal function and waste product excretion, means that even the ingestion of human milk is an "unphysiological" process for the very low birth weight preterm infant.

Feeding

Infants of less than 34 weeks gestation require specialised feeding methods. Enteral feeding is usually by a naso-gastric or orogastric feeding tube although on occasion transpyloric feeding (into the duodenum or jejunum) may reduce the frequency of vomiting and inhalation of stomach content. This method of feeding, however, is much less popular than previously as it may lead to complications including intestinal perforation, necrotising enterocolitis and diarrhoea. There is also some evidence that weight gain and growth is less satisfactory in infants fed nasojejunally. Continuous or bolus intragastric feeds may be given. Feeding with human milk should commence at about 2 hours of age to reduce the risk of hypoglycaemia and at a rate of about 60 ml/kg in the first day increasing to 150 ml/kg per day by the 4th day of life. Most infants weighing more than 1500 g will tolerate 3 hourly feeds but smaller infants will require to be fed hourly or even continuously. Preterm infants may reach an intake of 200 ml/kg per day by the end of the 2nd week of life. Very immature infants of 24-26 weeks gestation frequently require total parenteral nutrition with slower introduction of enteral feeding. The currently available foods recommended for preterm infants are mother's own "preterm milk", banked donor milk, human milk fortified with special preterm formulae or with concentrated extracts of human milk, standard infant cow milk or soya based formulae, special "preterm" infant formulae and parenteral nutrition either total or combined with enteral feeding. There is evidence that the use of fresh human milk with its protective effect against infection will provide important protection for the vulnerable preterm infant and reduce the incidence of necrotising enterocolitis. There is also a possibility that the use of human milk might protect against future allergic disease in preterm infants. At present it is probably wise to recommend the use of mother's own fresh milk complemented with a special preterm formula which contains increased concentrations of protein, energy, sodium, calcium, phosphorus, magnesium, copper, zinc, vitamins, essential and long-chain polyunsaturated fatty acids.

It is important to ensure that there is little or no separation of mother and infant as this may have adverse effects on the relationship between them. There are many strategies now developed to help mother overcome the enormous difficulties of achieving successful feeding and an intimate relationship in the intensive care situation. There are now findings to suggest that preterm infants who do not receive human milk and do not grow well in the first months of life are subsequently less intelligent, have poorer visual function and have a greater risk of ischaemic heart disease, chronic bronchitis, hypertension, stroke and non insulin dependent diabetes.

Key Learning Points

- The gut in term infants is only mature enough to digest and absorb human milk.
- The gut in a premature infant < 30 weeks gestation is frequently unable to digest human milk and parenteral nutrition is required.
- Premature delivery cuts short the transfer of copper, iron and other trace metals from mother to fetus leading to deficiencies after birth unless supplements are started early.
- Nutritional deficiencies in the preterm may interfere with the rapid brain growth and maturation occurring at this age, leading to poor brain function and low intellect in later life.

Respiratory Disorders

Prolonged respiratory pauses (greater than 20 seconds) in preterm infants may be associated with cyanosis and bradycardia. These are called apnoeic attacks and may be a sign of septicaemia, meningitis or intracranial haemorrhage but in the majority of instances are not associated with any obvious metabolic problem or illness. Neonatal convulsions may present as apnoeic episodes. Careful investigation for infection, hypoglycaemia, hypocalcaemia and intracranial haemorrhage should be undertaken and oxygen administered if the infant is hypoxic. When no trigger for apnoea is found, caffeine can be administered orally or intravenously as a central respiratory stimulant to help reduce the frequency of apnoeic attacks.

Respiratory Distress

Respiratory difficulties may result from perinatal asphyxia, which may cause primary atelectasis or aspiration of meconium and meconium stained amniotic fluid into the lungs. Postnatal aspiration of gastric contents particularly in the tube fed preterm infant may give rise to respiratory problems. Aspiration of foreign materials such as meconium or gastric content leads to severe lung congestion, oedema and haemorrhage with radiological evidence of patchy emphysema, secondary atelectasis and pulmonary oedema. Tachypnoea, costal recession and crepitations on auscultation are the clinical features. Severe meconium aspiration is more common in the more vigorous term infants who develop pneumomediastinum and/or pneumothorax. If there is persistent fetal circulation and standard techniques of ventilation prove inadequate, treatment with nitric oxide (NO) and/or extra corporeal membrane oxygenation (ECMO) and High Frequency Oscillation may prove life saving.

Transient tachypnoea of the newborn is a condition in which there is a moderate degree of intercostal retraction and respiratory difficulty related to poor or delayed clearing of normal lung fluid. Chest X-ray shows a slightly enlarged heart with streaky infiltrates radiating from the hilum of the lung. Treatment with supplemental oxygen is required for those infants whose arterial oxygen tensions fall below 50 - 60 mmHg (6.7 - 8.0 kPa). Arterial PO_2 should be maintained at 70 mmHg (9.3 kPa). Measurements of transcutaneous oxygen tension ($TcPO_2$) and oxygen saturation (SaO_2) are helpful in ensuring adequate oxygenation. Because of the shape of the haemoglobin dissociation curve, saturation monitors may increase the risk of hyperoxia. An increase in SaO_2 from 90 to 98% may represent an increase in PaO_2 of more than 50 mmHg. Measurement of $TcPO_2$ is safer in the care of the acute phase of respiratory support whereas measurement of transcutaneous SaO_2 is of greater value in older infants, e.g. chronic lung disease (CLD).

THE IDIOPATHIC RESPIRATORY DISTRESS SYNDROME (IRDS)

This condition is characterised by pulmonary resorption atelectasis associated with intense congestion, the presence of an eosinophilic hyaline membrane within dilated alveolar ducts and sometimes–intrapulmonary haemorrhage. The hyaline material is not always present and is probably the result of a transudate of fibrinous material. It is only found in infants who have lived for at least l hour and the condition is rarely found in mature infants. Predisposing factors are antepartum haemorrhage, caesarean section, maternal diabetes mellitus and severe rhesus immunisation. The aetiology is a deficiency of surfactant, a protein that reduces surface tension within the alveoli, facilitates lung expansion during inspiration and prevents atelectasis during expiration. Surfactant is synthesized in cells known as Type II pneumonocytes. Surfactant synthesis is inhibited by acidosis, hypothermia and hypoxia. There is a marked increase in surfactant production in the fetal lung from 32 weeks gestation. Its production may be enhanced in the fetal lung by administration of betamethasone to the mother before delivery.

Clinical Features

Tachypnoea (over 50 per min), which persists for longer than two hours after birth is a simple and significant observation, which almost invariably heralds some form of pulmonary insufficiency. Within a few hours there is inspiratory sternal intercostal and subcostal recession. Expiratory grunting is associated with violent inspiratory efforts, but breath sounds are greatly diminished. The respiratory rate increases to 75 per minute or greater. Greyish cyanosis may be present and oedema often becomes severe during the first 12 hours. Spells of apnoea occur with increasing frequency in deteriorating infants. Radiographs show a characteristic granular mottling. As this becomes more confluent the bronchial tree stands out clearly as an "air bronchogram." Severe respiratory acidosis and metabolic acidosis may result and the arterial PO_2 is reduced. The kidneys are unable to conserve base because of an inability to excrete phosphate permitting the bicarbonate concentrations in the plasma to decrease. Increased catabolism releases excess potassium, nitrogen, and phosphorus from damaged cells.

Treatment

The aim of treatment is to maintain the infant's tissue oxygenation until spontaneous recovery takes place when the Type II pneumocytes begin to synthesize surfactant. The best outcome for infants with RDS is obtained in regional intensive care units with a major expertise in neonatal medicine. The problems of treatment may be considered under several categories: (i) temperature control; (ii) feeding with fluid and electrolyte balance; (iii) acid-base homeostasis; (iv) oxygenation and respiratory support; (v) drug therapy. It is also necessary to stress that in these very ill infants handling and intervention procedures must be kept to a minimum.

i. *Temperature Control* should be achieved by placing the infant in an incubator, preferably equipped with servo control. Skin temperature should be kept within 36-37°C. Accurate temperature control is imperative to conserve the infant's utilization of oxygen.

ii. *Feeding* is a major concern because of the dangers of aspiration, the frequent development of paralytic ileus, and the fact that any handling, such as the passing of a nasogastric tube, is liable to cause sudden hypoxia. Calories can be supplied by parenteral nutrients given through peripheral veins or umbilical arterial catheters. It is important to avoid over-hydration, which may encourage persistence of the ductus arteriosus or the development of necrotising enterocolitis. A degree of intravenous fluid restriction may be necessary in the first few days but a balance between this and the damage caused by under-nutrition must be weighed. Plasma electrolytes should be assessed daily or more frequently and any electrolyte disorders corrected with appropriate supplements. Provided there is no abdominal distension and meconium has been passed. Nasogastric feeding may be introduced after the first 24 hours. When the infant cannot tolerate enteral feeding, total or partial parenteral feeding with amino acids, glucose, lipids, minerals and vitamins may be given although this procedure carries its own risks.

iii. *Acid base homeostasis.* Occasionally intravenous sodium bicarbonate may be required to correct base deficits. The quantity given may be calculated from the formula: base excess in mmol/l × body weight in kg × 0.35. It can be administered as 8.4 per cent solution (1 ml = 1 mmol) into a central vein at a rate not to exceed 0.5 mmol/min.

iv. *Oxygenation and respiratory support* constitute a top priority of treatment. Periodic sampling of aortic blood through an umbilical artery catheter for measurement of PaO_2 may not reflect the PaO_2 in vessels supplying the brain and retinae if there is right-to-left shunting through a patent ductus arteriosus. Medical and occasionally surgical closure of the ductus may be required to improve oxygenation. Samples obtained by puncture of a radial artery will obviate this problem but the necessary handling of the infant may result in undesirable fluctuations in the PaO_2. Transcutaneous PO_2 ($TcPO_2$) can be measured using a transcutaneous PO_2 electrode and monitor.

The objective in treatment is to maintain the PaO_2 above 50 mmHg (7.0 kPa) and below 90 mmHg (12.0 kPa). Swings above 120 mmHg (16.0 kPa) are associated with an increased the risk of retinopathy of prematurity. In addition to monitoring PaO_2 it is, of course, essential that the oxygen concentration in the incubator is measured with a suitable, preferably continuous recording, analyser. While a satisfactory Pao2 concentration can be achieved in mild cases with an oxygen concentration of 35 to 40%, in severe cases much greater oxygen concentrations are required. This will necessitate enclosure of the infant's head in a plastic hood when the oxygen flow should pass through a nebuliser and be warmed to 30-33° C. In the most severely affected infants, particularly those below 1,500 g, the regimen described above proves inadequate. This is characterized by PaO_2 values < 50 mmHg (7.0 kPa) in 90% oxygen, $PaCO_2$ values which increase to 70 mmHg (9.3 kPa) or higher and attacks of apnoea with marked bradycardia. In such infants intermittent positive-pressure ventilation (IPPV) is life saving. It is, however, not free from risks such as pneumothorax and pneumomediastinum, pulmonary interstitial emphysema, lung sepsis and the later development of chronic lung disease (bronchopulmonary dysplasia). There are a variety of techniques of IPPV and different types of ventilators have their protagonists. Peak inspiratory pressures should be kept as low as possible consistent with satisfactory PaO_2 values. It is an advantage if the ventilator has the facility for providing synchronised intermittent mandatory ventilation (SIMV) whereby inspiratory pulses are superimposed 5-20 times/ minute on a continuous gas flow and 2-5 cm H_2O of positive airways pressure. This technique is helpful in weaning infants off IPPV by allowing them to start some spontaneous respiration for themselves. Continuing positive airways pressure (CPAP) may be delivered to the infant airways through a facemask or more commonly by the use of nasal prongs. CPAP increases the PaO_2 and reduces the need for IPPV. It has its greatest application in infants less than 1,500 g but to be effective it must be instituted early in the course of the illness. A suitable indication for use is where the inspired oxygen concentration has to be increased above 60% to achieve a PaO_2 of 60 mmHg (8.0 kPa). Transpulmonary pressures of about 6 cm water should be used initially, and sufficient oxygen administered in the inspired air to give a PaO_2 above 60 mmHg (8.0 kPa). As in the case of IPPV, CPAP is not without its hazards, such as pneumothorax

v *Drugs:* Surfactant materials extracted from animal lungs and from human amniotic fluid or synthesised in the laboratory have been found of value in prophylaxis and in treatment of RDS. Surfactant is instilled into the lungs via the endotracheal tube. It has been shown to benefit infants of less than 30 weeks gestation when used prophylactily and has significantly improved the outcome when used therapeutically.

Apart from surfactant, drug therapies have limited but controversial roles in RDS. This applies for example to the routine prophylactic use of antibiotics in view of the difficulty, which may be experienced in differentiating early onset Group B, streptococcal sepsis from RDS the routine administration of penicillin is probably justified. Furthermore, as Gram-negative bacteria and penicillin resistant staphylococci may also produce rapidly fatal illness; in these immature preterm infants, we recommend the addition of an aminoglycocide or third generation cephalosporin.

Patent Ductus Arteriosus

There is often delay in spontaneous closure of the ductus in preterm infants, particularly VLBW infants. This is more likely in the presence of RDS and fluid overload. Patent ductus becomes clinically obvious usually at 5 to 7 days after birth when the peripheral pulses become full and collapsing and a systolic or continuous murmur can be heard at the base of the heart. Cardiac failure commonly develops with radiographic signs of cardiomegaly and pulmonary oedema. The size of the shunt can best be assessed by echocardiography.

In addition to restricting fluid intake to less than 100 ml/kg/24 hr, frusemide 2mg/kg may be given intravenously. Indomethacin (0.1mg/k/day IV x 6 doses), which is an inhibitor of prostaglandin synthetase, has been used to close the ductus. Its use is based upon the finding that prostaglandin E_1 relaxes the ductus arteriosus tending to keep it open. It should not be prescribed if there is any evidence of a bleeding tendency, thrombocytopenia or if the plasma bilirubin concentration is > 180 µmol/l (10.5 mg per 100 ml). There is some evidence that the earlier indomethacin is commenced the better the chance of closure of the ductus and it is seldom effective if used later than 2 weeks after birth. If this treatment fails and cardiac failure persists the ductus should be closed surgically.

Intraventricular Haemorrhage (IVH)

Spontaneous bleeding into one or both lateral ventricles is a complication of the prematurity particularly the infant who develops RDS. The development of real-time ultrasound scanning at the cot side has made accurate diagnosis of IVH possible during life. In infants < 1,500 g more than 40% suffer a degree of IVH. Whilst large intraventricular haemorrhages are likely to prove fatal ultrasound has shown that smaller haemorrhages into the germinal layer or ventricles are frequently compatible with survival. Some survivors develop post-haemorrhagic hydrocephalus, porencephalic cysts or neurodevelopmental handicaps but others appear to progress quite normally.

In an infant less than 33 weeks gestation, bleeding may start in the germinal layer, which lies just under the ependyma in the roof of the lateral ventricles. Haemorrhage may be confined to the germinal layer (GLH) or it may rupture into the ventricle (IVH). In some infants the haemorrhage disrupts the substance of the brain. The microvasculature of the germinal layer consists of an extensive arrangement of fine capillaries and also of large irregular thin-walled vessels, which form short connecting channels between the arterial and venous trees. These vessels readily rupture when exposed to sudden surges in pressure, which can be provoked, by hypoxaemia and hypercapnia. On the other hand, hyperoxaemia and hypocapnia can cause abrupt falls in cerebral blood flow so that in some instances ischaemia in the subependymal layer results in infarction and cerebral atrophy. The germinal layer involutes from 32 weeks gestation and it is presumed that IVH in older infants of > 2,000 g arises in the choroid plexus. Ultrasound reveals the frequency with which GLH and IVH develop in preterm infants and shows that survival in 30-50% of affected children is possible. IVH may occur within 6 hours of birth.

Clinical Features

GLH and IVH can apparently remain asymptomatic and even when attacks of apnoea or convulsions occur they do not necessarily reflect the presence of haemorrhage. Abnormal neurological signs have been shown to correlate with the appearance of GLH and IVH on sequential ultrasound scans. The degree of haemorrhage observed

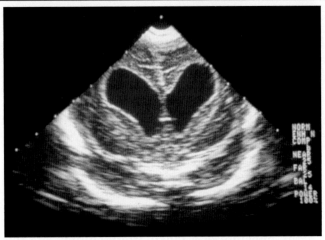

Fig. 3.1.5: Cranial ultrasound showing dilatation of both lateral ventricles

on ultrasound scanning can be graded as follows: grade 1–Germinal layer haemorrhage; grade 2–intraventricular haemorrhage; grade 3–intraventricular haemorrhage with ventricular distension; grade 4–haemorrhage into brain substance (Fig. 3.1.5).

Retinopathy of Prematurity (ROP)

This name is now preferred to retrolental fibroplasia because it takes account of the important fact that some cases are arrested early, before advancing to blindness. The disease first appeared in the USA in 1942 and in the UK in 1946. These dates coincided with the widespread use of incubators in both countries and this aroused early suspicion that oxygen therapy might have aetiological importance. Experimental proof of the role of oxygen came from a series of observations on newborn kittens. While the kittens were exposed to high concentrations of oxygen the retinal vessels underwent intense vasoconstriction. On subsequent transfer to air these vessels showed gross vasodilatation followed by the proliferation of new vessels in a completely disordered fashion. In the human infant the same sequence of events is directly related to the degree of immaturity, the arterial oxygen tension and the duration of exposure.

Clinical Features

This disorder is seen only in preterm infants. The acute stage is first seen between the ages of 3 and 6 weeks in the form of dilatation of retinal veins and arteries. This is followed by the growth, in a disorderly pattern, of new capillaries at the growing ends of the veins. Clusters of new capillaries may simulate haemorrhages. Subsequently, some of the new vessels begin to grow forwards into the vitreous towards the lens. Retinal oedema occurs and is followed by peripheral retinal detachment when the condition becomes irreversible. In the cicatricial stage there may be complete retinal detachment, leaving only a stalk of rolled-up retina connected posteriorly around the optic disc. Finally, there is a retrolental mass of fibrous tissue visible behind a clear lens with a naked eye. In severe cases the condition is bilateral with microphthalmos, a narrow anterior chamber, irregular small pupil and gross loss of vision. Squint is common and glaucoma frequent. There is also an increased incidence of learning disorder and cerebral palsy in these children.

Prevention

It is essential to prevent factors, which predispose to retinopathy of prematurity. The arterial PO_2 and/or transcutaneous oxygen should be monitored at all times while a premature baby is receiving oxygen therapy, which should not be continued a minute longer than is necessary.

The incidence of retinopathy of prematurity declined rapidly after the discovery of the causal role of oxygen it increased again in infants weighing between 501 and 1,500 g. It is important to examine routinely all infants weighing less than 1,500 g or 34 weeks gestational age for ROP. Larger infants who have required prolonged oxygen therapy may also be worth careful examination. Proper examination by an ophthalmologist skilled in the examination after pupil dilatation is required. Results are recorded using an International classification. Those found to have significant ROP are reviewed every one to two weeks until regression occurs or the threshold for treatment is reached. Cryotherapy of peripheral avascular retina and laser ablation of abnormal central retinal vessels has been shown to be effective in reducing the progression of the retinopathy. Severe visual impairment in early infancy may also be due to damage to the visual cortex. Electro physiological testing in such infants shows a normal electroretinogram but absent or abnormal visual evoked responses.

The Early Anaemia of Prematurity

This condition must be clearly differentiated from the hypochromic anaemia of iron-deficiency to which the preterm infant is susceptible after the age of 4 months. The latter condition may be thought of as the "late anaemia of prematurity". Unlike the early anaemia of prematurity it can be prevented or cured with iron.

The haemoglobin level at birth in venous blood of both term and preterm infants is high by adult standards (19-21 g per 100 ml). In all infants there is a fairly rapid decrease during the early weeks of life. This is because the oxygen saturation of blood increases at birth from a fetal level of 65% to the normal adult value of 95%, when the lungs take over the supply of oxygen from the placenta. There is, in consequence, a decrease in the need for circulating

haemoglobin and the bone marrow goes into a resting phase with relative erythropoietic inactivity. The decrease in red cell mass and circulating haemoglobin depends also on the infant's rate of growth. As preterm infants grow more rapidly than term in relative terms there is an exaggerated rate of fall in red cell mass and haemoglobin concentration. A value of 8 g per 100 ml is not uncommon at the age of 6-8 weeks. This early anaemia of prematurity is normochromic. Recovery tends to take place as the bone marrow responds to the low level of oxygenation in the tissues. However, as rapid growth also continues this spontaneous increase in haemoglobin concentration may be slow. It will be ill sustained unless adequate supplies of iron are made available from the age of 6-8 weeks.

Treatment

When the early anaemia of prematurity is aggravated by infection or haemorrhage blood transfusion is indicated. Treatment with erythropoietin has been shown to stimulate the marrow of preterm infants to produce more red cells and a higher haemoglobin concentration.

Key Learning Points
The relative polycythaemia present during fetal life is no longer needed after birth. The erythropoeitic drive in the bone marrow is reduced. The consequent drop in haemoglobin level is accentuated by rapid growth of the peterm baby and frequent venepunctures in the sick baby. Erythropoeitin administration may reduce the need for top-up transfusions.

Jaundice of Prematurity

There is an increased incidence of non-obstructive jaundice in preterm infants, particularly those who develop RDS. The pathogenesis of jaundice and its management are discussed subsequently.

INTRAUTERINE GROWTH RETARDATION

Approximately 30% of all infants weighing 2.5 kg or less at birth are light-for-date. As has already been suggested there are many important causes of infants being light for gestation and small for gestation. Small for gestation infants include those with congenital abnormalities such as the trisomies, microcephaly, and congenital heart disease; also infants who have acquired intrauterine infections such as rubella, cytomegalic inclusion disease, toxoplasmosis and syphilis. A feature of this group of infants is that they have smaller head circumferences than other light for dates infants.

Aetiology

When fetal growth retardation is detected from before 28 weeks by fetal ultrasound, it is likely that at birth the infant's weight and body size (length and OFC) will be small for date. Such small-for-dates (SFD) infants may have congenital abnormalities. It has been suggested that if smoking, hypertension and pre-eclampsia could be eliminated the number of light-for-date infants could be halved. The high level of light-for-date infants in socially deprived inner city areas highlights the need for the introduction of preventive strategies.

Whatever may be the precise aetiology, the light-for-dates infant has poor energy reserves of glycogen in liver, heart and skeletal muscle whilst the growth of the brain and mature lungs contrast with the shrunken liver. In the normal newborn infant the brain is about three times heavier than the liver whereas in the light-for-dates infant, the brain may be seven or eight times the weight of the liver. Pulmonary haemorrhage is a frequent postmortem finding in the severely growth restricted infant.

Clinical Features

In intrauterine growth retardation the infant may be born term or preterm and the growth retardation in length and head circumference may be less than indicated by body weight. The infant looks thin and wasted; the skin is dry and desquamating and often shows transverse cracks over the lower chest and abdomen and at the ankles and wrists; meconium staining of nails and cord may be present; and there is commonly a characteristic wide-awake expression which is not seen in the preterm low birthweight infant. Appearances in general reflect a fairly long period of malnutrition or under-nutrition in utero.

Management

The light-for-date infant is usually eager to feed and oral feeds should be commenced between 2 and 4 hours after birth to reduce the dangers of hypoglycaemia. Blood glucose concentrations should be determined every few hours by testing capillary blood with an indicator stix test, e.g. Dextrostix (Ames & Co). True blood glucose measurements should be performed if a reading of < 2.5 mmol/l (45 mg per 100 ml) is obtained on the stix test. Continued tachypnoea one or two hours after birth may indicate the presence of meconium aspiration. Core body temperatures should be recorded and precautions taken to avoid hypothermia.

COMPLICATIONS OF INTRAUTERINE GROWTH RETARDATION

Meconium Aspiration Syndrome

Whereas RDS is common in the preterm infant the usual cause of respiratory difficulties in the light-for-date infant is meconium aspiration. Meconium is intensely irritating to the bronchiolar epithelium. Radiographic appearances of the lung fields are different to those of RDS with coarser

streaking and varying degrees of collapse and emphysema. Treatment, however, is similar to that for RDS.

Transient Symptomatic Hypoglycaemia of the Newborn

This dangerous condition occurs more frequently in male light-for-date infants. If not promptly recognised and vigorously treated, permanent brain damage is a common sequel. The only complication of pregnancy known to increase the risk of spontaneous hypoglycaemia in the infant is pre-eclamptic toxaemia present in about half the cases. The pathogenesis is not yet clear although the extremely poor glycogen stores of the light-for-date infant is an important factor. There may be an insufficiency of glucose available for the relatively large glucose dependent brain and the metabolically active mature body.

Clinical Features

The infant usually appears well for a period, which may vary, from six hours to seven days after birth. Then various signs manifest themselves, such as jitteriness or twitchings, attacks of apnoea and cyanosis, pallor, reluctance to feed, limpness, apathy or generalized convulsions. When these manifestations occur in an infant showing the signs of intrauterine growth retardation the diagnosis of hypoglycaemia should be suspected and true blood glucose estimations arranged immediately. The diagnosis is confirmed when a blood glucose value of less than 1.1 mmol/l (20 mg per 100 ml) is detected. Values below 2.2 mmol/l (40 mg per 100 ml) should be used as the indication for increased glucose intake.

Treatment

An intravenous injection of 15% glucose in water, 2 ml per kg body weight, should be given immediately followed thereafter by continuous infusion of 10% glucose in water, 60-75 ml/kg/day. Oral feeds where tolerated should be increased to tolerance. If the intravenous 10% dextrose has to be given for longer than 24 hours it should be combined in quarter-strength physiological saline to prevent hyponatraemia. Occasionally it may be necessary to use corticosteroids such as oral hydrocortisone (5 mg per kg per day) in resistant cases. In some instances plasma calcium concentrations below 2 mmol/l (8 mg per 100 ml) may be found in which case the intravenous infusion of 3-5 ml of 10 per cent calcium gluconate should be given by slow intravenous injection. Long-term follow-up of such infants to assess development is essential.

It is common practice to monitor blood glucose values of all post term and light-for-date infants at 6 hourly intervals with one of the glucose test strip methods. This regimen will reveal a number of infants with blood glucose values below 1.1 mmol/l (20 mg per 100 ml) who are asymptomatic. It is important as stated earlier to increase glucose intake in any infant with blood glucose values below 2.2 mmol/l (40 mg per 100 ml). Glucose test strip screening of newborn infants may also reveal some pre-symptomatic cases of hypoglycaemia in infants with severe perinatal asphyxia, intracranial haemorrhage, haemolytic disease of the newborn and in the infants of diabetic mothers. Such infants are managed in the same way.

Case Study 2: Hypoglycaemia in a Light-for-date Infant

A female infant was born by elective LSCS at 37 weeks gestation weighing 1740 gm (2nd centile). Mother was hypertensive throughout the pregnancy and intrauterine growth retardation had been diagnosed on antenatal ultrasound from 32 weeks. The baby was meconium stained but cried at birth and needed minimal resuscitation. She was transferred to SCBU where blood sugar was checked using capillary blood and found to be 3.5 mmol/l at 30 min of age. She was offered her first feed at 1hour of age and sucked well. Her blood sugar was monitored using capillary blood at 3 hourly intervals before each feed. By 9 hours she was also put to the breast. At 12 hours she had a dusky episode and was noted to be jittery. Capillary blood sugar was 1.8 mmol/l confirmed on checking her true blood glucose. She was given a bolus of 10% dextrose IV (3ml/kg stat) and an IV infusion of 10% dextrose was continued at a rate of 3 ml/hr. Her capillary blood glucose increased to 2.5 mmol/l. Her colour improved but she remained lethargic and jittery on handling. IV 10% dextrose drip rate was increased to 4 ml/hr. Further checks showed a TBG of 3.2 mmol/l and a plasma calcium level of 1.7 mmol.l (low) and magnesium of 0.72 mmol/ml (normal). She was given oral calcium supplements and over the next 3 days the IV dextrose infusion was withdrawn and the calcium supplements stopped. She remained well demanding feeds every 2-3 hours and by day five had already started to gain weight.

NEONATAL INFECTIONS

Infections may be acquired prenatally, perinatally or postnatally. Development of intensive anti-infection measures has greatly reduced both mortality and morbidity from neonatal infections in developed countries during recent years. Nonetheless there are still significant numbers of deaths and handicaps resulting from such infections. Antibiotic resistance has assumed major importance and a more critical approach to their use is necessary.

Prenatal

During pregnancy infecting organisms pass from the maternal circulation to the intervillous spaces of the placenta and penetrate the fetal circulation. Viruses known to cross the placenta include rubella, poliomyelitis, coxsackie, variola, herpes, varicella zoster, human immunodeficiency virus and cytomegalovirus. Some of these, such as rubella, produce early damage to the developing embryo; others such as cytomegalovirus or Coxsackie produce late effects such as hepatitis or myocarditis in the newborn infant. Fetal damage from maternal viral infection during very early pregnancy can be severe. Many pregnancies abort but other fetuses survive with a continuing viraemia, which may indeed persist for two years or more after birth. It is recommended that all children, boys and girls are immunised against rubella at the age of 15 months with a combined mumps, measles, rubella immunisation in an attempt to eradicate the severe damage of congenital rubella. A surviving fetus may have congenital heart defects, deafness, cataracts and where the maternal infection is contracted later in pregnancy may present with purpura, thrombocytopenia, hepatosplenomegaly and radiological evidence of osteitis. Damage to the brain may result in severe learning difficulties. Eighty-five per cent of infants affected during the first 8 weeks of pregnancy will have multiple defects whereas 15% of infants affected in mid pregnancy may present with sensorineural deafness alone. Infections after pregnancy appear to carry less risk of damage.

Suspected rubella in a mother during pregnancy is an indication for testing maternal serum for haemaglutinin inhibition antibodies (HI). If the antibody concentration is increased within the incubation period of rubella the mother can be considered protected by previous infection or immunisation. If low titres are obtained a repeat serum sample should be obtained 2 - 3 weeks after first exposure. An increased titre confirms primary infection and a high risk of fetal damage. After birth the finding of specific rubella IgM antibody in the blood or rubella virus in the urine will confirm the diagnosis.

Cytomegalovirus is now the commonest congenital infection in the UK. Approximately 50% of pregnant women have antibodies to CMV and it is estimated that between 1 and 5% of pregnant women contract CMV infections with fetal involvement in about half of infected pregnancies. Mothers are usually asymptomatic and in most instances the infant appears normal. In severe infections the infant may be acutely ill, small for gestational age, have signs of meningoencephalitis, jaundice, petechiae, hepatosplenomegaly and feeding difficulties. The virus may be cultured from urine, upper respiratory tract secretions and cerebrospinal fluid. In milder cases in which there may be no clinical evidence of the disease there can be late sequelae such as neurodevelopmental delay, epilepsy and nerve deafness. Approximately 5% of infected infants have clinical signs at birth and most of these infants will have long-term sequelae. A further 5% will develop severe handicaps particularly deafness later in life. Presence of virus in the urine with raised CMV specific IgM antibody in the blood confirms the diagnosis. There is no value in routine screening for CMV in pregnancy. Termination cannot be justified on the basis of fetal infection, as 90% of infants will be unaffected. Also fetal infections can occur after primary or secondary CMV infections in pregnancy and fetal damage can occur from infection occurring at any time in pregnancy.

Human immunodeficiency virus (HIV) may be transmitted to the infant before, during or after birth. Maternal antibodies may persist in the infant up to 18 months of age and neonatal diagnosis is difficult in asymptomatic infants. There are varying estimates of the percentage of infected infants born to HIV positive mothers and these vary between 15 and 35%. With the spread of the virus into the heterosexual population a high index of suspicion and care in handling blood from mothers and newborn infants is necessary. Some infants progress rapidly to full blown AIDS and develop serious opportunistic infections during the first year of life whilst others may show features such as persistent lymphadenopathy, hepatospleno-megaly, chronic diarrhoea, unexplained fevers and failure to thrive. Postnatal infection may occur via the breast milk and in developed countries it is probably best to persuade known HIV positive mothers to avoid breastfeeding. In underdeveloped countries the other risks associated with artificial feeding probably outweigh the risks of the infant acquiring HIV infection from the mother.

HIV is covered in more detail in the section on Infectious Diseases (See chapter 26).

Maternal herpes *varicella zoster infection* in early pregnancy rarely affects the fetus but when it does there can be extensive scarring skin lesions, choroidoretinitis, cataracts and damage to the brain. When mother develops the chickenpox between 4 days before and 4 days after delivery, neonatal mortality from pneumonia can be high. This is because there is no time for protective transplacental antibodies to be acquired by the fetus. Infants born to a mother who develops chickenpox at this late stage should be given passive immunisation with zoster immune globulin as soon as possible after birth. Acyclovir may be given to infants showing clinical features of infection and any mother developing a perinatal rash should be isolated with barrier nursing of the infant and avoidance of breastfeeding until skin lesions have resolved.

Other viral infections such as Coxsackie, ECHO, myxo, parvo, and hepatitis B are amongst the viruses to be considered when meningoencephalitis, hepatitis, myocar-ditis, fetal oedema or hydrops, pneumonias, diarrhoea, jaundice and cataract are unexplained. Neonatal hepatitis B (HB) infections are more common in some populations than others, but world wide they are a major public health problem. Neonatal liver disease due to HB viraemia is very variable and can present as fulminant hepatic necrosis, chronic persistent hepatitis, mild focal necrosis or may be asymptomatic. Portal hypertension and primary liver cancers are later complications. The infant is most at risk when the mother has acute HB hepatitis during the third trimester and at delivery. Chronic HB surface antigen (HBs Ag) positive carrier mothers, particularly if they are also HBe Ag positive, HBe antibody negative or have high serum HBc Ab values are highly infective to their infants. In endemic areas, infants act as carriers and excreters of the virus. Protective immunisation of susceptible women of childbearing age and of infants within 48 hours of birth, particularly infants born to carrier mothers should be instituted in populations or sub-populations with high rates of HB virus infection.

Congenital syphilis can present in the newborn with hepatitis, splenomegaly, anaemia, thrombocytopenia, jaundice and oedema. There may be characteristic bone changes on X-ray. After three to four weeks a maculo-papular skin rash with mucocutaneous lesions, snuffles and pseudo-paralysis may develop. Most newborn infants with congenital syphilis remain well and there may be no manifestation of disease for several weeks when jaundice, anaemia, hepatosplenomegaly, oedema and signs of meningitis may develop. Adequate treatment of mothers with secondary syphilis detected by routine serological testing should reduce the incidence of congenital syphilis. Prompt treatment of affected infants with penicillin is indicated if there is clinical or radiological evidence of the disease or if cord blood serology is positive and the mother has not been adequately treated. If there is uncertainty about the presence of infection the infant should be given protective penicillin therapy and quantitative serological measurements and physical examinations made at monthly intervals. Infants with congenital syphilis require lumbar puncture and abnormal CSF is an indication to give crystalline penicillin G 50,000 units per kg by intramuscular or intravenous injection daily in two divided doses for a minimum of 10 days. Infants with normal cerebrospinal fluid should be given benzathine penicillin G 50,000 units per kg by intramuscular injection in a single dose.

Toxoplasma gondii is a protozoan transmitted to the fetus from the placenta in utero and is associated with intrauterine growth retardation, cerebral haemorrhage and microcephaly or hydrocephaly, intracranial calci-fication, choroidoretinitis, microphthalmia, thrombocy-topenia and jaundice. A combination of pyrimethamine given orally in a dose of 0.5 mg/kg twice daily and sulphadiazine given orally in a dose of 100 mg/kg per day is recommended for three to four weeks. Spiramycin is also reported to be effective. The organism may be cultured and the diagnosis confirmed by the indirect fluorescent antibody test in the maternal and infant serum. In the UK about 20% of women have toxoplasma antibodies and only a small percentage of women contract infection during the first trimester. The infection may be contracted by the ingestion of undercooked meat or from cat faeces. Pregnant women should avoid dealing with cat excreta.

Congenital malaria is rare except in non-immune mothers who, during pregnancy, have received inadequate protection. The malarial protozoan plasmodium in many parts of the world is a major cause of fetal damage. The degree of immunity to malaria possessed by an infant at birth is directly related to that of the mother, so that in spite of heavy or passive parasitisation of the placenta found in highly immune indigenous dwellers of endemic areas, the incidence of congenital malaria is rare. When it does occur fever, convulsions and severe haemolytic anaemia with jaundice, hepatosplenomegaly and brain damage with a high mortality are the result. In the partially immune child less severe infections occur and present with signs similar to that of bacterial septicaemia. In endemic areas transfused blood may be an important source of acquired infection in the newborn. Treatment includes a full therapeutic course of chloroquine or other relevant antimalarial drug for that area. Treatment of the infected newborn is usually with chloroquine 5 ml/kg by injection or 75 mg chloroquine base orally followed by 37.5 mg twice daily for two days.

Maternal infections with Listeria monocytogenes, a Gram-positive bacterium, may cause preterm labour or transplacental fetal infection. This organism flourishes in undercooked chicken and "cook-chill" foods, unpasteurised milk and soft cheeses causing a mild flu-like illness in the mother. After birth the infant may present with pneumonia, meningitis, septicaemia and a skin rash. The amniotic fluid has a characteristically offensive smell and there is 30% mortality. Infection can be acquired during delivery and there may be a later presentation with septicaemia and meningitis. Treatment with ampicillin and gentamicin of the mother and affected newborn is indicated.

Perinatal Infections

Infection acquired during the birth process or after rupture of the membranes is not uncommon. Premature membrane rupture before or during labour together with a long interval before delivery are important predisposing factors to the development of placentitis and infection of the amniotic fluid. Infection may also occur with intact membranes during prolonged labours especially when there has been excessive manipulation or sources of contamination. The fetus may inhale infected amniotic fluid resulting in a congenital pneumonia. Alternatively infection may spread from an infected placenta to the fetal circulation causing septicaemia. Infection of the eyes by gonococcus during delivery was once a major cause of blindness in childhood in the UK but is now rare. Unfortunately it persists in many parts of the world as a major cause of blindness. Frequent irrigation of the conjunctiva with antibiotic eye drops together with a course of systemic penicillin is recommended. Some organisms are resistant to penicillin and a broad-spectrum antibiotic is required. The maternal vulva and cervix may be infected with chlamydia trachomatis and this may be a cause of conjunctivitis and more rarely neonatal pneumonia in the newborn. Chlamydial pneumonitis may present 4 to 6 weeks after birth and is best treated with systemic erythromycin.

One of the most worrying organisms affecting newborn infants is the **Group B streptococcus** (GBS) which can produce severe fulminating pneumonia and septicaemia resulting in the death of infants within hours of birth. The clinical presentation is similar to that of the idiopathic respiratory distress syndrome and as it is more common in preterm low birthweight infants a high index of suspicion for infection should be maintained. The intrapartum administration of penicillin to mothers known to be colonised with the GBS significantly reduces the risk of infection being acquired by the baby. If there is any doubt the infant and mother should have bacteriological cultures of blood and vulva respectively and the infant treated with high dosage penicillin.

Herpes virus Type II infection may be transmitted to the fetus from a maternal cervicitis. The fetus may be aborted or delivered prematurely. The risk to the fetus is greatest if the maternal cervical lesion is primary rather than a reactivation lesion. Neonatal disease does not usually present until about a week after birth when there may be vesicular skin lesions, hepatosplenomegaly, jaundice, petechiae, encephalopathy and seizures associated with the generalised viraemia. Choroidoretinitis or cataract may be found at a later stage. Herpes virus antigen may be detected in fluid from blisters and treatment with intravenous acyclovir should be commenced immediately.

Postnatal Infections

Whilst intrapartum infection is an important cause of perinatal mortality, most fatal infections occur after birth. There has been a considerable change in the relative importance of different types of infection in hospital nurseries over the past 50 years. Puerperal fever with Group A β-haemolytic streptococcus caused severe morbidity in both mothers and infants. Epidemics of gastro-enteritis probably mainly bacterial in origin were a major problem in the 1940's when infections with the coagulase-positive staphylococcus aureus resistant to antibiotics such as benzylpenicillin, tetracycline, streptomycin and erythromycin made its appearance. The staphylococcus could cause sudden outbreaks of severe sepsis including pneumonia, osteitis and pyaemia. In addition there were problems of septic spots, paronychiae, conjunctivitis and umbilical sepsis. The marked fall in the incidence of staphylococcal lesions in newborn nurseries from the mid 1960's was related to improved standards of hand care and the introduction of hexachlorophane for skin cleansing. Although this seemed to help control the problems of the *staphylococcus aureus* the Gram- negative bacilli particularly *Escherichia coli*, *Proteus* and *Klebsiella* entered the arena. More recently the Group B streptococcus has colonised mothers and infants causing severe problems in the newborn.

Diagnosis

The diagnosis of infection during the neonatal period can be difficult. Localizing signs are frequently absent and the primary portal of entry is often not obvious. In fact the infection may so quickly become a generalised septicaemia or pyaemia as a result of the poor local resistance of the newborn tissues to micro-organisms that a "local diagnosis" has little relevance. Often the first indication in the term infant is a reluctance to finish feeds, vomiting, undue drowsiness sometimes alternating with excessive irritability, or a rise in the respiratory rate, which may rapidly progress, to dyspnoea. A sudden weight loss in an infant who has been progressing satisfactorily is significant. The infant may develop a characteristic greyish pallor and anxious face. Diarrhoea is not uncommon. Oedema, jaundice, purpura and other haemorrhages together with convulsions indicate severe sepsis. Hepatosplenomegaly is common in septicaemias. Fever may or may not be present. In preterm infants hypothermia and sclerema frequently accompany an infective process. The appearance of any of these manifestations should indicate the need for careful physical examination and relevant laboratory investigations. These may include urine analysis, blood culture, white cell count, C-reactive protein, lumbar puncture and radiography. They should precede treatment and there should be no delay in instituting the investigations and giving "best guess" therapy.

Case Study 3: An infant with septicaemia and severe hyperbilirubinaemia

A male infant was born at 31 weeks gestation weighing 1950 gm. Maternal membranes ruptured 8 days prior to delivery. Mother had received dexamethasone therapy to induce fetal lung maturation. The infant cried at birth and had an Apgar score of 8/10. He was given incubatoer care and initially seemed well. Blood cultures were taken and antibiotic cover started with penicillin and gentamicin because of prolonged rapture of membranes. At 12 hours of age he became tachypnoic and had frequent apnoeic episodes and desaturations. Umbilical artery and venous catheters were passed. Chest X-ray showed marked haziness of both lung fields suggestive of pneumonia. Assisted ventilation was started. Blood gases showed a persistent metabolic acidosis which was partly corrected by a sodium bicarbonate infusion.

He became jaundiced and phototherapy was started. Despite this unconjugated serum bilirubin continued to climb and reached 310 µmol/L at 30 hours. An exchange transfusion was indicated. He was cross matched and received an exchange transfusion at 34 hours. For each 10 ml aliquot of donor blood infused via the arterial catheter, 10 ml of the baby's blood was removed through the venous one until a total of 351 ml (180 ml/kg) had been exchanged. The procedure was done over 3 hours. At the end the SBR had dropped to 200 µmol/L. Phototherapy was continued. Blood cultures showed the presence of septicaemia with enterobacter resistant to both penicillin and gentamicin but sensitive to cefotaxime. The baby's general condition and jaundice stabilised after the change of antibiotics. IPPV was stopped on day 3 and phototherapy discontinued on day 5.

MAJOR INFECTIONS

1. Pneumonia in the Newborn

a. *Congenital (intrauterine) pneumonia* is often mistaken for asphyxia, respiratory distress syndrome or intracranial haemorrhage. Accurate diagnosis may be difficult because the affected infant is often apnoeic at birth and later shows the same type of grunting respiration with subcostal and sternal recession, and cyanosis as seen in IRDS. Pneumonia, however, is equally common in mature and preterm infants and should always be suspected when more than 24 hours have elapsed between rupture of the membranes and delivery particularly if the mother is febrile. The chest radiograph shows softer and more confluent opacities than in IRDS. Clinical signs over the lungs are usually few and unhelpful. Air entry may be poor and crepitations may be heard.

Treatment

Treatment with oxygen and intravenous antibiotics appropriate to the knowledge of the maternal microbiology and to the currently problematic micro-organisms in the nursery environment should be given. One combination, which gives wide spectral cover, is benzylpenicillin with gentamicin. In other nurseries the introduction of a third generation cephalosporin would be appropriate. This treatment will cover Group B haemolytic streptococci but occasionally organisms such as the enterobacter cloacae resistant to cephalosporins means that regular microbiological determination of organism sensitivities in each neonatal nursery must be determined.

b. *Staphylococcal pneumonia* is common in many neonatal nurseries throughout the world and may follow minor staphylococcal lesions such as paronichae. The staphylococcus produces massive lung consolidation in many infants and this may proceed to abscess formation, empyema or pyopneumothorax. Methicillin resistant staphylococcus aureus (MRSA) strains have come about through indiscriminate antibiotic therapy and occasionally neonatal wards have had to be closed because of an epidemic.

In addition to oxygen, intravenous infusion of flucoxacillin 25 mg per kg initially reducing to 12.5 mg per kg four times daily should be given.

c. *Streptococcal pneumonia* due to the Group B streptococcus has already been discussed. In addition to the characteristic features of respiratory distress, cyanosis and lethargy there may be either fever or hypothermia. In some infants there are signs of disseminated intravascular coagulation with thrombocytopenia, diminished plasma fibrinogen and raised serum fibrin degradation products. Both clinical features and radiographic appearance may closely mimic IRDS although in most cases the lung fields show coarser mottling. Blood cultures frequently yield a positive result.

Treatment

The drug of choice is benzylpenicillin given intravenously but until culture results have confirmed the streptococcal origin of the respiratory problem it is wise to add gentamicin.

Other pneumonias, which occur less commonly are caused by organisms including pneumococci, Group A β-haemolytic streptococci or *H.infuenzae* as in older infants, but in the newborn, organisms not usually associated with pneumonia may infect lung tissue, e.g. *E.coli*, enterococci, *enterobacter, proteus, pseudomonas and Chlamydia*.

2. Epidemic Diarrhoea of the Newborn

This name for infantile gastro-enteritis stresses the fact that in neonatal nurseries the disease tends to occur in explosive epidemics, which may have considerable mortality. Such outbreaks are reported less frequently in the UK in recent years and may reflect improved standards of care in newborn nurseries. It is important, however, to safeguard against the introduction of the E.coli with specific serotypes classified by their somatic (O) antigens. Outbreaks due to Salmonella group organisms are still seen. However, the most common aetiological agent in most neonatal nurseries today is the rotavirus.

Clinical Features

The illness may vary from a mild upset with lethargy, anorexia, slight loss of weight and loose stools to a fulminating outburst of severe diarrhoea and vomiting. In cases due to rotavirus there may be associated respiratory signs such as nasal discharge or inflamed tympanic membranes. The stools are large, fluid, green or orange coloured and losses of body water and electrolytes may be massive with resultant diminution in plasma volume. A severe metabolic acidosis may arise from the considerable losses of sodium and potassium, with renal failure due to the diminished blood flow through the kidneys. Within a few hours of the onset the infant may have developed the classical picture of severe dehydration with sunken eyes, depressed fontanelle, overriding sutures, scaphoid abdomen, glazed corneae and semi-coma. The extremities, lips and ears may be cold and cyanosed due to peripheral circulatory failure.

Treatment

Oral feeds should be discontinued and replaced with an oral rehydration fluid, although there is room for controversy as to its composition. Suitable solutions are the BPC sodium chloride and dextrose oral powder compound, small size, to be dissolved in 200 ml of water (per litre: Na 35 mmol, K 20 mmol, HCO, 18 mmol, dextrose 200 mmol); or Dextrolyte (ready-to-feed) (per litre: Na 35, K 13, lactate 18, dextose 200). The rehydration fluid should be given in small quantities every 1-2 hours (180 ml/kg/day). However, if the dehydration or vomiting is severe, fluid and electrolytes must be given by continuous intravenous infusion for 24-72 hours. A suitable fluid is 5 per cent dextrose in sodium chloride 0.18 % (120-150 ml/kg/day). If there is evidence of peripheral circulatory collapse, plasma diluted with equal parts of 10 % dextrose in water can be given (30 ml/kg over 30 min). Severe acidosis may require correction by slow intravenous infusion of 8.4% sodium bicarbonate under careful biochemical control. This is not often required and it is safer to restore the pH to no greater than 7.25 in the first instance. After 24-48 hours, milk feeds are re-started and gradually increased, the electrolyte fluids being correspondingly reduced. If potassium deficit is revealed by hypokalaemia after dehydration has been corrected potassium chloride may be given orally (l g twice daily) or intravenously (20 mmol/l of IV fluid). Antibiotics are of no value.

3. Pyogenic Meningitis

This grave infection of the newborn is most commonly due to Group *B streptococcus* or *E.coli*. Other organisms, which might be involved, include *salmonella, listeria,* pneumococci and staphylococci.

Clinical Features

The onset is insidious with loss of weight, drowsiness, apnoeic attacks, reluctance to feed and vomiting. Convulsive twitching is frequently seen. Significant signs are a bulging anterior fontanelle and head retraction. Nuchal rigidity and Kernig's sign do not occur in the newborn. The most important aid to diagnosis is a marked degree of suspicion when a newborn develops the general signs of severe infection and becomes excessively drowsy. Diagnosis must be confirmed by lumbar puncture. The cerebrospinal fluid is turbid due to large numbers of pus cells. Culture is required to determine antibiotic sensitivities.

Treatment

The mortality is high and many of the survivors suffer permanent brain and/or deafness. *E.Coli* meningitis may prove difficult to eradicate. Group B streptococcal meningitis carries a high risk of brain damage leading to cortical blindness, nerve deafness and spasticity.

Hydrocephalus may be a long-term complication. Early diagnosis and institution of antibiotic therapy with penicillin and cefotaxime is essential to minimise sequelae. These antibiotics can be later adjusted according to culture and sensitivity results.

4. Pyelonephritis

Gram-negative infections in the newborn seem to have a preference for settling in renal tissue when there has been a bacteraemia or septicaemia.

Clinical Features

The infant becomes ill with fever, and there is reluctance to feed, vomiting, greyish pallor and loss of weight. Diagnosis will be missed unless urine is obtained and subjected to microscopy and culture. In newborn a urinary white cell count is likely to be significant if it exceeds 15 per mm^3 in boys or 50 per mm^3 in girls. Urine for culture is much more reliably obtained by suprapubic bladder aspiration than by plastic bag. Pyuria may also be part of the clinical picture in a jaundiced baby suffering from Gram-negative septicaemia. In this event the pyelonephritis arises from the blood stream and sometimes there is also present a pyogenic meningitis. In such cases blood culture and sometimes lumbar puncture should be performed in addition to urine culture.

Treatment

A combination of ampicillin and gentamicin or third generation cephalosporin is likely to be effective and must be started without delay while awaiting culture results.

5. Acute Osteitis

Osteitis in the newborn is a metastatic lesion, which is usually due to a penicillin-resistant *Staph.aureus* but may occasionally be due to the haemophilus organism.

Clinical Features

In most cases the infant is seriously ill although fever is not always present. Localising signs are sometimes slow to appear and should be diligently sought in every ill infant. These are local swelling with or without discoloration; extreme irritability on handling the affected part or limb; or immobility of the affected limb (pseudoparesis). In the newborn, osteitis may involve multiple sites especially the superior maxilla and pelvis. When the maxilla is involved, retro-orbital cellulitis causes proptosis as a presenting sign. If diagnosis is delayed, extensive bone destruction and disorganisation of the neighbouring joint may lead to permanent crippling. In some infants general systemic illness is remarkably slight, when the dangers of late diagnosis are even greater.

Treatment

At attempt should be made to isolate the causal organism by blood culture. Aspiration of pus through a wide-bore needle from the effected bone site may be possible. An intravenous infusion of flucloxacillin 25 mg/kg 4 times a day may be required as the initial antibiotic treatment.

6. Tetanus Neonatorum

This topic is discussed in the chapter on infectious diseases (See chapter 26).

Necrotising Enterocolitis

Necrotising Enterocolitis (NEC) is a common neonatal emergency, still of unknown cause, which affects mainly premature neonates, although rarely it can occur in tern infants as well. It carries a high degree of morbidity and mortality. Its incidence is inversely related to birthweight and gestational age. It is rare in infants who have never been fed enterally and is much less common in breast fed babies or those babies receiving human breast milk.

The bowel becomes inflamed and ulcerated. Fluid exudes into the lumen resulting in hypotension and circulatory failure. Bleeding into the bowel lumen occurs together with the formation of gas bubbles within the bowel wall, which when extensive can result in the stripping of the intimal lining from the muscle which is a characteristic of the condition. Bowel perforation is a frequent and ominous complication.

NEC usually presents with rapid clinical deterioration, apnoeic spells, hypotension and abdominal distension. Blood in the stools may be noticed. The abdomen is tender and crepitus may be palpable in severe cases. X-ray abdomen may initially show a disappearance of intestinal gas but in most cases dilated loops of bowel are visible with the typical appearance of intramural gas, which confirms the diagnosis. Bowel perforation is signalled by the presence of free gas in the peritoneal cavity. In severe cases gas may be present in the portal venous system.

Treatment

Treatment is initially supportive. Oral feeds should be stopped and total parenteral nutrition started. After taking blood cultures antibiotic cover should be given with penicillin and gentamicin or cefotaxime. Metronidazole should be added to cover against anaerobic infection. Stool cultures should be arranged Intravenous N/2 saline fluid boluses and inotropic support might be needed if circulatory failure is present. Early review by a paediatric surgeon or transfer to a paediatric surgical unit should be arranged as perforation is a common complication and is a neonatal emergency.

Mild cases usually settle after one to two weeks, after which a gradual re-introduction of eneteral feeding should be attempted. Perforated bowel may require suturing or resection. Adhesions and bowel strictures are long-term complications in the survivors.

The cause of NEC is poorly understood but intestinal immaturity and poor motility, poor digestive ability and abnormal bacterial colonisation are thought to be predisposing factors.

JAUNDICE

In order to understand the investigation and management of a jaundiced infant it is useful to have some knowledge of the metabolism of the pigment bilirubin, which is the cause of the yellow discoloration of tissue known as jaundice. Bilirubin is a breakdown product of haem (ferro-protoporphyrin IX). The degradation of 1 gram of haemoglobin releases 600 μmol (35 mg) of bilirubin. The normal newborn infant during the first 2 - 3 weeks of life releases 135-137 μmol (8-10 mg) of bilirubin/kg body-weight/day. This is more than twice the adult output and probably reflects the relatively larger red cell mass, shorter red cell lifespan and possibly an increased turnover of hepatic haem. The bilirubin load to the liver is further increased by intestinal reabsorption of the excreted pigment from the small intestine. Prolonged jaundice occurring in some breastfed infants may be mediated by facilitation of intestinal absorption of bilirubin.

Hepatic Conjugation

Haem is oxidised by microsomal enzyme found in liver, spleen and macrophages. The bilirubin product (tetrapyrrole biliverdin) is transported in the plasma attached to albumin and is transported across the hepatocyte membrane via a specific membrane receptor. In the liver the bilirubin is conjugated by the microsomal enzyme uridyl diphosphate (UDP), glucuronyl transferase. This glucuronation effectively converts the bilirubin from a fat-soluble toxic substance to a non-toxic water-soluble substance, which can be excreted via the bile and kidney. Glucuronyl transferase activity can be increased by the use of microsomal enzyme – inducing drugs such as phenobarbitone. Several other substances important in medicine including steroids, salicylates, aniline and chloramphenicol are excreted by the same bilirubin conjugating system. The availability of glucose is of importance in bilirubin excretion. Other pathways of bilirubin excretion exist in addition to glucuronation and one of these is by conjugation to sulphate. In the newborn, this pathway does not seem to be available and cannot compensate for defective glucuronation. The excretion of conjugated bilirubin from the hepatocyte into bile is a process, which can be inhibited by organic ions and suggests a carrier-mediated system. Obstructive jaundice occurs when the liver is unable to excrete conjugated bilirubin into the gastrointestinal tract by the bile duct system. It may be caused by hepatic cell disorder or from obstruction of the intra-hepatic or extra-hepatic biliary ducts.

NON-OBSTRUCTIVE JAUNDICE

Causes of non-obstructing jaundice are shown in Table 3.1.5.

"Physiological" Jaundice

The serum "indirect" (unconjugated) bilirubin value is increased above the adult concentration (13.6 μmol/l; 0.8 mg per 100 ml) in most newborn infants. Some develop the yellow skin discolouration on the second or third day of life, are not unwell, show no evidence of excessive haemolysis and the jaundice fades some 7 to 10 days later. This has long been known as "physiological" jaundice although it is better regarded as a functional immaturity of glucuronyl transferase enzyme system. Preterm infants have a higher maximum bilirubin peaking on the 5th or 6th day with a prolonged period sometimes lasting weeks of relative hyperbilirubinaemia. There is some difficulty in deciding when non-physiological becomes pathological but in general any infant whose plasma bilirubin concentration exceeds 210 μmol/l (12 mg per 100 ml) by the 3rd day of life should be considered to have a non-physiological jaundice.

Bilirubin Encephalopathy

Unconjugated bilirubin can produce transient encephalopathy or irreversible brain stem damage. As brain damage increases twitching, convulsions and episodes of cyanosis occur. Kernicterus literally means nuclear jaundice and refers to damage to the basal nuclei. It can occur when the unconjugated bilirubin concentration

Table 3.1.5: Causes of non-obstructive jaundice
Immaturity of liver function
• Jaundice of immaturity
• Physiological jaundice
Inhibition of liver function
• Breast milk Jaundice
Haemolytic anaemias
• ABO incompatibility
• Rh incompatibility
• Glucose-6-phosphate-dehydrogenase (G-6-PD) deficiency
• Spherocytosis
• Haemoglobinopathies
• Severe infections
• Drug sensitivity
• Extravasated blood
Other rare causes
• Hypothyroidism
• Crigler-Najjar syndrome
• Pyloric stenosis
• Malrotation of the intestine
• Cystic fibrosis

exceeds 340 µmol/l (20 mg per 100 ml) from whatever cause. The affected brain is stained yellow but certain structures, the corpus striatum, thalamus, subthalamic nuclei, hippocampus, nucleus of the third nerve, mammillary bodies, red nucleus and nuclei on the floor of the fourth ventricle are intensely coloured. In older infants who survive the acute stage there is a marked loss of nerve cells and replacement gliosis. There are many factors which predispose an infant to kernicterus and these include hypoglycaemia, hypoproteinaemia, high plasma free fatty acid composition and the use of drugs which compete for albumin binding sites together with acidosis whether metabolic or respiratory. In the acute stage of kernicterus there may be rolling of the eyes, marked lethargy, convulsions, refusal to suck, increased muscle tone, head retraction or opisthotonus and coma. If the infant survives the period of intense jaundice, later in the first year he develops spasms of muscular rigidity, opisthotonus and sometimes seizures. After the age of 2 years the surviving infant may show the typical picture of athetosis with increased muscle tone. There may be pyramidal signs but extrapyramidal rigidity is more common. High-tone deafness is present and this leads to interference with the acquisition of speech and language. This in turn aggravates the learning difficulties of such children. In addition to the brain damage the hyperbilirubinaemia affects the growing tooth buds so that the first dentition may show an unwelcome green staining and sometimes a visible line of hypoplasia of the enamel and dentine between the antenatal and postnatal parts. It is likely that the bilirubin damage to neurones is related to the vulnerability of these cells, which in turn depend on metabolic state, the lipid composition of the neuronal membrane and the ability of the neurone to detoxify bilirubin with mitochondrial bilirubin oxidase. The only means of preventing kernicterus, of proved effectiveness is exchange transfusion. This removes bilirubin not only from the plasma but also from the tissue cells.

Case Study 4: Neonate requiring phototherapy

A male infant weighing 3.8 kg was born at term by ventouse delivery following failed progress. He had a markedly moulded head with a large chignon and scalp bruising. He became jaundiced by 24 hours when SBR was 170 µmol/l. Blood group was O Rh+ve Coombs –ve, same as the mother. The jaundice was thought to be due to the increased haemoglobin breakdown secondary to the extensive scalp bruising. Phototherapy was started at 26 hours of age. The baby was nursed in a cot, wearing only a nappy with eyes blindfolded to protect them from the strong light. Phototherapy was interrupted every 3 hours for 30 min at a time to allow breastfeeding. The baby was offered extra water in between breast feeds to ensure adequate hydration. SBR rose to a maximum of 315 µmol/l at 72 hours and gradually subsided. Phototherapy was stopped on day 4 when SBR dropped to 276 µmol/l The jaundice gradually cleared over the next 5 days.

BILIRUBIN PHOTOCHEMISTRY

When the skin of jaundiced infants is exposed to light in the spectrum of blue to green (420-450 nmol) bilirubin can be transformed into pigments, which can be excreted without conjugation. The water-soluble isomers of bilirubin produced in human infants undergoing phototherapy are bound to albumin before being excreted in bile or urine. In human infants bilirubin appears to be the major photodegradation product of the pyrrole rings, which make up the original porphyrin of the haem molecule. In the treatment of moderate to severe hyperbilirubinaemia, the standard method of reducing bilirubin concentrations in serum and tissues is by replacement (exchange) transfusion. The value of this technique in haemolytic disease of the newborn is proven but the indications for its use in the hyperbilirubinaemia of prematurity are less clearly defined. Not inconsiderable risks of the procedure in the preterm infant with poor coagulation function must be weighed against the risk of developing kernicterus. Infants with IRDS, relative hypoxaemia, acidosis or hypoglycaemia with lower levels of plasma albumin are at risk of kernicterus at lower values of plasma bilirubin than in the mature infant. Figure 3.1.6 gives a guideline to the criteria for exchange transfusion and phototherapy in preterm and term infants. Phototherapy is most readily carried out in an incubator with the infant fully exposed apart from the eyes, which should be covered by a mask made from non-irritant material. It is, however, possible to provide phototherapy in a cot, provided the naked infant is kept in a sufficiently heated environment. Phototherapy units providing an artificial source of light at the appropriate wave length

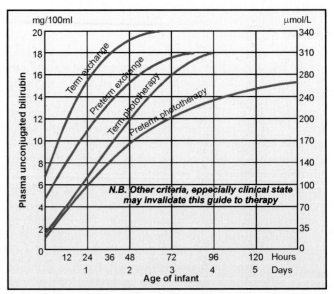

Fig. 3.1.6: Neonatal jaundice. Criteria for exchange transfusion and phototherapy

(425-475 nm) are most effective in reducing plasma bilirubin concentrations. Phototherapy is more effective in the prevention of an increase in bilirubin rather than reducing a high value. Treatment should be given to infants as soon as their unconjugated plasma bilirubin reaches 250 µmol/l (15 mg per 100 ml) in term infants and 170 µmol/l (10 mg per 100 ml) in preterm infants. Phototherapy is most suitable for the treatment of jaundice due to immaturity of liver function but may also be used prophylactically in infants with haemolytic anaemias. When haemolytic anaemias are treated in this way it is important to remember that the therapy has no effect on the underlying anaemia and a careful record of haemoglobin concentrations as well as unconjugated bilirubin must be kept. Infants treated with phototherapy lose an increased amount of water both through the skin and in the loose stools, which frequently develop. Fluid intake therefore should be well maintained during phototherapy. Early feeding with adequate fluid and carbohydrate intake will help reduce the risk of metabolic acidaemia and increase in free fatty acids which compete with bilirubin for albumin binding sites.

Key Learning Points

- The increased haemoglobin breakdown during the first week of life together with immaturity of liver enzymes results in the transient elevation of blood unconjugated bilirubin level known as 'physiological jaundice'.
- Unconjugated bilirubin is fat but not water-soluble and can lead to deafness and kernicterus if plasma level rises excessively.
- Conjugated bilirubin is water but not fat-soluble and does not carry a risk for kernicterus but its presence in the blood is always pathological.

HAEMOLYTIC ANAEMIAS

The earlier that jaundice appears and the longer it persists, the greater is the risk to the infant. Jaundice appearing on the first day of life should never be accepted as physiological and is highly suggestive of a haemolytic anaemia or of severe liver dysfunction. Similarly any jaundice, which persists for more than 10-14 days after birth, must be investigated thoroughly with particular reference to signs of obstructive jaundice and hypothyroidism. In European countries Rh incompatability was until the 1980's the most frequent cause of severe haemolytic anaemia. On a worldwide scale, incompatability of the fetus and mother for the ABO blood groups is the most frequent potential cause of haemolytic anaemia but fortunately it seldom results in severe degrees of jaundice. In Mediterranean peoples, black African and Far Eastern races deficiency of the enzyme glucose-6-phosphate dehydrogenase (G6PD) is a more common cause of haemolytic anaemia than Rh incompatability. Red cell membrane abnormalities such as thalassaemia associated

with unusual haemoglobins are a cause of haemolysis in certain racial groups. Antenatal detection of such haemolytic anaemias is now possible by the examination of fetal blood.

Blood Group Incompatibility

These occur when the fetus inherits from the father, a blood group such as the Rh factor, which is not present in the mother. If fetal cells should pass across the placenta into the mother in sufficient numbers she may develop antibodies to these "foreign" red cells which will destroy them within her circulation. Should the immunoglobulin (antibody) pass back to the fetus across the placenta it will cause haemolysis of fetal cells thus releasing haemoglobin and rendering the fetus anaemic. The bilirubin produced in this process will be transferred back across the placenta into the maternal circulation for conjugation by the maternal hepatic enzyme systems. Where extreme fetal haemolysis occurs the fetal anaemia can produce cardiac failure and severe fetal oedema (hydrops fetalis).

Rhesus Incompatibility

About 83% of Northern Europeans carry the rhesus antigen in their red cells (Rh positive). The remaining 17% do not possess this antigen and are referred to as Rh negative. When during pregnancy fetal red cells cross the placenta to sensitize the mother, or if mother has been previously sensitized to the Rh antigen by a transfusion of Rh incompatible blood or the miscarriage an Rh-positive fetus, any subsequent pregnancy with a Rh positive fetus is at risk of developing haemolytic anaemia. Although it is rare it is now recognised that a mother can be sensitized by her first rhesus positive fetus and that this fetus may develop a haemolytic disease (usually mild) during the first pregnancy. The Rhesus factor was first identified in 1940 and it has been shown to include at least 6 antigens (Cc, Dd, Ee which are determined by three allelomorphic pairs of genes similarly labelled). A mother may therefore be sensitized by any of these antigens, which she herself does not possess. The most important of these is the D antigen and those who possess it are Rh (D positive), whereas those who do not are Rh (D) negative. The three genes Cc, Dd and Ee are carried close together on the same chromosome and there are eight possible combinations of genes in descending order of frequency, CDe, cde, cDE, cDe, cdE, Cde, CDE and CdE. In somatic cells there are two autosomes carrying these genes and the commonest types in the UK are CDe/cde, CDe/CDe, cde/cde, CDe/cDE and cDE/cde. If the father is homozygous (D/D) with two D genes all his children must receive a D gene so that once haemolytic disease has made its appearance all subsequent children of the marriage will be similarly affected. When, however, the father is heterozygous Rh positive (D/d) half his children will inherit d. As they will also have inherited d from their Rh negative (d/d) mother they will be Rh (D) negative and so unaffected by the disease. The majority of cases of Rh sensitization involve D antigen but in some, the other antigens (e.g. c) are involved. These explain cases of haemolytic disease, which occur in the offspring of some Rh (D) positive women.

Clinical Features

a. *Fetus affected* – The disease develops severely during fetal life in only a minority of cases. It may then result in stillbirth, intrauterine death and the subsequent delivery of a macerated fetus, or in the birth of a living infant with hydrops fetalis.

   The hydropic infant is grossly oedematous with marked enlargement of liver and spleen, which are the site of extensive extramedullary erythropoieses. The placenta is large, pale and oedematous and the amniotic fluid – a deep yellow colour. The presence of hydrops fetalis may be recognised antenatally by ultrasonography.

b. *Infant affected* – In the majority of cases the infant is born apparently normal but subsequently develops signs of the disease. In its most severe form (icterus gravis) jaundice appears within minutes or hours of birth. It gradually deepens and develops a characteristic golden yellow colour. Purpura and haemorrhages may appear in the skin and liver and spleen become grossly enlarged. The peripheral blood shows anaemia, reticulocytosis, many erythroblasts and normoblasts and immature white cells of the granular series. If the condition remains untreated the unconjugated bilirubin concentration increases. There may develop in the later stages an increase in conjugated bilirubin with an obstructive element previously designated the inspissated bile syndrome. This term in fact is a misnomer and this obstructive type of jaundice reflects immaturity of the excretory function of the liver rather than blockage of the intercellular canaliculi by "inspissated" bile.

Diagnosis

In most instances it is possible to predict the appearance of haemolytic disease during pregnancy and by timely treatment to prevent most of the serious manifestations. The Rhesus and ABO blood groups of every pregnant woman should be determined early in pregnancy. In the case of Rh (D) negative women the serum should be tested for Rh antibodies periodically throughout the pregnancy. The finding of antibody is a strong indication that the infant may be affected and the mother should be delivered in a hospital with neonatal intensive care facilities. In women who have had previously affected infants the husband's Rh genotype must also be determined to help in more accurate prediction. The history of previous pregnancies gives an indication of the probable severity of the disease. In some families the disease pattern tends to be similar in each pregnancy; in others, succeeding infants show a worsening severity.

Antenatal Management

Spectrophotometric examination of amniotic fluid obtained by amniocentesis can be used to predict the probable severity of disease. The method gives an accuracy of prediction above 95% so permitting infants seriously at risk to be delivered before they are hydropic or moribund. The technique of amniocentesis and amniotic fluid optical density measurements is still used for "missed" third trimester problems. Improved methods of fetal monitoring have made this a less common necessity. Maternal Rh antibody concentrations are measured from 18 weeks gestation and rising values suggest increasing severity of haemolysis. Ultrasound measurements of placental thickness, umbilical vein diameter and fetal intraperitoneal volume and measures of cardiac output have proved unreliable in predicting the degree of anaemia. However, if fetal ascites appears this indicates a severe anaemia (Hb less than 4 g per dl). These methods are not entirely satisfactory as ascites is found in less than two thirds of fetuses with such low haemoglobin and at this level of haemoglobin the fetus may already be suffering from relative hypoxaemia. Fetal blood sampling allows direct assessment of the fetal haematocrit and haemoglobin concentration and will permit transfusion to be performed at the same procedure when anaemia is identified. Fresh Rhesus negative packed cells compatible with the mother are infused in a volume determined by the estimated fetal placental volume and the fetal and donor haematocrits. Transfusions are performed at between 2 and 4 weekly intervals thereafter based on the rates of fall of fetal haematocrit between the procedures. Survival rates of 80 - 90% have been achieved in severely affected fetuses by these methods.

Postnatal Management

A replacement blood transfusion is indicated in the infant where cord haemoglobin is below 12 g per 100 ml and/or the cord unconjugated bilirubin concentration about 85 µmol/l (5 mg per 100 ml). Clinical judgement will be required and lower criteria may be accepted in a preterm infant or where there has been a history of a previously severely affected infant or stillbirth. Confirmation of the diagnosis is seldom required but the Coombs' direct anti-human globulin test which detects antibody bound to the infant's red cells may be performed. Early exchange transfusion will correct anaemia, remove damaged and antibody-coated red cells from the circulation and remove unfixed antibodies. Donor blood should be Rh negative, preferably of the same ABO group as the infants and should also be compatible with the mother's serum by the indirect anti-globulin technique. The total volume of blood exchanged usually amounts to 175 ml per kg. Subsequent exchange transfusions may be required if the unconjugated bilirubin concentration increases again. Phototherapy can be used to help control the degree of hyperbilirubinaemia. It is important that the infant's haemoglobin is checked regularly for at least six weeks after birth as after these procedures the infant's red cell production may be suppressed for some time and quite severe anaemia may develop.

Prevention of Rh Haemolytic Disease

The incidence of haemolytic disease has been reduced from 6 per thousand in the UK to less than 1 per thousand by the introduction of a preventive programme. The programme is based on the fact that the "bleed" from Rh (D) positive fetus, which sensitizes the Rh (D) negative mother usually, occurs at the end of pregnancy or during labour and Rh antibodies take some weeks to develop. A very high degree of prevention of haemolytic disease is achieved by the intramuscular administration of anti-D immunoglobulin to the Rh-negative mother soon after the birth of her Rh-positive infant. Any fetal red cells, which have entered her circulation, are thus destroyed. The principal supply of anti-D immunoglobulin has been from naturally sensitized Rh (D) individuals. Mothers at greatest risk are those Rh (D) negative mothers who give birth to Rh (D) positive infants who are ABO compatible with their mothers. When the fetal cells are incompatible with the mothers in the ABO system, Rh sensitization only rarely occurs, because AB antibodies are already present in the blood of the mother, and if ABO incompatible fetal cells enter her circulation they are unlikely to survive for long enough to initiate the production of Rh antibodies. A protective dose of 100 micrograms anti-D immunoglobulin is now offered to all non-sensitized Rh (D) negative women delivered of Rh (D) positive infants irrespective of whether they are ABO compatible or incompatible. A smaller dose (50 micrograms) is offered to Rh (D) negative women having a pregnancy terminated, an amniocentesis, chorionic villus sampling or fetal blood sampling procedure or a spontaneous abortion. These measures have proved highly effective and there remain only a few some women who develop antibodies during their first Rh (D) positive pregnancy. Antenatal prevention has been used in some communities where anti-D immunoglobulin (100 micrograms) is given to all Rh-negative primagravidae at 28 and 34 weeks; a further dose being given after delivery if the infant is Rh (D) positive.

ABO Incompatibility

Cases of ABO incompatibility are probably more common than any other form of blood group incompatibility between mother and infant. Many are so mild that they are mistaken for "physiological" jaundice. The condition rarely leads to severe jaundice and anaemia but many cases produce sufficient jaundice to require phototherapy. Usually ABO antibodies are of the IgM variety rather than IgG (Rh antibodies are predominantly IgG) and therefore do not cross the placenta. Mothers of blood group O are more likely than those of Groups A or B to have IgG antibodies. In any infant developing jaundice within 24 hours of birth blood groups of both infant and mother should be determined and if they are potentially incompatible (e.g. mother O, infant A or B) the mother's serum must be examined for immune type antibodies specific for A and B antigens. In ABO incompatibility the direct Coombs' test in the infant is usually negative. Exchange transfusion is only required if the infant unconjugated bilirubin increases above 340 µmol/l (20 mg per 100 ml). Group O blood of homologous Rhesus group should be used.

Glucose-6-Phosphate Dehydrogenase (G-6-PD) Deficiency

Glucose-6-phosphate dehydrogenase catalyses the oxidation of glucose-6-phosphate to 6-phosphogluconate. Deficiency of this enzyme results in a block in the first stage of the pentose shunt pathway. Many different variants of G-6-PD have now been identified and all are determined by mutant alleles at a locus on the X chromosome. They differ from the normal enzyme in electrophoretic mobility and it is likely that each is related to a single amino acid substitution on the enzyme protein. The different alleles have been designated Gd^B, Gd^{A-}, Gd^A, $Gd^{Mediterranean}$, Gd^{Athens}, Gd^{Canton} and so forth. Some result in more severe deficiencies of enzyme activities than others.

In some parts of the world G-6-PD deficiency can cause a degree of haemolysis after the ingestion of drugs such as primaquine, sulphonamides and nitrofurantoin. It has long been recognised in Mediterranean countries that acute haemolytic anaemia can occur in some families following the ingestion of fava beans (favism). In some infants G-6-PD deficiency can cause a degree of haemolysis in the newborn sufficient to increase the unconjugated bilirubin to a level requiring exchange transfusion without obvious drug ingestion. In these neonatal cases jaundice has not been confined to hemizygous males or to hemizygous females and the X-linked gene seems to show great variability of expression in the heterozygous female. This variability in enzyme activities may be related to the Lyon hypothesis in which it is presumed that only one X-chromosome is genetically active in any cell during interphase.

Acholuric Jaundice (Congenital Spherocytosis)

It is uncommon for this hereditary disease, which is transmitted as a Mendelian dominant trait, to manifest itself during the neonatal period. When it does it may require splenectomy during early infancy because of persistent jaundice and anaemia. Whenever possible, however, splenectomy should be avoided during the first year of life because of the subsequent increased susceptibility to bacterial infections. Rarely, exchange transfusion is necessary in the neonatal period to prevent kernicterus. The spleen is enlarged; the blood shows anaemia with a reticulocytosis, some erythroblasts, increased fragility of the red cells and microspherocytosis. The plasma-unconjugated bilirubin is increased and there is urobilinogenuria.

NEONATAL HAEMORRHAGE

The newborn infant is liable to bleed under a variety of circumstances. These include anoxia, birth trauma, hypothermia, haemolytic anaemia, infections of bacterial, viral or protozoal origin and inadequacies of the blood clotting mechanisms.

Fetal Haemorrhage

Whereas haemorrhage in the newborn infant is usually visible and, when severe, accompanied by signs of shock and haemorrhage, in the fetus it is usually unheralded and undetected but may cause severe fetal damage. A variety of intracranial haemorrhages have been detected early in fetal development with ultrasonic examination. These may be subdural or intracerebral and may be associated with major CNS anomalies. Bleeding from the fetus may also occur when the placenta is accidentally incised during lower segment caesarean section for anterior placenta praevia. Rupture of a velamentous vessel overlying the cervix or a blood vessel on the fetal aspect of the placenta or indeed haemorrhage into the placenta itself may occur. Artificial rupture of the membranes may precipitate fetal placental haemorrhage, fetal placental blood loss and should be suspected whenever blood is obtained at this procedure.

The fetus may bleed across the placenta into the maternal circulation (fetomaternal transfusion). The factors, which predispose to transplacental bleeding, are unclear and although it has been associated with high rupture of the membranes, in most instances no abnormality of the placenta is obvious.

An intriguing situation arises when one monovular twin bleeds into the other so that one is anaemic and the other polycythaemic whilst one portion of the monochorionic placenta is pale and bloodless and the other purple and engorged. A monochorionic placenta is found in approximately 70% of twin pregnancies and a significant twin-to-twin transfusion occurs in at least 15 per cent.

Clinical Features

Fetal haemorrhage during labour should be suspected if there is a sudden flow of bright red blood from the introitus. The same applies to the appearance of blood during the artificial rupture of membranes. The fetal origin of the blood can be quickly confirmed by testing it for fetal haemoglobin, which is alkali-resistant. Early delivery and ligation of the umbilical cord should be instituted. The infant may be delivered in a state of oligaemic shock with severe pallor, but there will rarely be apnoea and the heart rate will be rapid in contrast to the bradycardia, which is usual in severe asphyxia. When bleeding has been less severe or has been taking place some time before birth, as in cases of fetal- maternal transfusion, the presenting sign is pallor alone. Indeed, this may not become manifest for some hours after birth. The infant will have a hypochromic anaemia, reticulocytosis and increased numbers of erythroblasts and normoblasts.

Diagnosis

Fetomaternal transfusion can be confirmed by differential agglutination provided there is a major blood group difference between mother and her infant but more usually the diagnosis of fetomaternal transfusion is made by the treatment of methanol-fixed blood films of the maternal blood with an acid buffer at pH 3.4. Fetal erythrocytes resist lysis by the buffer solution so that they react subsequently with ordinary haemoglobin stains whereas the adult maternal cells appear as ghosts. This test is known as the Kleihauer test.

Treatment

Blood transfusion can be life-saving. When the haemorrhage has taken place shortly before birth the infant haemoglobin concentration may not be much reduced, but as restoration of the blood volume takes place over the next few hours serial determinations will reveal a reducing haemoglobin concentration. Values of haemoglobin below 14 g per 100 ml are an indication for top-up transfusion. In the emergency situation Group O Rhesus negative blood should be given. In twin-to-twin transfusion the anaemic twin may require blood transfusion the recipient twin may suffer from respiratory distress and cerebral signs if polycythaemia is marked. In some instances the haemoglobin concentration is in the region of 30 g per 100 ml and the haematocrit 75 per cent. The relevant treatment in these circumstances is partial replacement transfusion with plasma, 30 ml per kg body weight.

HAEMORRHAGIC DISORDERS OF THE NEWBORN

Haemorrhagic disorders of the newborn may be associated with Vitamin K_1 deficiency, disseminated intravascular coagulation, deficiencies of other clotting factors or thrombocytopenia. The term haemorrhagic disease of the newborn was first used in the 19th century and was thought to be entirely explicable by deficiency of Vitamin K_1. The disorder is somewhat more complex and the term haemorrhagic disease of the newborn should be confined to infants in whom there is a temporary coagulation defect associated with spontaneous haemorrhage.

Vitamin K_1 Deficiency

Vitamin K_1 is essential for the synthesis of 4 of the factors involved in the clotting process – factors II (prothrombin), VII, IX, and X. These factors are present in the newborn but at lower concentrations than in the adult reaching a nadir on the 3rd day. The subsequent rise depends upon the provision of Vitamin K_1 in the diet or as a result of bacterial action in the bowel producing Vitamin K_1. Breast milk contains low concentrations of Vitamin K_1. "Haemorrhagic disease of the newborn" due to lack of dietary Vitamin K_1 is virtually confined to infants who have been breast-fed or who have had no oral feeds. Maternal anticonvulsant therapy may also lower the maternal breast milk supply of Vitamin K.

Clinical Features

The presenting feature is bleeding of varying severity. Most commonly it appears as melaena stools and in severe cases frank blood is passed per rectum and the infant may look shocked and pale. Haematemesis, haematuria, vaginal bleeding and haemorrhage from the umbilicus or into the skin may also occur. Visceral haemorrhages are uncommon but occasionally retroperitoneal haemorrhage, subcapsular haematoma of the liver and intracranial bleeding can occur. Diagnosis is confirmed by finding the infant's prothrombin time to be prolonged (normal 14-16 seconds) or the thrombotest low (normal 40-60%).

Treatment and Prevention

Treatment with blood transfusion or fresh frozen plasma may be required if the bleeding is severe. Otherwise treatment is with parenteral Vitamin K_1 1 mg by intramuscular injection. Haemorrhagic disease of the newborn can be prevented by providing all infants with Vitamin K_1 500 μg by intramuscular injection soon after birth. Preterm infants should be given 250 μg by intramuscular injection. Oral therapy with Vitamin K should be offered to those infants where intramuscular injections are contraindicated or refused by the parents.

Key Learning Points
• The main source of Vitamin K in the neonate comes from intestinal bacterial synthesis.
• Vitamin K deficiency occurs mostly in breastfed babies.
• Routine IM administration of Vit K at birth prevents haemorrhagic disease of the newborn.
• Oral Vit K administration is less effective but should be offered to babies when intramuscular administration is refused.

Disseminated Intravascular Coagulation (DIC; secondary haemorrhagic disease)

The process of DIC or consumptive coagulopathy results in a decrease in platelets, fibrinogen, factor V and factor VIII. There is often purpura or multiple bruising, intracranial haemorrhage, bleeding from mucous membranes or into internal organs. However, DIC is likely only to develop in a baby already unwell, e.g. Gram-negative septicaemia, severe asphyxia, hypothermia, renal vein thrombosis. Diagnosis is based on the finding of thrombocytopenia, reduced plasma fibrinogen levels and raised values for fibrin degradation products (FDP). The blood film contains fragmented red blood cells.

Treatment

The treatment of haemorrhagic disorders in the newborn period must be related to diagnosis of the specific cause of the bleeding tendency. Where bleeding is occurring and a haemorrhagic disorder suspected a prothrombin time or thrombotest and platelet count are essential investigations. When specimens have been taken 1 mg of Vitamin K_1 by slow intravenous injection should be given. This will prove effective only in haemorrhagic disease of the newborn but will do no harm in other conditions and will not obscure the diagnosis. Where the platelet count is below $40 \times 10^9/l$ a platelet transfusion may be indicated especially if there is bleeding. The use of heparin and exchange transfusion in the treatment of DIC has not been established but there are reports in favour of the controlled use of heparin.

Thrombocytopenia

When the platelet count is less than $100 \times 10^9/l$ there is significant thrombocytopenia and the range of causes shown in Table 3.1.6 must be considered (See chapter 15).

Maternal Idiopathic Thrombocytopenic Purpura (ITP)

Purpura in the newborn may be produced by thrombocytopenia or by capillary damage related to venous obstruction or hypoxia. In about half of the infants of mothers with ITP there is purpura, which may be

Table 3.1.6 Causes of thrombocytopenia in the newborn

Maternal factors involved
- Maternal idiopathic thrombocytopenic purpura
- Isoimmune thrombocytopenia
- Transplacental infection
- Severe rhesus incompatibility
- Thiazide diuretic given to mother
- Inherited thrombocytopenia

Other causes
- Infection acquired postnatally
- Disseminated intravascular coagulation
- Marrow hypoplasia
- Giant haemangioma

temporary and is apparently due to transplacental transfusion of maternal platelet IgG antibodies. It may occur even when mother's platelet count has returned to normal. It is usual to deliver such infants by caesaerian section because of the high risks of intracranial haemorrhage.

Alloimmune Thrombocytopenia

This is due to the transplacental passage of platelet antibody from a platelet antigen negative mother, who has been immunized either by blood from her platelet antigen positive fetus or previous blood transfusion, to a platelet antigen positive fetus. The outcome is similar to that found in Rhesus immunization. Ninety-eight per cent of all individuals are platelet antigen positive, only 2% antigen negative. The mother will have a normal platelet count. Other causes of thrombocytopenia are antenatal infections with syphilis, toxoplasmosis, rubella, cytomegalovirus and herpes virus. Thrombocytopenia has also been described in a number of infants born to mothers on prolonged courses of thiazide diuretics. Inherited thrombycytopenias are rarely manifested in the newborn. Severe postnatal infection, bacterial or viral, may be accompanied by purpura due to platelet deficiency and the thrombocytopenia may be a manifestation of DIC. Marrow depression from any cause such as drugs, congenital leukaemia and bone disorders may present as purpura due to thrombocytopenia. The platelet consumption, which occurs in giant haemangioma, may rarely be a cause of purpura in the newborn period.

Treatment

A platelet count of less than $40 \times 10^9/l$ is an indication in a bleeding infant for platelet transfusion. Where the cause is maternal ITP platelets will be consumed rapidly by the antibody and may require to be given frequently. Where there is iso-immune thrombocytopenia the platelets transfused must be platelet antigen negative. These can be obtained from the mother and "washed" prior to transfusion, or from other family members who are antigen negative. Steroid therapy is controversial.

Case Study 5: Neonatal Alloimmune Thrombocytopenia

A female infant was born at term weighing 2950 gm. Delivery was by SVD after a healthy pregnancy. Mother was a 26 year old primigravida with no past or family medical history. At 6 hours of age the baby was noted to have widespread petechiae on her face and trunk together with bruising over her left upper limb and was oozing from the umbilical cord. Examination showed an otherwise healthy infant with no hepatosplenomegaly or other signs of infection. Hb was 15.8 gm/dl, WCC 13400 x 10^9/L and platelets 23 × 10^9/L. CRP, U+E and LFT's were normal. Clotting screen was normal. Mother was found to be platelet antigen PIA$_1$-ve and the baby was PLA$_1$+ve. Anti -platelet antibodies were detected in the mother. An random donor platelet transfusion was administered which transiently increased the platelet count to 60 x 10^9/L and reduced the bleeding but within 24 hours fresh petechiae appeared and the platelet count had dropped to 27 × 10^9/L. A further platelet transfusion using platelets from a PLA$_1$-ve donor was given. The platelet count rose to 88 × 10^9/L and the bleeding stopped. The platelet count continued to rise gradually to normal levels over the next 4 days.

The Infant of a Diabetic Mother (IDM)

Poor glycaemic control in the diabetic mother leads to episodes of hyperglycaemia and sometimes hypoglycaemia. Low maternal blood sugars deprive he fetus of an important carbohydrate and energy source and can lead to fetal compromise and even sudden death, but tend to be short-lived. Hyperglycaemia frequently lasts longer. The fetal pancreas reacts to this increased glucose load by secreting large amounts of insulin which has an anabolic action. The IDM tends to be large because of increased subcutaneous fat deposition, a large body and a normal sized head, as the brain remains of normal size, giving the appearance of microcephaly. This macrosomia increases the chances of obstructed labour, instrumental delivery, birth trauma and intrapartum hypoxia. The excess production of insulin leads to a risk of severe hypoglycaemia during the first 3 days of life. IDMs tend to behave more immaturely than their healthy counterparts, having an increased risk of transient tachypnoea, respiratory distress syndrome, poor feeding and severe and/or prolonged jaundice partly due to polycythaemia. Exposure to the diabetic intrauterine environment is thought to be the main cause of the increased risk of congenital malformations in particular congenital heart disease (most commonly ventricular septal defects, transposition of great arteries) sacral agenesis, myelomeningocoele and vertebral dysplasia. Good glycaemic control of the diabetic mother before conception and throughout the pregnany is very important in reducing these risks to the fetus and neonate.

Maternal Drug and Alcohol Misuse

Any drug ingested by the mother is likely to cross the placenta and affect the fetus. Drugs taken for therapeutic purposes frequently have teratogenic effects of varying severity. The historic example always quoted is that of **thalidomide**, given to the mothers as a sedative and hypnotic agent during the 1960's, which caused severe phocomelia. Other drugs known to have less severe effects are **anticonvulsants** and the anticoagulant **warfarin**. It is fair to say that no drug is completely safe when taken during pregnancy.

Other drugs ingested by the mother for pleasure purposes, are addictive, so that drug misuse frequently continues throughout the pregnancy, with serious consequences to the fetus. **Heroin** and **dihydrocodeine** are two such drugs together with **methadone**, prescribed to the mother to prevent withdrawal symptoms. **Barbiturates** and **diazepam** are frequently misused drugs as well. Sudden withdrawal of these drugs during the pregnancy can result in withdrawal symptoms in both mother and fetus with serious consequences and even a risk of intrauterine death. The most frequent problems are encountered after birth when the drug supply from the mother is suddenly terminated with cord clamping.

Withdrawal symptoms manifest themselves at varying time intervals after birth depending on the half life of the drug taken by the mother. Heroin has a half life of about 12 hours while methadone has a half life of 48-72 hours so that withdrawal symptoms may not start until day 3-4. The baby becomes irritable and restless, turning around in its cot and crying incessantly. It cannot be placated by lifting. The cry is characteristically shrill, accompanied by increased tone, tremor, tachypnoea, pyrexia and even convulsions. The baby is frequently very hungry wanting fed all the time and taking far more milk that its daily requirements. Some babies are so irritable that they are hungry but cannot feed. Yawning, sniffles, sneezing, vomiting and increased stool frequency are other manifestations of maternal drug withdrawal.

These babies can be very demanding especially on nursing time. Sedation with oral morphine has been found to be helpful in calming them down. This may be required for several days or weeks until withdrawal symptoms settle down.

Cocaine and Crack cocaine are particularly dangerous to the fetus. They are powerful vasoconstrictors and stimulants of placental contraction, causing placental abruption and preterm labour. The babies are frequently growth retarded and have an increased risk of congenital malformations resulting from intrauterine blood vessel constriction such as limb reduction defects, microcephaly, cerebral infarction and intestinal atresias, single or multiple.

Alcohol has to be included under this heading. The Fetal Alcohol Syndrome has long been recognised as a consequence of alcohol ingestion during pregnancy whether on a regular basis or binge drinking and no amount of alcohol can be considered safe in a pregnant woman. These babies are usually small-for-dates with mild microcephaly and a typical facial appearance including a flat nasal bridge, thin upper lip and a long simple philthrum. They remain small and short and frequently need special schooling because of a borderline low IQ.

Maternal smoking is another addictive habit exposing the fetus and the neonate to the action of nicotine and other chemicals in cigarette smoke. Although not teratogenic, nicotine causes significant vasoconstriction of the placental bed leading to intrauterine growth retardation. The baby has a small head circumference, abdominal girth and reduced femur length. These babies are at increased risk of wheezing and asthma later on in life especially if maternal smoking continues after birth. There is also an increase risk of sudden infant death. Studies have shown an association between maternal smoking and mild developmental delay.

3.2 Newborn Health in Developing Countries

INTRODUCTION

Each year an estimated 4 million babies die before they reach the age of one month, and another 4 million more are stillborn, dying between 22 weeks of pregnancy and birth. 98% of these newborn deaths take place in developing countries, and for the most part these newborn deaths occur at home in the absence of any skilled health care (Fig. 3.2.1). Thus, developing a better understanding of home care practices, leading to effective behaviour change communication strategies to promote healthy behaviours while discouraging harmful practices, is a priority.

WHO estimates that 40% to 60% of neonatal deaths are potentially preventable and it may be possible to save over 2 million newborn infants through basic low-cost interventions. More epidemiological research is needed to make available more accurate data on risk factors and causes of neonatal morbidity and mortality, and improved and validated neonatal verbal autopsy instruments are needed in order to collect accurate data.

Most newborn deaths are largely due to infections (36%), birth asphyxia and injuries (23%), and consequences of prematurity and congenital anomalies (34%). Infections may account for approximately half of newborn deaths at the community level. Low birth weight (LBW) is an overriding factor in the majority of the deaths (Fig. 3.2.2).

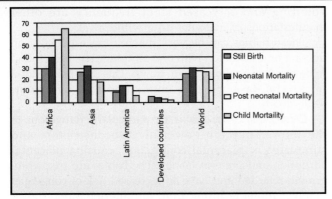

Fig. 3.2.1: Child mortality rates and rates of stillbirths per 1000 births *(Source: World Health Organisation)*

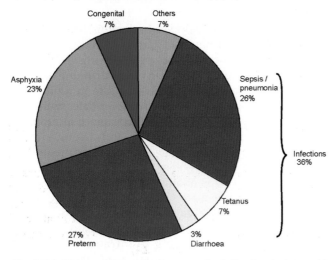

Fig. 3.2.2: Major problems affecting neonates in the developing world

Birth Asphyxia

Failure to breathe at delivery is probably the mechanism responsible for asphyxia secondary to some acute crisis such as an antepartum hemorrhage or cord prolapse. Affects mainly cortical and sub cortical gray matter of the brain (Table 3.2.1).

Table 3.2.1 Aetiology and risk factors

- *Antenatal:* Maternal diabetes, Pre-eclampsia
- *Intrapartum:* Breech presentation, cord compression, placental abruption, maternal shock, infection
- *Postnatal:* Congenital heart disease, respiratory failure

Epidemiology

Intrapartum asphyxia is a single most important cause of perinatal and neonatal morbidity and mortality. An estimated 4 to 9 million cases of birth asphyxia occur each year in the developing world, accounting for 24% to 61% of all perinatal mortality and an estimated 1.2 million new-

borns die annually of birth asphyxia. Sarnet and Sarnet introduced a grading system to describe the neurological dysfunction which was modified by Levene et al (Table 3.2.2).

Table 3.2.2: Grading system to describe the neurological dysfunction

Grade I (Mild)	Grade II (Moderate)	Grade III (Severe)
Irritability	Lethargy	Comatose Severe
Mild hypotonia	Relative hypertonia	hypotonia
Poor suck	Tube feeds	Failure to maintain spontaneous respiration
No seizures	Seizures	Prolong seizures

Diagnosis

The diagnosis of birth asphyxia is based on clinical as well as biochemical findings (Table 3.2.3).

1. Tricuspid regurgitation murmur may be audible early in the course of disease.
2. Arterial blood gas shows acidosis, high pCO_2, and low pO_2.
3. Lactic acid provides a sensitive measure of end organ perfusion.
4. EEG may show seizures and background slowing.
5. Drop in hematocrit may indicate intracranial bleed.

Table 3.2.3: Diagnostic criteria

- Profound metabolic acidosis (PH < 7.0) and base deficit > 12 on arterial sample
- Apgars score of 0-3 for longer than 5 minutes
- Neurologic manifestation, e.g. seizures, coma, or hypotonia
- Multisystem organ dysfunction, e.g. cardiovascular, gastrointestinal, pulmonary or renal systems.

Prevention

At delivery, most neonates can be successfully resuscitated by simple techniques such as tactile stimulation and, in some cases, clearing of upper airway secretions using a gauze-covered finger or simple mucus extractor. The need for bag-mask ventilation is exceptional, and can be accomplished using room air. Routine caesarean section for preterm babies presenting by the breech is much more controversial. There is yet no randomized control trial for the benefit and hazards of such intervention to prevent birth asphyxia.

Neonatal Resuscitation

Extensive efforts to train physicians in neonatal resuscitation are needed, for example using WHO and American Academy of Pediatrics-American Heart

Association Neonatal Resuscitation Program materials, are underway in many developing countries, and are showing encouraging results in influencing behaviour. Few studies, however, especially community-based studies have evaluated appropriate methods to train health workers and family members at the community level to recognise birth asphyxia and provide simple interventions and support. (Figs 3.2.3 and 3.2.4).

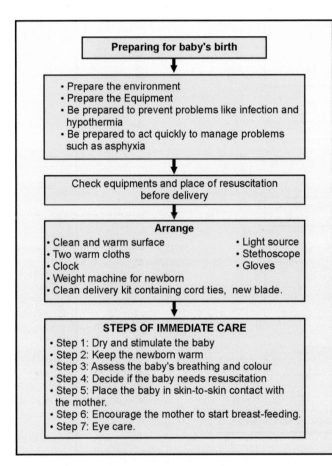

Fig. 3.2.3: Algorithm of immediate or routine care of newborn at birth

Goals of Management

Unsupervised, unskilled delayed and complicated deliveries that characterise obstetrics in developing countries and the high frequency of low birthweight babies contribute to a high prevalence of birth asphyxia and birth trauma. The aim should be to provide these equipment and training of doctors and nurses for essential neonatal care at primary health centre.

Medical Management

- Maintain adequate oxygenation and ventilation. Avoid hyperventilation. Keep O_2 sats > 90% and pco_2 between 35 and 50 mmHg
- Inotropes for maintenance of adequate blood pressure
- Fluid restriction to treat SIADH
- Delay gastric feeding until adequate gut perfusion is ensured
- Treat seizures if necessary with phenobarbitol
- Treat hypoglycemia.

Prognosis

Prognosis can be predicted by recovery of motor function and sucking ability. There are case reports in the past established that babies who had suffered a severe and clear insult some time before labour could be neurologically abnormal in the neonatal period and end up with cerebral palsy. Early onset of seizures and use of multiple medications predict worse prognosis. Severely affected infants often require G-tube for feeding and tracheotomy with home ventilation (Table 3.2.4).

NEONATAL INFECTIONS

Epidemiology

Infections account for 30% to 50% of all neonatal deaths in developing countries, with pneumonia, tetanus, sepsis and diarrhoea the most common causes. Knowledge of the aetiology of infectious diseases in neonates in developing countries is based almost entirely on studies of hospitalized infants or on retrospective, verbal autopsy-

		< 2501 g			> 2500 g			
Time (min.)	Number of live-born	Death by 1 year (%)	Number known to 7 years	Cerebral palsy (%)	Number of live-born	Death by 1 year (%)	Number known to 7 years	Cerebral palsy (%)
1	428	25.5	257	1.9	1729	3.1	1330	0.7
5	163	55.2	56	7.1	286	7.7	217	0.9
10	67	67.2	15	6.7	66	18.2	43	4.7
15	51	84.3	8	0	23	47.8	11	9.1
20	139	95.7	7	0	39	59	14	57.1

Table 3.2.4: Outcome associated with very low apgar score (0-3)

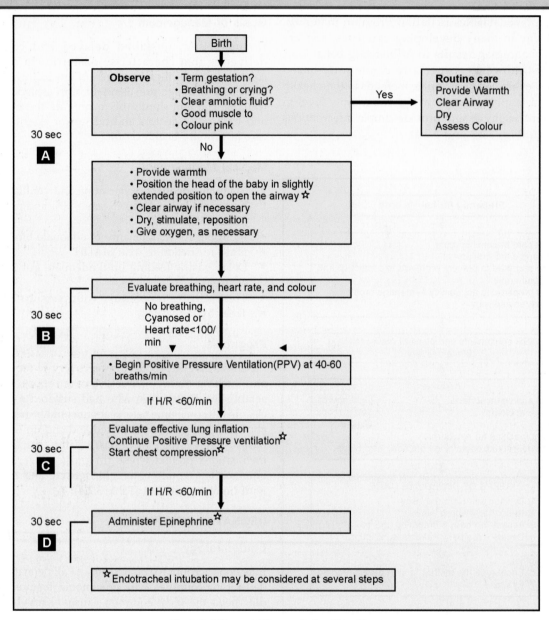

Fig. 3.2.4: Neonatal Resuscitation Flow Chart

based surveys in the community, neither of which may accurately reflect the true burden of disease in the community.

The reported incidence of neonatal sepsis varies from 7.1 to 38 per 1000 live birth in Asia, from 6.5 to 23 per 1000 live births in Africa, and from 3.5 to 8.9 per 1000 live births in south America and Caribbean. The WHO's recommended clinical criteria for diagnosing sepsis and meningitis in neonates are given in Table 3.2.5. The main organisms causing sepsis in developing countries are shown in Fig. 3.2.5.

Prevention

In developing countries, 90% of mothers deliver babies at home without skilled health professional present. Simple low-cost interventions, notably tetanus toxoid vaccination, exclusive breast-feeding, counseling for birth preparedness, breast-feeding promotion through peer counselors and women's groups, have been shown to reduce newborn morbidity and mortality. Alcohol-based antiseptics for hand hygiene are an appealing innovation because of their efficacy in reducing hand contamination and their ease of use.

Table 3.2.5: World Health Organization's recommended clinical criteria for diagnosing sepsis and meningitis in neonates*

Sepsis	Meningitis
Symptoms	**General Signs**
Convulsions	Drowsiness
Inability to feed	Reduced feeding
Unconsciousness	Unconsciousness
Lethargy	Lethargy
Fever (more than 37.7°C or feels hot)	High pitched cry
Hypothermia (less than 35.5°C or feels cold)	Apnea
Signs	**Specific Signs**
Severe chest in-drawing	Convulsions
Reduced movements	Bulging fontanelle
Crepitations and Cyanosis	

* The more symptoms a neonate has, the higher the probability of the disease.

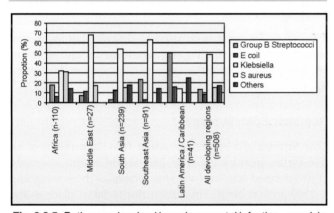

Fig. 3.2.5: Pathogens involved in early neonatal infection < week in hospitals of developing countries

The most effective strategies for preventing and treating neonatal infections in developing countries is to devise simple, inexpensive management strategies for reducing the morbidity and mortality of neonatal infections, risk factors, historical information, and clinical signs and symptoms predictive of serious neonatal infections (pneumonia, sepsis and meningitis) must be identified for use in first-line healthcare facilities and at home by trained caregivers and healthcare workers.

The Role of Breastfeeding

A wide variety of benefits of breastfeeding have been well documented, including reduced risk of hypothermia, hypoglycemia, necrotizing enterocolitis, omphalitis, acute respiratory infections, diarrhoea, septicemia, and mortality, particularly in the late neonatal period. Although breastfeeding is common, immediate and exclusive breastfeeding, despite its benefits, is not normal practice in many developing countries, particularly for LBW newborns. Breastfeeding also provides a variety of immune and non-immune components that accelerate intestinal maturation, resistance to and recovery from infection.

Role of Umbilical Cord and Skin Care

Little is known, however, about traditional umbilical cord practices in the community. Application of antiseptics such as chlorhexidine, has been shown to be effective against both gram-positive and gram-negative bacteria and shown in the community studies to reduce rates of cord infection and sepsis in the newborn. In rural Pakistan, application of ghee heated with cow dung to the umbilical stump was associated with neonatal tetanus, but in studies, in which topical antimicrobial agents were applied to promote wound healing, instead of ghee, suggests that promotion of antimicrobial applications as a substitute for ghee might be an effective strategy.

A randomized controlled trial of topical application of sunflower seed oil to preterm infants in an Egyptian NICU showed that treated infants had substantially improved skin condition and half the risk of late onset infection.

Diagnosis

The danger signs are shown in Table 3.2.6.

Table 3.2.6: Newborn danger signs of infection

- Breathing problems
- Feeding difficulties/unable to suck
- Cold body temperature/Hypothermia
- Fever
- Redness swelling or pus around the cord
- Convulsions/Fits
- Jaundice

Investigations

- Blood cultures (may be negative if antibiotics were administered to the mother).
- Urine cultures
- CSF studies (protein, glucose, cell count, and cultures)
- Complete blood count with differential
  - Immature to total neutrophil ratio >30% should raise suspicion of sepsis.
  - A drop in platelet count is often a late sign.
- C- reactive protein is a non-specific marker of infection
- Chest X-ray to distinguish pneumonia from respiratory distress syndrome
- Hypoglycemia
- Metabolic acidosis

Patient Group	Likely Etiology	Antimicrobial choice	
		Developed countries	Developing countries
Sepsis			
Immunocompetent children	Developed Countries Streptococcus (Group B) E. coli Developing Countries Klebsiella Pseudomonas Salmonella	Ampicillin/Penicillin Plus aminoglycoside Gentamicin	Ampicillin/Penicillin Plus aminoglycoside Or Co-trimoxazole plus Gentamicin
Meningitis Immunocompetent children (age < 3 Months)	Developed countries Streptococcus (Group B) E. coli L. monocytogenes* Developing countries S. pneumoniae E. coli	Ampicillin plus Ceftriaxone or Ceftrizxime	Ampicillin plus Gentamicin
Immunodeficient	Gram negative organisms L.monocytogenes	Ampicillin plus Ceftazidime	

Table 3.2.7: Antibiotic treatment of neonatal meningitis and sepsis

Medical Treatment

Knowledge of the antimicrobial resistance patterns of common neonatal bacterial pathogens is essential for planning empiric antimicrobial therapy for the treatment of neonatal infections.

Currently, WHO recommends that acutely infected neonates less than 2 months of age be treated in a health care facility capable of administering parenteral antibiotics (e.g. benzylpenicillin or ampicillin plus, an aminoglycoside, such as gentamicin). Every attempt should be made to deliver this standard of care. Hospitalization and parenteral treatment of neonates is not feasible in many communities, however. Thus, alternative treatment strategies are needed, including the feasibility and efficacy of therapy in the home and treatment with oral antibiotics. Guidelines for integrated Management of childhood illness (IMCI) have been widely implemented as the main approach for addressing child health in health systems Table 3.2.7 shows the antibiotic treatment of sepsis and meningitis.

Following the demonstration of significant reduction in neonatal mortality with the use of oral cotrimoxazole and injectable gentamicin by community health workers this strategy could be employed in circumstances where referrals are difficult.

Prognosis

Gram-negative sepsis has a high mortality rate. Associated meningitis may result in long-term developmental abnormalities (e.g. hearing loss).

Term IUGR / LBW

Various terms have been used to describe babies whose weight is low for their gestational age including intra-uterine growth retardation or restriction, fetal malnutrition, light-for-dates and small-for-dates.

Regional Epidemiology

Low birthweight babies constitute 16% (20 million) of all live births world wide. The 29th world health assembly (1976) defined low birthweights infants as those weighing < 2500 gms at birth. The vast majority takes place in the developing world ranging from 33% in south Asia to 67% in Africa. Much higher frequencies for small for gestational age infants are reported from India (77–90%). The aetiology of IUGR babies is summarized in Fig. 3.2.6 and Fig. 3.2.7.

Problems in Low birthweights babies (Table 3.2.8)

Table 3.2.8 Problems in low birthweight babies	
1. Breathing problems	2. Hypothermia/Hypoglycemia
3. Feeding problems	4. Infections
5. Jaundice	6. Coagulopathy
7. Polycythemia	

Prevention and Recurrence

Small case reports suggested low-dose aspirin prophylaxis during pregnancy may reduce the risk of recurrent IUGR in women at high-risk, subsequent large randomized

Classification of IUGR

Symmetrical ↓

The baby's head and body are proportionately small. May occur when the foetus experiences a problem during early development.

Asymmetrical ↓

Baby's brain is abnormally large when compared to the liver. May occur when the foetus experiences a problem during later development

Fig. 3.2.6: In a normal infant, the brain weighs about three times more than the liver. In asymmetrical IUGR, the brain can weigh five or six times more than the liver

Maternal Risk Factors:
- Drugs (Anticoagulants, Anticonvulsants).
- Cardio-vascular disease–pre-eclampsia, hypertension, cyanotic heart disease, diabetic vascular lesions.
- Chronic kidney disease
- Chronic infection–UTI, Malaria, TB, genital infections
- Antiphospholipid syndrome, SLE.

Fetal Risk Factors:
- Exposure to rubella, cytomegalovirus, herpes simplex, tuberculosis, syphilis, or toxoplasmosis,Parvo virus B19.
- A chromosome defect: Trisomy-18 (Edwards' syndrome), Trisomy 21(Down's syndrome), Trisomy 13, and XO (turner's syndrome).
- A chronic lack of oxygen during development (hypoxia).
- Placenta or umbilical cord defects.

Placental Factors:
- *Uteroplacental insufficiency resulting from:*
  - Inadequate placentation in the first trimester.
  - Lateral insertion of placenta.
  - Reduced maternal blood flow to the placental bed .
- *Foetoplacental insufficiency due to:*
  - Vascular anomalies of placenta and cord.
  - Small placenta, abruptio–Placenta, placenta previa, post term pregnancy.

Fig. 3.2.7: Etiology of intrauterine growth retardation

trials have not confirmed significant risk reduction. Antihypertensive therapy of hypertensive women does not improve fetal growth.

In subsequent pregnancies, any potential treatable causes of IUGR, e.g. thrombophilic disorder should be treated promptly.

Diagnostic Strategies

Clearly, from what has been said, the assessment of gestational age can be performed by doing complete history and physical examination to look for maternal, placental, or fetal disorders associated with impaired fetal growth (e.g. alcohol abuse, inherited or acquired thrombophilia, maternal vascular disease). Additional imaging and laboratory evaluations are also directed toward determining an etiology.

Management

The management strategies for growth restricted babies in the developing countries would be their prevention by reducing teenage pregnancies, increasing the birth interval, improving maternal nutrition, treating anemia and prompt treatment of maternal infections. These measures would promote significant increase in the birthweights and would break the vicious cycle of growth retarded females who become stunted-adults and produce growth retarded babies.

Prognosis

The preponderance of intrauterine growth retarded infants in the developing world related to the observation that such infants grow into adults with an increased risk of death from ischemic heart disease. Congenital malformations, perinatal asphyxia, and transitional cardio-respiratory disorders contribute to the high mortality rate in term IUGR infants.

Poor developmental outcome has been associated with IUGR that involved poor head growth (symmetric IUGR). Impairments of verbal outcome, visual recognition memory and general neurodevelopmental outcome have been found to be altered at and years. Cognitive disabilities are seen more frequently than motor disabilities.

It is hoped that the recognition of the intrauterine growth restricted babies antenatally and in the neonatal period as a special high risk infant, and the prompt institution of both therapeutic and prophylactic measures, will result in an improved outlook for this group of growth restricted infants.

Congenital Malformations and Inherited Disorders

The birth prevalence of congenital anomalies in developing countries is similar to that observed in developed countries. However, the health impact of birth defects is higher because of a lack of adequate services for the care of affected infants and a higher rate of exposures to infections and malnutrition although, as a proportion of infant deaths it is greater in wealthier countries (Table 3.2.9).

Table 3.2.9: Major birth defects and inherited disorders in the developing world
- Down syndrome
- Thalasaemia
- Sickle cell disease
- G6PD Deficiency
- Oculocutaneous Albinism
- Cystic fibrosis
- Phenylketonuria
- Neural tube defects and hydrocephalus
- Congenital heart disease
- Cleft lip and plate
- Developmental dysplasia of hip

A number of successful measures for the prevention of congenital anomalies are being taken in a number of developing nations. Primary prevention programs are based on public education about preconceptional and prenatal risks. Prevention based on reproduction options includes teratogen information services and prenatal screening for fetal anomalies.

In addition, programmes for the detection of congenital malformations at birth, followed by early treatment, are contributing to secondary prevention. Prevention of congenital anomalies in the developing world requires:

1. Good epidemiological data on the prevalence and types of birth defects and genetic disorders
2. Educating health professionals in the goals and methods of preventing birth defects at low cost but with high impact.
3. Expansion of family planning and improvement of antenatal care combined with educational campaigns to avoid the risks for birth defects.

Prematurity

Preterm birth refers to a birth that occurs before 37 completed weeks (less than 259 days) of gestation. A very preterm birth is generally defined as less than 32 weeks of gestation and late preterm between 34 and < 37 weeks gestation. Preterm birth is the second leading cause of infant mortality, after congenital anomalies, and a major determinant of neonatal and infant morbidity.

On the basis of an international disease classification system, 61% of the early neonatal deaths were due to prematurity/LBW in developing countries. It is difficult or meaningless to compare the survival statistics of developed and developing countries when the latter have insufficient facilities and equipment. Poor infection control results in serious infections that rank very high as the cause of neonatal death in such countries. The complications associated with prematurity are shown in Table 3.2.10.

Table 3.2.10 Complications associated with prematurity
• Respiratory Distress Syndrome
• Hypothermia
• Hypoglycemia
• Hemorrhagic and Periventricular White Matter Brain Injury
• Bronchopulmonary Dysplasia
• Necrotising Enterocolitis
• Apnea/Anemia of Prematurity

Respiratory Distress Syndrome

Respiratory distress syndrome (RDS) is a common cause of neonatal mortality in many parts of the world. Developed countries spend a vast expenditure on equipment, training and research for babies with RDS. Such expenditure would be inconceivable in developing countries.

Reports of RDS in developing countries are seldom an overall incidence from any one country but rather from various hospital studies. For reasons to be discussed this incidence may increase with improvements in perinatal care. Largely, the major determinant of the incidence of RDS is the proportion of deliveries which are preterm. Common pulmonary conditions that need to be differentiated from RDS are transient tachypnea of newborn, pneumonia, pneumothorax and persistent pulmonary hypertension. The factors associated with RDS are shown in Table 3.2.11.

Table 3.2.11 Factors associated with RDS
• Higher male incidence
• Caesarian section without labour
• Second twin
• Maternal diabetes

The diagnosis of RDS is made from the combination of clinical and radiological findings. It is rarely occurs over 38 weeks gestation. There is a tachypnoea, grunting, retraction of chest wall in moderate to severe cases. Multiple randomized, controlled clinical trials indicate the benefits of surfactant replacement therapy, including reduction in the severity of RDS.

The overall mortality of the RDS has now been reduced to between 5 and 10%. Up to 50% of babies weighing less than 1.5 kg and who survives RDS will require readmission to a general Paediatric ward within first year of life.

Hypothermia and Hypoglycemia

Hypothermia and hypoglycemia may be prevented through simple and inexpensive interventions. Risk factors for hypoglycemia include birth asphyxia, prematurity and hypothermia. Hypothermia is common in developing countries, affecting more than half of all newborns in many communities, and is associated with an increased risk of mortality. Hypothermia also is associated with increased rates of morbidity, including increased risk of neonatal infections, coagulation defects, acidosis, delayed fetal-to-newborn circulatory adjustment, hyaline membrane disease, and intraventricular hemorrhage.

Hypothermia can be prevented by simple measures such as ensuring a warm environment during delivery; early breastfeeding and skin-to-skin contact with the mother; proper bathing, drying and swaddling; and prompt identification and rewarming of hypothermic neonates. Basic knowledge and practice of thermal control, however, generally are inadequate among health care providers and families in developing countries. The effects of hypothermia on babies are shown in Table 3.2.12.

Table 3.2.12: Effects of hypothermia on babies

- Lethargy
- Poor feeding / weak cry
- Peripheral edema
- Marked facial edema (may give false impression of healthy infant)

Hemorrhagic and Periventricular white Matter Brain Injury (PVL)

The germinal matrix is a weakly supported and highly vascularized area that is prone to rupture upon fluctuations in cerebral blood flow. This condition remains the commonest cause of death in very low birthweight neonate ventilated for RDS. Most intraventricular hemorrhage (IVH) occurs in the first 72 hours after birth.

The incidence and severity of IVH is inversely proportional to gestational age and rare after 32 weeks postconceptional age. The development of large IVH is usually associated with subtle clinical deterioration in a ventilated child with increase in ventilatory support, anaemia, fall in blood pressure, acidosis and neurological signs. Cranial ultrasonography is the most frequent imaging modality used to diagnose IVH. The classification of IVH is shown in Table 3.2.13.

Table 3.2.13: Classification of IVH [volpe]

Grade I:	Hemorrhage of germinal matrix
Grade II:	Intraventricular Hemorrhage without ventricular dilatation
Grade III:	Intraventricular hemorrhage with ventricular dilatation
Grade IV:	Intraventricular hemorrhage with parenchymal involvement

To, date no single intervention has been found to prevent IVH although many approaches have been tried. Best approach would be to minimize the hemodynamic instability during the perinatal period. Uncomplicated IVH has a good prognosis. About 30% of infants with IVH went on to develop post hemorrhagic ventricular dilatation and have the highest risk of adverse neurodevelopmental outcome. Prognosis for the white matter brain injury is even more difficult to ascertain as not all brain injuries are hemorrhagic but there is no doubt that PVL is the most powerful predictor of cerebral palsy.

BIBLIOGRAPHY

1. Adair LS, Popkin BM. Low birth weight reduces the likelihood of breastfeeding among Filipino infants. J Nutr 1996; 126:103-12.
2. Bang AT, Bang RA, Baitule SB, Deshmukh MD & Reddy MH. Burden of morbidities and the unmet need for health care in rural neonates — a prospective observational study in Gadchiroli, India. Indian Pediatrics 2001;38:952-64.
3. Bennett J, Macia J, Traverso H et al. Neonatal tetanus associated with topical umbilical ghee: covert role of cow dung. Int J Epidemiol 1999;28:1172-75.
4. Bhutta ZA, Darmstadt, GL, Hasan B, Haws R. Community-Based Interventions for Improving Perinatal and Neonatal Outcomes in Developing Countries: A Review of the Evidence Pediatrics 2005;115(2):520-603.
5. Christensson K, Ransjo-Arvidson AB, Kakoma C, et al. Midwifery care routines and prevention of heat loss in the newborn: a study in Zambia. J Trop Pediatr 1988;34: 208-12.
6. Costello A, Manandhar D. Current state of the health of newborn infants in developing countries. In Costello A, Manandhar D, editors, Improving Newborn Health in Developing Countries. London, Imperial College Press 2000;3-14.
7. Ellis M. Birth asphyxia in developing countries: epidemiology, sequellae and prevention. London Imperial college press; 2000;233-72.
8. Huffman SL, Zehner ER, Victora C. Breastfeeding and Neonatal Mortality. LINKAGES Washington, DC: Academy for Educational Development, 1999.
9. Hyder AA, Morrow RH, Wali S, McGuckin J. Burden of Disease for Neonatal Mortality in South Asia and Sub-Saharan Africa Washington, DC: Save the Children Federation-US, 2001; 1-93.
10. Johanson RB, Spencer SA, Rolfe P, Jones P, Malla DS. Effect of post-delivery care on neonatal body temperature. Acta Paediatr 1992;81: 859-63.
11. Moss W, Darmstadt GL, Marsh DR, Black RE, Santosham M. Research priorities or the reduction of perinatal and neonatal morbidity and mortality in developing country communities. J Perinatol 2002;22(6):484-95.
12. Mutch L, Newdick M, Lodwick A, Chalmers I. Secular changes in re-hospitalization of very low birth weight infants. Pediatrics 1986 ;78:164-71.
13. Newborn Care in South-East Asia Region (WHO/SEAR). Report of Regional Expert Group Meeting 1998;14: (November 16-17).
14. Zaidi AK, Huskins WC, Thaver D, Bhutta ZA, Abbas Z, Goldmann DA. Hospital-acquired neonatal infections in developing countries The Lancet - Vol. 365, Issue 9465, 26 March 2005;1175-88.

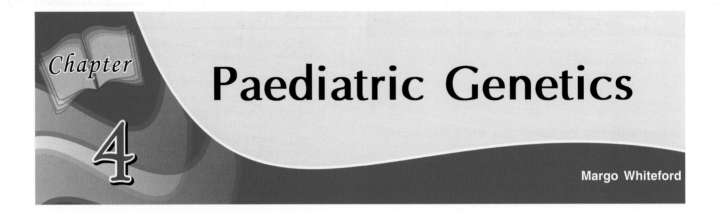

Chapter 4

Paediatric Genetics

Margo Whiteford

INTRODUCTION

With the improvements in treatment of infectious diseases in the developed world, conditions, which are either wholly or partially genetic in their aetiology, have become more prominent as a cause of childhood morbidity and mortality. It is estimated that around one third of admissions to paediatric wards are due to conditions with some genetic component and therefore an understanding of basic genetic principles is becoming increasingly important.

The field of medical genetics is an ever expanding one and within the context of this text it is not possible to cover all areas of the speciality in detail. Instead, this chapter tries to provide enough basic genetic information to allow understanding of the aspects of medical genetics encountered during day to day paediatric practice.

In practice, clinical genetics does not differ from any other speciality, in that the clinician's ability to make a diagnosis relies on the same skills; i.e. the ability to take a detailed history, including pregnancy and family history, perform a physical examination, arrange appropriate investigations and interpret the results. However, the emphasis may be slightly different with more time being taken over the family history and the physical examination may extend to other members of the family as well as the child who is the patient.

Taking the History and Patterns of Inheritance

A detailed history of a child's illness is always required when a child is seen as an outpatient or admitted to hospital. Obviously if a child is admitted acutely unwell then treating the current illness is paramount, but if a genetic cause for the illness is suspected it is important, once the child's condition is stable, to return to asking questions about the child's previous health, growth and development in much more detail.

In addition to trying to ascertain genetic factors which may have contributed to the child's illness it is equally important to look for non-genetic factors which may offer an explanation and allow a genetic cause to be excluded: for instance a history of significant perinatal asphyxia in a child with severe microcephaly and seizures or the ingestion of teratogens such as alcohol or anti-epileptic medication during pregnancy if a child has multiple congenital anomalies.

Care has to be taken when drawing family trees in order to get the correct information without causing offence or distress to the family. For instance, many parents feel guilty if their child has been diagnosed with a genetically inherited condition and worry that it may have been inherited from their side of the family. In the developed world it is not unusual for a woman to have had children by several different partners and sensitivity must be used while obtaining this information. Similarly, in other populations, asking questions about consanguineous (related) marriages may also cause concern.

Within the genetics clinic, family trees or 'pedigrees' are usually drawn to at least three generations. An example of various family trees is shown in Figure 4.1. The child, who brings the family to medical attention is usually known as the 'proband' with his parents being referred to as 'consultants'. By convention, males are represented by squares and are drawn to the left of a couple and females are represented by circles. 'Affected' individuals are shaded in, while carriers of recessive disorders and chromosome translocations are half shaded and female carriers of X-linked disorders are indicated by a central dot. Other commonly used family tree symbols are listed in Figure 4.1

Well before people were interested in human genetics, patterns of inheritance had been recognised both in animal breeding and plant crossing experiments. In the 19th century Gregor Mendel was the first person to propose the idea of 'recessive' genes to explain why some traits appeared to 'skip generations'. Nowadays many patterns of inheritance are recognised and often by drawing a family tree it is possible to predict the 'risk' to offspring of subsequent generations even in situations where no specific genetic diagnosis has been made.

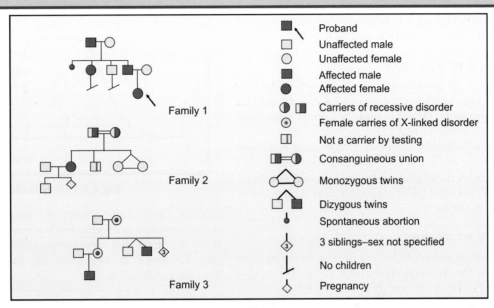

■ (with arrow)	Proband
□	Unaffected male
○	Unaffected female
■	Affected male
●	Affected female
◐ ▣	Carriers of recessive disorder
⊙	Female carries of X-linked disorder
◫	Not a carrier by testing
■—●	Consanguineous union
○△	Monozygous twins
□△	Dizygous twins
◦	Spontaneous abortion
◇3	3 siblings–sex not specified
⊥	No children
◇	Pregnancy

Family 1
Family 2
Family 3

Fig. 4.1: Patterns of Inheritance

Autosomal Dominant Inheritance

With conditions which are autosomal dominantly inherited the condition typically appears to occur in all generations of a family and males and females are equally affected (see Family 1—Fig. 4.1). The important point to note with dominantly inherited conditions is that males can pass the condition to their sons and this can be a useful feature for distinguishing an autosomal dominant condition from an X-linked condition where females are sometimes 'affected'.

The clinical status of an individual is usually referred to as 'phenotype' whereas their genetic constitution is the 'genotype'. Some autosomal dominant conditions are not fully penetrant, which means that not all individuals, who inherit the mutant gene, will be clinically affected and others may be so mildly affected that the condition is not immediately noticed. For this reason an autosomal dominant condition may appear to 'skip' a generation and then return. Thus, when a condition is known to have variable penetrance it is important to exercise caution when determining the risk to the next generation, even when an individual has a normal phenotype.

Males and females affected by an autosomal dominant condition will transmit the condition to 50% of their sons and 50% of their daughters

Autosomal Recessive Inheritance

Typically autosomal recessive conditions only affect individuals in one generation of a family (see Family 2—Fig. 4.1) but exceptions to this will occur when the carrier frequency of the gene in a population is high, e.g. 1:10 people of Caucasian origin are carriers of a haemo-chromatosis gene mutation and therefore it is not uncommon for a person who is affected by haemo-chromatosis to have a partner who is a carrier of the condition, resulting in the possibility of their offspring also being affected. This phenomenon is known as 'pseudo-dominance'. Autosomal recessive conditions may also occur in more than one generation of a family if there are many consanguineous marriages within the family.

When both parents are carriers of an autosomal recessive condition they will transmit the condition to 25% of their children whether they are male or female and 50% of their children will be carriers. A person affected by an autosomal recessive condition will have a low risk of having an affected child, provided that their partner is not a relative and that the carrier frequency of the condition in the population is low.

X-linked Recessive Inheritance

X-linked recessive conditions generally only affect males and never pass from father to son (see Family 3—Fig. 4.1). However, occasionally a female may be affected by an X-linked recessive condition if she only has one X-chromosome (as a result of also having Turner syndrome), if she has a skewed X inactivation pattern (see later) or if she has inherited a mutant gene on both of her X-chromosomes, which may occur if (a) her father is affected by the condition and her mother is a carrier (b) a new mutation arises in the gene on one X-chromosome and her other X-chromosome is inherited from a parent who is affected or a carrier.

Female carriers of an X-linked recessive condition will have a 25% chance of having an affected son and a 25% chance of having a carrier daughter. All of the daughters of a male affected by an X-linked recessive condition will be carriers and none of his sons will be affected.

X-linked Dominant Inheritance

X-linked dominant conditions also affect both males and females and occur in several generations of a family but their distinguishing feature is that they never pass from father to son.

A female affected by an X-linked dominant condition will transmit the condition to 50% of her sons and 50% of her daughters. A male affected by an X-linked dominant condition will transmit the condition to all of his daughters and none of his sons.

Mitochondrial Inheritance

Although the majority of DNA inherited from parents occurs within the chromosomes in the nucleus of cells, a small amount of DNA also occurs within the mitochondria, which are the organelles responsible for cell energy production. As sperm do not contain any mitochondria, conditions, which occur as a result of mutations in mitochondrial DNA, are always maternally transmitted.

The proportion of mitochondria containing the mutant gene varies from cell to cell in all tissues of the body and therefore an individual's phenotype will also vary depending on the proportion of mutant mitochondria in relation to normal or 'wild-type' mitochondria. It can be extremely difficult to predict the chance of a woman having an affected child, if she is either affected by or a carrier of a mitochondrial condition. The various possibilities arising in this situation are illustrated in Figure 4.2.

Polygenic Inheritance

Many congenital anomalies and later onset diseases, e.g. diabetes and hypertension occur more commonly in some families than would be predicted from the population incidence of the disorder, but do not follow the patterns of single gene inheritance, described above. Such conditions are referred to as 'polygenic' or 'multifactorial' and their aetiology involves both genetic and environmental factors. In this situation the disorder only occurs if an individual

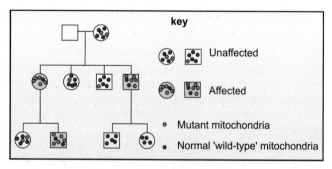

Fig. 4.2: Mitochondrial Inheritance

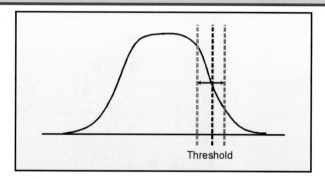

Fig. 4.3: Threshold effect

inherits a sufficient quantity of 'susceptibility' genes and is also exposed to specific environmental factors. Many of these multifactorial conditions exhibit a threshold effect (Fig. 4.3) and it is only when this threshold is exceeded that the condition occurs.

For the majority of multifactorial disorders neither the susceptibility genes nor the specific causative environmental factors are known. The exception to this is perhaps illustrated with neural tube defects where the result of the MRC multivitamin trial published in 1991, concluded that the risk of neural tube defects occurring could be reduced by 60-70% with peri-conceptual folic acid supplementation. This in effect moved the 'threshold' to the right of the curve. Conversely, it is well-recognised that taking folic acid antagonists, such as some anti-epileptic drugs, during pregnancy increases the risk of neural tube defect and in this case the threshold is shifted to the left of the curve (Fig. 4.4).

In order to predict the recurrence risk for multifactorial conditions, geneticists rely on population studies which provide 'empiric' recurrence risks. For most of the congenital anomalies the risk figures lie between 2-5%. If a couple have a second affected child the risk increases, since it is more likely that for this particular family genetic factors are involved.

Clinical Examination and Dysmorphology

The clinical examination of a child within the genetics clinic does not differ in any way from that carried out elsewhere, but making a 'genetic diagnosis' often relies on the recognition of patterns of clinical features and symptoms. It is only with experience that the more common 'syndromes' become easily recognised and often it is a facial 'gestalt', i.e. overall appearance, rather than individual features which suggests a likely diagnosis. For instance the child with Down's syndrome (Fig. 4.5) is easily identified by people who have no medical knowledge, because it is a relatively common condition. It is impractical to memorise the features of hundreds of genetic syndromes and modern day geneticists frequently use computerised

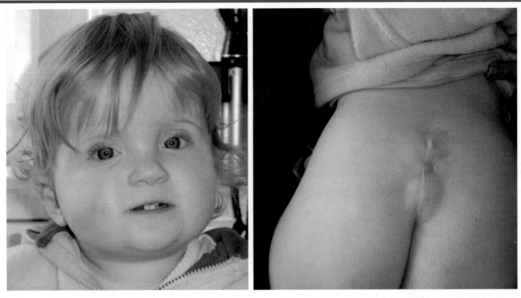

Fig. 4.4: Repaired neural tube defect in a girl who also has facial features of 'foetal valproate syndrome' (flat nasal bridge, hypertelorism, infra-orbital crease, long smooth philtrum)

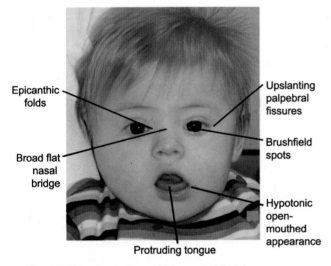

Epicanthic folds

Broad flat nasal bridge

Upslanting palpebral fissures

Brushfield spots

Hypotonic open-mouthed appearance

Protruding tongue

Fig. 4.5: Down's syndrome (Trisomy 21) facial appearance

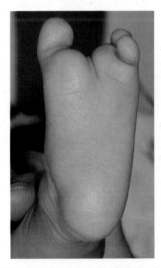

Fig. 4.6: Ectrodactyly (Split-foot)

dysmorphology databases to aid diagnosis. These databases contain information on the clinical features of syndromes compiled from the published literature and by searching on a patient's key clinical features it is possible to obtain a list of suggested diagnoses, which aids the direction of further investigations in order to confirm or exclude a particular diagnosis. Clinical features may be regarded as 'hard handles' if they only occur with a small number of conditions, e.g. ectrodactyly (Fig. 4.6), whereas features such as single palmar creases and hypoplastic nails (Fig. 4.7) are 'soft signs', which occur with many different genetic diagnoses. Features such as marked asymmetry of any part of the body (Fig. 4.8) or patchy abnormalities of skin pigmentation are suggestive of 'mosaicism' and a skin biopsy should be considered.

INVESTIGATIONS

The diagnosis of many genetic disorders can be made on the basis of biochemistry results, e.g. sweat electrolytes in the case of cystic fibrosis or urinary glycosaminoglycans in the case of the mucopolysaccharidoses. Similarily, radiographs are an essential tool for the diagnosis of inherited skeletal dysplasias (see Chapter 32). However the investigations specific to the field of genetics are chromosome

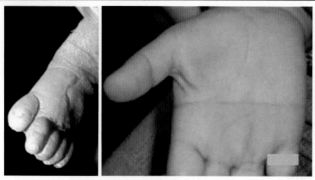

Figs 4.7A and B: A. Hypoplastic nails **B.** Single palmar crease

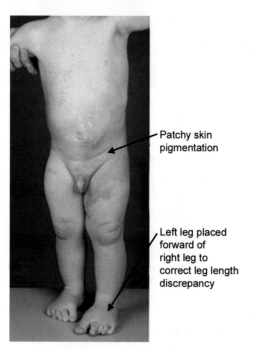

— Patchy skin pigmentation

— Left leg placed forward of right leg to correct leg length discrepancy

Fig. 4.8: Asymmetry

tests ('cytogenetics') and DNA analysis (molecular genetics), which are discussed in more detail below.

Cytogenetics

The study of chromosomes was perhaps the earliest branch of Medical Genetics to develop, with Hsu and Levan being the first to accurately observe human chromosomes in 1952 and the correct human chromosome number being recorded, in 1956, by Tjio and Levan.

Chromosomes are the structures in the nucleus of the cell into which DNA is packaged. In humans there are 46 chromosomes in all nucleated cells except the gametes. The 46 chromosomes occur as 23 pairs, with one copy of each pair being inherited from the mother and the other from the father. The first 22 pairs of chromosomes are the same whether an individual is male or female and are known as 'autosomes' and the remaining pair are the 'sex

chromosomes'. Females have two X sex chromosomes while males have one X and one Y sex chromosome. The chromosome constitution of an individual is usually referred to as their karyotype and the normal karyotype for a female is denoted 46,XX and for a male 46,XY.

The chromosomes can only be examined in dividing cells and are best seen during the metaphase stage of mitosis. For this reason it usually takes around 1 week to get the result of a chromosome test. Various staining techniques can be used to examine chromosomes with the light microscope in order to show the 'banding pattern' along the length of each chromosome. The stain most commonly used is Giemsa which reveals dark and light regions of chromosomes rather like a bar-code (Fig. 4.9) and by searching for variations in the pattern created by these bands, trained cytogeneticists are able to identify structural abnormalities along the length of any chromosome. The chromosomes are photographed and then arranged in their pairs starting with the largest autosome to the smallest and finally the sex chromosomes. The diagrammatic representation of a chromosome (Fig. 4.10) shows that the chromosome is divided into two arms, the 'p' short-arm and the 'q' long-arm, by the narrowed centromere region. With the larger chromosomes the 'short arms' are almost as long as the 'long arms'.

Numerical Chromosome Abnormalities

Soon after the correct number of human chromosomes was determined it was recognised that numerical abnormalities of chromosomes were associated with clinical disorders. Numerical abnormalities can arise with both the autosomes and sex chromosomes.

- **Numerical Abnormalities of Autosomes**
  Extra or missing copies of any of the autosomes can arise as a result of non-dysjunction occurring during meiosis, which is the process by which the total chromosome number is halved during gamete formation. Numerical abnormalities of chromosomes are known as 'aneuploidy' and most autosome aneuploidies are incompatible with survival, leading to spontaneous abortions of affected pregnancies. The exceptions to this are trisomies of chromosomes 13, 18 and 21 and the clinical features of these conditions are summarised in Table 4.1.

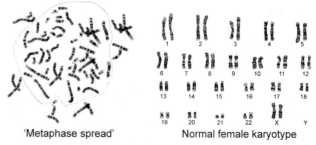

'Metaphase spread'   Normal female karyotype

Fig. 4.9: Giemsa-Banded chromosomes

Trisomy	Name	Approximate birth incidence	Main clinical features
		Table 4.1: Autosomal trisomies	
13	Patau's syndrome	1:5000	Cleft lip and palate, microcephaly, holoprosencephaly, seizures, severe learning disability, scalp defects, colobomata, microphthalmia, cardiac defects, exomphalos, polydactyly
18	Edward's syndrome	1:3000	Low birth weight, female preponderance, small facial features, prominent occiput, severe learning disability, low set malformed ears, cardiac defects, renal anomalies, flexion deformities of fingers, rocker-bottom feet
21	Down's syndrome	1:700	Hypotonia, flat occiput, up-slanting palpebral fissures, epicanthic folds, Brushfield spots, flat nasal bridge, protruding tongue, learning disability, cardiac defects, intestinal atresia, imperforate anus, Hirschsprung's disease

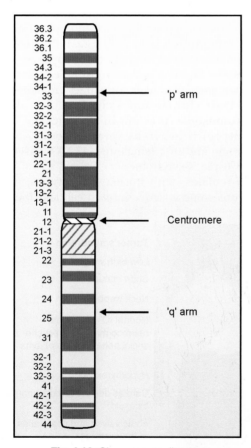

Fig. 4.10: Chromosome diagram

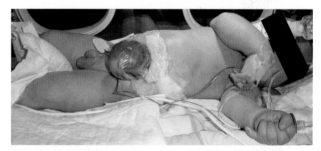

Fig. 4.11: Trisomy 13—note exomphalos and polydactyly

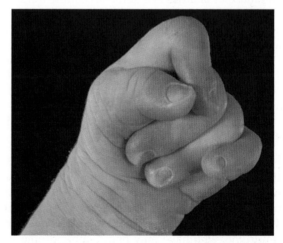

Fig. 4.12: Trisomy 18—typical overlapping fingers

Trisomy 13 (Fig. 4.11) and trisomy 18 (Fig. 4.12) are both associated with multiple congenital anomalies and the majority of babies born with these conditions die within the first year of life. These autosomal trisomies occur with increased frequency with increasing maternal age and tables are available for advising women of their age related risk of having a liveborn baby with an autosomal trisomy. After a couple have had a child with an autosomal trisomy, the risk of recurrence for future pregnancies is around 1% and prenatal diagnosis could be offered in the form of chorionic villus sampling or amniocentesis.

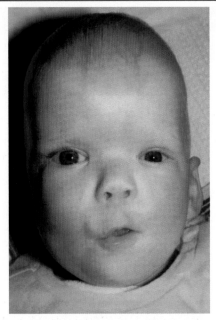

Fig. 4.13: Mosaic trisomy 22—note marked facial asymmetry

Table 4.2: Pallister - Killian syndrome clinical features	
Pallister-Killian syndrome	
Neurological features	Profound learning disability, seizures profound hypotonia
Dysmorphic facial featues	General 'coarse' appearance, high forehead, sparseness of hair in frontal region in infancy, hypertelorism, epicanthic folds, flat nasal bridge, large mouth with down turned corners, macroglossia, abnormal ears
Other featues	Pigmentary skin anomalies, short neck, diaphragmatic hernia, supernumerary nipples

The most frequent autosomal trisomies found in tissue from spontaneous abortions are trisomy 16 and trisomy 22, but these are generally only found in live born babies in the mosaic state i.e. the situation where only a proportion of the patient's cells have the chromosome abnormality (Fig. 4.13). Such mosaic aneuploidies are often only identified by carrying out chromosome analysis of a fibroblast culture from a skin biopsy. Analysis of skin chromosomes should always be considered if a patient has marked asymmetry or if a diagnosis of Pallister-Killian is being considered. Pallister-Killian arises as a result of mosaic tetrasomy 12p i.e. some cells have two additional copies of the short arms of chromosome 12 joined together to form an additional chromosome. The clinical features of Pallister-Killian syndrome are summarised in Table 4.2.

- **Numerical abnormalities of sex chromosomes**

  It is unusual for abnormalities of the sex chromosome number to be detected in newborn babies as they are not usually associated with physical abnormalities. The exception to this may be girls affected by Turner's syndrome, who have only one X-chromosome (i.e. a 45,XO karyotype) and who may have congenital malformations (Fig. 4.14). Even in the absence of structural malformations, a diagnosis of Turner's syndrome may be suspected in a newborn infant because of intrauterine growth retardation and the presence of lymphoedema. This can, on occasions, persist into adulthood (Fig. 4.14).

  A 47,XYY karyotype is often detected by chance when chromosomes are being checked for an unrelated reason, e.g. a family history of a structural chromosome abnormality, as this chromosome abnormality is not usually associated with any phenotypic effect. There are some studies which suggest that behaviour abnormalities are more common in boys with 47, XYY karyotypes, but this probably just reflects the fact that boys with behavioural abnormalities are more likely to have their chromosomes checked. An additional X-chromosome present in a male (i.e. 47,XXY karyotype) is generally referred to as Klinefelter syndrome and in a female (i.e. 47,XXX karyotype) is called triple X-syndrome.

  In females, with normal karyotypes, only one X-chromosome is active in each cell and the other is

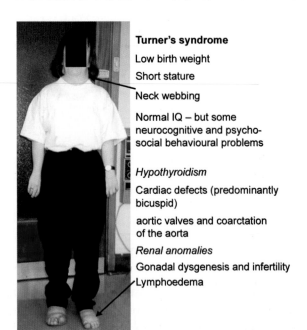

Turner's syndrome

Low birth weight

Short stature

Neck webbing

Normal IQ – but some neurocognitive and psycho-social behavioural problems

Hypothyroidism

Cardiac defects (predominantly bicuspid)

aortic valves and coarctation of the aorta

Renal anomalies

Gonadal dysgenesis and infertility

Lymphoedema

Fig. 4.14: Clinical features of Turner's syndrome

condensed into a structure called a 'Barr body'. The X chromosome which is active varies from cell to cell, usually with the maternal X being active in 50% of cells and the paternal X being active in the remaining 50%. If this is not the case it is referred to as 'skewed X-inactivation'. In children with additional copies of the X-chromosome, only one X-chromosome remains activated and the additional copies are inactivated to form extra Barr bodies.

Males with Klinefelter syndrome are usually diagnosed in adulthood as they are taller than would be predicted from their parental heights and have hypogonadism, resulting in infertility.

Females with Triple X syndrome are also taller than average and some may experience fertility problems. Around 30% of girls with Triple X syndrome have significant learning difficulties and mild learning difficulties may occur in a small proportion of males with 47,XXY or 47,XYY karyotypes. Multiple extra copies of the sex chromosomes can also occur e.g. 48,XXYY, 48,XXXX or even 49, XXXXY karyotypes. In general higher numbers of additional X chromosomes are associated with significant learning difficulties.

The frequency of Turner's syndrome is around 1:3000 female births, while the frequency of Klinefelter syndrome, Triple X syndrome and 47,XYY is around 1:1000 livebirths.

Sex chromosome aneuploidies are not associated with increased maternal age and the recurrence risk for future pregnancies is not increased.

Structural Chromosome Abnormalities

Structural chromosome abnormalities are termed 'unbalanced' if there is loss or gain of chromosomal material and 'balanced' if the overall amount of chromosomal material remains unchanged. Generally speaking balanced chromosome abnormalities are unlikely to cause any adverse effect. The main categories of structural chromosome abnormalities are listed below and illustrated in Figure 4.15:

- **Robertsonian Translocations**
  A Robertsonian translocation is the fusion of two of the smaller chromosomes at their centromeres. During this process the short arms of the chromosomes are lost, but as these contain no essential genetic material, no harmful effect occurs. A carrier of a balanced Robertsonian translocation will have a total of 45 chromosomes as the two fused chromosomes are counted as one. Similarly, the correct cytogenetic nomenclature for a person with an unbalanced Robertsonian translocation, describes them as having 46 chromosomes, but they will of course have three copies of the long arms of one of the chromosomes involved in the translocation.

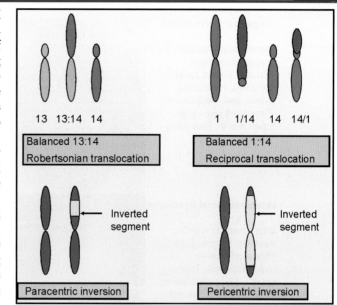

Fig. 4.15: Structural chromosome rearrangements

Carriers of balanced translocations are at risk of having children with unbalanced chromosomes. The actual risk varies depending on; (a) the chromosomes involved in the translocation—highest when chromosome 21 is involved and (b) the sex of the parent who is a carrier - higher when it is the mother. It is important to recognise that all of the children of a carrier of a 21:21 Robertsonian translocation, will be affected by Down's syndrome.

- **Reciprocal Translocations**
  A reciprocal translocation is the exchange of segments of chromosomal material between non-identical chromosomes, usually two chromosomes are involved but complicated exchanges between several chromosomes can occasionally occur. This is detected by there being a disruption to the normal banding pattern along the length of the chromosomes involved.

  Carriers of balanced reciprocal translocations are healthy but as they produce a proportion of chromosomally abnormal gametes they may present with infertility, particularly in males, or recurrent miscarriages. Sometimes an individual will be identified as being a carrier of balanced reciprocal translocation following the birth of child with congenital malformations, dysmorphism or learning disability, if investigations reveal the unbalanced form of the translocation in the child. The birth of a liveborn child with chromosomal imbalance arising from a reciprocal translocation, is more likely to occur if the length of the chromosomal segments involved in the translocation represent less than 5% of the overall length of all 46 chromosomes.

Angelman's syndrome

Severe learning disability,
Happy disposition,
Virtually absent speech,
Seizures, Hypotoinia,
Ataxic gait, Microcephaly,
Prominent jaw, Large
open mouth, Protruding
tongue

Prader-Willi syndrome

Mild-moderate learning
disability, Severe neonatal
hypotonia, Poor suck and
weak cry, Hypogonadism,
Hyperphagia and obesity in
childhood, short stature,
Small hands and feet,
Bitemporal narrowing of the
skull, 'Almond' shaped eyes,
Up-slanting palpebral
fissures, Stabismus

Velocardiofacial Syndrome

Mild-moderate learning
disability, Cardiac defects,
Palatal anomalies,
Hypocalcaemia, Thymic
aplasia, Myopathic facies,
Short palpebral fissures,
Long nose, Broad nasal
tip, Ear anomalies, Long
Slender fingers

Williams Syndrome

Moderate learning disability,
Characteristic outgoing
personality, Heart defects
(supravalvular aortic
stenosis most commonly),
Renal anomalies,
Hypercalcaemia,
Hyperacusis, Short stature,
'Elfin' facies, full cheeks,
Thick lips, Stellate irides,
Features coarsen with
incresing age

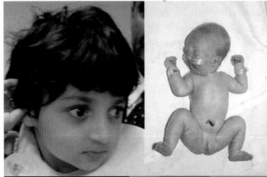
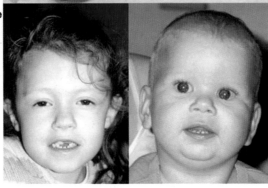

Fig. 4.16: Clinical features of some chromosome microdeletion syndromes

- **Inversions**

  An inversion is the term used to describe a segment of chromosome, which has broken away and then rejoined in the same position but rotated through 180°. If the inverted segment is confined to one arm of the chromosome it is termed a 'paracentric inversion' and if the segment spans the centromere it is termed a 'pericentric inversion'. Chromosomal inversions usually have no phenotypic effect, but they interfere with meiosis and again may result in chromosomally abnormal gametes being produced. The chromosome abnormalities arising from paracentric inversions are unlikely to be compatible with survival and are therefore more likely to result in recurrent early miscarriages. Pericentric inversions, on the other hand, may result in small chromosomal deletions or duplications and can result in liveborn children with malformations or learning disability arising from chromosomal imbalance.

- **Chromosomal Deletions and Duplications**

  Deletions or duplications of chromosomal segments may arise and most of these are unique to the individuals in whom they are identified. However, there are some regions of chromosomes which are more prone to deletions or other rearrangements. These are termed 'sub-telomeric' if they occur at the ends of the chromosomes and 'interstitial' if they occur elsewhere. It is now clear that many of these recurrent rearrangements give rise to recognisable dysmorphic syndromes (see Table 4.3 and Fig. 4.16) and that some of the variability in the features of these syndromes is due to the size of the deletion and the number of genes which are missing as a result.

  Many chromosomal deletions are visible when observing chromosomes with the light microscope but others are too small to be seen and require a specialised technique, called fluorescent *in situ* hybridisation (FISH) to be detected. FISH is basically a molecular genetic

Table 4.3: Chromosomal deletion syndromes

Chromosome segment	Syndrome
4p16.3	Wolf-Hirschorn's syndrome
5p15.2	Cri-du-Chat syndrome
5q35	Soto's syndrome
7q11.23	Williams' syndrome
11p15.5	Beckwith-Wiedeman's syndrome
13q14.11	Retinoblastoma
15q12	Angelman and Prader-Willi's syndromes
16p13.3	Rubinstein-Taybi's syndrome
17p11.2	Smith-Magenis' syndrome
22q11.2	Di George/Velocardiofacial syndrome

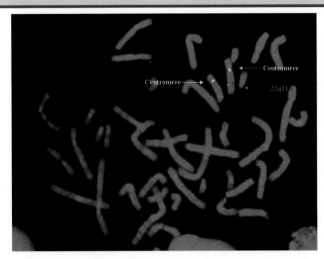

Fig. 4 17: Photograph of FISH technique used to detect the 22q 11.2 deletion associated with velocardiofacial syndrome

technique (see later) whereby a fluorescent probe is attached to the region of interest of the chromosome. In the normal setting two fluorescent signals should be seen, i.e. one on each of the chromosome pair, but if that particular region of chromosome is deleted, only one signal will be seen. In practice two different probes of different colours are used—one purely to identify the particular chromosome of interest and the other for the specific region (Fig. 4.17).

Uniparental Disomy and Imprinting

Uniparental disomy (UPD) is a relatively recently recognised form of chromosome abnormality. It is defined as the 'inheritance of a pair of homologous chromosomes from one parent', with no copy of that chromosome being inherited from the other parent. There are various mechanisms by which UPD can arise but it is thought that it most commonly occurs as a result of 'trisomic rescue', i.e. the loss of one copy of a chromosome during early cell division in an embryo which was originally destined to be trisomic for that chromosome.

With most autosomal genes, both the paternal and maternal copies of the gene are expressed, but a small number of genes are 'imprinted', which means that only the maternal or paternal (depending on the particular gene) copy is expressed. Therefore, although UPD can occur without clinical effect, for certain chromosomes it can mimic a deletion of an imprinted gene e.g. Angelman syndrome can arise as a result of a deletion of the maternal copy of the chromosome region 15q12, but it will also occur if a child has paternal UPD of chromosome 15, since there will be no maternal copy of 15q12 present. Other conditions arising as the result of abnormalities of imprinted genes are summarised in Table 4.4. 'Isodisomy' is a form of UPD where a child inherits two identical copies of the same

Table 4.4: Syndromes due to abnormalities in the expression of imprinted genes
Angelman's syndrome
Prader-Willi's syndrome
Beckwith-Wiedeman Syndrome
Russel-Silver syndrome
Transient neonatal diabetes

chromosome from one parent and 'heterodisomy' is the inheritance of a homologous pair of chromosomes from one parent. Thus, another consequence of UPD may be the occurrence of an autosomal recessive disorder in a child, when only one of the parents is a carrier of the disorder. The first case of UPD reported was in fact a child with short stature and cystic fibrosis, which occurred as a result of maternal isodisomy of chromosome 7.

Another consequence of UPD of certain chromosomes is a recognisable pattern of congenital malformations e.g. UPD of chromosome 16 can give rise to intrauterine growth retardation, cardiac defects, imperforate anus, scoliosis, hypospadias and herniae (Fig. 4.18).

Molecular Genetics

Before discussing the more clinical aspects of molecular genetics, it is useful to review some basic genetic principles. Deoxyribose nucleic acid (DNA) is the genetic template required to construct all the enzymes and proteins, which are necessary for the formation and function of the human body. DNA consists of strands of nucleic acids, containing the bases, adenosine, guanine, cytosine and thymine, held together by a sugar, phosphate backbone (Fig. 4.19). Each DNA molecule exists as two of these strands wrapped around each other to form a 'double helix'. The variable part of the DNA chain is the order of the bases along the backbone and the two strands of DNA are linked by hydrogen bonds between these bases. As a result of their shapes adenine always pairs with thymine and cytosine always pairs with guanine.

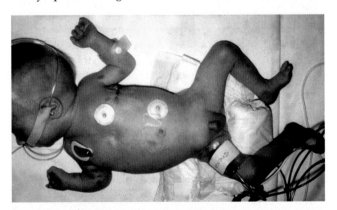

Fig. 4.18: Infant with multiple congenital anomalies due to maternal UPD 16

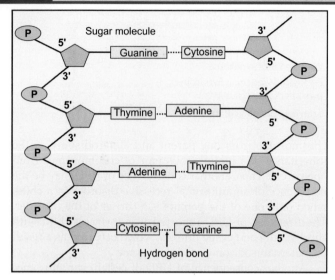

Fig. 4.19: DNA structure

It is the order of the DNA bases which form the 'genetic code' required for the production of amino acids and subsequently proteins. The code is a triplet code, as each three bases codes for an amino acid or provides the instruction 'stop' at the end of a peptide chain. As there are 4^3 i.e. 64 possible combinations of these bases and only 20 amino acids, the code is said to be 'redundant' and more than one triplet may code for the same amino acid. This can obviously be useful when it comes to DNA mutations arising since not all base substitutions will alter the sequence of amino acids in a protein and therefore the protein function will not be lost. Such harmless substitutions are referred to as 'harmless' or 'benign' 'polymorphisms'.

In order to understand how this system works it is necessary to look at the DNA molecule, shown in Figure 4.19, more closely. The deoxyribose sugars of the DNA backbone each have two hydroxyl groups, which occur at the 3 prime and 5 prime positions (denoted 3' and 5' respectively). The phosphate molecules join the sugar molecules together by forming a phosphodiester bond between the 3' hydroxyl group of one deoxyribose molecule and the 5' hydroxyl group of another. This gives the DNA strand a direction, running from the free 5' hydroxyl group of the first deoxyribose molecule to the free 3' hydroxyl group of the last. The two strands of DNA will of course be 'complimentary' in view of the base pairing, with one strand running in one direction an the other in the opposite direction.

DNA replication is an extremely complicated process, whereby the strands of DNA are separated and copied to produce new daughter strands. The process is initiated by the enzyme DNA polymerase and as the initial strands are separated, new deoxyribonucleoside triphosphates are added in a 5' to 3' direction. The process is said to be semi-conservative as each new DNA molecule will consist of one of the initial 'parent' strands bound to a new 'daughter' strand.

It was originally thought that genes consisted of a length of DNA providing the triplet code for the necessary amino acids to form a peptide chain. However, it is now recognised that this is not the case and the DNA sequence of each gene contains regions in between its protein coding sequence, known as intervening sequences (IVS). The nomenclature generally used are 'exons' (protein coding sequences) and 'introns' (intervening sequences). There are particular DNA codes which herald the start (TAG) and end of protein synthesis (TAA, TAG or TGA). Similarly, the dinucleotides GT and AG are found at the start and end of introns, respectively. Other particular nucleotide codes, which may be some distance away from the first exon of a gene, are also important for protein synthesis and are known as promoter regions.

The first stage of protein synthesis is known as transcription and involves the processing of messenger RNA (mRNA). DNA acts as a template for the production of mRNA and is read in a 5' to 3' direction. The process is initiated by enzymes known as RNA polymerases, which separate the strands of DNA. As with DNA replication the order of bases along the strand of mRNA, which is produced, are complimentary to the original DNA bases. The only difference between DNA and RNA is that the backbone sugar is ribose rather than deoxyribose and in RNA the base thymine is replaced by the base uracil. The primary transcript of mRNA, which is produced, contains the entire DNA coding region, including introns and exons. The mRNA then undergoes a number of processing steps, which result in the introns being cleaved out and the exons being spliced together (Fig. 4.20). Finally, the mRNA is modified by the attachment of various adenylic acids and protein molecules, which serve to protect the mRNA as it passes from the nucleus into the cytoplasm, in preparation for protein synthesis.

The process of protein synthesis also involves several different steps, namely 'initiation', whereby the ribosome is assembled on the mRNA, 'elongation', where complimentary tRNA molecules attach to each codon in turn, resulting in the addition of amino acids to the growing peptide chain and finally 'termination' when the polypeptide is released into the cytoplasm.

Not surprisingly with such a complicated process, errors (mutations) can arise and this results in the genetically inherited single gene disorders. There are various different types of mutation and these are summarised in Table 4.5.

Molecular Genetic Investigations

Southern Blotting

This is one of the older techniques used for DNA analysis, but it is still sometimes needed for detecting large genomic rearrangements, such as the large trinucleotide repeats which can occur in patients with myotonic dystrophy.

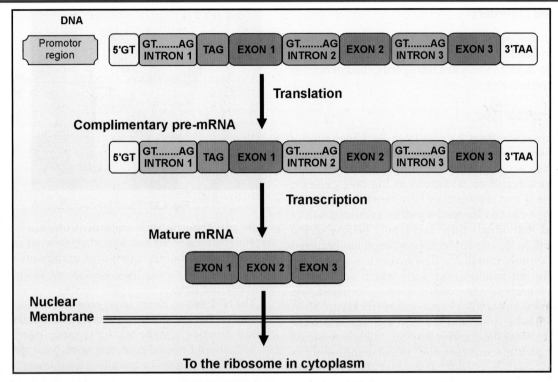

Fig. 4.20: DNA translation and transcription

Table 4.5: Types of mutation

Type of mutation	Outcome
Point mutation	A single base substitution
a. Missense mutation	Base change results in different amino acid
b. Nonsense mutation	Base change results in 'stop' and a shortened protein
Insertion or deletion	Alteration of the reading frame. If a complete codon is deleted an amino acid will be missing from the protein, which may or may not affect function
Trinucleotide repeat expansion	After a particular threshold is reached protein function is altered. Severity of the disorder is generally related to the size of the expansion

The Southern blotting technique is labour intensive and it can take several weeks to obtain results when this process is used.

Polymerase Chain Reaction

For many single gene disorders 'polymerase chain reaction' (PCR) is now the method of choice for DNA analysis. This process allows the analysis of short sequences of DNA which have been selectively amplified and tests looking for common recurring mutations, such as in cystic fibrosis, or known familial mutations which have previously been detected by other methods, can provide results within 48 hours.

DNA Sequencing

This type of testing reveals the specific sequence of bases within a region of DNA and compares them to reference sequence data in order to determine if any substitutions, deletions, etc have occurred. Much of this type of DNA testing is now computerised but it can still take lengthy periods of time to get results, particularly if the gene being investigated is large.

Multiple Ligand Probe Amplification

Multiple Ligand Probe Amplification (MLPA) is a new high resolution technique for detecting copy number variation of a large number of DNA segments simultaneously and it can therefore be used to provide a rapid screen for deletions and duplications at a number of sites throughout the genome. For instance it can be used to screen for very small chromosomal deletions or duplications in children with learning disability and dysmorphism, in whom conventional cytogenetic testing has failed to reveal any abnormality.

Single Gene Disorders

The clinical features of many of the single gene disorders will be discussed in other chapters throughout this text, but it may be useful to look at a few specific disorders from a genetics perspective.

Neurofibromatosis Type 1

Neurofibromatosis Type 1 (NF1) [Von Recklinghausen's Disease] is one of the most common genetically inherited disorders, having an incidence of approximately 1:3000. It occurs as a result of mutations in the NF1 gene on chromosome 17 and is essentially fully penetrant, although the phenotype can be extremely variable. In around half of the affected individuals there is a family history of the condition and in the remainder the condition has occurred as a result of new mutations. The main clinical features are:- café au lait patches (Fig. 4.21) which are usually present by 5 years of age, cutaneous neurofibromata, iris Lisch nodules and axillary and groin freckling. Most affected individuals are shorter than average and have larger than average head circumferences. Mild to moderate learning difficulties are common. Regular follow-up is required as a small proportion of people with NF1 develop more severe complications such as pseudoarthroses (present from birth), plexiform neurofibromata of the head and neck (usually present within the first year of life), optic gliomata (usually present by 6 years of age), plexiform neurofibromata of other parts of the body as seen in Figure 4.22 (usually present before puberty) and scoliosis (usually present between age 6 years to puberty).

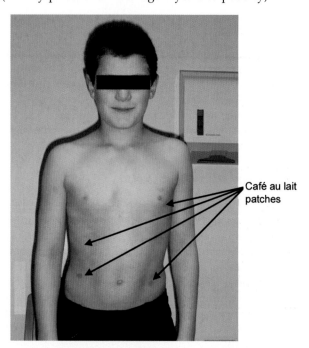

Fig 4.21: Boy with neurofibromatosis type 1

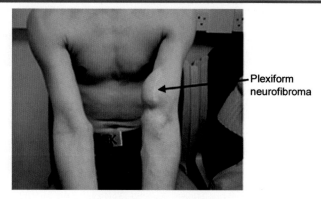

Fig. 4.22: Plexiform neurofibroma

In adulthood, other complications such as hypertension (both essential and secondary to renal artery stenosis or phaeochromocytoma) and malignant peripheral nerve sheath tumours may also occur so follow-up is generally life long.

The NF1 gene is a very large gene and mutation analysis is possible, but as NF1 can usually be easily diagnosed on clinical grounds, genetic testing is rarely necessary.

NF1 should not be confused with Neurofibromatosis Type 2 (NF2), which is a completely separate disorder due to a gene on chromosome 22. Although patients affected by NF2 may have café au lait patches, they seldom have six or more and they do not have the axillary and groin freckling found in NF1. The most common presenting feature is bilateral vestibular schwannomas.

Tuberous Sclerosis

Tuberous sclerosis complex (TSC) occurs with an incidence of 1:5000-6000. It can occur as a result of mutations in two different genes, TSC1 (located on chromosome 9) and TSC2 (located on chromosome 16). The condition is now thought to be fully penetrant and recurrences which have occurred when parents are apparently unaffected are now recognised to be due to one of the parents having minimal clinical features such as peri-ungual fibromata (Fig. 4.23) and the phenomenon of 'gonadal mosaicism', whereby one of the parents is a carrier of the mutation only in their gametes.

TSC is a multisystem disorder with extreme variability in the phenotype, even within one family. The clinical features are divided into major features (facial angiofibromata, ungal and periungal fibromata, forehead plaques, hypomelanotic macules, shagreen patches (connective tissue naevi), multiple retinal hamartomata, cortical tubers, subependymal nodules, subependymal giant cell astrocytomata, cardiac rhabdomyomata, lymphangiomyomatosis and renal angiomyolipomata) and minor features (dental enamel pits, hamartomatous rectal polyps, bone cysts, cerebral white matter radial migration lines, gingival fibromata, non-renal hamar-

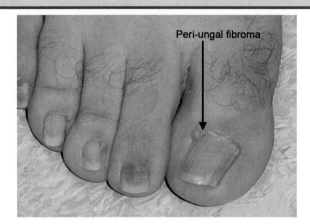

Fig. 4.23: Peri-ungual fibroma in patient with tuberous sclerosis

tomata, retinal achromic patches, 'confetti' skin lesions and multiple renal cysts). The clinical diagnosis is based on the presence of two major or one major plus two minor features. In the most severe cases TS can present with infantile spasms and such children can remain profoundly handicapped with difficult to control seizures throughout their lives. In milder cases mild to moderate learning disability may be present but some individuals affected by TS have completely normal intelligence. Regular follow-up is again important particularly with regard to the possibility of renal complications.

Mutation analysis is available for both TSC1 and TSC2 and prenatal diagnosis is possible if a mutation is identified.

Marfan's Syndrome

Marfan's syndrome has an incidence of 1:5000-10000 and in the majority of affected individuals the condition is due to mutations in Fibrillin1 (FBN1) on chromosome 15. It is a disorder of collagen and is therefore also a multisystem disorder affecting primarily the eye, the skeletal system and cardiovascular system. Individuals affected by Marfan's syndrome are usually dispropor-tionately tall with long limbs and arachnodactyly (long fingers and toes) (Fig. 4.24). However, as many people who are tall with long arms and legs do not have Marfan's syndrome it is necessary that patients meet strict clinical criteria, known as the Ghent's Criteria, before the diagnosis can be made. The main clinical features included in the Ghent's Criteria are: disproportionate stature, pectus excavatum or carinatum, long fingers, flat feet, protrusion acetabulae (an abnormality of the hip identified by X-rays), dental crowding, joint hypermobility, flat cheek bones, ectopia lentis and other eye abnormalities, dissection or dilatation of the ascending aorta, mitral valve prolapse and spontaneous pneumothoraces.

Although the ocular complications and aortic root dilatation and dissection, associated with this condition, are more common in adulthood long-term follow-up is required from the time of diagnosis. The diagnosis of Marfan syndrome in the past was mainly based on clinical features but mutation analysis can now be used in combination with clinical features and in families where a mutation is identified prenatal diagnosis is possible.

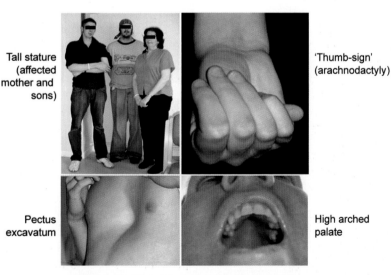

Tall stature (affected mother and sons)

'Thumb-sign' (arachnodactyly)

Pectus excavatum

High arched palate

Fig. 4. 24: Clinical features of Marfan's Syndrome

Myotonic Dystrophy

Myotonic dystrophy (Dystrophia myotonica) has an incidence of around 1:8000 and as the name suggests is a muscle wasting disease. However, it too, is a multisystem disorder and can be of very variable severity. The majority of people affected by myotonic dystrophy have myotonic dystrophy type 1 (DM1) due to abnormalities of the DMPK gene on chromosome 19. Myotonic dystrophy type 2 (DM2) is due to abnormalities of the ZNF9 gene on chromosome 3 and is much rarer. DM1 is an example of a condition due to a *triplet repeat expansion*. Other trinucleotide repeat disorders which may be encountered in paediatric practice are Fragile X syndrome, Friedreich's Ataxia and juvenile onset Huntington's disease.

In the case of myotonic dystrophy the repeated trinucleotide is CTG and the normal size is 5-35 repeats. In very general terms the age of onset and severity of symptoms relates to the size of the expansion of this repeat, although it is not possible to predict with accuracy an individual's prognosis from their expansion size. Like other triplet repeat disorders, myotonic dystrophy exhibits the phenomenon of *anticipation*. Anticipation is seen because the expanded trinucleotide region is unstable and therefore expands further as it passes from one generation to the next, resulting in symptoms occurring earlier and with greater severity in each successive generation. For this reason it is particularly important to take a detailed three-generation family history as the older, more mildly affected relatives may only have single symptoms, such as cataracts or diabetes, which may otherwise be overlooked.

The clinical features of DM1 are: muscle disease (muscle weakness and myotonia [difficulty in relaxing the muscles after contraction]), GI tract symptoms (as smooth muscle is also affected patients often complain of constipation, colicky abdominal pain and problems with bowel control), cardiovascular disease (conduction defects may lead to sudden death), respiratory problems (alveolar hypoventilation due to diaphragmatic and probably also a central component, postanaesthetic respiratory depression can be significant and care should be taken), ocular problems (subcapsular cataracts and retinal abnormalities), CNS (major cognitive dysfunction is unusual with adult onset disease but personality traits such as apathy, with marked daytime sleepiness and stubbornness are well-recognised) and endocrine problems (testicular atrophy - sometimes resulting in male infertility, recurrent miscarriages, diabetes mellitus, frontal balding).

Congenital myotonic dystrophy is a severe form the disorder and almost always occurs when the condition is transmitted by the mother and generally only if the mother has symptomatic disease. Affected neonates have profound hypotonia and usually require prolonged ventilatory assistance. Survivors have learning disabilities in addition to the physical features of the disease.

BIBLIOGRAPHY

1. Rimoin DL, Connor JM, Pyeritz RE, Korf BR, Eds (2007) Principles and Practice of Medical Genetics, 5th edn, Edinburgh, Churchill Livingstone.

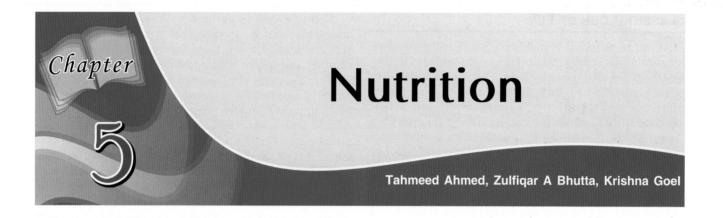

Chapter 5

Nutrition

Tahmeed Ahmed, Zulfiqar A Bhutta, Krishna Goel

5.1: Protein-energy Malnutrition and Micronutrient Deficiencies in Childhood

PROTEIN-ENERGY MALNUTRITION

Protein-energy malnutrition (PEM) is one of the most common childhood illnesses. Almost 30 percent of under-five children in the developing world suffer from PEM. On a blueprint agreed to by all countries to overcome the pervasive problems of poverty, malnutrition, diseases, and inequity, the United Nations has set the Millennium Development Goals (MDG) to be achieved by the year 2015. The non-income poverty component of the MDG 1 is to reduce by half the proportion of people suffering from hunger (and malnutrition). The fourth MDG is to reduce by two-thirds the mortality rate among under-five children. Neither of these goals will be achieved unless meaningful and concerted efforts are made to combat and control childhood PEM. The prevalence of child malnutrition in countries of Sub-Saharan Africa is less than that in many countries in Asia, but it is gradually increasing which is a matter of great concern.

Marasmus, a type of PEM characterised by wasting, has been recognised for centuries. Hinajosa in Mexico published the earliest account of kwashiorkor, a severe form of PEM characterised by oedema, in 1865. The acuteness of kwashiorkor has been the focus of attention of nutritionists and as many as 70 names have been given to this condition in different parts of the world. Cicely Willliams first introduced the name kwashiorkor in 1935, which in the Ga language of West Africa means "the disease of the deposed child". This literally refers to the child who develops oedema after being weaned with starchy gruels following the birth of a sibling who is breastfed.

CAUSES OF PEM

Malnutrition due to primary lack of food and interplay of infections is known as primary malnutrition, which is responsible for most of the 112 million children suffering from moderate malnutrition in the developing world. Malnutrition occuring as a result of chronic diseases such as chronic kidney, liver, or heart disease is known as secondary malnutrition. Although lack of food and repeated infections including diarrhoea and pneumonia are the immediate, precipitating causes of malnutrition, the root causes are political in nature interlaced with issues of social and gender inequity particularly of income and education (Fig. 5.1.1).

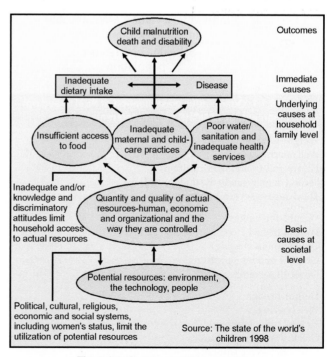

Fig. 5.1.1: Causes of child malnutrition

CLASSIFICATION OF PEM

PEM can be classified best on the basis of anthropometric measurements (comparing body weight and/or height/length with that of reference data of healthy children). The reference data so far used is the National Centre for Health Statistics median. The WHO has introduced a new standard in 2005, which is based on data of children from Asia, Africa, North and Latin America who were exclusively breastfed up to six months of age, and therefore is more representative of a true standard for children globally. Weight-for-age (WA), height-for-age (HA), and weight-for-height (WH) are the three anthropometric indices used in assessing nutritional status (Table 5.1.1). Classification according to WA is known as Gomez classification. Classification by WH or by HA is also called Waterlow classification. A low WA indicates under-nutrition, a low WH wasting or acute malnutrition, while a low HA indicates stunting or chronic malnutrition. Although assessment by WA involves the measurement of weight only and is convenient, a disadvantage of using WA is that the age of children is not reliably known in many communities. Wasting and stunting are commonly seen in children between the ages of 1-2 years, but by 3 to 4 years of age, children are more stunted than wasted. This indicates that these children have stopped growing in height but may have a normal WH.

Nutritional status is also expressed in terms of standard deviation (SD) or z score of an anthropometric index such as WH. This score indicates deviation of a child's nutritional status from median reference values.

$$SD\ score = \frac{Individual's\ value - Median\ value\ of\ reference\ population}{SD\ value\ of\ reference\ population}$$

Table 5.1.1: Quantitative classification of PEM based on percentage of NCHS median reference values

Weight-for-age		
Well nourished	:	90-120%
First degree (mild undernutrition)	:	75-89%
Second degree (moderate undernutrition)	:	60-74%
Third degree (severe undernutrition)	:	<60%
Weight-for-height		
Well nourished	:	90-120%
Grade I (mild wasting)	:	80-89%
Grade II (moderate wasting)	:	70-79%
Grade III (severe wasting)	:	<70%
Height-for-age		
Well nourished	:	95-110%
Grade I (mild stunting)	:	90-94%
Grade II (moderate stunting)	:	85-89%
Grade III (severe stunting)	:	<85%

Malnutrition is defined as less than o2 standard deviations from the median (<o2 z scores). WA, HA and WH less than -3 z constitute severe underweight, severe stunting and severe wasting respectively.

The Wellcome classification is a clinical classification for children admitted to a hospital or a nutrition unit. It is based upon WA and the presence or absence of nutritional. A child with a WA <60% and no oedema is said to have marasmus while a child with WA >60% and has kwashiorkor. Marasmic kwashiorkor is the condition where WA is <60% and there is severe weight reduction, gross wasting of muscle and tissue beneath the skin, stunting, and no characterised marasmus, usually seen in infancy. In a severe case, the body appears to have only skin and bones with wrinkling of the skin, the head looks proportionately large, and the ribs are markedly visible (Table 5.1.2). Usually the child is irritable. Marasmus occurs as a result of severe deficiency of energy, protein, vitamins and minerals, although the primary cause is inadequate energy intake. This deficiency often results when there is a decrease or absence of breastfeeding, feeding diluted milk formula, or delay in introducing solid foods in the diet. In marasmus, the body generally adapts itself to the deficiency of energy and protein. The muscles provide amino acids leading to the production of adequate amounts of proteins including albumin and beta-lipoprotein. Adequate amounts of albumin and beta-lipoprotein prevent the development of oedema and fatty enlargement of the liver in marasmus.

Kwashiorkor, which occurs mostly in children 1-3 years of age, results from a deficiency of dietary protein and is usually associated with an infection. However, Gopalan in India did not find any difference in diets of children developing marasmus or kwashiorkor. He emphasized that the two conditions are interconvertible and the outcome is determined not by the diet but by the child's response. Marasmus according to C. Gopalan is an adapted state and kwashiorkor occurs when there is dysadaptation. Typically there are skin lesions (pigmented

Table 5.1.2: Difference between marasmus and kwashiorkor

Factors	Marasmus	Kwashiorkor
Age	1st year	2nd and 3rd years
Weight-for-age	<60%	60-80%
Oedema	-	+
Skin changes	Less common	Common
Hair changes	Rare	Common
Mental changes	Uncommon (irritability)	Common (loss of interest)
Face	Monkey like	Moon face
Muscle wasting	+++	+
Enlarged liver	+/-	+
Adaptation	Good	Poor
Appetite	Usually good	Poor

or depigmented areas with or without ulceration), scanty lustreless hair, an enlarged fatty liver, loss of interest in the surroundings, and loss of appetite. The oedema is usually noticed in the feet but can also occur in other parts of the body. There is a decrease in blood albumin level, which is partly responsible for development of oedema. Beta-lipoprotein is not produced in adequate amounts, resulting in impaired transport of fat and an enlarged fatty liver.

The child with marasmic kwashiorkor has clinical findings of both marasmus and kwashiorkor. The child has oedema, a WA <60%, gross wasting and is usually stunted. There may be mild hair and skin changes and an enlarged, fatty liver.

A new term, severe acute malnutrition (SAM), is now used to describe the acutely malnourished children (WHO). A child is said to have SAM if any of the following is present:
- Weight-for-height <70% or <-3z
- Bipedal oedema
- Mid upper arm circumference (MUAC) <11 cm (for children between the ages of 1-5 years)

MANAGEMENT OF MILD OR MODERATE MALNUTRITION

Mild and moderately malnourished (underweight or stunted) children account for the major burden of malnutrition in any developing country. Management of these children is, therefore, very important from a public health perspective. These children are managed at the household and community levels. The focus is on counselling of parents on health and nutrition education, care during common illnesses including diarrhoea, micronutrient supplementation, and in many countries periodic deworming. A commonly used strategy in developing countries is growth monitoring and promotion (GMP) where under-five children are weighed at regular intervals and a package of interventions provided at the contacts. Potential strengths of GMP are that it provides frequent contact with health workers and a platform for child health interventions. However, the success of GMP depends on how sincerely the program is carried out.

FACILITY-BASED MANAGEMENT OF SAM

According to the World Health Organisation, a death rate of >20% is unacceptable in the management of severely malnourished children, 11-20% is poor, 5-10% is moderate, 1-4% is good, and <1% is excellent. The reason for the high death rates among severely malnourished children is believed to be faulty case-management. Appropriate feeding, micronutrient supplementation, broad-spectrum antibiotic therapy and judicious use of rehydration fluids (particularly intravenous fluids) are factors that can reduce death, morbidity and cost of treatment of these children. A severely malnourished child having any of the following features should be admitted to a nutrition unit having appropriate facilities and trained staff or referred to a hospital. But these criteria are flexible and may be modified according to local conditions, such as availability of trained staff and facilities. Criteria for referral of a child with SAM to a hospital include:
- Signs of circulatory collapse: cold hands and feet, weak radial pulse, not alert (may be due to severe dehydration or septic shock)
- Convulsion/unconsciousness
- Cyanosis of lips, tongue or finger tips
- Inability to drink
- Chest indrawing
- Fast breathing (60 breaths/min or more in an infant <2 months, >50/min in a child 2 months-1 year, >40/min in a child 1-5 years old)
- Wheezy breathing
- Hypothermia (body temperature <35.5°C)
- High fever (>39.0°C)
- Very severe pallor or anaemia (haemoglobin <5 g/dl)
- Persistent diarrhoea (diarrhoea for >14 days)
- Persistent vomiting (>3 episodes per hour)
- Bloody mucoid stools
- Loss of appetite
- Severe vitamin A deficiency (keratomalacia)
- Jaundice
- Purpura
- Distended, tender abdomen
- Age less than 1 year.

Evaluation of the Severely Malnourished Child

If the child with SAM is acutely ill and requires immediate treatment, details of the history and physical examination should be delayed. History taking should include the following:
- Usual diet given before the present illness
- History of breastfeeding
- Food and fluids taken in the past few days
- Duration, frequency and nature of diarrhoea or vomiting
- Time when urine was last passed
- Recent sinking of the eyes
- Duration and nature of cough
- History of fever
- Contact with measles or tuberculosis
- Major past illness
- Any deaths of siblings
- Milestones reached (sitting, standing, etc)
- Immunisations
- Socio-economic history.

A thorough physical examination should be done, that includes:

- Temperature (for diagnosing fever and hypothermia)
- Respiratory rate and type of respiration (for diagnosing pneumonia and heart failure)
- Signs of circulatory collapse (cold hands and feet, weak/absent radial pulse, not alert)
- Weight, and height or length. Length is measured for children aged <2 years, <85 cm tall, or those who cannot stand.
- Hydration status
- Pallor
- Oedema
- Abdominal distension, bowel sounds
- Enlarged or tender liver, jaundice
- Vitamin A deficiency signs in eyes
- Pus in eyes
- Signs of infection in mouth, throat, ears
- Signs of infection in and around the genital organs
- Appearance of stools (consistency, presence of blood, mucus, or worms).

Laboratory Investigations

Laboratory tests are not essential for management. The following tests should be done if facilities are available:
- Blood glucose if the child is not alert
- Hemoglobin if the child is severely pale
- Urine for pus cells if urinary tract infection is suspected
- X-ray chest if *severe* pneumonia, or if tuberculosis (TB) is suspected
- Mantoux test if TB is suspected (an induration of >5 mm indicates a positive test in a severely malnourished child)

Reductive Adaptation in SAM

Children with SAM undergo physiological and metabolic changes to conserve energy and preserve essential processes. This is known as reductive adaptation. If these changes are ignored during treatment, hypoglycemia, hypothermia, heart failure, untreated infection can cause death. This can be illustrated by the reasons for not giving iron during the initial acute phase treatment of SAM. The child with SAM makes less hemoglobin than usual. Giving iron early in treatment leads to 'free iron' that can cause problems:
- Free iron is highly reactive and promotes formation of free radicals which can damage cell membranes
- Promotes bacterial growth and can make infections worse
- The body tries to convert it into ferritin, the storage form of iron. This uses up essential energy and amino acids.

Therefore, iron should not be given during the acute phase of management of SAM.

PHASES OF MANAGEMENT OF SAM

The management of children with severe malnutrition can be divided into three phases:

Acute Phase

Problems that endanger life, such as hypoglycemia (a low blood glucose level) or an infection, are identified and treated. Feeding and correction of micronutrient deficiencies are initiated during this phase. Broad-spectrum antibiotics are started. Small, frequent feeds are given (about 100 kcal/kg and 1-1.5 g protein/kg per day). The main objective of this phase is to stabilise the child. Case fatality is highest during this phase of management, the principal causes being hypoglycemia, hypothermia, infection, and water-electrolyte imbalance. Most deaths occur within the first 1-2 days of admission. This phase usually takes about 4-5 days.

Nutritional Rehabilitation Phase

The aim of this phase is to recover lost weight by intensive feeding. The child is stimulated emotionally and physically, and the mother is trained to continue care at home. Around 150-250 kcal/kg and 3-5 g protein/kg are provided daily during this phase. Micronutrients, including iron, are continued. Treatment remains incomplete without health and nutrition education of the mothers. This phase takes 2-4 weeks if the criterion of discharge is WHZ -2 without oedema.

Follow up

Follow up is done to prevent relapse of severe malnutrition, and to ensure proper physical growth and mental development of the child. The likelihood of relapse into severe malnutrition is more within one month of discharge. Follow up visits should be fortnightly initially and then monthly until the child has achieved WHZ >-1. Nutritional status and general condition are assessed and the caregivers counselled. Commonly occurring illnesses are treated and health and nutrition education for the caregivers reinforced.

These phases of management can be carried out through the 10 steps of treatment:

STEP 1: TREAT/PREVENT HYPOGLYCEMIA

Hypoglycemia and hypothermia usually occur together and are signs of infection. The child should be tested for hypoglycemia on admission or whenever lethargy, convulsions or hypothermia are found. If blood glucose cannot be measured, all children with SAM should be assumed to be are hypoglycemic and treated accordingly.

If the child is conscious and blood glucose is < 3 mmol/l or 54 mg/dl give:

- 50 ml bolus of 10% glucose or 10% sucrose solution (5 g or 1 rounded teaspoon of sugar in 50 ml or 3.5 tablespoons water), orally or by nasogastric (NG) tube. Then feed starter diet F-75 (see step 7) every 30 min for two hours (giving one quarter of the two-hourly feed each time).
- Two-hourly feeds, day and night for first 24-48 hours (see step 7).

If the child is unconscious, lethargic or convulsing give:

- IV sterile 10% glucose (5 ml/kg) or 25% glucose (2 ml/kg), followed by 50 ml of 10% glucose or sucrose by NG tube.
- Then give starter F-75 as above.

STEP 2: TREAT/PREVENT HYPOTHERMIA

If the axillary temperature is <35.0°C or the rectal temperature is <35.5°C:

- Start feeding right away (or start rehydration if needed)
- Rewarm the child by clothing (including head), covering with a warm blanket or placing the child on the mother's bare chest (skin to skin) and covering them. A heater or lamp may be placed nearby. During rewarming rectal temperature should be taken two hourly until it rises to >36.5°C (half-hourly if heater is used). The child must be kept dry and away from draughts of wind.

STEP 3: TREAT/PREVENT DEHYDRATION

The WHO-ORS (75 mmol sodium/l) contains too much sodium and too little potassium for severely malnourished children. They should be given the special **Re**hydration **So**lution for **Mal**nutrition (ReSoMal) Table 5.1.3. It is difficult to estimate dehydration status in a severely malnourished child. All children with watery diarrhoea should be assumed to have dehydration and given:

- Every 30 minutes for first 2 hours, ReSoMal 5 ml/kg body weight orally or by NG tube, then
- Alternate hours for up to 10 hours, ReSoMal 5-10 ml/kg/h (the amount to be given should be determined by how much the child wants, and stool loss and vomiting). F-75 is given in alternate hours during this period until the child is rehydrated.
- After rehydration, continue feeding F-75 (see step 7).

If diarrhoea is severe then WHO-ORS (75 mmol sodium/l) may be used because loss of sodium in stool is high, and symptomatic hyponatremia can occur with ReSoMal. Severe diarrhoea can be due to cholera or rotavirus infection, and is usually defined as stool output >5 ml/kg/hr.

Return of tears, moist mouth, eyes and fontanelle appearing less sunken, and improved skin turgor, are signs that rehydration is proceeding. It should be noted that many severely malnourished children would not show these changes even when fully rehydrated. Continuing rapid breathing and pulse during rehydration suggest coexisting infection or overhydration. Signs of excess fluid (over hydration) are increasing respiratory rate and pulse rate, increasing oedema and puffy eyelids. If these signs occur, fluids are stopped immediately and the child reassessed after one hour. Intravenous rehydration should be used only in case of shock, infusing slowly to avoid overloading the heart.

STEP 4: CORRECT ELECTROLYTE IMBALANCE

All severely malnourished children have excess body sodium even though serum sodium may be low. Deficiencies of potassium and magnesium are also present and may take at least two weeks to correct. Oedema is partly due to these imbalances and must never be treated with a diuretic.

Give:

- Extra potassium 3-4 mmol/kg/d
- Extra magnesium 0.4-0.6 mmol/kg/d
- When rehydrating, give low sodium rehydration fluid (e.g. ReSoMal)
- Prepare food without salt.

The extra potassium and magnesium can be prepared in a liquid form and added directly to feeds during preparation (Table 5.1.3 for a recipe for a combined electrolyte/mineral solution).

STEP 5: TREAT/PREVENT INFECTION

In severe malnutrition the usual signs of infection, such as fever, are often absent, and infections often hidden. Therefore give routinely on admission:

- Broad-spectrum antibiotics
- Measles vaccine if child is > 6m and not immunised (delay if the child is in shock)

If the child appears to have no complications give:

- Oral amoxycillin 15 mg/kg 8-hourly for 5 days

If the child is sick looking or lethargic or has complications (hypoglycaemia, hypothermia, skin lesions, respiratory tract or urinary tract infection) give:

- Ampicillin 50 mg/kg IM/IV 6-hourly for 2 days, then oral amoxycillin 15 mg/kg 8-hourly for 5 days, and
- Gentamicin 7.5 mg/kg IM/IV once daily for 7 days

If the child fails to improve clinically by 48 hours or deteriorates after 24 hours, a third-generation cephalosporin (e.g. ceftriaxone 50-75 mg/kg/d IV or IM once daily may be started with gentamicin). Ceftriaxone, if available, should be the preferred antibiotic in case of septic shock or meningitis. Where specific infections are identified, add:

- Specific antibiotics if appropriate

Table 5.1.3: Rehydration solution for malnutrition	
Ingredient	*Amount*

Recipe for ReSoMal

Water (boiled and cooled)	2 litres
WHO-ORS	One 1 litre sachet
Sugar	50 g
Electrolyte/mineral solution (see below)	40 ml

ReSoMal contains approximately Na <45 mmol/L, K 40 mmol, and Mg 3 mmol /litre.

Recipe for electrolyte/mineral solution

Weigh the following ingredients and make up to 2500 ml. Add 20 ml of electrolyte/mineral solution to 1000 ml of milk feed.

	g	*molar content of 20 ml*
Potassium chloride	224	24 mmol
Tripotassium citrate	81	2 mmol
Magnesium chloride	76	3 mmol
Zinc acetate	8.2	300 μmol
Copper sulphate	1.4	45 μmol
Water up to	2500 ml	

Note: Add selenium if available and the small amounts can be measured locally (sodium selenate 0.028 g) and iodine (potassium iodide 0.012g) per 2500 ml.

Preparation: Dissolve the ingredients in cooled boiled water. Store the solution in sterilised bottles in the refrigerator to retard deterioration. Make fresh each month and discard if it turns cloudy. If the preparation of this electrolyte/mineral solution is not possible and if premixed sachets are not available, give K, Mg and Zn separately.

Potassium
- Make a 10% stock solution of potassium chloride (KCl), 100 g in 1 litre of water
- For oral rehydration solution, use 45 ml of stock KCl solution instead of 40 ml electrolyte/mineral solution
- For milk feeds, add 22.5 ml of stock KCl solution instead of 20 ml of the electrolyte/mineral solution

Magnesium
- Give sterile magnesium sulphate (50% w/v) intramuscularly once daily (0.1 ml/kg up to a maximum of 2 ml) for 7 days.

Zinc
- Prepare a 1.5% solution of zinc acetate (15 g zinc acetate in 1 litre of water). Give the zinc acetate solution orally, 1 ml/kg/day.

- Antimalarial treatment if the child has a positive blood film for malaria parasites.

If anorexia still persists, reassess the child fully, checking for sites of infection and potentially resistant organisms, and ensure that vitamin and mineral supplements have been correctly given.

STEP 6: CORRECT MICRONUTRIENT DEFICIENCIES

All severely malnourished children have vitamin and mineral deficiencies. Although anemia is common, do not give iron initially but wait until the child has a good appetite and starts gaining weight (usually by the second week), as giving iron can make infections worse.

Give:
- Vitamin A orally on Day 1 (for age >12 months, give 200,000 IU; for age 6-12 months, give 100,000 IU; for age 0-5 months, give 50,000 IU) unless there is definite evidence that a dose has been given in the last month. If the child has xerophthalmia, the same doses of vitamin A are repeated on days 2 and 14 or on day of discharge.

Give daily for the entire period of nutritional rehabilitation (at least 4 weeks):
- Multivitamin supplements
- Folic acid 1 mg/d (5 mg on day 1)
- Zinc 2 mg/kg/d
- Copper 0.3 mg/kg/d
- Iron 3 mg/kg/d but only when gaining weight (start after the stabilisation phase is over).

A combined electrolyte/mineral/vitamin (CMV) mix for severe malnutrition is available commercially. This can replace the electrolyte/mineral solution and multivitamin and folic acid supplements mentioned in steps 4 and 6, but still give the large single dose of vitamin A and folic acid on Day 1, and iron daily after weight gain has started.

STEP 7: START CAUTIOUS FEEDING

During the stabilisation phase a cautious approach is required because of the child's fragile physiological state and reduced capacity to handle large feeds. Feeding should be started as soon as possible after admission. WHO-recommended starter formula, F-75, contains 75 kcal/100 ml and 0.9 g protein/100 ml (Table 5.1.4). Very weak children may be fed by spoon, dropper or syringe. Breastfeeding is encouraged between the feeds of F-75. A recommended schedule in which volume is gradually increased, and feeding frequency gradually decreased is:

Days	Frequency	Vol/kg/feed	Vol/kg/d
1-2	2-hourly	11 ml	130 ml
3-5	3-hourly	16 ml	130 ml
6-7+	4-hourly	22 ml	130 ml

If intake does not reach 80 kcal/kg/d despite frequent feeds, coaxing and re-offering, give the remaining feed by NG tube.

Criteria for increasing volume/decreasing frequency of F-75 feeds:
1. If vomiting, lots of diarrhoea, or poor appetite, continue 2-hourly feeds
2. If little or no vomiting, modest diarrhoea (less than 5 watery stools per day), and finishing most feeds, change to 3-hourly feeds
3. After a day on 3-hourly feeds – if no vomiting, less diarrhoea and finishing most feeds, change to 4-hourly feeds.

In case of SAM infants less than 6 months old, feeding should be initiated with F-75. During the nutritional rehabilitation phase, F-75 can be continued and if possible re-lactation should be done.

STEP 8: ACHIEVE CATCH-UP GROWTH

During the nutritional rehabilitation phase feeding is gradually increased to achieve a rapid weight gain of >10 g gain/kg/d. The recommended milk-based F-100 contains 100 kcal and 2.9 g protein/100 ml (Table 5.1.4). Modified porridges or modified family foods can be used provided they have comparable energy and protein concentrations.

Readiness to enter the rehabilitation phase is signaled by a return of appetite, usually about one week after admission. A gradual transition is recommended to avoid the risk of heart failure, which can occur if children suddenly consume huge amounts.

To change from starter to catch-up formula:
1. Replace F-75 with the same amount of catch-up formula F-100 every 4 hours for 48 hours then,

2. Increase each successive feed by 10 ml until some feed remains uneaten. The point when some remains unconsumed after most feeds is likely to occur when intakes reach about 30 ml/kg/feed (200 ml/kg/d).

If weight gain is:
- Poor (<5 g/kg/d), the child requires full reassessment for other underlying illnesses e.g. TB
- Moderate (5-10 g/kg/d); check whether intake targets are being met, or if infection has been overlooked
- Good (>10 g/kg/d), continue to praise staff and mothers.

STEP 9: PROVIDE SENSORY STIMULATION AND EMOTIONAL SUPPORT

In severe malnutrition there is delayed mental and behavioral development. Just giving diets will improve physical growth but mental development will remain impaired. This is improved by providing tender loving care and a cheerful, stimulating environment. The play sessions should make use of toys made of discarded material.

STEP 10: PREPARE FOR FOLLOW-UP AFTER RECOVERY

A child who has achieved WHZ -2 SD can be considered to have improved. At this point, the child is still likely to have a low weight-for-age because of stunting. Good feeding practices and sensory stimulation should be continued at home. Parents or caregivers should be counseled on:
- Feeding energy- and nutrient-dense foods
- Providing structured plays to the children
- To bring the child back for regular follow-up checks
- Ensure that booster immunisations are given
- Ensure that vitamin A and antihelminthic drugs are given every six months.

TREATMENT OF COMPLICATIONS

Shock in Severely Malnourished Children

Shock may be due to severe dehydration or sepsis, which can coexist and difficult to distinguish from one another. Children with dehydration will respond to IV fluids while those with septic shock and no dehydration may not. Emergency treatment is started with:
- Oxygen inhalation
- Sterile 10% glucose (5 ml/kg) IV
- Infusion of an isotonic fluid at 15 ml/kg over 1 hour
- Measure and record pulse and respiration rates every 10 minutes
- Give broad-spectrum antibiotics (step 5).

Table 5.1.4: Recipes for F-75 and F-100

If you have cereal flour and cooking facilities, use one of the top three recipes for F-75:

Alternatives	Ingredient	Amount for F-75
If you have dried skimmed milk	Dried skimmed milk	25 g
	Sugar	70 g
	Cereal flour	35 g
	Vegetable oil	30 g
	Mineral mix*	20 ml
	Water to make 1000 ml	1000 ml**
If you have dried whole milk	Dried whole milk	35 g
	Sugar	70 g
	Cereal flour	35 g
	Vegetable oil	20 g
	Mineral mix*	20 ml
	Water to make 1000 ml	1000 ml**
If you have fresh cow's milk, or full-cream (Whole) long life milk	Fresh cow's milk, or full-cream (whole) long life milk	300 ml
	Sugar	70 g
	Cereal flour	35 g
	Vegetable oil	20 g
	Mineral mix*	20 ml
	Water to make 1000 ml	1000 ml**

If you do not have cereal flour, or there are no cooking facilities, use one of the following recipes for F-75:   *No cooking is required for F-100*

Alternatives	Ingredient	Amount for F-75	Amount for F-bo
If you have dried skimmed milk	Dried skimmed milk	25 g	80 g
	Sugar	100 g	50 g
	Vegetable oil	30 g	60 g
	Mineral mix*	20 ml	20 ml
	Water to make 1000 ml	1000 ml**	1000 ml**
If you have dried whole milk	Dried whole milk	35 g	110 g
	Sugar	100 g	50 g
	Vegetable oil	20 g	30 g
	Mineral mix*	20 ml	20 ml
	Water to make 1000 ml	1000 ml**	1000 ml**
If you have fresh cow's milk, or full-cream (Whole) long life milk)	Fresh cow's milk, or full-cream (whole) long life milk	300 ml	880 ml
	Sugar	100 g	75 g
	Vegetable oil	20 g	20 g
	Mineral mix*	20 ml	20 ml
	Water to make 1000 ml	1000 ml**	1000 ml**

**Important note about adding water: Add just the amount of water needed to make 1000 ml of formula. (This amount will vary from recipe to recipe, depending on the other ingredients). Do not simply add 1000 ml of water, as this will make the formula too dilute. A mark for 1000 ml should be made on the mixing container for the formula, so that water can be added to the other ingredients up to this mark.

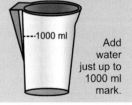

Add water just up to 1000 ml mark.

If there are signs of improvement (pulse and respiration rates fall):
- Repeat infusion 15 ml/kg over 1 hour; then

- Switch to oral or nasogastric rehydration with ReSoMal, 10 ml/kg/h in alternate hours up to 10 hours; Give ReSoMal in alternate hours with starter F-75, then continue feeding with starter F-75

If the child fails to improve (pulse and respiration rates fall) after the first hour of treatment with an infusion 15 ml/kg, assume that the child has septic shock. In this case:

- Give maintenance IV fluids (3 ml/kg/h) while waiting for blood,
- When blood is available transfuse fresh whole blood at 10 ml/kg *slowly* over 3 hours.

Very Severe Anemia in Malnourished Children

A blood transfusion is required if:

- Hb is less than 4 g/dl or packed cell volume < 12%
- Or if there is respiratory distress and Hb is between 4 and 6 g/dl

The child is given whole blood 10 ml/kg body weight slowly over 3 hours and furosemide 1 mg/kg IV at the start of the transfusion. If the severely anemic child has signs of cardiac failure, transfuse packed cells (5-7 ml/kg) rather than whole blood.

In all cases of anemia, oral iron (elemental iron 3 mg/kg/day) should be given for two months to replenish iron stores. This should not be started until the child has begun to gain weight.

Vitamin A deficiency

If the child shows any eye signs of deficiency, give orally:

- Vitamin A on days 1, 2 and 14 (for age >12 months, give 200,000 IU; for age 6-12 months, give 100,000 IU; for age 0-5 months, give 50,000 IU).

    If there is corneal clouding or ulceration, give additional eye care to prevent extrusion of the lens:

- Instil chloramphenicol or tetracycline eye drops (1%) 2-3 hourly as for 7-10 days in the affected eye
- Instil atropine eye drops (1%), 1 drop three times daily for 3-5 days
- Cover with eye pads soaked in saline solution and bandage.

Children with vitamin A deficiency are likely to be photophobic and keep their eyes closed. It is important to examine the eyes very gently to prevent damage and rupture.

Dermatosis

Weeping skin lesions are commonly seen in and around the buttocks of children with kwashiorkor. Affected areas should be bathed in 1% potassium permanganate solution for 15 minutes daily. This dries the lesions, helps to prevent loss of serum, and inhibits infection.

Parasitic Worms

- Give albendazole 400 mg orally, single dose (if > 2 years old)
- Give albendazole 200 mg orally, single dose (if 1 to 2 years old)

This treatment should be given only during the nutritional rehabilitation phase.

Lactose Intolerance

Most children with SAM and diarrhoea respond to the initial management. Diarrhoea due to lactose intolerance in SAM is not common. In exceptional cases, milk feeds may be substituted with yoghurt or a lactose-free formula.

Osmotic diarrhoea may be suspected if diarrhoea worsens substantially in young children who are given F-75 prepared with milk powder (this preparation has slightly higher osmolarity). In such a situation, use F-75 prepared with cereal powder may be helpful.

Tuberculosis

If TB is strongly suspected (contact with adult TB patient, poor growth despite good intake, chronic cough, chest infection not responding to conventional antibiotics):

- Perform Mantoux test (false negatives are frequent in severe malnutrition)
- Chest X-ray if possible.

If test is positive or there is a strong suspicion of TB, treat according to national TB guidelines.

COMMUNITY-BASED MANAGEMENT OF SAM

In countries with a heavy burden of SAM, facilities and resources for taking care of such children are far from being adequate. It is now agreed that children with SAM who have good appetite but no complications can be treated at the community level. Because the number of facilities is always sub-optimal in developing countries, facility-based treatment cannot cater to the huge numbers of severely malnourished children living in the community. Moreover, feeding therapeutic diets including F-75 and F-100 at home is not recommended because of the propensity of these liquid diets to become contaminated in the home environment. To overcome this problem, ready-to-use-therapeutic food (RUTF) has been developed and used in field situations. It is now being used in emergency relief programs. If prepared as per prescription, RUTF has the nutrient composition of F-100 but is more energy dense and does not contain any water. Bacterial contamination, therefore, does not occur and the food is safe for use also in home conditions. The prototype RUTF is made of peanut paste, milk powder, vegetable oil, mineral and vitamin mix as per WHO recommendations. It is available, as a paste in a sachet, does not require any cooking and children can eat directly from the sachet. Local production of RUTF has commenced recently and several studies have concluded that local RUTF is as good as the prototype RUTF.

RUTF seems to play an important role in the management of severe malnutrition in disaster and emergency settings. A supplementary feeding program providing food rations to families of the affected child should be in place. So should be a stabilisation centre for taking care of acutely ill severely malnourished children who need facility-based care based on WHO guidelines. For countries in Asia including India, Bangladesh and Pakistan, which have the highest burden of child malnutrition, there is a need for research on cost-effectiveness and sustainability of management of severe malnutrition using ready-to-use-therapeutic food (RUTF).

Micronutrient Deficiencies in Childhood

Micronutrients represent specific nutrients that impact on health and nutrition outcomes when consumed in small quantities. These micronutrients represent essential ingredients necessary for homeostasis and are affected by a variety of factors including maternal nutrition status, dietary intake, existing morbidity and body losses (Fig. 5.1.2).

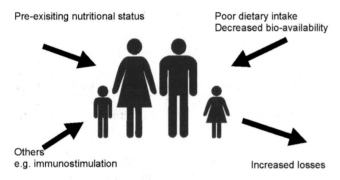

Fig. 5.1.2: Determinants of micronutrient status

Of various micronutrient deficiencies of relevance to children, vitamin A deficiency, iron and zinc deficiency represent the few for which there is considerable body of evidence for adverse outcomes and intervention strategies.

Vitamin A Deficiency in Childhood

Vitamin A is essential for the functioning of the immune system and the healthy growth and development of children. Vitamin A deficiency (VAD) is a public health problem in more than half of all countries, especially in Africa and South-East Asia, hitting hardest young children and pregnant women in low-income countries. VAD is the leading cause of preventable blindness in children and increases the risk of disease and death from severe infections. Globally, it is estimated that 140–250 million children under five years of age are affected by vitamin A deficiency. These children suffer a dramatically increased risk of death, blindness and illness, especially from measles and diarrhoea. While severe ocular manifestations of vitamin A deficiency such as Bitot's spots, xerophthalmia and keratomalacia are fortunately rare, sub-clinical

deficiency of vitamin A is relatively common in poor communities.

For pregnant women in high-risk areas, VAD occurs especially during the last trimester when demand by both the unborn child and the mother is highest. The mother's deficiency is demonstrated by the high prevalence of night blindness during this period. In pregnant women VAD causes night blindness and may increase the risk of maternal mortality.

Vitamin A is also regarded as crucial micronutrient for maternal and child survival and it has been shown that supplying adequate vitamin A in high-risk areas can significantly reduce mortality. Conversely, its absence causes a needlessly high risk of disease and death. Based on these findings a number of preventive and therapeutic strategies are in place for the prevention and treatment of vitamin A deficiencies

Preventive and Therapeutic Strategies

Vitamin A is a crucial component for health throughout the life cycle. In areas with high rates of maternal malnutrition and vitamin A, adequate supply of maternal vitamin A (as well as other nutrients) in pregnancy is a fundamental measure. Since breast milk is a natural source of vitamin A, promoting breastfeeding is the best way to protect babies from VAD.

For deficient children, the periodic supply of high-dose vitamin A in swift, simple, low-cost, high-benefit interventions has also produced remarkable results. It is estimated that this has the potential or reducing child mortality by 23% overall and by up to 50% for those with measles infection.

These measures must be supplemented with measures to promote adequate feeding and dietary diversification. For vulnerable rural families, for instance in Africa and South-East Asia, growing fruits and vegetables in home gardens complements dietary diversification and fortification and contributes to better lifelong health. Where this may be difficult, food fortification is a cost effective measure for providing daily minimal needs for vitamin A. Food fortification, for example sugar in Guatemala, has been shown to adequately maintain population level vitamin A status, especially for high-risk groups and needy families.

Combining the administration of vitamin A supplements with immunisation is an important part of this effort. Since 1987, WHO has advocated the routine administration of vitamin A with measles vaccine in countries where vitamin A deficiency is a problem. Great success and many millions of children have been reached by including vitamin A with National Immunisation Days (NIDs) to eradicate polio. High-dose vitamin A should be avoided during pregnancy because of the theoretical risk of teratogenesis (birth defects). From a programmatic perspective, high-dose vitamin A supplementation must occur during the safe infertile period immediately after delivery. Accordingly, high-dose vitamin A supplementation can be provided safely to all postpartum mothers within six weeks of delivery, when the chance of pregnancy is remote. For breastfeeding mothers, the safe infertile period extends up to eight weeks after delivery. The first contact with the infant immunisation services provides an excellent opportunity to supplement postpartum mothers and improve the vitamin A content of their breast milk.

Provision of vitamin A supplements every four to six months is an inexpensive, quick, and effective way to improve vitamin A status and save children's lives. The Beaton Report concluded that all-cause mortality among children aged 6–59 months was reduced by 23% through vitamin A supplementation in areas where vitamin A deficiency was a public health problem. However, comprehensive control of vitamin A deficiency must include dietary improvement and food fortification in the long term.

Immunisation contacts offer unrivalled opportunities for delivering vitamin A to children who suffer from deficiency. Studies show that vitamin A does not have any negative effect on sero-conversion of childhood vaccines. As well as routine immunisation services, national immunisation days for polio eradication, measles, and multi-antigen campaigns have been used safely and successfully to provide vitamin A to a wide age range of children at risk.

There is a well-established scientific basis for the treatment of measles cases with vitamin A supplementation that is recommended by WHO as part of the integrated management of childhood illness. The recommended doses of vitamin A supplementation for the prevention of vitamin A deficiency are indicated in the following Table 5.1.5.

Iron Deficiency in Childhood

Iron is an important dietary mineral that is involved in various bodily functions, including the transport of oxygen in the blood, essential in providing energy for daily life. Iron is also vital for brain development. Infants, toddlers, preschoolers and teenagers are at high risk of iron deficiency, mainly because their increased needs for iron may not be met by their diets. Without intervention, a child whose dietary intake is inadequate in providing enough iron or has excessive losses through the intestine e.g. with hookworm infestation, will eventually develop iron deficiency (Table 5.1.6).

Causes of Iron Deficiency in Children

Major risk factors for the development of iron deficiency in children include:

Table 5.1.5: Strategies for vitamin A supplementation with immunisations		
Potential target groups and immunisation contacts in countries with vitamin A deficiency Target group	*Immunisation contact*	*Vitamin A dose*
All mothers irrespective of their mode of infant feeding up to six weeks postpartum if they have not received vitamin A supplementation after delivery	BCG, OPV-0 or DTP-1 contact up to six weeks	200 000 IU
Infants aged 9-11 months Children aged 12 months and older	Measles vaccine contact	100 000 IU 200 000 IU
Children aged 1-4 years	Booster doses* Special campaigns* Delayed primary immunisation doses*	200 000 IU

* The optimal interval between doses is four to six months. A dose should not be given too soon after a previous dose of vitamin A supplement: the minimum recommended interval between doses for the prevention of vitamin A deficiency is one month (the interval can be reduced in order to treat clinical vitamin A deficiency and measles cases).

1. Prematurity and low birth weight
2. Exclusive breastfeeding beyond six months
3. Introduction of cow's milk as the main drink before 12 months
4. High intake of cows milk
5. Low or no meat intake and poor quality diet in the second year of life
6. Possible gastrointestinal diseases including coeliac disease and persistent diarrhoea.

Infants, children and teenagers greatly increase their iron requirements during the period of rapid growth spurts, which also increase their need for iron.

Signs and Symptoms

The signs and symptoms of iron deficiency anaemia in children can include:

- Behavioural problems
- Recurrent infections
- Loss of appetite
- Lethargy
- Breathlessness
- Increased sweating
- Strange 'food' cravings (pica) like eating dirt
- Failure to grow at the expected rate.

Table 5.1.6: Iron requirements and recommended iron intakes by age and gender group					
Groups	Age (years)	Mean body weight (kg)	Required iron intake for growth (mg/day)	Median iron losses (mg/day) Basal	Mens-trual
Children	0.5 - 1	9.0	0.55	0.17	
	1 - 3	13.3	0.27	0.19	
	4 - 6	19.2	0.23	0.27	
	7 - 10	28.1	0.32	0.39	
Adolescent boys					
	11 - 14	44.0	0.55	0.62	
	15 – 17	65.4	0.60	0.90	
	18 +	75.0		1.05	
Adolescent girls					
	11 – 14*	46.1	0.55	0.65	
	11 - 14	46.1	0.55	0.65	0.48
	15 - 17	56.4	0.35	0.79	0.48
	18 +	62.0		0.87	0.48

*Non-menstruating

Preventive and Therapeutic Strategies

Suggestions to prevent or treat iron deficiency in babies less than 12 months of age include the following measures:
- Eating an iron-rich diet during pregnancy. Red meat is the best source of iron.
- Regular use of iron folate supplements in pregnancy to ensure adequate iron stores.
- Delayed cord clamping at birth, especially in preterm infants to ensure adequate trans-placental transfer of blood and iron supplies.
- Exclusive breastfeeding for the first six months with the possible introduction of iron drops in preterm or low birth weight infants by 3-4 months of age.
- Avoidance of cow's milk or other fluids that may displace iron-rich solid foods before 12 months of age.
- Timely introduction of good quality complementary foods at six months of age and promotion of iron and zinc containing foods (especially minced meat, liver, poultry etc).
- If affordable, fortified baby cereals may also be used along with pureed fruit and vegetables. Vitamin C helps the body to absorb more iron, so make sure your child has plenty of fruit and vegetables.
- In vegetarian populations, offer good sources of non-haem iron like peas, broccoli, spinach, beans etc.
- In populations at high risk of nutritional anemia other strategies such as the use of Sprinkles with micro-encapsulated iron may also help prevent and treat anemia. However, care must be exercised when using iron supplements in malaria endemic areas as iron

supplementation may increase morbidity and risk of hospitalisation.
- Excessive intakes of tea and coffee may interfere with iron absorption and should be avoided in children.
- Prevention and treatment of infections is an important strategy for anemia prevention as infection is a frequent underlying cause of mild anemia in children.

Zinc in Child Health

Zinc is widely recognised as an essential micronutrient with a catalytic role in over a 100 specific metabolic enzymes in human metabolism. The role of zinc in human health has been recognised for almost half a century with the discovery of the syndrome of zinc deficiency, delayed sexual development and growth failure among adolescents in Iran. Zinc is one of the most ubiquitous of all trace elements involved in human metabolism and plays multiple roles in the perpetuation of genetic material, including transcription of DNA, translation of RNA, and ultimately cellular division. It is thus critical to understand the role of zinc in health and disease, especially during the vulnerable periods of growth and development.

Unlike other essential micronutrients such as iron and vitamin A, there are no conventional tissue reserves of zinc that can be released or sequestered quickly in response to variations in dietary supply. It is recognised that the equivalent of approximately one-third (~450 mg) of total body zinc exchanges between the blood stream and other tissues. The major source of zinc intake is through diet, with the trans-cellular uptake occurring in the distal duodenum and proximal jejunum, potentially facilitated by specific transporters. The intestine also serves as the major conduit for zinc elimination from the body with almost 50% of the daily zinc losses occurring in the gut. However, much of the zinc that is secreted into the intestine is subsequently reabsorbed, and this process serves as an important point of regulation of zinc balance. Other routes of zinc excretion include the urine, which accounts for approximately 15% of total zinc losses, and epithelial cell desquamation, sweat, semen, hair, and menstrual blood, which together account for approximately 17% of total zinc losses.

Table 5.1.7 below indicates the average daily requirements for zinc from a variety of diets.

Growth and Development

Given the multiple metabolic roles of zinc and the earlier reports of the clinical association of zinc deficiency, there has been considerable interest in the potential growth benefits of zinc. Although the primary mechanisms whereby zinc influences growth are uncertain, there is a large body of literature indicating that zinc depletion limits growth and development. These include several studies of zinc supplementation among low birth weight infants

Table 5.1.7: Estimated average requirement (EAR) for zinc by life stage and diet type				
Age	Sex	Reference body weight (kg)	Estimated average Requirement for zinc (mg/d)	
			Mixed or refined vege-tarian diets	Unrefined, cereal-based diets
7-12 months	M+F	9	3	4
1-3 years	M+F	12	2	2
4-8 years	M+F	21	3	4
9-13 years	M+F	38	5	7
14-18 years	M	64	8	11
14-18 years	F	56	7	9

(LBW) in developing countries indicating significant benefits on weight gain and some benefit on linear growth. Subsequent trials in Bangladesh have likewise found greater weight gain among severely malnourished inpatients who received supplemental zinc (10 mg/kg/day up to a maximum of 50 mg/day) during the course of nutritional rehabilitation.

However, there have been relatively fewer reports of a positive effect of zinc supplementation on children's linear growth during recovery from severe malnutrition perhaps related to the duration of supplementation and pre-existing zinc status. A recent meta-analysis of 33 randomised intervention trials evaluating the effect of zinc supplementation on the growth of pre-pubertal children concluded that zinc supplementation produced highly significant positive responses in linear growth and weight gain (mean effect sizes of 0.30-0.35 SD units), with comparatively greater growth responses in children with low initial weight-for-age or height-for-age Z-scores.

Effect of Zinc on Diarrhoea

Given the association and biological plausibility of the role of zinc in intestinal mucosal injury and recovery, a number of randomized controlled trials have demons-trated significant reduction in the incidence and duration of acute and persistent diarrhoea in zinc-supplemented children compared to their placebo-treated counterparts. A pooled analysis of randomised, controlled trials of zinc supplementation performed in nine low-income countries in Latin America and the Caribbean, South and Southeast Asia, and the Western Pacific, demonstrated that supplemental zinc led to an 18% reduction in the incidence of diarrhoea and a 25% reduction in the prevalence of diarrhoea. While the pooled analysis did not find differences in the effect of zinc by age, baseline serum zinc status, presence of wasting, or sex, the relevance of zinc supplementation to various geographic regions of the

world remained unclear. Recent studies from Africa using zinc supplementation in young children indicate significant benefit on diarrhoea burden indicating that the effect may be consistent across various geographical regions and even if zinc is administered with oral rehydration solution. Recent studies in Bangladesh of using zinc in the treatment of diarrhoea in a community setting have also demonstrated substantial reduction in concomitant use of antibiotics by health-care providers, thus suggesting that there may be additional benefits to the use of zinc in the treatment of diarrhoea. It is also anticipated that the forthcoming World Health Assembly will also ratify a joint UNICEF WHO statement that will strongly endorse the use of zinc supplements in young children with diarrhoea.

Respiratory Infections

Despite advances in the recognition and management of acute respiratory infections (ARI), these account for over 20% of all child deaths globally. In preventive trials of zinc supplementation, a significant impact has been shown on the incidence of acute lower respiratory infections. The recent pooled analysis of trials conducted in India, Jamaica, Peru and Vietnam indicated an overall 41% reduction in the incidence of pneumonia among zinc-supplemented children. More recently, the administration of zinc to children hospitalized with pneumonia in Bangladesh has been shown to reduce the severity and length of hospitalisation.

Malaria

The benefits of zinc supplementation on the severity of disease and outcome of malaria are less straightforward. Bates et al administered 70 mg zinc twice weekly for eighteen months to children in Gambia and were able to show 32 % reduction in clinic visits due to *P. falciparum* infections. Similarly a trial undertaken in Papua New Guinea among pre-school children indicated a 38% reduction in clinic visits attributable to *P. falciparum* parasitemia as well as heavy parasitemia. In contrast a recent trial in Burkina Faso did not find any reduction in episodes of falciparum malaria among children who received daily supplementation with 10 mg zinc for six months. This variable effect of zinc in malarial areas may be related to an impact on the severity of disease rather than the incidence.

Preventive and Therapeutic strategies

Although there is considerable potential for zinc for improving child health in public health settings, there are few intervention strategies to address this at scale. There is a real need for large effectiveness trials in representative settings that may help understand and develop mechanisms for the use of zinc in health systems in a replicable and sustainable manner. Presently the most effective strategies for improving zinc status are improved maternal nutrition in pregnancy, exclusive breastfeeding. dietary diversification during the weaning period and the use of zinc for the treatment of diarrhoea.

BIBLIOGRAPHY

1. Ahmed T, Ali M, Ullah M, Choudhury IA, Haque ME, Salam MA, Rabbani GH, Suskind RM, Fuchs GJ. Mortality in severely malnourished children with diarrhoea and use of a standardised management protocol. Lancet 1999;353:1919-22.
2. Ahmed T, Begum B, Badiuzzaman, Ali M, Fuchs G. Management of severe malnutrition and diarrhoea. Indian Journal of Pediatrics 2001; 68:45-51.
3. Beaton GH, Martorell R, L'Abbé, et al. Effectiveness of vitamin A supplementation in the control of young child morbidity and mortality in developing countries. UN, ACC/SCN State-of-the-art Series, Nutrition policy Discussion Paper No. 13, 1993.
4. Bhutta ZA, Ahmed T, Black RE, Cousens S et al. What works? Interventions to affect maternal and child undernutrition and survival globally. Lancet (2007 in press).
5. Bhutta ZA. Effect of infections and environmental factors on growth and nutritional status in developing countries. J Pediatr Gastroenterol Nutr. 2006 Dec;43 Suppl 3:S13-21.
6. Bhutta ZA. The role of zinc in child health in developing countries: taking the science where it matters. Indian Pediatr. 2004;41:429-33.
7. Collins S. Treating severe acute malnutrition seriously. Arch Dis Child 2007;92:453–461.
8. Jones G, Steketee RW, Black RE, Bhutta ZA, Morris SS. How many child deaths can we prevent this year?. Lancet 2003;362:65:65-71.
9. WHO/UNICEF/IVACG. Vitamin A supplements: a guide to their use in the treatment and prevention of vitamin A deficiency and xerophthalmia (2nd edition.) Geneva: World Health Organisation; 1997.
10. World Health Organization, Management of the child with a serious Infection or severe malnutrition. Guidelines for care at the first-referral Level in developing countries. Geneva: World Health Organisation, 2000 (WHO/FCH/CAH/00.1).
11. World Health Organization, Management of severe malnutrition. A manual for physicians and other senior health workers. Geneva: World Health Organisation, 1999.

5.2: Other Disturbances of Nutrition

VITAMIN D DEFICIENCY

Rickets is a metabolic disturbance of growth, which affects bone, skeletal muscles and sometimes the nervous system. The disorder is due primarily to an insufficiency of vitamin D3 (cholecalciferol), which is a naturally occurring steroid. It can be formed in the skin from 7-dehydrocholesterol by irradiation with ultraviolet light in the wavelengths 280-305 nm; or it can be ingested in the form of fish-liver oils, eggs, butter, margarine and meat. The most important natural source of vitamin D is that formed from solar irradiation of the skin. Ultra-violet irradiation of ergosterol produces vitamin D2 (ergocalciferol), which, in humans, is a potent antirachitic substance. It is, however, not a natural animal vitamin and may have some adverse effects. Less vitamin D is made in the skin of dark-skinned people than white skinned people.

VITAMIN D METABOLISM

Cholecalcificerol (D3) is converted in the liver to 25-hydroxyvitamin D3 (25-OHD3) by means of enzymatic hydroxylation in the C25 position. This metabolite circulates in the plasma with a transport protein, which migrates with the alphaglobulins. It is then 1α-hydroxylated in the kidney to 1,25-dihydroxyvitamin D3 (1,25 (OH)2 D3) by the action of 25-hydroxyvitamin D hydroxylase. Its production appears to be regulated by several factors, including the phosphate concentration in the plasma, the renal intracellular calcium and phosphate concentrations, and parathyroid hormone. It acts on the cells of the gastrointestinal tract to increase calcium absorption and on bone to increase calcium resorption. In the kidney it improves the reabsorption of calcium whilst causing a phosphate diuresis. It also acts on muscle, with the ability to correct the muscle weakness often associated with rickets.

Vitamin D deficiency causes a fall in the concentration of calcium in extracellular fluid, which in turn stimulates parathormone production. The phosphate diuresis effect of a raised parathyroid hormone level results in lowering of the plasma phosphate. This produces the low (Ca) x (P) product, which is such a characteristic feature of active rickets. This stage is quickly followed by an increase in the plasma alkaline phosphatase concentration and then by radiological and clinical features of rickets.

Aetiology

Deficiency of vitamin D, which once resulted in so much infantile rickets, with its toll of permanent deformities and death during childbirth, arose principally because of the limited amount of sunshine and skyshine in northern latitudes. Furthermore, in large industrial cities the sky shine contained very little ultra-violet light after filtering through dust, smoke and fog. The need in a cold climate for heat-retaining clothing and the tendency to remain indoors in inclement weather further deprived infants of ultra-violet radiation. The natural diet of the human infant contains little vitamin D, especially if fed artificially on cow's milk. Cereals, which are commonly used, have a rachitogenic effect because the phosphorus in cereals is in an unavailable form, phytic acid (inositol-hexaphosphoric acid) that combines with calcium and magnesium in the gut to form the complex compound, phytin. It is essential to fortify the infant's diet with vitamin D if rickets is to be avoided. This would not be necessary in the wholly breast-fed infant living in a sunny land.

Another important causative factor, necessary for the development of rickets, is growth. The marasmic infant does not develop rickets when vitamin D deficient until re-fed and growth commences. The preterm low birth weight infant who grows rapidly is particularly prone to develop rickets. There is evidence that hydroxylation of vitamin D in the liver of preterm infants is impaired and this together with dietary phosphate deficiency is an important factor in the osteopenia of preterm infants.

Pathology

In the normal infant there is a zone of cartilage between the diaphysis and the epiphysis the epiphyseal plate. At the epiphyseal end this cartilage is actively growing (proliferative zone); whereas at the diaphyseal end, where mature cartilage cells are arranged in orderly columns, osteoblasts lay down calcium phosphate to form new bone. In rickets the cartilage near the diaphysis (resting zone) shows a disordered arrangement of capillaries and although osteoblasts are numerous normal calcification does not take place. This is called osteoid tissue. In the meantime active growth of the proliferative zone continues so that the epiphyseal plate is enlarged and swollen. Osteoid tissue instead of normal bone is also formed under the periosteum. There is also, in severe cases, a general decalcification of the skeleton so that curvatures and deformities readily develop.

The diagnosis of infantile rickets is not difficult but its rarity in developed countries has resulted in its being unfamiliar to many doctors. A careful dietary history with especial reference to the ingestion of vitamin D fortified milks and cereals and of vitamin supplements will reveal the child who is at risk In the case of mothers with osteomalacia from their own malnutrition, rickets has been present in their infants at birth, as the fetal requirements of 25-OHD3 are obtained directly from the maternal pool. In congenital rickets the presenting feature is usually a hypocalcaemic convulsion although typical bone changes

are to be expected in radiographs. Subclinical maternal and fetal vitamin D deficiency has also been found in white mothers and infants, particularly in infants born in early spring. It causes compensatory maternal hyperpara-thyroidism, and dental enamel defects in the infant's primary dentition. Such infants are predisposed to neonatal tetany if fed on unmodified cow's milk.

There are few subjective signs of rickets. Head sweating is probably one. General muscular hypotonia encourages abdominal protuberance; this can be increased by flaring out of the rib margins and by fermentation of the excess carbohydrate so commonly included in the diets of nutritionally ignorant people. The rachitic child commonly suffers from concomitant iron deficiency anaemia. His frequent susceptibility to respiratory infections is related more to the poor environment and overcrowding rather than to the rickets. The same applies to the unhappy irritable behaviour which rachitic children sometimes exhibit.

Key Learning Points

- Vitamin D deficiency leads to rickets in children, which is due to undermineralisation of bone.
- There are few rich sources of vitamin D and it is unlikely that requirements of infants can be met without the use of supplements or food enrichment.
- Some infants are especially sensitive to hypercalcaemia due to vitamin D toxicity.

The objective signs of rickets are found in the skeleton. The earliest physical sign is craniotabes. This is due to softening of the occipital bones where the head rubs on the pillow. When the examiner's fingers press upon the occipital area the bone can be depressed in and out like a piece of old parchment or table tennis ball. Another common early sign is the "rachitic rosary" or "beading of the ribs" due to swelling of the costochondral junctions. The appearance is of a row of swellings, both visible and palpable, passing downwards and backwards on both sides of the thorax in the situation of the rib ends (Fig. 5.2.1). Swelling of the epiphyses is also seen at an early stage, especially at the wrists, knees and ankles.

In severe cases the shafts of the long bones may develop various curvatures leading to genu varum, genu valgum and coxa vara (Fig. 5.2.2). A particularly common deformity, shown in Fig. 5.2.2, is curvature at the junction of the middle and lower thirds of the tibiae. This is often due to the child, who may have "gone off his feet", being sat on a chair with his feet projecting over the edge in such a fashion that their weight bends the softened tibial shafts. Bossing over the frontal and parietal bones, due to the subperiosteal deposition of osteoid, gives the child a broad square forehead, or the "hot-cross-bun head". The anterior fontanelle may not close until well past the age of eighteen months, although this delay can also occur in hypo-thyroidism, hydrocephalus, and even in some healthy

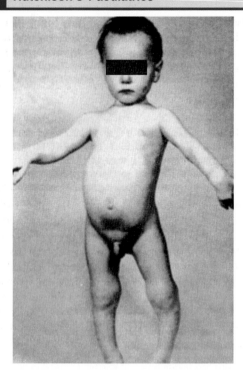

Fig. 5.2.1: Twenty-month-old child with rickets. Note swollen radial epiphyses, enlarged costochondral junctions, bowing of tibiae and lumbar lordosis

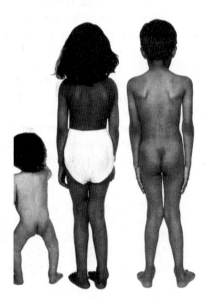

Fig. 5.2.2: Rickets-showing genu valgum (knock knee) and genu varum (bowleg)

children. Another deformity affecting the bony thorax results in Harrison's grooves. These are seen as depressions or sulci on each side of the chest running parallel to but above the diaphragmatic attachment. This sign, however, may also develop in cases of congenital heart disease, asthma and chronic respiratory infections. Laxity

of the spinal ligaments can also allow the development of various spinal deformities such as dorsolumbar kyphoscoliosis. In children who have learned to stand there may be an exaggerated lumbar lordosis. The severely rachitic child will also be considerably dwarfed. Pelvic deformities are not readily appreciated in young children but in the case of girls can lead to severe difficulty during childbirth in later years. The pelvic inlet may be narrowed by forward displacement of the sacral promontory, or the outlet may be narrowed by forward movement of the lower parts of the sacrum and of the coccyx.

Radiological Features

The normally smooth and slightly convex ends of the long bones become splayed out with the appearance of fraying or "cupping" of the edges. The distance between the diaphysis and the epiphysis is increased because the metaphysis consists largely of non-radioopaque osteoid tissue. Periosteum may be raised because of the laying down of osteoid tissue, and the shafts may appear decalcified and curved. In the worst cases greenstick fractures with poor callus formation may occur. The earliest sign of healing is a thin line of preparatory calcification near the diaphysis (Figs 5.2.3 (a) and (b) followed by calcification in the osteoid just distal to the frayed ends of the diaphysis. In time both the ends and shafts of the bone usually return to normal.

BIOCHEMICAL FINDINGS

Typical findings are a normal plasma calcium concentration (2.25-2.75 mmol/l; 9-11 mg per 100 ml) whereas the plasma phosphate (normally 1.6 - 2.26 mmol/l; 5-7 mg per 100 ml) is markedly reduced to between 0.64 and 1 mmol/l (2-3 mg per 100 ml). The normal plasma calcium

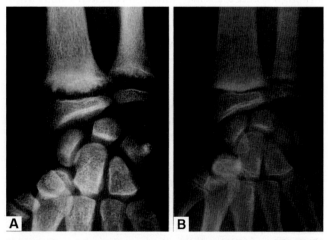

Fig. 5.2.3A and B: A. Florid rickets showing splaying and fraying of ends of the long bones **B.** Radiograph of the same case as in Rickets had healed

in the presence of diminished intestinal absorption of calcium is best explained on the basis of increased parathyroid activity, which mobilizes calcium from the bones. Plasma phosphate diminishes due to the phosphaturia, which results from the effects of parathyroid hormone on the renal tubules. A plasma calcium x phosphorus product (mg per 100 ml) above 40 excludes rickets, while a figure below 30 indicates active rickets. This formula is useful in clinical practice but it has no real meaning in terms of physical chemistry. The plasma alkaline phosphatase activity (normal 56-190 IU/litre) is markedly increased in rickets and only returns to normal with effective treatment. It is, in fact, a very sensitive and early reflection of rachitic activity but can be raised in a variety of unrelated disease states such as hyperparathyroidism, obstructive jaundice, fractures, malignant disease of bone and the "battered baby" syndrome. The mean 25-OHD3 levels in healthy British children are 30 nmol/l (12.5 mg/l), although considerably greater concentrations are reported from the USA. In children with active rickets, the level of 25-OHD3 may fall below 7.5 nmol/l (3 mg/l). However, it is not possible to equate the presence of rickets with particular absolute values for 25-OHD3, although its measurement can provide the most sensitive index of the vitamin D status of a population. Plasm 1, 25 $(OH)_2$ D can also be measured but is a specialized investigation.

Differential Diagnosis

Few diseases can simulate infantile rickets. In hypophosphatasia some of the clinical and radiological features resemble those seen in rickets, but their presence in the early weeks of life exclude vitamin D deficiency. Other features such as defective calcification of the membranous bones of the skull, low plasma alkaline phosphatase and hypercalcaemia are never found in rickets. The characteristic features of achondroplasia - short upper limb segments, large head with relatively small face and retroussé nose, trident arrangement of the fingers, lordosis, waddling gait, and X-ray evidence of endochondral ossification - are unmistakenly different from anything seen in rickets. The globular enlargement of the hydrocephalic skull is quite distinct from the square bossed head of severe rickets. The bone lesions of congenital syphilis are present in the early months of life and are associated with other characteristic clinical signs such as rashes, bloody snuffles, hepatosplenomegaly and lymphadenopathy. In later childhood the sabre-blade tibia of syphilis shows anterior bowing and thickening which is different from rachitic bowing. Some healthy toddlers show an apparent bowing of the legs due to the normal deposition of fat over the outer aspects; this is unimportant and temporary, and there are no other signs of skeletal abnormality. Other normal young children have a mild,

and physiological, degree of genu valgum due to a mild valgus position of the feet; in rachitic genu valgum there will be other rickety deformities. Other types of rickets due to coeliac disease and renal disease must be excluded by appropriate investigations. Their existence is almost always indicated in a carefully taken history.

Prevention

It is important to keep a degree of awareness of the problem of rickets, as the feeding pattern of many adolescents in inner city areas would indicate that they are unaware and/ or unconcerned of the need to ensure an adequate vitamin D status for themselves and for their children. Departments of health are striving hard to maintain a public awareness of the importance of nutrition to health and through the supply of vitamin D fortified foods are endeavouring to prevent the recrudescence of this preventable disorder. The United States Institute of Medicine estimates 'adequate intakes' (AI) of vitamin D for those with no sun-mediated synthesis in the skin.- for ages 0-50 years (including pregnancy and lactation), the AI is 5µg/day.

Treatment

Although rickets can be healed by exposure to ultraviolet light it is more practicable and reliable to administer vitamin D in adequate dosage by mouth. A suitable dose is 1600 - 2000 International Units (IU) orally (1 mg calciferol = 40,000 IU). This can be achieved using the BP or a proprietary concentrated preparation. Although calcium deficiency *per se* very rarely has caused rickets there should be an adequate amount of calcium in the infant's diet (approx 600 mg/day). This is contained in l pint (600 ml) of milk per day. An alternative method of treatment, especially useful where it is suspected that the parents are unreliable and unlikely to administer a daily dose of vitamin D, is the oral or intramuscular administration of a massive dose of vitamin D ("Stoss therapy") (300,000 - 600,000IU). It is, however, uncertain how much of such a large dose the body can utilize although rapid healing of rickets can be confidently expected. Some children are unusually sensitive to vitamin D and a rare condition with elfin facial appearance, William syndrome can occur.

Even major deformities will disappear with adequate treatment in the young child and surgical correction is rarely required. The child should be kept from weight bearing until X-rays show advanced healing, to prevent aggravation of the deformities. The parent of a rachitic child requires education in nutrition and childcare. They should be urged to take the child, after treatment, for regular supervision by their family doctor or at a local child health clinic.

VITAMIN C (ASCORBIC ACID)

Aetiology

The primary cause is an inadequate intake of vitamin C (ascorbic acid), a vitamin that the human unlike most other animals is unable to synthesize within his own body. It is rare in the breast-fed infant unless the mother has subclinical avitaminosis C. Cow's milk contains only about a quarter of the vitamin C content of human milk and this is further reduced by boiling, drying or evaporating. Scurvy is particularly common in infants who receive a high carbohydrate diet. The suggested recommended dietary allowance is 35 mg/day.

Pathology

Vitamin C deficiency results in faulty collagen, which affects many tissues including bone, cartilage and teeth. The intercellular substance of the capillaries is also defective. This results in spontaneous haemorrhages and defective ossification affecting both the shafts and the metaphyseo-epiphyseal junctions. The periosteum becomes detached from the cortex and extensive sub-periosteal haemorrhages occur; these explain the intense pain and tenderness, especially of the lower extremities.

Clinical Features

Increasing irritability, anorexia, malaise and low-grade fever develop between the ages of 7 and 15 months. A most striking feature is the obvious pain and tenderness which the infant exhibits when handled, e.g. during napkin changing. The legs are most severely affected and they characteristically assume a position ("frog-position") in which the hips and knees are flexed and the feet are rotated outwards. Gums become swollen and discoloured and may bleed; this is seen only after teeth have erupted and the teeth may become loose in the jaws. Periorbital ecchymosis ("black eye") or proptosis due to retro-orbital haemorrhage is common but haemorrhages into the skin, epistaxis or gastrointestinal haemorrhages are not commonly seen in infantile scurvy. The anterior ends of the ribs frequently become visibly and palpably swollen but this does not affect the costal cartilages as in rickets; the sternum has the appearance of having been displaced backwards. Microscopic haematuria is frequently present.

RADIOLOGICAL FEATURES

The diagnosis is most reliably confirmed by X-rays. The shafts of the long bones have a "ground-glass" appearance due to loss of normal trabeculation. A dense white line of calcification (Fraenkel's line) forms proximal to the epiphyseal plate and there is often a zone of translucency due to an incomplete transverse fracture immediately proximal to Fraenkel's line. A small spur of bone may project from the end of the shaft at this point ("the corner sign"). The epiphyses, especially at the knees, have the appearance of being "ringed" by white ink. Subperiosteal haemorrhages only become visible when they are undergoing calcification but a striking X-ray appearance is then seen (Fig. 5.2.4).

Diagnosis

Measurement of vitamin C in serum and leukocytes is the common means of assessing vitamin C status. For practical purposes, measurement of vitamin C in serum is preferred over leukocyte measurement. Measurement of urinary vitamin C in patients suspected of scurvy can provide supportive diagnostic information. There are no reliable functional tests of vitamin C.

Key Learning Points
• Vitamin C deficiency manifests as scurvy.
• Vitamin C status is assessed by plasma and leukocyte concentrations.
• At intakes above 100 mg/day the vitamin is excreted quantitatively with intake in the urine.
• There is little evidence that high intakes have any beneficial effects, but equally there is no evidence of any hazard from high intakes.

Treatment and Prevention

The most rapid recovery can be obtained with oral ascorbic acid, 200 mg per day. There is no advantage in parenteral

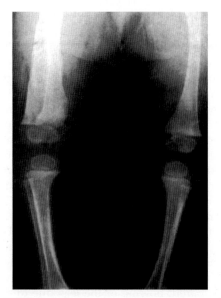

Fig. 5.2.4: Radiograph from a case of infantile scurvy in the healing stage with calcified subperiosteal haematoma. Note also "ringing of epiphyses, Fraenkels' white lines and proximal zone of translucency

administration. Excess vitamin C is excreted in the urine and there is no evidence that vitamin C is in any way poisonous. In developed countries the usual cause of vitamin C deficiency is ignorance of the parents of the need to supply adequate amounts of vitamin C or alternatively some obsessive parents boil fruit juices, which would normally supply adequate vitamin C to the child, but the act of boiling destroys the ascorbic acid.

Vitamin B Deficiencies

The B vitamins are widely distributed in animal and vegetable foods. Deficiency of one of the B group vitamins is commonly associated with deficiencies of the others. The main functions of B vitamins are as cofactors for metabolic processes or as precursors of essential metabolites. Deficiencies occur when there is severe famine, where there are dietary fads, where diets are severely restricted or where there has been inappropriate preparation of the food. Many B vitamins are destroyed by cooking.

Thiamine (Vitamin B₁) Deficiency

Thiamine, as are all the B vitamins, is water soluble and readily destroyed by heat and alkali. It is necessary for mitochondrial function and for the synthesis of acetylcholine. It is present in a wide variety of foods but deficiency states have been particularly common in communities where polishing rice and refining flour has removed the vitamin B containing husks. Beri-beri is now rare in the countries where it was originally described – Japan, Indonesia and Malaysia.

Clinical Features

Deficiency of thiamine (beri-beri) causes clinical manifestations in the nervous and cardiovascular systems predominantly although all tissues are affected. There is degeneration of peripheral nerve fibres and haemorrhage and vascular dilatation in the brain (Wernicke encephalopathy). There can be high output cardiac failure and erythemas. Signs of the disease develop in infants born to thiamine deficient mothers at the age of 2 to 3 months. They appear restless with vasodilatation, anorexia, vomiting and constipation and pale with a waxy skin, hypertonia and dyspnoea. There is peripheral vasodilatation and bounding pulses with later development of, hepatomegaly and evidence of cardiac failure. The is due to a combination of the peripheral vasodilatation and decreased renal flow. This is known as the "wet" form of beri-beri. There is reduction of the phasic reflexes at knee and ankle.

In older children "dry" beri-beri or the neurological complication of thiamine deficiency results in paraesthesia and burning sensations particularly affecting the feet. There is generalised muscle weakness and calf muscles are tender. Tendon reflexes may be absent, a stocking and glove peripheral neuritis develops and sensory loss accompanies the motor weakness. Increased intracranial pressure, meningism and coma may follow.

Key Learning Points

The classical thiamine deficiency disease beri-beri, affecting the pripheral nervous system, is now rare. Thiamine status is assessed by erythrocyte transketolase activation coefficient.

Diagnosis

There are few useful laboratory tests although in severe deficiency states the red blood cell transketolase is reduced and lactate and pyruvate may be increased in the blood, particularly after exercise.

Treatment

The usual thiamine requirement is 0.5 mg per day during infancy and 0.7 - 1 mg daily for older children. Pregnant and lactating women should have a minimal intake of 1 mg per day. Treatment of B₁ deficiency is 10 mg per day for infants and young children increasing to 50 mg per day for adults. In the infant with cardiac failure intravenous or intramuscular thiamine (100 mg daily) can be given. The response can at times be dramatic. There is no evidence of any toxic effect of high intakes of thiamine, although high parenteral doses have been reported to cause anaphylactic shock.

RIBOFLAVINE (VITAMIN B₂) DEFICIENCY

Clinical Features

Deficiency is usually secondary to inadequate intake although in biliary atresia and chronic hepatitis there may be malabsorption. Clinical features are those common to a number of B group deficiency states namely cheilosis, glossitis, keratitis, conjunctivitis, photophobia and lacrimation. Cheilosis begins with pallor, thinning and maceration of the skin at the angles of the mouth and then extends laterally. The whole mouth may become reddened and swollen and there is loss of papillae of the tongue. A normochromic, normocytic anaemia is secondary to bone marrow hypoplasia. There may be associated seborrhoeic dermatitis involving the nasolabial folds and forehead. Conjunctival suffusion may proceed to proliferation of blood vessels onto the cornea

Diagnosis

Urinary riboflavine excretion of less than 30 mg per day is characteristic of a deficiency state. There is reduction of red cell glutathione reductase activity.

Treatment

Riboflavine is present in most foods although the best sources are milk and milk products, eggs, liver, kidney, yeast extracts and fortified breakfast cereals. However, riboflavine is unstable in ultraviolet (UV) light, and after milk has been exposed to sunlight for 4 hours, up to 70% of riboflavine is lost.

In childhood the daily requirement for riboflavine is 0.6 mg per 4.2 mJ (1000 kcal) and treatment of a deficiency state requires 10 mg oral riboflavine daily. In some circumstances riboflavine 2 mg three time per day can be given by intramuscular injection until there is clinical improvement.

Key Learning Points
• Riboflavine deficiency is relatively common.
• Phototherapy for neonatal hyperbilirubinaemia can cause iatrogenic riboflavine deficiency.

Pellagra (Niacin Deficiency)

Niacin is the precursor of nicotinamide, adenine dinucleotide (NAD) and its reduced form NADP. It can be synthesised from trytophan and pellagra tends to occur when maize, which is a poor source trytophan and niacin, is the staple diet. Niacin is lost in the milling process. Communities where millet, which has a high leucine content, is consumed also have a high incidence of pellagra.

Clinical Features

The classical triad for pellagra is diarrhoea, dermatitis and dementia although in children the diarrhoea and dementia are less obvious than in the adolescent and adult. There is light-sensitive dermatitis on exposed areas, which can result in blistering and desquamation of the skin. On healing the skin becomes pigmented (Fig. 5.2.5). The children are apathetic and disinterested and feed poorly because of an associated glossitis and stomatitis.

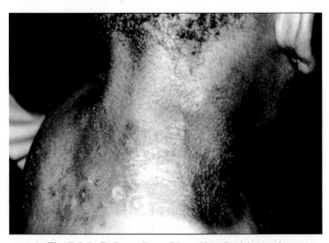

Fig. 5.2.5: Pellagra-"casal's necklace" on the neck

Diagnosis

The two methods of assessing niacin deficiency are measurement of blood nicotinamide nucleotides and the urinary excretion of niacin metabolites, neither of which is wholly satisfactory.

Treatment

The normal requirement for niacin in infancy and childhood is 8 to 10 mg per day when the tryptophan intake is adequate. Deficiency states can be treated with up to 300 mg per day given orally but care must be taken, as large doses will produce flushing and burning sensations in the skin. There is almost always other associated vitamin B deficiencies and these should be supplied during the treatment of pellagra. Because of the intimate involvement of the three major B vitamins described in intermediary metabolism the requirement is best determined in relation to energy intake. Recommended intakes on this basis are: thiamine 0.4 mg per 4.2 mJ (l00 kcal); riboflavine 0.55 mg per 4.2 mJ; niacin 6.6 mg per 4.2 mJ.

Vitamin B$_6$ (Pyridoxine Deficiency)

Vitamin B$_6$ occurs in nature in three forms: pyridoxine, pyridoxal and pyridoxamane, which are interconvertible within the body. The principal one in the body and in food is pyridoxal.

There may be inadequate intake of dietary pyridoxine when there is prolonged heat processing of milk and cereals or when unsupplemented milk formulae or elemental diets are used. There can be inadequate absorption in coeliac disease and drug treatment with izoniazid, penicillamine and oral contraceptives will aggravate deficiency states.

The disorder has to be differentiated from pyridoxine dependency in which pyridoxine dependent convulsions and anaemia are secondary to a genetic disorder of the apo enzyme. Deficiency on its own is rare; it is most often seen with deficiencies of other vitamins, or with protein deficiency.

Clinical Features

Pyridoxine deficiency states result in convulsions, peripheral neuritis, cheilosis, glossitis (as in riboflavine deficiency), seborrhoea and anaemia and impaired immunity. The anaemia is microcytic and is aggravated when intercurrent infections complicate the clinical picture. There may be oxaluria with bladder stones, hyperglycinaemia, lympho-penia and decreased antibody production.

Diagnosis

There is increased xanthurenic acid in the urine after an oral dose of the aminoacid tryptophan. Glutamine-oxalo acetic acid transaminase is reduced in the red cells.

Treatment

The usual requirements for non-pyridoxine dependent individuals are 0.5 mg per day in infancy and 1 mg per day in children.

Vitamin B$_{12}$

If maternal vitamin B$_{12}$ status is satisfactory the reserves of B$_{12}$ in the term newborn infant should last throughout the first year of life especially if the infant is breastfed. Dietary deficiency of vitamin B$_{12}$ is unusual except amongst the strict vegans who consume neither milk nor eggs. Absorption of B$_{12}$ requires a gastric intrinsic factor, which promotes absorption in the terminal ileum. Deficiency of intrinsic factor, secondary to gastric achlorhydria is rare in childhood. It has been reported secondarily to the development of gastric parietal cell antibody but this is extremely rare. Familial pernicious anaemia is secondary to a series of autosomal recessively inherited defects in B$_{12}$ metabolism or in the function of B$_{12}$ binding proteins. Resection of the terminal ileum or Crohn's disease will predispose children to B$_{12}$ deficiency unless B$_{12}$ supplementation is given.

Clinical Features

Pallor, anorexia and glossitis are common features. Paraesthesia with loss of position and vibration sense is a disorder of adolescence rather than childhood. There is a megaloblastic anaemia with neutropenia, thrombocytopenia and hypersegmentation of polymorphonuclear leucocytes. The bone marrow shows a megaloblastic, erythroid picture with giant metamyelocytes.

The neurological signs of subacute combined degeneration of the cord with peripheral neuritis; degeneration of the dorsal columns and corticospinal tract is a late phenomenon as is retrobulbar neuropathy.

Diagnosis

Serum vitamin B$_{12}$, normal levels range from 200 to 900 pg/ml or over 150 pmol/L. Deficiency is indicated by values below this. Elevated serum or urinary excretion of methylmalonate and raised plasma homocysteine are the other biochemical tests indicating low B$_{12}$ status. Schilling test is used to confirm the diagnosis of pernicious anaemia. It measures oral absorption of vitamin B$_{12}$ labelled with radioactive cobalt on two occasions, the first without and the second test with intrinsic factor (IF).

Key Learning Points

Dietary deficiency of vitamin B$_{12}$ occurs only in strict vegans; there are no plant sources of the vitamin B$_{12}$.

Treatment

In the rare instance of dietary deficiency oral supplementation is satisfactory. Where there is inadequate absorption intramuscular injections, initially of 1 mg per day reducing to 1 mg at three monthly intervals in the light of clinical improvement is the usual management in older children and adolescents Hydroxocobalamine has completely replaced cyanocobalamin as the form of vitamin B$_{12}$ of choice for therapy; it is retained in the body longer than cyanocobalamin and thus for maintenance therapy can be given at intervals of up to 3 months. Treatment is generally initiated with frequent administration of intramuscular injections to replenish the depleted body stores.

Folate Deficiency

The word folic is from the Latin 'folia' (leaf), coined in 1941 for an early preparation of this vitamin from spinach leaves.

Deficiency of folic acid is widespread in many communities and is a known factor in the aetiology of neural tube defects. Although found widely in plant and animal tissues the vitamin is easily destroyed by cooking and storage processes. Requirements for growth during fetal and neonatal life and childhood are high. Deficiency states are likely to occur during childhood particularly when there is excessive cell turnover such as occurs in the haemolytic anaemias and in exfoliative skin conditions such as eczema. Folic acid is the precursor of tetrahydrofolate, which is intimately involved in a series of enzyme reactions of aminoacid, purine and intermediary metabolism. Folate is absorbed in the duodenum and in malabsorptive states including coeliac disease folate deficiency is common. In some situations where the small intestine is colonised by bacteria (blind loop syndrome) folate is diverted into bacterial metabolism. Some anticonvulsants and antibacterial agents either increase the metabolism of folate or compete with folate.

Clinical Features

Megaloblastic anaemia and pancytopenia together with poor growth are the result of the cessation of cell division, which comes about when nucleoprotein formation is interrupted because of the lack of synthesis of purines and pyrimidines.

Diagnosis

The blood picture is one of a megaloblastic anaemia with neutropenia and thrombocytopenia. The neutrophils contain large hypersegmented nuclei and bone marrow is hypercellular because of erythroid hyperplasia. Although the reticulocyte count is low nucleated red cells appear in the peripheral blood. Red cell folate measurements are < 75 ng/ml.and it gives a better idea of cellular status. There is a close interaction of B_{12} and folic acid in the synthesis of tetrahydrofolate and formyltetrahydrofolate, which are required for purine ring formation. With isolated folate deficiency there are none of the neuropathies associated with the megaloblastic anaemia of B_{12} deficiency.

Treatment

Response to treatment with oral or parenteral folic acid 2-5 mg per day is usually rapid. If there is a combined folate and B_{12} deficiency folic acid alone may cure the megaloblastic anaemia but the subacute combined degeneration of the cord will persist until B_{12} is given. In order to reduce the risk of neural tube defect it is recommended that all women should ensure an intake of 0.4 mg folic acid/day from before conception and throughout pregnancy. Any woman giving birth to an infant with a neural tube defect should have 4 mg folic acid from before conception and throughout pregnancy. Folinic acid is also effective in the treatment of folate-deficient megaloblastic anaemia but it is normally only used in association with cytotoxic drugs; it is given as calcium folinate.

Key Learning Points
• Dietary folate deficiency is not uncommon; deficiency results in megaloblastic anaemia.
• Low folate status is associated with neural tube defects, and periconceptional supplements reduce the incidence.
• Folate status can be assessed by measuring plasma or erythrocyte concentrations.

Vitamin E

Vitamin E deficiency except in the preterm infant is rare. In the preterm vitamin E deficiency is occasionally associated with haemolytic anaemia and may contribute to the membrane damage associated with intraventricular haemorrhage and bronchopulmonary dysplasia. Vitamin E is essential for the insertion and maintenance of long chain polyunsaturated fatty acids in the phospholipid bilayer of cell membranes by counteracting the effect of free radicals on these fatty acids. When the essential fatty acid content of the diet is high, vitamin E is required in increased amounts. Plant foods high in fat, particularly polyunsaturated fat, are the best sources of vitamin E. Natural sources of vitamin E are oily fish, milk, cereal, seed oils, peanuts and soya beans. Children with abetalipoproteinaemia have steatorrhoea and low circulating levels of vitamin E associated with neurological signs. More recently older children and adults with cystic fibrosis have developed neurological signs similar to those

in abetalipoproteinaemia due to vitamin E deficiency. In any child with fat malabsorption it would be important to give supplementary vitamin E in addition to correcting the underlying fat malabsorption where possible. The most commonly used index of vitamin E nutritional status is the plasma concentration of á-tochopherol. From the plasma concentration of á-tochopherol required to prevent haemolysis in vitro, the average requirement is 12 mg/day.

Key Learning Points
Premature infants have inadequate vitamin E status and are susceptible to haemolytic anaemia.

Vitamin K

Vitamin K is necessary for the production of blood clotting factors and proteins necessary for the normal calcification of bone. Osteocalcin synthesis is similarly impaired, and there is evidence that undercarboxylated osteocalcin is formed in people with marginal intakes of vitamin K who show impairment of blood clotting. Treatment with warfarin or other anticoagulants during pregnancy can lead to bone abnormalities in the fetus the so-called fetal warfarin syndrome, which is due to impaired synthesis of osteocalcin.

Because vitamin K is fat soluble, children with fat malabsorption, especially in biliary obstruction or hepatic disease may become deficient. Neonates are relatively deficient in vitamin K and those who do not receive supplements are at risk of serious bleeds including intracranial bleeding. Therefore newborn babies should receive vitamin K to prevent vitamin K deficiency bleeding (haemorrhagic disease of the newborn).

Key Learning Points
• Dietary deficiency of vitamin K is rare.
• Newborn infants have low vitamin K status and are at risk of severe bleeding unless given prophylactic vitamin K.
• Vitamin K status is assessed by estimation of prothrombin time.

BIOTIN AND PANTOTHENIC ACID

Biotin is a coenzyme for several caboxylase enzymes. Biotin deficiency is very rare as biotin is found in a wide range of foods, and bacterial production in the large intestine appears to supplement dietary intake.

Pantothenic acid is part of CoA and of acyl carrier protein (ACP). Spontaneous human deficiency has never been described. As pantothenic acid is so widely distributed in foods, any dietary deficiency in humans is usually associated with other nutrient deficiencies.

Copper Deficiency

Copper is the third most abundant dietary trace metal after iron and zinc and is found at high levels in shellfish, liver, kidney, nuts and whole grain cereals. In 1962, copper deficiency was reported in humans.

Copper is also an important constituent of many enzyme systems such as cytochrome oxidase and dismutase yet clinical copper deficiency states are rare except in very low birthweight infants, in states of severe protein energy malnutrition and during prolonged parenteral nutrition. The term infant is born with substantial stores of liver copper largely laid down in the last trimester of pregnancy bound to metallothionein. Preterm infants will therefore be born with inadequate liver stores of copper and may develop deficiency in the newborn period unless fed foods supplemented with copper. No estimated average requirement (EAR) or recommended dietary intake (RDI) has been estimated for copper. However, it is thought that the daily requirement for copper in term infants is 0.2 mg per day increasing to 1 mg per day by the end of the first year of life hereafter the requirement for copper is between 1 and 3 mg per day. Human milk contains about 0.6 mmol (39 mg) per 100 ml copper but cow's milk only contains 0.13 mmol (9 mg) per 100 ml. Many infant formulae are supplemented with copper. In soya-based infant formulas, phytate binding prohibits absorption and additional copper supplementation is required. Percentage absorption of copper is increased in deficiency states although, like iron, absorption is partly dependent on the form in which copper is presented to the gut. Other trace elements such as iron, zinc, cadmium, calcium, copper, sulphur and molybdenum interfere with copper absorption. After absorption the copper is bound to albumin in the portal circulation. Caeruloplasmin is formed in the liver and is the major transport protein for copper. Frank copper deficiency can be determined by the measurement of plasma copper concentrations, or plasma caeruloplasmin or by determination of the activities of copper – dependent enzymes such as superoxide dismutase. Therefore plasma copper has been used as a measure of copper deficiency but caeruloplasmin also acts as an acute-phase reactant and will increase in stress situations particularly during infections. The normal plasma copper concentration is 11-25 mmol/l, (0.7 - 1.6 mg/l) and caeruloplasmin 0.1-0.7 g/l. These values are decreased in deficiency states.

Clinical Features

In preterm infants there may be severe osteoporosis with cupping and flaring of the bone ends with periosteal reaction and submetaphyseal fractures. Severe bone disease has been reported in older infants on bizarre diets.

It has been argued that subclinical copper deficiency may account for some of the fractures in suspected non-accidental injury. It is most unlikely that copper deficiency in an otherwise healthy child could result in unexplained fracture. To suggest that copper deficiency develops without obvious cause and results in bone fractures without other evidence of copper deficiency is at best unwise.

Menkes steely- hair or kinky-hair syndrome is a rare X-linked disorder associated with disturbed copper metabolism. There is gross osteoporosis and progressive neurological impairment. Scalp hair is sparce and brittle with pili torti on microscopic examination. The disorder does not respond to copper therapy.

Selenium Deficiency

Muscular dystrophy in lambs and calves has been reported in parts of the world where there is deficiency of selenium in the soil. In humans Keshan disease has been reported in China. Selenium is essential for glutathione peroxidase activity which catalyses the reduction of fatty acid hydroperoxides and protects tissues from peroxidation. Thus selenium is important in maintaining the fatty acid integrity of phospholipid membranes and reducing free radical damage. It is found in fish, meat and whole grain and reflects the soil selenium content of the region. Vitamin C improves the absorption of selenium.

Clinical Features

In China an endemic cardiomyopathy affecting women of childbearing age and children known as Keshan disease has been reported. The condition responds to selenium supplementation. In New Zealand low selenium concentrations in the soil result in low plasma levels and in children with phenylketonuria on a low phenylalanine diet low plasma levels of selenium have been reported. There is no obvious clinical abnormality in the New Zealand population although poor growth and dry skin has been reported in the selenium deficient PKU children Increasingly, epidemiological evidence as well as data from animal studies points to a role for selenium in reducing cancer incidence. However, it should be noted that while selenium is an essential micronutrient and supplementation or fortification of foods may in many cases be advantageous, in excess selenium is exceedingly toxic. The margin between an adequate and a toxic intake of selenium is quite narrow. Symptoms of selenium excess include brittle hair and nails, skin lesions and garlic odour on the breath due to expiration of dimethylselenide. Lack of dietary selenium has also been implicated in the aetiology of cardiovascular diseases, but the evidence is less convincing than for cancer.

Chromium

Chromium may be involved in nucleic acid metabolism and is recognised as a cofactor for insulin. It is poorly absorbed and there is some evidence that in the elderly, glucose tolerance can be improved by chromium supplementation. Chromium deficiency has been reported in severely malnourished children and in children on prolonged parenteral nutrition. Weight gain and glucose tolerance in such children has been reported to improve after chromium supplementation. In long-term parenteral nutrition peripheral neuropathy and encephalopathy have also been reported to respond to chromium administration.

Iodine Deficiency

Endemic goitre has been recognised for many centuries in mountainous regions of the world. The Andes, Himalayas, mountains of Central Africa and Papua, New Guinea as well as Derbyshire in the U.K, are areas where the condition has been recognised. Minimal requirements are probably less than 20 mg/day in infants and young children increasing to 50 mg/day during adolescence. Breast milk contains up to 90 mg/l. Goitre occurs when the iodine intake is less than 15 mg/day and results in a reduced serum thyroxine (T_4) but a decreased tri-iodothyronine (T_3). Thyroid stimulating hormone (TSH) values increase. The introduction of iodised salt to areas of endemic goitrous and cretinism has largely eradicated goitre cretinism in these regions. Thus at present this is best achieved through iodine fortification of foods. Some plants including brassicas, bamboo shoots act as goitrogens by inhibiting iodine uptake by the thyroid gland.

Key Learning Points
Iodisation of salt is the preferred way and >60% of families in affected regions now have access to fortified salt.

Fluoride

Fluoride is present in most foods at varying levels and also in drinking water, either naturally occurring or added deliberately. Fluoride content of teeth and bones is directly proportional to the amount ingested and absorbed from the diet. Fluoride has been recognized as an important factor in the prevention of caries. Where the fluoride content of the drinking water is less than 700 micrograms per litre (0.7 parts per million), daily administration of fluoride tablets or drops is a suitable means of supplementation. It is now considered that the topical action of fluoride on enamel and plaque is more important than the systemic effect. Systemic fluoride supplements should not be prescribed without reference to the fluoride content of the local water supply. Infants need not receive fluoride supplements until the age of 6 months. Tooth paste or powder which incorporate sodium fluoride or monofluorophosphate are also a convenient source of fluoride.

Higher intakes of fluoride are (10 mg/l) of fluoride are toxic and leading to fluorosis. However, fluorosis is common in parts of Southern Africa, the Indian subcontinent and China where there is a high fluoride content in the subsoil water, which enters the food chain either directly or via plants.

Other Trace Minerals

Manganese, molybdenum and cadmium are known to be necessary for health in animals but no clear human evidence of deficiency states are known to man. Following recent experience with zinc, copper and chromium, it seems likely that future research will lead to the identification of specific deficiencies of some of these other trace elements in infants and children.

Chapter 6

Respiratory Disorders

Anne Devenny

HISTORY AND EXAMINATION

A careful history and physical examination is vital in respiratory medicine. When a child presents with respiratory symptoms, e.g. cough, the following are some of the questions that should be asked:

1. When did the cough start?
2. Is it there all the time?
3. What makes it better or worse?
4. Is the cough productive of sputum? If so is it green or blood stained? (Remember young children commonly swallow sputum rather than coughing it up). A persistent productive cough in a child can be a sign of bronchiectasis.
5. Is it worse at night? (In asthmatics night cough is a common problem)
6. Are there other associated symptoms, e.g. wheeze, breathlessness, fever or lethargy?
7. What treatments have been tried and what do the parents feel helped?

Past Medical History

Previous operations and hospital admissions
Presence of other conditions, e.g. eczema, cerebral palsy.

Birth History

1. Was the infant born preterm?
2. Did they have respiratory difficulties?
3. Birth weight.

Family History

1. Who lives with the child?
2. Are there family members with respiratory illness, e.g. asthma?
3. Is there a family history of hay fever or eczema?

Social History

1. Is there anyone in the house who smokes?
2. Are there housing problems, e.g. dampness?
3. What pets do they have?
4. What recent travel have they had?

Vaccination History

Have all vaccines been given?

RESPIRATORY INVESTIGATIONS

1. *Chest imaging,* - e.g. chest radiograph, chest CT scan and MRI of chest.
2. *Lung function studies*—Includes spirometry and plethysmography. Figures 6.1 to 6.3 show a normal flow volume loop, an obstructed flow volume loop and a restrictive flow volume loop respectively. Figure 6.4 shows a plethysmograph. These are similar to the studies performed in adults and usually children need to be at least 5 years old for them to do the manoeuvres needed. Exercise testing and Histamine Challenge is also performed.
3. *pH studies* - This uses placement of an oesophageal probe to measure acidity.

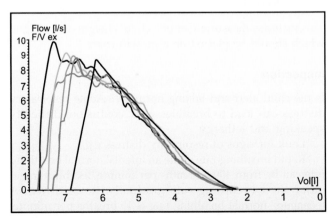

Fig. 6.1: Normal flow volume loop

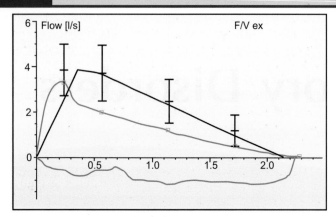

Fig. 6.2: Obstructed flow volume loop

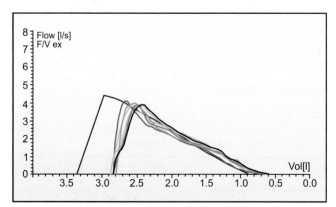

Fig. 6.3: Restrictive flow volume loop

4 *Barium swallow* - performed for gastro-oesophageal reflux and also helps to identify the presence of vascular rings that compress the oesophagus and trachea.
5 *Video-fluoroscopy of swallowing* - this is a test used to look for swallowing problems, particularly aspiration.
6 Flexible Bronchoscopy
7 Skin Prick Testing for common allergens
8 Sweat test - used for cystic fibrosis

EXAMINATION

This includes measurement of a child's height and weight, which should be plotted on a growth chart

Inspection

Is the child alert and talking normally? Acute respiratory distress can lead to breathlessness, confusion, difficulty speaking and lethargy

Look for signs of respiratory distress e.g.

Rapid breathing rate - note an infants' normal breathing rate can be from 40-60 breaths per minute, as children get older their breathing rate gradually slows down. A teenagers' normal breathing rate is 15 breaths per minute.

Is there use of accessory muscles of respiration? In an infant you may see tracheal tug and head bobbing, in an

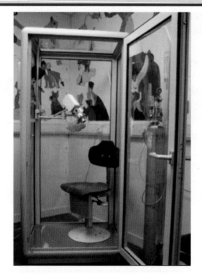

Fig. 6.4: Body plethysmograph – Used to measure lung volumes

older child there may be sub-costal recession and use of their sternocleidomastoid muscles

Is there central cyanosis or finger clubbing? Are there scars or central venous access devices?

Is the chest hyper inflated? Is there Harrison sulci evident?

Palpation

Chest excursion—can be difficult in a young infant.

Feel for apex beat and tracheal deviation - again this can be difficult in a young infant as they often have short necks.

Percussion

Percuss the chest for areas of dullness.

Auscultation

Is air entry equal on both sides?

Are the breath sounds normal?

Are there added sounds such as crackles, wheeze or stridor?

Examination of Ear, Nose and Throat

These should be inspected directly with an auroscope. Children need to be held correctly for this to allow for proper inspection.

THE RESPIRATORY TRACT IN CHILDREN

At birth the lungs have the same number of conducting airways, e.g. bronchial divisions as adults though they are much smaller. The number of alveoli present is only one third to one half of the total adult number. Lung growth occurs by increasing the number of alveoli and their size and by increasing the size of the airways. The upper and lower airways in children are small and therefore prone to obstruction.

Infants use diaphragmatic breathing rather than using their intercostal muscles, as these are underdeveloped. Children's ribs lie more horizontally and do not contribute as much to expansion of their chests. Their rib cage is less bony than in adults and is therefore more compliant and this can also make them more prone to respiratory difficulties.

Congenital abnormalities of the respiratory tract are rare. They can be divided into abnormalities of the upper airways, e.g. larynx and above and of the lower respiratory airways.

CONGENITAL ABNORMALITIES OF THE UPPER RESPIRATORY TRACT

Choanal Atresia

Choanal atresia is a narrowing or blockage of the nasal airway by membranous or bony tissue. It is thought to result from persistence of the membrane between the nasal and oral spaces during fetal development. It can be complete or partial, bilateral or unilateral, bony or membranous. The newborn is an "obligate nose breather," meaning it must breathe through its nose. In fact, almost the only time an infant does not breathe through its nose is when it is crying.

Bilateral choanal atresia causes acute breathing problems and cyanosis soon after birth. The cyanosis is typically relieved when the baby cries. There can also be persistent green thick nasal secretions. The diagnosis may be suggested by failure to pass a nasogastric tube down the nose. Nasal endoscopy and a CT scan of the choanal area can also help delineate how severe the atresia is. Choanal stenosis can lead to noisy breathing and difficulty feeding. The management of choanal atresia is surgical.

It is well recognized that approximately 47% of children with choanal atresia can have other congenital abnormalities - the "CHARGE" association in which there are 7 main types of abnormalities noted. Coloboma, Heart defects, Atresia [choanal], Retardation [mental and growth], Genital anomaly, Ear anomaly and deafness. This is an association caused by a developmental defect involving the midline structures of the body, specifically affecting the craniofacial structures. Children need to have abnormalities of at least 4 out of the 7 organs to have the CHARGE association. The severity of abnormalities can vary.

Therefore a child with choanal abnormalities should be examined carefully and investigated to look for these other features.

Laryngomalacia

This is a common condition of unknown cause where the larynx is floppier than normal, the epiglottis is large and differently shaped, the arytenoids are also floppy and on inspiration the larynx collapses inwardly obstructing the airway causing stridor. Stridor is usually present from soon after birth. It is louder on inspiration, on crying and when there is an upper respiratory tract infection. Laryngomalacia does not usually cause difficulty breathing or feeding unless severe but it can be associated with apnoea if severe. There can be sub costal recession due to the obstruction to airflow. The baby's voice should be normal.

Diagnosis is made by history and clinical findings of a well child with stridor. Infants with difficulty breathing or feeding do need visualisation of their upper airways by flexible laryngoscopy. This can be done without sedation. In fact the dynamic airway is best seen this way. Laryngomalacia rarely needs treatment and infants usually grow out of it. If severe then aryepiglottoplasty can be used.

However, normal laryngoscopy in a child with persistent stridor warrants flexible or rigid bronchoscopy of the entire bronchial tree, as there may be subglottic or tracheal stenosis.

Subglottic Stenosis

This can occur as a primary problem, e.g. Subglottic web. However, it is more often seen in infants who have had previous episodes of intubation. It can be life threatening. Treatment can include tracheal reconstruction using a cartilage graft. Infants may initially need a tracheostomy.

Haemangiomas of the Airways

These are rare. The abnormal blood vessels can obstruct the larynx. They can shrink in response to steroids, which may have been given in the mistaken thought that the infant's stridor was due to croup. Treatment can include surgical removal of the lesions, laser therapy and direct injection of corticosteroids. Again tracheostomy may be needed.

Laryngeal Papillomatosis

A rare condition where infection with the Human Papilloma virus, leads to papillomata in the larynx, which causes hoarseness and stridor. The infection is usually acquired peri-natally. Treatment involves laser therapy of the lesions. Anti-viral treatment with Cidofovir can also be used.

Tracheobronchomalacia

This is a condition where the trachea, one particular bronchus or the whole bronchial tree is floppy and fails to maintain airway patency due to an abnormality of the cartilaginous ring and hypotonia of the myoelastic elements. There is collapse of the affected area on inspiration. It can occur in extreme prematurity or when there is an aberrant vessel, e.g. pulmonary artery sling pressing on the airways. These aberrant vessels can also press on the oesophagus. It can present with stridor or with apparent life threatening events or ALTE's. Investigations include barium swallow, bronchoscopy, cardiac echo, and magnetic resonance imaging of the great vessels. The treatment of this condition is dependent on the cause.

Tracheal Stenosis

Congenital tracheal stenosis is a rare condition where there is focal or diffuse complete tracheal cartilage rings. This results in narrowing or stenosis of the trachea. It can occur on its own or in association with a vascular ring, e.g. pulmonary artery sling –where the left pulmonary artery comes off the right pulmonary artery and encircles the right main stem bronchus and trachea. Acquired tracheal stenosis can occur secondary to prolonged intubation or infection in the trachea. Tracheal stenosis can present with breathing difficulties and stridor on inspiration and expiration. It has significant morbidity and can have significant mortality if severe. Tracheal reconstruction is often needed.

Tracheal Oesophageal Fistula with Oesophageal Atresia

In this condition there is a failure of embryonic development of the trachea and oesophagus. In oesophageal atresia the oesophagus is a blind ending pouch. This presents soon after birth when the infant cannot swallow its own secretions or milk and often will choke. It will be difficult to pass a nasogastric tube. Any fluid aspirated from the nasogastric tube will not contain acid so the pH paper which is used to check the position of the tube will not turn red. A tracheo-oesophageal fistula (TOF) is an abnormal connection between the trachea and oesophagus, which can occur along with an oesophageal atresia. A TOF usually presents early on with recurrent choking with feeds associated with desaturations. Treatment is surgical. The airways of babies with TOF can be malacic and babies post-repair can have ongoing respiratory difficulties.

In 25% of cases other gastrointestinal malformations e.g. as imperforate anus, pyloric stenosis, and duodenal atresia occur. The "VACTERL" complex is a condition where children have vertebral, anal, cardiovascular, tracheoesophageal, renal, radial, and limb malformations.

Pulmonary Agenesis / Pulmonary Hypoplasia

In pulmonary agenesis there is failure of development of the bronchi and lung tissue of one or both lungs. Bilateral agenesis is incompatible with life. Babies born with one lung can have a normal life expectancy. These abnormalities are rare. More common is pulmonary hyoplasia where one or both lungs fail to develop properly –they have reduced bronchial branches, alveoli and blood vessels. Bilateral pulmonary hypoplasia is found in Potter syndrome where there is renal agenesis and oligohydramnios. The severity of the hypoplasia is dependent on what gestational age the arrest of development occurs. The earlier this occurs the worse the outlook. Most cases of pulmonary hypoplasia are seen as a secondary consequence of congenital diaphragmatic hernia.

Congential Diaphragmatic Hernia

In the first few weeks of fetal life there is communication between the pleural and peritoneal cavities via the pleuroperitoneal canal. This usually closes between 8 and 10 weeks gestation. Failure of this closure results in a defect in the diaphragm. The abdominal contents can then herniated through into the chest compressing the intrathoracic structures leading to poor lung development. 85% of congenital diaphragmatic hernias are left sided. They occur in 1 in every 2500-3000 births.

The mortality rate from this condition is high about 40%. The mortality occurs from the pulmonary hypoplasia and also the elevated pulmonary artery pressures (pulmonary hypertension). Larger defects are associated with worse herniation and more severe hypoplasia. 10% of children will have other abnormalities. This condition can be detected antenatally by ultrasound - if detected the infant should be delivered in a unit where there is a neonatal surgical team on site.

An infant with a large diaphragmatic hernia usually presents within the first few hours after birth with breathing difficulties and cyanosis. If the hypoplasia is severe the baby may have obvious difficulties and cyanosis just after birth. Treatment involves resuscitation with intubation and ventilation. A CXR will confirm the diagnosis showing herniation of the bowel into the chest and usually mediastinal displacement (Fig. 6.5). A nasogastric tube should be passed to decompress the stomach. Surgery is then performed to repair the defect. Nitric oxide, ECMO (Extracorporeal Membrane Oxygenation) and high frequency oscillation have all been used to try to stabilize infants prior to surgery.

OTHER CONGENITAL LUNG ABNORMALITIES

Congenital Lobar Emphysema

This is a rare condition where there is over expansion of a pulmonary lobe with resultant compression of the remaining ipsilateral lung (Fig. 6.6). This is caused by an abnormally narrow bronchus where there is weakened or absent bronchial cartilage, so that there is air entry when by the CCAM, which affects venous return to the heart causing low cardiac output and effusions. The CCAM can also press on the parts of the lung, which are growing normally and cause them to be hypoplastic leading to respiratory difficulties. Large CCAM's can be detected by antenatal ultrasound. Small CCAM's may go unnoticed for years until someone has a chest radiograph for another reason or until they become infected. Treatment is usually surgical excision.

Congenital Pulmonary Sequestration

In this condition there is an abnormal development of primitive lung tissue, which does not communicate with the bronchial tree and receives its blood supply from one or more systemic vessels rather than the pulmonary circulation. It can present with cough and recurrent chest infections. Treatment is surgical excision.

ACQUIRED ABNORMALITIES

UPPER RESPIRATORY TRACT

Upper Respiratory Tract Infection (URTI)

URTI are common in children and usually viral in origin caused by rhinoviruses and adenovirus. Bacterial pathogens include *Streptococcus and Haemophilus influenzae*. The child will usually have fever, cough, and nasal discharge and may be lethargic and refuse feeds. Common examination findings include an inflamed throat and often inflamed tympanic membranes. Cervical lymphadenopathy may also be present. Treatment is supportive with fluids and anti-pyretics such as paracetamol.

Investigations can be taken such as throat swabs for virology and bacterial culture. If the child is not improving antibiotics may be needed e.g. Penicillin V. If breathing or feeding difficulties are evident children should be referred to hospital for further management.

Tonsillitis

This is where the tonsils are enlarged and inflamed, purulent exudates may be evident. The child may have difficulty swallowing and can need admitted for intravenous fluids. Throat swabs can be taken if symptoms are not resolving. SIGN Guidelines for the management of sore throats can be found at http://www.sign.ac.uk. The indications for tonsillectomy are the following: that the episodes should have occurred over at least a one year period, that they should be tonsillitis and not pharyngitis, that there should be 5 or more episodes per year and the episodes should be interfering with normal life. *Streptococcus pyogenes* is the commonest pathogen isolated and is treated with penicillin V or erythromycin if penicillin

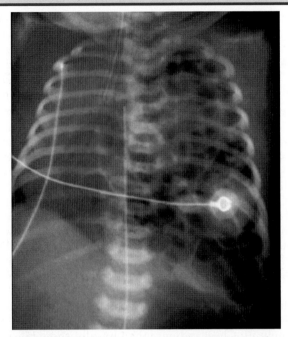

Fig. 6.5: Left sided congenital diaphragmatic hernia

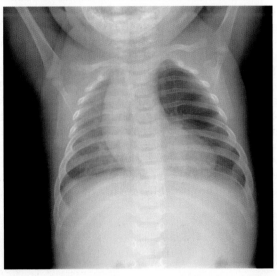

Fig. 6.6: Congenital lobar emphysema of left upper lobe

the baby breathes in but collapse of the narrow bronchial lumen during expiration. This can present with breathing or feeding difficulties and treatment is surgical excision of the affected lobe.

Congenital Cystic Adenomatoid Malformation of the Lung (CCAM)

In this condition there is an abnormal cystic development of lung tissue during weeks 7 to 35 of gestation. Large CCAM's may be associated with hydrops fetalis in as many as 40%, which has a significant mortality. Hydrops is thought to arise from compression of the inferior vena cava allergy is present. Remember glandular fever caused by Epstein-Barr virus can cause significant throat infla-mmation and cervical lymphadenopathy, which will not respond to antibiotics.

Acute Otitis Media and Otitis Media with Effusion (AOM and OME)

This is inflammation of the middle ear—It can be acute or chronic and can also be accompanied by fluid in the middle ear - so called otitis media with effusion. Acute and chronic otitis media are very common presentations in children. Acute otitis media (AOM) usually presents with fever and pain in the ears. Young children who cannot yet speak may just be irritable and febrile and their parents may note them rubbing their ears. If the infection causes the tympanic membrane to burst the parents may notice a yellow discharge and often the pain improves as the pressure is released. Hearing loss may also be present. Again SIGN Guidelines exist www.sign.ac.uk. On inspection of the tympanic membranes in AOM they may be bulging and red with fluid evident behind the tympanic membrane. In otitis media with effusion the tympanic membrane may not be inflamed but there is fluid evident. The main management of AOM is supportive with analgesia and fluids –if there is no improvement within a few days or a child gets worse then oral antibiotics, e.g. penicillin can be used. Children with more than 4 episodes of AOM in 6 months need referred to an ENT specialist. In OME the child needs its hearing assessed. If hearing loss is found a child should be referred to ENT should be referred as persistent hearing loss can cause speech delay. There is no place for antibiotics or decongestants in OME.

Croup-laryngotracheobronchitis

This is viral induced inflammation of the larynx and trachea. Symptoms include a barking cough, inspiratory stridor and fever of rapid onset. Children may also have difficulty breathing when it is severe. They may also show signs of respiratory distress with subcostal recession. The management of this is high flow oxygen if needed, paracetamol and prednisolone or dexamethasone. If there are signs of significant distress nebulised adrenaline 5 ml of 1 in 1000 should be given and anaesthetic help should be obtained.

Acute Epiglottitis

This is bacterial inflammation of the epiglottis usually caused by *Haemophilus influenzae*. There is significant toxicity with high fever, drolling, stridor and difficulty breathing. It has become less common due to the introduction of the HIB vaccination. Management of this should be prompt induction of anaesthesia, intubation and intravenous antibiotics.

ACQUIRED LOWER RESPIRATORY TRACT PROBLEMS

COMMUNITY ACQUIRED PNEUMONIA

Viral Pneumonias

Respiratory syncitial virus is the single most important cause of viral lower respiratory tract infection in infancy and childhood worldwide. Classically it causes bron-chiolitis and it is prevalent in the winter months. RSV causes inflammation and destruction of the airways leading to airway narrowing and air trapping.

Common symptoms are fever, coryza, cough, wheeze and difficulty breathing and feeding. Babies with bronchiolitis can have signs of respiratory distress with bilateral crackles on auscultation, low oxygen saturation levels, fever and dehydration. Many of these babies can be managed at home with frequent small feeds and anti-pyretics when needed.

Indications for admission include significant feeding problems and those needing oxygen or those who are severely ill. Chest radiographs typically show bilateral hyperinflation with increased lung markings bilaterally. They can show consolidation of one or more lobes of the lung in severe disease (Fig. 6.7). Premature infants and those with haemodynamically significant congenital heart disease are more at risk of severe disease.

There is a monoclonal antibody preparation called Palvizumab "Synagis" which has been shown to reduce hospitalization in children less than 6 months of age who were born at 35 weeks gestation or less, those less than 2 years with chronic lung disease of prematurity and those with congenital heart disease. In some centres this is given to babies in those high-risk groups in the hope it will prevent severe RSV infection. SIGN guidelines for the management of bronchiolitis are currently being developed.

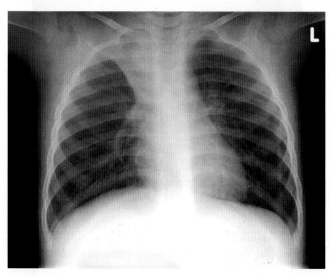

Fig. 6.7: Right upper lobe collapse/consolidation

Bacterial Pneumonia

The mortality from bacterial pneumonia is very low in developed countries in stark comparison to the high mortality rates in the developing world.

The most common bacterial pathogen is *Streptococcus pneumoniae* followed by *Mycoplasma pneumoniae*. In 20-60% of cases a pathogen is not identified and in fact there is often a mixture of pathogens. Evidence Based Guidelines can be found on the British Thoracic Society website www.brit-thoracic.org.uk

Bacterial pneumonia usually presents with fever, cough and fast breathing or grunting. The child can be breathless at rest with signs of distress. On auscultation signs can include crackles and bronchial breathing. Lower lobe pneumonia can present with abdominal pain and fever. Many bacterial pneumonias are managed in the community with oral antibiotics, e.g. amoxycillin. Those who fail to respond to this will need further investigation and management. This can include chest radiography, blood cultures, full blood count, nasopharyngeal aspirate for viral culture for those under 2 years and acute serology for respiratory pathogens, e.g. Mycoplasma. A right middle lobe pneumonia is shown in Figure 6.8.

Children who have significant difficulty breathing, those who can not feed, who are dehydrated, who need supplemental oxygen or who are systemically unwell should all be admitted. They may need intravenous antibiotics, e.g. Amoxycillin and intravenous fluids. Children with community-acquired pneumonia do not need routine follow up chest radiographs. However, those who have a round pneumonia on their radiograph and those with lobar collapse should have a follow up radiograph done at 6 weeks. Continuing symptoms despite treatment should also have a repeat chest radiograph performed.

Pleural Infection in Children

Bacterial pneumonia in children can cause fluid in the pleural space (para-pneumonic effusions) which can become infected causing pus in the pleural space (empyema). They are rare but the incidence is increasing and the reason for this is not clear. They are a significant cause of morbidity in children but mortality is rare unlike empyema in adults. Guidelines have been developed for the management of empyema in childhood and they are available at www.brit-thoracic.org.uk.

The most common bacteria responsible is Streptococcus pneumoniae. Such pleural collections usually present with persistent fever, cough and difficulty breathing. The children may already be on antibiotics for a chest infection. If the collection is large they may have dullness to percussion on the affected side with reduced air entry. A large pleural collection will show as a complete "white out" of one lung (Fig. 6.9). An example, of a smaller collection is shown in Figure 6.10. With an empyema the white cell count and the c reactive protein (CRP) are usually significantly raised. If the chest radiograph is suggestive of an effusion an ultrasound of the chest should be done to assess the amount of fluid present and look for loculation. Children should be treated with intravenous antibiotics which will cover *Streptococcus pneumoniae* e.g. amoxycillin or cefotaxime. Close observation is needed.

Blood cultures should be taken. Larger collections causing difficulty breathing and those with persistent fever should be drained. Chest drains in children are inserted under anaesthetic. The pleural fluid should be sent for

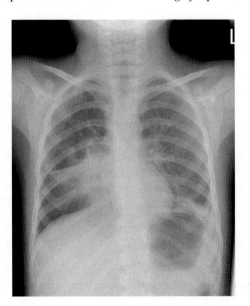

Fig. 6.8: Right middle lobe pneumonia

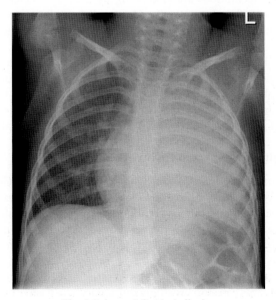

Fig. 6.9: Large left sided effusion

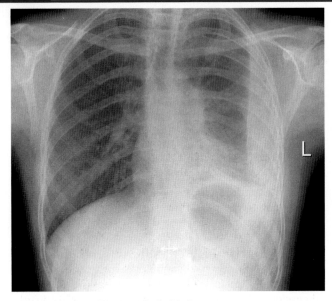

Fig. 6.10: Left sided empyema

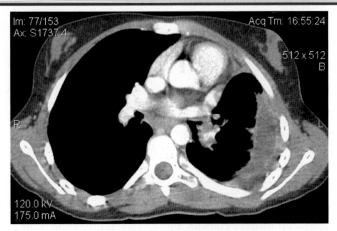

Fig. 6.11: CT scan showing left sided empyema

culture. Children need good pain relief afterwards to ensure early mobility. The chest drain usually stays in until it has stopped draining fluid. The majority of children with empyema responds well to intravenous antibiotics and drainage and makes a complete recovery. Intrapleural Fibrinolytics, e.g. Urokinase and Tissue Plasminogen Activator can be instilled into the pleural space to try to break down the adhesions present in the pleural fluid.

Children who fail to respond may require further imaging, e.g. computer assisted tomography (CT) of the chest (Fig. 6.11) and may need more invasive thoracic procedures, e.g. decortication. Video assisted thoraco-scopic techniques are also being used to try to clear the pus from the pleural cavity. Once well enough to go home children need a follow up chest X-ray at approximately 6 weeks to ensure that there are no complications.

Children without fever who present with a pleural effusion are of more concern as malignancies particularly lymphoma and leukaemia may present this way. In these children a chest CT is indicated sooner and the pleural fluid drained should be sent for cytological examination.

Gastro-oesophageal Reflux (GOR)

Reflux of the stomach contents into the oesophagus (GOR) is a common condition and classically in infants presents as recurrent non-bilious vomiting. Infants usually continue to gain weight unless the reflux is severe. Infants with reflux can also be very irritable with feeding and can refuse feeds. GOR can also cause respiratory symptoms with chronic cough, wheeze and aspiration. In severe reflux the infants can stop breathing due to laryngospasm causing Apparent life Threatening Events or ALTE's. GOR is also

found in association with other respiratory conditions such as asthma and cystic fibrosis and if found is treated, but unfortunately does not always improve the respiratory symptoms. Children with severe cerebral palsy can also have significant problems with GOR and are also more prone to chest problems.

Diagnosis

This is based on the clinical history and examination findings. Oesophageal pH monitoring and a barium swallow are also used. If there is a suggestion that a child has difficulty swallowing then a barium swallow is indicated to exclude an oesophageal stricture. In more difficult and severe reflux cases upper GI endoscopy and biopsy of the oesophageal and gastric mucosa is indicated.

Treatment

Simple reflux treatment in infants includes attention to posture by elevating the child's head in bed by placing a blanket or similar underneath the mattress. Feed thickeners such as Carobel can also be used. Infant Gaviscon sachets can also be added to feeds to reduce acidity. H_2 blockers, e.g. Ranitidine and Proton Pump inhibitors, e.g. Losec are also used. Domperidone a dopamine antagonist that stimulates gastric emptying and low dose erythromycin can also be used to stimulate gastric motility.

Severe cases unresponsive to medical management may require surgical intervention using the Nissen Fundoplication procedure where the fundus of the stomach is wrapped around the lower oesophagus, strengthening the lower oesophageal sphincter.

Aspiration Pneumonia

This is a condition where the contents of the pharynx or oesophagus spill over into the larynx and bronchial tree causing cough, fever and irritant pneumonias. This can occur in previously normal children who have a reduced conscious level and can therefore not protect their own airway by coughing and closing their larynx e.g. those with a head injury or coma from any cause. More often it is seen in children with chronic neurological conditions e.g. cerebral palsy. Gastro-oesophageal reflux where the stomach contents reflux back into the oesophagus can also predispose to aspiration, particularly in the significantly neurologically handicapped children.

It can present in a child who coughs and chokes during feeds but it can also occur silently until enough aspiration has occurred to cause symptoms of chronic cough, breathlessness and fever. It should be suspected in neurologically handicapped children who have reduced muscle power and developmental delay who present with recurrent severe chest infections. Recurrent aspiration can cause severe chronic lung disease.

Investigation of Aspiration Pneumonia

This can be difficult. A chest X-ray can show changes of aspiration but these are often non-specific. Often in aspiration it is the right lung, which is worst affected. A barium swallow or a pH study can be done to look for reflux. A videofluoroscopy where screening is done during the child eating and drinking is very helpful and can show direct aspiration of the swallowed foods.

Management of Aspiration Pneumonia

The acute treatment is to manage the chest infection with antibiotics, chest physiotherapy and oxygen if needed. GOR should be treated. Children who are shown to be aspirating should have a gastrostomy tube placed and consideration should be given to gastrostomy tube placement in children with cerebral palsy, with feeding difficulties, who have recurrent aspiration pneumonia.

ASTHMA

Asthma is one of the commonest chronic conditions affecting children. In some studies nearly one in four children have had a diagnosis of asthma. Asthma increased in prevalence in the 1980's and 1990's but is now showing signs of decreasing in prevalence. It causes significant morbidity and there are still asthma deaths in childhood. Asthma is a chronic inflammatory condition of the airways where there is mast cell activation and infiltration of inflammatory cells, e.g. eosinophils, airway macrophages , neutrophils, lymphocytes -usually TH$_2$ and interleukins. These cause oedema of the airways, disruption of the epithelium and mucus hypersecretion. There is reversible airways obstruction due to smooth muscle constriction in response to various trigger factors. This leads to the clinical symptoms of wheeze, nocturnal cough and difficulty breathing – a child sometimes will complain of chest tightness or chest pains.

The most common trigger in childhood is viral upper respiratory tract infections. Other common precipitating factors include exercise, emotion, cold weather and smoking. Children with asthma may have other atopic conditions such as hay fever and eczema. Atopy involves the capacity to produce IgE in response to common environmental proteins such as house dust mite, grass pollen, and food allergens. There is often a family history of atopy. There is ongoing research into genetic causes of asthma—the most investigated location for atopy has been the 5q 31–33 region of the chromosome, which includes the genes for the cytokines IL-4, -5, -9, and -13.

The diagnosis of asthma is a clinical one based on history taking and examination. It can be difficult in young children. Some children can have recurrent virus induced wheeze but no symptoms in between. There is constant debate as to whether this is asthma or not or whether they are two ends of the same spectrum of disease. It can be difficult to separate out and often these children are initially treated with asthma medication until the situation becomes clearer. Additional tests can help such as peak flow measurement in the over 5 years, lung function testing with reversibility and histamine challenge, exercise testing to see whether the bronchospasm can be induced and skin tests to check for common allergens.

Examination Findings

During an acute asthma episode the child will show signs of respiratory distress depending on the severity of the attack. These include tachypnoea, hyperinflation, and subcostal recession, and tracheal tug, use of accessory muscles of respiration. If severe, the child may be hypoxic or confused. On auscultation there is usually wheeze, which is often bilateral and reduced air entry. Crackles can also be heard. The child with severe acute asthma may have a silent chest. Routine chest radiographs are usually not needed in asthma, however they usually show marked hyperinflation (Fig. 6.12).

Severe chronic asthma can lead to chest deformity of the lower part of the chest, i.e. Harrison sulci and/or a barrel shaped chest. If a child with recurrent respiratory symptoms has finger clubbing then further investigations are needed. Finger clubbing in children is associated with chronic suppurative lung conditions such as cystic fibrosis and bronchiectasis.

Asthma Management

The management of acute and chronic asthma depends on the severity of the symptoms. The British Thoracic Society has evidence-based guidelines on the management of asthma (www.brit-thoracic.org.uk). There is strong support for asthmatics, their carers and professionals from

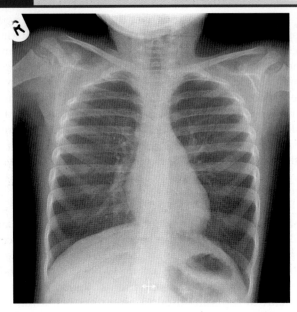

Fig. 6.12: Acute severe asthma with marked hyperinflation

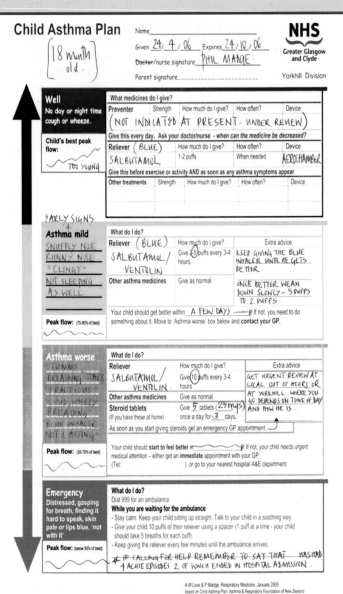

Fig. 6.13: Child asthma management plan for 18-month-child (Adapted from the asthma management plans from the Asthma and Respiratory Foundation of New Zealand)

various lung charities e.g. Asthma UK (www.asthma.org.uk) and the British Lung Foundation (www.lunguk.org).

Education and Management Plans

The key to good asthma management is education. This should include education of the parents and of the child if they are old enough. Parents need to know the early warning signs such as runny nose, cough, dark circles under their child's eyes progressing to the classical symptoms of persistent coughing, wheezing and difficult breathing. Often if you ask parents they will tell you exactly what they notice when their child is becoming unwell. Asthma management plans are very useful particularly in the management of asthma attacks (Fig. 6.13). They document a child's individual symptoms and signs of their asthma, what their medication is, when to give it and when to call for help.

Parents who smoke should be given stopping smoking advice. Asthma education should occur in general practice and in hospital. It is important that nurses, doctors and allied health professionals in fact all professionals looking after children with asthma, have asthma education. Many hospitals and general practices in the UK have nurses with a special interest in Paediatric asthma. Their role is very important in helping parents and children cope with their asthma. Advice is also given about minimizing exposure to other allergens, e.g. house dust mite. An example of our asthma education leaflet is shown in Figure 6.14. Electronic interactive asthma education packages are available. Asthma management plans are very useful particularly in the management of asthma attacks.

Drug Treatment of Asthma

Inhalers are the main form of treatment for asthma. In children these are usually metered dose inhalers given using a spacer device (Fig. 6.15). Dry powder devices, activated by sucking, such as turbohalers and accuhalers can be useful in children over 8 years.

Children with mild intermittent asthma symptoms (step 1 of British Thoracic Society guidelines) require inhaled beta agonists, e.g. Salbutamol as required. This provides rapid relief for bronchospasm.

Children with more persistent asthma symptoms (step 2) should be treated with an inhaled steroid, e.g.

Yorkhill Children's Services

Asthma

A Guide for Parents

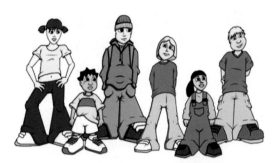

Fig. 6.14: Asthma – A guide for parents.

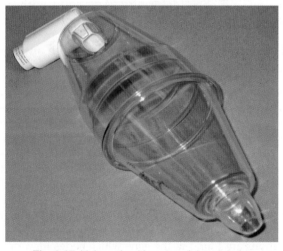

Fig. 6.15: Volumatic with metered dose inhaler

becotide or budesonide at as low a dose as possible to maintain symptom control, e.g. 100 microgram twice daily. Children need to wash their mouths out afterwards.

High dose inhaled steroids have been shown to cause adrenal suppression in a number of children. Some children may need high dose inhaled steroids to keep their asthma under control. They are at increased risk of systemic absorption of the steroids, which can cause suppression of the adrenal glands and adrenal insufficiency. They should have a Syncathen test perfomed and a management plan discussed with the parents and their own doctor as to what to do if their child became unwell. These children

would be at risk of adrenal crises with hypoglycaemia, coma and death should they develop intercurrent illness.

Children with moderate asthma symptoms, not controlled on low dose inhaled steroids (step 3) can have their dose of inhaled steroids increased to 200 microgram twice daily of beclomethasome or equivalent. A long acting beta 2 agonist e.g. Salmeterol or Formoterol or a leukotriene receptor antagonist e.g. Montelukast can also be tried.

Step 4 of the guidelines suggests that if asthma control is inadequate with inhaled steroids (children: 400 microgram/day) plus long-acting B_2 agonist, then consideration should be given to increasing the inhaled steroid dose to 800 mcg/day, adding a leukotriene receptor antagonist and oral theophylline children fail to improve, then the drug should be stopped and the child referred on to specialist care. If increasing the dose of inhaled steroid has not helped, then this should be put back down to its previous dose.

If asthma symptoms persist and children are having frequent exacerbations, the next step is daily oral steroids. This can have significant side effects, e.g. weight gain and immune suppression. Prior to starting this, many children will have further investigations to try to make sure that this is difficult to control asthma and not another problem such as cystic fibrosis or gastro-oesophageal reflux. Other medications for difficult asthma include subcutaneous Bricanyl infusions, anti IGE antibody therapy, cyclosporin or methotrexate.

In the under 5 years the management of asthma is somewhat different as there is more evidence for the effectiveness of Montelukast. It should be tried in addition to low dose inhaled steroids before long acting beta agonists. Young children with difficult asthma symptoms should be referred for further investigation and management.

Management of Acute Asthma Attack

This very much depends on the severity of the attack. The child needs to be assessed quickly and efficiently. There are courses run worldwide by resuscitation organisations e.g. the Advanced Paediatric Life Support Course run by the Advance Life Support Group (www.alsg.org). These provide an excellent way to manage paediatric emergencies.

The approach is based on assessment of airway, breathing and circulation. Is the child's airway open? What is their work of breathing? What is their circulation (normal skin colour, capillary refill time less than 2 seconds)?

A child who is alert, talking easily with a normal respiratory rate is less concerning than a child who is too breathless to talk, has significantly increased work of breathing and who appears confused or looks exhausted and pale.

The following should be considered in a child with acute asthma episode

1. Assess and manage: Arway, breathing and circulation –if unwell with respiratory distress start high flow oxygen.
2. Check oxygen saturation level and if less than 94% start oxygen.
3. If over 5 years and if able to check peak flow – if less than 50% this is a moderately severe attack, if less than 33% of normal this is a life threatening exacerbation.
4. Give salbutamol 10 puffs via a spacer device – this is called Multidosing– this can be repeated half hourly until benefit seen. Arterial blood gases are not performed in acute asthma - they can cause further distress. Capillary blood gases can be done in those causing concern – they will give a useful CO_2 level.
5. Children with severe distress who cannot multidose, should be given nebulised salbutamol (2.5 mg in those under 5 years and 5mg in those over 5 years). The nebuliser can be given continuously in severe attacks.
6. Give oral prednisolone 2 mg/kg per day up to maximum of 40 mg per day
7. Reassess –if child not improving or getting worse obtain intravenous access, start IV hydrocortisone. Consider IV aminophylline infusion –bolus should be given if child not on theophylline. IV Salbutamol and IV Magnesium can also be added for severe attacks. Paediatric centres vary in their first choice of IV treatment for asthma.

Unwell children should be moved to a high dependency area if available, for close observation and cardiac monitoring. If children with life threatening asthma deteriorate despite these measures with increasing CO_2 levels and increasing oxygen requirement then non invasive ventilatory support can be given by way of a face mask and either continuous positive airway pressure (CPAP) or bi level ventilatory support (BIPAP) where both inspiration and expiration are supported by the ventilator. Very rarely do children need invasively ventilated for asthma. Indications for this would be respiratory failure not responding to all other measures and respiratory arrest. As with many other causes of arrest in children out of hospital arrests have a very poor prognosis. Most children respond well to Multidosing with salbutamol, oxygen and steroids.

BRONCHIECTASIS

Bronchiectasis is a condition where the bronchi are irregularly shaped and dilated (Fig. 6.16). Pulmonary secretions do not drain properly and are prone to infection. This causes further inflammation and scarring with airways obstruction. Congenital bronchiectasis is rare. Most are acquired from genetic conditions such as cystic fibrosis, primary ciliary dyskinesia and immunodeficiency

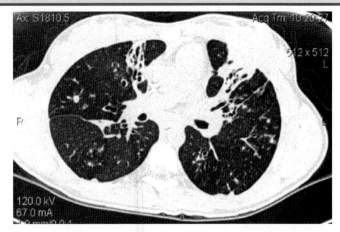

Fig. 6.16: CT scan showing severe bilateral bronchiectasis

syndromes. Post-infectious bronchiectasis can occur following pneumonia, measles or whooping cough. It can also occur secondary to recurrent aspiration or to foreign body aspiration. Often no cause is found. Bronchiectasis causes chronic cough and sputum production. Recurrent exacerbations can occur causing breathlessness and significant morbidity.

The clinical features of bronchiectasis include finger clubbing and chest deformity. Any child with bronchiectasis needs investigations to try to find and treat the cause. The mainstay of treatment is chest physiotherapy and prompt treatment of exacerbations with antibiotics. Sputum cultures aid in choice of antibiotics.

CYSTIC FIBROSIS

This is a very common genetic condition in Caucasians. In the UK the carrier rate is approximately 1 in 25. It is rare in the African American population but is found in the Asian population particularly those of Pakistani and Indian origin. It has autosomal recessive inheritance caused by mutations on the CF gene, which is located on the long arm of chromosome 7. There are over 1000 causative mutations the most common one being Delta F508. The mutations are found in the gene which codes for a protein - the Cystic Fibrosis Transmembrane Regulator protein , CFTR which is made up of 1480 amino acids. This protein is a chloride channel regulator and mutations in it cause defects in salt and water absorption across cells. There are 5 main classes of severity of CF mutations as shown in Figure 6. 17. They can result in different problems with CFTR function from Class 1 nonsense mutations causing the CFTR protein not to be made properly in the first instance, to the CFTR being made properly but not transported to the cell membrane where it is needed. Individuals who are homozygotes with Class 1 or Class II mutations are associated with more severe disease.

The different combinations of mutations lead to different levels of functioning CFTR protein. Classic CF

Classes of Mutations of CFTR Protein
CLASS 1 G542X, W1282X, 1078 DELTA T, 621+1G-t, R553X
CLASS 2 DF508, S549N
CLASS 3 G551D, R560T
CLASS 4 R117H, G85E, R347P
CLASS 5 3849+10KbC-T

Fig. 6.17: Classes of severity of CF mutations of CFTR protein

disease with failure to thrive, severe bronchiectasis and pancreatic insufficiency is usually only clinically apparent where the levels of CFTR protein are extremely low. The parts of the body, which are most reliant on the functioning of the CFTR protein, are the vas deferens, the pancreas, lungs and bowel. Interestingly there are other genes called "disease modifiers" and they are thought to explain the findings that you can have 2 children from the same family with the same CF mutations who have different disease severity.

Presentation of Cystic Fibrosis

"Mild CF" may only present in adulthood with male infertility and sinusitis whereas "Classic CF" where 2 of the more severe mutations are involved presents in childhood with recurrent chest infections, malabsorption and failure to thrive due to pancreatic exocrine insufficiency.

CF should be suspected in children with frequent chest infections, particularly those with diarrhoea. Finger clubbing may be present as well as chest deformity, crackles and wheeze. Abdominal distension and malabsorptive signs should also prompt further investigation.

Cystic fibrosis can also present as neonatal gut obstruction where the bowel is obstructed by inspissated meconium. This causes small bowel obstruction and can be associated with micro colon (Figure 6.18). The small bowel distension can be detected on antenatal ultrasound. The affected bowel can be necrotic and frequently the affected bowel is resected and stomas created and then reconnected when the bowel has healed. Bowel dysfunction is common and it can take some time for the bowel to absorb feeds normally. Specialist input from dieticians and gastroenterology is needed as these babies can require TPN for several months until their bowel recovers.

Screening for Cystic Fibrosis

In some countries where CF is common neonatal screening has been introduced. The process is based on measuring the immunoreactive trypsin level (IRT) in the newborn screening blood spot which is taken at day 5 of life. If the IRT level is significantly elevated then the blood is sent for genetic analysis for the 30 common CF mutations. If the

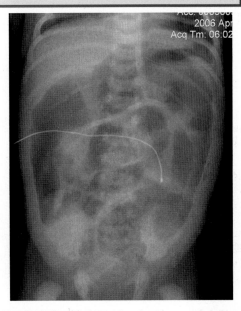

Fig. 6.18: Bowel obstruction due to meconium ileus

baby is found to have CF it is hoped that earlier diagnosis could lead to a better prognosis.

Cystic Fibrosis Diagnosis

The gold standard for the diagnosis of CF is the sweat test. This involves obtaining a sample of sweat induced by Pilocarpine and measuring the amount of sodium and chloride present. The weight of sweat needed is 100 mg of sweat and a sweat chloride concentration over 60 mmol/kg is diagnostic of CF. Often the sodium levels are elevated as well. False positive and false negative sweat tests do occur and usually 2 or 3 sweat tests are done. If the sweat test is positive then the child's blood is sent for CF gene mutation analysis.

Additional tests that can help include measurement of the faecal fat, which is often positive in malabsorption, and measuring faecal chymotrypsin levels which are low.

Disease Progression

CF is a life-shortening disease with no cure. Many treatments are available which can help to improve life expectancy but the average life expectancy of a child born today with CF is to the late 30's. Thirty years ago children with cystic fibrosis rarely survived into adulthood. CF specialists continue to look for new therapies and potential cures, e.g. Gene therapy to try to replace the defective gene. Cystic fibrosis causes tenacious respiratory secretions, lung infection and inflammation. The repeated infections and inflammation cause destruction of the airways with obstruction and bronchiectasis (Fig. 6.19). Ultimately this causes respiratory failure. Such children should be considered for referral for double lung transplant.

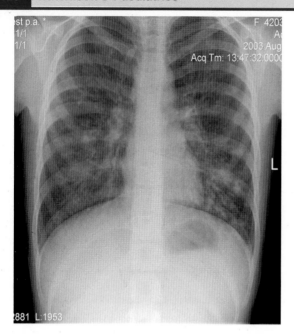

Fig. 6.19: Severe cystic fibrosis lung disease with hyperinflation, central peribronchial thickening and bronchiectasis

However, this is not without risk and consideration needs to be taken of what organisms the child recurrently cultures from their sputum, whether the child is significantly underweight and how compliant patients and their parents are with treatment. Unfortunately there is a significant shortage of organs, particularly for children.

There are several charitable organizations worldwide for cystic fibrosis which have valuable information on their websites (www.cftrust.org.uk, www.cff.org).

Common Respiratory Pathogens in CF

The CF lung is susceptible to infection and damage from a number of organisms. These include *Staphylococcus aureus*, *Pseudomonas aeruginosa*, *Haemophilus influenzae* and *Burkholderia cepacia*. UK centers have most children on prophylactic anti-staphylococcal antibiotics. *Pseudomonas aeruginosa* and *B. cepacia* are organisms that are ubiquitous in the environment. *Pseudomonas aeruginosa* colonization, where *Pseudomonas* is recurrently isolated from cough swabs or sputum has been shown to adversely affect the outcome in CF. If *Pseudomonas* is isolated, even if a child is well, eradication measures are started including oral, nebulised and intravenous anti-pseudomonal antibiotics. This is to try to prevent colonization with *Pseudomonas*.

Epidemic subtypes of the *B.cepacia* organism have caused significant increased mortality. Many centres are now segregating both inpatients and outpatients to try to reduce the spread of organisms from one patient to another.

Management of Cystic Fibrosis

This is multidisciplinary and involves specialist physiotherapists, dieticians, dedicated nursing, medical and surgical staff, social workers, psychologists, pulmonary physiologists and geneticists. The cornerstones of therapy are chest physiotherapy, nutritional support, prophylactic antibiotics and prompt antibiotic treatment of increased respiratory symptoms.

Physiotherapy

Physiotherapy in CF has 2 main goals the first being secretion clearance and the second being improving overall fitness. Various techniques are used such as the use of PEP masks; flutter devices and specific breathing exercises with vibration. Chest physiotherapy should be performed twice daily. Chest percussion and drainage are rarely used now. Daily activity is encouraged in children and should be as fun as possible, e.g. use of trampoline.

Nutrition

The aim in CF is to achieve normal growth. This can be difficult in cystic fibrosis due to the combination of pancreatic insufficiency and the fact that recurrent infections lead to poor appetite and increased basal metabolic rate. Normal growth has been shown to improve lung function and survival in cystic fibrosis. Usually for this to occur the child's intake often needs to be more than a child of their age would normally have. This can mean larger portions and consumption of foods higher in calories. In children who are pancreatic insufficient, pancreatic enzymes need to be given with all meals and most snacks to help with food digestion and absorption. Malabsorption can still occur despite pancreatic enzymes. Other medications, e.g. ranitidine can be added to their treatment to try to reduce gastric acidity and improve the functioning of the enzymes. Children may need calorie supplements and also gastrostomy feeding. Children with advanced lung disease can continue to lose weight despite all of these measures. Fat- soluble vitamins are given daily usually in multivitamin preparations.

Antibiotics

In the UK prophylactic antibiotics are given usually against *Staphylococcus aureas* e.g. Flucloxacillin. Mild pulmonary exacerbations are treated with additional oral antibiotics. Moderate to severe exacerbations are managed with intravenous antibiotics usually with 2 drugs e.g. Ceftazidime and tobramycin, which are active against *Pseudomonas* as well as a number of other bacteria for 2 weeks. Physiotherapy is also increased in frequency. Many parents can do some of the intravenous antibiotic therapy

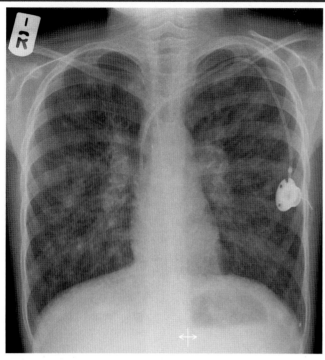

Fig. 6.20: Advanced bronchiectasis in cystic fibrosis with a Port-a cath

at home. Some children with difficult intravenous access require semi-permanent subcutaneous central venous access e.g. Port-a-cath (Fig. 6.20). This allows frequent drug administration without repeated venepuncture. Nebulised antibiotics e.g. "Colomycin" and "Tobi (neubiliser solution, tobramycin)" are also used in the management of *Pseudomonas aeruginosa*.

Azithromycin is also increasingly being used in patients with CF who recurrently grow *Pseudomonas*. It has been shown in several studies to reduce the number of exacerbations. It is thought to have an anti-inflammatory effect.

Other CF Therapies

Pulmozyme, a nebulised preparation that breaks down the DNA in respiratory secretions is used in some patients to aid sputum expectoration. Nebulised Hypertonic saline has also been shown to help with sputum clearance.

CF COMPLICATIONS

CF Gut Disease

CF affects gut function and can cause chronic constipation and occasionally distal intestinal obstruction (DIOS). The treatment of constipation includes dietary interventions and laxatives, e.g. Lactulose and Movicol. Obstruction

requires admission to hospital and further management with gastrograffin.

CF Liver Disease

Focal biliary cirrhosis is the commonest form of liver disease in cystic fibrosis. It is often asymptomatic. Cirrhosis with portal hypertension is only reported in 2-3% of children with CF and 5% of adults. However, liver disease is the second most common cause of death. There is increased incidence in those who have had meconium ileus but otherwise it is unrelated to genotype. Liver disease is three times more common in boys. The pathogenesis of liver disease in CF is not entirely understood. It is thought to be due to defects in biliary chloride transport, leading to diminished bile salt production. The liver often has fatty infiltrates as well. Stasis and obstruction in the biliary tree then ensue. Also intrahepatic bile ducts are often abnormally narrow and gallbladder abnormalities are common. The diagnosis of liver disease is difficult as liver enzymes may only be mildy elevated. Annual liver ultrasounds are the best way of picking up early changes. The treatment includes Ursodeoxycholic acid, attention to nutrition and Vitamin K for those with abnormal coagulation studies.

Cystic Fibrosis Related Diabetes (CFRD)

Again this is a rare complication in childhood but affects up to 30% of adults with CF. Untreated it causes increased morbidity and mortality. Its onset is often insidious and it needs to be thought of in a child who is not doing well and losing weight for no apparent reason. Its exact pathogenesis is not understood but there is fibrosis and fatty infiltration of the pancreas with resulting loss of islet cells. However, there are people with CF who appear to have similar levels of pancreatic damage but one is diabetic and one is not. There is therefore thought to be an additional genetic predisposition. Insulin is used in the management of CFRD.

PRIMARY CILIARY DYSKINESIA

The respiratory tract is lined by ciliated mucosa. Mucociliary clearance plays an important role in defending the lungs against bacteria. PCD is a rare autosomal recessive condition in which the cilia beat abnormally and are structurally defective. This results in abnormal mucus clearance that causes frequent chest infections with chronic cough and bronchiectasis. Males are also infertile. Ear infections are common. Kartagener first described it in 1933 as a syndrome of bronchiectasis, situs inversus (where the heart and abdominal organs are located on the opposite sides of the body to normal and sinusitis. The diagnosis is made by biopsy of the nasal mucosa and the material analysed for cililal movement and structure. Treatment of this condition includes chest physiotherapy and prompt treatment of infections with antibiotics.

PULMONARY TB

Tuberculosis is caused by infection with *Mycobacterium tuberculosis*. Tuberculosis is most common in the developing countries of the world and is sustained in areas of poverty and deprivation. TB notifications steadily decreased in the 20th Century but have not decreased in the past decade. Significant cause or morbidity and mortality worldwide.

In children the infection is spread from an adult who is infected and so called "sputum positive" i.e. has Mycobacterium in their sputum. Children are rarely contagious as they rarely expectorate infected sputum. Spread is more common with close household or school contacts. Pulmonary TB is caught by inhaling respiratory secretions from an infected person when they cough or sneeze. The bacteria then grow over several weeks and stimulate the immune system as the body tries to kill the bacteria. In about one fifth of infected individuals this process is not effective and the bacteria remain in a latent form. The *Mycobacterium tuberculosis* can reactivate at any time leading to TB disease. Pulmonary TB disease causes cough, night sweats and weight loss. Full Guidelines for the management of TB can be found at www.nice.org.uk.

All children who are known contacts of someone with sputum positive TB should be seen and have a Mantoux and chest X-ray performed. Blood tests for TB are based on detecting Tuberculous Antigens, e.g. Early Secretions Antigen Target 6 (ESAT-6) and Culture Fibrate Protein (CFP-10).

Children with positive Mantoux test and chest X-ray changes are usually admitted for 3 early morning gastric washings. This is the best way of obtaining an organism in a child. Young children are particularly at risk of TB meningitis. Rifampicin, Isoniazid, Pyrazinamide and Ethambutol are common dugs used in TB. They are used in combination usually 3 drugs for 2 months and then Rifampicin and Isoniazid are continued for a further 4 months. In parts of the world where resistance to these drugs is a problem then other agents, e.g. Streptomycin is used. Close follow up is needed and frequently children are put on Directly Observed Therapy or "DOTS" where nursing staff observe the therapy being given three times a week.

BRONCHIOLITIS OBLITERANS

Bronchiolitis obliterans is rare in children. It is a result of an injury to the bronchioles and smaller airways. Repair of this leads to excessive granulation tissue that block airways. The airways then become obliterated by nodular masses of granulation and fibrosis.

In children the majority of cases are post infectious, e.g. adenovirus 3, 7 and 21, Measles, Influenza, Mycoplasma and Pertussis. It can also occur post lung transplant. In many no obvious injury can be found. The symptoms of bronchiolitis are usually persistence of cough, wheeze and breathlessness following viral like illness. Affected children usually have persisting wheeze and crackles on auscultation. They can significant hypoxia with cyanosis. It can also cause bronchiectasis and chronic respiratory failure.

The chest radiograph findings vary from normal to areas of hyperlucency, hyperinflation, to bronchial wall thickening consolidation and bronchiectasis. The changes may be bilateral or unilateral. The diagnosis of bronchiolitis obliterans relies on high-resolution chest CT scan where areas of hyper aeration, mosaic ground glass appearance and bronchial wall thickening are seen. The treatment of bronchiolitis obliterans in children is difficult. In some cases prednisolone has been used and appears to be of benefit. Other reports suggest spontaneous remission. Some children still die of respiratory failure. Poor prognostic factors are age –children who are older do worse, atopy and also those who present in the winter. The reasons for these differences are not known.

PNEUMOTHORAX

Air in the pleural space is called pneumothorax. A tension pneumothorax is one where the air collection gets larger with each breath and causes mediastinal shift to the opposite side of the chest. The clinical signs of this are hyperresonance and decreased air entry on the affected side with tracheal shift to the opposite side. This is a life-threatening emergency, which requires immediate resuscitation and needle decompression by placement of an intravenous cannula in the second intercostal space in the midclavicular line on the affected side. A formal chest drain connected to an underwater seal should then be inserted usually in the 5th intercostal space in the mid axillary line on the affected side.

Rarely spontaneous pneumothoraces do occur –they can be associated with chest pain on the affected side and breathlessness. Some of these may be due to rupture of previously undiagnosed congenital lung bullae. Small pneumothoraces do not need drained, as many will resolve spontaneously.

Most pneumothoraces in children are secondary to other problems. They can occur secondary to chest trauma, acute severe pneumonia, cystic fibrosis, as a complication of chest drain insertion for pleural effusion or central line insertion or to foreign body inhalation. The chest X-ray in Figure 6. 21 shows the appearance of a pneumothorax with the loss of lung markings and free air round the lung.

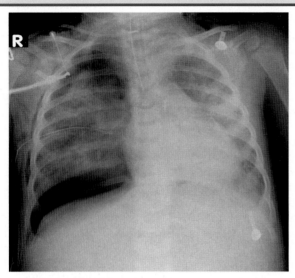

Fig. 6.21: Severe pneumonia with a large right sided pneumothorax in an intubated child

In some severe pneumonic processes the pleural air can actually be in pockets around the lung and sometimes more than one chest drain is needed.

SLEEP DISORDERED BREATHING IN CHILDREN

Sleep disordered breathing is increasingly recognized in children. When asleep the normal child's breathing control changes and there is reduced muscle tone in the intercostal muscles and the pharyngeal dilator muscles. This increases airways resistance. Children with e.g. adeno-tonsillar hypertrophy who can breathe satisfactorily when awake then develop significant obstruction to air flow when asleep. Hypoventilation can also occur when asleep, particularly children with neuromuscular weakness. The most serious form of hypoventilation is congenital central hypoventilation syndrome (CCHS) where the infant's ventilatory drive is impaired and when the infant falls asleep they stop breathing. This condition is fatal without treatment with ventilatory support.

OBSTRUCTIVE SLEEP APNOEA (OSA)

This is thought to affect 0.7-3% of children with the majority being under 5 years. It is thought to result from a combination of problems with ventilatory drive, neuro-muscular control and anatomical factors. The classical features are loud snoring, pauses in breathing with gasping breaths at the end of an apnoea and abnormal chest movement. This is associated with partial awakening. Children with OSA are often restless. The disturbed sleep leads to daytime sleepiness, irritability and poor concentration. Severe OSA in a young child can cause failure to thrive. OSA in young children is usually due to adenotonsillar hypertrophy. Upper airway congenital abnormalities e.g. cranio facial abnormalities can also cause OSA. Older children with OSA are often morbidly obese –either from eating too much, or secondary to other conditions which cause excess weight gain.

Children with suspected OSA need clinical examination and further investigation. This can include an overnight oxygen saturation study which will document periods of hypoxia to full polysomnography where oxygen saturation levels, respiratory muscle movement, eye movements, airflow, heart rate and EEG are recorded.

Children whose OSA is due to adenotonsillar hypertrophy usually respond well to adenotonsillectomy. They start to sleep better and most of the behaviour and concentration problems improve. There are some concerns however that there may be lasting neurodevelopmental consequences. Children with underlying conditions and those obese children who fail to lose weight need further treatment. Untreated OSA with recurrent hypoxia and hypercapnia leads to hypertension, left ventricular hypertrophy, cor pulmonale and death. Pulmonary hypertension can also occur.

Treatment involves ventilatory support at night with non-invasive ventilation using either a nasal or face mask and ventilator. Usually BIPAP support is used. This method gives additional pressure support to aid breathing in both inspiration and expiration. This is usually well tolerated in children and significantly improves sleep quality by correcting the hypoxia and hypercapnia. It can be difficult to institute in children with significant neurological handicap, particularly those with behaviour problems.

NEUROMUSCULAR CAUSES OF SLEEP DISORDERED BREATHING

There are many neuromuscular disorders which cause sleep disordered breathing from a combination of either neurological insult, severe muscle weakness or hypotonia, e.g. Downs syndrome, Duchenne's muscular dystrophy (DMD), spinal muscular atrophy, cerebral palsy, CCHS and children with impaired breathing following spinal cord damage. The treatment of these children is based on their individual needs and their prognosis from their underlying condition. Children with DMD will ultimately die from respiratory failure, however non-invasive ventilation using BIPAP at night has been shown to improve life expectancy.

SUDDEN INFANT DEATH SYNDROME

This can be defined as the sudden unexpected death of an infant for which no apparent cause can be found despite careful investigation and postmortem. It is the most common cause of post neonatal infant death in the United States and Canada. The cause of SIDS is not understood however there are documented postmortem findings such as evidence of low-grade asphyxia in the lungs and structural and neurotransmitter abnormalities in the brain stem. The incidence of cot death fell dramatically with the "Back to Sleep" campaign where evidence had shown that infant who were laid prone to sleep had an increased chance of SIDS so advice was given to lay all infants on their back. Maternal and antenatal risk factors include maternal smoking, alcohol use in pregnancy, illegal drug use and poverty. Infant risk factors include age – SIDS peaks at 2-4 months, male sex, prematurity and exposure to tobacco smoke. Losing an infant to SIDS can have devastating effects on families and there are several charities offering support and funding ongoing research into SIDS such as the Foundation for the Study of Infant Deaths (www.sids.org.uk).

CHEST INJURY

Chest trauma in children is rare and in younger children it is usually accidental, e.g. road traffic accident. In older children and teenagers deliberate violence, such as stabbings and gun shot wounds, can cause significant injury. Children's chest walls have increased elasticity in comparison to the adult bony thorax. They can sustain chest trauma with damage to internal thoracic organs without rib fractures. Therefore if the history of the accident is such that significant force has been involved, then it should be assumed that there is underlying internal organ damage until proven otherwise. If the chest wall is significantly damaged, e.g. flail chest then this is tolerated less well in children in comparison to adults. Chest injuries seen in children include tension pneumothorax, open pneumothorax, haemothorax, pulmonary contusions, and cardiac tamponade; flail chest and disruption of the great vessels. The priority in managing a child with trauma is establishment and protection of the airway; assessing breathing and dealing with life threatening problems, e.g. needle decompression of tension pneumothorax and then assessing the circulation and giving fluid resuscitation. Children with significant trauma should have 2 large bore cannula inserted and blood should be taken for immediate cross-matching so it is available when needed.

FOREIGN BODY INHALATION

This is a fairly common problem in paediatrics, particularly in the preschool child. It occurs when a child accidentally inhales a foreign object, which is often food. Usually this leads to choking and coughing, which nearly always dislodges the object from the larynx and expels it.

Children who fail to clear the object and who are choking and having difficulty breathing need urgent measures to clear the blockage – if the object is visible in the mouth it should be removed. If the child can cough they should be encouraged to cough. If the cough is ineffective and a child is conscious then a combination of back blows and abdominal thrusts and the Heimlich manoeuvre can be used in the older child. In young infants abdominal thrusts should not be used because of the possible damage to internal organs. Emergency help should be sought. In the unconscious child who has choked, airway opening manoeuvres should be performed, rescue breaths given and cardio-pulmonary resuscitation started if there are no signs of improvement.

Smaller inhaled objects e.g. peanuts can pass through the larynx and lodge in the trachea or one of the bronchi. This can lead to persistent coughing and on auscultation you may hear unilateral wheeze. A chest radiograph could show hyperinflation of one lung, caused by partial obstruction to the flow of air on that side, i.e. air can get into that lung but not get out. Peanuts are also very irritant and can lead to a secondary pneumonia. If a child is suspected of foreign body inhalation then they require a rigid bronchoscopy to remove the offending object.

QUESTIONS

1. A fourteen-week-old baby presents with a 1 week history of intermittent stridor. She had been admitted twice previously and had been diagnosed as having croup and had been given oral steroids, which did appear to help. On examination she is alert and has marked inspiratory stridor with mildy increased work of breathing, her oxygen saturation is 98% in air. What further investigations does she need?

2. What pattern of lung disease do the following lung function results suggest? What 2 diseases could result in this picture?

FEV1	1.35 predicted 1.80
FVC	1.90 predicted 1.86
TLC	3.0 predicted 2.76
RV/TLC	40% predicted 24%

3. A 2-year-old boy is admitted to the surgical wards with his fourth rectal prolapse.
   He is thriving with weight on the 50th centile and height on the 50th centile.
   He has a very good appetite and eats as much as his 5 year old brother. He passes 2- 3 pale loose stools per day. He has an occasional cough.
   His full blood count and urea and electrolytes are normal.
   What investigations are needed?

4. A 5-year-old boy is admitted with a severe choking episode requiring resuscitation. He recovers well.
   However, he had a history of recurrently choking with feeds from early infancy. He had a hoarse voice. At 6 months he had a chest X-ray and barium swallow which were normal. He was allowed home and apart from one admission with croup was not unwell enough to require admission. His parents report

that the choking with fluids has been an ongoing problem. He is thriving and has no problems swallowing. What other investigations does he need?

What is the management of this condition?

5. A two-month-old baby girl is admitted with two days of snuffles, cough and difficulty feeding. On examination her temperature is 37.9 degrees, her respiratory rate is 60, she has moderate subcostal recession and crackles evident bilaterally. Her oxygen saturation is 89%

What is the most likely diagnosis?

What would your management be?

What investigations are needed?

6. A twelve-year-old girl is admitted with several days of cough and fever. An X-ray shows partial left lower lobe pneumonia. As she is systemically well she is commenced on oral antibiotics and is allowed home. Four days later she is readmitted with recurrence of fever and difficulty breathing. There is decreased air entry at the left base.

What further investigations would you do?

Her white cell count is 25; her urea and electrolytes are normal. Her chest X-ray shows a left sided effusion.

What investigation would you do next?

What is the management now?

7. A twelve year old boy is referred with chest tightness on exercise and breathlessness. His asthma control had previously been well controlled on Flixotide 250 mcg twice daily via spacer and ventolin as needed. His inhaler technique is good and you are fairly certain he takes his inhalers! What treatment would you add?

8. A 5-year-old girl is reviewed as an emergency with an exacerbation of asthma

She is breathless, wheezy and pale

What would you do?

ANSWERS

1. This baby should have a barium swallow performed to look for a vascular ring. If this is negative then she should have a bronchoscopy performed to rule out the presence of an anatomical abnormality of her airway or laryngeal haemangiomas.

2. The results suggest an obstructive lung disease pattern such as that caused by severe asthma or cystic fibrosis.

3. With the history given the possibility of cystic fibrosis needs to be investigated, e.g. child needs a sweat test in the first instance.

4. He requires a bronchoscopy to look for a tracheo-oesophageal fistula. The management of this is surgical repair of the fistula. This is a real case and postoperatively the child remained well with no cough.

5. The most likely diagnosis is bronchiolitis. The management is to give oxygen, start NG feeds or IV fluids and obtain an NPA for virology. This baby requires close observation of temperature, pulse and respiratory rate and oxygen saturation

6. Initial investigations would be FBC, Blood cultures, Electrolytes, Mycoplasma Serology and chest X-ray. The abnormal chest X-ray should be followed by chest ultrasound to assess the amount of effusion present. The management would be insertion of a chest drain under general anaesthetic and instillation of a Fibrinolytic agent, e.g. Tissue Plasminogen Activator.

7. There are several options here – you could add in an inhaled long acting beta agonist, start a combination preparation of an inhaled steroid and a long acting beta agonist or add a leukotriene receptor antagonist.

8. Give oxygen, multi-dose with ventolin 10 puffs via spacer and repeat as needed depending on patient response. Give oral prednisolone 2 mg/kg up to max of 40 mg per day.

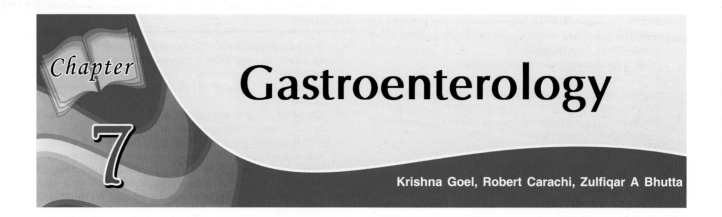

Chapter 7

Gastroenterology

Krishna Goel, Robert Carachi, Zulfiqar A Bhutta

7.1: Gastrointestinal and Liver Disease

INTRODUCTION

The alimentary tract is a complicated viscus extending from the mouth to the anus with structural differentiation and adaptation according to the specific function needed. The oesophagus is a passage from the pharynx to the stomach, where digestion begins. Food then moves into the small intestine, where further digestion and absorption occurs. The large intestine reabsorbs 95% of water and completes absorption of digested products leaving the residue to be expelled intermittently from the rectum.

The most common signs of alimentary tract disorders are vomiting, abdominal distension and disorders of defaecation. In the older infant and child abdominal pain becomes the most common symptom indicating dysfunction of the gut and requires investigation of its cause. An adequate history from the parents and child is most helpful in arriving at the correct diagnosis, and this may be followed by examination and investigations. Many of the causes of abdominal pain are discussed later in the differential diagnosis of acute appendicitis. Most newborn babies vomit a few times in the first weeks of life. A small quantity of milk is often regurgitated when wind is "broken" during or after feeding. Persistent vomiting and vomiting in the older child is usually a significant sign and may be associated with a wide variety of pathological conditions. Infections of the alimentary tract such as gastroenteritis, result in the infant or child presenting with vomiting, which is also a common non-specific, sign in other infections e.g. meningitis, urinary tract infection or septicaemia. Vomiting is the most consistent sign of obstruction in the newborn. It usually starts in the first day of life and becomes progressively more frequent. The vomit usually contains bile, as it is rare for the obstruction to be above the ampulla of Vater. Bile stained vomiting in the absence of an organic cause is rare and infants and children with bile stained vomit should be investigated in hospital.

Normal infants should pass meconium within 24 hours of birth. Delay to do so or failure to pass meconium is an important sign, which should not be overlooked. Failure to pass meconium may be due to an organic obstruction but subsequent passage may be a sign of disease such as hypothyroidism or Hirschsprung's disease.

The infant normally settles into a pattern of having one, two or more bowel actions daily but diarrhoea, increased frequency of passage of stools which become more liquid, or constipation are presenting signs of a variety of disorders. In the early stages of intestinal obstruction there may be little abdominal distension, and any such distension may be difficult to distinguish from the naturally protuberant abdomen of the newborn. Visible loops of bowel and peristalsis are abnormal in the term or older infant, but in the thin walled premature infant may not be indicative of obstruction. For surgical paediatric problems see chapters 10 and 11.

> **Key Learning Point**
>
> Bile–stained vomiting in the absence of an organic cause is rare and infants and children with bile–stained vomit should be investigated in hospital.

GASTRO-OESOPHAGEAL REFLUX (GOR)

Reflux of gastric contents is a physiologic occurrence that takes place more often during infancy and decreases with advancing age. The vast majority of infants with GOR who are symptomatic of vomiting during the first year of life resolve their overt symptoms between the ages of nine and twenty four months. Because most infants with symptoms of GOR are thriving and healthy, they require no diagnostic or therapeutic measures other than a careful history and physical examination, with appropriate reassurance to the parents if they are worried. However, infants and older children who have significant neurologic deficits or psychomotor retardation often have significant GOR and may suffer from serious sequela secondary to GOR. Recurrent pneumonia or blood loss from erosive oeso-phagitis in these children is not uncommon. These children usually require aggressive or definite treatment, such as fundoplication, to reduce their likelihood of peptic oesophagitis with bleeding, aspiration pneumonia, or both.

Abnormal posturing with the tilting of the head to one side and bizarre contortions of the trunk has been noted in some children with GOR. These symptoms are often referred to as Sandifer syndrome.

The barium swallow is a sensitive way of detecting reflux but has a very low specificity rate because many infants who have little or no clinical symptoms of reflux experience reflux of some barium into the oesophagus. However, a 24-hour pH probe study can give fairly reproducible information on the amount of reflux that is occurring in an infant. Now pH monitor can be done on children as outpatients with the ambulatory device being read by an automatic system at a later date.

Treatment of GOR is by keeping the baby propped up upright in a baby seat and this gives a gravitational effect, which may help to decrease the vomiting. Thickening of feeds decreases vomiting without causing significant delay in gastric emptying.

GASTROINTESTINAL HAEMORRHAGE

The paediatrician who is confronted with a child with gastrointestinal haemorrhage faces one of the most difficult diagnostic and management problems in clinical practice of paediatrics. In spite of the availability of sophisticated diagnostic tools, many paediatric patients with gastro-intestinal haemorrhage remain undiagnosed. However, differentiating upper gastrointestinal from lower gas-trointestinal bleeding will guide the sequence of diagnostic tests.

Haemetemesis is obviously a marker of upper gastro-intestinal haemorrhage and melena a marker of lower gastrointestinal bleeding. The term melena signifies the passage of dark stools stained with blood pigments or with altered blood (maroon stool). It is vital that only after exclusion of upper gastrointestinal bleeding one should consider a colonic lesion in the case of melena. On the other hand hematochezia i.e. the passage of bloody stools (not dark or maroon) points to a colonic source of blood. Small intestinal bleeding may manifest as either melena or hematochezia. The causes of gastrointestinal haemo-rrhage are shown in Table 7.1.1.

Diagnosis

A history of haemetemesis is suggestive of an upper gastrointestinal bleeding lesion. Therefore upper GI

Table.7.1 1: Causes of Gastrointestinal Bleeding in Children

- Haemorrhagic disease of the newborn
- Swallowed maternal blood (neonate)
- Infectious diarrhoea
- Oesophageal varices
- Mallory-Weiss tear
- Gastric and duodenal ulcers
- Meckel's diverticulum
- Intussusception
- Duplication cysts
- Ulcerative colitis
- Crohn disease
- Nonsteroidal anti-inflammatory drugs (NSAIDs)
- Vascular malformations
- Anal fissure
- Haemorrhoids
- Henoch-Schönlein purpura
- "Unexplained"

endoscopy should be carried out and it may lead to the diagnosis. Massive lower gastrointestinal bleeding in children is uncommon. The presence of leukocytes in the stool suggests an infectious or inflammatory diagnosis. Thus a stool specimen should be sent for culture and identification of parasites. After anal inspection, a flexible sigmoidoscopy is indicated. If this is negative a colono-scopy should be done to visualise the entire colon and the terminal ileum. If melena (dark stool) is the presenting feature and upper GI endoscopy is negative, colonoscopy should be the next step. However, if the diagnosis remains unclear, a Meckel's scan may suggest a bleeding site, to be confirmed by angiography during active bleeding.

Treatment

Treatment of a massive GI haemorrhage is aimed at resuscitating the patient, localising the site of bleeding, and deciding on a treatment plan to stop the haemorrhage. Treatment for mild bleeding depends on the lesions found.

OESOPHAGEAL VARICES

Bleeding from oesophageal varices (Fig. 7.1.1) may be sudden and profuse and cause exsanguination of the patient. Rapid and adequate transfusion is necessary. Emergency endoscopy should be undertaken in an attempt to establish this diagnosis and injection of varices with sclerosant agents may be commenced. If this is impossible, then control of the bleeding may be achieved by giving intravenous infusions of vasopressin or somatostatin. Tamponading of the oesophageal and gastric varices may be possible with the Sengstaken tube. Someone experienced in proper positioning of the balloons should do insertion of this tube and it should be done under imaging control. The oesophageal balloon is blown up to a pressure of 40 mmHg. This pressure will have to be released

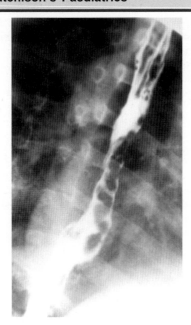

Fig. 7.1.1: Barium swallow demonstrating oesophageal and gastric varices.

intermittently to prevent pressure necrosis. This measure should only be undertaken in an attempt to resuscitate the patient prior to more definitive treatment, which may include surgical transection of the oesophagus of hemitransection or the stomach (Tanner's operation). Emergency portocaval or splenorenal shunting is rarely necessary in children. Most patients with portal hypertension and variceal bleeding can be managed by repeated injections of sclerosants into the varices, thus allowing collaterals to develop and improve the drainage from the portal venous system.

PEPTIC ULCER

Although rare in infancy and childhood, gastric and duodenal ulcers may occur. Secondary ulcers (Curling) associated with severe infections or extensive burns have become rare.

Clinical Features

Some of the vague abdominal pains, which are so common in childhood, may be due to undiagnosed peptic ulcer. Indeed, many of these patients may have paid several visits to the hospital and seen several consultants, and eventually referred to the psychiatric department before an underlying peptic ulcer may be diagnosed. While the disease may run a silent course in infancy, in the older child the clinical picture is similar to that in adult life. There is epigastric pain or discomfort relieved by eating; pain at night is common. Vomiting an hour or two after food may follow pylorospasm or actual scarring of the pylorus. There may be evidence of malnutrition. The

disease may present with recurrent or severe haemorrhage or with perforation into the peritoneal cavity, which is very rare. Endoscopy is usually diagnostic although barium meal is less invasive and if indicated may not always reveal a peptic ulcer. During endoscopy, biopsies of the pyloric antrum and the duodenal mucosa are examined to establish the presence of *Helicobacter pylori*. The typical appearance of nodular gastritis is highly suggestive of *H.pylori* infection, especially in the paediatric population. The urea breath test is the most reliable of the non-invasive tests for *H. pylori* infection. If *H. pylori* are present, then the association between them and peptic ulceration is quite high and treatment should be given. Eradication of *H.pylori* infection reduces the recurrence of primary duodenal ulcers in children.

Treatment to eradicate *H. pylori* infection in children consists of: one-week triple-therapy regimen that comprises omeprazole, amoxicillin, and either clarithromycin or metronidazole. There is normally no need to continue antisecretory treatment (with a proton pump inhibitor or H_2-receptor antagonist) unless the ulcer is complicated by haemorrhage or perforation. Resistance to clarithromycin or to metronidazole is much more common than to amoxicillin and can develop during treatment. A regimen containing amoxicillin and clarithromycin is therefore recommended for initial therapy and one containing amoxicillin and metronidazole for eradication failure. Lansoprazole may be considered if omeprazole is unsuitable. Treatment failure usually indicates antibacterial resistance or poor compliance. Two-week triple-therapy regimens offer the possibility of higher eradication rates compared to one-week regimens, but adverse effects are common and poor compliance is likely to offset any possible gain.

Key Learning Point
Long-term healing of gastric and duodenal ulcers can be achieved rapidly by eradicating *Helicobacter pylori*.

Antacids have been used for many years in the treatment of ulcer disease in infants and children. H_2 receptor antagonists have made substantial impact on the clinical practice of treating peptic ulcer disease.

BLOOD PER RECTUM

Passage of blood from the rectum is common in paediatric practice. The diagnosis may be straightforward and the cause obvious, but in many the cause of bleeding is never found even after full investigation including laparotomy. Serious underlying causes have to be excluded as outlined in Table 7.1.1.

Most children seen in the outpatient department with rectal bleeding pass only small quantities of blood after defaecation. Anal fissure is the most common cause but it may be due to rectal prolapse and proctitis. Acute anal fissure is the most common cause of rectal bleeding. There is usually a history of constipation and generally pain on defaecation. The bleeding is usually small in amount, bright red, streaked on the outside of the stool and occurs during or just after defaecation. The fissure is usually in the midline posteriorly. Perianal redness and shallow fissures may be the first sign of a granulomatous proctitis sometimes associated with Crohn disease. Most fissures are easily seen and digital rectal examination without anaesthesia, which may be very painful, is unnecessary and should be avoided. The management of anal fissures includes stool softening and the short-term use of a topical preparation containing a local anaesthetic. Children with chronic anal fissures should be referred to a hospital specialist for assessment and treatment with a topical nitrate, or for surgery.

Moderate or extensive bleeding is infrequent but the common lesions are rectal polyps, enteritis or enterocolitis, intussusception, Meckel's diverticulum, volvulus, duplication of the alimentary tract, haemangiomas in the bowel, systemic haemorrhagic disease and in the neonate, necrotising enterocolitis and haemorrhagic disease of the newborn.

Digital rectal examination, proctoscopy, sigmoidoscopy colonoscopy or barium enema may show up the lesion which can then be treated appropriately. A Technetium scan may be necessary to demonstrate a Meckel's diverticulum or a duplication of the bowel but a negative scan does not exclude either, as it is dependent on the presence of ectopic gastric mucosa.

Key Learning Point

Acute anal fissure is the most common cause of rectal bleeding.

RECTAL PROLAPSE

Rectal prolapse may be partial when the mucous membrane only is prolapsed or complete when there is protrusion of the entire rectal wall (Fig. 7.1.2). The 1 to 3 year age group is the usual age. Mucosal prolapse is more common and occurs in children with chronic constipation and is usually initiated by prolonged straining. Prolapse is sometimes the presenting sign of cystic fibrosis. Complete prolapse occurs in debilitated or malnourished children. It is also seen in children with paralysed pelvic floor muscles as in myelomeningocele.

Parents usually notice the red mucosa coming out of the anus after defaecation. The prolapse has usually reduced before the doctor sees the patient. On rectal examination the anal sphincter is found to be very lax and redundant folds of rectal mucosa often follow the withdrawn finger. The child presenting for the first time with a rectal prolapse should have a sweat test performed to exclude cystic fibrosis.

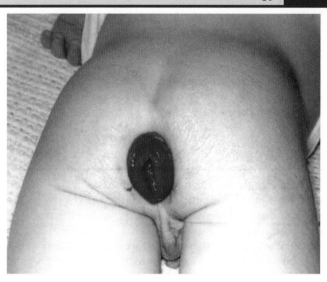

Fig. 7.1.2: Rectal prolapse in a child subsequently confirmed as having cystic fibrosis

To the parent a prolapse may be a terrifying event and it is important that the anxious parents are reassured. The prolapse may be reduced by simple pressure or by elevating the foot of the cot, or raising the buttocks on a pillow. Reversion to nappies instead of squatting on the pot should be advised for 3 months from the last prolapse but reassurance that this will not interfere with long-term defaecation control is necessary. For persistent or frequently recurring prolapse the buttocks may be strapped together and the child given a laxative. In most instances once the stool is softened, the prolapse becomes less of a problem and rectal prolapse in children is usually a self-curing condition. Only very rarely is it necessary to treat this surgically with injection of phenol in olive oil into the submucosa of the rectum or by a perianal stitch.

Key Learning Point

A child presenting for the first time with a rectal prolapse should have a sweat test to exclude cystic fibrosis.

INTESTINAL POLYPS

A solitary rectal polyp is a common cause of bleeding from the rectum. This low polyp is easily felt on digital rectal examination. The polyp is a granulomatous hamartoma of the mucous membrane, which becomes pedunculated and may protrude at the anus like rectal mucosa prolapse. Polyps high in the rectum and lower colon require sigmoidoscopy under general anaesthesia and may be removed by snaring. Occasionally, juvenile polyps are multiple and may be demonstrated by double contrast studies. True familial polyposis is very rare under the age of 12 years, but the rectum and colon can be carpeted with polyps, which histologically are papillomas or adenomas of the adult type. This disease is usually carried as a Mendelian dominant and cancer of the colon develops in young adult life. Peutz-Jegher's syndrome is a familial condition in which polyps of the small intestine are accompanied by brown pigmentation of the lips, buccal mucosa. Symptoms and signs include repeated episodes of abdominal pain due to transient intussusceptions, blood loss from the intestinal tract and anaemia.

INFANTILE COLIC

Infantile colic is defined as excessive crying in an otherwise healthy infant. The crying usually starts in the first few weeks of life and ends by four to five months. The cause is unclear. It may represent part of the normal pattern of infantile crying. Other possible explanations are painful intestinal contractions, lactose intolerance, gas or parental misinterpretation of normal crying. Infantile colic improves with time.

RECURRENT ABDOMINAL PAIN IN CHILDREN

Recurring and unexplained abdominal pain often presents a difficult problem to the family doctor and to both the paediatric physician and surgeon. Most of these patients do not have underlying disease; however they often require evaluation and treatment to allay fears and improve their quality of life. The pain may amount to little more than discomfort. It may be accompanied by nausea and vomiting. Physical examination should be complete and not only directed toward the abdomen. It is unusual to find any definite signs on abdominal examination and it may be difficult to assess the severity of the pain. Questions, which should be asked, of the pain are:
1. What is the duration of each attack?
2. Is the child ever sent home from school because of the pain?
3. Does it interfere with games or does it become worse when there
   are household chores to be done or errands collected?
4. Does the pain ever waken the child from sleep?

Constipation should always be eliminated in these cases and the presence of dysuria, increased frequency of micturition, pyuria or haematuria call for urological investigation. Plain X-rays of abdomen may be useful to reveal a faecolith in an appendix, calcification in mesenteric glands, or calculus formation in the renal tract. Barium meal or barium enema examination may reveal such lesions such as polyps, peptic ulceration or malrotation, which can be a cause of chronic abdominal pain. In the female, recurrent abdominal pain may precede by many months the onset of the first menstrual period (menarche). When organic disease has been reasonably excluded, the proportion of patients who are found to be suffering from emotional disorders is related to the degree of skill and experience in the diagnosis. The term abdominal migraine covers a group of patients who suffer from recurrent attacks of acute, midline abdominal pain, vomiting and headache, photophobia during episodes, family history of migraine with intervening symptom-free intervals lasting weeks to months

Management of the child with recurrent abdominal pain after treatable causes have been excluded is by reassurance to the patient and parents that there is no serious underlying disease and that symptomatic treatment until the child outgrows the problem is indicated.

APPENDICITIS

Acute appendicitis is the most common lesion requiring intra-abdominal surgery in childhood. The disease runs a more rapid course in children and the criteria for establishing a diagnosis and for treatment are different. Under the age of four, the diagnosis is difficult and in 90% the infection has spread transmurally to the peritoneal cavity or the appendix has ruptured.

Pathology

There is marked variation in the anatomy of the appendix. The appendix is attached to the posterior medial quadrant of the caecum. In childhood, the appendix lies in a retrocaecal position in 70% of patients. Obstructive appendicitis is common in childhood, the obstruction being caused by a kink, a faecolith, or the scar of a previous attack of inflammation. When inflammation occurs, there is an accumulation of purulent exudate within the lumen and a closed loop obstruction is established. Blood supply to the organ is diminished by distension or by thrombosis of the vessels and gangrene occurs early in children. Fluid is poured into the peritoneal cavity as a result of irritation, and within a few hours this fluid is invaded by bacteria from the perforated appendix or from organisms translocating the inflamed but still intact appendix. Peritoneal infection may remain localised by adhesions between loops of intestine, caecal wall and parietal peritoneum. There is danger in administering a purgative in these children because it increases intestinal and appendicular peristalsis and perforation and dissemination of infection are more likely to occur.

Appendicitis may present as:
1. Uncomplicated acute appendicitis.
2. Appendicitis with local peritonitis.
3. An appendix abscess or diffuse peritonitis.

The onset of symptoms is vague and initially may be of a general nature. Only a third of younger patients are seen in hospital within 24 hours of onset of abdominal symptoms, and the appendix has ruptured in a high percentage of these young patients before admission. The diagnosis is made late in many cases. One reason for delay in diagnosis is failure to suspect appendicitis in a child less than 4 years of age and the other is the poor localisation of pain by the younger child. Although often not severe, the pain appears to come intermittently and irritability, vomiting and diarrhoea may result in the mistaken diagnosis of gastroenteritis. Psoas spasm from irritation of the muscle by the inflamed appendix may cause flexion of the hip resulting in a limp, thus distracting attention from the abdomen and directing it to the hip joint. Vomiting occurs in most patients. The child is usually pyrexial but the temperature is only moderately elevated to between 37°C and 38.5°C. Temperatures higher than this usually suggest upper respiratory tract infections or occasionally diffuse peritonitis from appendicitis. A history of constipation is uncommon and in many patients there is a history of diarrhoea.

The clinical features in the older child are similar to those in the adult. Abdominal pain is usually followed by nausea and vomiting. The pain begins centrally and later shifts to the right iliac fossa. If the appendix is retrocaecal, abdominal pain and tenderness may be slight. If the child has a pelvic appendix then tenderness may again be slight, or absent, or elicited only on rectal examination. Anorexia is a common accompanying sign.

Clinical Examination

The child with acute appendicitis is usually anorexic, listless and does not wish to be disturbed. There is often a characteristic fetid odour from the tongue, which is furred.

The child is usually irritable, crying and unco-operative. Low-grade pyrexia is usual but the temperature seldom exceeds 38.5°C. Inspection alone may be very informative while attempting to gain the child's confidence. The most important physical sign on abdominal examination is the area of maximum tenderness located in the right iliac fossa and the presence of rebound tenderness. If this is not defined, then a gentle digital rectal examination should be made and tenderness may be elicited or a mass felt in the pelvis in patients with a pelvic appendix.

Urine should be checked for presence of bacteria or white cells and also to exclude glycosuria or significant proteinuria. Leucocytosis is usually present in children with acute appendicitis but a normal white cell count does not exclude the diagnosis. The child with diffuse peritonitis may have a low white cell count. Plain X-ray of the abdomen often gives useful signs of acute appendicitis (Fig. 7.1.3).

The sensitivity and specificity of ultrasound examination for appendicitis can be quite variable. The examination must be the part of the whole clinical picture in deciding upon operative intervention. Also a negative ultrasound examination does not exclude appendicitis. Use of CT scan of abdomen in the evaluation of difficult

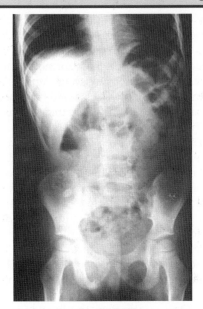

Fig. 7.1.3: X-ray of abdomen showing faecolith, scoliosis with psoas spasm, dilated loops of bowel with fluid level and loss of fat line cell.

cases of abdominal pain has been reported. The CT findings suggestive of appendicitis include appendiceal wall thickening, presence of inflammatory changes in the periappendiceal fat, or the presence of an abscess.

Differential Diagnosis

Differential diagnosis includes numerous other disorders the commonest of which is upper respiratory tract infection. Presence of a common cold, sinusitis, acute tonsillitis, pharyngitis may all be associated with acute non-specific mesenteric lymphadenitis. This is the most common condition to be differentiated from acute appendicitis. The presence of enlarged glands elsewhere in the body accompanied with an upper respiratory tract infection may suggest this condition. Fever may be absent but temperature can be very high. The presence of abdominal tenderness is not as acute as that in appendicitis. It is usually more generalised and not localised to the right iliac fossa and there is no rebound tenderness. The presence of a cough, increased respiratory rate and runny nose may suggest a respiratory infection. Examination of the chest is mandatory to pick up any signs of consolidation as right lower lobe pneumonia may result in referred pain occurring in the right lower quadrant of the abdomen. Constipation can cause abdominal pain, nausea and vomiting, with tenderness over the distended caecum. It can be easily mistaken for acute appendicitis. Faecal masses may be felt per abdomen or on digital rectal examination. Usually following a suppository, satisfactory evacuation of the colon and rectum will bring rapid relief in patients whose symptoms are caused by constipation.

Urinary tract infection can usually be differentiated by a higher temperature, pus cells in the urine, and tenderness over one or other kidney in the renal angle.

Abdominal trauma, accidental or non-accidental may cause injury to the abdominal viscera. A plain X-ray of the abdomen and a serum amylase should be done to exclude the presence of traumatic or idiopathic pancreatitis and a pneumoperitoneum.

In gastroenteritis and dysentery there may be severe cramping and abdominal pain. The pain and tenderness may be more marked over the distended caecum. Other members of the family may have similar symptoms or diarrhoea. Rectal examination can help differentiate between a pelvic appendicitis and appendicitis with pelvic peritonitis from gastroenteritis

Infective hepatitis may occur in epidemic form but in an isolated case may simulate appendicitis. The temperature is usually elevated and the child complains of a headache with nausea, vomiting, abdominal pain and tenderness. On examination, the liver is enlarged and tender. The child may or may not be jaundiced depending on whether he is seen in the prodromal phase of the disease. Examination of the urine usually reveals the presence of bile salts, but urobilinogen may be present.

Intestinal obstruction may be due to incarceration of a hernia, secondary to anomalies, e.g. a volvulus around a vitello-intestinal remnant, or adhesions following previous abdominal operations. Vomiting, abdominal colic, abdominal distension and constipation are the usual signs. After a thorough clinical examination plain X-ray of the abdomen in the erect and supine positions should be carried out to differentiate intestinal obstruction from appendicitis.

Primary peritonitis is an uncommon diagnosis and almost always affects the female. There is a diffuse infection of the visceral and parietal peritoneum usually due to a pneumococcus. With the peritonitis there is exudation of fluid to the peritoneal cavity. Mesenteric lymph nodes are swollen. Diffuse abdominal pain, vomiting, dehydration and a high fever are the main features and diarrhea may be present initially, but is usually followed by constipation. Rectal examination usually is suggestive of a pelvic appendicitis as there is diffuse tenderness and heat present. The white blood cell count is usually grossly elevated between 20,000 to 50,000 per cu mm. The diagnosis is usually made at laparotomy when peritonitis is found but the appendix is normal.

Severe abdominal pain and vomiting may occur during passage of a renal calculus. Hydronephrosis due to blockage of the pelviureteric junction by stricture, stone or aberrant vessel may present with abdominal pain and nausea. The pain and tenderness are maximal in the flank. Red or white cells may be found in the urine.

Haemolytic Uraemic syndrome may present with acute abdominal pain and may be confused with acute appendicitis. The presence of fragmented red blood cells on a blood film and also the presence of oliguria is suggestive of this disease.

Crohn disease is an uncommon diagnosis in childhood but the incidence is increasing in Western countries. It can present with all the symptoms of acute appendicitis and at operation the terminal ileum is found to be acutely inflamed and thickened. A biopsy reveals the diagnosis and barium meal and follow-through very often indicates the presence of other areas of the affected gut.

In torsion of the right cord or testis, confusion with acute appendicitis may occur whereas this is less likely with torsion of the left testis. Routine examination should always include the inguinal regions and the scrotum. Inflammation of Meckel's diverticulum and intussusception in older children may simulate acute appendicitis. Other medical conditions, which should be considered, are those of diabetes mellitus, cyclical vomiting and Addison's disease. The onset of menstruation may simulate appendicitis and many girls have recurring attacks of lower abdominal pain, sometimes for a year before menstruation actually begins. Pain associated with torsion of an ovary or an ovarian cyst may also present with signs similar to those of acute appendicitis.

It is not uncommon for children to harbour threadworms (pinworms) without noticeable symptoms. Many symptoms and signs have been ascribed to the presence of threadworms including weight loss, poor appetite, nausea, vomiting and chronic abdominal pain.

Carcinoid tumour in the appendix is rare in childhood but the tumour may obstruct the lumen of the appendix and lead to obstructive appendicitis. It is far more common to find this as an incidental finding on histopathology of the removed appendix. When it is present in the tip of the appendix, no further follow-up is necessary in these cases. In older children, if a carcinoid exists in the caecal region there is a chance of invasive disease with subsequent evidence of the carcinoid syndrome. Treatment should include a right hemicolectomy and careful follow-up with MIBG scan and measurement of 5-H.I.A.A.

Treatment

The treatment of the child with acute appendicitis is early operation. In the toxic child with peritonitis, time may be profitably spent in combating toxaemia and dehydration. It is important to resuscitate the patient and start intravenous antibiotics before surgery is undertaken. In such cases, metronidazole, Ceftazidime and Cefotaxime should be given intravenously. The institution of intravenous antibiotics given as three doses pre-per and post-operatively with peritoneal lavage in children with peritonitis has considerably reduced the incidence of post-operative complications. In children, early appendicectomy is indicated in the child with appendix abscess.

This hastens the recovery period and allows much earlier discharge from hospital.

The best access to the appendix with the minimal disturbance of the peritoneal cavity is through a gridiron or lance incision and appendicectomy is performed. There is an increasing trend to perform appendicectomy by minimal invasive surgical techniques rather than "open" operation.

Post-operative complications. Wound infection is the most common complication following appendicitis. Since the introduction of metronidazole and Cefotaxime given routinely to patients who have appendicectomy, the incidence of wound infection has dropped significantly. Evidence of infection may be obvious within a day or two of the operation or may be delayed for several weeks. There is a rise in temperature, local tenderness of the wound, and redness and swelling. Pus may be released by inserting sinus forceps into the edge of the wound to allow it to be discharged.

Localised intraperitoneal abscesses may form after the subsidence of a diffuse peritonitis particularly in the pelvis. Fever may fail to resolve and there is usually lower abdominal pain, tenderness and even diarrhoea with increased frequency of micturition. There may also be abdominal distension due to an associated ileus affecting the terminal ileum. On digital rectal examination, a tender swelling is felt anteriorly. Many pelvic collections resolve on intravenous antibiotics, and very occasionally pus may be evacuated spontaneously through the rectum. Alternatively, drainage through the original incision under a general anaesthetic and insertion of a Penrose drain to maintain a route to the surface will help clear the pelvic collection. There is no evidence to substantiate the claim that pelvic peritonitis in the young female may lead to sterility in adult life. Subphrenic collections have become extremely rare in children even in those who have had diffuse peritonitis.

Early post-operative intestinal obstruction is usually due to impaired motility of matted loops of ileum lying in pus in the pelvis. Treatment is by antibiotics, intravenous fluids and continuous nasogastric suction. With this conservative management resolution is usual and very few require surgical intervention. If there is volvulus or a closed loop situation then earlier surgical intervention is mandatory in order to relieve the distension and prevent devascularisation of part of the bowel.

Respiratory complications are seldom severe. Mild atelactasis is not uncommon and infection of a collapsed area should be prevented with help from physiotherapists and breathing exercises. Faecal fistula is rare and may be due to necrosis of part of the caecal wall. The fistula usually closes spontaneously with conservative treatment. Rarely a faecolith may have escaped from the necrotic appendix at the original operation and lie in the peritoneal cavity.

This causes persistence of a fistula until the faecolith is removed.

FOREIGN BODIES

Children frequently place objects in their mouth and occasionally accidentally swallow them. Most pass down the alimentary tract and out of the anus in 24 to 48 hours, but occasionally the coin, pin or toy may stick in the oesophagus. This causes discomfort and inability to swallow freely. The offending foreign body may be removed by passing a catheter beyond the foreign body, inflating a balloon on the distal end of the catheter, prior to withdrawing the catheter and the object proximal to it. If this fails, removal under direct vision through an endoscope under anaesthesia is the preferred method. Most foreign bodies, which reach the stomach ultimately, pass spontaneously. Two exceptions to the "wait and see" approach are the hairball and batteries. The formation of a hair ball (trichobezoar) may be followed by poor health and vague abdominal pain as the gastric lumen becomes partially occluded by a dense mass. The history of hair eating (trichotillomania) is rarely given spontaneously by the child or the parents. A mass may be palpated in the epigastrium. Diagnosis is confirmed by endoscopy or X-ray after a barium swallow. The hairball may be passed spontaneously but gastrostomy may be required. Children swallow small alkaline batteries and the gastric juice may interact with them and if left may cause severe ulceration. These should not be allowed to remain in the stomach for more than 48 hours and may be removed endoscopically or by gastrotomy under anaesthesia. All other swallowed foreign bodies pass uneventfully through the gastro-intestinal tract once they have reached the stomach.

Key Learning Point
Ingested Foreign Bodies "Wait and See" Most ingested foreign bodies, which reach the stomach ultimately, pass uneventfully through the gastrointestinal tract.

NECROTISING ENTEROCOLITIS (NEC)

Necrotising enterocolitis (NEC) is a severe disease of the gastrointestinal tract. Prematurity or low birth weight is the most commonly associated factors and occurs in 90% of babies with this disease. Term infants are affected to a lesser extent and constitute about 10% of the affected group. Hypovolaemia and hypoxia result in damage within the mucosa cells initiating the NEC. It is often multifactorial in origin, resulting in loss of integrity of the gut mucosal barrier with passage of bacteria into the wall of the bowel.

Prematurity, respiratory distress syndrome (RDS), congenital cardiac malformations, umbilical vessel catheterisation, exchange transfusions, hypoglycaemia, polycythemia, post-operative stress and hyperosmolar feeds have all been implicated in the aetiology. Bacterial infection has been implicated in NEC and from time to time one sees some confirmation of this because of the clustering of the disease in neonatal units. There are protective antibodies in breast milk, which decreases but does not completely protect babies at risk from NEC.

The incidence of this disease varies from country to country. There is a very low incidence in Japan and a high incidence in the United States. The severity of the disease is variable from a minor form seen in many cases, which are managed entirely in the Neonatal Units, to a fulminating type of the disease with perforation, peritonitis and death.

Initially, one sees a preterm infant with signs of sepsis, vomiting of feeds, abdominal distension and frequently the passage of blood or mucus in the stools. Clostridial infections have been associated with some outbreaks of NEC. If the disease continues to progress peritonism develops and this is often appreciated first by nursing staff observing abdominal distension.

Examination of the abdomen may show signs of inflammation, redness, oedema of the abdominal wall with localised or generalised tenderness, and if the baby has a patent processus vaginalis, free fluid or even gas or meconium is occasionally seen in the scrotum. If a perforation has occurred then one loses the area of superficial dullness of the liver on percussion of the abdomen. Palpation may reveal crepitus from the intramural gas, which can be palpated among the coils of distended loops of bowel, and this is an important sign of NEC.

A plain X-ray of abdomen (Figs 7.1.4. A to C) may show pneumatosis intestinalis (gas within the bowel wall) and gas in the portal vein and liver. This sign is often an ominous one with a very high mortality. The extent of the NEC may be localised to an area of the bowel, very often the colon, but in extensive disease the whole of the gastrointestinal tract may be involved.

The differential diagnosis early in this disease may be difficult and one should consider the following diagnoses.
1. Septicaemia from other causes
2. Volvulus neonatorum
3. Hirschsprung's enteritis
4. Infarction of the bowel

Management

Most babies with NEC are managed medically and relatively few require surgical care. Management consists of stopping all oral intake, nasogastric aspiration and instituting intravenous fluids to counteract the hypovolaemia, dehydration and acidosis. Infants with NEC tend to lose a lot of fluid, which is very rich in protein and in electrolytes into the tissues and into the lumen of the bowel. Anaemia, if present, needs to be corrected by blood transfusion, and the fluids, electrolytes and protein replaced. The baby must be maintained normovolaemic with a good peripheral perfusion. On the basis that there is a septic element involved, a broad-spectrum antibiotic is given. Following stabilisation of circulation and ventilation when indicated, total parenteral nutrition is commenced. When the physical signs have reverted to normal, the oral intake is started and gradually built up over several days until full feeds are again established.

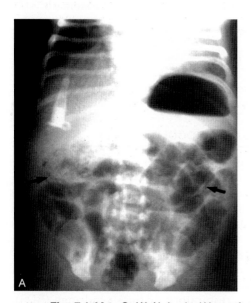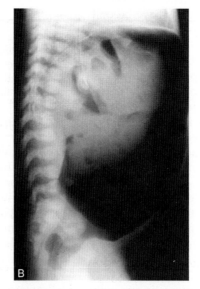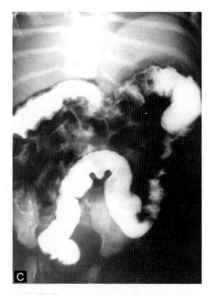

Figs 7.1.4A to C: (A) Abdominal X-ray of premature infant showing pneumatosis (see arrows). (B) The free air in peritoneal cavity indicates perforation. (C) Barium enema showing extensive pneumatosis coli.

Surgical Management

If there is a persistent acidosis, which often indicates progressive disease or a perforation of the bowel, then surgical intervention is very often necessary. Perforation is detected by seeing free gas in the peritoneal cavity in an erect or lateral abdominal X-ray. In very low birth weight (under 500 g) infants percutaneous drainage has been used in preference to laparotomy. This is performed by means of applying a local anaesthetic to the right lower quadrant of the abdomen, and then a 10 to 12 French gauge catheter is inserted into the abdominal cavity to drain air, meconium and faecal material which has leaked from perforated bowel.

TODDLER'S DIARRHOEA

Toddler's diarrhoea is the commonest cause of chronic diarrhoea without failure to thrive in childhood, but its pathogenesis remains unclear. Stool in children with toddler's diarrhoea classically contains undigested food materials because of rapid transit and often is referred to as "peas and carrots" stool.

Diagnosis is based on the history and the clinical criteria: age of onset between 6 and 36 months, diarrhoea during waking hours, and no failure to thrive. Treatment usually is not necessary. Dietary adjustments with elimination of fruit juices and other drinks with high osmotic load may be helpful.

INFECTIOUS DIARRHOEA IN CHILDHOOD
(See Section 7.2)

FERMENTATIVE DIARRHOEA
(Disaccharide Intolerance)

In the healthy child the disaccharide sucrose is split into the monosaccharides, glucose and fructose by small intestinal sucrase-isomaltase enzyme and the disaccharide lactose into the monosaccharides glucose and galactose by the enzyme lactase. Failure of any of these enzyme systems will result of an excess of disaccharide in the intestine where bacteria will ferment the sugars to produce acid and an increased osmotic bowel content. This results in fermentative diarrhoea with the passage of highly acid watery stools. Symptoms are relieved when the offending disaccharide is removed from the diet. Lactase deficiency inherited as an autosomal recessive disorder causes persistent diarrhoea from birth because both human and cows' milk contains lactose. When there is a delay in the onset of symptoms this suggests a sucrase-isomaltase deficiency, as sucrose and starch are not usually added to the diet in the first weeks after birth. In addition to the autosomal recessive inheritance of the deficiency there can be transient disaccharide intolerance acquired secondarily

to gastroenteritis or other intestinal mucosal insult. Investigations, which help to confirm disaccharide intolerance, include the pH of the fresh stool less than 5.5 and the presence of reducing sugars revealed by the Clinitest and by the identification of faecal sugars on thin-layer chromatography. Removal of all disaccharide from the diet and replacement with monosaccharide will result in a resolution of the diarrhoea. Re-introduction of the disaccharide will result in the return of the diarrhoea and there will be a failure of the normal increase in blood glucose of at least 2.8 mmol/l (50 mg per 100 ml) expected in the normal subject. Rarely a monosaccharide malabsorption syndrome (glucose - galactose malabsorption) can occur. Jejunal biopsy will allow direct measurement of enzyme activity in the jejunal mucosa. The diarrhoea in infants with the hereditary forms of the disorder can be abolished by total exclusion from the diet of the offending carbohydrate.

Systemic Illness

In addition to the acute diarrhoea caused by food poisoning from food toxins or bacterial toxins, viral, bacterial and protozoal bowel infections there are a number of systemic illnesses, which are complicated by acute diarrhoea, and vomiting. Septicaemia, meningitis, pneumonia and infectious hepatitis may be accompanied by diarrhoea and vomiting. Abdominal distension with bloody diarrhoea may suggest an acute surgical condition or the haemolytic uraemic syndrome. Hospital admission is indicated if significant dehydration (more than 5%) is present, when there is doubt about the diagnosis, when hypernatraemia is suspected, when an underlying medical condition such as adrenogenital syndrome or chronic renal insufficiency is present or when outpatient management has failed or is thought to be inappropriate due to adverse social or other circumstances.

PARASITIC INTESTINAL INFECTION

It is estimated that between 800 million and one thousand million people in the world are suffering from at least one type of worm infection. The most important intestinal worms are nematodes and cestodes.

NEMATODES

These are round elongated, non-segmented worms with differentiation of the sexes.

Roundworm (Ascaris lumbricoides)
Mode of infection

Infection arises from swallowing ova from soil contaminated with human excreta. The ova are not embryonated

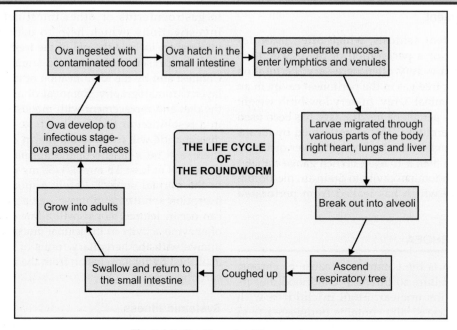

Fig. 7.1.5: The life cycle of the roundworm

when passed in the faeces but they become infective in soil or water. When swallowed by man the hatched larvae penetrate the intestinal wall and pass via the liver and lungs to the trachea, oesophagus, stomach and intestine where they grow into mature worms (Fig. 7.1.5).

Clinical Effects

A few roundworms in a well-fed patient usually produce no ill effects and are not noticed until a worm is either vomited or passed in the stool. Typical clinical features include: a protuberant abdomen, intermittent intestinal colic, digestive disturbance, general debility, loss of appetite and insomnia. In heavy infections worms may migrate into and block the bile duct producing jaundice while similar blocking of the appendix can cause appendicitis. In very heavy infections intestinal obstruction can occur from a tangled ball of roundworms. The presence and extent of roundworm infection is readily detected by microscopical examination of the stools for ova.

Piperazine citrate in a single oral dose of 75-mg/kg to a maximum single dose of 5 g will clear roundworm from 75% of patients. Two doses on successive days give a marginally higher cure rate. Piperazine citrate has minimum adverse effects - very occasionally unsteadiness and vertigo. Mebendazole is active against threadworm, whipworm and as well as roundworm infections and can be safely recommended for children over the age of 2 years. A dose of 100 mg twice daily for 3 days is effective.

(Ankylostoma duodenale; Necator americanus)

There are two types of hookworms, Ankylostoma duodenale being most commonly found in Egypt, Africa, India, Queensland and also in the Southern USA, while Necator americanus is found in the Americas, the Philippines and India. These two species differ in small anatomical details but their life cycles are identical (Fig. 7.1.6). The male and female worms live chiefly in the jejunum. The worm attaches itself to the intestinal mucosa by its teeth and sucks blood. The ova, passed in the faeces, hatch out in water or damp soil and larvae penetrate the skin of the buttocks or feet. They reach the heart and lungs by the lymph vessels and blood stream, penetrate into the bronchi, are coughed up into the trachea and then pass down the oesophagus to mature in the small intestine.

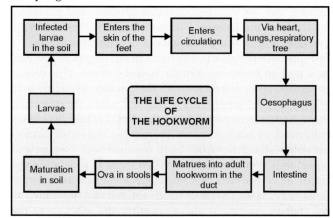

Fig. 7.1.6: The life cycle of the hookworm.

Clinical Effects

The main clinical picture of disease is caused by prolonged loss of blood. Therefore the clinical manifestations of infection depend on the number of worms present and the nutritional state of the patient. A few hookworms in a fairly well fed person produce no disease as the small blood loss in constantly being replaced. In children whose diet is inadequate and the worm load heavy severe anaemia may stunt growth, retard mental development and in very severe cases result in death through heart failure. Infection is diagnosed by microscopical examination of the stools for eggs, the number of which indicates the severity of infection (72,000 ova/g = significant infection).

Treatment

Children with severe anaemia and malnutrition should have blood transfusion and nutritional support before definitive worm therapy is started. Mebendazole has a useful broad-spectrum activity, and is effective against hookworms; the usual dose for children over one year of age is 100 mg twice daily for three days. Levamisole is also effective.

Strongyloidiasis: (Strongyloides stercoralis)

These worms are fairly widespread in warmer climates and may be found concurrently with hookworm infection. Incidence is often highest in children and the usual mode of infection is penetration of the skin by infective larvae present in the soil. Migration through the lungs also occurs and can produce respiratory signs and there may be abdominal distension, bloody diarrhoea and anaemia. Creeping eruptions, particularly around the buttocks, can develop as a result of the reinfection. Diagnosis is made by identification of larvae in the faeces.

Thiabendazole (50 mg/kg divided into two doses given morning and evening) is the most effective treatment. Albendazole is an alternative with fewer side-effects; it is given to children over two years of age in a dose of 400 mg once or twice daily for three days, repeated after three weeks if necessary. Invermectin given to children over five years in a dose of 200 micrograms/kg daily for two days may be the most effective drug for chronic Strongyloides infection.

Threadworm: (Enterobius vermicularis-oxyuriasis; pinworm or seatworm)

The male worm is about 3 mm in length and the female, which looks like a small piece of thread is about 10 mm. The female, lives in the colon. Eggs are deposited on the perianal skin by the female contaminating the fingers of the child who may then reinfect himself. The ova after ingestion hatch in the small intestine. The male worm also fertilizes the female in the small intestine, after which the male dies while the female migrates to the caecum. It is common for this infestation to affect all members of a family because the ova can be found on many household objects. The initial infection may also be acquired from contaminated water or uncooked foodstuffs (Fig. 7.1.7).

Clinical features of enterobiasis are mainly perianal, perineal and vulval pruritus, which can interfere with sleep. Scratching leads to secondarily infected dermatitis and to reinfection through contaminated fingers. Heavy infestations could be associated with episodes of severe abdominal pain. The association of appendicitis with threadworms is exceptionally rare. Diagnosis is made by direct examination of the worms or ova trapped by "sellotape" applied sticky side to the anal skin early in the morning and then stuck on to a glass slide.

Mebendazole is the drug of choice for treating threadworm infection in children over six months. It is given as a single dose as reinfection is very common, a second dose may be given after two weeks. Piperazine is also effective. Measures to break the cycle of reinfection should be taken and these include scrupulous personal hygiene, boiling all infected linen and the wearing of occlusive clothing to prevent scratching. Treatment should also be given to other members of the family and it should be reinstituted when symptoms recur and eggs are again found in the perineal area.

Larva Migrans

Cutaneous variety (Creeping eruption)

Cutaneous larva migrans is caused by the infective larvae of various dog hookworms. These larvae can penetrate the human skin and finding themselves in an unsuitable habitat wander around in the epidermis for several weeks. Their progress is marked by a characteristic itching and a serpiginous urticarial track. The infection is more common in children than in adults and is occasionally seen in people recently returned from tropical countries.

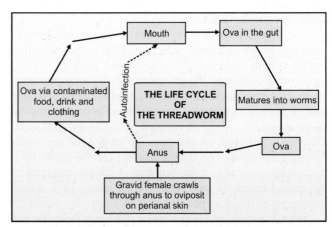

Fig. 7.1.7: The life cycle of the threadworm.

Treatment by freezing the advancing end of the track with dry ice or liquid nitrogen is no longer recommended. Applications of topical 15% thiabendazole powder in water-soluble base with or without diethylcarbamazine 5 mg/kg/day for 7 days will eliminate the larvae.

Visceral variety

This is caused by various species of the nematode Toxocara, usually *T. canis* the common roundworm of the dog. The larvae may penetrate the intestinal wall but are unable to migrate to the lungs of their unnatural host and pass through or become encysted in liver, lungs, kidneys, heart, muscle, brain or eye, causing an intense local tissue reaction. The child may fail to thrive, develop anaemia and become pyrexial with a cough, wheeze and hepatosplenomegaly. There is usually a marked eosinophilia and there can be CNS involvement. In addition to this generalized form of the disorder there may in the older child (7-9 years old), there may be the isolated loss of sight in one eye associated with ocular toxocariasis. The diagnosis can only be established with certainty from a tissue biopsy; generally taken from the liver and the Toxocara ELISA test is a useful screen.

Recently thiabendazole 50-mg/kg body weight for three to five days has been shown to kill encysted larvae and is especially useful for early ocular lesions. Normally the visceral variety is self-limiting and requires no treatment. Regular and routine deworming of puppies and pregnant bitches with mebendazole, prevention of face licking by dogs and the need to wash hands carefully after handling pets are preventative health measures. Multiple infections respond to invermectin, albendazole or tiabendazole by mouth.

CESTODES

Cestodes (tapeworms) of importance to humans are Taenia saginata (beef tapeworm), Taenia solium (pork tapeworm), Hymenolepis species (dwarf tapeworm), and Taenia echinococcus (hydatid cyst).

The ingestion of raw or inadequately cooked beef or pork can result in human infection. Man is the definitive host for both the beef (*T.saginata*) and pork (*T.solium*) tapeworms. Although the infections may be asymptomatic, epigastric discomfort, increased appetite, dizziness and loss of weight sometimes occur. These features may be more marked in children and debilitated persons. Diagnosis is based on the passage of gravid segments through the anus. The differentiation can be made by a microscopical study of the number of lateral branches in the gravid uterus of each segment, the uterus of *T. solium* having about 10 branches and that of *T. saginata* about 20.

With *T. solium* infection a major danger is the ingestion of eggs from an infected person (heteroinfection) or self-ingestion of eggs (autoinfection). This can give rise to cysticercosis where cysticerci develop almost anywhere including brain, skin, muscle and eye.

Taenia echinococcus (hydatid cyst)

The definitive host of Taenia echinococcus is the dog, wolf, fox or jackal. Man and sheep may become the intermediate host by swallowing the ova from the dog and this is especially likely in sheep-rearing countries. The adult worm in the dog is very small (0.5 cm) but the ingested ovum when swallowed by man liberates a six-hooked onchosphere into the small intestine. This penetrates to the tissues, usually the liver but sometimes lung, bones, kidneys or brain to form a hydatid cyst. This has a three-layered wall - an outer layer of host fibrous tissue, a laminated middle layer and an inner germinal layer that produces many daughter and granddaughter cysts.

Clinical Effects

These are largely due to local pressure effects. The liver may be greatly enlarged and there may be a palpable rounded swelling over which the classical "hydatid thrill" can be elicited. Ultrasound and CT scanning can reveal the cystic nature of the lesions. Eosinophilia may be marked. The diagnosis may be confirmed by complement fixation, haemagglutination or latex-slide agglutination tests but the hydatid ELISA test and improved immunoelectrophoresis tests are likely to prove more specific.

Treatment

The only measure is surgical incision. The cyst must never be tapped as a leakage of hydatid fluid into the tissues can cause shock or death. The outlook is grave if suppuration occurs within the cyst. Spontaneous recovery can occur if the cyst dies, inspissates and calcifies. Medical treatment for this most important tapeworm infecting man is generally unsatisfactory but albendazole is used in conjunction with surgery to reduce the risk of recurrence or as primary treatment in inoperable cases. Albendazole is given to children over two years of age in a dose of 7.5 mg/kg (maximum 400 mg) twice daily for 28 days followed by 14-day break and then repeated for up to 2-3 cycles. Careful monitoring of liver function is particularly important during drug treatment.

Hymenolepis (dwarf tapeworm)

Mild infestations due to Hymenolepis (dwarf tapeworm) cause no symptoms, but heavy infestations can sometimes cause diarrhoea, irritability and fits. Diagnosis is made by finding the typical ova in the faeces.

Clinical Features	Ulcerative Colitis	Crohn Disease
Location	Rectum and colon (variable)	Ileum and right colon
Diarrhoea	Severe	Moderate
Mucus blood	Frequent	Infrequent
Rectal involvement	Always	Infrequent
Fistula in ano	Absent	Infrequent
Perirectal abscess	Absent	Infrequent
Abdominal wall fistula	Absent	Infrequent
Toxic megacolon	Infrequent	Absent
Arthritis	Rare	Common
Eye pathology	Rare	Iridocyclitis, granuloma
Proctoscopic appearance	Diffuse, ulceration	Cobblestone
Small bowel involvement	Absent	Frequent
Microscopic appearance	Mucosal ulceration	Transmural granulomas

Table 7.1.2: Clinical features of ulcerative colitis and Crohn disease

Treatment

Niclosamide is the most widely used drug for tapeworm infections and side effects are limited to occasional gastrointestinal upset light-headedness and pruritis. It is not effective against larval forms. A laxative may be given two hours after the dose; an antiemetic may be given before treatment.

Praziquantel is as effective as niclosamide and is given to children over four years of age as a single dose of 10-20 mg/kg after a light breakfast (or as a single dose of 25 mg/kg for Hymenolepis nana).

INFLAMMATORY BOWEL DISEASE (IBD)

The term inflammatory bowel disease includes two clinical conditions in children, ulcerative colitis and Crohn disease (Table 7.1.2). On the whole the prognosis of chronic inflammatory bowel disease in childhood is good.

ULCERATIVE COLITIS

Aetiology

The aetiology is unknown. It is fortunately rare in children. Over the past decade it would appear that there has been little change in the incidence of ulcerative colitis but Crohn disease has increased. The reason for the change is not clear.

Severe behavioural problems in some of the affected children and their families has sometimes led physicians to regard the disease as a psychosomatic disorder, but the evidence in support of this hypothesis is extremely slender. Food allergy has been suspected, but only a small group of patients respond to withdrawal of milk. Boys and girls are equally affected. The mean age of onset is about 10 years. There is no clear-cut inheritance pattern but ulcerative colitis is more common in first-degree relatives than in the general population.

Pathology

The mucous membrane of part or all of the colon and sometimes of the terminal ileum becomes hyperaemic, oedematous and ulcerated. The lesion is continuous rather than patchy and usually involves only the mucosal and submucosal layers. The earliest lesion in many cases is a crypt abscess (Fig. 7.1.8). Granuloma formation is rare. In some cases oedema may give rise to pseudopolypoid nodules. Ulceration may extend through the muscularis and perforation of the colon can occur. Usually perforation is preceded by toxic megacolon with dilatation of an ulcerated segment of the large bowel. Carcinoma is a common late complication. Hepatic complications such as sclerosing cholangitis and chronic active hepatitis can occur with ulcerative colitis in childhood.

Clinical Features

The onset is sudden with diarrhea and the frequent passage of small stools containing blood and mucus. This tends to be most severe during the early morning but may also be

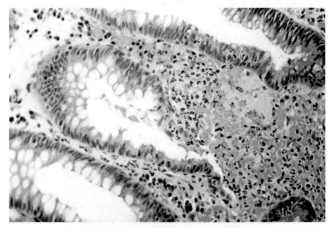

Fig. 7.1.8: Ulcerative colitis. Rectal biopsy with crypt abscess formation (obj x 25).

nocturnal. There may be abdominal pain, anorexia, weight loss or poor weight gain. Tenesmus is common.

Hypochromic anaemia due to chronic blood loss is almost invariably present. Hypoproteinaemic oedema may develop. Associated extraintestinal manifestations of the disease are more common in children than in adults. They may include erythema nodosum, aphthous stomatitis, conjunctivitis, iridocyclitis, haemolytic anaemia, arthralgia or arthritis, pyoderma gangrenosum and finger clubbing.

After exclusion of infective causes of bloody diarrhea the diagnosis should be confirmed by rectosigmoidoscopy, mucosal biopsy and barium enema. The last shows loss of normal haustrations in the colon and the so-called lead-pipe appearance (Fig. 7.1.9). Colonoscopy may allow the examination of the whole colonic mucosa and thus the extent of the disease. Radiologically differentiation of Crohn disease from ulcerative colitis can be made on the basis that Crohn disease can affect any part of the gastrointestinal tract and is patchy in distribution, whereas ulcerative colitis is a continuous lesion affecting only the rectum, colon and occasionally the terminal ileum ('Backwash ileitis'). It is worth remembering that early in the course of disease no X-ray abnormality may be found.

Ulcerative colitis frequently runs an acute course in the child. The cumulative risk of carcinoma of the colon is 20% per decade after the first decade of the illness. Dysplastic changes in the colonic epithelium are considered to be pre-malignant.

CROHN DISEASE

Aetiology

This disorder like ulcerative colitis is not common in children and it is of unknown cause.

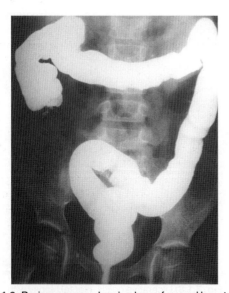

Fig. 7.1.9: Barium enema showing loss of normal haustrations (lead-pipe appearance in the colon) in ulcerative colitis.

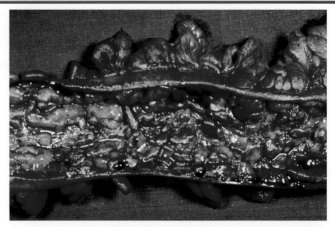

Fig. 7.1.10: Crohn disease. Open loop of ileum showing typical cobblestone appearance of the mucosa.

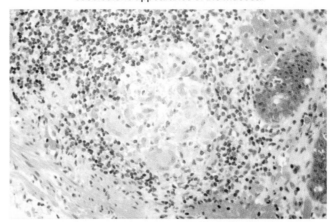

Fig. 7.1.11: Crohn disease showing a diagnostic granuloma in the lamina propria of a colonic biopsy with a central collection of epithelioid and multinucleate cells surrounded by a cuff of lymphocytes and plasma cells (obj x 25).

Pathology

Crohn disease may affect any part of the gastrointestinal tract but most commonly the terminal ileum and proximal colon. Although any part of the gastrointestinal tract from mouth to anus may be affected. The lesions are basically chronic granulomatous and inflammatory with a tendency towards remissions and relapses. The histological changes are transmural, i.e. affecting all layers of the bowel wall with oedema and ulceration of the mucosa, fissures, submucosal fibrosis and many inflammatory foci of mononuclear and giant cells (Figs 7.1.10 and 7.1.11). Perforation, haemorrhage and fistula formation are uncommon complications in childhood.

Clinical Features

In Crohn disease the diarrhoea is much less severe than in ulcerative colitis; it is often intermittent and there may be little or no obvious blood or mucus in the stools. Crohn disease presents with less specific signs and symptoms than ulcerative colitis hence the delay in diagnosis often found in Crohn disease.

General manifestations commonly include anaemia, loss of weight, growth failure, pubertal delay, erythematous rashes and a low-grade fever. Other associated features are: erythema nodosum, pyoderma, iridocyclitis, arthralgia or arthritis, spondylitis, finger clubbing, anal skin tags, fissures and fistulae. Quite frequently the disease presents with oral ulceration and this may progress to extensive involvement of the buccal mucosa, which becomes oedematous and granulomatous sometimes years before there is evidence of intestinal involvement. There is no single gold standard for the diagnosis of Crohn disease. The diagnosis is made by clinical evaluation and a combination of endoscopic, histological, radiological and biochemical investigations. Sigmoidoscopy is only helpful when the left side of the colon is involved. A barium meal or enema typically shows segmental involvement of the small bowel and/or colon, sometimes with intervening areas of normal bowel (Fig. 7.1.12). Crohn disease shows a segmental lesion while ulcerative colitis is diffuse. The appearances vary from a "cobblestone appearance" due to thickened oedematous mucosa to narrowing of the lumen with the so- called "string sign". There may be fistulous tracts to adjacent loops of bowel. Biopsy of a perirectal lesion or even of the involved buccal mucosa may reveal diagnostic granulomatous changes. Colonoscopy and biopsy may provide an immediate diagnosis.

Prognosis

Crohn disease is a lifelong condition, with periods of active disease alternating with periods of remission.

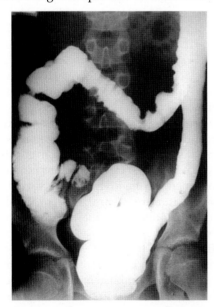

Fig. 7.1.12: Barium meal and follow through illustrating segmental involvement of the same bowel (Crohn disease).

Treatment of Ulcerative colitis and Crohn disease

To date, the standard therapies for Crohn disease and ulcerative colitis have been similar and in general can be classified as anti-inflammatory, or immunosuppressive therapy. 5-Aminosalicylic acid compounds, antibiotics, and nutritional therapy usually are considered as anti-inflammatory, whereas 6-mercaptopurine, azathioprine, cyclosporin A, and methotrexate have immunosuppressive properties. Some therapies, such as corticosteroids have both.

The general principle of IBD treatment mainly depends on the disease severity and it aims with the treatment that has the best possible chance of obtaining clinical remission with the fewest side effects. However, depending on the child's therapeutic responses or lack thereof, additional medications are added to the therapeutic regimen. Some of the differences in therapy between Crohn and ulcerative colitis include surgical intervention, antibiotics, and nutritional therapy. The surgical intervention is used in both ulcerative colitis and Crohn disease but is only curative in ulcerative colitis and is reserved exclusively for localised Crohn disease such as strictures and fistulas. The antibiotic therapy is beneficial in Crohn disease, whereas it has been used rarely in ulcerative colitis. The nutritional therapy is vital from the growth perspective in both diseases but is shown to be effective in the control of Crohn disease symptoms only.

Recently advances in immunology have led to discovery of several new immunotherapies referred to as biologics. Together with infliximab, which has been approved for the treatment of Crohn disease, other biologic therapies may be available in the near future.

COELIAC DISEASE (Gluten-Sensitive Enteropathy)

Aetiology

Coeliac disease (CD) is now regarded as an autoimmune type of chronic inflammatory condition and may have its onset at all ages. It is apparent that the harmful substance is in the gliadin fraction of gluten in wheat, barley and rye flour. The immune-mediated enteropathy is triggered by the ingestion of gluten in genetically susceptible individuals. Gluten is a mixture of structurally similar proteins contained in the cereals wheat, rye and barley. Coeliac disease is associated strongly with HLA class 11 antigens DQ2 and DQ8 located on chromosome 6p21. Coeliac disease is frequent in developed world and increasingly found in some areas of the developing world e.g. North Africa and India.

Pathology

Histological features have been defined mainly from study of jejunal biopsy specimens. The most characteristic appearance is called total villous atrophy in which the

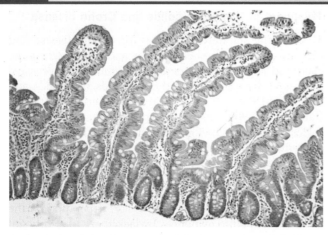

Fig. 7.1.13A: Normal jejunal biopsy: long finger –shaped villi, short crypts, scattered chorionic inflammatory cells in the lamina propria and occasional lymphocytes in intraepithelial spaces (obj x 10).

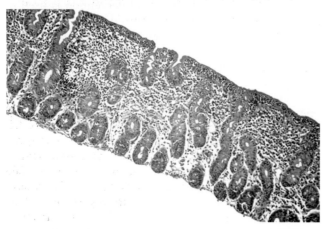

Fig. 7.1.13B: Total villous atrophy with loss of villi, elongated hyperplastic crypts, dense plasmacytic infiltrate in the lamina propria and increased number of surface intra-epithelial lymphocytes (obj x 10).

mucosa is flat and devoid of normal villi but the underlying glandular layer is thickened and shows marked plasma-cell infiltration (Figs 7.1.13A and B). Absence of villi has been confirmed by electron microscopy. In other cases, however, there is subtotal villous atrophy in which short, broad and thickened villi are seen. Children with dermatitis herpetiformis also have an intestinal lesion similar to that of coeliac disease.

Clinical Features

These do not develop until gluten-containing foods are introduced into the infant's diet. In many cases the first signs are noted in the last three months of the first year of life, but the child may not be brought to the doctor until the second year. Delayed introduction of wheat containing cereals into the diet of infants in recent years has resulted in the later onset of coeliac disease.

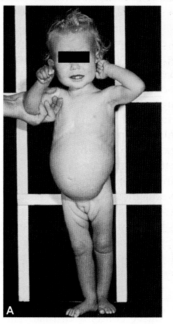
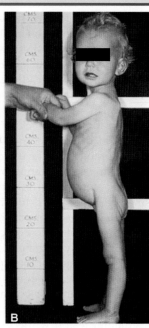

Figs 7.1.14A and B: (A) Fourteen- month –old girl with untreated coeliac disease. Note abdominal distension and gross tissue wasting (B) Lateral view of the same patient.

Affected children become fractious and miserable with anorexia and failure to gain weight. Stools are characteristically of porridgy consistency, pale, bulky and foul smelling, but in some children this feature is not very marked. In others, however, the illness may start with vomiting and watery diarrhoea. The abdomen becomes distended as a result of poor musculature, altered peristaltic activity and the accumulation of intestinal secretions and gas. This contrasts with the child's wasted buttocks and thighs and produces the so-called coeliac profile (Fig. 7.1.14A and B). A small number of children may be desperately ill with profuse diarrhoea leading to dehydration, acidosis and shock (coeliac crisis). In the worst cases malabsorption of protein can lead to hypoproteinaemic oedema.

Various other defects in absorption may become clinically manifest. Iron deficiency anaemia is common. There is usually diminished absorption of folic acid as revealed by a reduced red cell folate concentration. If there is ileal involvement, serum B$_{12}$ may be decreased. Although deficiency of vitamins A and D is probably always present, rickets is quite rare (due to lack of growth) and xerophthalmia is almost unknown. However, rickets may develop after starting treatment with a gluten free diet if supplements of vitamin D are omitted while active growth continues. Hypoprothrombinaemia is often present.

There has been a change in the clinical presentation of the disease since a large fraction of affected patients mainly adults remain undiagnosed due to atypical or vague symptoms, or even the absence of symptoms. We should be especially aware of the disease in certain risk groups, i.e. first-degree relatives of patients with diagnosed disease, patients with autoimmune diseases such as type 1 insulin dependent diabetes and child with Down syndrome.

Diagnostic Tests

While the definitive diagnosis of coeliac disease must rest upon jejunal biopsy, the procedure is unpleasant and requires admission to hospital. A variety of screening tests has been developed. The use of serological markers i.e. serum anti-gliadin (AGA), anti-endomysial (EMA) and anti-tissue transglutaminase (tTG) antibodies of IgA isotype for case finding and epidemiological studies is mandatory. However, IgA deficiency must be excluded.

A barium meal and follow-through examination will reveal an abnormal coarsening of the mucosal pattern of the small bowel, jejunal dilatation and possibly delay in the passage of barium to the colon. The bones may become osteoporotic and ossification delayed.

No investigation apart from small intestinal biopsy is 100% diagnostic of children who have coeliac disease.

Key Learning Point
Diagnosis of Coeliac Disease The only diagnostic test for coeliac disease at present is small intestinal biopsy while the child is on a gluten containing diet "The Gold Standard for Diagnosis".

Treatment

Coeliac disease is a gluten-sensitive enteropathy and the results of treatment with a gluten free diet are impressive. This is first apparent as a striking improvement in personality soon to be followed by rapid growth, while the stools more slowly return to normal. Strict supervision is essential and the child's height and weight should be recorded at regular intervals.

The parents should be supplied with a comprehensive list of the many foodstuffs which contain gluten and are, therefore, forbidden; also a list of the gluten free foods which are freely permitted. Bread and biscuits made from gluten free wheat starch are commercially available. It is also possible to home bake gluten-free bread, biscuits and cakes with recipes supplied by dieticians.

An adequate intake of vitamins and especially of Vitamin D is important. Iron deficiency anaemia may be corrected with oral preparations such as Sytron 5 ml thrice daily or Ferromyn Elixir 5 ml thrice daily. When the red cell or whole blood folate value is low folic acid should be prescribed in a dose of 5 mg daily.

Key Learning Point
Treatment of coeliac disease Effective treatment for coeliac disease is available through lifelong adherence to a strict gluten-free diet, i.e. exclusion of all foods containing wheat, rye or barley.

As long as the child remains on a gluten free diet growth and development will be entirely satisfactory, and the mortality rate for coeliac disease is nowadays negligible. It is, however, recognised that adults who have been successfully treated for coeliac disease in childhood and who have gone back to an ordinary diet, may later relapse. It is therefore desirable to confirm the persistence of true gluten intolerance in these so called "coeliac children" before recommending a life long gluten free diet. There is in addition the risk that the poorly treated adult coeliac may in time develop a lymphoma or gastrointestinal carcinoma.

The therapeutic trial of a gluten free diet without a prior biopsy is a dangerous practice and should be abandoned.

CYSTIC FIBROSIS

Aetiology

Cystic fibrosis (CF) is an autosomal recessive hereditary multi-organ disease caused by mutations in the CF transmembrane conductance regulator gene. The gene, which codes for this protein is located on chromosome 7 and the most common so far described is at the ΔF 508 locus and accounts for about 74% of cases in Caucasians. Although the incidence varies considerably between ethnic groups and populations, CF seems to be present in every population studied. CF is much less common in native African and native Asian populations.

Pathology

Although the gene defect is present in all nucleated body cells it is only in those cells where the gene requires to be activated for normal cell function that abnormalities are recognised. It is not surprising that the disease has variable clinical manifestations given the range of gene defects. The pancreas is abnormal in over 90% of the cases. A constant change is fibrosis with atrophy of the exocrine parenchyma. Cystic dilatation of acini and ducts is common but not invariable. Islet tissue, however, is rarely involved until later childhood or adolescence. Mucous glands throughout the body are grossly distended and they secrete abnormal viscid mucus. Stagnation of mucus in the smaller bronchioles usually leads to infection, which in turn stimulates further mucus secretion. The non-resolving neutrophilic inflammatory response to chronic infection in turn causes progressive and permanent airway damage, such that bronchiectasis and respiratory failure are the common findings in end-stage CF lung disease. The liver shows a focal type of biliary cirrhosis, most marked under the capsule, which may progress to produce portal hypertension.

Clinical Features

While most CF patients present disease symptoms at birth or in early infancy, some may not be diagnosed until adulthood.

The symptoms tend to occur in a more or less ordered fashion and the diagnosis is not often unduly difficult. In about 10% the illness presents in the neonatal period in the form of meconium ileus in which inspissated meconium causes intestinal obstruction. The most common presentation, however, is in the form of an intractable respiratory infection dating from the early weeks or months of life. Indeed, cystic fibrosis of the pancreas should always be suspected when a respiratory infection in infancy fails to respond promptly to adequate antibiotic therapy. In the early stages of the disease radiographs of the chest may show only increased translucency of the lung fields; later heavy interstitial markings appear; then multiple soft shadows representing small lung abscesses. In other cases there may be lobar consolidation, empyema or pyoneumothorax. In children who survive the early months of life, the respiratory picture may become that of bronchiectasis, increasing emphysema, and clubbing of the fingers. Sputum culture in such cases will most often show the predominant organisms to be *Staphylococcus* aureus and *Pseudomonas aeruginosa* and other gram-negative bacteria (e.g. Burkholderia cepacia complex, Stenotrophomonas maltophilia, Achromobacter xylosoxidans) often dominate the clinical picture. (For respiratory manifestations of CF see chapter 6).

In a minority of cases the respiratory infection is less prominent than the presence of semi-formed, greasy, bulky and excessively foul smelling stools. These features coincide with the introduction of mixed feeding. After the first year of life the history of abnormal and frequent stools occurring in association with abdominal distension and generalised tissue wasting may simulate coeliac disease. The differential diagnosis can, however, almost always be made on clinical grounds alone. In cystic fibrosis a careful history will elicit that signs first appeared in the early weeks of life, whereas coeliac disease rarely presents before the age of six months. The excellent, often voracious appetite in cystic fibrosis contrasts sharply with the unhappy anorexia of the coeliac child. Chronic respiratory infection of some degree, often severe, is an invariable accompaniment of cystic fibrosis but it is not a feature of coeliac disease. Furthermore, the diagnosis of cystic fibrosis may be suggested by a history that previous siblings have the disease.

If the affected infant survives the first year, childhood seems often to bring a period of improvement in the chest condition. All too frequently, however, the approach to puberty is associated with cor pulmonale. Less commonly, in about 10% during the second decade, biliary cirrhosis and portal hypertension develop and may lead to massive gastrointestinal haemorrhage. In recent years as an increasing proportion of sufferers from cystic fibrosis survive insulin dependent diabetes mellitus has been found in some as they approach puberty. A further important manifestation, which seems to present in a majority of male survivors into adulthood is aspermia and sterility. This has been shown to be due to absence of the vas deferens. Women have only slightly reduced fertility associated with abnormal tubal ciliary movement and cervical mucus.

Key Learning Point
The vast majority of men with CF (98%) are infertile due to abnormalities in the development of structure derived from the Wolffian duct.

Some children with cystic fibrosis can develop distal small bowel obstruction. This disorder is due to viscid mucofaeculent material obstructing the bowel causing recurring episodes of abdominal pain, constipation and acute or sub acute intestinal obstruction. The cardinal sign is a soft, mobile, non-tender mass palpable in the right iliac fossa. Mild cases can be treated by increasing the intake of pancreatic enzyme. If the condition is not improved oral N-acetylcysteine 10 ml four times a day or one or two doses of oral Gastrografin 50 to 100 ml taken with 200 to 400 ml of water may relieve the patient discomfort and obstruction. Toddlers with cystic fibrosis may sometime present with rectal prolapse. Also the incidence of nasal polyps in patients with cystic fibrosis is about 70%.

Diagnostic Tests

The sweat test is still sufficient to confirm the diagnosis in typical cases but gene screening for known mutations is now becoming routine in many centres. The sweat test can be carried out from the third week of life on, provided the infant weighs more than 3kg, is normally hydrated and without significant illness. There are various methods of obtaining sweat for analysis but the most accurate and widely used technique is stimulation of local sweating by pilocarpine iontophoresis. One should try to achieve the collection of at least 100 mg of sweat. To minimise diagnostic errors, two reliable sweat tests confirmed in a laboratory used to performing the test should be obtained. Diagnostic levels of sodium and chloride are 60 mmol/kg. In patients with atypical disease manifestations, the sweat test is often equivocal. Additional diagnostic tests will be necessary to substantiate the diagnosis: CFTR mutation analysis and, at times, CFTR bioassays.

In neonates, there is a reliable method of screening which is based on the serum concentration of immuno-reactive trypsin (IRT). Serum IRT levels are abnormally high (> 80 ng/ml) during the first few months of life, although in older children they fall to subnormal values. Prenatal diagnosis by chorionic villus biopsy obtained at 9 - 12 weeks post conception will allow termination of affected fetuses. As there is still no curative treatment for CF the introduction of screening has to be considered regionally, in close cooperation with CF centres.

Key Learning Point

A sweat chloride concentration of >60 mmol/l confirms the clinically suspected diagnosis of CF.

A majority of patients with cystic fibrosis have pancreatic insufficiency which if inadequately treated could result in fat, vitamin and protein malnutrition. The most important factors in the treatment are control of lung infection and maintenance of adequate nutrition; indeed upon the success of these efforts depends the prognosis. Persistent bacterial infection is a major problem for children with cystic fibrosis; the four bacterial pathogens involved being *Staphylococcus aureus*, *Pseudomonas aeruginosa*, *Haemophilus influenzae* and *Berkholderia cepacia*.

The intensive long-term antibiotic treatments, deve-loped at many centres, have resulted in problems with resistant strains. Different treatment strategies have been developed, most focusing on preventing colonisation with gram-negatives, mainly *P. aeruginosa*. The strategies contain generalised pulmonary mucus-dissolving agents, physical therapy and antibiotics.

Antibiotic treatment with intravenous antimicrobial drugs at signs of exacerbation of the pulmonary symptoms has been the most widely used treatment modality. In the struggle to keep the infectious load as low as possible more or less continuous inhalation therapy has been more common in recent years. The cost of intravenous therapy can also be kept relatively low by teaching parents and patients to perform home intravenous antibiotic therapy, which also gives the family more freedom and acceptance of treatment.

Patients should be considered for lung transplantation when there lung function is impaired to a FEV1.0 of <30% of the predicted values.

All children with cystic fibrosis should receive pertussis, measles, *Haemophilus influenzae* and influenza vaccinations.

The services of a surgeon may be required at several stages of the disease, e.g. for meconium ileus in the neonatal period, for distal small bowel obstruction, for lobectomy in bronchiectasis or for portacaval anastomosis if portal hypertension is severe.

There has been amazing success in the treatment of CF, a condition that was once frequently fatal in the first year of life. Identification of CFTR (CF transmembrane conductance gene) has been a key step in understanding pathophysiology at a molecular level and establishing the degree to which variation in CFTR function influences the outcome of CF.

Key Learning Point

Most patients with CF die from end-stage pulmonary disease; therefore emphasis is on prevention and treatment of pulmonary infections. Most patients would benefit from improved nutrition, including refined pancreatic supplementation therapy and essential fatty acid status.

CONSTIPATION

Terminology is a problem, which causes confusion in communication between doctors and patients. It is important that the doctor be sure of the patients understanding of the terms used. Constipation may be defined as a difficulty or delay in defaecation that causes distress to the child and the parents. The infrequent passage of stools with no distress does not fall into this category. Encopresis or faecal soiling is the frequent passage of faecal matter at socially unacceptable times. This is discussed in Chapter 31. Psychogenic causes are the most frequent. Faecal continence is the ability to retain faeces until delivery is convenient. Ingestion of fluid or food stimulates the gastrocolic reflex and results in two or three mass colonic propulsive activities per day. This process delivers faecal material to a normally empty rectum. On distension of the rectum, stretch receptors start a rectal contraction and a reflex inhibition is sent to the anal canal. This is mediated via the myenteric plexus of nerves in the submucosa and the plexus of nerves between the outer longitudinal and inner circular smooth muscle layers. The process produces sensation since the upper part of the anal canal has sensitive sensory receptors as well as stretch receptors. The motor element of the external sphincter and the puborectalis muscle make up the striated sphincter together with the smooth muscle of the internal sphincter. The striated sphincter is able to contract strongly to prevent the passage of a stool at an inconvenient time. This however, can only function for 30 seconds, i.e. long enough to contain a rectal contraction wave till it passes. The internal sphincter can maintain persistent tonic activity so preventing leakage of stool between periods of rectal activity by maintaining closure of a resting anal canal. Clinical experience suggests that the external sphincters are of much less importance than the puborectalis sling and the internal sphincter. Defaecation occurs by inhibiting the activity of the puborectalis sling and the sphincter mechanism of the anus, thus allowing faeces to pass from the rectum into the anal canal. This is augmented by voluntarily increasing intra-abdominal pressure using the abdominal wall musculature as well as the diaphragm as accessory muscles for defaecation. There are two main clinical states, the acute and the chronic state, which must be differentiated.

Key Learning Point

Hirschsprung's disease, CF, anorectal anomalies and metabolic conditions such as hypothyroidism are rare organic causes of childhood constipation.

Acute Constipation

Acute constipation usually occurs in a child after a febrile illness with a reduced fluid intake. This situation arises when convalescing after an illness or in the immediate post-operative period. There is a danger that this acute state of constipation may progress to a chronic state if it is not identified early enough. Treatment with a laxative, suppositories or an enema usually corrects the problem initially but the child must be encouraged to return to a good diet and adequate fluid intake.

Chronic Constipation

Chronic constipation is distressing to the child and the parents. An early diagnosis is essential to prevent a prolonged and persistent problem. In chronic constipation the rectum is overstretched and ballooned. The sensory receptors are inactive and the bowel is flaccid and unable to contract effectively. A greater amount of water is absorbed from the faecal stream. The stool becomes harder, more solid and more difficult and painful to pass. The faecal mass increases in size and spurious diarrhoea can also occur from stercoral ulceration of the distended rectal mucosa.

History is important as failure to pass meconium within 24 hours of birth in the term infant born normally, makes it likely that there may be some underlying problem. Infants, for whom childbirth has been abnormal, take longer to establish a normal defaecation pattern. The delay in establishing normal stooling may be a sign of other disorders, not only Hirschsprung's disease or anal stenosis, but systemic disorders such as hypothyroidism Psychogenic causes are the commonest origin of constipation in childhood often due to inappropriate toilet training and this aspect is also discussed in Chapter 31.

In older infants and children the distress caused by constipation may be related to pain. There may be abdominal discomfort, usually a dull ache, which may or may not be related to defaecation. Occasionally the pain may be localised to the right iliac fossa due to a distended caecum filled with stool. The pain may be in the anal region, particularly when an anal fissure has occurred and bleeding may result from the mucosal tear.

There are occasions when there is no complaint of constipation but the parents may notice a distended abdomen, and may even at times feel a mass arising out of the pelvis.

A full dietary history must be obtained. This should include a detailed account of a typical day's breakfast, lunch, supper and any in-between snacks, noting the amount of fluid taken, any dietary fads and the amount of fruit and vegetables and cereals ingested.

An accurate account of drugs given and other remedies tried by the parents before presenting at the clinic is documented.

Examination

A full examination of the child is important noting the presence of any dysmorphic features, height and weight as well as any signs of failure to thrive. Inspection of the abdomen noting any abdominal distension or the presence of localised swelling. The abdomen is then palpated in routine fashion, feeling for any abdominal mass. A faecal mass can usually be indented through the abdomen, although at times the impacted mass may be so hard as to make it quite impossible to indent, and may mislead one into thinking it is a malignant mass. A loaded, impacted colon with a megarectum can in turn cause retention of urine resulting in a full bladder, which may or may not distress the child if this is a chronic situation.

Digital rectal examination must be carefully explained to the parents and the child before proceeding, explaining the importance of deciding whether constipation is a problem especially in the presence of diarrhoea, which may be spurious in nature. It is helpful to have a nurse in attendance to position the child in the left lateral position with knees bent in the fetal position. It is useful to carry on conversation during this investigation to relax an otherwise tense atmosphere and also explaining to the parent and the child what is being done. While the child is in this position, it is important to examine the spine and the sacrum for any sign of spina bifida occulta. The position of the anus as well as its size should be noted to exclude the possibility of an anterior ectopic anus or an anal stenosis. The skin around the anus should look normal. Erythema may indicate the presence of candida or streptococcal infection or may be due to topical applications by the parents. The presence of puckering of the anus as well as the presence of a skin tag may indicate an underlying anal fissure, which could be the result of the vicious cycle of retention of stool, chronic constipation and painful defaecation. The presence of soiling should be noted and the consistency and volume of stool, if it is hard or soft or liquid in form, as well as whether there is any blood present.

Investigations

A plain X-ray of the abdomen in a child with a distended abdomen and constipation may indicate the degree of

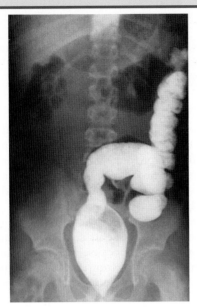

Fig. 7.1.15: Barium enema of a child demonstrating gross rectal dilatation and obstruction with mass of faeces ("terminal reservoir").

constipation and may also detect underlying bony abnormalities such as spina bifida occulta or sacral abnormalities. Barium enema (Fig. 7.1.15) may be carried out in a few children with chronic constipation where there is a suspicion of Hirschsprung's disease but in most children radiological investigations are not required if an adequate history is taken. These children must not be prepared by bowel washout prior to the barium enema because this will obscure the X-ray appearance.

Management of Acute Constipation

It is important to explain the mechanism of acute constipation to the parents and the child and to emphasise the benign nature of this condition. It is treated by increasing the fluid and fibre content of the diet or, if necessary, a bulk agent to restore the normal pattern of defaecation of the child.

Management of Chronic Constipation

The management of this condition involves getting the co-operation of the child, the parents, as well as the general practitioner and the nurse. An explanation of the cause of the intractable problem should be given to the parents. Dietary measures with a high fluid intake and an adequate dietary residue should be commenced. Bran should be added to the cereal in the morning. In addition to this it is necessary to dislodge the faecal masses with oral preparations of laxatives. Stool softeners and laxatives are titrated according to the clinical response. A phosphate enema is sometimes necessary. During the period of impaction, soiling is often worse and this has to be explained to the parents so that they are not disheartened.

The period of regulation of bowel habits to food and fluid intake may take several months to achieve. Occasionally manual evacuation under general anaesthesia is necessary to dislodge firm impacted faecal masses; before continuing with prolonged dietary and medicinal management.

Some children require referral for psychological help to treat underlying problems of a psychogenic nature, but this should be only done once other disease processes have been excluded (see chapter 31).

PROTEIN-LOSING ENTEROPATHY (PLE)

The intestinal loss of proteins may be greatly increased in many diseases, not only diseases which primarily affect the gastrointestinal tract but many other more generalised disorders such as cystic fibrosis, coeliac disease and anaphylactoid purpura.

Little is known about the mechanisms by which the plasma proteins reach the lumen of the gut. In inflammatory and ulcerative conditions local exudation of protein seems the obvious explanation. In other conditions such as lymphangiectasia, retroperitoneal fibrosis and congestive cardiac failure, the loss may be accounted for by disturbance of lymphatic drainage. For the most part the mechanism remains obscure. The classification in Table 7.1.3 includes those found in children.

Gastrointestinal protein loss is non-selective. Serum proteins are lost 'in bulk' irrespective of molecular size. Although all serum proteins may be reduced the abnormality is most obvious in the reduction in concentration of albumin, IgG, IgA, and IgM. Abnormal intestinal protein loss may occur without any clinical manifestations.

Table 7.1.3 Diseases associated with protein-losing enteropathy
• Invasive bacterial infection (e.g. Salmonella, Shigella)
• Crohn disease
• Ulcerative colitis
• Intestinal tuberculosis
• Sarcoidosis
• Intestinal lymphangiectasia
• Retroperitoneal fibrosis
• Neoplasia affecting mesenteric lymphatics
• Thoracic duct obstruction
• Congestive cardiac failure
• Menetrier disease
• Cystic fibrosis
• Milk and Soy-induced enteropathy
• Henoch-Schönlein purpura
• Giardiasis
• Kwashiorkor
• Veno-occlusive disease
• Necrotising enterocolitis
• Tropical sprue
• Graft-versus host disease

However, at serum levels below 4 g per 100 ml there is an increasing risk of peripheral oedema, which may then become a major or even the presenting complaint.

Protein-losing enteropathy may be suspected in any case of unexplained hypoproteinaemia or oedema especially in the presence of gastrointestinal symptoms. Suspicion is strengthened by the demonstration of particularly low levels of albumin and immunoglobulins. The diagnosis is proved by the use of such tests as the use of ^{51}Cr-labelled serum proteins. The measurement of faecal α_1 antitrypsin can be used to document protein loss and to potentially localise the site of loss. Diagnosis is not complete without the demonstration of excess intestinal protein loss. It is necessary to determine the nature of the causative disease. Treatment is the treatment of that disease.

WILSON'S DISEASE
(Hepatolenticular degeneration)

Caeruloplasmin is a copper – containing α_2 globulin, which functions as a transport mechanism for copper in the plasma. Deficiency of caeruloplasmin is associated with copper deposition in many tissues resulting in Wilson's disease.

Clinical Features

Wilson's disease may present any time from early childhood to the fifth decade. In early childhood, hepatosplenomegaly, jaundice and acute hepatitis or nodular cirrhosis of the liver are the most common findings. This disease should always be considered in such cases. A brown or green ring around the corneal limbus – the Kayser-Fleischer ring – is caused by copper deposited in Descemet's membrane. It is only found in this disease. The ring is often not present under the age of seven.

Urine, plasma and tissue concentrations of copper are high and serum caeruplasmin (or copper oxidase activity) is usually low, although rare families with normal caeruloplasmin levels have been reported. Plasma caeruloplasmin levels are very low in the normal newborn, rising to normal by about 2 years of age.

Diagnosis

Tissue copper is high but serum copper and caeruloplasmin are low, although rare forms are known in which the caeruloplasmin level may be normal although its functional activity is impaired. In these cases, liver biopsy or radioactive copper uptake may be required to make the diagnosis. Some heterozygotes have reduced caeruloplasmin levels; others can be distinguished by measuring caeruloplasmin uptake of radioactive copper. Slit lamp examination may be needed to see the KF rings.

Treatment

It is important to diagnose the disease early since treatment can prevent the onset of symptoms, and can result in striking clinical improvement. Oral D-penicillamine is the drug of choice. The drug should be continued for life. Trientine is used for the treatment of Wilson's disease only, in patients intolerant of D-penicillamine.

Zinc prevents the absorption of copper in Wilson's disease. Symptomatic patients should be treated initially with a chelating agent because zinc has a slow onset of action. When transferring from chelating treatment to zinc maintenance therapy, chelating treatment should be co-administered for two to three weeks until zinc produces its maximal effect.

Liver transplantation has also been reported to reverse all the neurologic and biochemical abnormalities.

JAUNDICE

Jaundice occurs either when there is excess haemolysis increasing the load of bilirubin, when the diseased liver is not able to cope with the normal load or when there is obstruction to excretion of bilirubin. Jaundice can be classified into haemolytic (prehepatic), hepatocellular (hepatic) and obstructive (post-hepatic) varieties. In this chapter we shall discuss only virus hepatitis, chronic active hepatitis, and cirrhosis of the liver. Neonatal jaundice has been discussed in Chapter 3.1 and obstructive jaundice in Chapters 11 and 13.

VIRAL INFECTIONS OF THE LIVER

HEPATITIS A

Hepatitis A virus (HAV) is present in the blood and stool of a patient for 2-3 weeks before clinical symptoms occur and it persists in stool for up to 2 weeks after disease onset. The primary mode of transmission is faecal-oral route. Common source outbreaks occur with contamination of water or food. In developing countries with inadequate hygiene and poor sanitation HAV infection is endemic and most children are infected in the first years of life.

Clinical Features

Hepatitis A virus infection is usually an acute self-limiting illness. The mean incubation period is 30 days. In infants and young children, the infection could be entirely asymptomatic. Jaundice is rare in this age group. In older children, there may be a prodromal period of several days in which fever, headache and malaise predominate, followed by the onset of jaundice, abdominal pain, nausea, vomiting and anorexia. Pruritis may accompany the jaundice.

Clinical examination may reveal a mildly enlarged tender liver and occasionally splenomegaly is noted.

Serum aminotransferase values usually are often 20 to 100 times the upper limit of normal and they decrease rapidly within the first 2 to 3 weeks.

Diagnosis

The diagnosis of HAV infection is made by detection of the immunoglobulin M antibody to HAV (IgM and anti-HAV).

Prevention

Hepatitis A vaccine should be considered for children with chronic liver disease including chronic hepatitis B or chronic hepatitis C; prevention of secondary cases in close contacts of confirmed cases of hepatitis A, within 7 days of onset of disease in the primary case. Protection against hepatitis A is recommended for travellers to high-risk areas. Hepatitis A vaccine is preferred as compared to immunoglobulin and it is likely to be effective even if given shortly before departure. Intramuscular normal immunoglobulin is no longer recommended for routine prophylaxis in travellers but it may be indicated for immunocompromised patients if their antibody response to vaccine is unlikely to be adequate. In unimmunised children, transmission of hepatitis A is reduced by good hygiene.

HEPATITIS B

Hepatitis B virus (HBV) is relatively uncommon in Caucasians but has a high prevalence in Southeast Asia and parts of Africa where highly infective carriage of HBV is common. The incubation period is 90-120 days. Hepatitis B virus is found in high concentration in the blood of infected individuals and in moderate concentrations in semen, vaginal fluid and saliva. Risk factors for acquisition of HBV infection include parenteral exposure to blood or blood products. Risk factors in children include perinatal exposure (vertical) being born to an HbsAg seropositive mother. Horizontal spread is by living in a household with a chronic HBV carrier.

The hepatic injury that occurs with HBV infection is mediated by the host immune response. Most instances of HBV infection are acute and self-limited. In some individuals HBV is not cleared by the host immunologic response, and chronic infection results.

Clinical Features

After an incubation period of 30-180 days, patients with HBV infection may develop a prodrome that consists of malaise, fatigue, nausea, low-grade fever, or even a serum – sickness like illness. Papular acrodermatitis of childhood may be the major or only manifestation of HBV in infants and young children. Patients who manifest these prodromal symptoms are already seropositive for HbsAg.

Within a week or two of the prodrome, clinical hepatitis is seen with jaundice, pruritis, nausea and vomiting. Clinical examination reveals mild hepatomegaly and liver tenderness and mild splenomegaly may also be noted. Serum bilirubin and aminotransferase levels decrease over several weeks to normal. However, in those children who will develop fulminant hepatitis, the typical features of coagulopathy and encephalopathy will appear. In patients who develop chronic HBV infection, jaundice clears, but alanine transaminase (ALT) and aspartate transaminase (AST) may or may not return to normal.

Chronic HBV infection is often completely asymptomatic and may not be diagnosed if the patient has not had an acute icteric illness. Chronic hepatitis may manifest as a complication of cirrhosis or portal hypertension. Chronic HBV infection is highly associated with the risk of developing hepatocellular carcinoma.

Diagnosis

The diagnosis of acute HBV infection is made by detection of HbsAg and IgM anti-HBc; although HbeAg confirms active replication, its presence is not essential to confirm the diagnosis. Chronic HBV infection is defined by the presence of HbsAg for more than 6 months; typically it persists for many years. In chronic HBV infection, HbeAg persists, often for many years, indicating ongoing viral infection.

Treatment

Treatment for acute hepatitis B is mainly supportive and most patients recover fully. Chronic HBV infection is a rare indication for liver transplantation in the paediatric age group.

Prevention

Hepatitis B vaccine is used in individuals at high risk of contracting hepatitis B. They include:

- Close family contacts of a case or carrier
- Babies whose mothers have had hepatitis B during pregnancy or are positive for hepatitis B surface antigen (regardless of e – antigen markers)
- Children with chronic liver disease, chronic renal failure including those on haemodialysis
- Parenteral drug abusers and their household contacts

HEPATITIS C

Hepatitis C virus (HCV) was discovered in sera from patients with post-transfusion hepatitis, and is now the predominant cause of transfusion associated non-A non-B hepatitis in the world. However, since the institution of screening donors for antibody to HCV (anti-HCV) and thus eliminating positive blood/blood products, the risk of HCV from transfusion has diminished. On the other hand the proportion of cases associated with intravenous drug abuse has increased. However, exposure to blood products and perinatal exposure have been the most consistent risk factors for HCV acquisition in children. The incubation period for post-transfusion HCV infection ranges from 2 to 26 weeks.

Clinical Features

Many acute HCV infections are clinically asymptomatic but those who become icteric show a modest rise in aminotransferase levels. Some patients have symptoms of acute hepatitis, such as anorexia, malaise, fatigue and abdominal pain. In most instances, chronic HCV infection is asymptomatic.

Treatment

At present there are no widely accepted recommendations for treatment of acute HCV infection in children. Interferon has been used with some success in chronic hepatitis C infection.

HEPATITIS D (Delta Hepatitis)

Delta hepatitis is caused by the hepatitis D virus (HDV). It occurs only in conjunction with hepatitis B infection. In general, HDV infection does not have specific features to distinguish it from ordinary HBV infection. Testing for HDV infection is recommended in any child with chronic HBV and unusually severe liver disease. Several antiviral drugs have been studied in Delt hepatitis, but the only treatment that has had a beneficial effect is $1F_N$-α. Passive or active immunisation against HDV infection is not available.

HEPATITIS E

Hepatitis E virus (HEV) infection is also called enterically transmitted non-A non-B hepatitis. The symptoms and signs are similar to those of hepatitis A. At present, the diagnosis depends on the detection of anti-HEV IgM. Prevention is by improving standards of hygiene. No therapy or prophylaxis currently exists.

HEPATITIS G

The clinical significance of hepatitis G virus (HGV) remains uncertain. This virus has not been implicated in acute non-A non-E hepatitis or fulminant hepatic failure in children.

Hepatitis Caused by Other Viral Agents

Hepatitis viruses A, B, C, D, and E are the agents of most viral hepatitis. Other viruses that can cause hepatitis as part of a generalised illness (CMV, herpes virus, EB virus, human parvovirus B 19, rubella, coxsackie B, yellow fever hepatitis and dengue haemorrhagic fever) will not be discussed here.

CIRRHOSIS OF THE LIVER

Aetiology

Hepatic cirrhosis is uncommon in children in the United Kingdom and the histological differentiation into "portal" and biliary" types tends to be less well defined than in adults. A pathological picture similar to that of Laënnec portal cirrhosis may follow neonatal hepatitis, blood group incompatibility, the de Toni-Fanconi syndrome and it may be the form of presentation of Wilson's hepatolenticular cirrhosis. Infective hepatitis-B may also lead to hepatic cirrhosis. Other rare causes of cirrhosis of the liver include galactosaemia, Gaucher's disease, Niemann-Pick disease and xanthomatosis. Pure biliary cirrhosis is seen invariably in congenital biliary atresia and a focal type is very common in cystic fibrosis of the pancreas.

Indian childhood cirrhosis (ICC) is a common and fatal disease, which appears to be restricted to India. There is a positive family history in about 30% of cases. It is not found in Indian expatriates in other parts of the world. It usually presents between the ages of nine months and five years and has characteristic histological features in liver biopsy material. These have been called "micro-micronodular cirrhosis" which includes necrosis and vacuolation of liver cells, aggressive fibrosis both intralobular and perilobular and a variable inflammatory infiltrate. The liver contains an exceedingly high copper content and the hepatocytes contain multiple, coarse, dark brown orcein-staining granules, which represent copper-associated protein. The pathogenic role of chronic ingestion of copper was supported by the finding of a much greater use of copper utensils to heat and store milk by families of affected than unaffected children. Since then, the use of copper pots has reduced, and the disease has largely disappeared from many parts of India. Recently a copper-binding factor has been identified in Indian childhood cirrhosis, liver cytosol. This factor may play a role in hepatic intracellular copper accumulation. Penicillamine given before the terminal stages has reportedly reduced mortality from 92 to 63%.

In Jamaica a form of cirrhosis called veno-occlusive disease of the liver, in which there is occlusion of the small hepatic veins, is due to the toxic effects of an alkaloid in bush tea compared from plants such as Senecio and Crotalaria.

Chronic active hepatitis is an autoimmune disorder characterised by hepatic necrosis, fibrosis, plasma cell infiltration and disorganisation of the lobular architecture In the young adult, often female, associated disorders include thyroiditis, fibrosing alveolitis and glomerulonephritis. Some cases are related to chronic virus B hepatitis (positive HBsAg). In chronic active hepatitis smooth muscle antibodies are found in the serum in two thirds of cases, antinuclear factor in about 50 per cent, and the gamma globulin level is markedly elevated.

Clinical Features

The child usually presents with abdominal swelling due to enlargement of the liver, which has a firm edge, sometimes smooth, often nodular. Anorexia, lack of energy and slowing of growth are common complaints. Splenomegaly develops if there is portal hypertension In most cases jaundice makes its appearance sooner rather than later. Spontaneous bleeding is usually due to hypoprothrombinaemia. Orthochromic anaemia is common. When ascites develops the outlook is grave; it is usually associated with hypoproteinaemia and portal hypertension. The latter may result in massive gastrointestinal haemorrhage. In other cases death occurs from hepatic encephalopathy with flapping tremor, mental confusion, extensor plantar responses and coma. Spider naevi and "liver palms" are uncommon in children, but clubbing of the fingers may develop. Hypersplenism may produce leucopenia and thrombocytopenia. Various derangements of liver function can be demonstrated biochemically, e.g. raised direct bilirubin levels, hypoalbuminaemia, and raised serum gamma globulin. In hepatic encephalopathy the blood ammonia level is high. Diagnosis should be confirmed by liver biopsy.

Treatment

Specific treatment is available only for the few cases due to metabolic errors such as Wilson's disease or galactosaemia. Life can be prolonged with a high protein diet, plus a liberal intake of the B vitamins and oral vitamin K, 10 mg per day. Ascites should be treated with frusemide and a low-sodium diet. Hypokalaemia may require supplements of potassium chloride. In resistant cases diuresis may be improved by giving (along with frusemide) an aldosterone antagonist such as spironolactone, 25 mg four times daily. Paracentesis abdominis should be avoided whenever possible. When signs of hepatic failure supervene protein should be completely eliminated from the diet and the therapeutic regimen already described for this emergency should be started. There is little basis for the use of corticosteroids save in chronic active hepatitis where they do probably slow down the progress of the disease. An alternative but more dangerous therapy is immunosuppression, e.g. with azathioprine.

Obstructive Jaundice (see chapter 11)

Cholecystitis

Cholecystitis is uncommon in childhood and rarely presents as an acute emergency. Cholelithiasis is less common in infancy and childhood. It presents with recurrent upper abdominal pain, nausea and vomiting. It is often associated with congenital spherocytosis. The stones are usually bile pigment stones and should be looked for whenever laparotomy is carried out for removal of the spleen in this condition. Most gallstones are clinically silent. Ultrasonography is the most sensitive and specific method to detect gallstones. Cholecystotomy has been preferred to cholecystectomy when the gallbladder is not diseased.

PANCREAS

Pancreatic disorders are uncommon in childhood except that which is part of the generalised disease of cystic fibrosis Pancreatitis presents as an acute abdominal emergency but the signs and symptoms are less dramatic than in adults. Single, self-limited attacks, or recurrent attacks of acute pancreatitis are, by far the most frequent feature of this disease in childhood. Chronic pancreatitis is quite rare in children. Based largely upon clinical and epidemiological observations, a broad spectrum of underlying conditions has been associated with acute pancreatitis. According to one series, trauma, structural disease, systemic diseases, drugs and toxins are the major etiological factors. A variety of systemic infectious agents have been implicated in the aetiology of acute pancreatitis. The mumps virus is an important cause of acute pancreatitis in children. Acute pancreatitis has been reported in association with a variety of connective tissue disorders. Abdominal pain and vomiting are the most consistent signs. Abdominal tenderness is more marked in the upper abdomen. There is a lack of a "gold standard" diagnostic test for acute pancreatitis. However, considerable diagnostic importance has been placed on the total serum levels of amylase or lipase, but the specificity and sensitivity of these tests is unsatisfactory. Ultrasonography is now the most commonly used test in the preliminary evaluation of children with abdominal pain when pancreatitis is suspected. Abdominal CT should be reserved where ultrasound examination is technically unsatisfactory.

Treatment

It consists of the treatment of pancreatic disease symptoms and complications. Most specific therapeutic interventions are of questionable or unproven benefit.

JUVENILE TROPICAL PANCREATITIS

The syndrome of chronic pancreatitis with pancreatic calculi and diabetes has been reported from many countries such as Uganda, Nigeria, Sri Lanka, Malaysia, India, and Bangladesh. The exact aetiology has not yet been established; malnutrition is an important epidemiologic association.

The cardinal manifestations of juvenile tropical pancreatitis are recurrent abdominal pain, followed by diabetes mellitus, and pancreatic calculi, and death in the prime of life. The management of this condition consists of the alleviation of abdominal pain, the treatment of diabetes, the prevention of complications and the correction of nutritional problems.

Key Learning Point
Juvenile Tropical Pancreatitis Abdominal pain followed by diabetes in an emaciated teenager and the radiologic demonstration of calculi in the pancreatic duct are the hallmark of the disease.

LIVER TRANSPLANTATION

Paediatric liver transplantation should be considered at an early stage in babies and children dying of end-stage liver failure. With increasing experience, there are fewer contraindications to liver transplantation. Liver transplantation for children with life-threatening acute or chronic liver disease has proven to be durable with high success rates. The majority of paediatric liver recipients can now expect to enjoy a good quality of life with normal growth and development. Life-long immunosuppressive therapy is required. The circumstances in which liver transplantation should be considered are:

• Chronic liver disease
• Liver based metabolic disorders
• Acute liver failure
• Unresectable hepatic tumours
• Poor quality of life due to chronic liver disorders

7.2: Infectious Diarrhoea in Childhood

Diarrhoea is a common manifestation of infection of the gastrointestinal tract and can be caused by a variety of pathogens including viruses, parasites and bacteria. The most common manifestations of such infections are diarrhoea and vomiting, which may also be associated with systemic features such as abdominal pain, fever etc. Although several non-infectious causes of diarrhoea are well recognized, the bulk of childhood diarrhoea relates to infectious disorders.

Epidemiology of childhood diarrhoea

Despite considerable advances in the understanding and management of diarrhoeal disorders in childhood, these still account for a large proportion (18%) of childhood deaths globally with an estimated 1.9 million deaths. Although the global mortality of diarrhoea has reduced, the overall incidence remains unchanged with many children in developing countries averaging about 3.2 episodes per child year.

Although information on aetiology specific diarrhoea mortality is limited, it is recognized that rotavirus infections account for at least one-third of severe and potentially fatal watery diarrhoea episodes, with an estimated 440,000 deaths in developing countries. A similar number may also succumb to *Shigella* infections especially *S. dysenteriae* type 1 infections. In other parts of the world periodic outbreaks of cholera also account for a large number of adult and child deaths. The peak incidence

of diarrhoea as well as mortality is among 6-11 months old infants.

Although there is very little information on the long-term consequences of diarrhoeal diseases, recent data suggest that diarrhoeal illnesses especially if prolonged, may significantly impair psychomotor and cognitive development in young children.

Aetiology of diarrhoea

The major factor leading to infectious diarrhea is infection acquired through the faeco-oral route or by ingestion of contaminated food or water. Hence this is a disease largely associated with poverty, poor environmental hygiene and development indices. Table 7.2.1 lists the common pathogens associated with diarrhea among children. Enteropathogens that are infectious in a small inoculum [*Shigella, Escherichia coli* (*E.coli*) enteric viruses, *G. lamblia, C. parvum,* and *E. histolytica*] may be transmitted by person-to-person contact, whereas others such as cholera are usually a consequence of contamination of food or water supply. In developed countries episodes of infectious diarrhea may occur by seasonal exposure to organisms such as rotavirus or by exposure to pathogens in settings of close contact e.g. in day care centers.

Table 7.2.2 details the incubation period and common clinical features associated with infection with various organisms causing diarrhoea. Globally *Escherichia coli* are the most common organisms causing diarrhoea, followed

Table 7.2.1: Common pathogens causing diarrhea in children

Bacteria producing inflammatory diarrhea	Bacteria producing non-inflammatory diarrhea	Viruses	Parasites
Aeromonas	Enterotoxigenic *Escherichia coli*	Rotavirus	Giardia lamblia
Campylobacter jejuni	Vibrio cholerae 01 and 0139	Enteric adenovirus	*Entamoeba histolytica*
Clostridium difficile	Enteropathogenic *Escherichia coli*	Astrovirus	*Balantidium coli*
Enteroinvasive E. coli	Enterotoxigenic *Escherichia coli*	Norwalk agent–like virus	*Cryptosporidium parvum*
E. coli O157:H7	Vibrio parahaemolyticus	Calicivirus	*Strongyloides stercoralis*
Salmonella	*Staphylococcus aureus*		*Trichuris trichiura*
Shigella			
Yersinia enterocolitica			
Vibrio parahaemolyticus			
Clostridium perfringens			

Table 7.2.2: Diarrhea pathogens and clinical syndromes in children

Pathogen	Incubation period	Clinical features
Enteropathogenic *Escherichia coli* EPEC	6-48 hours	Self limiting watery diarrhea Occasional fever and vomiting
Enteroinvasive *Escherichia coli* EIEC	1-3 days	Watery diarrhea, occasionally bloody diarrhea
Enteroaggregative *Escherichia coli* EAEC	8-18 hours	Watery, mucoid diarrheaBloody diarrhea in a third of cases
Enterohemorrhagic *Escherichia coli* EHEC	3-9 days	Abdominal pain, vomiting, bloody diarrhea, Hemolyic uremic syndrome in 10% of cases
Enterotoxigenic *Escherichia coli* ETEC	14-30 hours	Watery diarrhea, fever, abdominal pain and vomiting.
Diffusely adherent *Escherichia coli*	6-48 hours	Mild watery diarrhea
Shigella	16-72 hours	Mucoid and Bloody diarrhea (may be watery initially), fever, toxicity, tenesmus,
Yersinia enterocolitica	4-6 days	Watery or mucoid diarrhea (bloody in < 10%) with abdominal pain, fever, bacteremia in young infants
Campylobacter	2-4 days	Abdominal pain (frequently right sided), watery diarrhea (occasionally mucoid and bloody), fever
Rotavirus	1-3 days	Mostly in young children. Typically watery diarrhea with upper respiratory symptoms in some children. May cause severe dehydrating diarrhea

by Rota virus, *Shigella* species, and non-typhoidal *Salmonella* species.

Risk factors for gastroenteritis

In addition to the obvious sources of environmental contamination and increased exposure to enteropathogens, there are a variety of factors that increase susceptibility to infection. These risk factors include young age, immune deficiency, measles, malnutrition and lack of exclusive or predominant breastfeeding. In particular, malnutrition has been shown to increase the risk of diarrhoea and associated mortality several folds. The risks are particularly higher with micronutrient malnutrition. To illustrate, in children with vitamin A deficiency, the risk of dying from diarrhoea, measles, and malaria is increased by 20–24%. Likewise, zinc deficiency increases the risk of mortality from diarrhoea, pneumonia, and malaria by 13–21%.

It is recognized that most diarrhoeal disorders form a continuum, with the majority of cases resolving within the first week of the illness. However, a smaller proportion of diarrhoeal illnesses may fail to resolve and persist for longer duration. Persistent diarrhoea has been defined as episodes that began acutely but lasted for at least 14 days and identifies a subgroup of children with a substantially increased diarrhoeal burden and between 36-54% of all diarrhoea-related deaths. Such episodes may account for between 3% and 20% of all diarrhoeal episodes in children under 5 years of age and up to half of all diarrhoea-related deaths.

Clinical Manifestation of Diarrhoea

Most of the clinical manifestations and clinical syndromes of diarrhoea are related to the infecting pathogen and the dose/inoculum. A number of additional manifestations depend upon the development of complications (such as dehydration and electrolyte imbalance) and the nature of the infecting pathogen. Usually the ingestion of pre-formed toxins (such as those of *S. aureus*) is associated with the rapid onset of nausea and vomiting within 6 hrs with possible fever, abdominal cramps, and diarrhoea within 8–72 hrs. Watery diarrhoea and abdominal cramps after an 8–16 hr incubation period are associated with enterotoxin-producing *Clostridium perfringens* and *B. cereus*. Abdominal cramps and watery diarrhoea after a 16–48 hr incubation period can be associated with calicivirus, several enterotoxin-producing bacteria, Cryptosporidium, and Cyclospora. Several organisms including *Salmonella, Shigella, C. jejuni, Y. enterocolitica,* enteroinvasive *E. coli,* and *V. parahaemolyticus* are associated with diarrhoea that may contain faecal leukocytes, abdominal cramps, and fever, although these organisms can cause watery diarrhoea without fever. Bloody diarrhea and abdominal cramps after a 72–120 hr incubation period are associated with infections due to Shigella and also Shiga toxin–producing *E. coli,* such as *E. coli* O157:H7.

Although many of the manifestations of acute gastroenteritis in children are non-specific, some clinical features may help identify major categories of diarrhea and could facilitate rapid triage for specific therapy (Table 7.2.2). However, it must be underscored that there is considerable overlap in the symptomatology and if facilities and resources permit, the syndromic diagnosis must be verified by appropriate laboratory investigations. Table 7.2.3 indicates some of the features that help characterize diarrhoea severity and associated dehydration

Complications

Most of the complications associated with gastroenteritis are related to the rapidity of diagnosis and of institution of appropriate therapy. Thus unless early and appropriate rehydration is provided, most children with acute diarrhea would develop dehydration with associated com-plications. In young children such episodes can be life threatening. In other instances, inappropriate therapy can lead to prolongation of the diarrhoeal episodes with consequent malnutrition and complications such as secondary infections and micronutrient deficiencies such as those with iron and zinc.

Diagnosis

The diagnosis of gastroenteritis is largely based on clinical recognition of the disorder, an evaluation of its severity by rapid assessment and confirmation by appropriate laboratory investigations.

Clinical evaluation of diarrhoea. The most common manifestation of gastrointestinal tract infection in children is with diarrhoea, abdominal cramps, and vomiting. Systemic manifestations are varied and associated with a variety of causes. The following system of evaluation in a child with acute diarrhea may allow a reasonably rapid assessment of the nature and severity of the disorder

1. Assess the degree of dehydration and acidosis and provide rapid resuscitation and rehydration with oral or intravenous fluids as required.
2. Obtain appropriate contact or exposure history to determine cause. This can include information on exposure to contacts with similar symptoms, and intake of contaminated foods or water, childcare center attendance, recent travel to a diarrhea endemic area, use of antimicrobial agents.
3. Clinically determine the etiology of diarrhea for institution of prompt antibiotic therapy. Although nausea and vomiting are nonspecific symptoms, they are indicative of infection in the upper intestine. Fever is suggestive of an inflammatory process and also occurs as a result of dehydration. Fever is common in patients with inflammatory diarrhea, Severe abdo-minal pain and tenesmus are indicative of involvement of the large intestine. Features such as nausea and vomiting, absent or low grade fever with mild to moderate periumbilical pain and watery diarrhea are indicative of upper intestinal tract involvement.

Table 7.2.3: Clinical features associated with dehydration			
	Minimal or none (<3% loss of body weight)	*Mild to Moderate (3-9% loss of body weight)*	*Severe (>9% loss of body weight)*
Mucous membrane	Moist	Dry	Parched
Eyes/Fontanelle	Normal	Sunken	Deeply sunken
Skin pinch	Normal	Skin pinch goes back slowly 1-2 sec	Skin pinch goes back very slowly >2 sec
Tears	Present	Decreased	Absent
Extremities	Perfused	-/+ delayed cap. refill	Delayed cap. refill>2 secCold, mottled
Mental status	well, Alert	Normal, Irritable, lethargic	Lethargic, apathetic,unconscious
Pulse volume/H. rate	Normal	Rapid	Thready, Weak, impalpable
BP	Normal	Decreased	Hypotensive or unrecordable (in shock)
Urine output	Normal	Decreased	Absent for > 8hr
Breathing	Normal	Fast	Rapid /deep

Stool examination. Microscopic examination of the stool and cultures can yield important information on the etiology of diarrhea. Stool specimens should be examined for mucus, blood, and leukocytes. Fecal leukocytes are indicative of bacterial invasion of colonic mucosa, although some patients with shigellosis may have minimal leukocytes at an early stage of infection, as do patients infected with Shiga toxin–producing *E. coli* and *E. histolytica.* In endemic areas stool microscopy must include examination for parasites causing diarrhea such as *Giardia lamblia* and *E. histolytica.*

Stool cultures should be obtained as early in the course of disease as possible from children with bloody diarrhea, in whom stool microscopy indicates fecal leukocytes, in outbreaks, with suspected hemolytic-uremic syndrome (HUS), and in immunosuppressed children with diarrhea. Stool specimens for culture need to be transported and plated quickly and if the latter is not quickly available, may need to be transported in special media. The yield and diagnosis of bacterial diarrhea can be significantly improved by using molecular diagnostic procedures such as PCR techniques and probes.

Treatment

A clinical evaluation plan and management strategy for children with moderate to severe diarrhea as per the WHO/UNICEF IMCI strategy is outlined in Figs 7.2.1 and 7.2.2. The broad principles of management of acute diarrhoea in children include the following

1. Oral rehydration therapy

Children, especially infants, are more susceptible than adults to dehydration because of the greater basal fluid and electrolyte requirements per kilogram and because they are dependent on others to meet these demands. This must be evaluated rapidly and corrected within 4-6 hours according to the degree of dehydration and estimated daily requirements. A small minority, especially those in shock or unable to tolerate oral fluids, may require intravenous rehydration but oral rehydration is the preferred mode of rehydration and replacement of on-going losses. While in general the standard WHO oral rehydration solution (ORS) is adequate, recent evidence indicates that low-osmolality oral rehydration fluids may be more effective in reducing stool output. Compared with standard ORS, lower sodium and glucose ORS (containing 75 milliequivalents of sodium and 75 millimoles of glucose per litre, with total osmolarity of 245 milliosmols per liter) reduces stool output, vomiting, and the need for intravenous fluids.

2. Enteral feeding and diet selection

It is now well recognized that continued enteral feeding in diarrhoea aids in recovery from the episode and thus continued appropriate feeding in diarrhoea is the norm. Once rehydration is complete, food should be reintroduced while oral rehydration can be continued to replace ongoing losses from stools and for maintenance. Breastfeeding of infants should be resumed as soon as possible. The usual energy density of any diet used for the therapy of diarrhoea should be around 1 kcal/g, aiming to provide an energy intake of minimum 100 kcal/kg/day, and a protein intake of between 2-3 g/kg/day. With the exception of acute lactose intolerance in a small proportion with diarrhoea, most children are able to tolerate milk and lactose containing diets. Thus in general withdrawal of milk and replacement with specialized (and expensive) lactose-free formulations is unnecessary. Administration of a lactose load exceeding 5 g/kg/day is associated with higher purging rates and treatment failure in children with diarrhoea and alternative strategies for feeding such children may include the addition of milk to cereals as well as replacement of milk with fermented milk products such as yogurt.

Rarely when dietary intolerance precludes the administration of cow's milk based formulations or milk, it may be necessary to administer specialized milk-free diets such as a comminuted or blenderised chicken-based diet or an elemental formulation. It must be pointed out that although effective in some settings, the latter are unaffordable in most developing countries. In addition to rice-lentil formulations, the addition of green banana or pectin to the diet has also been shown to be effective in the treatment of persistent diarrhoea. Fig. 7.2.3 indicates a suggestive algorithm for the management of children with prolonged diarrhoea.

3. Zinc supplementation

There is now strong evidence that zinc supplementation among children with diarrhoea leads to reduced duration and severity of diarrhoea and WHO and UNICEF now jointly recommend that all children (> 6 months of age) with acute diarrhoea should receive oral zinc in some form for 10 to 14 days during and after diarrhoea (10-20 milligrams per day).

4. Appropriate Antimicrobial therapy

Timely antibiotic therapy is critical in reducing the duration and severity of diarrhea and prevention of complications. Table 7.2.4 lists the commonly recommended antibiotics for use in infections with specific pathogens. While these agents are important to use in specific cases, their widespread and indiscriminate use may lead to the development of antimicrobial resistance. There is no role for anti-secretory or anti-motility agents in the treatment of acute gastroenteritis in children.

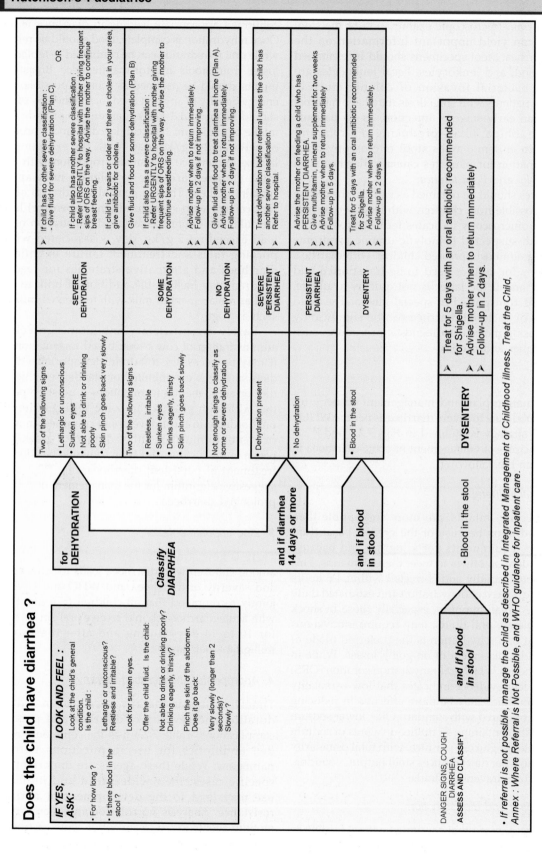

Fig. 7.2.1: IMCI protocol for the recognition and management of diarrhea

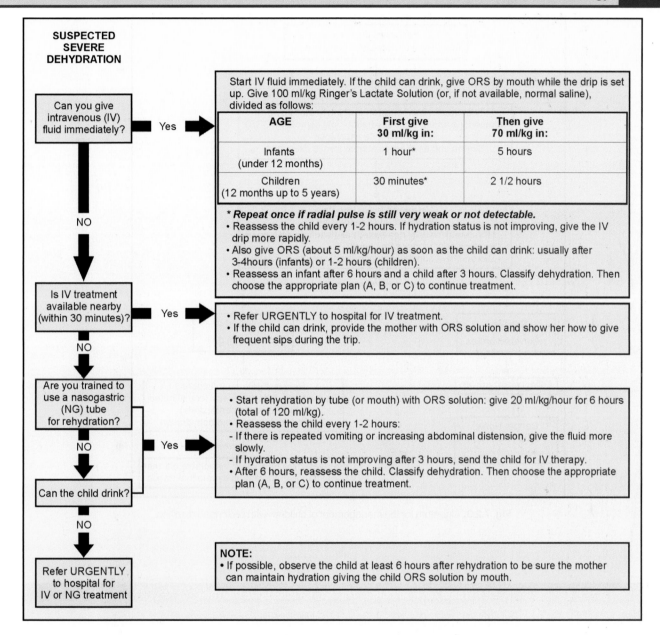

SUSPECTED SEVERE DEHYDRATION

Can you give intravenous (IV) fluid immediately? — Yes →

Start IV fluid immediately. If the child can drink, give ORS by mouth while the drip is set up. Give 100 ml/kg Ringer's Lactate Solution (or, if not available, normal saline), divided as follows:

AGE	First give 30 ml/kg in:	Then give 70 ml/kg in:
Infants (under 12 months)	1 hour*	5 hours
Children (12 months up to 5 years)	30 minutes*	2 1/2 hours

* **Repeat once if radial pulse is still very weak or not detectable.**
- Reassess the child every 1-2 hours. If hydration status is not improving, give the IV drip more rapidly.
- Also give ORS (about 5 ml/kg/hour) as soon as the child can drink: usually after 3-4hours (infants) or 1-2 hours (children).
- Reassess an infant after 6 hours and a child after 3 hours. Classify dehydration. Then choose the appropriate plan (A, B, or C) to continue treatment.

NO ↓

Is IV treatment available nearby (within 30 minutes)? — Yes →

- Refer URGENTLY to hospital for IV treatment.
- If the child can drink, provide the mother with ORS solution and show her how to give frequent sips during the trip.

NO ↓

Are you trained to use a nasogastric (NG) tube for rehydration? — Yes →

- Start rehydration by tube (or mouth) with ORS solution: give 20 ml/kg/hour for 6 hours (total of 120 ml/kg).
- Reassess the child every 1-2 hours:
- If there is repeated vomiting or increasing abdominal distension, give the fluid more slowly.
- If hydration status is not improving after 3 hours, send the child for IV therapy.
- After 6 hours, reassess the child. Classify dehydration. Then choose the appropriate plan (A, B, or C) to continue treatment.

NO ↓

Can the child drink?

NO ↓

Refer URGENTLY to hospital for IV or NG treatment

NOTE:
- If possible, observe the child at least 6 hours after rehydration to be sure the mother can maintain hydration giving the child ORS solution by mouth.

Fig. 7.2.2: Management of severe dehydration

Preventive Strategies for reducing diarrhoea burden and improving outcomes

In developing countries with high rates of diarrhoea in children, a wider approach to diarrhoea prevention is required in addition to improved case management. These include

Improved Water and Sanitary Facilities and Promotion of Personal and Domestic Hygiene

Diarrhoea is a disease of poverty and much of the reduction in diarrhoea prevalence in the developed world has been a result of improvement in standards of hygiene and improved water supply. Several studies that hand washing promotion, access to soap as well as water purification strategies can significantly reduce the burden of diarrhoea in population settings.

Promotion of Exclusive Breastfeeding

Exclusive breastfeeding protects very young infants from diarrhoea through the promotion of passive immunity and through reduction in the intake of potentially contaminated food and water. There is now evidence that even in HIV

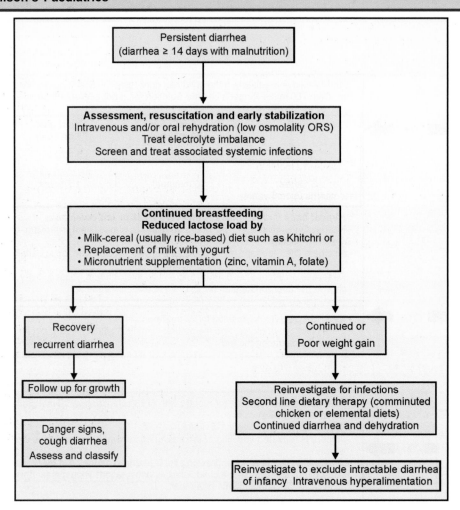

Fig. 7.2.3: Algorithm for the management of children with prolonged diarrhea

Table 7.2.4: Antibiotic Therapy for Infectious Diarrhea		
Organism	*Drug of Choice*	*Dose and Duration of Treatment*
Shigella (severe dysentery and EIEC dysentery)		ciprofloxacin Ciprofloxacin=20-30mg/kg/d divided bd for 7-10days
EPEC, ETEC, EIEC	Trimethoprim sulfamethoxazole (TMP/SMX) or ciprofloxacin	10 mg/kg/d of TMP and 50 mg/kg/d of SMX divided bid for 5 d20-30mg/kg/d qid for 5-10days
Campylobacter jejuni	Erythromycin or azithromycin	50 mg/kg/d divided qid for 5 d
Giardia lamblia	Metronidazole	30-40 mg/kg/d divided tid for 10 d
Entamoeba histolytica	Metronidazole	30-40 mg/kg/d divided tid for 7-10 d
Cryptosporidium species	Paromomycin or azithromycin	25-35mg/kg/d divided tid for 5-10d
Entamoeba histolytica	Metronidazole followed by iodoquinol	Metronidazole 30-40mg/kg/d divided tid x7-10d
Blastocystis hominis	Metronidazole or iodoquinol	Metronidazole 30-40mg/kg/d divided tid x 7-10d

EIEC = Enteroinvasive *E. coli;*TMP = trimethoprim; SMX = sulfamethoxazole; bid = 2 times a day; qid = 4 times a day; tid = 3 times a day.

endemic populations in developing countries, exclusive breastfeeding may reduce the risk of mortality without enhanced rates of mother to child transmission of the virus through breast milk and so this recommendation is indeed universal.

Safe Complementary Feeding Practices

Complementary foods in developing countries are generally poor in quality and frequently heavily contaminated, and thus are a major predisposing factor for diarrhoea after weaning. Contamination of complementary foods can be potentially reduced through caregiver's education in hygiene and sanitation, improving home food storage and strategies such as fermentation.

Rotavirus Immunization

Almost all infants acquire rotavirus diarrhoea early in life, and given the burden estimates of rotavirus infections and mortality, an effective rotavirus vaccine would have a major effect on reducing diarrhoea mortality in developing countries. Two recent Rotavirus vaccines have shown remarkable protective efficacy in diverse settings and are being incorporated in national vaccine strategies.

Other vaccines that could potentially reduce the burden of severe diarrhoea and mortality in young children are vaccines against Shigella and ETEC.

BIBLIOGRAPHY

1. Ashkenazi S. Shigella infections in children: New insights. Semin Pediatr Infect Dis. 2004;15:246-52.
2. Bhutta ZA, Black RE, Brown KH, Gardner JM, Gore S, Hidayat A, et al. Therapeutic effect of oral zinc in acute and persistent diarrhea in children in developing countries: pooled analysis of randomized controlled trials". Am J Clin Nutr 2000;72:1516-22.
3. Bhutta ZA, Ghishan F, Lindley K, Memon IA, Mittal S, Rhoads JM. Persistent and chronic diarrhea and malabsorption: Working Group report of the second World Congress of Pediatric Gastroenterology, Hepatology, and Nutrition. J Pediatr Gastroenterol Nutr. 2004; Suppl 2:S711-6.
4. Bhutta ZA. "Persistent Diarrhea" in Guandalini S (editor). Text book of Gastroenterology. Taylor and Francis, 2004.
5. Denno DM, Stapp JR, Boster DR, Qin X, Clausen CR, Del Beccaro KH, Swerdlow DL, Braden CR, Tarr PI. Etiology of diarrhea in pediatric outpatient settings. Pediatr Infect Dis J. 2005;24:142-8.
6. Hahn S, Kim Y, Garner P. Reduced osmolarity oral rehydration solution for treating dehydration due to diarrhea in children: systematic review. BMJ 2001; 323: 81-85.
7. Jones G, Steketee RW, Black RE, Bhutta ZA, Morris SS. "How many child deaths can we prevent this year?". Lancet 2003;362:65:65-71.
8. O'ryan M, Prado V, Pickering LK. A millennium update on pediatric diarrheal illness in the developing world. Semin Pediatr Infect Dis. 2005;16:125-36.
9. Thapar M, Sanderson IR. Diarrhea in children: an interface between developing and developed countries. Lancet 2004; 363:641–53.

Chapter 8

Paediatric Cardiology

Trevor Richens

INTRODUCTION

Disorders affecting the cardiovascular system in childhood can as always be split into congenital and acquired. Over the last fifty years the congenital forms of heart disease have evolved from a group of conditions for which no treatment was available to a set of abnormalities, the vast majority of which are treatable if recognised early.

As a group, heart disorders constitute the commonest congenital abnormality with incidences quoted between 6/1000 and 9/1000. In the developed world the incidence seems to be declining largely as a result of increased fetal diagnosis and subsequent termination of pregnancy. This effect however, appears less marked in Asia.

The aetiology of congenital heart disease remains poorly understood. It is well known that many syndromic abnormalities have associated heart defects, and that exposure to certain drugs or toxic agents in utero can result in malformations of the heart (Table 8.1). The incidence of congenital heart disease is also known to be higher in siblings or offspring of those already affected. The incidence rises from 6-9/1000 to 30-40/1000 for siblings of affected children. Unfortunately the genetic basis for this remains largely unknown however it is the subject of intense ongoing research.

Of the acquired forms of heart disease in childhood, those resulting from rheumatic fever remain the commonest in Asia. Conversely, rheumatic heart disease is now rare in the developed world, where viral infections are the commonest type of acquired heart disease.

Congenital heart disease can be classified in a number of ways. From a clinical standpoint the most straightforward is to split them into acyanotic and cyanotic before further subdividing on the basis of precise anatomical diagnosis (Table 8.2). Acyanotic congenital heart disease is by far the commonest group, comprising ventricular septal defect, atrial septal defect, atrioventricular septal defect, arterial duct, coarctation of the aorta, pulmonary stenosis and aortic stenosis. Together this group account

for about 90% of congenital heart disease. The principal cyanotic lesions are tetralogy of Fallot, transposition of the great arteries, pulmonary atresia, tricuspid atresia and Ebsteins anomaly, altogether comprising about 5% of congenital heart disease. Other rare conditions such as total anomalous pulmonary venous drainage, hypoplastic left heart syndrome and other forms of univentricular heart constitute the remaining 5%. Conveniently it is this classification I will use to discuss the individual lesions.

GENERAL PRINCIPLES OF DIAGNOSIS

Despite the huge improvements in cardiac echocardiography (echo), there remains no substitute for accurate clinical assessment possibly aided by a 12 lead electrocardiogram (ECG). Echo should be used to confirm and refine the clinical diagnosis, and then for follow up assessment of abnormalities. The ECG remains an extremely important adjunct to the history and clinical examination. It is a simple, cheap, non-invasive tool that can often confirm or refute a diagnosis. The routine use of a chest X-ray is more controversial. Whilst more widely available than echo, it does involve a radiation dose and should probably be confined to children where the suspicion of heart disease is high, and the availability of echo low.

EXAMINATION

Inspection

A complete cardiovascular examination should start with careful inspection of the child asking five questions.

1. Is the child breathless? If a child is breathless as a result of a cardiac abnormality it suggests pulmonary vascular engorgement, usually caused by heart failure (Table 8.3). This may result from increased pulmonary blood flow as in the case of a left to right intracardiac shunt – VSD, PDA, AVSD – or because of pulmonary venous engorgement – mitral regurgitation, dilated

Table 8.1: Conditions associated with congenital heart disease	
Association	*Defect(s)*
Chromosomal Abnormality	
Trisomy 21	VSD, AVSD (in 50%)
Trisomy 18	VSD, PDA, pulmonary stenosis (in 99%)
Trisomy 13	VSD, PDA, dextrocardia (in 90%)
5p – cri du chat	VSD, PDA, ASD (in 25%)
XO (Turner)	Coarctation, aortic stenosis, ASD (in 35%)
XXXXY (Klinefelters)	PDA, ASD (in 15%)
Syndrome	
Noonans	Dysplastic pulmonary stenosis
Williams	Supravalve aortic stenosis, branch pulmonary stenosis
Di George	VSD, Tetralogy, Truncus, aortic arch abnormality
CHARGE	VSD, Tetralogy
VATERL	VSD, Tetralogy
Holt - Oram	ASD
Friedreich Ataxia	Hypertrophic cardiomyopathy, heart block
Apert	VSD, Tetralogy
Ellis van Creveld	Common atrium
Pompe (GSD II)	Hypertrophic cardiomyopathy
Leopard	Pulmonary stenosis, cardiomyopathy, long PR interval
Muscular dystrophy	Dilated cardiomyopathy
Tuberous sclerosis	Cardiac rhabdomyomata
Pierre Robin	VSD, PDA, ASD, coarctation, Tetralogy
Long QT syndrome	Long QT interval and torsades de pointes
Maternal Conditions	
Rubella	PDA, branch pulmonary stenosis
Diabetes	VSD, Hypertrophic cardiomyopathy (transient)
SLE (anti Ro/La positive)	Congenital heart block
Phenylketonuria	VSD
Lithium	Ebsteins
Sodium valproate	Coarctation, HLHS
Phenytoin	VSD, coarctation, mitral stenosis
Alcohol	VSD

Table 8.2: Classification of congenital heart disease in childhood
Acyanotic Defects
Increased Pulmonary blood flow
Atrial septal defect
Ventricular septal defect
Atrioventricular septal defect
Patent arterial duct
Normal pulmonary blood flow
Pulmonary stenosis
Aortic stenosis
Coarctation of the aorta
Cyanotic Defects
Normal or reduced pulmonary blood flow
Tetralogy of Fallot
Transposition of the great arteries
Critical pulmonary stenosis
Ebsteins anomaly
Pulmonary atresia
Tricuspid atresia
Single ventricle with pulmonary stenosis
Increased pulmonary blood flow
Total anomalous pulmonary venous drainage
Hypoplastic left heart syndrome
Truncus arteriosus
Single ventricle without pulmonary stenosis

Table 8.3: Causes of heart failure by age	
First week	– Left heart obstruction (HLHS, Aortic stenosis, Coarctation), arrhythmia
First month	– Left to right shunt (VSD, AVSD, PDA, truncus arteriosus), arrhythmia
Thereafter	– Rheumatic fever, dilated cardiomyopathy, myocarditis, endocarditis, arrhythmia

cardiomyopathy, obstructed total anomalous pulmonary venous return, pericardial effusion.

2. Is the child cyanotic? Although the absence of clinical cyanosis does not exclude cyanotic congenital heart disease, if it is present it limits the potential diagnoses to a relatively small group of abnormalities. In the newborn most commonly it would suggest transposition of the great arteries or severely obstructed pulmonary blood flow (tetralogy of Fallot, critical pulmonary stenosis, pulmonary atresia, tricuspid atresia). In infancy tetralogy is the commonest cause, although transposition with ventricular septal defect and other rare forms of complex congenital heart disease can also present at this age. In older children, a

presentation with cyanosis would suggest pulmonary vascular disease complicating a VSD or PDA. Untreated, the high pulmonary pressures ultimately damage the pulmonary vasculature resulting in high pulmonary resistance and a reversal of the intracardiac shunt (right to left) with subsequent cyanosis. Rarely tetralogy and other complex forms of congenital heart disease can present in later life.

3. Is the child dysmorphic? Many children with congenital syndromes have cardiac abnormalities, the principal ones of which are outlined in Table 8.1. Thus prompt recognition of a syndrome may alert the clinician to search for a particular abnormality.

4. Is the child failing to thrive? There are many causes of failure to thrive in infancy of which heart disease is a relatively minor one. The predominant group of cardiac disorders causing poor weight gain are those resulting in breathlessness and poor feeding. These include VSD, AVSD and PDA. Whilst some children with cyanotic abnormalities also fail to grow this is far less common.

5. Does the child have any thoracic scars? If the child has had previous heart surgery the type of scar may give clues to its nature. A median sternotomy scar suggests an open-heart procedure during which the heart would have been stopped and opened. All major intracardiac abnormalities requiring a surgical repair are corrected in this manner. A right lateral thoracotomy scar is usually only used for a right modified Blalock Taussig shunt. During this procedure a tube is interposed between the right subclavian artery and the right pulmonary artery, providing an alternative source of pulmonary blood flow in children who have an obstructed native pulmonary blood flow (tetralogy of Fallot, pulmonary atresia, tricuspid atresia). A left thoracotomy scar is used in the repair of aortic coarctation, ligation of patent arterial ducts, a left Blalock Taussig shunt and occasionally a pulmonary artery band (a ligature placed around the main pulmonary artery to protect the lungs from high pressures in children with large ventricular septal defects).

Palpation

Always start the examination by feeling the femoral and brachial pulses simultaneously. A reduction in volume, or absence of the femoral pulse is strongly suggestive of coarctation of the aorta and should prompt closer examination and investigation. Although classically textbooks talk of radio-femoral delay this really only becomes appreciable as the child reaches adult size. Some children who have had previous procedures have an absent femoral pulse on one side only. It is therefore advisable to examine both femoral pulses.

Palpation for an enlarged liver should then be undertaken. The liver enlarges in heart failure and can reach below the umbilicus in some children. The liver is often quite soft and difficult to feel in infants, particularly if the child is struggling so great care must be taken.

The heart enlarges in response to any chronic volume load. This may arise because of a right to left shunt – ASD, VSD, PDA, AVSD – because of valve dysfunction – mitral regurgitation, aortic regurgitation, pulmonary regurgitation – or because of a primary myocardial abnormality – viral myocarditis, dilated cardiomyopathy. In younger children this can be felt as a sub-xyphoid heave by palpating just below the inferior end of the sternum. In children of all ages with a volume loaded heart a parasternal heave can also be felt with the palm of the hand on the left side.

Finish off palpation by carefully placing your index finger in the suprasternal notch feeling for a thrill. If one is present it is strongly suggestive of aortic stenosis, although rarely pulmonary stenosis and a PDA can produce this sign.

Auscultation

Auscultation is often difficult in children. The combination of fast heart rate, noisy breathing and a poorly co-operative child make it the most challenging part of the examination. To ensure nothing is missed you should follow a fixed pattern when listening to a childs heart. I would suggest listening with the diaphragm at all points over the left side of the praecordium, followed by the right upper sternal edge and at the back. At each point it is important to listen to systole, diastole and the heart sounds in turn. All can provide vital diagnostic information that is easy to miss when distracted by a loud, obvious systolic murmur. Murmurs are classically graded to permit easy comparison, systolic murmurs out of 6 and diastolic out of 4 (Table 8.4).

A full discussion of the auscultatory findings associated with different abnormalities will follow under the specific abnormalities.

Innocent Murmurs

By definition an innocent murmur has no associated heart disease however it is an extremely common finding and some clarification is needed. Innocent murmurs can be heard in up to 80% of children at some point. They can cause considerable diagnostic confusion so if you are in doubt get a more experienced opinion. Innocent murmurs have an otherwise normal cardiovascular examination, are systolic, often vary with posture and usually have a characteristic quality. Some murmurs are soft, short and heard only at the lower left sternal edge, others have a typical vibratory quality much like humming and can be quite loud. These are known as Still's murmurs. A venous hum is also common, particularly when a child is examined standing up. It is heard beneath either clavicle and extends through systole into diastole sometimes sounding like an arterial duct. Unlike a duct however a venous hum disappears as a child rotates his head.

Table 8.4: Grading of heart murmurs						
Murmur	1	2	3	4	5	6
Systolic	Barely audible	Quiet	Easily audible	Associated with thrill	Audible without stethoscope	Audible from end of bed
Diastolic	Quiet	Easily audible	Associated with thrill	Audible without stethoscope		

All innocent murmurs allow the examining doctor to be very reassuring with the parents that the heart is structurally normal.

Investigations

Many heart conditions result in failure to thrive in infancy, therefore height and weight should always be measured and plotted on a centile chart. To complete the examination the child's saturation should be measured using a pulse oximeter. When using this equipment care should be taken to ensure the child's peripheries are warm, well perfused and the oximeter should be left in place on the child for at least 30 seconds to allow stabilisation of the reading. Measurement of the right brachial blood pressure should be made using the correctly sized cuff for the child. If coarctation is a possibility many advocate the comparison of blood pressure measurements between arm and leg. In my experience I have found this comparison misleading and do not place great emphasis on its importance. If there is any suspicion of endocarditis, a urine sample should be analysed for haemolysed blood and proteinuria.

Electrocardiography

Electrocardiography is a simple non-invasive tool that records the electrical activity of the heart. A study is performed by attaching recording electrodes to specific sites on the skin to obtain raw recordings of cardiac electrical activity. These recordings are then processed to produce recognised "leads" that are printed out for examination. The electrical activity associated with each heart beat can be seen as a sequence of waves denoted P, Q, R, S and T (Fig. 8.1). These different leads look at the heart from different angles allowing information to be obtained from most areas. By analysing the electrical activity of the heart the precise heart rate and rhythm can be identified, the electrical axis can be measured, as can the heights and durations of the various waves. These measurements give information about the size and thickness of the various heart chambers, about areas of ischaemic or infarction, and about abnormalities of conduction that might predispose the child to arrhythmias.

Echocardiography

Echocardiography is essentially ultrasound of the heart. The differences compared with conventional ultrasound are the hardware and software settings that are configured to view the rapidly moving structures within the heart. Four main types of imaging are produced that look at various aspects of cardiac function. 2-dimensional or cross-sectional echo produces conventional ultrasound-type images of the heart structures, moving in real time (Fig. 8.2). This modality facilitates accurate anatomical diagnosis of heart conditions by imaging how the various structures relate to each other. M-mode echo takes a single line through the heart and plots all the information obtained against a time axis (Fig. 8. 3). This mode is used for measurements and calculations particularly concer-

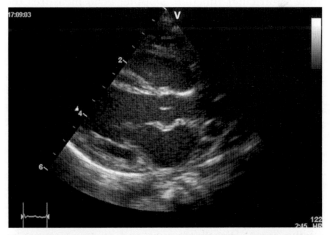

Fig. 8.2: Normal para-sternal long-axis echocardiogram

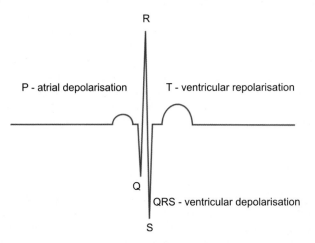

Fig. 8.1: ECG complex diagram

R

P - atrial depolarisation   T - ventricular repolarisation

Q

QRS - ventricular depolarisation

S

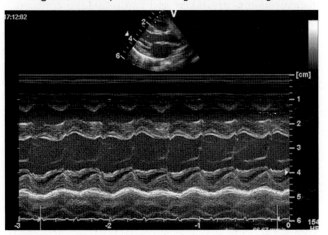

Fig. 8.3: Normal M mode echocardiogram through left ventricle

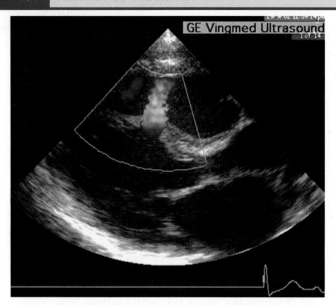

Fig. 8.4: Colour flow Doppler echocardiogram demonstrating small mid-septal muscular ventricular septal defect

ning ventricular function. Doppler echo measures the velocity of blood moving through the heart and great arteries. Using this data it is possible to estimate pressure differences at various points in the heart such as the aortic or pulmonary valve, and thus measure the severity of any narrowing. Colour Doppler superimposes Doppler information on a 2-dimensional image, representing the flow direction and velocity with different colours (Fig. 8.4). This mode allows identification of valve leaks or heart defects that might not be seen on 2-dimensional imaging alone.

Cardiac Catheter

Cardiac catheterisation is both a diagnostic and treatment tool. Long thin plastic tubes (catheters) are introduced into a vein or artery and threaded though the various chambers of the heart. Direct pressure and oxygen saturation measurements are taken and radio-opaque contrast is injected into the heart to outline various structures and abnormalities. This technique has evolved over recent years to permit many common cardiac anomalies to be treated using this minimally invasive approach. Suitable atrial septal defects, patent arterial ducts, ventricular septal defects, stenotic pulmonary and aortic valves as well as aortic coarctation can all be treated by the transcatheter route using specialised techniques.

CONGENITAL HEART ABNORMALITIES

ACYANOTIC CONGENITAL HEART DISEASE

Ventricular Septal Defect (VSD)

Ventricular septal defect is the commonest single congenital heart abnormality accounting for a third of all lesions. It is caused by a defect in the septum that divides the two ventricles. Defects can exist in the muscular septum (muscular defects) or in the membranous septum (perimembranous defects). The symptoms and signs result from the flow of blood between the two ventricles through the defect. At birth the resistance to flow through the lungs is equal to the resistance to flow to the body i.e. the pulmonary vascular resistance (PVR) is equal to the systemic vascular resistance (SVR). Consequently little blood will pass through the VSD and no murmur will be audible. Over the first few days of life the PVR falls resulting in a drop in right ventricular pressure facilitating flow through a VSD. When a VSD is present blood can exit the left ventricle through both aorta and VSD. The VSD flow will increase the overall pulmonary arterial flow and thus venous return to the left atrium (Fig. 8.5). The left heart therefore has to cope with increased volumes and enlarges producing a characteristic heave. Defects vary widely in size and position, as do the clinical features. The majority of defects are small communications between the two ventricles through the muscular septum. These usually present as asymptomatic murmurs and require only reassurance and antibiotic prophylaxis for dental and surgical procedures. Clinically they can be recognised by the typical high-pitched, harsh pansystolic murmur, often well localised over the left praecordium. The exact position of the murmur is dependent on the location of the defect within the septum. The absence of a precordial or subxyphoid heave confirms the lack of a significant left to right shunt, and normal intensity of the second heart sound demonstrates normal pulmonary artery pressure.

Small perimembranous defects can be indistinguishable from muscular defects although the murmur tends to be higher on the left parasternal border. When a perimembranous defect is suspected the early diastolic murmur of aortic regurgitation must be excluded, as this would constitute an indication for repair.

Moderate sized defects, either muscular or perimembranous, result in a gradual increase in murmur intensity often with a corresponding reduction in pitch. As the volume of blood flowing through the defect increases, so the stroke volume of the left ventricle must increase producing a parasternal heave. In even larger defects, blood flow through the VSD becomes less turbulent and the murmur quietens becoming silent with completely unrestrictive defects although the heave is usually marked. As the size of defect increases so does the pulmonary artery pressure resulting in a loud pulmonary component of the second heart sound.

Infants with moderate to large defects develop the classical signs of heart failure as the PVR falls and the shunt increases. Typically they fail to thrive and feed poorly because of breathlessness and gut oedema. On examination they are tachypnoeic, tachycardic, sweaty, have hepatomegaly a marked heave, variable systolic

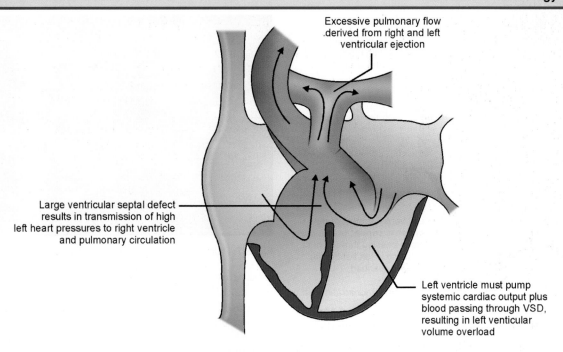

Excessive pulmonary flow derived from right and left ventricular ejection

Large ventricular septal defect results in transmission of high left heart pressures to right ventricle and pulmonary circulation

Left ventricle must pump systemic cardiac output plus blood passing through VSD, resulting in left venticular volume overload

Fig. 8.5: Ventricular septal defect –diagram demonstrating left heart volume overload

murmur, loud second heart sound and a summation gallop (combined third and fourth heart sounds producing a noise similar to a horse galloping).

With a significant VSD the ECG may show evidence of biventricular hypertrophy and a sinus tachycardia. The chest X ray will show cardiomegaly and plethoric lung fields. Diagnosis can be confirmed by echocardiogram which will demonstrate the position and size of the defect, exclude or confirm additional lesions, measure the size of the left ventricle which will reflect the degree of left to right shunt, and using Doppler estimate the pulmonary artery pressures to reveal any pulmonary hypertension.

Management

Treatment is aimed at stabilisation and encouragement of growth prior to surgical repair. The mainstays of therapy include nasogastric feeding to maximise caloric intake and minimise the energy spent trying to suck a feed. Diuretics treat the compensatory salt and water retention that is a consequence of heart failure. Angiotensin converting enzyme inhihibtors (ACEi) such as captopril reduce left ventricular afterload and encourage systemic flow. Digoxin combats excessive tachycardia and maximises ventricular contraction. Oxygen can cause pulmonary vasodilatation effectively worsening heart failure. Ultimately the majority of children will require surgical closure of the defect. Where open cardiac surgery is available repair will usually be undertaken within 6 months to prevent the development of pulmonary vascular disease. Where only closed procedures are possible a pulmonary artery band can be

applied to protect the lungs from excessive blood flow and high pressure, and permit later closure.

Children with small to moderate defects may need no therapy at all if the haemodynamic shunt is small. Others may slowly develop left heart overload and require repair later in life, a number of these being suitable for transcatheter closure using one of the growing number of catheter deployable devices. A small number of children with sub aortic defects will develop aortic regurgitation, which is also an indication for repair.

Untreated infants with large defects may die, usually from concomitant respiratory infections. Alternatively the symptoms may resolve from 6 months onwards as PVR increases due to inflammation and thickening of the pulmonary arterioles. These changes usually become irreversible at approximately 6 – 12 months, tending to slowly worsen thereafter. When the effective PVR becomes greater than the SVR the haemodynamic shunt through the VSD will reverse and the child will become cyanosed. This situation is known as Eisenmengers syndrome and will not improve with correction of the original cardiac defect.

Patent Ductus Arteriosus (PDA)

The arterial duct is a vital fetal structure that connects the main pulmonary artery to the aorta. In utero it allows blood to pass directly to the aorta from the pulmonary artery avoiding the high resistance pulmonary circulation. This "right to left" shunt exists because the PVR exceeds the SVR. At birth the rise in blood oxygen concentration

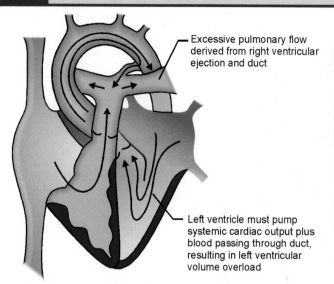

Fig. 8.6: Patent ductus arteriosus –diagram demonstrating left heart volume overload

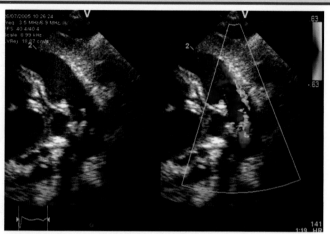

Fig. 8.7: Patent ductus arteriosus- colour Doppler echocardiogram

together with a reduction in circulating prostaglandins usually causes spasm of the duct with eventual permanent closure. Ongoing patency of the duct beyond the immediate neonatal period results in the development of a "left to right" shunt from aorta to pulmonary artery as the PVR drops (Fig. 8.6). The significance of this to the child varies depending upon the size of the child and size of the duct.

Preterm infants have an increased risk of PDA. In this group the flow of blood through the duct results in excessive pulmonary blood flow, increased pulmonary venous return to the left heart, with subsequent chamber enlargement.

The infant is often breathless, may have high ventilation requirements; will have high volume pulses, a left precordial heave and a systolic or continuous murmur. Term infants with a significant PDA may present with failure to thrive, together with signs of left heart overload and a murmur. The murmur is continuous (extends throughout systole and into diastole), heard best below the left clavicle and has a "machinery" character. Usually older children have small ducts that are only detected during auscultation at a routine childhood medical check.

Because the haemodynamic effects are similar to those seen in a child with a VSD, the ECG and chest X-ray findings are similar. Echocardiogram allows an appreciation of the size of the duct (Fig. 8.7), as well as assessment of the shunt by the left heart chamber size (often comparing the left atrium to the aorta), and the pulmonary artery pressure using Doppler.

Management

Preterm infants with large ducts require duct closure. This can often be accomplished using non-steroidal antinflammatory drugs, the most frequently used of which is

intravenous indomethacin (three to six doses, 0.1 – 0.2 mg/kg, 12-24 hours apart). Intravenous ibuprofen has also been used recently with similar success rates and a lower adverse effect rate. If these drugs fail to achieve permanent closure, surgical ligation can be used with a high success rate and low complication rate. In symptomatic children beyond term the duct can be closed either surgically or more commonly by the transcatheter route. Prior to closure symptomatic improvement can be achieved by the use of diuretics with or without digoxin. In the asymptomatic child closure is only indicated where a murmur is heard. In most cases this is done to reduce the risk of endocarditis, as the possibility of left heart enlargement is small. In children where there is no murmur and the PDA is only detected by echocardiogram, no treatment (including antibiotic prophylaxis) is indicated.

Atrial Septal Defect (ASD)

Isolated ASDs rarely cause symptoms in childhood. The most common type of ASD is the secundum defect, which is formed by a gap in the centre of the atrial septum. Less common is the primum type (also called a partial or incomplete atrioventricular septal defect - see below), where a gap exists low down in the atrial septum adjacent to the mitral and tricuspid valves. In some primum defects there is also a gap, or cleft, in the anterior mitral valve leaflet which can result in valve regurgitation. The left to right shunt at atrial level seen in ASD produces enlargement of the right heart (Fig. 8.8).

An ASD may produce no detectable signs however with a significant haemodynamic shunt a palpable heave may be present and flow murmurs across the pulmonary (systolic) or tricuspid (diastolic) valves in addition to a fixed widely split second heart sound may be heard.

The ECG in a secundum defect will show right axis deviation whereas it will be leftward, or superior with a primum defect. As the right ventricle enlarges a partial right bundle branch block pattern will develop (RSR' in

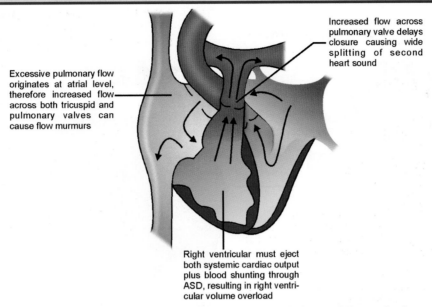

Excessive pulmonary flow originates at atrial level, therefore increased flow across both tricuspid and pulmonary valves can cause flow murmurs

Increased flow across pulmonary valve delays closure causing wide splitting of second heart sound

Right ventricular must eject both systemic cardiac output plus blood shunting through ASD, resulting in right ventricular volume overload

Fig. 8.8: Atrial septal defect –diagram demonstrating right heart volume overload

V4R and V1). The chest X ray will reveal cardiomegaly resulting from enlargement of the right heart structures. Echo confirms size and position of the defect, allows assessment of the shunt size by measuring the right ventricle and excludes any other lesions.

Management

ASDs do not require antibiotic prophylaxis provided there is no other co-existing lesion. Because they rarely produce symptoms in childhood medical therapy is rarely required, although untreated the atrial enlargement can cause arrhythmias and heart failure in adulthood. Unlike VSDs, spontaneous closure is rare and closure is indicated where the right ventricle is enlarged. Interventional catheter techniques can now be used to close many secundum ASDs although open surgery remains the treatment of choice for all primum and the remainder of secundum defects.

Atrioventricular Septal Defect (AVSD)

AVSD results from a failure of fusion of the endocardial cushions in the centre of the heart. Defects are said to be complete where a ventricular defect is present and incomplete where the defect is restricted to the atria (Fig. 8.9). These defects are particularly common in Downs syndrome where they may be associated with Tetralogy of Fallot.

Incomplete AVSD as with all types of ASD usually presents as an asymptomatic murmur. The atrial defect will cause right heart overload resulting in right-sided chamber enlargement detectable as a heave. The systolic and diastolic murmurs are similar to other forms of ASD,

however if there is significant mitral regurgitation through the cleft, left ventricular enlargement is likely together with an apical systolic murmur. The presentation of complete AVSD will vary according to the size of the ventricular component. Small ventricular component defects present in a very similar way to incomplete defects, however large ventricular components present with heart failure and failure to thrive in a similar way to large VSD's. It is not surprising that it can often be difficult to distinguish clinically between VSD and AVSD.

The characteristic finding on electrocardiography is leftward or superior deviation of the QRS axis. This permits distinction from secundum ASD and VSD. Chest X ray findings depend largely on the size of ventricular defect present and effective left to right shunt. Typically it will show an enlarged cardiac silhouette and plethoric lung fields.

Management

No AVSD will resolve spontaneously and all need surgical repair as well as antibiotic prophylaxis. Where a child

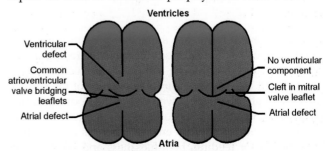

Ventricular defect

Common atrioventricular valve bridging leaflets

Atrial defect

Ventricles

No ventricular component

Cleft in mitral valve leaflet

Atrial defect

Atria

Fig. 8.9: Atrioventricular septal defect – complete vs. incomplete AVSD

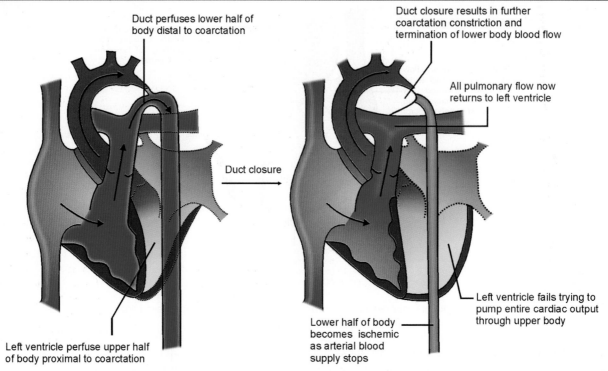

Duct perfuses lower half of body distal to coarctation

Duct closure results in further coarctation constriction and termination of lower body blood flow

All pulmonary flow now returns to left ventricle

Duct closure

Left ventricle fails trying to pump entire cardiac output through upper body

Lower half of body becomes ischemic as arterial blood supply stops

Left ventricle perfuse upper half of body proximal to coarctation

Fig. 8.10: Aortic coarctation – diagram demonstrating effect of duct closure

presents with heart failure due to a large ventricular component the medical management is as described for VSD. The timing of surgery depends on the lesion; large ventricular components need repair within the first six months whereas if the pulmonary artery pressures are normal, providing the mitral leak is not severe, surgery can often be deferred many years.

Coarctation of the Aorta

The arterial duct joins the aorta at the distal portion of the aortic arch and it is at this point that coarctation occurs. A coarctation is an area of narrowing of the aorta that restricts flow. Broadly speaking children with coarctation comprise two groups; those that present in heart failure in infancy and those that present as asymptomatic children or adults with a murmur or hypertension.

Infants

The more severe forms are those that present within the first few weeks of life. In these children closure of the duct results in sub-total or even complete obstruction to the aorta (Fig. 8.10). The left heart fails because of the sudden increase in afterload, the lower half of the body including liver, kidneys and gut become ischaemic and a severe metabolic acidosis rapidly ensues. There is a very short history of poor feeding, breathlessness and poor colour. The infant will be grey, peripherally shut down, poorly responsive, cold, tachypnoeic, tachycardic, sweaty, have absent femoral pulses, hepatomegaly, a summation gallop and may or may not have a murmur.

This situation constitutes a medical emergency. The child should be resuscitated and vascular access obtained by whatever means possible. As a priority the child should be started on a prostaglandin E (0.01 – 0.1 microgram/kg/min) infusion as well as dopamine (5 – 20 microgram/kg/minute). Prostaglandin E is used to open the arterial duct and also reduce the severity of the coarctation by relaxing the ductal tissue that may extend into the aortic wall. An unfortunate effect of prostaglandin E is that it can cause apnoea at therapeutic doses and the child may need intubation and ventilation. Once the child has been resuscitated a detailed assessment can be made including ECG, chest X ray and echo to both confirm the clinical diagnosis and exclude any associated lesion. At this age surgical repair is the only option and should take place as soon as the child is stable. Prostaglandin should not be discontinued until repair.

Older Child

Older children with coarctation present at routine examination with either reduced femoral pulses or hypertension. The narrowing is usually milder and will have progressed over a longer period of time allowing the child's circulation to adjust by developing collateral arteries around the obstruction. In some smaller children there may be a history of failure to thrive but usually they are symptom free. Examination will show a well, pink

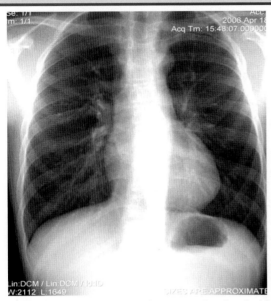

Fig. 8.11: Aortic coarctation – chest x-ray showing double aortic knuckle and rib notching

child with reduced or absent femoral pulses, a loud second heart sound and a systolic murmur heard over the back at the left hand side. Hypertension may be present and four-limb blood pressure recording may reveal an arm/leg gradient, although its absence does not exclude the diagnosis.

ECG will show evidence of left ventricular hypertrophy, particularly if the coarctation is longstanding and chest X-ray may show characteristic features such as double aortic knuckle and rib notching (Fig. 8. 11). An echo-cardiogram will confirm the diagnosis, allow assessment of the severity and also exclude associated abnormalities such as a bicuspid aortic valve or a VSD.

Management

Hypertension can be treated carefully, taking care not to reduce the blood pressure excessively as this may precipitate renal failure. Classically coarctation has always been repaired surgically, however recently balloon angioplasty has proved successful in selected cases. In older children or adults, metal stents can be implanted at the time of angioplasty to reduce the re-coarctation rate. Children with aortic coarctation should receive antibiotic prophylaxis as appropriate for dental and surgical procedures.

Aortic Stenosis

Obstruction of the left ventricular outlet usually occurs at the level of the valve. Less commonly a fibrous ring or membrane can cause sub valve obstruction, and rarely the obstruction can occur above the valve (e.g. Williams Syndrome associated with branch pulmonary stenosis, hypercalcaemia, mental retardation and Elfin facies). Valve

obstruction is more common in boys and results from either a bicuspid valve, or fusion of the valve cusps with or without dysplasia of the valve tissue. Whilst it is often an isolated lesion, aortic stenosis is a key feature of hypoplastic left heart syndrome.

As with most lesions presentation depends on severity. Mild aortic stenosis is usually due to a bicuspid valve and produces no symptoms. It will only be detected in childhood as an asymptomatic murmur, usually preceded by a characteristic ejection click that helps to distinguish it from sub aortic stenosis. The murmur is heard at the upper left sternal edge, radiates to the neck and is often associated with a thrill in the suprasternal notch. If severe obstruction occurs early on in fetal life there is accumu-lating evidence it will progress to hypoplastic left heart syndrome at birth, however most commonly severe aortic stenosis presents in the newborn period as a duct dependent lesion (in such children the arterial duct permits blood to flow from right to left effectively providing or augmenting the systemic cardiac output) (Fig. 8.12). The child will be cyanosed, possibly with a drop in saturations between upper and lower limbs, and have the characteristic ejection systolic murmur and ejection click (short sharp sound heard immediately before the murmur). Upon closure of the duct the child may develop a low cardiac output state with poor pulses, cool peripheries, tachypnoea, tachycardia and hepatomegaly.

Children have moderate aortic stenosis usually present with an asymptomatic murmur. The degree of stenosis gradually progresses as the child grows causing exertional dyspnoea and possibly angina or syncope. These late symptoms are associated with a risk of sudden death and require urgent investigation and treatment.

Although the chest X ray maybe normal even in quite severe aortic stenosis, the ECG will usually show evidence of left ventricular hypertrophy often with the characteristic ST changes of left ventricular strain (Fig. 8.13). Echo-cardiogram will confirm the diagnosis and also estimate its severity using Doppler. In addition, it will demonstrate any associated aortic regurgitation.

Management

All children with aortic stenosis require antibiotic prophy-laxis. The indications for treating aortic stenosis are either symptoms such as angina or syncope, or evidence of left ventricular hypertrophy and strain. Where symptoms exist patients should be advised to restrict physical activity and avoid exertion. There is no form of medical treatment indicated and relief of obstruction can be achieved by balloon valvuloplasty, surgical valvotomy or valve replacement. The problem with valvotomy and valvuloplasty is the risk of converting a stenotic valve into a regurgitant one. Although aortic regurgitation is well tolerated in terms of symptoms it will in time produce enlargement of the left ventricle requiring a valve replacement.

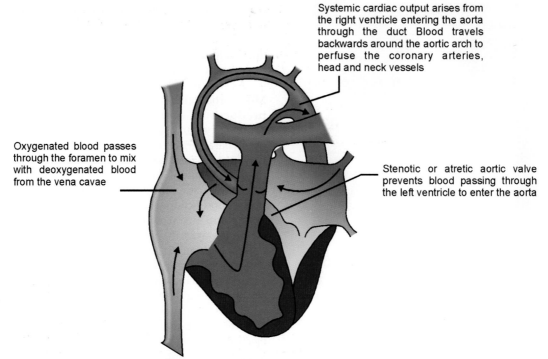

Systemic cardiac output arises from the right ventricle entering the aorta through the duct Blood travels backwards around the aortic arch to perfuse the coronary arteries, head and neck vessels

Oxygenated blood passes through the foramen to mix with deoxygenated blood from the vena cavae

Stenotic or atretic aortic valve prevents blood passing through the left ventricle to enter the aorta

Fig. 8.12: Duct dependent systemic circulation

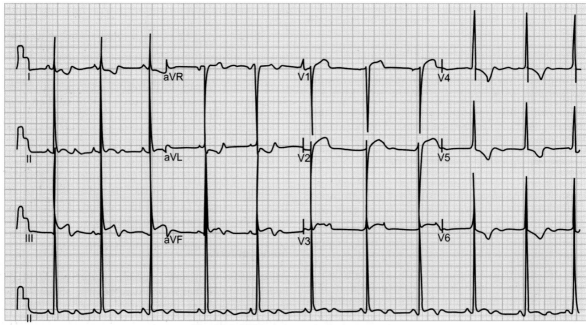

Fig. 8.13: ECG – left ventricular hypertrophy

Pulmonary Stenosis

As with aortic stenosis, pulmonary stenosis most commonly occurs at the valve itself but can be seen below the valve (e.g. Tetralogy of Fallot), above the valve or in the pulmonary branches. Valve stenosis results from fusion or dysplasia of the valve cusps and in isolation is a relatively common abnormality.

Mild pulmonary valve stenosis presents with an asymptomatic ejection systolic murmur and click. The murmur tends to be heard more to the left than with aortic stenosis, may radiate to the back and is not usually associated with a suprasternal thrill. The second heart sound is often quiet and a heave will only be present in the more severe lesions. Mild or even moderately severe pulmonary stenosis can improve in childhood, thus a

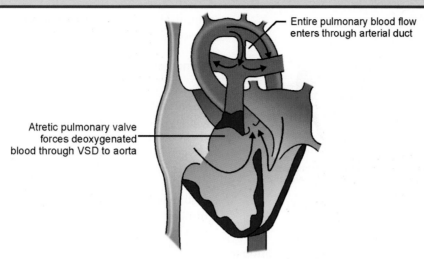

Entire pulmonary blood flow enters through arterial duct

Atretic pulmonary valve forces deoxygenated blood through VSD to aorta

Fig. 8.14: Duct dependent pulmonary circulation

"wait and see" approach is often appropriate at presentation.

Severe pulmonary stenosis will present in the newborn, lesion, as a duct dependent lesion. Whereas in aortic stenosis the arterial duct allows the systemic circulation to be augmented by the pulmonary side, in pulmonary stenosis the converse is true and pulmonary blood flow is derived largely from the aorta (Fig. 8.14). Prior to the duct closure the infants will be cyanosed (because of a right to left shunt at atrial level), have a characteristic systolic murmur and click but be otherwise well. Duct closure will herald hypoxia, acidosis and an abrupt deterioration in the child.

The ECG will demonstrate right axis deviation and right ventricular hypertrophy. In more severe cases P pulmonale and partial right bundle branch block will be present. Chest X ray may show post stenotic dilation of the pulmonary artery as a bulge around the left hilum together with oligaemic lung fields. As with aortic stenosis echocardiography will confirm the diagnosis and estimate severity using Doppler.

Management

Antibiotic prophylaxis is only required for both severe stenosis, although this policy is subject to ongoing argument. Transcatheter balloon valvuloplasty is now the treatment of choice for this lesion, producing good results with a very low requirement for re-intervention. The exception to this is in Noonan's syndrome where the pulmonary valve is often severely thickened and classically unresponsive to valvuloplasty. In such cases open surgical valvotomy is still indicated.

CYANOTIC CONGENITAL HEART DISEASE

Tetralogy of Fallot

Tetralogy is the commonest form of cyanotic congenital heart disease comprising 10% of all lesions. It is associated with Downs's syndrome, deletions of chromosome 22 (DiGeorge syndrome), and VACTERL (vertebral defects, anal atresia, tracheo-oesophageal atresia, sacral aplasia, renal and limb abnormalities) although it usually occurs in isolation. Classically it was described as the tetrad of VSD, right ventricular outflow tract obstruction, aorta overriding the crest of the ventricular septum and right ventricular hypertrophy. In effect only two of these factors are important in the pathogenesis; a VSD large enough to be completely unrestrictive and significant obstruction to pulmonary blood flow (Fig. 8.15).

Presentation depends on the degree of obstruction to pulmonary blood flow. The level of obstruction varies but usually comprises a degree of muscular sub valve (infundibular) obstruction together with either valve or supravalve stenosis. Because the VSD is large and does not restrict flow, if there is mild to moderate pulmonary obstruction there will be no net flow through the VSD and the child will be in a balanced state, sometimes called a "Pink Tetralogy". With more severe obstruction deoxygenated blood will flow right to left across the defect resulting in cyanosis. The obstruction tends to progress as the infundibular muscle hypertrophy increases culminating in a behaviour known as "spelling". During a hypercyanotic spell without warning the cyanosis becomes acutely worse. This may occur when the child has just been fed, is falling asleep, waking up or when upset. It is likely a reduction in the systemic vascular resistance causes an increase in right to left shunt. This leaves the right ventricle underfilled permitting increased systolic contraction and consequent worsening of the muscular subpulmonary stenosis. The cycle is self-perpetuating and may result in hypoxic syncope and convulsions. Children with this problem often develop a behaviour known as squatting, during which they crouch down; effectively increasing the systemic vascular resistance as well as increasing venous return.

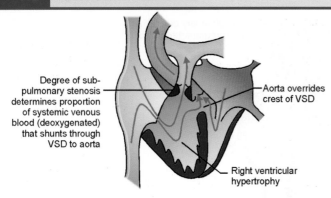

Degree of sub-pulmonary stenosis determines proportion of systemic venous blood (deoxygenated) that shunts through VSD to aorta

Aorta overrides crest of VSD

Right ventricular hypertrophy

Fig. 8.15: Tetralogy of Fallot – diagram

On examination infants with Tetralogy have a characteristic ejection systolic murmur of pulmonary stenosis radiating through to the back with no ejection click and a right ventricular heave is invariably present. The degree of cyanosis varies in newborns, but tends to worsen as the child grows and if prolonged cyanosis will result in clubbing of the digits and the plethoric facies of polycythaemia. The child's growth may be affected, although in isolated tetralogy is often normal. ECG demonstrates right axis deviation and right ventricular hypertrophy. Chest X ray typically shows a "boot-shaped" heart with upturned apex and oligaemic lung fields (Fig. 8.16). The diagnosis together with the level and severity of the pulmonary obstruction can be determined by transthoracic echo, which can help to exclude associated anomalies such as AVSD and right aortic arch.

Untreated Tetralogy has a poor prognosis. Progressive sub-pulmonary obstruction results in increasing cyanosis, poor exercise tolerance, increasingly frequent hyper-cyanotic spells and syncope. The obligatory right to left

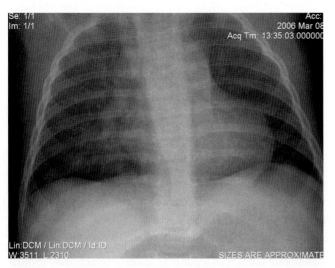

Se: 1/1
Im: 1/1
Acc:
2006 Mar 08
Acq Tm: 13:35:03.000000

Lin:DCM / Lin:DCM / Id:ID
W:3511 L:2310
SIZES ARE APPROXIMATE

Fig. 8.16: Chest x-ray, Tetralogy of Fallot showing a "boot shaped" heart with upturned apex and oligaemic lung fields

shunt also causes an increased susceptibility to brain abscesses.

Management

When a child presents with a hypercyanotic spell it is important not to panic in front of the mother or child. Calmly tuck the child's knees up to their chest and place them on the parents' chest in the tucked position. Waft oxygen into the child's face but try not to upset them. If this is ineffective then venous access must be obtained and the child given volume (10 mls/kg), morphine (100 microgram/kg) and propanolol (10 microgram/kg) intravenously.

Children with Tetralogy can either be surgically palliated or repaired. Palliation involves placing a modified Blalock Taussig shunt between the subclavian artery and the pulmonary artery, usually on the right side. This allows blood to flow into the pulmonary circulation irrespective of any intracardiac obstruction. The age at which full repair is undertaken varies but is usually between 6 to 12 months. Full repair requires closure of the VSD, resection of the subpulmonary muscle and enlarge-ment of the pulmonary valve orifice. Where the pulmonary valve annulus is small a patch is required to enlarge it, unfortunately rendering it regurgitant and introducing the possibility that a pulmonary valve replacement will be required later in life. Although the repair can be complex and requires full cardiopulmonary bypass it now carries an operative mortality of less than 5% in most centres.

Transposition of the Great Arteries (TGA)

Although overall less frequent than tetralogy, in neonates with cyanosis TGA is the most common underlying cause. It is more common in male infants, and is not usually associated with any non-cardiac abnormality.

In TGA the pulmonary artery is connected to the left ventricle and the aorta to the right. Consequently deoxygenated blood circulates around the systemic circulation and oxygenated blood around the pulmonary circulation with mixing between the two circulations occurring through the foramen ovale and the arterial duct (Fig. 8.17). Following birth mixing continues and the child is usually well but cyanotic. Aside from cyanosis typically cardiovascular examination will be normal although the second heart sound may be loud and a systolic murmur present from the duct. When the duct shuts, mixing is only possible through the persistent foramen ovale (PFO). This is usually inadequate and the child becomes hypoxic and acidotic. They are unlikely to survive without urgent medical intervention. An exception to this is where a significant VSD is also present. The VSD may permit more than adequate mixing to the extent that the child may have

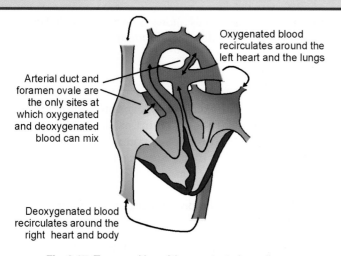

Oxygenated blood recirculates around the left heart and the lungs

Arterial duct and foramen ovale are the only sites at which oxygenated and deoxygenated blood can mix

Deoxygenated blood recirculates around the right heart and body

Fig. 8.17: Transposition of the great arteries – diagram

oxygen saturations in the low 90's even after the duct has shut. The natural history of TGA/VSD differs from that of uncomplicated TGA. Untreated the children may develop heart failure as the pulmonary vascular resistance drops but will not die of hypoxia and so are unlikely to die in the newborn period.

Chest X ray demonstrates a typical egg-on-side appearance with a narrow mediastinum and usually increased pulmonary vascularity although oligaemia can be present (Fig. 8.18). ECG shows right axis deviation and right ventricular hypertrophy. Echocardiogram confirms the diagnosis in addition to showing patency of the arterial duct, adequacy of the foramen ovale, coronary artery positions and also any defects in the ventricular septum.

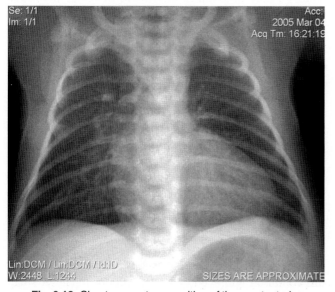

Fig. 8.18: Chest x-ray – transposition of the great arteries

Management

If the infant is unwell it is likely the arterial duct is narrow or closed. An infusion of prostaglandin E should be started urgently at a dose of 50 – 100 nanogram/kg/min, accepting that the child may become apnoeic and require intubation. If the child improves at this dose it can be reduced to 5 – 10 nanogram/g/min facilitating extubation. In addition to prostaglandin E most infants will require augmentation of the foramen ovale by balloon atrial septostomy. This can either be performed through the umbilical vein or the femoral vein. A specialised balloon septostomy catheter is introduced into the right atrium and manipulated across into left atrium using echo guidance. Once in position the balloon is inflated with up to 4 ml of normal saline and jerked back across the septum using a sharp but controlled tug. The "jump" as the septum tears is usually palpable. Although the pullback may be repeated several times in practice I rarely pull the balloon back more than once.

Surgical repair of transposition usually takes place at 1–2 weeks of life. This allows the infant to gain a little maturity, but does not permit the left ventricle to "detrain" by pumping to the low resistance pulmonary circulation for too long. The vast majority of infants with TGA now undergo an arterial switch procedure. This affords a complete anatomical repair by detaching the aorta, coronary arteries and pulmonary artery above the valve, and reanastomosing them to the anatomically appropriate ventricles. Where the coronary artery positions are favourable this produces an excellent repair with a risk of <5% in most Western centres.

Although deeply cyanosed most children will survive into infancy without an arterial switch providing an adequate septostomy has been performed.

Tricuspid Atresia

This rare form of cyanotic congenital heart disease comprises less than 2% of all infants with a cardiac anomaly. Absence of normal RV filling in utero, results in poor development of the right ventricle and pulmonary valve to develop normally. Systemic venous return passes through the foramen ovale to mix with the pulmonary venous return before entering the left ventricle. The mixed blood then passes through the aortic valve to the systemic circulation where a proportion will pass to the pulmonary artery via the arterial duct (Fig. 8.19). A VSD is usually present permitting anterograde flow through the right ventricle to the pulmonary artery. In 30% the great arteries are transposed and the aorta arises from the hypoplastic right ventricle. Some children, including all without a VSD, have significant obstruction to pulmonary blood flow and are duct-dependent. Others have adequate flow at birth however with growth obstruction may develop rapidly either at VSD level or in the subpulmonary area such that

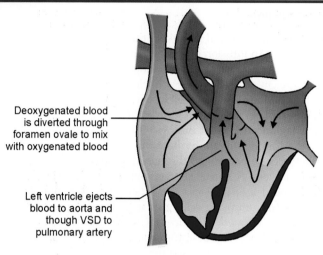

Deoxygenated blood is diverted through foramen ovale to mix with oxygenated blood

Left ventricle ejects blood to aorta and though VSD to pulmonary artery

Fig. 8.19: Tricuspid atresia – diagram

cyanosis becomes a major problem. A small number never develop obstruction and progress to heart failure when the PVR drops.

Usually cyanosis is obvious from birth and deepens with time. Such infants may fail to thrive, develop finger clubbing and untreated are unlikely to survive more than 12 months. A systolic murmur at the mid left sternal edge may be present from the VSD or sub-pulmonary obstruction and the second heart sound will be single. Electrocardiography shows left axis deviation, which in a cyanotic child is virtually diagnostic of tricuspid atresia (Fig. 8.20). Chest X ray typically shows a "box" like cardiac silhouette with pulmonary oligaemia. Echo will confirm the diagnosis and show with great detail the VSD and

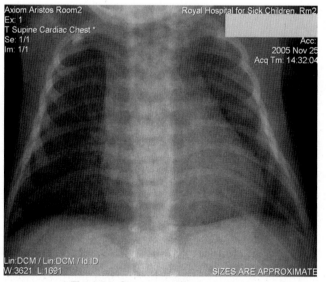

Fig. 8.20: Chest x-ray tricuspid atresia

sub-pulmonary area. This allows a tentative prediction to be made regarding the development of obstruction to pulmonary flow.

Management

Early palliation in excessively cyanotic infants is by modified Blalock Taussig shunt as described under tetralogy of Fallot. Further palliation follows the Fontan-type pattern and will be summarised later in the univentricular heart section.

Total Anomalous Pulmonary Venous Drainage (TAPVD or TAPVC)

This rare, cyanotic abnormality accounts for less than 1% of all congenital heart disease, however with recognition and early surgical repair it is curable. Although there are three main forms, each with their own peculiarities, all share a common pathophysiology. In fetal life the pulmonary venous confluence fails to fuse with the left atrium. The pulmonary veins drain to the heart, through either an ascending vein to the superior vena cava, a descending vein to the inferior cava or directly to the coronary sinus and right atrium (Fig. 8.21). As both pulmonary and systemic venous return enters the right atrium these children are dependent on adequacy of the foramen ovale for the entire systemic cardiac output. Obstruction at this level or any other impairs venous return causing a rise in pulmonary venous pressure with accompanying pulmonary hypertension and pulmonary oedema. Obstruction can be present in the first few days as the pulmonary vascular resistance drops but in other children may take many months to develop. If venous return is unobstructed these infants have mild cyanosis, are slow to grow but often have no other physical signs. As obstruction develops cyanosis deepens and the child becomes acidotic causing tachypnoea and tachycardia. The infant will have hepatomegaly, a gallop rhythm and a right ventricular heave.

ECG demonstrates right axis deviation, right ventricular hypertrophy and P pulmonale. Chest X ray shows pulmonary venous congestion and in chronic supra-cardiac TAPVD the widened superior mediastinum gives the mediastinal silhouette a "figure of eight" appearance. Echo is usually diagnostic, will clarify the type of drainage and show any area of obstruction.

Management

There is no effective medical therapy and all children with this condition will eventually die without repair. A small

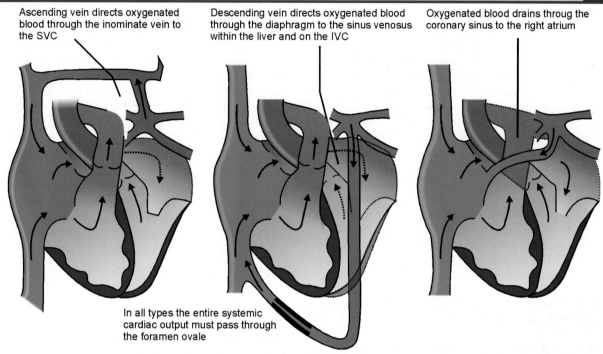

Ascending vein directs oxygenated blood through the inominate vein to the SVC

Descending vein directs oxygenated blood through the diaphragm to the sinus venosus within the liver and on the IVC

Oxygenated blood drains throug the coronary sinus to the right atrium

In all types the entire systemic cardiac output must pass through the foramen ovale

Fig. 8.21: Total anomalous pulmonary venous drainage – diagram

percentage of children will go on to develop pulmonary vein obstruction even after successful early repair.

Pulmonary Atresia (PAt)

Pulmonary atresia is a widely varying condition, however all infants are cyanosed and most are duct-dependent.

There are three main groups; PAt/Intact ventricular septum, PAt/Ventricular septal defect and confluent pulmonary arteries, PAt/Ventricular septal defect and major aortopulmonary collateral arteries (MAPCAs) (Fig. 8. 22).

All children are cyanosed at birth. The second heart sound will be single but there may be no murmurs unless

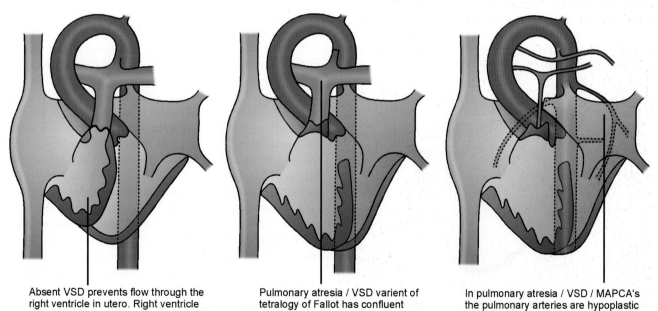

Absent VSD prevents flow through the right ventricle in utero. Right ventricle becomes hypoplastic often with coronary arteries draining into it through sinusoids.

Pulmonary atresia / VSD varient of tetralogy of Fallot has confluent pulmonary arteries of good size

In pulmonary atresia / VSD / MAPCA's the pulmonary arteries are hypoplastic and often not confluent. Pulmonary blood flow is derived from collaterals arising from the aorta (MAPCA's)

Fig. 8.22: Pulmonary atresia – variants diagram

MAPCAs are present in which case continuous murmurs are often heard throughout the chest.

Where no VSD is present the absence of flow through the right ventricle in utero results in a hypoplastic right ventricle. Most children with this condition require a modified Blalock Taussig shunt in the neonatal period followed by a Fontan type repair when older (discussed later). Where a VSD is present and the pulmonary arteries are confluent the child will still need initial palliation with a modified Blalock Taussig shunt however at a later stage the VSD can be closed and a tube interposed between the right ventricle and the pulmonary arteries. Both of these types of PAt are duct-dependent requiring prostaglandin E infusion to maintain ductal patency without which infants will die upon duct closure. Prognostically the worst anatomy is pulmonary atresia with MAPCAs. In these children MAPCAs arise directly from the aorta and supply individual segments of lung often with little communication between them or with any rudimentary main pulmonary artery. Extensive surgery is often required to create a pulmonary artery big enough to get a graft (Blalock Taussig or RV – PA conduit) onto and even then further surgery is usually required to further increase pulmonary blood flow prior to VSD closure.

Ebsteins Anomaly

In this rare abnormality the tricuspid valve arises in part from the right ventricular wall. In effect part of the right ventricle functions as an atrium, the right ventricular cavity is significantly reduced; the tricuspid valve is abnormal often with significant regurgitation and the right ventricular outflow tract maybe obstructed (Fig. 8.23). In severe cases the abnormality causes huge enlargement of the right atrium in utero such that the sheer size of the heart impedes lung development and the child dies in the newborn period. In less severe cases blood struggles to

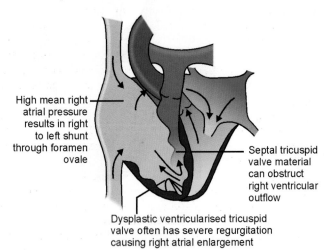

High mean right atrial pressure results in right to left shunt through foramen ovale

Septal tricuspid valve material can obstruct right ventricular outflow

Dysplastic ventricularised tricuspid valve often has severe regurgitation causing right atrial enlargement

Fig. 8.23: Ebsteins anomaly – diagram

enter the pulmonary artery and tends to shunt right to left across the atrial septum causing cyanosis and poor exercise ability. Mild cases are virtually asymptomatic and present late in life with either right heart failure or arrhythmias.

Clinically there is variable cyanosis and the neck veins may be distended and demonstrate prominent V waves because of the tricuspid regurgitation. A systolic murmur and sometimes a late diastolic murmur are heard at the lower left sternal edge often with a gallop rhythm. The ECG shows notched P waves signifying right atrial enlargement, right bundle branch block (Fig. 8.24), and may reveal the short PR interval and delta wave of associated pre-excitation (Wolf Parkinson White syndrome). Chest X ray often shows a much increased cardiothoracic ratio composed primarily of right atrial enlargement in addition to oligaemic lung fields. Echo will again confirm the diagnosis and help assess the degree of tricuspid regurgitation and atrial shunting.

Management

Medical treatment is useful only for arrhythmia management. Surgical intervention is difficult and controversial with a significant risk. The exact procedure must be tailored to the individual case and will be determined mainly by the adequacy of the right ventricle.

Hypoplastic Left Heart Syndrome (HLHS) and Other Forms of Univentricular Heart

HLHS is the broad term given to describe inadequacy of the left ventricular size in combination with stenosis or atresia of the mitral and aortic valves and hypoplasia of the aortic arch. Coarctation is a common association. As with aortic stenosis, the systemic circulation is dependent on flow through the arterial duct, thus duct constriction causes a low cardiac state with severe acidosis and hypoxia. Such children require resuscitation and prompt administration of prostaglandin E as described previously. Despite these measures, infants with HLHS cannot survive without radical surgical palliation in the form of a Norwood procedure. Briefly, this operation bypasses the left heart by removing the atrial septum, detaching the pulmonary artery from above the valve and connecting it to the systemic circulation using a shunt. The pulmonary artery is then connected to the side of the ascending aorta and the aortic arch enlarged using a patch such that blood entering the right ventricle is pumped to the systemic circulation through the pulmonary artery to aortic anastomosis (Fig. 8.25).

Such surgery carries a significant risk even in the best centres and is only the first of three operations that will be needed. It is not therefore surprising that after appropriate

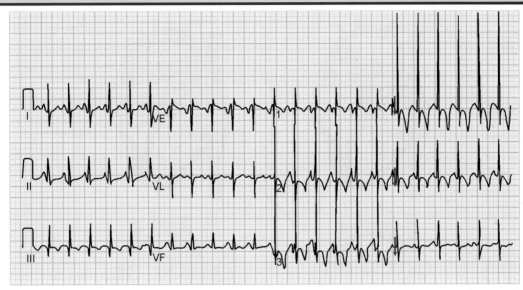

Fig. 8.24: ECG Ebsteins anomaly

counselling many families elect not to proceed to surgical palliation but to allow the child to die.

Other forms of heart disease where only a single functioning ventricle exists do not require such radical early palliation. The key to presentation and early management is pulmonary blood flow. If this is obstructed the child will usually have a duct-dependent circulation, present early with cyanosis and require a modified Blalock Taussig shunt to increase effective flow to the pulmonary artery. Alternatively if there is no obstruction to pulmonary blood flow, the child will present with tachypnoea and failure to thrive as the pulmonary vascular resistance drops and flow increases. Such children often benefit from having a restrictive band placed around the pulmonary artery to limit flow.

Long-term palliation for all single ventricle circulations requires to volume load to be removed from the heart. This involves diverting the systemic venous drainage around the heart and allowing it to drain directly to the pulmonary artery. This circuit is usually achieved in 2 parts. At the first procedure the superior vena cava is disconnected from the right atrium and reconnected directly to the pulmonary artery, reducing the volume load on the heart but leaving the child still cyanosed. At a second and final procedure the inferior vena caval flow is redirected to the lungs, usually by means of an extra-cardiac conduit, thus all deoxygenated blood is now oxygenated as it passes through the lungs before finally draining to the heart (Fig. 8.25).

The long- term prognosis of children with univentricular forms of heart disease is constantly improving as the techniques for repair continue to improve. Currently life expectancy without a cardiac transplant is in the third decade, and quality of life reasonable accepting reduced physical capacity. Clearly given the resources required to palliate children with univentricular circulations for what appears to be a relatively short period of time, harsh decisions must be made regarding appropriateness of treatment.

Vascular Ring

Numerous abnormalities of great artery development can occur, most of which are rare and many insignificant. The commonest is a right sided aortic arch which although more common in Di George syndrome has no pathological significance in isolation. Similarly aberrant right subclavian artery from the descending aorta is common but rarely causes problems. A small number of abnormalities can however constitute a ring around the trachea and oesophagus, and so cause airway obstruction with stridor and/or swallowing difficulties. A double aortic arch constitutes just such an abnormality where the trachea and oesophagus are caught in a ring between the two arches. It should be noted that only one of the arches might have flow throughout its course. Another type of ring is that formed by a right aortic arch, duct or ductal ligament from left subclavian artery and the pulmonary artery, which similarly encloses the trachea and oesophagus (Fig. 8.26).

These types of abnormalities are best diagnosed by barium swallow where the pattern of indentation seen on the posterior aspect of the oesophagus indicates the type of ring (Fig. 8.27). Further evidence can be obtained from bronchoscopy, CT or MRI scans. Echocardiography is less reliable in these situations as at least part of the anatomical substrate often has no lumen or flow.

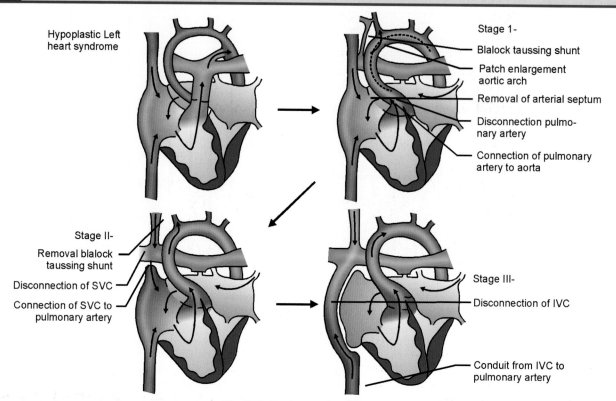

Hypoplastic Left
heart syndrome

Stage 1-
Blalock taussing shunt
Patch enlargement
aortic arch
Removal of arterial septum
Disconnection pulmo-
nary artery
Connection of pulmonary
artery to aorta

Stage II-
Removal blalock
taussing shunt
Disconnection of SVC
Connection of SVC to
pulmonary artery

Stage III-
Disconnection of IVC

Conduit from IVC to
pulmonary artery

Fig. 8.25: Fontan repair - diagram

Oesophagus
Trachea

Ring formed by
left subclavin artery
Arterial duct
Right aortic arch
Pulmonary artery

Fig. 8.26: Vascular ring – diagram

Treatment is surgical and usually requires simple division of the ligamentous portion of the ring.

ACQUIRED HEART DISEASE

Rheumatic Heart Disease

Outside North America and Europe rheumatic fever is the commonest cause of acquired heart disease in childhood. In the acute phase, rheumatic fever is a systemic disorder that causes cardiac morbidity and mortality from acute valve dysfunction and myocardial involvement. Evolution of the valve abnormality to its more chronic form can lead to problems both in late childhood and adult life.

The pathology seen in the heart results from an immune reaction triggered in certain individuals by exposure to Lancefield-A Streptococci, usually acquired through an upper respiratory tract infection. Not all group A Streptococci cause rheumatic fever; conflicting evidence suggests that those belonging to certain M serotypes may be responsible however this is probably an over-simplification. There also seems to be a familial tendency to develop the disease and the expression of certain HLA groups on a hosts B cells may make them more susceptible to rheumatic fever.

Antibodies produced in response to a streptococcal throat infection in a susceptible host react to both the streptococcal M protein and the myosin and laminin filaments within the hosts' heart. It is the reaction to host myosin that causes the myocarditis and laminin the endocarditis and valve dysfunction that is characteristic of acute rheumatic heart disease.

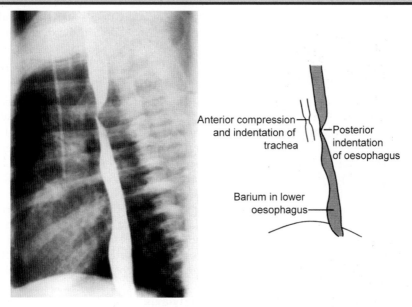

Fig. 8.27: Vascular ring due to double aorta (lateral view barium swallow)

Peak incidence occurs between 10 and 14 years but rheumatic fever can be seen in children as young as 3 years and adults as old as 30 years, although it is under 5 years that carditis is most marked.

Acutely the carditis always involves the endocardium, usually the myocardium and occasionally the pericardium. Late sequelae are most commonly related to mitral or aortic valve damage.

Typically the first signs of carditis are a tachycardia and a new murmur. Although the most common murmur seen in acute rheumatic fever is the apical systolic murmur of mitral regurgitation, systolic murmurs are very common in children particularly when a tachycardia is present so the appearance of a soft diastolic murmur at the apex is much more suggestive of early carditis. These findings in a child with other manifestations of rheumatic fever should prompt urgent further investigation as unrecognised or untreated carditis can result in arrhythmias and heart failure.

Electrocardiography confirms a sinus tachycardia and often shows lengthening of the PR interval, a characteristic finding in acute rheumatic fever. Echocardiography may show early valve dysfunction, usually regurgitation of the left heart valves, reduced ventricular function or a pericardial effusion. Serology will show evidence of Streptococcal infection with a raised antistreptolysin O (ASO) titre greater than 200U/ml and often much higher. DNase B is a more sensitive indicator of streptococcal infection but will not start to rise for 1 – 2 weeks. Other non-specific indicators of a systemic inflammatory process will also be raised including C-reactive protein (CRP) and erythrocyte sedimentation rate (ESR).

Management

Management has four distinct aims:

1. The infection that triggered the inflammatory response must be eradicated to remove the immune stimulus. High dose intravenous or intramuscular benzyl penicillin should be given for three days followed by high dose oral treatment for a further 10 days. Dose will be dependent on weight.

2. The acute inflammatory response must be suppressed. Bed rest and high dose aspirin are the mainstays of treatment. Some centres advocate the use of corticosteroids although there is limited evidence for their use. Acute inflammation can be monitored by measuring the ESR on a daily basis. When this has normalised bed rest can be stopped and moderate exercise positively encouraged. Similarly high dose aspirin (100mg/Kg/day in four doses) is usually given until at least 2 weeks after the ESR has returned to normal to prevent any rebound inflammation. Whilst using high dose aspirin it is sensible to measure serum levels to avoid overdose, maintaining a level of 2mmol/l (24-30mg/100ml).

3. Further Streptococcal infections must be prevented. This is adequately achieved using moderate dose oral phenoxymethylpenicillin (250mg BD) and encouraging compliance. Where compliance is questionable an alternative would be intramuscular benzathine penicillin. Currently it is recommended that prophylaxis be continued throughout childhood and adolescence up to 21 years of age.

4. Treatment of co-existing cardiac dysfunction is largely supportive with diuretics, digoxin and ACEi. It is best

to avoid surgical intervention in the acute phase, although occasionally this is required. Ultimately chronic valve dysfunction will often require repair or replacement.

Infective Endocarditis (IE)

Whenever bacteria enter the blood stream of a child with a structural heart abnormality there is a possibility-localised infection may occur around the site of the lesion. Structural heart lesions cause areas of turbulence and stagnant flow where bacteria can dwell and attach/infect the area concerned. This may be at the site of the lesion such as in the case of a regurgitant mitral valve or where the resultant jet hits the myocardium such as where a VSD jet strikes the opposing right ventricular wall. Bacteria can enter the circulation from a variety of sources although poor dental hygiene and dental procedures are perhaps the commonest cause, during which Streptococcus viridans may enter the blood. Staphylococcus aureas is another common causative organism, usually entering through skin lesions (e.g. infected eczema) or during tattoos or piercings. When bacteria infect the endocardium they can form vegetations (small lumps attached to the endocardium by flexible stalks) or they can invade the myocardium causing abscess formation.

IE should be suspected in any child with a known structural heart abnormality and an unexplained febrile illness. Classically IE has been described as sub acute bacterial endocarditis (SBE). This name derives from the pre-antibiotic era where the disease often went un-diagnosed for many weeks and the child demonstrated signs of chronic infection such as finger clubbing, painful embolic nodes in the finger tips (Oslers nodes), micro-emboli in the nail beds (splinter haemorrhages), embolic infarctions in the retina (Roth spots) and anaemia of chronic disease. These findings are now rarely seen, and more commonly the child will present with a fever, tachycardia, changing or new murmur, splenomegaly, possibly splinter haemorrhages and haematuria.

Investigation

The most important management step in any child with suspected IE is avoidance of antibiotics before blood cultures are taken. At least 3 and preferably 6 sets should be obtained from different venepuncture sites. The microbiologist must be made aware of the suspected diagnosis, as occasionally causative organisms can be very difficult or slow to grow in culture. Blood should also be taken for white cell count, haemoglobin, ESR and CRP. An ECG should be recorded as occasionally IE around the aortic valve can result in heart block and a transthoracic or even transoesophageal echo should be obtained. It must be emphasised that the absence of vegetations on echocardiography does not exclude endocarditis, however when seen they confirm the diagnosis.

Management

Appropriate intravenous broad-spectrum antibiotics can be given after blood cultures have been taken. The agents used can be modified once the target organism and its sensitivities have been identified. Usually parenteral therapy is continued for six weeks to ensure eradication of deep-seated infection as judged clinically and by inflammatory markers (CRP and ESR). Surgical excision of vegetations may be required where they pose a serious risk in case of embolism or they are affecting cardiac function. Severe valve dysfunction may also require surgical treatment acutely, however it is best to "sterilise" the area first using prolonged antibiotic therapy prior to attempting to repair or replace a damaged valve.

Prophylaxis

Antibiotic prophylaxis is generally recommended for any child with an "at risk" cardiac lesion undergoing an invasive dental or surgical procedure likely to cause a significant bacteraemia. All cardiac lesions producing a high velocity jet or turbulent flow are considered at risk of endocarditis. These include aortic stenosis, mitral regurgitation, VSD, and PDA. Antibiotic prophylaxis is not required for low velocity lesions such as ASD, mild pulmonary stenosis or 6 months following complete repair of lesions such as VSD or PDA.

Mucocutaneous Lymph Node Syndrome (Kawasaki syndrome)

Kawasaki syndrome is an idiopathic vasculitis that is often difficult to diagnose but is important because of potential coronary artery involvement. Key features of presentation are persistent fever, a miserable and irritable child, conjunctivitis, lymphadenopathy, swelling of the lips, tongue, hands and feet followed later by desquamation. Coronary artery inflammation results in aneurysm formation with intraluminal thrombus that may occlude the artery causing myocardial infarction. Early recognition of the disease together with prompt administration of immunoglobulin has reduced the incidence and severity of coronary artery involvement and its potentially fatal sequelae. If aneurysms are present long-term treatment with aspirin should be offered, as the risk of future coronary artery disease is raised.

Pericarditis

Inflammation of the pericardium with the accumulation of fluid around the heart may occur for a variety of reasons. Tuberculosis remains an important if less common cause than previously. Similarly, with the widespread use of antibiotics, bacterial pericarditis usually secondary to pneumonia is also now rare. Pericarditis resulting from viral infections, rheumatic fever, end stage renal failure, malignancy or systemic inflammatory disorders such as juvenile chronic arthritis now constitutes the bulk of cases.

Clues to the cause of the pericarditis will often be gained from the history. Most children will have some degree of chest pain that will vary in intensity with cause and degree of fluid accumulation (pain often eases as the volume of pericardial fluid increase or when the child leans forward). A fever is often present as is general malaise and lethargy. Symptoms attributable to pericardial fluid accumulation depend on both volume and rate of accumulation. A small amount of fluid entering the pericardium suddenly (e.g. an intravascular cannula perforating the right atrium) will be more disabling than a considerable volume accumulating over time (e.g. tuberculosis). In general as more fluid accumulates the child will become increasingly breathless with worsening exercise tolerance. The child will often be more comfortable sitting forward. The cardinal signs are a pericardial friction rub (a scratching sound varying as much with respiration as it does with the cardiac cycle), and muffled heart sounds. With significant pericardial fluid accumulation signs of tamponade will be present including raised jugular venous pulsation, pulsus paradoxus, tachycardia and hepatomegaly.

ECG will usually show sinus tachycardia, reduced voltage complexes and "saddle" shaped ST segment elevation. If the effusion is significant the heart may "swing" with respiration causing a variation in complex morphology with the respiratory cycle. Chest X ray may demonstrate a globular, enlarged cardiac silhouette (Fig. 8. 28) and the diagnosis is confirmed by echocardiogram (Fig. 8.29) which will also allow estimation of the size and whether it is impairing venous return (tamponade). Further investigations revolve around establishing the cause, ASO titre, viral titres, CRP and ESR should routinely be sent and a Mantoux test performed. Where pericardiocentesis is indicated examination of the fluid aspirated will usually confirm the diagnosis.

Management

In the absence of tamponade most cases of pericarditis will settle with appropriate treatment of the underlying cause and supportive therapy such as bed rest, oxygen and analgesia. Where tamponade is present the pericardial fluid should be aspirated and if necessary a drain left in situ.

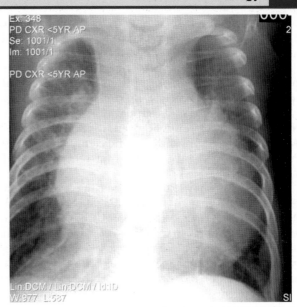

Fig. 8.28: Chest x-ray – showing pericardial effusion

Myocarditis

Myocarditis can be caused by viral infection or rarely as part of autoimmune systemic inflammatory disorder. Viral myocarditis results from infection by a wide variety of agents including enteroviruses (particularly Coxsackie B), adenovirus, hepatitis C and HIV. It is unclear why in the majority of children myocarditis is a mild, transient illness, whereas in others it can be rapidly fatal. The degree to which an individual is affected ranges considerably from asymptomatic ECG evidence of myocarditis during viral epidemics to fulminant cardiogenic shock a few days following a usually unremarkable viral illness. Just as viral myocarditis varies widely in its severity so do signs at presentation. Some children demonstrate only a minor tachycardia and summation gallop; whilst others are shut

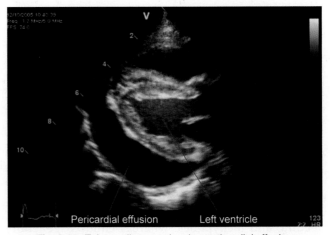

Fig. 8.29: Echocardiogram showing pericardial effusion

down peripherally (cold, grey and clammy), have low volume pulses, a marked parasternal heave and hepatomegaly.

Patients with myocarditis have a variable outcome. Those with only minor symptoms will usually fully recover, as surprisingly will those with fulminant myocarditis if they can be supported through the acute illness. Those children who present with moderate to severe impairment of ventricular function have the worst prognosis, with many having long-term ventricular dysfunction.

ECG usually shows low voltage complexes and may demonstrate ST changes, QT prolongation and possibly ectopic beats or sustained arrhythmias. Chest X ray usually demonstrates pulmonary plethora however the cardiac outline may or may not be enlarged (acutely, although ventricular function is poor the ventricle may not have had time to dilate). Blood serology for commonly responsible viral agents should be sent and a metabolic screen should be considered in younger children to exclude rare but treatable causes. The gold standard investigation to confirm the myocarditis is myocardial biopsy however many centres rely on a clinical diagnosis with or without serological confirmation of viral infection.

Management

All children with this disease need appropriate treatment for ventricular dysfunction. This will range from diuretics and angiotensin converting enzyme inhibitors for those with moderate symptoms, up to full intensive care with inotrope support and even mechanical assist devices (if available) for children with fulminant heart failure. Many specific treatments to address the myocarditic process itself have been tried including steroids, pooled immunoglobulin and other more aggressive forms of imunosupression. Currently there is no convincing evidence that any are of benefit.

Dilated Cardiomyopathy

Dilated cardiomyopathy is usually idiopathic although approximately 10% are the end result of viral myocarditis. Other causes are familial inheritance, previous anthracycline chaemotherapy, a metabolic derangement such as acyl-carnitine deficiency and others are part of a systemic myopathic process such as Duchenne muscular dystrophy. Whatever the underlying process the left ventricular function is impaired resulting in enlargement that in turn reduces function further. With increasing enlargement the mitral valve annulus dilates causing regurgitation, which further strains the failing left ventricle.

Infants typically present with failure to thrive, poor feeding and tachypnoea, whereas children generally complain of a gradual decline in exercise tolerance, often culminating in orthopnea and resting tachypnoea.

Examination will demonstrate the classical triad of tachypnoea, tachycardia and hepatomegaly. In addition there may be a marked heave, gallop rhythm and the apical systolic murmur of mitral regurgitation.

Diagnosis is confirmed on echo and further investigation revolves around finding a treatable cause. In most cases none is found and treatment is supportive and symptomatic. Children are usually started on diuretics and digoxin, with the addition of angiotensin converting enzyme inhibitors and beta-blockers such as carvedilol now being commonplace. Some form of anticoagulation is often required to prevent thrombus formation in the ventricular chamber.

It is unusual for there to be a significant improvement in function and most will deteriorate with time. Where possible a cardiac transplant may be the only long-term solution.

Hypertrophic Cardiomyopathy

Hypertrophic cardiomyopathy is usually inherited in an autosomal dominant manner although sporadic cases do occur. Thickening of the left ventricular wall may be concentric or predominantly within the septum (asymmetrical septal hypertrophy). These changes result in impaired filling of the left ventricle and where asymmetrical hypertrophy is present sub-aortic obstruction develops. Unfortunately all forms are at risk of ventricular arrhythmias and sudden death particularly on exercise.

Many children are asymptomatic at presentation and discovered during screening where another family member is affected or where a murmur has been detected and referred for investigation. Other children may present with exertional dyspnoea, chest pain, dizziness or syncope.

Diagnosis is by echocardiogram. Whilst the ECG may show changes of hypertrophy and strain, a normal test does not exclude the diagnosis. When a diagnosis has been made, screening should be offered to first-degree relatives.

If significant hypertrophy is present intense exercise should be avoided and Beta-blockers may be used for symptom control. Although many treatments including surgical resection of the muscle have been tried the only measure shown to be of benefit in these patients is an implantable defibrillator.

HEART RHYTHM ABNORMALITIES

Normal

Normal heart rate, like blood pressure, varies with age. A neonate should have a rate of 110 – 150 beats per minute (BPM), infants 85 – 125 bpm, 3 – 5 years 75 – 115 and over 6 years 60 – 100 bpm. The heart rate in infants may rise as high as 220 bpm when febrile. Sinus arrhythmia is common in children and can produce a marked drop in heart rate during expiration. Extra beats are also common in childhood. Atrial or junctional ectopic beats can be recognised as narrow complex and may have a preceding abnormal P wave. They are benign and require no further investigation. Ventricular ectopics are broad complex and also occur in healthy children however occasionally they can indicate underlying myocardial disease, electrolyte dysfunction or drug ingestion. When they can be shown to disappear on exercise they require no further investigation. Three types of rhythm abnormality deserve further attention; supraventricular tachycardia (SVT), ventricular tachycardia (VT) including torsades de pointes and complete heart block (CHB).

Supraventricular tachycardia (SVT)

SVT in childhood is a narrow complex tachycardia, with rates usually of between 200 and 300. There are many different underlying mechanisms but most fall into two groups.

1. Re-entry arrhythmias. These arrhythmias are by far the commonest and are caused by an electrical circuit developing either through the AV node (e.g. Wolf Parkinson White) or within the atria (e.g. atrial flutter)

(Fig. 8.30). The electrical impulse passes around the loop repeatedly sending off an action potential to atria and ventricles with each circuit. In most childhood SVT including Wolf Parkinson White syndrome it occurs through the AV node and an accessory pathway (extra piece of conduction tissue connecting the atria to ventricles). These arrhythmias tend to be paroxysmal in nature and usually have rate of 200–250 bpm. In atrial flutter the circuit occurs within the atria often around the foramen ovale and the atrial rate is faster ranging from 400 bpm in the newborn to 300 bpm in adolescents (usually only alternate beats are conducted to the ventricles).

2. Automatic Tachycardias. These arrhythmias are also known as ectopic tachycardias. They arise from increased automaticity of a group of cells within the myocardium (Fig. 8. 30). Essentially this group of cells depolarises at a faster rate than the sinus node, thus taking over the role of pacemaker. If the rate of depolarisation exceeds normal for the child concerned it is designated a tachycardia. These forms of tachycardia tend to be incessant and have lower rates of 160–220 bpm.

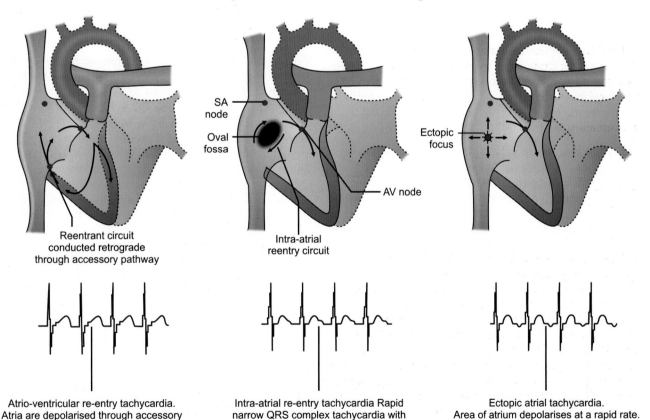

SA node

Oval fossa

AV node

Ectopic focus

Reentrant circuit conducted retrograde through accessory pathway

Intra-atrial reentry circuit

Atrio-ventricular re-entry tachycardia. Atria are depolarised through accessory pathway after ventricles, therefore P wave is buried in the ST segment

Intra-atrial re-entry tachycardia Rapid narrow QRS complex tachycardia with P wave visible in preceeding T wave

Ectopic atrial tachycardia. Area of atrium depolarises at a rapid rate. P wave has unusual morphology and short PR interval

Fig. 8.30: Supraventricular tachycardia—mechanism diagram

Presentation

Infants are unable to communicate symptoms of palpitation. Because of this, SVT lasting less than 24 hours may remain undiagnosed. When prolonged however, symptoms of heart failure (poor feeding, sweating, poor colour) develop, raising awareness of the problem. Incessant, automatic tachycardias tend to have slower rates and cause less haemodynamic compromise. They usually take longer to present and often do so with a form of dilated cardiomyopathy. In contrast to infants, older children will complain of odd feelings, thumping or fluttering within the chest after relatively short episodes. More rapid forms can be associated with chest pain, breathlessness and dizziness, particularly when prolonged.

Investigation

The paroxysmal nature of many tachycardias makes accurate diagnosis difficult. A baseline ECG may reveal the short PR interval and delta wave of Wolf Parkinson White (Fig. 8. 31), or may show a prolonged QT interval suggesting a ventricular tachycardia is responsible for the symptoms (next page). Ideally a 12 lead ECG should be recorded during the tachycardia that will provide the optimum information for an accurate diagnosis. With infrequent episodes obtaining a 12 lead ECG may prove impossible in which case ambulatory recordings can be obtained using one of the many systems now available. An echocardiogram is also normally performed to exclude structural heart disease.

Management

Acutely, re-entry forms of tachycardia may respond to vagal manoeuvres. In infants immersing the face in ice-cold water for 5 seconds may be tried. Older children can be taught to perform a Valsalva manoeuvre. If these measures fail, intravenous adenosine is a very effective alternative. Because it has a very short half-life in the circulation it should be injected through a large cannula in a proximal vein with a rapid bolus and flush. By convention a small dose is used initially (0.05 mg/kg) which is increased in steps to 0.25 mg/Kg (max 12mg)). If this fails it is likely the arrhythmia is automatic in nature. Acutely automatic tachycardias are harder to control and often require preloading with an anti-arrhythmic agent such as amiodarone prior to synchronized electrical cardioversion (0.5 – 1 J/Kg).

Chronically many children with infrequent short episodes of SVT require no treatment and adequate explanation is sufficient to reassure them and their parents. Where episodes are infrequent but of long duration, patients can be offered a "pill in pocket" form of treatment. This involves the child carrying a supply of verapamil or beta-blocker to take only when an attack starts. The medication is designed to terminate the attack rather than prevent it. Where episodes are frequent many families prefer preventative treatment, usually with digoxin, beta-blockers or verapamil. If the baseline ECG demonstrates Wolf Parkinson White, digoxin is considered contraindicated at most ages and should be avoided (can theoretically accelerate conduction through the accessory pathway allowing rapid ventricular depolarisation and raising the chance of ventricular tachycardia or fibrillation). If arrhythmias persist despite medical treatment, trans-catheter radiofrequency ablation of the accessory pathway can be offered to abolish the arrhythmia.

Ventricular Tachycardia/Fibrillation

Ventricular arrhythmias are very rare in childhood even after congenital heart surgery. The most common abnormality that predisposes to ventricular tachycardia is long QT syndrome. Long QT syndrome is a group of disorders characterised by a long QT interval when measured on the ECG and a predisposition to a particular type of ventricular tachycardia called torsades de pointes. Torsades de pointes can be triggered in one type of long QT syndrome by exercise, another type by stress (particularly loud noises) and in an unlucky few by sleep. On the ECG it appears as a polymorphic broad complex tachycardia with a rotating axis. Long QT interval is a group of disorders some of which are inherited in an autosomal dominant manner and others recessive. Subsequently when an affected individual is identified, family members should be screened by ECG.

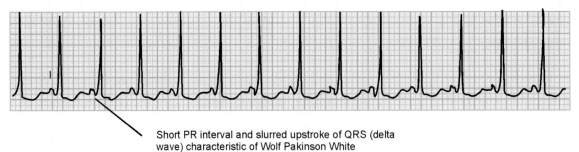

Short PR interval and slurred upstroke of QRS (delta wave) characteristic of Wolf Pakinson White

Fig. 8.31: ECG showing Wolff Parkinson White syndrome

The main risks in long QT syndrome are syncope and sudden death. Treatment is with beta-blockers or pacemakers, although in severely affected individuals an implantable defibrillator is indicated where available.

Complete Heart Block

In complete heart block the electrical activity of the atria is isolated from that of the ventricles. Therefore the atria beat at one rate whilst the ventricular rate (effective heart rate) is slower (Fig. 8. 32). This is a rare condition. The congenital form is usually seen in newborns when the mother has systemic lupus erythematosus with circulating anti-la and anti-Ro antibodies. These antibodies cross the placenta and damage the heart particularly targeting the conduction system. Occasionally congenital heart block can also be seen rare forms of congenital heart disease such as congenitally corrected transposition of the great arteries and in atrial isomerism. The commonest cause of acquired heart block is following heart surgery when the conduction system is damaged. Often this is a transient problem lasting no more than a few weeks however in some children it can persist requiring a pacemaker. Bacterial endocarditis particularly around the aortic valve can destroy the junctional tissue and also cause heart block.

In the congenital form if an infant's heart rate is greater than 55 bpm and there is no heart failure, no treatment is indicated and the outlook is reasonable. Where the heart rate is slower or heart failure co-exists then a pacemaker may be required. In acquired forms, where the block is permanent a pacemaker is always indicated.

CASE STUDIES

1. Infant VSD

A 4-week-old child presents with failure to complete feeds, poor weight gain and sweating. On examination a cachectic child is noted with a respiratory rate of 60, moderate sub costal in drawing, normal pulses, an enlarged liver, a marked sub-xyphoid heave and loud second heart sound. There is a 2/6 systolic murmur audible at the upper left sternal edge and radiating to the lower left sternal edge.

Name three possible diagnoses?
VSD, AVSD, Truncus arteriosus. Not PDA as murmur wrong, note loud PSM not a constant finding in large VSDs.

What investigations are required?
ECG, Echo.

What medical treatment measures would you take?
Introduce high calorie nasogastric feeds, start a loop diuretic such as frusemide together with spironolactone, refer for surgical correction before 6 months of age (risk of irreversible pulmonary hypertension thereafter).

2. Cyanosed newborn

A 3-day-old child is found to be cyanosed on pre-discharge check. The child is otherwise well, with no dyspnoea and only a mild tachycardia of 160bpm. On examination there are normal femoral pulses, no hepatomegaly, no heave, loud second heart sound and no murmurs.

Name three possible diagnoses?
Transposition of the great arteries, pulmonary atresia, tricuspid atresia. Not tetralogy as a significant murmur would be present if cyanosed and not atretic.

VSD

• A VSD murmur may not be heard at birth
• Loudness of the murmur does not correspond to the size of the defect
• Small VSD often need no treatment
• Large VSD are the commonest cause of heart failure in infants

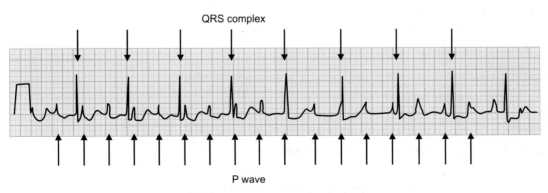

QRS complex

P wave

Fig. 8.32: ECG –Complete heart block

- Large VSD should be repaired before 6 months to protect pulmonary arterioles
- VSDs place an increased volume load on the left heart.

Heart Failure in Infants

- Nasogastric feeding removes work of feeding and maximises caloric intake
- Diuretics, digoxin and ACEi constitute medical treatment
- Aim to identify and treat cause
- Oxygen therapy may worsen heart failure

ASD

- ASD commonly have no symptoms
- Signs may be minimal in childhood
- ASD can cause fixed, wide splitting of the second heart sound
- ASD place an increased volume load on the right heart
- ASD do not require antibiotic prophylaxis

PDA

- PDA produce a continuous "machinery" murmur
- PDA is common in prematurity where they can cause heart failure
- Indomethacin can be used to close PDA in prematurity
- Most PDA in childhood can be closed by a transcatheter technique

AVSD

- Complete AVSD usually present as heart failure in infancy
- AVSD is common in Downs's syndrome
- AVSD cause left (superior) axis on the ECG
- The atrioventricular valves are often regurgitant
- Complete AVSD require repair within 6 months

Coarctation of the aorta

- Infants with coarctation present with heart failure at 3 – 10 days when the arterial duct closes
- Always examine the femoral pulses during routine clinical examination
- Older children with coarctation present with hypertension or a murmur at the back

Aortic Stenosis

- Clinical assessment of the severity of aortic stenosis can be difficult
- Aortic stenosis causes left ventricular hypertrophy
- Neonates with severe aortic stenosis depend on the arterial duct for the systemic circulation

- Older children with severe aortic stenosis are at risk of syncope and sudden death
- Aortic stenosis can be treated by balloon valvuloplasty or surgery

Pulmonary Stenosis

- Pulmonary stenosis causes right ventricular hypertrophy
- Neonates with severe pulmonary stenosis depend on the arterial duct for the pulmonary circulation
- Moderate pulmonary stenosis in infancy can improve with growth
- The treatment of choice for pulmonary stenosis is balloon valvuloplasty

Tetralogy of Fallot

- Suspect Tetralogy in any infant with a harsh systolic murmur and cyanosis
- The key lesions in tetralogy are the degree of sub-pulmonary stenosis and the VSD
- Cyanosis worsens with growth
- Hypercyanotic spells are a feature of severe sub-pulmonary obstruction
- A Blalock Taussig shunt can be used to palliate children with Tetralogy

Transposition of the great arteries

- Suspect transposition in an asymptomatic cyanosed neonate with no murmur
- Transposition is a "duct-dependent" lesion and should be treated with prostaglandin E
- Prostaglandin E can cause apnoea
- Most children with transposition require an atrial septostomy

Tricuspid atresia

- Suspect tricuspid atresia in any cyanotic infant with left axis deviation on the ECG
- Cyanosis is usually progressive, requiring early palliation
- Ultimately children with tricuspid atresia will require a Fontan-type repair

Pulmonary atresia

- Infants with pulmonary atresia are dependent on arterial duct flow
- Where the ventricular septum is intact the right ventricle is hypoplastic

- Management is often complicated requiring several procedures

Univentricular Heart

- All infants with a single functional ventricle require regulation of the pulmonary blood flow
- Ultimately a child with a single ventricle will require a Fontan-type repair
- A Fontan–type repair directs the systemic venous drainage directly to the pulmonary artery, bypassing the heart.
- In the long term single ventricles fail.

Rheumatic Fever

- With widespread use of antibiotics, the initial presentation of rheumatic fever can be atypical
- ASO and anti-Dnase will always rise
- Eradication of the streptococcus with penicillin is a crucial first step in management
- Following recovery long-term prophylaxis should be given to prevent further attacks

Infective Endocarditis

- Consider endocarditis in any child with a heart lesion and unexplained fever
- Avoid antibiotics until several sets of blood cultures have been taken
- Echocardiography cannot exclude the diagnosis
- Prolonged parenteral antibiotic therapy is mandatory

Kawasaki Disease

- Coronary artery involvement is common in Kawasaki disease if untreated
- Early immunoglobulin therapy prevents coronary aneurysm formation
- Aneurysm can give rise to coronary ischaemia and infarction both acutely and later in life

Pericarditis

- Consider pericarditis in a child with chest pain and a large heart on X ray

- A pericardial rub may be absent where significant fluid has accumulated
- Tamponade depends on how quickly fluid accumulates, not how much

Myocarditis

- Myocarditis is usually caused by a viral infection, most commonly Coxsackie B
- Although many children are only mildly affected, some develop fulminant myocardial failure
- Even in severe myocardial failure, a good recovery is possible
- Some children with moderate myocarditis will develop a dilated cardiomyopathy

Hypertrophic cardiomyopathy

- Most children have no symptoms when diagnosed
- Chest pain, dizziness or syncope on exercise are worrying symptoms
- Close family members should be screened
- Intense exercise should be avoided

SVT

- In SVT the heart rate is usually over 200 bpm and difficult to count on examination
- Infants with SVT may not present until myocardial function is affected by prolonged tachycardia
- Re-entry forms of SVT can be terminated by vagal manoeuvres and adenosine
- Automatic tachycardias can be resistant to treatment and cause cardiomyopathy
- Children with Wolf Parkinson White syndrome should not receive digoxin
- Most SVT carries a good prognosis

Heart Block

- Congenital heart block is associated with maternal anti Ro and La antibodies
- A pacemaker is indicated if the mean heart rate is less than 55 or there is heart failure

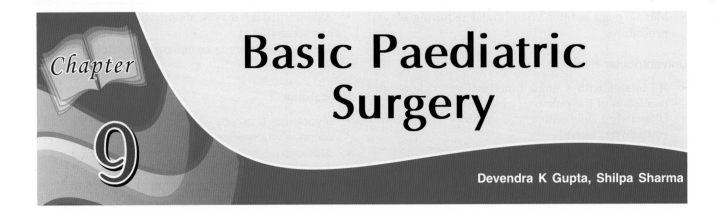

Basic Paediatric Surgery

Chapter 9

Devendra K Gupta, Shilpa Sharma

INTRODUCTION AND HISTORY TAKING OF PAEDIATRIC SURGICAL PATIENTS

Introduction

This chapter provides a bird's eye view about the paediatric diseases and about the bedside history taking skill in paediatric patients. Indiscriminate and injudicious prescription of drugs in paediatric age group results in adverse reactions and toxicity though drugs play pivotal role in protection and restoration of health. To get fruitful effect and to avoid toxicity it should be based on per kilogram body weight and the division of per day requirement may vary with drug used, which a paediatric medical practitioner should be aware.

A child manifesting with a disease may be having other occult problem involving other system of the body which all can be explained by a single cause called as the sequence for example Pierre Robin sequence is a condition in which there is cleft palate, micrognathia and glosso-ptosis. The presence of these entire three problems is due to a small size mandible, which causes the tongue to fall back and prevent closure of the two halves of secondary palate during the developmental period. If all the group of disorder cannot be explained by single etiology then it is called as syndrome. Some innocuous superficial mani-festation may really be representative of severe dreadful underlying disease in paediatric age group. For example, white-eye in an adult is due to senile cataract where as in a child it may be due to retinoblastoma.

It is a must for every medical practioner to know about paediatric surgical illness for timely detection, management and safe transportation and referral to higher centres for complicated illnesses needing tertiary level care. Either a surgeon or a physician caring for children should be aware of technique and art of basic life support and advanced life support. The aim of these text articles is to provide basic idea of paediatric surgical illnesses, their manifestation, and diagnosis and to emphasize on the pre-treatment emergency care and timely referral for saving life of future pillars of a country.

History Taking

Though there is tremendous advance in the field of medical science and technology during the last few decades but none of these advances can replace a proper history taking and bedside clinical examination. They lead the treating doctor to the illness concerned and reduce the gap between time of presentation and finalizing the diagnosis by streamlining the investigation and excluding the conditions having similar manifestation. It also avoids unnecessary investigation and helps the proper and economic usage of available manpower and health resources thus over all reducing the national health care cost without compromising the quality of care given. As a student it is mandatory to learn the art of methodical history taking and examination, which plays a pivotal role in further dealing with patients and improving the future career.

History taking should be methodical to prevent losing important history. After obtaining the history it should be recorded in the record sheet of the patients, which is important for others to understand and for our future review. Throughout the history taking the parents and child should be encouraged. The history is obtained and recorded in the following headings.

History of Present Illness

In this what problem made the parents to bring the child to hospital is obtained and recorded in non- medical terms in descending order of severity and chronological order. The relevant leading questions can be asked to parents to rule out the conditions having the same presentation. Enquiry should also be made to know the possible etiology and also to know how much the parents are aware of their kid's problem. From this detailed history itself we can come to conclusion about the possible system affected and the possible differential diagnosis.

History of Past Illness

By knowing about the past illness it may be possible to correlate the present problem if related one. Enquiry about any complications during the previous anaesthesia and surgery provides an opportunity to remain alert in the future. Any associated medical illness present should also be taken care during the surgical treatment.

Family History

Since certain illness run in families by enquiring about family members having similar illness we can arrive at diagnosis, the risk of other family members being affected with similar illness and need for screening asymptomatic cases can be ascertained. For example, a child presenting with bleeding per rectum with multiple colorectal polyps may be suffering from familial adenomatous polyposis.

Antenatal History

History of severe medical illness, febrile conditions, abortion, anti-teratogenic exposure in the form of radiation, drugs, etc. are enquired. Any problem to the mother like polyhydramnios (in congenital gut obstruction) oligo-hydramnios (in posterior urethral valve) gives suggestion about any congenital illness, antenatal ultrasonogram which is an integral part of antenatal screening detects fetal anomalies and helps to plan about, MTP, planning time and mode of delivery and early postnatal care for fruitful outcome.

Birth History

The time of delivery (term or preterm), place of delivery (hospital or home delivered) and mode of delivery (vaginal or cesarean) are to be enquired which all carry importance during management.

Developmental History

About the milestones achieved and mental age and chronological age are ascertained by examining the anthropometrical chart maintained by the paediatrician.

Immunization History

To know about the immunization status the vaccines administered with reference to national immunization schedule is enquired and entered in the case record.

Nutritional History

About the duration of breastfeeding, weaning administered, amount of food material consumption now are recorded.

Summary

By getting detailed history it may be possible to exclude many conditions mimicking each other, and avoid unnecessary investigation and in short reduce the medical care cost and reduce the time between presentation and onset of treatment.

CLINICAL EXAMINATION

Preparing the child for the physical examination helps reduce anxiety and minimizes trauma. It also enhances your ability to perform a comprehensive examination. Make an effort to increase the child/adolescent's sense of control and suggest relevant coping strategies. In addition, throughout the examination, reassure the child and encourage him by sweet words or morale. Assess the child level of fearfulness before the examination. This information will be helpful in determining appropriate preparation strategies.

Bedside manners, which have to be followed during history taking and examination

Before entering knock at the door of the suite in which patient is staying, always introduce yourself to parents and the child, have a smiling face and never stare at the child.

- Use simple language when communicating with the parents, pay attention to their words, and nod head for their response, maintain eye-to-eye contact.
- Wear light colour dress and some suggest even avoiding large white coat, which may panic the child.
- Be aware of fears specific to age or developmental level and be familiar with some management techniques.
- Attach toys to the stethoscope; the outpatient cubicle should be clean and free of large medical appliance, cast, specimen, etc. that may be annoying to the child.
- Examine in good natural lighted room, get the permission of the parents before examining the child, and warm your hands before touching the child in cold countries, best time to examine a child is when the baby is feeding or sleeping which should be made use of whenever feasible.
- Proper positioning is essential for painless examination and for detecting clinical signs, Examine always gently without jerky forceful manipulation.
- Examine in single attempt thoroughly keeping all the differential diagnosis in mind.
- Explain the examination in child-friendly language that uses developmentally appropriate words.
- Remember that children often interpret statements very literally.
- Provide toys, music, and pacifying speech during examination.
- Avoid the use of medical restraints or force of any kind during the examination. Allow children and

adolescents to choose whether they would like a parent or care giver present during the examination. Examine the painless area first, encourage the child during examination and build their self confidence during history taking and examination, never do painful procedure in front of other child, keep parents throughout the examination bedside, keep the mental agony of the family due to sick child in mind.

- It is unusual to use sedation or anaesthesia for the examination. The use of medication should be restricted to situations where suspected major injuries require assessment or surgical repair. If sedation or anaesthesia must be used, carefully explain the procedures to the child/adolescent and parent or care giver and obtain consent. Express empathy and give assurance to the parents, based on scientific evidence.

- The typical head to feet examination system may not be feasible in children and hence modification of the examination system may be needed in some uncoope-rative children. Examine the relevant things first and avoid causing pain during examination. Apart from examination of the major systems like respiratory system, cardiovascular system, central nervous system and abdomen, detailed examination about the nutri-tion and development by anthropometry is also needed.

PRE AND POSTOPERATIVE CARE

Preoperative assessment is an important evaluation that provides wide information about the child's disease status, family circumstances, making good rapport for future follow up. It also provides the child and parents to get accustomed to new surgical environment. Before the surgery, focused history with regards to previous surgical procedure, bleeding problems, anaesthetic complication and drug allergies gives valuable information for better care and planning for early discharge. The pre anaesthetic evaluation includes examination of major organ systems and emphasis on any recent illness like respiratory infection, which is important from anaesthetic point of view. This is evidenced by the observation that operating on a child with acute recent respiratory infection will increase the adverse events by seven folds during induction of anaesthesia and extubation.

Associated Medical Problems

In children undergoing surgical procedures there can be associated many medical illnesses, which need special consideration while undertaking surgery in those high-risk patients. Patients may be taking medications for the medical illness. There are some drugs, which have to be continued till the morning of the day of surgery for example steroids, thyroxin, antiepileptics etc. There are some drugs, which can interact with anesthetic agents and may need

to be changed to safer drugs or discontinued if there is no contraindication for stopping the drug. For example tricyclic antidepressants are ideally to be stopped at least two weeks before surgery and aspirin has to be stopped 6 weeks before. Apart from the medications there is also concern in preparing those patients for uneventful good outcome. In patients with congenital heart disease or valvular heart disease prophylactic antibiotics with ampicillin and gentamycin in general surgical procedure and added metronidazole for colorectal surgery is mandatory to prevent dreaded sub acute infective endocarditits. Patients with major organ disease are not candidates for out patient's surgery because it is to prevent an early intervention of postoperative calamities

There is also major issue about the preoperative routine laboratory investigations in pediatric age group. The American Society of Anesthesiologists stated that routine preoperative investigation is not needed in pediatric age group. Decisions regarding the need for routine preope-rative investigation should be based on the individual patients and the proposed surgical procedure. This avoids, mechanical trauma to the child by difficult venipuncture, unnecessary investigation causing manpower and economic loss.

Pre-anaesthetic Medication

Usage of certain medications before the induction and preceding to surgery makes anesthesia smooth and avoids anxiety and preoperative complications like aspiration pneumonitis. Anxiolytics like diazepam, midazolam, ranitidine, analgesics like fentanyl or pethidine and atropine to reduce secretions and prevent bradycardia is suggested in pre- anesthetic medications. However in an emergency situation the patient is resuscitated and taken for surgery.

Preoperative Antibiotics

The policy of administration of pre- induction antibiotics reduces the infection rate to almost nil and avoids unnecessary prolonged administration of antibiotics in clean surgery. In clean case only three doses of antibiotics are recommended. In cases with frank sepsis it is based on severity and culture and sensitivity. In special occasions a longer course of antibiotics may be needed for example in urological surgeries. Patients with cardiac problems and metallic implants (in joints and valves) need prophylactic antibiotics. In children there is no need for prophylactic administration of heparin to prevent deep vein thrombosis, as it is uncommon except in cases with congenital predisposition like protein S or protein C deficiency.

Transportation of Patients

In case of newborns proper maintenance of temperature and safe transport in transport incubator to operation suite is mandatory to prevent hypothermia and cardio-respiratory depression. In patients with central venous line or intra-arterial line continuous flushing with heparinised saline is essential to prevent blockage of line. In very sick patients continuous monitoring with pulse oxymeter, uninterrupted respiratory support with battery back up, emergency resuscitation drugs should accompany.

Securing Intravenous Access

Safe secure intravenous line is essential component in the surgical management of patients. It is mandatory to learn the technique of safe insertion and safeguarding the line by proper immobilization with splints and dressings because finding and getting intravenous access may be difficult. Difficult cases may need open venesection or central venous access. Local anaesthetic EMLA cream may be applied half to one hour before the intravenous access for painless insertion of intravenous line. In very uncooperative patients inhalation induction done with halothane or sevoflurane and then intravenous access and intubations can be done.

Postoperative Analgesia

Non-steroidal anti-inflammatory drugs (NSAIDs) along with local anaesthesia are the mainstay of postoperative pain relief in paediatric day case surgery. They have several advantages over opioid analgesics including a lack of respiratory depression and sedation. They do not cause nausea or vomiting. NSAIDs have been found to be very effective analgesics in older children. However, use of these agents is not recommended below one year of age due to the possibility of immature renal function and hepatic metabolism. Paracetamol (acetaminophen) Diclofenac, ibuprofen and Ketorolac are the most commonly used agents. Administration of these agents before surgery as a pre-medication provides optimal analgesia due to their anti-inflammatory activity.

Opioids are not ideal for paediatric day case surgery as they may produce respiratory depression, excessive sedation and postoperative nausea and vomiting. With some procedures however, opioids are required during and after surgery to control pain. Shorter acting opioids are ideal - Fentanyl (1-2 micrograms/kg) is commonly used. Longer acting opioids (morphine/pethidine) may be required if postoperative pain is unexpectedly severe. Although the procedure may have been planned on a day case basis unexpected hospital admission may be required for control of severe pain.

Outpatient Surgery

In patients with minor paediatric surgical illness 70 % of cases can be managed as outpatient ambulatory cases. In selecting cases for outpatient management needs consideration about the disease concerned because major procedure involving opening of cavities cannot be discharged after the procedure and associated severe medical illness, preterm, previous anaesthetic complications, no access for emergency problem are considered contraindication for out patient office procedure. From the time of invention of laparoscopy the chances of early discharge is possible with less postoperative pain.

Planning Discharge and Follow-up

Patient's condition should be assessed thoroughly before thinking of discharge. Parents should be instructed as early as possible and provide time for them to prepare for situation. Assistance should be provided in arranging for transport, issue of medications for further use. The warning signs of any complications should be mentioned to parents for early review to the emergency. The family physician or periphery district hospital of the locality should be communicated about the patient about the type of procedure done and follow-up instructions and any warning signs for early referral.

Patients detailed contact address, phone number; electronic mail address is recorded properly in the discharge registry for future contact and follows-up. The drugs to be administered, instruction to be followed and frequency of follow up are to be provided before discharged. The advice in the local language or the language, which parents can understand easily helps in gaining good rapport and compliance. Contact number of the hospital and the consultant or near by family physician should be given to patients for any emergency contact.

FLUID AND ELECTROLYTE MANAGEMENT

Introduction

This section focuses on the normal physiology of child, fluid requirement, and factors influencing it and assessment and correction of dehydration. From the time of origin of fetus there are dynamic changes in the fluid and electrolytes. Soon after delivery there is a change in the amount of fluid in the intracellular fluid into the extracellular. Fluid management in the preoperative period is divided into replacing the preoperative fluid deficit, ongoing maintenance requirements and replacement of intra-operative losses, continuing into the postoperative period. For elective patients the deficit before surgery should be minimal because oral fluids may be safely given until 2 hours before surgery. For the emergency patient, the degree of dehydration must be assessed and corrected, along with any electrolyte disturbance. During surgery we need to give maintenance fluid to replace insensible and obligatory losses, along with replacing blood loss and loss of fluid into the third space due to the trauma of surgery. The maintenance fluid we use needs to have an appropriate dextrose and electrolyte content to maintain homeostasis. The commonest electrolyte disturbance in the postoperative period is hyponatraemia, usually as a result of inappropriate anti-diuretic hormone secretion, often in combination with the use of hypotonic solutions with a low sodium concentration.

Children have more fluid per meter square body surface area than adults. In adults 60% of the body weight is due to water whereas in a newborn the water constitute 80% of the total body weight. In adults 20 % of the water is extracellular and 40% as intracellular, whereas in newborns it is 45% extracellular and 35 % intracellular. The significance of this difference is that in cases of dehydration due to any reason because of the large extracellular fluid the loss may not be obvious till a late stage by which time the child would have lost significant volume.

The amount of fluid loss through skin is also more and hence the overall fluid requirement per square meter of body surface area is also more. In newborns the kidney is not fully mature to handle fluid load and there is loss of fluid and sodium. Therefore pathological changes can lead to changes that lead to disturbance of homeostasis leading to drastic irreversible changes. A healthy full-term newborn loses about 10 % of their total body water in their first one week of life because pre-term infants have an increased total body water content and extracellular compartment. They lose on an average of about 15% of their weight after birth in the first week of life. There is a pre-diuretic phase in the first day of life, followed by diuretic phase in the second to third day and then the post-diuretic phase from the fourth day onwards.

There are also changes in the intracellular solute. Potassium is the major intracellular compartment cation and sodium is the major extracellular cation. Changes in the osmolality of extracellular compartment are reflected as net movement of water in and out of the cells.

Regulation of Solute and Fluid

Starling's law regulates the exchange of fluids between the intravascular and extravascular compartment. Under physiological conditions the balance between hydrostatic force and oncotic pressure determine the amount of fluid moving across the capillary membrane. Under various pathological conditions this balance can be disturbed leading to expansion of interstial compartment at the expense of the circulating intravascular compartment. In health, a balance is struck between intracellular and extracellular osmotic forces and interstitial and intravascular oncotic forces, which in turn govern fluid distribution between the intracellular, extracellular and interstitial fluid compartments. The use of hypo- and hypertonic electrolyte solutions has major effects on brain cells, which can be detrimental or beneficial.

The sodium and potassium maintenance is important for critical cell function. They are maintained by kidney, blood and bone buffers. Hormones like steroids, ADH (ant diuretic factor, ANP (atrial natriuretic factor) and aldosterone play dominant role in sodium maintenance. Reduction of serum level of sodium (hyponatraemia) is mostly due to loss of gastrointestinal fluid, diuretics, burns, pancreatitis, adrenal insufficiency, etc. It manifests with lethargy, perioral numbness and convulsions. The correction is to be done slowly otherwise demyelination of nervous system occurs. The total deficit is calculated by using the formula-sodium deficit in mEq/L is 0.6 X weight in kilogram X (135- serum sodium). Potassium the major intracellular cation, homeostasis is maintained both by renal and extrarenal mechanisms. In kidney the increase in serum potassium level stimulates aldosterone, which in turn acts upon distal convoluted tubule to reabsorb sodium in exchange for potassium thereby excrete potassium to maintain electroneutrality. Extrarenal homeostasis is also maintained by aldosterone by causing potassium loss in the colon, saliva and sweat. Following three factors enhance the movement of potassium into the cell. Alkalosis causes an efflux of H^+ from the cells and in exchange K^+ moves intracellularly. Insulin increases K^+ uptake by the cells by directly stimulating Na-ATPase activity independent of cyclic AMP. Beta agonists act by stimulating cyclic AMP via adenylate cyclase, which in turn activates Na-K^+ ATP ase pump.

Calcium homeostasis is maintained mainly by the parathormone secreted by the parathyroid gland and calcitonin secreted mainly by parafollicular C cells of thyroid and some amount by parathyroid gland.

The body water deficit can be estimated on the basis of the degree of dehydration. The water deficit is calculated from the degree of dehydration as 10 % of intravascular fluid is lost in mild dehydration, 25% lost in moderate dehydration and up to 50 % is lost in severe dehydration.

Clinical Signs of Dehydration

CVS	Moderate: Tachycardia collapsed veins, collapsed pulse Severe: Decreased BP, cold extremity, distant heart sounds
GIT	Moderate: Decreased food consumption, Severe: nausea, vomiting, silent ileus, and distention
Tissues	Moderate: Wrinkled tongue with longitudinal wrinkling Severe: Atonic muscles, sunken eyes

CNS	Moderate: Excess sleepiness, apathy, and slow response
	Severe: Decreased tendon reflexes.
Metabolism	Moderate: Mild decrease in temperature (97-9° F)
	Severe: Marked decrease in temperature (95-98°F)

Type and Rate of Administration of IV Fluid

The type of fluid, rate of administration is decided by the cause and degree of dehydration. Fluid of choice for postoperative maintenance is 0.45% NaCl in 5% Dextrose. Fluid of choice for insensible loss is 5% Dextrose. Better Initial fluid in case of resuscitation to be Ringer's lactate and for maintenance be Normal saline In upper gastro-intestinal fluid loss normal saline with addition of potassium after passage of urine, Normal saline or Ringer's lactate for lower GI loss and Ringer's lactate and plasma for burns loss is the ideal. Blood loss up to 20 % of the blood volume can be managed with fluids without replacing the blood loss. The recommended dose of IV fluid to be given is based on weight and the degree of dehydration. The maintenance fluid for the first 10 kg weight is 100 ml per kg per day and hence 1000 ml if child is 10 kg weight. For weight between 11 to 20 kg, 1000 ml and 40 ml per every kg per day over 10 kg, thus 1400 ml for 20 kg weight child. From 20 to 30 kg 20 ml per every kg per day is added to 1400 ml for children above 30 kg weight add 10 ml per every kg excess of 30 kg to 1600 ml for the 30 kg. The rate of administration is 4 ml per kg per hour for their first 10 kg, 2 ml per kg per hour for weight between 11to 20 kg is added to 40 ml per hour for the first 10 kg and for children over 20 kg add 1 ml per every kg excess of 20 kg to 60 ml per hour. Based on the degree of dehydration the deficit is added to the maintenance fluid. In general shorter and acute the loss the correction should also be quick. Fast correction can lead to volume overload, cerebral oedema and convulsions. Generally 50 % of the total required fluid is given over the first eight hours and remaining in next sixteen hours. Initial rehydration should be fast using large bore needle until pulse is well felt. If dehydration is not improving then IV drip should be more rapid. Periodic assessment is essential so as to avoid dehydration as well as over hydration. Rehydration should be continued till all the signs of dehydration have disappeared.

Signs of Overhydration

1. **CVS** Increased venous pressure, pulmonary oedema, and distention of peripheral veins, bounding pulse, high pulse pressure, increased cardiac output.
2. **Tissues** Earliest of all the sign to be weight gain and oedema of eyelid, subcutaneous pitting, anasarca and basal rales.

It is important to have an idea about the composition of IV fluid used in clinical practice (Table 9.1).

Blood Transfusion

Child's blood volume is 80 ml/kg 20 ml/kg is a quarter of blood volume. Small amount of blood loss leads to shock e.g. by the time the loss reaches 15 ml/kg – need to replace blood.

In the acute situation – give bolus of 20 ml/kg of blood by syringe until circulation is restored.

In the elective situation for correction of anaemia packed red cells at 10-15 ml/kg over 4-6 hours.

3 ml/kg of packed red cells raised Hb × 1. 10 ml raises × 3 and 15 ml raises × 5 (Table 9.2).

Hb Transfusion Formula

Desired Hb – Present Hb × body weight kg × 80 = ml whole blood
Hct = 50% (packed red cells 50% of whole blood)

Energy Requirements for Infants

Basal metabolism	— 50 cal/kg/day
Growth	— 25 cal/kg/day
"Energy thermogenesis"	— 45 cal/kg/day
Total	= 120 cal/kg/day

Acid Base Status

pH	— 7.25-7.43
pCO_2	— 32-45 mmHg
pO_2	— >50 mmHg
Base deficit/excess	— Minus 4, plus 3 mmol/L
Standard HCO_3	— 18 - 25 mmol/L

Table 9.1: Composition of Commonly Used IV Fluids						
	pH	*Na+*	*Cl-*	*K+*	*Ca 2+*	*other components*
Ringer's lactate	6.5	130	109	4	3	Lactate 28 mEq/L
Normal Saline (NS)	4.5	154	154	0	0	-
5% Dextrose	5	–	–	–	–	Dextrose 50 g/L

Table 9.2: Blood Volume According to Body weight		
Premature baby (26 weeks)	Term baby (40 weeks)	Adult
Body wt 800 g	3,500 g	60,000(F) 70,000(M)
10% body weight -Blood vol.	8% body weight -Blood vol.	7% body weight -Blood vol.
Blood vol. 80 ml	280 ml	4,200 ml

Correction of Acidosis

Body weight (kg) × base deficit × 0.3 = mmolNaHCO$_3$
8.4% NaHCO$_3$ 1 ml = 1 mmol

Non-respiratory Acidosis

Body weight (kg) × base deficit × 0.3 = mmol NaHCO$_3$
8.4% NaHCO$_3$ 1 ml = 1mmol

Non-respiratory Alkalosis

½ normal saline (77 mmol/L Na, 77 mmol/L)
If urine output is good add KCL 1 gm – 13 mmol to each 500ml

BURNS

Burns are the most devastating type of trauma that the human beings suffer. The post-burn scars leave behind indelible blemishes, and the victims may suffer till the end of their lives. The incidence of burn injuries is increasing and today children suffer from burns more and mortality is also high. Significant morbidity in terms of burn complications such as functional, cosmetic, social and psychological impairment is also seen. Children are at high risk because of their natural curiosity, their mode of reaction, their impulsiveness and lack of experience in calculating the risk of the situation.

Epidemiology

Children unfortunately are the innocent victims of circumstances that result in major fire accidents. Superficial flame burns rate the highest amongst the aetiological factors. Scalds due to hot liquids in the domestic setup ranks next in the aetiology. More serious types of scalding occur when older children 2 -4 years fall into the hot water or hot milk kept on the floor for cooling under the fan. Neonates suffer burns due to hot water bottles, which are used as warmers.

Electrical burns are very common in the domestic setup, when children place their fingers into open plug socket and suffer low voltage burns. Playing near dish antenna on the top of multistoried buildings could result in serious high voltage electrical burns in the upper limbs. Contacts with live wires are a common type of electrical burn when children play and try to retrieve kites. These could result in major burn injuries with wound of entry and wound of exit.

Acid burns are not very common in children, but corrosive esophageal injury occurs due to accidental ingestion of acid, which is kept in kitchen closets for cleaning purposes. Children sometimes are innocent victims of homicidal acid burns.

Pathophysiology of Burns

Problems in the paediatric burns are mainly due to physiological immaturity; this is especially true in infants. The temperature regulating mechanism is labile as the ratio of surface area of the body to weight is more. Rapid shifts in the core temperature occur. Deep burns occur rather rapidly due to the thin skin of the infant that has scant dermal appendages, which are close to the surface, permitting the burn to penetrate into the depths easily. Children are also more susceptible to fluid overload and dehydration. Infants require higher energy and their peripheral circulation is labile. Their metabolic demands are also on the higher side. With all these special problems, the children with burns present a special management issue.

Burn shock is consequent to the massive fluid shifts that occur soon after burn injury. Direct thermal injury results in changes in the microcirculation and capillary permeability increases. Multiple inflammatory mediators are also secreted which increase the vascular permeability throughout the capillary vascular bed all over the body. This results in the leak of intravascular fluid into the extra-vascular spaces resulting in burn oedema, which is maximum at the end of 12 hours post-burn in minor burns and lasts till 24 hours in major burns. Hypovolaemia occurs due to the fluid shifts at the expense of circulating blood and plasma. This results in burn shock with reduced cardiac output, increased heart rate, increased pulse rate, oliguria, acidosis and air hunger. The inflammatory mediators that are responsible are Bradykinin, Histamine, Prostaglandins, Leukotrienes and hormones. Products of platelet degradation, and Interleukin 1 and 6 also act as mediators of burn shock.

In burnt patients the levels of sodium adenosine triphoshphate are reduced in the tissues, which alters the cell transmembrane potential and the concentration of sodium increases in the extra-vascular compartment. This also contributes to burn oedema.

Classification of Burns

Classification of burns can be done according to the agent inducing the injury and according to depth and extent of the total body surface area involved (TBSA).

Agents Causing Burn

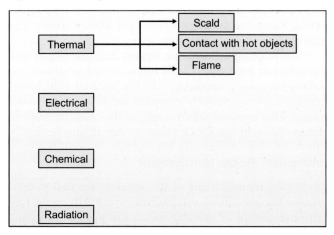

Depth

A clear understanding of the depth and structure of the skin is needed to understand the grades of burn.

First Degree Burn (Superficial)

Only the superficial epithelium is involved. There is always varying degree of erythema and regardless of the type of therapy used, this type of burn heals without scar formation. For about six to ten hours, burn is painful and then gradually it becomes less painful. Sunburns and flame burns are generally of this type.

Second Degree Burn (Partial Thickness)

Here the entire epidermis and a variable depth of dermis is involved. These are commonly seen due to splashes of hot liquids, flash burns, longer contact with flames and limited exposure to chemicals. Depending upon the extent of dermal involvement it is further divided into superficial and deep partial thickness burn.

The superficial type is painful and has blisters. Since sweat glands and hair follicles are spared the healing is satisfactory and scarring does not occur. These heal in 2-3 weeks time and are painful during healing phase due to regeneration of nerve fibres.

The deeper variety is not very painful and is generally without blisters, but since the reticular layer of the dermis is involved these usually do not heal spontaneously, and when it heals after several weeks, it does so with hypertrophic scarring. The appearance will be almost like third degree burn. A sterile 'pin-prick test' with a hypodermic needle can be very valuable in assessing the depth of the burn.

Third Degree Burn (Full Thickness)

Here the entire thickness of the skin and adnexae are involved. The burn is not very painful and is parchment like in appearance. These do not heal spontaneously and have to be excised and grafted. When the third degree burn is extensive, it gives rise to a systemic response, which may result in shock. If it is allowed to heal by itself, it may result in crippling contractures. These are seen due to prolonged contact with any of the agents causing second-degree burns as seen above.

Fourth Degree Burn

Involvement of tissues and structures beneath the skin such as muscles and bones signifies a fourth degree burn. These are obviously insensate and a charred appearance is seen. Classically seen due to molten metal, high voltage electrical burns and prolonged contact with flames.

Extent of Burn

TBSA burnt should be quantified early in assessment; it is the single most important factor for management and prognosis. There are various methods to calculate it:
1. **Rule of nines:** According to this algorithm-head and neck comprise 9% of BSA, front and back of trunk - 20% each, each arm-9%, front and back of leg-9% each and the remaining 1% is made up by the genitalia. This rule is quite reliable in patients who are >15 years old but is not suitable for use in children.
2. **According to palm hands:** A rough estimate of the BSA burnt can be made by the number of palm hands of the patient required to cover the area. Palm surface area roughly equals 1% across all age groups.

Burn Wound Healing

Skin is the largest organ in the body, with multi-structural and multi-functional components with regional variations. The ischaemic, hypoxic and edematous burn wound takes a very slow course for healing compared to a traumatic wound. Unique characteristics of burn wound healing requires a thorough understanding of normal wound healing which is a very complex and dynamic process consisting of many coordinated cellular, biochemical molecular processes. The wound healing goes through phases of angiogenesis, granulation tissue formation, processes of matrix formation, remodeling and epithelialisation to the formation of a scar.

Epithelialization

In a regular wound epithelialisation begins within hours after injury. In superficial and superficial partial thickness burns epithelialization occurs spontaneously from the dermal remnants of hair follicle and sebaceous glands. In deep partial thickness burns the epidermal cells undergo phenotypic alteration at the margins of the normal skin and loose their adherence to one another and to the basement membrane, which allows for the lateral movement of epidermal cells. The migrating epidermal cells dissect the wound space separating the eschar from viable tissue guided by an array of integrins, which the migrating cells express on their cell membrane. One or two days after injury the epidermal cells at the wound margin begin to proliferate behind the actively migrating cells. The stimulus for proliferation and migration of epidermal cells is epidermal growth factor. If the area of the burn is large, re-epithelialization may not completely cover the raw wound and split skin grafting may be necessary to hasten the wound healing. In smaller burn areas, within ten to twelve days, epithelialization is complete and the burn wound gets closed.

Pathophysiology of Burn Shock

A clear understanding is necessary to plan the treatment in paediatric burns and to organize the resuscitation schedule.

Burns shock is the result of vascular changes that take place immediately after burns. Direct thermal injury result in changes in the microcirculation and capillary permeability. The latter increases and alterations in the transcell membrane potential occur. These occur due to certain mediators like Bradykinin and Histamine. This increased capillary permeability results in massive fluid shifts from the intravascular to extravascular compartment. The total body fluid volume may remain unchanged, but the volume of each compartment gets altered. For normal maintenance of ionic gradient across the cell membrane, adequate levels of Na-adenosine Triphosphatase are required. In burns the levels of Na-ATPase decreases and consequently sodium concentration in the cells increases and intracellular oncotic pressure increases. This results in massive oedema in the burnt tissue, hypovolaemia and oliguria, which are the components of shock. Intracellular and interstitial volume increases at the expenses of plasma and blood volume. Other mediators, which have been identified in this process, are products of platelet degradation, prostaglandins, leukotrienes, interleukins 1, 6 and TNFα. The formation of oedema is maximum by the end of 12 hours post-burn in minor burns and lasts till 24 hours in major burns.

Immunological Response to Burn Injury

Today it has been realized that in massively burnt patients (>40% TBSA) chaotic cytokine array is responsible for higher mortality rate and not infection as was thought earlier. The appropriate term for the immunological failure that is seen is 'Systemic Inflammatory Response'. As soon as burn injury occurs, macrophage margination and activation occurs. This results in the release of three cytokines ILI, IL6 and TNF-alpha. Macrophages also produce products of lipid peroxidation namely leuko-

trienes and prostaglandins. All these are very toxic to the patient and these produce T cell failure, inhibit lymphocytes, haemoglobin synthesis and also depress the granulocyte colony formation.

Skin is recognized as the largest immune organ and the effect of heat could well figure in the origin of the pathophysiology encountered. The area of skin burnt quantitatively is related to mortality and cellular functional failure. This immune failure could be the cause of death in children during the shock phase, rather than infection.

Emergency Room Management

The initial management of the severely burned patient follows the guidelines established by the Advanced Life Support course of the American College of Surgeons according to which, like any other trauma, airway and breathing assume the highest priority.

Airway and Breathing

Airway management is the first and the foremost priority as there is high incidence (up to 30%) of associated inhalation injury in a severely burnt patient which can be immediately life threatening. Inhalation injury may be present with minimal cutaneous burns and may not be evident at presentation but can develop rapidly. Inhalation injury should be suspected if there is any history of exposure to smoke in a confined space, loss of consciousness, impaired mental status or disorientation and obtundation. Important clinical signs to be looked for are - any hoarseness of voice, stridor (impending airway obstruction), facial burns, singed nasal hair, wheezing and expectoration of black carbonaceous sputum. Affected patients should be given 100% oxygen by mask (to wash out carbon monoxide), oxygen saturation should be monitored and equipment kept ready for intubation. Ideally fibreoptic bronchoscopy should be done on any suspicion and signs such as airway oedema, mucosal necrosis, haemorrhages, ulcers and pseudomembranous casts should be looked for. If any of these are present the patient should be intubated and respiratory care protocol established. The final point to be remembered is the fact that the burn patient could also be a victim of associated trauma, hence decreased levels of consciousness or oxygen desaturation should not be blamed only on burn shock or inhalation injury, but could be due to associated head injury.

Circulation and Intravenous Access

It is important to start two intra-venous portals, one for infusing fluids and the other for giving drugs through the unburnt skin. Central line though ideal, may invite sepsis and could be disastrous and hence should be inserted only if required urgently. If the child has already gone into shock with falling blood pressure, then a central line must be started. Adequate fluid resuscitation should be started and a Foley's catheter should be placed. A nasogastric tube should be placed to drain the stomach.

Eliciting History for Medicolegal Purpose

To ensure proper epidemiological documentation and also for medico-legal records, a detailed history should be elicited from the conscious patient and in the case of children from the parents. This would enable implementation of preventive programme.

Recording of the Weight of the Patient

Recording of the weight of the burnt child is important for calculating and administering fluids and drugs. Ideally weight is recorded as soon as possible at the emergency room.

Investigations

When the iv portals are started, blood is drawn for serum chemistry and a sample is refrigerated for grouping and cross matching.

Escharotomy and Fasciotomy

Burn eschar may act an inelastic constricting tourniquet impairing circulation and even respiration. This is seen generally in extremity and chest burns though can occur in neck and abdominal wall burns also. This phenomenon is seen only with deep second and third degree burns only. The constricting effect may not be there initially and develop later on during resuscitation; 8-24 hours period is most critical period. A frequent assessment of the peripheral perfusion can help in early diagnosis. Parameters to be checked are capillary filling time, pulses and oxygen saturation. Doppler can aid the diagnosis in difficult cases. For prevention, extremities with deep burns should be kept elevated and splinted in a functional position. If signs of vascular insufficiency appear then escharotomy should be performed without delay. This procedure involves an incision through the burn eschar to relieve the constriction caused by it. This procedure can be done at the bedside with an electrocautery with the patient under sedation, as the eschar is insensate. A rapid restoration of the circulation suggests a successful procedure; if the blood flow is still not restored then a consideration should be given to fasciotomy, i.e. incision of the deep fascia to alleviate the compartment syndrome.

Fluid Resuscitation in Paediatric Burns

It is important to bear in mind that a burnt child continues to be a special challenge, since resuscitation therapy must be more precise than that for an adult with a similar burn. Important point to bear in mind is the fact that a burnt child requires intravenous resuscitation for a relatively smaller TBSA (10-20 %) unlike an adult. Primary goal of resuscitation is to support the child throughout the initial 24 to 48 hours period of hypovolaemia that sets in due to extravascular fluid sequestration during post-burn shock period.

Calculation of the Requirements

Cope and Moore in 1947 gave the first rational scheme of fluid resuscitation in burn patients. Though their formula is no longer in use all the modern formulas derive their basic scheme from their formula, i.e. requirements are calculated according to the extent of the burn and the weight of the patient, initially for the first 24 hours. Half of this amount is given in the initial 8 hours and the rest over next 16 hours. Though for adults Parkland's formula is the one that is in most common use, the only formula for calculation in paediatric burn patients is the one devised by Shriners Burn Hospital. According to this formula:

For first 24 hours – Total fluid requirement is 5000 ml/m² TBSA burn + 2000 ml/m² as maintenance, 50% of this volume is given in initial 8 hours and the rest in ensuing 16 hours. Ringer's lactate is the fluid used for resuscitation.

Thereafter – 3750 ml/m² + 1500 ml/m² is used for next 24 hours; a part of total of it may be made up by the enteral feeds. Urine output of >1-ml/kg/hr and stable vitals signify an adequate replacement.

Place of Colloid

There is a controversy regarding the use of colloids in the initial resuscitation scheme. It is known that the plasma proteins are extremely important in the circulation since they generate the inward oncotic force that counteracts the outward capillary hydrostatic force. But protein solutions are not given in the initial 16 hours, as they also leak through the dilated capillaries, and are no more effective than more salt water. After 16 hours, if colloids are added to the crystalloid regimen, the reversal from shock is phenomenal. Either fresh frozen plasma 0.5 to 1 ml/kg TBSA or 5% albumin can be given. A reasonable indication of giving albumin early on, i.e. after 8 hours is serum albumin less than 2 g%.

Place of Whole Blood

In extensive third degree electric burns or in third degree burn over 50% TBSA, actual entrapment of RBCs and cell death results in severe hypoxia. This situation can be reversed by whole blood transfusion and preferably fresh blood improves the situation better. Fresh whole blood transfusion is usually given. This can be combined with crystalloids.

Urine Output Monitoring

Measured volume bags are preferably used. Child should void 1 ml/kg/hr of urine if resuscitation is adequate. Diuretics are generally not indicated during acute resuscitation period. But in children sustaining high voltage electrical burns with myoglobinuria/haemoglobinuria, there is increased risk of renal tubular obstruction. Forced alkaline diuresis is indicated in such situations with urine output as high as 3-5 ml/kg/hr. To alkalinize the urine, sodium bicarbonate is added, while an osmotic diuretic like mannitol achieves a high urine output.

Problems in Resuscitation

It is important to identify acidosis. Electrolyte estimation must be done periodically and acidosis must be corrected without delay. There is a risk of hyponatraemia and hyperkalaemia early on.

Thermal injury results not only in massive fluid shifts that cause hypovolaemia, but also in release of inflammatory mediators from burn wounds. These mediators deleteriously affect cardiovascular function and lead to burn shock. The end result of a complex chain of events is decreased intravascular volume, increased systemic vascular resistance, decreased cardiac output, end organ ischaemic and metabolic acidosis. Without early and full resuscitation therapy these derangements progress to acute renal failure, cardiovascular collapse and death.

Resuscitation in itself is not without complications. Burn oedema is worsened with resuscitation, particularly crystalloid solutions. The above given formulae are generalizations only; each child should get individualized treatment to avoid complications.

Infection Control

Infection is the most common complication seen in the burn patients. Initially gram-positive organisms are the ones that cause sepsis but as early as 3 days post-burn gram-negative organisms start predominating. Systemic antibiotics are not recommended in burn patients for prevention of burn wound sepsis, as the burn tissue is a poorly perfused tissue. Also this practice leads to the emergence of resistant strains. They are certainly recommended in special circumstances such as:

- Peri-operatively—Around the time of burn wound excision to limit the incidence of bacteraemia. They should be guided by the quantitative burn wound cultures.

- Autografting- At the time of autografting to prevent local loss of the graft and also to prevent infection at the donor site. A first generation oral cephalosporin is good enough till the first dressing change if the cultures are not available.
- Infection elsewhere—In the presence of infection elsewhere such as pneumonitis, thrombophlebitis, urinary tract infection and sepsis, systemic antibiotics are obviously indicated.

Topical therapy is all that is required for most of the burn wounds. Appropriate topical therapy reduces microbial growth and chances of invasive sepsis. It should be soothing in nature, easy to apply and remove and should not have systemic toxicity. Such an ideal antimicrobial probably does not exist.

DRESSINGS: Option of closed dressing and open dressing methods are available. In open method, topical antimicrobials are applied and the wound is left open to warm dry air. *Pseudomonas* infections are rare but this method requires a strict environmental control and is painful. The fluid requirements also increase due to greater evaporative losses. This method is useful for facial and scalp burns. In closed dressings topical antimicrobial creams are applied and then covered with gauze dressings. This method is less painful though more labor intensive. Closed dressings are preferred for the extremities and over the back.

Surgical Management of the Burn Wound

A proper assessment of the burn wound guides the choice of the surgical therapy.

First-degree burn: As there is minimal loss of the barrier function of the skin, the infection and fluid loss are not common. Management aims at providing pain relief and optimal conditions for wound healing. Topical salves and oral analgesics are the only medications required.

Superficial Second-degree burns: These require daily dressings with topical antimicrobials till spontaneous re-epithelialization occurs in 10-21 days. Alternatively, temporary biological or synthetic dressings can be used.

Deep Second-degree and Third-degree burns: Early burn wound excision has been shown to be beneficial in these types of burns. Advantages are:
- Decreased rates of infection as dead and devitalized tissue is removed.
- Removal of source of inflammatory mediators.
- Decreased scarring and more functional rehabilitation.
- Decreased stay in hospital.
- Early excision (<48 hours) is associated with less blood loss.

Two types of burn wound excisions are described:
1. *Tangential Excision:* Implies sequential excision of burnt skin layers to reach the viable tissue layer. It is more time consuming and is associated with more blood loss and requires a certain experience.

2. *Fascial Excision:* This involves removal of all tissue down to the level of deep fascia. This procedure is technically easier and is associated with comparatively less blood loss. As this procedure is cosmetically disfiguring it should be used in only compelling situations- such as life threatening burn wound sepsis. Blood loss during surgery can be controlled by use of tourniquets, elevating the limb and local application of thrombin solution or epinephrine soaked pads.

WOUND COVERAGE: After burn wound excision, the tissue bed consists of dermis and the subcutaneous fat. It is necessary to cover this raw area to promote healing and to provide for better cosmetic and functional outcome.

1. *Autograft:* Ideal coverage is the patient's own skin. It is generally possible to get enough split skin autograft in <40% TBSA burns. Meshing allows more area to be covered and also allows for seepage of the exudates in the postoperative period. Maximum meshing allowed is 4:1. More meshing ultimately leads to more scarring; for this reason the grafts to be used on face and joints should preferably be not meshed.

2. *Autograft with Allograft Overlay:* If the autograft is inadequate a 4:1 or even 6:1 meshed autograft is used and over it 2:1 meshed allograft is placed. Allograft falls away as the autograft epithelializes underneath. In massively burnt patients, rejection is not a major issue as there is profound immunosuppression. It is mandatory to screen the donor for HIV, CMV, HBV and HCV before using these grafts.

3. *Allograft:* Allograft can be used for temporary coverage of the wound till the donor sites heal and further grafts can be taken from them. Such situations can arise in massively burnt patients (>40% TBSA).

4. *Xenograft:* Porcine skin is readily available and it resembles human skin morphologically. It adheres well to the dermis and then is gradually degraded; the main drawback is its inability to prevent infection.

5. *Amniotic membrane:* Amniotic membrane can provide an excellent temporary biological coverage till more autograft is available. It is freely available, is non-antigenic and has some infection resisting properties. Cord blood sample should be tested for HIV, CMV, HBV and HCV prior to its use.

6. *Synthetic dressings:* Various biologically engineered membranes such as keratinocyte sheets, silicon mesh with porcine or human collagen and silicon mesh with fetal keratinocytes are available in the west but their cost and availability still precludes common clinical use.

Reasons for the non take-up of grafts:
1. Fluid collections underneath the grafts - meticulous haemostasis, meshing and good pressure dressings help prevent this complication.

2. Shearing stress on the grafted surfaces – can be prevented by proper immobilization and splinting.
3. Infection – Good peri-operative antibiotic cover based on cultures should be used.
4. Residual necrotic tissue in the bed – Adequate excision takes care of this aspect.

Proper care of the donor sites to allow for reuse cannot be overemphasized, as every inch of the skin is precious. Donor area if not properly cared for behaves in the same way as a second-degree burn.

Hypermetabolic Response and Nutrition

Hypermetabolic response:
Burns >40% TBSA cause a tremendous increase in the resting energy expenditure amounting to even 50-100%. The following factors contribute
• Increased release of IL1, IL2, TNF-alpha, thromboxane.
• Increased release of stress hormones such as catecholamines, glucagon and cortisol.

All these promote systemic vasoconstriction and may lead to renal and mesenteric ischaemia. This hypermetabolic response can be modified to improve the outcome:
1. Ambient temperature should be kept between 28-30° C.
2. Early enteral nutrition in the post-burn period reduces the incidences of bacterial translocation and counters the catabolic state.
3. Beta-blockers can block the deleterious effects of catecholamines to decrease the heart rate and the cardiac output.
4. Growth hormone has also been shown to help in catch up growth by fostering a positive nitrogen balance. It also improves immunity and helps in faster healing at the donor sites.
5. Adequate pain relief also helps in decreasing the stress response. Specially during dressing changes intravenous pethidine can make dressing changes less distressful for these sick children.

Nutrition: Early establishment of enteral feeds as soon as the child is stabilized via a nasogastric tube decreases the metabolic rate, gastric atrophy, stress ulceration and bacterial translocation. Parenteral nutrition leads to more chances of systemic sepsis, thus enteral route with all its advantages is preferred. An adequate calorie intake provided as 40-70% carbohydrates, 10-20% fats and 20-40% protein should be the goal. Calorie requirement is calculated according to the Shriners Burn Institute formulas.
• Infant formula –1800 kcal/m^2 maintenance + 1000 kcal/m^2 area burnt
• For 1-11 years-1800 kcal/m^2 maintenance + 1300 kcal/m^2 area burnt
• >12years-1500 kcal/m^2 maintenance + 1500 kcal/m^2 area burnt

Complications and Rehabilitation

Apart from the myriad acute metabolic and systemic complications the burn patient might experience, the following complications, which deserve a special mention.

1. Burn wound sepsis: Burn wound sepsis is indicated by change of the colour to black or dark brown, haemorrhage of the subeschar fat, progression of the partial thickness injury to full thickness, dirty foul smelling exudates, premature separation of eschar or appearance of eruptions. Treatment involves change of topical antibiotics, systemic antibiotics and excision of the burn wound.
2. Pulmonary complications: Inhalation injury as such and other conditions like profound immunosuppression, systemic sepsis and ventilation predispose the burnt patient to pneumonia. Management includes judicious use of antibiotics, aggressive physiotherapy and respiratory care.
3. Gastrointestinal complications: Hypokalaemia in the acute phase, sepsis, hypovolaemia all contribute towards ileus in the post-burn period. Management includes nasogastric suction and correction of underlying aetiology. Gastric ulceration and bleeding-Curling's ulcers are also common due to impaired perfusion and the stress response. Antacids are no longer recommended for prevention as these increase gastric pH and colonization of the stomach. Sucralfate and early enteral feeds are the strategies that are most helpful.
4. Orthopaedic complications: Osteomyelitis, non-healing fractures, ulcers and heterotrophic calcification are also common.

Long-term Complications

Hypertrophic scar: It is the phase of redness and induration that is seen during the healing phase of deep second degree and third degree burns. Spontaneous resolution occurs in most of the cases. Pruritus associated with these scars can be managed by local application of emollients, 1% hydrocortisone ointment, local triamcinolone injection or systemic anti-histaminics. Pressure garments also help in fast resolution.

Contractures: Burns occurring at the flexor aspects of joints and if deep are especially prone to develop contractures during the healing phase. All scars and split skin grafts have a tendency to shrink, and this tendency is more with thin grafts. Contractures are best prevented by:
- Use of thick grafts at the joints.
- Splinting the joints for three months in a functional position after grafting (while keeping in mind that prolonged splinting may cause peri-articular fibrosis and joint capsule contractures).

- Pressure garments and silicone gel dressings provide a uniform pressure over the healing area and thus may help in prevention of contractures.
- Established contractures require surgical management:
- Local re-arrangement of skin as single or multiple Z plasties.
- Free grafts – A thick free graft can be placed after the excision of the contractures is small. For a large contracture a relaxing incision is given at the site of maximum tension and a free graft is placed in the resulting defect.
- Flaps – Full thickness flaps that can be pedicled or mucocutaneous flaps can be utilized to release the contractures.
- Tissue expanders – Can be used to expand the nearby normal full thickness skin which can then be used as a rotational flap to release the contracture.

Rehabilitation

Burns produce a severe psychological set back in many individuals and especially in children. Their proper growth and development depends upon their psychological rehabilitation. Nurses and medical staff must be children friendly.

Social rehabilitation also has to be emphasized. They must be accepted by the society at large. Occupational therapy and rehabilitation form an integral part of burn therapy.

PAEDIATRIC TRAUMA

Trauma is the most frequent cause of death in children beyond infancy. The management has improved considerably over the past decades; effective early management by those who are familiar with the management of paediatric trauma patients can significantly reduce morbidity and mortality. A common systematic approach to all children's resuscitation has been developed which begins treatment of life threatening injuries/problems as soon as they are detected. The anatomy and physiology of children differs significantly from that of adults.

Body proportions, structures, normal physiological parameters change with age.

Head

Children have a large head to body size ratio that needs to be considered, in relation to heat loss, and surface area of burns patients. The head is 19% of surface area at birth, reducing to 9% at the age of 16 years. The neck must not be over extended as trachea is short and soft, and over-extension may cause tracheal compression.

Upper Airway

Infants less than 6 months are obligate nasal breathers. Narrow airways are often obstructed by mucus, loose teeth are at risk of being lost into the bronchial tree, and adenotonsillar hypertrophy is frequently present between 3-8 years, adding to the difficulties of securing the airway. The epiglottis is more U shaped in a child, projecting posteriorly at 45 degrees.

The larynx is cephalad and anterior at cervical vertebrae C2-3 in the infant, as compared with C5-6 in the adult. It is therefore easier to intubate children younger than 12 months with a straight bladed laryngoscope. The narrowest point of the upper airway is the cricoid ring, which is lined with pseudostratified ciliated epithelium, which is prone to oedema if cuffed tubes are used for intubation. Uncuffed tubes are used for all children who have yet to reach puberty, and the sizing of the tube should allow a small leak of gas past the tube during inflation of the lungs.

The trachea is short, in neonates 4-5 cm, in infants 7-8 cm and therefore tubes can easily become displaced accidentally or during transport, entering the relatively straight right main bronchus.

Neck

In children the interspinous ligaments and joint capsules are more flexible, the vertebral bodies are wedged anteriorly so tend to slide forward with flexion and the vertebral facet joints are flat. Cervical spine radiograph in children can cause some concern due to normal physiological appearances mimicking fracture or dislocation. It is important to link clinical examination and radiological findings. It is unusual to find a fracture without physical signs.

Skeletal growth centres can be confused with fractures. The basal odontoid synchrondrosis has a radiolucent area at the base of the dens in children less than 5 years whilst the tip of the odontoid epiphyses appears separate in children age 5-11 years. The growth centre of the spinous process can be mistaken for a fracture of the spinous processes.

Spinal injuries in children are rare but can occur. Spinal cord injury without radiological abnormality (SCIWORA) occurs almost exclusively in children < 8 years old. It affects the C-spine and to a lesser frequency the thoracic spine, and is commoner in the upper C-spine segments due to the increased mobility of this region. Seriously injured children should be immobilised until full neurological assessment is possible. MRI may have to be used.

Fractures

Skeletal injuries in children can be difficult to detect, with only minor signs visible.

In the early stages of resuscitation fractures should be thought of as a potential source of volume loss. Grossly displaced fracture/dislocations should be reduced. The blood loss from a long bone or pelvic fractures is proportionately greater in a child than adult. The majority of children's fractures heal rapidly and well. Whilst the bones are still growing there is a good capacity for bone remodelling, so some angulation of a reduced fracture can be accepted. Fractures of the soft springy immature bones in children are often the classic greenstick fracture. Some injuries such as crush injuries to the epiphysis are very difficult to diagnose radiologically, yet they can have serious consequences on the future growth and therefore symmetry of the limbs.

Physiological Parameters

The cardiovascular system in children has an increased physiological reserve compared to adults and is able to tolerate significant blood loss without obvious distress, there may only be subtle signs of severe shock. Hence early assessment and recognition of shock is essential for appropriate management of the injured child. Tachycardia and reduced capillary refill are frequently the only signs available.

The child's heart has a limited capacity to increase stroke volume so cardiac output is mostly dependent on heart rate. With a typical blood volume of 80 ml/kg, an amount of blood, which would otherwise be considered a minor blood loss in an adult, could severely compromise a child.

The child initially responds to reductions in intra-vascular volume by increased heart rate, and vaso-constriction with a low pulse pressure.

Shock in a child is difficult to recognise below 25% volume loss, but may be suggested by a weak thready pulse and an increased heart rate, lethargy and irritability, and cool clammy skin. There would be a slight reduction in urine output if measured.

As volume loss approaches 25 – 45% the heart rate remains raised, but there is a definite reduction in consciousness and a dulled response to pain. The skin becomes cyanotic, with reduced capillary refill time (CRT) and the extremities become cold. If measured there would be minimal urine output.

Finally above 45% volume loss the child can no longer compensate and there is a point at which the child becomes hypotensive and bradycardiac, and the child is comatose.

An idea of a child's normal parameters is required. (Table 9.3)

As an approximate guide systolic BP = 80 mm Hg + age (years) x 2

Other useful guides:
Weight = 2 x (age + 4)
Blood volume = 80 ml × weight in kg
Volume of dehydration = weight in kg × % of dehy-
dration x 10

Age	WeightKg	Heart rateper min	Blood pressure mmHg	Respiratory Breath/min	Urinary output ml/kg/hr
0 – 6 months	3 – 6 kg	180 – 160	60 – 80	60	2
Infant	12	160	80	40	1.5
Preschool	16	120	90	30	1
Adolescent	35	100 – 50	100	20	0.5

Table 9.3: Normal physiological parameters

Approach to the Injured Child

The approach is to be found in greater detail in the manuals of the Advanced Trauma and Life Support – (ATLStm), Paediatric Advanced Life Support (PALStm) and Advanced Paediatric Life Support (APLStm).

The Primary Survey

The aim is a rapid assessment to identify immediate life threatening problems and prevent secondary injury.
A Airway and cervical spine control
B Breathing and ventilation
C Circulation and control of haemorrhage
D Disability
E Exposure and control of environment

Endotracheal tube size (mm) = 4 + age (years) / 4 which should be close to the diameter of the little finger or the size of the nares. An uncuffed tube is used which sits in position at the cricoid ring.

Children's normal ventilatory rate varies and reduces with age. Tidal volume is of the order 7-10 ml/kg. Care should be taken when assisting ventilation to match these parameters without using excessive force, which can cause barotrauma to young lungs.

Assessment of parameters to gauge the stage of shock includes pulse, systolic blood pressure, capillary refill time, skin colour, temperature, respiratory rate and mental status.

Capillary refill time (CRT) is measured by squeezing and elevating an extremity, great toe or thumb, above heart level, for 5 seconds, then releasing it.

CRT >2 seconds, skin mottling, and low peripheral temperature are signs of shock.

When shock is suspected 20ml/kg of warmed crystalloid solution is used. Failure to improve suggests either ongoing haemorrhage or gross fluid depletion. This 20 ml/kg represents 25% of blood volume, but as this volume becomes distributed into other body fluid compartments up to three boluses of 20 ml/kg may be necessary to achieve 25% blood volume replacement. If a third bolus is being considered then blood replacement should be considered.

Disability is assessed by pupil size, reactivity and conscious level as alert, responsive to voice, responsive to pain and unresponsive.

All surfaces of the child need to be inspected during the course of the primary survey, but this can be done region by region to avoid distress and heat loss.

Secondary Survey

The secondary survey is a head to toe assessment, including Reassessment of vital signs.

A complete neurological exam including the GCS should be carried out.

A brief medical history needs to be recorded.

Standard trauma blood investigations are taken during IV access and primary survey.

Radiological investigations are required as an adjunct.
Bloods   Baseline
Full blood count (FBC), electrolytes (UandE), glucose (Glu), amylase (Amy)
Blood for group and save (GandS) or Urgent cross match (XM)

Arterial blood gases (ABGs)
X-ray   Trauma series   Chest
C-spine
Pelvis
Additional investigations are taken when the patient is stabilised.

Emergency Treatment

Emergency treatment is that required to stabilise the child prior to transfer to an appropriate referral centre, theatre for operative treatment or the ward for conservative expectant observation.

Head Trauma

Head injury is the most common reason for hospital admission in children, and the most common cause of death in children after the age of 1 year. Fortunately many injuries are trivial and their admission to hospital is mainly to reassure parents and cover the hospital.

The standard trauma and resuscitation approach is used in the assessment and early treatment of these patients and the aim of emergency treatment is directed at preventing secondary brain injury, and referring early to a neurosurgical unit for definitive treatment.

Primary and Secondary Brain Injury

Neurosurgical referral is indicated if there is a deteriorating conscious level or coma score <12, focal neurological signs, depressed skull fracture or penetrating injury, or basal skull fracture. Definitive treatment is directed at the cause of the raised intracranial pressure or injury. This may involve the evacuation of haematoma or elevation of depressed fracture in addition to other intensive care measures.

Any child with a Glasgow Coma Scale (GCS) of 8 or less should be intubated and ventilated with rapid sequence anaesthesia.

If the conscious level deteriorates rapidly despite all other supportive measures then urgent referral is indicated and measures intended to increase cerebral perfusion in the short term are used. These include the use of:
1. IV mannitol 0.5 to 1 g/kg
2. Hyperventilation to a $PaCO_2$ of 3.5-4.0 kPa
3. 20 degree head up position to promote venous drainage
4. Plasma expanders to avoid cerebral hypotension

A focal seizure is considered as a focal neurological sign.

Generalised fits are of less concern but should be controlled if they have not stopped within 5 mins. IV diazepam is preferred.

In many cases the head injury is limited to minor scalp haematoma, limited vomiting with normal neurology. If the head injury appears stable a period of close observation for 24 hours is appropriate.

The assessment of head injuries in children depends on the age of the child, their ability to describe the mechanism of injury, and the history obtained from reliable witnesses. Potentially serious injuries are suggested by significant energy transfer, e.g. road traffic accident (RTA) or fall from height > 2 m, loss of consciousness (LOC), an altered state of consciousness, obvious neurology, or penetrating injury. The conscious level should be documented using the appropriate scale for the age of the child and the time noted.

Thoracic Trauma

Children have elastic ribs and significant amounts of energy can be absorbed by the thoracic region without obvious external signs of injury. An apparently normal chest radiograph cannot exclude significant thoracic injury.

The presence of rib fractures therefore suggests a very significant transfer of energy and other associated organ injuries should be suspected.

The provision of high flow oxygen via a reservoir mask allows FiO_2 of greater than 60% to be achieved and should be used routinely in chest trauma.

Chest injuries which can occur include those which can be immediately life threatening and those which become apparent later.

1. Tension pneumothorax

Air is drawn into the pleural space compressing the mediastinum and compromising venous return to the heart. Cardiac output reduces, so that the child becomes hypoxic and shocked, and the jugular veins become distended.

There will be hyperresonance and reduced air entry on the lung field on the side of the pneumothorax. As the mediastinum is pushed to the opposite side the trachea is said to deviate away from the side of the pneumothorax.

Treatment should be immediate, needle thoracocentesis in the 2nd intercostals space mid clavicular line, relieving the tension and converting the injury into a simple pneumothorax. Definitive treatment is the insertion a chest drain.

2. Major haemothorax

Bleeding into the pleural space from damage to the lung vessels or chest wall can be a source of a large volume of blood loss, in addition to the reduction in lung volume, shock and hypoxia may be evident if significant blood volume has been lost. There will be reduced chest movement, reduced air entry and reduced resonance to percussion on the side of a haemothorax.

Treatment requires volume replacement and the insertion of a large bore chest drain.

3. Open Pneumothorax

The presence of penetrating wounds to the upper body, between umbilicus and root of the neck must alert one the possibility of an open pneumothorax.

There will be reduced chest movement, reduced breath sounds and hyperresonance on the side of the pneumothorax. Air may be heard to suck and blow through the wound. Treatment requires the creation of a flap valve using a air tight dressing secured on three of four sides, to allow air out but not in, preventing a tension pneumothorax developing and converting the injury into a simple pneumothorax. A chest drain is required, followed by surgical exploration, debridement and repair.

4. Flail Segment

In the child a flail chest is a very significant injury due to the amount of energy required to create it and the degree of underlying lung injury. Abnormal chest movement may be seen over the flail segment and crepitus may be felt. The early involvement of an anaesthetist is advised. Treatment should consist of endotracheal intubation and ventilation.

5. Cardiac Tamponade

Injury, which causes bleeding into the pericardial sac, reduces the volume available for cardiac filling. As the pericardial sac fills with more blood the cardiac output is reduced. Shock develops, the heart sounds become muffled and the neck veins may become distended. Treatment is pericardiocentesis, which may need to be repeated.

Abdominal Trauma

The abdomen is more exposed in children than in adults. The soft elastic rib cage offers less protection to the liver kidneys and spleen. The pelvis is shallow and the bladder is intra-abdominal in the younger child. The most common organs to be damaged following blunt trauma are in order, spleen, liver, kidney, gastrointestinal tract, genitourinary tract and pancreas. Penetrating trauma most commonly affects the gastrointestinal tract, liver, kidneys and bloods vessels. The significant morbidity and mortality following splenectomy has led to a more conservative approach to possible splenic trauma. Experience has shown that the majority of abdominal injuries can be treated conservatively provided they receive close observation, repeated assessment and monitoring. Attention should be paid to vital signs, fluid balance and blood factors. A paediatric surgeon should be available during this period if required.

Operative intervention is required in:
1. Haemodynamically unstability after the replacement of 40 ml/kg of fluid.
2. Penetrating abdominal injury
3. A non-functioning kidney is demonstrated on contrast study (remembering the warm ischaemic time for the kidney is a maximum of 60 mins)
4. Signs of bowel perforation

The abdomen is only considered in the primary survey under C circulation if shock does not respond to volume replacement, if no other obvious site of haemorrhage can be found. In children a naso/oro gastric tube should passed as air swallowing occurs during crying and can cause significant gastric distension. Gastric distension can cause splinting of the diaphragm making breathing and/ or ventilation difficult.

During the secondary survey the abdomen is inspected for bruising, laceration, penetration. The external genitalia must also be examined and the external urethral meatus inspected for blood. If blood is seen this is an indication for retrograde urography and passage of urethral catheter must not be attempted by anyone other than a Consultant Urologist. Rectal examination on children is carried out only if it is considered appropriate by the paediatric surgeon who would be operating.

Child Abuse

Child abuse can take many forms, physical, sexual, emotional, or neglect. It is important to have a high index of suspicion of the possibility of abuse and be aware of the patterns of presentation, explanations and injury seen.
Factors which should alert the doctor to the possibility of non-accidental injury (NAI) include, odd times of presentation for treatment, delayed presentation, presenting without the prime carer, inconsistent and imprecise times and accounts of the mechanism of injury. The injury may not be compatible with the mechanism of injury, or the parents' attitude or focus of concern does not seem right. Perhaps the child's interaction with the adult is abnormal, or their behaviour seems inhibited or withdrawn.

Injuries seen in NAI include head injuries, including occipital fractures and intracranial injury. Fractures of long bones, and particularly multiple fractures at different stages of healing may be seen. Bruising and finger marks in a hand print distribution, burns, scalds, cigarette burns, belt, bite marks should all be carefully examined.

Sexual abuse may present as frank injury, genital infection, or may present with odd inappropriate behavioral or other emotional problems.

Assessment of any child with suspected child abuse needs great care and sympathy, and the involvement of seniors at the earliest point of concern.

Trauma scores

Trauma scores are used as a predictor of survival and for comparative purposes.
They include the following (Table 9.4)

Table 9.4: Paediatric Trauma Score			
	Coded value		
Patient factors	+2	+1	–1
Weight (kg)	> 20	10 - 20	< 10
Airway	Normal	Maintained	Not maintained
Systolic BP	> 90	50 - 90	< 50
CNS	Awake	Obtunded	Coma
Open wound	None	Minor	Major
Skeletal trauma	None	Closed	Open / multiple

Revised Trauma Score

This is a physiological scoring system consisting of a weighted combination of Glasgow Coma Scale, Systolic blood pressure and Respiratory Rate.

Glasgow coma scale score	Systolic blood pressure	Respiratory rate	Coded value
13 – 15	> 89	10 – 29	4
9 – 12	76 – 89	> 29	3
6 – 8	50 – 75	6 – 9	2
4 – 5	1- 49	1 – 5	1
3	0	0	0

RTS = 0.94 GCS + 0.73 Systolic BP + 0.29 Respiratory Rate
The RTS can be in a range between 0 to 7.84.
When RTS is plotted against survival a sigmoid shaped curve is produced.

BIBLIOGRAPHY

1. Advanced Life Support Group. Advanced Paediatric Life Support – The Practical Approach 2nd Edition. BMJ Publishing Group 1997.
2. Lloyd-Thomas AR Anderson I. ABC of Major Trauma Chapter 18 Paediatric Trauma. BMJ Publishing Group 1996.
3. Seminars in Pediatric Surgery Vol4 no2 May 1995. Editor: Jay L Grosfeld, W. B Saunders Company.

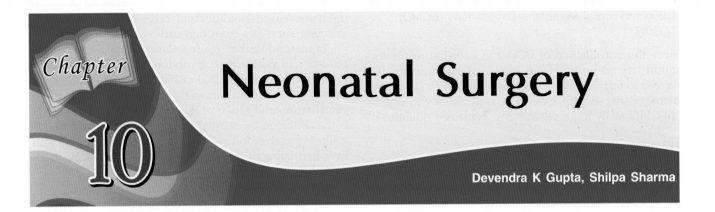

Devendra K Gupta, Shilpa Sharma

CONGENITAL DIAPHRAGMATIC HERNIA

It is a congenital defect in the diaphragm usually posterolateral in location through which intra-abdominal contents protrude into the thorax and may cause respiratory compromise.

The earlier the baby presents, the worse is the prognosis.

Embryology

It is still believed that the defect in CDH results from failure of closure of pleuroperitoneal canal at the end of embryonic period. Using scanning electron microscopy and a new animal model, the nitrogen rat model, crucial steps of development of CDH formation have been studied for the first time.

Pulmonary hypoplasia is central to the pathophysiology of CDH. Structural abnormalities of pulmonary vasculature can result in acute pulmonary vasoconstriction. Failure of transition from the fetal to newborn circulation results in pulmonary hypertension.

Diagnosis

Diagnosis of CDH is often made on a prenatal ultrasonography and is accurate in 40-90%.

Polyhydramnios is present in 80% of pregnancies. USG diagnosis is suggested by fluid filled bowel loops in thorax, absence of stomach and other viscera in abdomen. Fetal USG can be misinterpreted with oesophageal disease, cystic lung bud anomalies. After birth symptoms are dependent on the degree of hypoplasia and hypertension. Classically, these infants have scaphoid abdomen and funnel chest. Most severely affected ones, present with respiratory distress at birth, whereas a large majority will present within 24 hrs. Diagnosis can be confirmed with plain X-ray abdomen. The location of gastric bubble can be confirmed by placement of an NG tube. Rarely a contrast study may be required. About 10-20% of infants may present late with mild respiratory distress, CPD, pneumonia, effusion, empyema or gastric volvulous.

Differential diagnosis includes eventration, anterior diaphragmatic hernia of Morgagni, oesophageal hiatal hernia, cystic disease of pulmonary parenchyma and agenesis of lungs.

Associated Anomalies

Cardiac anomalies may contribute to right to left shunt, pulmonary hypertension and circulatory instability in CDH. Hypoplastic heart and ASD are most common. Even in the absence of anatomic defects, left ventricular mass is decreased in patients with CDH. There is a significant reduction in post ductal PO_2 in patients with CHD so a low post ductal PO_2 should prompt a search for hidden cardiac defects.

Treatment Options

Though the mainstay of treatment is surgery, yet the prognosis depends upon the preoperative stabilisation and degree of hypoplasia of the lung. Thus many therapies have been explored to improve the survival.

1. Pulmonary Vasodilators

Numerous agents have been tried to treat pulmonary hypertension including Tolazoline, Prostacycline and inhaled nitric oxide.

2. Ventilator Strategies

a. Hyperventilation
b. Permissive Hypercapnia
c. High Frequency Ventilation
d. Liquid ventilation with perfluorocarbon

3. Surfactant

Patients with CDH may also possess a relative surfactant deficiency. This therapy still remains inconclusive.

4. Extracorporeal Membrane Oxygenation (ECMO) IN CDH

Since the introduction of ECMO in neonatal respiratory failure, its use in CDH has increased significantly. It is offered to infants with high risk of dying. It can be offered before or after surgery. It can be venoarterial or venovenous. If ECMO really improves survival, remained doubtful.

Fetal Surgery

Fetal surgery for CDH is controversial. The rationale for fetal intervention remains as compelling today as it was a decade ago. To answer the question, one must decide whether the benefit to an individual fetus justifies the risk to the life and future reproductive function of an innocent bystander, the mother.

Prenatal Selection

1. Gestational Age at Diagnosis

Bulk of data suggests early prenatal diagnosis as a poor prognostic indicator. If age at diagnosis is less than 24 wks, prognosis is uniformly bad.

2. Fetal Cardiac Ventricular Disproportion

There is now abundant evidence that in addition to pulmonary hypoplasia there is also cardiac hypoplasia. The pathogenesis is postulated to be either direct effect of compression or a secondary effect of altered haemodynamics. Aortic to pulmonary artery ratio is also predictive with a significantly larger ratio in survivors.

3. Lung to Head Circumference Ratio

Metkus et al reported that the single most predictive factor was the right lung area to head circumference ratio. Survival was 100% when this ratio exceeded 1.5 and 0% when it was less than 0.6.

4. Liver Herniation

The presence of left lobe of liver is a poor prognostic marker. If herniation is present survival is < 60%. So the patients diagnosed before 24 wks of gestation, with massive mediastinal shift, when associated with ventricular disproportion and liver herniation, have dismal prognosis. This is the population for which the best argument for fetal surgery can be made. Two techniques available are – in utero repair, in utero tracheal ligation.

Surgery

CDH is not a surgical emergency and preoperative stabilisation is a prerequisite. Deferred surgery has not in itself increased the survival rates but has helped in selecting survivors from non-survivors.

Trans-abdominal route is used because (1) easier reduction of viscera through abdominal route, (2) accurate visualisation of abdominal viscera and correction of any associated intestinal anomaly is possible, (3) accurate visualisation and repair of defect possible, (4) can enlarge is the abdomen by manual stretching and construction of a silo is possible. In case of a right-sided defect with only liver herniating, a thoracotomy approach could be used.

- Subcostal incision is given
- Gentle reduction of viscera is done
- Rolled up posterior margin of diaphragm is identified to release the posterior rim
- Closure of the defect is done in single layer, non absorbable suture starting medially
- For large defects synthetic mesh repair or muscle flaps could be used
- Additional procedures like Ladd's could be done if patient is stable
- Abdominal wall closure only after ensuring no respiratory compromise where only skin closure, patch repair or silo construction should be used
- Chest tube is placed under vision and kept clamped and used only if needed, although use of chest tubes is controversial
- The overall survival is around 60%.

OESOPHAGEAL ATRESIA

The incidence varies from 1 in 3000 to 1 in 4500. The improved survival of these neonates reflects the advancement in neonatal care and anesthesia over the years. The first successful primary repair is credited to Cameron Haight in 1941.

Embryology

The embryology of EA and TEF is poorly understood because no animal model of the malformation was available until recently. Now the new adriamycin model has shown great promise. Recent studies by Kluth suggest that the larynx begins to develop and the trachea and oesophagus simply grow and elongate side by side after the tracheobronchial diverticulum appears. Defects or failure in the mesenchyme separating the two structures or an aberrant position of either component, may explain most of the anomalies encountered. The events leading to this malformation are likely to occur between 4-6 weeks of fetal life.

Anatomy and Classification

Various classification have been proposed
The most simple and commonly used classification is by Gross who divides it into 7 types (Fig. 10.1).

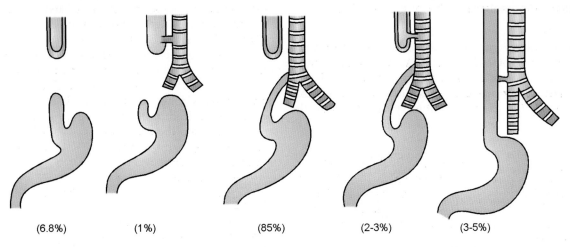

(6.8%)   (1%)   (85%)   (2-3%)   (3-5%)

Fig. 10.1: Gross classification for oesophageal atresia with tracheoesophageal fistula

a. EA without fistula (6-8%)
b. Upper oesophageal fistula with distal atresia
c. Upper pouch atresia with distal fistula (85%)
d. Upper and lower pouch fistula
e. H type (N type) tracheoesophageal fistula (3-5%)
f. Esophageal stenosis
g. Membranous atresia
   B, D, F, G comprises 3-5% of all these anomalies.

Clinical Features

- At birth, oesophageal atresia should be suspected when there is excessive salivation, with bubbling of mucus out of mouth and nose. The breathing is noisy because of overflow of pharyngeal secretions into the trachea. Episodes of cyanosis or choking may be present. If feedings are attempted, the choking and coughing will be aggravated.
- Fever, trachycardia, pallor and listlessness are late signs of pneumonitis with sepsis. With mechanical ventilation required, abdominal distension can develop rapidly, since there is free passage of air from fistula to stomach. Gastric rupture may occur particularly when obstruction of the stomach from duodenal atresia or malrotation is present. With a pure oesophageal atresia the abdomen is flat as no air can pass into stomach.
- Abdominal distension may be marked in a baby with patent distal fistula. However, the presence of a scaphoid abdomen in these neonates is strongly suggestive of a pure oesophageal atresia without a distal fistula.

Diagnosis

Antenatal

With improved obstetrical ultrasonography, the diagnosis can often be suspected in the fetus. Polyhydroamnios is present in nearly all cases of pure oesophageal atresia and 60% of cases with distal fistula. The fluid filled stomach, seen easily after sixtenth weeks of gestation, may appear smaller than usual or may escape visualisation, especially with pure oesophageal atresia. Polyhydroamnios and non-visualization of the stomach, of course, may also occur in conditions such as diaphragmatic hernia, facial cleft and others.

Postnatal

- An infant with excessive oropharyngeal mucus, choking spell, recurrent cough and dyspnea must have a chest X-ray at the earliest. The best examination is the 'babygram' – a radiograph of the whole body that includes the neck, chest, abdomen and pelvis. Just before the X-ray is taken, the mucus should be aspirated and air insufflated through the red rubber catheter. The upper pouch is then easily seen. The upper oesophageal pouch is sometimes better seen on lateral chest radiograph.

- The presence or absence of gas in the abdomen is an important finding. If no gas is seen, and an oesophageal obstruction has been confirmed by catheter, the diagnosis of pure oesophageal atresia can be confidently made, although rarely the distal fistula may be occluded.

- The plain film is also examined for the presence of vertebral anomalies; right sided aortic arch and signs of other anomalies like duodenal atresia, cardiac defect.

- The passage of a firm catheter (at least 8 French) through the mouth or nose into the oesophagus confirms the diagnosis. The catheter usually blocks at about 10 cm from the alveolar margins.

- Echocardiography is further recommended preoperatively to identify cardiac anomalies, which are present in 20-30% of the patients.

Associated Anomalies

They involve nearly every part of the body. Cardiovascular, musculo-skeletal gastrointestinal and genitourinary defects are most common. VSD, PDA and right aortic arch are most common of cardiovascular lesions. Imperforate anus, malrotation and duodenal atresia are the lethal anomalies of the gastrointestinal system. Among the genitourinary; hydronephrosis, renal agenesis, uterine or vaginal anomalies are most common.

Combination of anomalies is frequent and form various syndrome. These are VATER (or VACTRL) association, seen in roughly 10% of the cases. The eponym stands for vertebral defects, anorectal malformation cardiovascular anomalies, tracheoesophageal, renal and limb malformations. The CHARGE syndrome is much less common and has a more guarded prognosis.

Management

In the past many surgeons used the classification proposed by Waterston to establish treatment plan. Advances in neonatal care have affected the prognostic usefulness of the Waterston classification.

Preoperative Management

The surgical repair of EA is not an emergency and it is far important to stabilize the neonate and complete preoperative evaluation before taking up the baby for surgery. The preoperative care involves

1. Continuous or intermittent upper pouch low pressure suctioning. A replogle sump catheter is placed in upper pouch and connected to low pressure (< 5 mmHg) suction to avoid "Gas-steal".
2. The neonate is to be nursed in prone or lateral head up position.
3. Hypothermia is avoided using overhead warmer and keeping the handling of the baby to minimum.
4. The respiratory rate and saturation are monitored with blood gas parameters to assess the need for supplemental oxygen or ventilation.
5. Good intravenous access is established for intravenous fluids and antibiotics. Babies with pneumonia or sepsis may require 24-48 hours of antibiotics, chest physiotherapy and ventilation.

Operative Technique

The infant is placed in standard right posterolateral thoracotomy position. A subscapular muscle cutting incision is used.

Thorax is entered through 4th intercostals space.

The extrapleural dissection is done.

Azygous vein is divided between ligatures for better exposure.

Lower pouch is identified and looked up.

The fistula is ligated and divided. The closure is checked for air leak. The upper pouch is identified with the help of the anesthetist pushing down on a preoperatively placed tube in upper pouch. After adequate mobilization, a single layer, interrupted end-to-end anastomosis is done. The anastomosis is completed after passing a # 5 feeding tube through the nose across the anastomosis into the stomach.

Postoperative Care

The baby is shifted to ICU after extubation or with the tube in situ of elective ventilation is planned. With the anastomosis under severe lesion elective ventilation with paralysis and neck flexion may be of benefit. Tube feeds can be started 24-48 hours postoperatively with concomitant use of H_2 blockers and prokinetic agents. The postoperative dye study is carried out around one week following the repair to assess the anastomotic site for narrowing or leak and confirm the patency of distal esophagus. Feeds are started gradually after the dye study and progress slowly because of poor swallowing and sucking reflexes. The chest tube is removed and antibiotic discontinued. In the presence of leak the transanastomotic tube and drain is kept for 7-10 days and a repeat dye study is done to confirm spontaneous closure of leak.

Complications

A. Early

1. Anastomotic leak (5-50%)
    -   Incidental – small radiological leak, no symptoms
    -   Minor – saliva in chest tube but clinically well
    -   Major – mediastinitis, abscess, empyema, tension pneumothorax
2. Anastomic stricture 30%
3. Recurrent fistula (3-5%)
4. Swallowing incoordination: Aspiration

B. Delayed

1. Tracheomalacia
2. Gastroesophageal reflux (50-70%)
3. Motility disorder
4. Asthma, bronchitis
5. Scoliosis, chest wall deformities (Late)

Pure Oesophageal Atresia/Long Gap Atresia

There is no precise definition of 'long gap' atresia and the term is applied when the two ends of esophagus cannot be brought together with ease despite adequate mobilization. Some authors consider a gap of > 2 vertebral bodies

as long gap and > 6 vertebral body as ultra long gap atresia.
A. At the initial procedure
   1. Anastomosis under tension with or without elective paralysis/ventilation
   2. Tension relieving techniques – Myotomy (single, multiple, spiral)
   3. Flap technique
   4. Suture fistula technique
B. Delayed primary anastomosis (6-12 weeks)
   1. With bougenage – proximal, proximal and distal, electromagnetic
   2. Esophageal lengthening techniques – flaps, myotomy, lesser curve elongation (Scharli)
   3. Foker's technique to bring both ends together with sutures.
   4. Kimura's technique - serial extra thoracic lengthening of upper pouch.
C. Transmediastinal thread
   1. With or without thread
   2. Kato method
D. Esophageal replacement in newborns
   1. Gastric transposition
E. Diversion and Later replacement

Prognosis and Long-term Outcome

The decline in mortality associated with esophageal atresia is the major success story in the annals of pediatric surgery. The factors contributing to early mortality include those related to surgery, late presentation and inadequate transport, problems of prematurity, and associated anomalies. Mortality after discharge from hospital is less common but in the first year of life may be related to (1) congenital heart disease (2) recurrent pneumonia (3) tracheomalacia or gastroesophageal reflux (GER) related sudden infant death syndrome (SIDS).

INFANTILE HYPERTROPHIC PYLORIC STENOSIS

Infantile hypertrophic pyloric stenosis (IHPS) is a common cause of gastric outlet obstruction in infants. The prevalence of IHPS ranges from 1.5 to 4.0 in 1000 live births among whites but is less prevalent in African-Americans and Asians. It is more common in males with a male: female ratio of 2:1 to 5:1.

Although obstructing pyloric muscular hypertrophy is occasionally found in still borns, cases have been reported with intra-uterine gastric distension associated with pyloric hypertrophy. This disorder generally evolves during the first postnatal week and become clinically significant only after two to four or more weeks of life. For these reasons the entity should be considered acquired rather than congenital.

Anatomy and Aetiology

The appearance of the pylorus in IHPS is that of enlarged muscle mass measuring 2-2.5 cms in length and 1-15 cm in diameter. Histologically the mucosa and adventitia are normal. There is marked muscle hypertrophy primarily involving the circular layer, which produces partial or complete luminal occlusion.

There is genetic predisposition to the development of IHPS. In addition to the variability among races and clear male preponderance, there is an increased risk to the first born infants with a positive family history and certain ABO blood types, elevated gastrin levels, higher concentrations of neurotransmitter substance P and a decrease in nerve supporting cells in muscle layers have all been implicated in pylorospasm and muscle hypertrophy.

Clinical Presentation

The cardinal symptom is vomiting after 3-4 weeks of age. The initial emesis is mild but within one to several days, it increases in its frequency, its amount and its forcefulness until typical projectile vomiting has developed. Affected babies are usually vigorous and not obviously dehydrated. Although they remain hungry they begin to refuse breast or the bottle feeds as the stenosis becomes more severe. They continue to urinate until late in the course of disorder, but the stools are usually diminished in their number and amount.

About 20% of the infants begin to vomit shortly after birth. A second group has an abrupt onset of vomiting after the first weeks or two of life. The "Classical" history is that of increasing emesis at two to four weeks of age, in a first born male, seen in less than 20% of the cases.

Haematemesis is a symptom of variable frequency. The bleeding is oesophageal in origin due to erythema and friability of the distal one-third of the oesophagus.

Gastritis with gastric ulceration can occur late in the disease because of distension and stasis.

Jaundice is seen in a significant number of babies and is associated with depression of the enzyme hepatic gluconyl transferase.

Diagnosis

Nonbilious projectile vomiting, visible gastric peristalsis and hypochloremic hypokalemic metabolic alkalosis are cardinal features of IHPS. A definitive diagnosis can be made in 75% of the infants with IHPS by careful physical examination alone but this is becoming more of a lost skill. Frequently, imaging procedures are requested in lieu of careful physical examination. To be successful in palpating the pyloric olive, the infant must be calm and co-operative. The examiner should be ready to commit

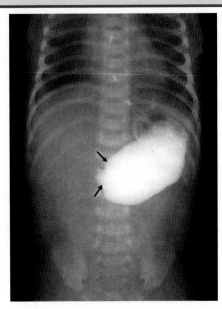

Fig. 10.2: Upper gastrointestinal tract contrast study in hypertrophic pyloric stenosis

5-15 minutes for proper examination. Examination with a pacifier or just after feeds could be more successful.

Ultrasonography is the most common imaging technique for the diagnosis. The commonly used criteria on ultrasonography include a pyloric muscle thickness of 4 mm and a pyloric channel length of 16 mm or more.

A barium upper gastrointestinal examination is highly effective in making the diagnosis. An elongated pyloric channel and two indentations at the distal end of antrum are suggestive of IHPS (Fig. 10.2).

Laboratory Studies

The classical findings in advanced pyloric stenosis are a raised haematocrit, an increased urinary specific gravity and severe hypochloraemic alkalosis. In severely depleted infants, the hepatic glycogen content is markedly reduced and serum glucose levels are precarious.

Differential Diagnosis

Medical conditions, which can be responsible for repeated emesis in small babies, include subdural haematoma, meningitis, adrenal insufficiency, milk intolerance hepatic enzyme defects, and other inborn errors of metabolism. Surgical causes include other causes of gastric outlet obstruction.

Initial Management

Most of the babies are severely depleted and must be treated vigorously. It is not essential that the pyloric obstruction be relieved immediately. The slow replacement of potassium chloride and sodium and the replenishment of glycogen and protein in the liver and muscles may require several days. A nasogastric tube should not be placed routinely because it removes additional fluid and hydrochloric acid from the stomach. The electrolyte replacement is based upon the well-known loss of K+ as compared to the Na+. An associated decrease in K+ in both the intracellular and vascular compartments will lead to the paradoxical renal excretion of the acid urine in the face of serum alkalosis. This is because ammonium and hydrogen ions are substituted for sodium and potassium in the urine when these are seriously depleted.

The preoperative fluid treatment of infants with pyloric stenosis requires maintenance fluids plus replacement of the estimated losses. Intravenous fluid resuscitation with 5% dextrose in 0.45 normal saline containing 20-40 mEq/L of KCl is the optimal solution for fluid and electrolyte replacement.

Surgical Treatment

The key to successful operation is the extramucosal operation of the pyloric muscle from near the pyloro-duodenal junction well onto the normal stomach.

Classical Pyloromyotomy (Ramstedt Operation)

The serosa on the anterior wall of the hypertrophied pylorus is incised with a scalpel from just proximal of the pyloric vein to the antrum just proximal to the area of the hypertrophied muscle.

Perforation during pyloromyotomy should be a rare event. If this occurs the submucosa should be approximated and a portion of omentum placed over the site. The pylorus should be rotated 180° and a myotomy done on posterior wall. Laparoscopy has also been described and is becoming more and more popular.

Postoperative Management

Most infants can be started on oral feeds 6-8 hours after surgery. If the duodenum has been entered and has been repaired, feeds are withheld for 24-36 hours. Vomiting occurs to some degree in 50-80% of babies after surgery. This is due to narrowing and edema of the pyloric canal. The main cause of vomiting however is GOR. A failed myotomy is very rare. No infant should be considered for re-operation until two or three weeks have passed.

MALROTATION

Anomalies of intestinal differentiation rotation and fixation are common, occurring in 1:200 to 1:500 live births. Although newborns and small infants are more likely to present symptoms from these anomalies, chronic abdominal problems or acute bowel obstruction resulting from malrotation are also seen in older children, adolescents and adults. The symptoms are often deceptive and the findings at operation confusing, unless the surgeon has a clear understanding of the embryology.

Embryology

Normal rotation and fixation may be described according to the way in which it affects the two ends of intestinal tract, the proximal duodenojejunal loop and the distal cecocolic loop. The intestinal development can be divided into eight stages.
1. Formation of straight intestinal tube.
2. Formation of body stalk (umbilicus).
3. Progression of duodenum into mesenchyme beneath intestine vessels.
4. Withdrawal of jejunum and ileum (preductal) intestine into abdomen on right pressing colon to left side.
5. Withdrawal of terminal ileum and caecum to sub-pyloric area.
6. Growth of abdomen, with ascent of liver and growth of ascending colon.
7. Migration of caecum and ascending colon to right gutter.
8. Fixation of mesenteries – ascending, descending colon and small bowel.

Malrotation in a Newborn

Persistent vomiting is the regular symptom. If emesis is due to rotational anomaly bile is almost always present. Diarrhoea with blood streaking or even frank haemorrhage, may occur as a result of mesenteric vascular congestion depending upon the time the vessels have been occluded. Abdominal distension and tenderness, toxicity and increasing pallor and cyanosis are progressive manifestations of sepsis gangrene of bowel.

Malrotation in Older Infants and Children

After early infancy, malrotation is more likely to present with irritability, recurrent abdominal pain, nausea, bilious vomiting and periodic abdominal distension. Small children manifest with failure to thrive from malabsorption due to longstanding lymphatic and vascular obstruction while other children develop chylous ascites. Large foul, fat containing stools are also characteristic of malabsorption.

Catastrophic volvulus is possible at any time of life. Young adults with unusual types of malrotation present with right lower quadrant pain, fever, tenderness and leukocytosis.

Diagnosis

Laboratory Studies

The usual laboratory studies are normal until prolonged vomiting or bowel ischaemia occurs. Children with volvulus develop haemoconcentration, high urinary specific gravity and leukocytosis. Since bacterial infection should always be anticipated. Therefore blood and urine cultures should be obtained before any operative procedure. Jaundice occurs readily and hyperbilirubinemia is usually present.

Radiologic Studies

X-ray of abdomen is of utmost importance in a study of any baby with bilious vomiting.

Plain X-rays can usually differentiate between high, middle and low intestinal obstruction. In malrotation the duodenum is partially or completely occluded, the stomach and duodenum are distended, and only small amounts of gas or contrast material are seen in the lower duodenum.

Examination of upper intestinal tract with contrast study is also important. In the usual case of malrotation the stomach and duodenum are found to be excessively distended. Some contrast may pass into jejunum but very little is seen in lower bowel. To exclude malrotation conclusively the duodenojejunal junction must be located to the left of spine at the level of the duodenal bulb in a position half way between the lesser and greater curvature of the stomach.

Ultrasonography has become very useful in detecting malrotation with midgut volvulous with a whirlpool flow pattern in the superior mesenteric vein and mesentery around a superior mesenteric artery; best seen on colour Doppler.

Treatment

Radiologically identified rotational anomalies (mixed) are known to produce serious sequel in 40-50% of cases. For this reason, these should be corrected whenever their presence is confirmed. The base of mesentry should be widened to avoid recurrence.

Preoperative

If malrotation has been identified by radiological analysis the determination must be made as to whether or not immediate operation is necessary. When there is simple obstruction, but no evidence of ischemia, nutritional evaluation and measures to improve the general state of infant should be undertaken prior to surgical exploration.

With volvulus the transvascular losses are accelerated. If the fluid losses have not been replaced and general circulation is already inadequate because of hypovolemia, severe hypotension may result intraoperatively. If there is any question of volvulous, rapid resuscitation and operative correction must be done expeditiously. Operations for malrotation often lead to shock because of unrecognized severe hypovolemia. A moderate degree of over hydration and a modest increase in normal expected blood volume are safety factors, which should not be neglected.

Surgical Technique

It is now agreed that Ladd's operation is the best treatment of almost all forms of malrotation. The temptation to fix the bowel in normal position with the cecum in the right lower quadrant and small bowel on its left side-should be resisted. Ladd's procedure consists of following steps, which should be carried out in proper sequence.

1. Evisceration of the midgut and inspection of mesenteric root.
2. Counter clockwise derotation of midgut volvulus.
3. Lysis of Ladd's peritoneal bands with straightening of duodenum along the right paracolic gutter.
4. Appendectomy widering the base of mesentry.
5. Placement of cecum in left upper quadrant.

When the intestine appears viable, simple Ladd's procedure suffice. A localized gangrenous segment, with ample remaining bowel, may be resected and primary anastomosis done.

A simple enterotomy is preferred when the bowel remains obviously ischemic at ends or with areas of marginal viability. Second look surgery is usually performed when there are multiple areas of questionable viability or when entire midgut appears nonviable.

Postoperative Care

Majority of infants can be expected to experience early return of gastrointestinal function. If there has been severe congestive ischemia, feedings should be withheld for one to two weeks. The antibiotics should continue for 7-10 days in an effort to eliminate bacteria, which may be sequestered in lymphatics.

Long-term Results

- Most authors report permanent cure of infants and children after operation.
- There may be pattern of abdominal pain in few children after Ladd's procedure. Although recurrent volvulus is unusual continued venous and lymphatic obstruction can certainly occur.

HIRSCHSPRUNG'S DISEASE

Hirschsprung's disease is characterized by an absence of ganglion cells in the intermuscular (Auerbach's) and submucosal (Meissner's) plexuses of the intestine usually the large intestine starting distally from Ano-rectum proximally, to a varying distance, leading to constipation.

The aetiology is unknown. The enteric ganglion cells migrate from the neural crest, along the course of the vagus nerves, to the intestine. The rectum is innervated by the twelfth week of gestation. The passive migration and neuronal differentiation appears to depend on the intercellular matrix.

The conventional theory is that migration is incomplete. Failure of ganglion cell precursors to differentiate and mature would result in similar findings. The distal aganglionic bowel remains tonically contracted and does not exhibit normal peristalsis.

At present two genes have been implicated in strongly increasing the susceptibility to Hirschsprung's disease, and doubtless others will come to light in the near future. The RET gene encodes a tyrosine kinase transmembrane receptor whose ligand is a neurotrophic factor. The manner in which the gene abnormality contributes to aganglionosis is unclear. Mutations of the RET proto-oncogene have been found in 50% of those with familial Hirschsprung's disease but were not related to the length of the aganglionic segment. The second gene, which has been implicated, is termed the endothelin-B receptor gene (EDNRB). This gene has been localised to chromosome 13q22.

The incidence of Hirschsprung's disease is 1 in 4,500 to 1 in 5,000. The male/female ratio is about 4:1, but this disparity diminishes to 1.5 to 2:1 with total colonic disease.

Associated anomalies include urological anomalies (2.2%), anorectal malformations and colonic atresia (4.5%), small bowel atresia (1%), deafness (2.2%) and cardiovascular anomalies (5.6%). Also included was Down's syndrome (2.8%).

An absence of ganglion cells in the intermuscular (Auerbach's) and submucosal (Meissner's) plexuses is the hallmark of Hirschsprung's disease. Thickened nerve trunks are seen in the intermuscular plane and in the submucosa. The length of the aganglionic segment varies.

The junction between ganglionic and aganglionic bowel is called the transition zone and usually corresponds to the area of tapering or coning between dilated and non-dilated bowel seen on X-ray or at laparotomy. With long segment disease however, false cones are known to occur so the gross appearance is not a reliable guide to the presence or absence of ganglion cells.

Histologically the transition zone is considered to show reduced numbers of ganglion cells and an increase in nerve fibres. The length of the transition zone varies from a few millimetres to many centimetres.

Clinical Presentation

About 94-98% of normal full term newborn infants will pass meconium within the first 24 hours of life. It is unusual for a normal baby not to have passed meconium by 48 hours. A history of delayed passing of meconium is considered a common feature of Hirschsprung's disease. The presence of abdominal distension is usual unless the baby has had a rectal examination or rectal washout. Bilious vomiting and poor feeding are also common.

The majority of infants who present within the neonatal period have signs of low intestinal obstruction - distension, bilious vomiting and little or no passage of stool.

Examination will reveal generalised distension, active bowel sounds and a narrow empty rectum on rectal examination. Withdrawal of the finger may be followed by passage of gas and meconium.

Plain abdominal X-ray will show many loops of distended gas filled bowel with typically, an absence of gas in the rectum. The differential diagnosis includes causes of low intestinal obstruction in addition to Hirschsprung's disease such as intestinal atresia, meconium ileus, small left colon and meconium plug syndromes.

The second type of acute presentation is with enterocolitis. X-rays show gross distension with thickened bowel wall.

The third and least common acute mode of presentation is with intestinal perforation. The risk of perforation is higher with total colonic disease; the perforation is usually in the aganglionic bowel. With short segment disease, the perforation is proximal to the aganglionic zone.

In older infants and children the history is of long standing constipation and distension, sometimes associated with failure to thrive. The clinical picture is of massive abdominal distension and marasmus and is managed with a combination of laxatives, suppositories and enemas but with only partial success.

Types

1. Short segment or Classical rectosigmoid- Involving rectal and rectosigmoid. Comprises 70% cases.
2. Long segment Hirschsprung's disease. Involving more than the classical segment, reaches upto descending colon
3. Subtotal Hirschsprung's disease. Involves upto mid transverse colon
4. Total Colonic Aganglionosis- involves entire large colon
5. Total intestinal Aganglionosis – extending to ileum and even jejunum.
6. Ultrashort segment Hirschsprung's disease – limited to distal 2-3 cm of rectum.

Initial Management

The management for those presenting with neonatal intestinal obstruction is the same as for any other form of obstruction - intravenous fluids, nasogastric decompression and consideration of antibiotics. If rectal examination produces gas and meconium then causes of complete mechanical obstruction, such as atresia, have been out-ruled. If no gas or meconium are produced after rectal examination then a single rectal washout with saline is performed. The aim is to establish if there is gas in the distal intestine to narrow the range of differential diagnoses. If there is no gas after the washout, a contrast enema is performed. This will show the colonic anatomy, may demonstrate the presence of a meconium plug or a small left colon, and if the contrast reaches gas filled intestine then intestinal continuity is confirmed. It is usual for children with Hirschsprung's disease to pass large amount of gas and meconium after a washout or a contrast enema and the infant's clinical condition will then improve.

If the presentation is with enterocolitis then urgent decompression is necessary. A rectal examination and rectal washouts are employed and are usually successful. Failure to decompress under these circumstances will indicate a need for surgery. If decompression is successful then surgery should be deferred until a time of greater physiological stability. All these children should receive oral Vancomycin as well as broad-spectrum intravenous cover.

For those infants and children presenting with a history of constipation, the need for urgent investigation is less pressing. Recourse to enemas and washouts will alter the appearance of the bowel on a contrast enema.

Diagnosis

There is no substitute for a tissue diagnosis. Reliance on contrast enemas or manometry is less secure and less accurate. Clinical impression needs confirmation.

Rectal suction biopsy has been proved satisfactory and reliable in the hands of expert pathologists Regardless of the method used, the biopsies should be taken from the posterior rectal wall, at least 25 mm above the dentate line. The bowel below this level is hypoganglionic and the failure to see ganglion cells may not be pathological.

Various methods of punch biopsy obtaining biopsies have been described. Suction biopsy instruments are widely used in young infants. Rectal biopsy may be followed by complications like bleeding and perforation.

Anorectal manometry assesses the relaxation of the internal anal sphincter in response to rectal distension. A failure of the sphincter to relax, or indeed an increase in tone, is a feature of Hirschsprung's disease.

Contrast enemas are widely used, both to make the diagnosis and to establish the position of the transition zone. Not infrequently contrast enemas are requested in the presence of intestinal obstruction in newborns to more clearly define large bowel anatomy. Subsequent to the enema marked decompression may be achieved and the infant's condition improved.

When specifically looking for Hirschsprung's disease the recommendation is to use 50% dilute barium sulphate. The irregular contracted rectum and distal sigmoid colon with a transition cone into dilated proximal bowel will be seen. With standard length Hirschsprung's disease the contrast enema appearance will usually correspond with the histological findings. With long segment or total colonic disease the appearance on the enema may not be reliable and false cones are known to occur.

A delayed X-ray film taken at 24-48 hours may demonstrate retention of contrast, lending support to a diagnosis of Hirschsprung's disease. The cardinal features included a transition cone, irregular bizarre contractions of the aganglionic zone and barium retention. However, high false positive rates of diagnosing Hirschsprung's disease by barium enema in infancy have been reported.

Ache Study Rarely Used

Operations:

- Staged (colostomy, pull through, colostomy closure)
- Single stage pull through (without colostomy)
- Laparoscopic assisted pull through.

Treatment

Once the diagnosis has been established there are many options for treatment.

The first decision is whether or not to bring out a stoma. Many infants can be managed for a weeks or months by means of daily saline rectal washouts. However, some children with extensive disease will not achieve satisfactory decompression by this means. If washouts are unsatisfactory then a stoma will be necessary.

The next consideration is where to site the stoma. For many years the approach to Hirschsprung's disease was a three-stage reconstruction - right transverse colostomy, pull-through at 6-9 months of age and colostomy closure some weeks later. Others have used a two-stage procedure - fashioning the stoma above the transition zone and then using the stoma as the apex of the pull-through. In many cases, a single stage reconstruction is safe and effective.

Single stage procedures can only be accomplished if reliable frozen section histology is available.

In attempting to define the length of the aganglionic bowel, biopsies may be sent from the apex of the sigmoid colon, distal descending colon, splenic or hepatic flexures and appendix of terminal ileum. Given the unpredictable anatomy of the transition zone it is unwise to take biopsies closer than at these intervals. In addition, each of these sites can be brought to the anus.

Three pull-through operations and their variants are in common use throughout the world and will be described here. These are the Swenson, Duhamel and Soave procedures. All are modified from the original descriptions but in each case the original concept is valid.

When performed by open operation the initial approach is similar for each operation. The patient is placed in semi-lithotomy position and a bladder catheter is inserted. Various incisions are used but it is essential to be in a position to dissect deep in the pelvis and this can only be achieved if the incision is close to the symphysis. A lower mid line incision is the most adaptable. The site chosen for the pull-through is chosen on the basis of histological evaluation either by frozen section or standard formalin-fixed tissue histology.

The Swenson operation entails dissection of the rectum from its attachments in a plane on the rectal muscle wall. The dissection may be commenced on the wall of the distal sigmoid or upper rectum. The dissection advances distally, dissecting the full circumference of the rectum. Deep in the pelvis it is important to remain close to the rectum on its anterior aspect. When the dissection has reached to within 2 cm of the dentate line anteriorly and 1 cm posteriorly this phase is complete. The distal extent of the dissection is judged by inserting a finger in the anus. At this stage the bowel is divided at the level chosen for the pull-through and the two ends sutured closed.

The anal phase of the dissection then commences. The apex of the dissected rectum is drawn out through the anus, everting the rectum. If the dissection has been adequate the anus may be partially everted. An incision is made from 9 to 3 o'clock anteriorly through the rectal wall, 1-2 cm above the dentate line. Only the bottom of the dentate line can be identified with any certainty and this is the point from where measurements are made.

Through this opening in the rectum the ganglionic colon is pull through with care to avoid torsion. The colon is opened at its apex and sutured full thickness to the cut edge of anorectum with interrupted absorbable 4/0 sutures.

The incision of the rectum is then completed in stages, as is the anastomosis.

Posteriorly in the 6 o'clock position the suture line should be about 1cm from the dentate line. The rectum is now free and should be sent for histological examination.

The commencement of the Duhamel procedure is identical. The early phase of rectal dissection is also the same. The dissection proceeds circumferentially until within 3-4 cm of the dentate line. This level is well below the pelvic peritoneum.

The anal phase then commences. It is best to partially evert the anus for this phase. This is easily accomplished by using tissue forceps at the 3 and 9 o'clock positions. An incision is then made along the dentate line from 4 to 8 o'clock and a retrorectal tunnel developed initially with scissors and then with a long clamp. This tunnel should quickly reach the level of the abdominal dissection. The tunnel is then widened to accommodate the pull-through bowel.

The previously divided and sutured bowel is then pulled through with care to avoid torsion. The open end is sutured to the anal incision with interrupted absorbable 4/0 sutures. Finally, the double wall between rectum and colon is stapled and divided with a linear stapler. Alternatively, a crushing clamp can be left attached.

Within the abdomen, the open end of rectum is then closed with a running extramucosal 4/O suture.

At the level chosen the muscle coat is divided with scissors circumferentially to enter the submucosal plane. This plane is then dissected with gauze pledgets or with artery forceps. The dissection is easier in young infants. The submucosal dissection progresses to a level about 1cm above the dentate line and the mucosal tube is then everted.

Once the dissection has been completed the mucosal tube is divided 1-2 cm above the dentate line and the ganglionic bowel is pulled through and sutured at this level. There seems little reason to perform the original Soave operation which left the pull through bowel outside the anus and most now perform the Boley modification. The catheter is usually removed after 24 hours and enteral feeding resumed once intestinal function is established.

In the presence of a defunctioning stoma a contrast study should be performed after two weeks. If the appearances are satisfactory the stoma may then be closed.

Complications

Surgery for Hirschsprung's disease is associated with all the usual complications that may follow major intestinal surgery. These include leakage, wound infection, dehiscence and postoperative bleeding. The early mortality was 3.3%.

Long-term complications include varying degrees of faecal incontinence, recurrent enterocolitis intractable strictures and fistulae.

ANORECTAL MALFORMATIONS

Anorectal malformations account for the most common congenital anomalies dealt by paediatric surgeons all over the world. To understand the present treatment options of the varied forms of this anomaly, it would be interesting to briefly go through the historical developments of the treatment options for anorectal malformations.

Although the absence of a normal anus was recognized by the Greek, Romans and Arabic physicians in ancient history, it was in the seventh century that Paulas Aeginata described a method of treatment by passing a bistoury through the perineum followed by dilatation with bougies. In 1710, the use of colostomy was described for these malformations.

Denis Browne described these malformations as high and low depending on whether the gut ended above or below the levator ani.

The aim of management is now from saving life to ensuring a normal quality of life. Management is now based on accurate scientific information and the surgery is performed by trained paediatric surgeons.

Embryology

The anus, lower rectum and urogenital system become differentiated between 5th –8th weeks of embryonic life.

The allantoic duct is in communication with the hindgut in a cavity known as cloaca, closed to the exterior by the cloacal membrane.

This cavity is divided by the urorectal septum into urogenital tract anteriorly and posteriorly by 2 processes. First there is the Torneaux's septum which stops its downgrowth at the level of the verumentanum or the mullerian tubercle. It is here that most rectourethral fistulas occur in the male. Below this point, the urorectal septum consists of an ingrowth of mesenchyme from a lateral direction that fuses in the midline. This is called Rathke's fold.

An ingrowth of mesoderm divides the cloacal membrane into the urogenital membrane ventrally and the anal membrane dorsally. The perineum is formed by a continued ingrowth of this mesoderm between the two membranes.

The urogenital portion acquires an external opening by the 7th week.

The anus develops by an external invagination, the proctodeum, which deepens to the rectum but is separated from it by the anal membrane. At the 8th week, the anus acquires an external opening by the rupture of the membrane.

In the female, the mullerian ducts which form the uterus and vagina descend in the urorectal fold long after the portioning of the cloaca by the urogenital septum so that the rectal fistulous connections usually occur in the vagina and not in the bladder or urethra as in the male. If the portioning fails to occur in the female, the mullerian ducts relentlessly descend on the undivided cloaca and carry through to the perineum. Thus, the rectum is carried along with the descent of the mullerian ducts to arrive at or very near the perineum.

The external sphincter muscle is derived from the regional mesoderm (although sphincter muscle fibres are present in all cases, there may be a good deal of variation in the size of the muscle bundle).

The puborectalis plays a key role in maintaining the angle between the anal canal and rectum and hence is essential for preservation of continence.

Incidence and Aetiology

The worldwide incidence of the anomaly is 1 : 5000 live births. The anomaly is more common among male infants (55-65%).

The exact cause is still unknown but these malformations are thought to be the result of arrests or abnormalities in the embryological development of the anus, rectum and urogenital tract.

Genetic predisposition has been seen rarely in some families. Sex linked and autosomal dominant inheritances have been suggested. Apparently there is no racial predilection.

Classification

There are two main classifications as given in Tables 10.1 and 10.2. Wingspread Conference Classification and Krickenbeck International classification.

Clinical Presentation

Local examination

The anomaly is usually characterized by the absence of anal opening at its normal site though a varied spectrum of anomalies is seen depending upon the extent of anorectal

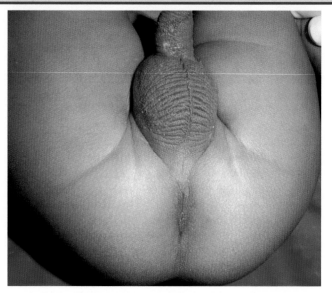

Fig. 10.3: Absent anal opening in a case of anorectal malformation

Table 10.1: Types of Anorectal Malformations (Wingspread Conference Classification)

Male	Female
1. HIGH	
Anorectal agenesis	Anorectal agenesis
(a) With rectoprostatic urethral fistula	(a) With rectovaginal fistula
(b) Without fistula	(b) Without fistula
(c) Rectal atresia	(c) Rectal atresia
Rare malformation (Rectovesical fistula)	Rare malformation (cloacal malformation)
2. INTERMEDIATE	
(a) Recto bulbar fistula	(a) Rectovestibular fistula
(b) Anal agenesis without fistula	(b) Rectovaginal fistula
(c) Anal agenesis without fistula	
3. LOW	
(a) Anocutaneous fistula	(a) Anovestibular fistula
(b) Anal stenosis	(b) Anal stenosis
	(c) Anocutaneous fistula

Table 10.2: International Classification (Krickenbeck - 2005)

Major clinical groups	Rare/regional variants
Perineal (cutaneous) fistula	Pouch colon
Rectourethral fistula	Rectal atresia/stenosis
- prostatic	Rectovaginal fistula
- bulbar	H-fistula
Rectovesical fistula	Others
Vestibular fistula	
Cloaca	
No fistula	
Anal stenosis	

agenesis and the presence or absence of associated genitourinary fistula (Fig. 10.3).

The key to successful clinical diagnosis in case of anorectal malformation is very careful examination, which may need to be repeated in babies seen only few hours after birth as it takes 12-18 hours for swallowed air to reach the terminal part of the colon.

The following tell tale signs should be looked for:

• Gross abdominal distension after 24 hours of life may be seen in a patient without fistulous communication or with a tiny fistulous communication with the genitourinary tract.

• Abdominal distension with redness over the abdomen in a sick baby could be due to perforation peritonitis in delayed presentations after 36 hours.

• Meconeum stain over the thighs is usually seen if carefully looked for in a case with fistulous communication.

• Frank meconurea is seen in a case of large fistulous communication with the bladder, as in cases of congenital pouch colon associated with anorectal agenesis.

• The anocutaneous reflex needs to be elicited.

• The perineum needs to be examined for presence of sacral agenesis which is usually associated with high anorectal anomaly, gluteal muscles and most importantly the bulge at the site of normal anal opening seen and felt on making the baby cry.

• Associated urethral anomalies in males like megalourethra, hypospadias, urethral duplication and congenital urethral fistula need to be identified.

Perineum

The perineum in a *normal neonate is convex and broad*, the anal opening is placed centrally within the sphincter complex and in males the median raphe is very faint.

In rectal atresia, the perineum is normal appearing.

In low anomalies in males, the perineum is convex and broad but the median anogenital raphe is hypertrophied across the perineum and scrotum. Meconeum bleb may be seen at the site of fistula and the anocutaneous tract may be seen filled with meconeum.

In high anomalies in males, the perineum is short or inconspicuous and the scrotum is in close proximity to the anal pit. The anal pit is covered by heaped up dermal mound of variegated appearance. The median anogenital raphe beyond the anal pit across the perineum is uniformly faint.

1. A visible abnormal anal opening

If there is a visible opening in the perineum near the normal site of anus, it has to be examined in detail carefully.

Anal Stenosis - The anal opening may be small and at the normal anal site. It may be covered by a bridge of skin resembling a bucket handle. Bowel of normal caliber is generally found close to the surface, but occasionally it may be higher up with a long narrow tract when named it is called anorectal stenosis.

Ectopic Anus - The anal opening may be sited anteriorly. In boys, it is generally found between the normal anal site and the posterior limit of the scrotum, but may extend anteriorly on the penile shaft. Rarely the anus may be located posteriorly in the midline. It may be in the midline or slightly deviated.

Anocutaneous fistula - The anal opening may be ectopic and stenotic and a meconium filled tract may be seen in the midline behind it. The meconeum may be milked out on applying pressure over the tract. On passing a bougie, it is felt almost horizontally backwards and bowel of normal caliber is usually found fairly close to the surface.

Rectoperineal fistula - The bougie in the visible opening passes more vertically and bowel of normal caliber is higher up.

In girls, the opening may be in the perineum, but is more commonly seen in the vestibule. The anatomy can be recognized in the same manner with the help of a bougie after identifying three separate openings in the vestibule.

Anovestibular fistula - The opening is in the vestibule and on passing a metallic bougie, it takes a posterior route towards the normal anal site and it can be felt percutaneously.

Rectovestibular fistula - The opening is in the vestibule and on passing a metallic bougie, it takes a cranial route towards the vagina and it cannot be felt percutaneously

Vulval anus - it is lined by mucosa anteriorly and by skin posteriorly.

However, there are shades of gray between the classical types in both sexes. Clinically, if the baby is symptomatic with straining at stools or remains constipated, the opening is inadequate and possibly a fistula exists requiring a preliminary colostomy.

2. No visible anal opening

In boys, the passage of meconium through the urethra may sometimes be noted. The bowel commonly terminates in either the prostatic or the bulbar urethra, but it may terminate blindly or at the bladder base. Thus the anomaly in males may be

a. ARM with rectoprostatic urethral fistula
b. ARM with rectobulbar urethral fistula
c. ARM with bladder neck fistula
d. ARM without fistulous connection

In girls, meconium may be seen emerging from the orifice of the vagina or of a common urethrovaginal canal or cloaca. The level of the terminal bowel can be established by ultrasonography, invertogram, CT scan and MRI scan as described above or by a lateral vaginogram or a cloacogram if there is a large fistula.

The anatomy of the pelvic organs of girls who have normal urethral and vaginal orifices is relatively easy to unravel, but if there is a common urethrovaginal canal, the anatomy can be bizarre.

If there are two openings in the vestibule the lesion may be:

a. Rectovaginal fistula which may be high or low
b. Anorectal agenesis without fistula
c. Anal agenesis without fistula

If there is one opening in the vestibule the lesion may be Rectocloacal fistula which may be high or low.

As mentioned earlier there may in both sexes be shades of gray between the classical types.

3. Rectal atresia

A normal anal opening without continuity with the bowel above.

Systemic Examination

Complete physical examination, including passage of a nasogastric tube to rule out an esophageal atresia should be done in all cases.

The abdomen should be examined for any palpable enlargement of the kidneys or bladder, other associated congenital anomalies like major cardiac malformations, major vertebral and craniocerebral defects and Down's syndrome.

It is possible today to exclude or confirm the presence of all these malformations in a reasonably short time by a careful clinical examination, ultrasonography including echocardiography, plain skiagram of the chest, abdomen and spine.

Associated anomalies which need to be identified before the baby is discharged include
(a) Obstructive uropathies and severe vesicoureteric reflux
(b) Ambiguous external genitalia and deformities of male and female genitalia
(c) Other renal, limb and ocular anomalies.

Investigations

The gold standard Wangensteen and Rice invertogram whether done in the standard head down position or the prone cross table lateral position is still the most widely used investigation of choice (Figs 10.4A and B). It is reliable only after at least 18-20 hours after birth as it takes this much time for the swallowed gas to reach the lower rectal pouch. Once filled with air or contrast, the blind rectal

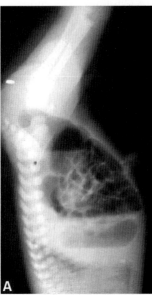

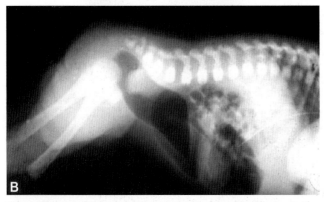

Figs 10.4A and B: (A) invertogram showing an anorectal malformation. Note marker at the anal pit (B) Cross table lateral invertogram showing an anorectal malformation

pouch is located in relation to the pubo coccygeal line or the I-point of Ischium. If the sacrum is poorly developed, the (P-C) line may be determined by commencing from the midpoint of the pubis anteriorly and transecting the junction of the upper and lower three quarters of Ischium (Figs 10.5A and B).

Supralevator lesions are identified when the blind rectal pouch ends above the P-C line (Fig. 10.6A). The bowel in intermediate lesions extends to a line drawn through the most inferior portion of the Ischium, parallel to the P-C line (Fig. 10.6B).

A gap of ≥ 1 cm between gas shadow and skin usually represents a high anomaly (A gap <5 mm usually represents a low lesion.

The level of the terminal bowel can also be determined by ultrasonography. The relation of the terminal bowel to the sacrum, the urogenital organs and the surface can thus be visualized.

A lateral X-ray taken after instillation of radio-opaque dye through a catheter in the urethra will delineate the terminal bowel if there is a relatively large urethral fistula. Voiding cystogram may be obtained to demonstrate a fistula, ureteral reflux, urethral stricture or connection between the ureter and vas deferens. This is usually not done in the newborn period as the main criteria to decide at that time is whether or not a colostomy will be required.

Table 10.3: Treatment plan for Intermediate and High Anorectal malformations

In Males:	Rectourethral fistula (bulbar and prostatic) – PSARP
	Recto-bladder neck fistula – AbdominoPSARP/ Abdominoperineal pullthrough
	Imperforate anus without fistula – blind end of rectum is located at same level as bulbar urethral fistula ! PSARP
	Pouch Colon – Abdominoperineal pullthrough/ AbdominoPSARP
	Rectal atresia and stenosis – The rectum and anal canal are usually separated by a few millimetre of fibrous tissue – Rectum is mobilized and end-to-end anastomosis performed.
In Females:	Anovestibular fistula – Anal Transposition/ASARP
	Rectovestibular fistula – PSARVP
	Rectovaginal fistula – PSARVP
	Rectal atresia and stenosis – PSARP and end to end anastomosis
	Pouch Colon –Abdominoperineal pullthrough/ AbdominoPSARP
	Persistent cloaca - < 3 cm common channel – PSARVP > 3 cm common channel (very high vagina)
	Abdominoperineal pullthrough with vaginal replacement or augmentation maneuver
	Small or no vagina – Vaginal replacement or augmentation manoeuvre
	Vagina may be replaced with a segment of bowel.

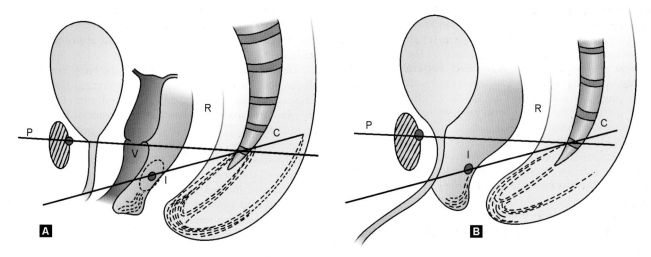

Figs 10.5A and B: A line diagram showing the conventional understanding of the pelvic anatomy in (A) Female and (B) Male, showing relationship of PC and P1 lines (I)

In cases that have undergone colostomy in the newborn period, a distal cologram is performed to delineate the fistulous communication.

The newer imaging modalities, namely CT scan and MRI scan are not really essential for managing a neonate, though their information is valuable in delineating the anatomy in complicated cases or those requiring a redo surgery.

Management

Low ARM

Perineal procedures can be carried out safely on all neonates with a very low lesion.

1. Anal stenosis. – Dilatations - Minimal stenosis can be cured by repeated dilatations.
   Y-V plasty - a posterior V flap of sensitive perianal skin is sutured into the posterior wall of the anal canal after this is opened up.
   Limited posterior sagittal anoplasty can achieve the same objective.
2. Imperforate anal membrane can be perforated easily.
3. A low anocutaneous fistula can be opened up by a cutback to the normal anal site and the operation completed as a Y-V plasty or a limited sagittal anoplasty.
4. Anterior ectopic anus - Anal Transposition
   - Limited PSARP (posterior sagittal anorectoplasty)
5. Vestibular anus- PSARP/ Anal transposition

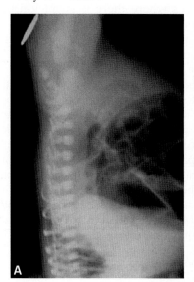
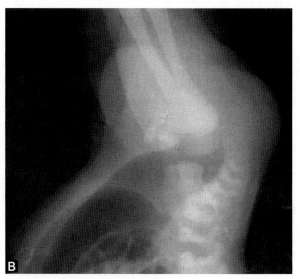

Figs 10.6A and B: Invertogram showing A) a high anorectal anomaly above PC line
B) an intermediate anorectal anomaly between PC and PI lines

Anal transposition. A circumferential incision is made around the opening; the bowel is separated posteriorly and laterally from the surrounding levator sling, and anteriorly from the posterior surface of the vagina until bowel of normal caliber is reached. Separation is easily achieved in the relatively low lesions but is difficult if there is a long tract adherent to the whole length of the vagina and dissection has to be continued up to the level of the peritoneal reflection.

ASARP- Anterior sagittal anorectoplasty dividing all the muscles between the posterior wall of the vestibule and the normal anal site strictly in the midline, and repairing the muscles after placing the bowel in the normal position have claimed equally good results.

Perineal fistula in both boys and girls is also similarly treated, namely by anal transposition or by sagittal anorectoplasty; the latter is more commonly performed. The procedure is generally easier but is difficult in boys who have a long perineal tract densely adherent to the posterior wall of the urethra; in these patients the dissection has to be continued up to the bladder base and the peritoneal reflection.

High and Intermediate Level ARM

Colostomy

It is usually performed as a first stage in a new born with high anomaly. Transverse loop colostomy is simple to perform and close loop stoma is suitable in neonates when early reconstruction and closure is contemplated. Author prefers a high sigmoid loop colostomy in newborns with ARM, but a right transverse colostomy for cases with common cloaca, so that the adequate distal colon is available for future pull through.

Colostomy should be urgently performed on the neonate who presents without a visible opening of the bowel, with low birth weight, with bilious vomiting and abdominal distension and with a life threatening associated anomaly. The colostomy should generally be done at the most proximal part of the sigmoid colon by a left lower quadrant incision. This loop of bowel is exteriorized and the site for colostomy is carefully selected. Both the limbs of the loop are approximated for about 2 cm, so as to form a dividing spur between the two loops. The cut margins of the peritoneum and the abdominal wall muscles are sutured to the seromuscular coat of the exteriorized colon; this is then opened and both loops are emptied of meconium. The mucosa of the bowel is sutured to the skin margins. The site of the colostomy has to be modified when there is associated pouch colon.

Anorectal Reconstruction

Posterior Sagittal Anorectoplasty (PSARP)

The description of the posterior sagittal anorectoplasty by deVries and Pena (1982) is a landmark achievement in the recent times to develop a new approach in surgery of this region. It is the operation of choice for almost all types of ARM cases. However, in cases of difficulty to achieve mobilization, an additional abdominal approach can be added.

The operation is performed with the baby in the knee-elbow position. The parasagittal and vertical fibres of the striated muscle complex are identified and stay sutures are placed to mark the anterior and posterior limits of the vertical fibers. The parasagittal and the posterior half of the vertical fibers are incised in the midline and the coccyx is split also in the midline. A right angle clamp is introduced into the presacral space. The levator ani is then exposed and incised in the midline. The rectal pouch is identified and opened. The urethral fistula if present is identified; a circumferential incision is made on the bowel mucosa around it and the fistula closed. The anterior wall of the bowel is then dissected until the peritoneal reflection is reached; the posterior wall is mobilized by opening up the retrorectal space. The fibrovascular bands are divided and the bowel can then be pulled to reach the normal anal site. It is sutured in place and the divided muscles repaired. Bowel tapering is optional. A urethral catheter is left in the bladder for a few days.

In girls without a fistula or with a rectovaginal or low rectocloacal fistula, a similar operation is performed.

An end-to-end anastomosis can be carried out through a similar approach for Rectal Atresia if the gap between the two parts of bowel is small (up to 1 cm).

Abdomino PSARP

It is done either in

a. Doubtful cases where one is not sure of finding the rectal pouch by PSARP route
b. In cases with higher level of fistula
c. In cases where there is suspicion of pouch colon preoperatively
d. As a planned procedure by some as they feel the anatomic postoperative location of the rectal pouch is better by this procedure.

In AbdominoPSARP, the first stage of the operation is done as for PSARP in prone position and then a red rubber catheter of adequate size as that of the expected rectal pouch is placed as a tunnel and the muscles are approximated around it.

The patient is then turned in the lithotomy position, redraped and a curved left lower abdominal incision is given. The bowel is identified, the fistula is divided and closed if not done earlier by the PSARP route. The bowel is prepared for pullthrough by dividing blood vessels in the mesocolon as necessary.

Abdominoperineal pullthrough

This is required for the high anorectal malformations as an alternate to PSARP. In lithotomy position, the abdomen is opened with a curved lower abdominal or suprapubic incision. The bowel is mobilized, the fistula is identified, divided and repaired. The bowel is prepared for pull-through by dividing blood vessels in the mesocolon preserving an arcade of vessels to maintain the blood supply of the mobilized loop.

The operation then shifts to the perineal route and an incision is given over the proposed anal site. Dissection is done strictly in the midline upto the peritoneal dissection. A tunnel is made between the urogenital organs and the levator sling and the bowel is pulled through to reach the normal anal site. The bowel is fixed in place by seromuscular stitches followed by mucocutaneous anastomosis taking care to avoid mucosal prolapse or retraction. It is also taken care that the anastomotic line is inverted inside the new anal opening so as to look like the normal lower end of the anal canal which is skin lined.

In girls with cloacal malformations, the urethral passage may be narrow and urine may accumulate both in the bladder and in the vagina; this urocolpos aggravates obstructive uropathy by external pressure on the ureters.

Continence

Good bowel control is usually achieved after correction of low anomalies in about 90% of patients. In case of high anomalies, it depends on the sacral, muscular and sphincteric development. After Pena's PSARP, the reported results of continence have markedly improved worldwide.

Summary

Anorectal agenesis has a varied spectrum of anomalies and each case should be examined carefully with a wide knowledge of the anatomical variations and identification of rare anomalies when encountered so that the best possible treatment option can be adopted to have the best continence results. In the author's experience, colostomy is performed in most neonates with ARM presenting after 48 hrs or so with distension of abdomen. However, if the baby is presented early and the distal bowel is not much dilated, we prefer a single stage PSARP in the newborn period without a covering colostomy.

NEURAL TUBE DEFECTS

The incidence of apparent neural tube defects also known as spina bifida aperta is approximately 0.8-1 per 1000 live births, but there is a wide geographical variation. A decrease in incidence has been noted as a result of improved maternal nutrition and antenatal diagnosis with elective termination.

Definition

There are three main types of spina bifida aperta.

Meningocoele: A meningocoele is a skin-covered lesion, which consists of cerebrospinal fluid, meninges and skin. There is usually no associated neurological deficits or hydrocephalus.

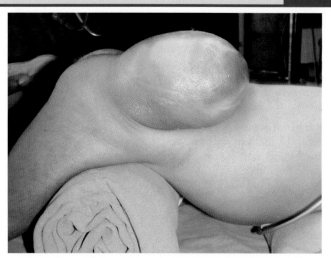

Fig. 10.7: Lumbosacral meningomyelocoele

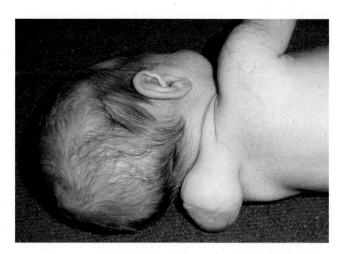

Fig. 10.8: Cervical meningomyelocoele

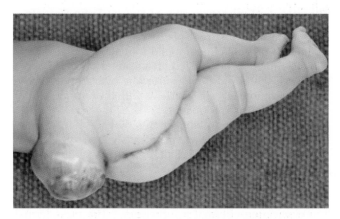

Fig. 10.9: Sacral meningomyelocoele with gross deficits; paresis, neurogenic bladder and bowel

Myelomeningocoele: A myelomeningocoele is a parchment membrane covered lesion that in addition to CSF and meninges also contains the neural plaque, which is usually an abnormal conus medullaris. Associated hydrocephalus is noted in 75-90% patients and neurological deficits are common (Figs 10.7, 10.8 and 10.9).

Rachischisis refers to a large neural placode with open central canal without any encasing meninges. It is usually associated with severe hydrocephalus and neurological deficits.

Embryology

The primitive streak appears at the caudal end of the embryo in stage 6 (Day 13-15) and elongates cranially. The Hensen's node is at the cranial end of the primitive streak. The epiblast cells migrate through the primitive groove and form the endoderm and mesoderm (gastrulation) during stage 6. As the primitive streak regresses the notocord is formed which has a central canal. The notocord induces the overlying ectoderm to form the neural plate, the lateral ends of which form neural folds that fuse in the midline to form the neural tube (neurulation - stage 8-12, 18-27 days). The formation of the neural tube starts from the cervical region and proceeds cranially and caudally. The anterior and posterior neuropores close at about 23 and 25 days of gestation respectively. The superficial ectoderm fuses in the midline and mesenchymal cells migrate between the neural tube and skin to form the meninges, neural arches and muscles.

By day 25, the caudal end of the neural tube blends into the caudal cell mass. Small vacuoles form in the caudal cell mass, which coalesce and eventually connect with the central canal of the cord by a process called canalization. The distal spinal cord then involutes (retrogressive differentiation) to form the filum terminale and the differential growth causes the conus medullaris to ascend. The conus lies at the L 2-3 interspace at birth and reaches the adult position (L1-2) by 3 months of age.

Theories on Embryogenesis of Neural Tube Defects

a. Simple non-closure: This theory postulates that the normal process of neural fold formation and closure is interrupted in a localized area leading to a NTD.
b. Overgrowth and nonclosure: The overgrowth of the neural epithelial cells interferes with the normal folding and neural tube formation.
c. Reopening: This theory states that the neural tube reopens after closure as a result of degenerative changes at the junction of the ectoderm and neural tissue.
d. Overgrowth and reopening: The overgrown dorsal caudal neural plate is exposed after normal closure has taken place.
e. Primary mesodermal insufficiency - The mesodermal defect is the primary event that leads to the neural tube defect.

Etiology

Etiologic factors implicated in neural tube defects include alcohol, drugs like Carbamazepine and Valproate, malnutrition and folate deficiency

Epidemiology

Myelomeningocele is the single most common congenital defect of the central nervous system. Relation with maternal age and nutrition, parity, seasonal variation and a host of other environmental factors have all been implicated as etiologic factors. The risk of recurrence is believed to be around 3-5%.

Prenatal Diagnosis and Prevention

a. Screening - Maternal serum AFP levels at 16-18 week gestation, if raised, suggests a neural tube defect but this test has a sensitivity of around 75% only and is not expected in skin covered lesions. Elevated amniotic fluid AFP and acetylcholinesterase measurement also suggests NTD but false positive results can be expected.
b. Fetal ultrasonography may visualize the spinal placode or splaying of the posterior elements or vertebral anomalies. Indirect signs of myelomeningocoele are more easily detected and include the banana sign (elongated appearance of the cerebellum secondary to the Chiari malformation) and the lemon sign (inward appearance of the frontal bones). The lemon signs detect 80% of NTD as compared to 93% with the banana sign. Ventriculomegaly (>10mm lateral ventricular atrium diameter) is usually more common after 24 weeks of gestation.
c. Up to 14% of fetuses with NTD detected in the 2nd trimester have associated trisomy 13 or 18 and therefore it is mandatory to do a chromosomal analysis prior to taking a decision regarding further management.

The risk of recurrence is around 1-3% and it is mandatory that mothers with one affected child be started on 5 mg/d of folic acid 3 months prior to a planned pregnancy. Prenatal repair of myelomeningocele in utero has been attempted to decrease the risk of neurological deficits as a result of trauma or amniotic fluid exposure.

Caesarean section or continuation of pregnancy is contraindicated in presence of chromosomal abnormality, associated anomaly, advanced hydrocephalus, flat lesion at or below plane of the back and absent knee and ankle movements.

Associated Anomalies in Myelomeningocoele

1. Hydrocephalus 80- 90%
2. Chiari Malformation
   Nearly 100%
   Clinically significant - 10-20%
3. Brain
   Micropolygyria
   Cerebellar dysgenesis

Corpus callosum agenesis

Cysts

4. Vertebral anomalies

Fusion defect

Hemivertebrae

Butterfly vertebrae

5. Scoliosis / kyphosis (30%)

6. Genitourinary

Undescended testes

Vesicoureteric reflux

Hydronephrosis

7. Club feet

8. Others - cardiovascular anomalies, cleft palate, congenital dislocation of hip, hernias

Clinical Assessment

- **Evaluation of the lesion**

a. Size, shape of lesion; presence of scoliosis / kyphosis; laxity of surrounding skin to plan surgery

b. Evidence of CSF leak or infection

c. Transillumination to assess the amount of neural tissue in sac

- **Evaluation of lower limb power, tone and reflexes**

a. There is usually flaccid paralysis with lumbosacral meningomyelocoeles. In cervical/ and some of the thoracic lesions there may be features of spasticity.

b. Deformities of the foot and evidence of flexion contractures.

c. Note grade of muscle power in limbs by stimulating upper abdomen or chest.

- **Evaluation of hydrocephalus**

Note the initial head circumference, fullness of anterior fontanelle, squamo- parietal sutural diastasis and 'setting-sun sign.'

- **Evaluation of lower cranial nerves and brainstem function:**

Look for regurgitation, difficulty in feeding, stridor, apnea, Hypotonia, which suggests a significant Chiari malformation

(Poor prognostic factor).

- **General paediatric assessment**

To rule our associated anomalies or chromosomal anomalies (club feet, Congenital heart disease, cleft palate, hernias, congenital dislocation of the Hips, genitourinary abnormalities).

- **Evaluation of the bladder/bowel**

a. Elicit the anocutaneous reflex and bulbocavernous reflex

b. Palpate for bladder/kidneys and check if bladder is expressible; note urinary stream. It is important to note that if one leg is normal, bladder function can be expected to be normal.

Clinical Examination and Investigations

Motor examination	Nerve roots
a) Hip flexion	L1-3
b) Hip adduction	L2-4
Knee extension	
c) Hip abduction	L5-S2
Hip extension	
Knee flexion	
d) Plantar flexion	S1

Investigations

1.	Ultrasound	- Sac
		- Head
		- Kidney
		- Post void residue
2.	CT/MRI	- CNS abnormalities
		- Hydrocephalus
		- Other vertebral anomalies
3.	Routine preop workup	

Counselling and Selection Criteria

The following factors help the surgeon in arriving at a decision and counselling the parents:

1. Age and general condition at presentation

2. Size, shape and level of defect

3. Presence of infection or CSF leak

4. Status of lower limbs and sphincters

5. Presence of hydrocephalus

6. Socio-economic status of parents and family history

The Parents are Explained Regarding

1. Prognosis in terms of ambulation, mental development and continence of urine and feces.

2. Need for shunt surgery in up to 75-80% cases with its associated complications and revisions

3. Need for urological and bowel treatment with repeated follow up and surgical intervention as needed.

4. Risk of surgery and chances of secondary tethered cord later.

It is important to understand that the parents should ultimately decide regarding the management, but it is the duty of the surgeon to give the correct picture in detail. Also, it must be remembered that not all untreated children die and may present later with a far worse neurological status. A few of them may require surgery of the large sac for better nursing care.

Preoperative Care

Besides maintaining normothermia and the standard neonatal care, these children have to be nursed prone. The lesion is covered with sterile and saline soaked dressings. A deep head ring may be helpful for nursing. Preoperative antibiotics are used routinely in anti-meningitic doses.

Principles of Operation

- Proper positioning, adequate intravenous lines, temperature control are vital.
- Use of bipolar coagulation and optical loupes are advisable.
- Sac mobilized from the skin and subcutaneous tissues and neck delineated.
- Central membrane and placode separated by sharp dissection from the sac. Cord detethered by dividing arachnoid adhesions and epithelial elements trimmed from the placode.
- Neural placode retubularized by 7-0 interrupted sutures on the pia-arachnoid tissues.
- Dura dissected from the sac and areolar tissue, closed with continuous 5-0 prolene or Vicryl.
- Third level closure using fascial flaps or preferably using the left over viable sac elements.
- Wide mobilization of the skin and subcutaneous tissues till the lateral abdominal wall (if necessary) and also superiorly/caudally.
- Closure of subcutaneous tissue (4th layer) and skin (5th layer).
- Tight barrier dressing.

Postoperative Care

- Routine antibiotics, nurse prone.
- Mannitol for 3 doses followed by oral diamox (50-100 mg/kg/day) the next day.
- Monitoring of head circumference and serial ultrasound for hydrocephalus.
- Watch for Chiari malformation complications.
- Monitor postoperative neurological status.
- CSF leak is managed by increasing diamox dose, and CSF shunting.
- Barrier dressing at all times to prevent infection.
- Monitor post void residue; institute Clean Intermittent Catheterization or anticholinergics early.
- Explain postoperative care; follow up protocols, physiotherapy, expected complications and long-term problems in detail.

HYDROCEPHALUS

Hydrocephalus is defined as a dilatation of the cerebral ventricles caused by a discrepancy between cerebrospinal fluid production and absorption.

The incidence of infantile hydrocephalus is around 3- 4 : 1000 live births. Congenital hydrocephalus comprises about one third of all congenital malformations of the nervous system.

Cerebro Spinal Fluid (CSF) Production

1. **Choroid plexus:** Eighty percent of the CSF is formed by the choroid plexus of the lateral, third and fourth ventricles by an active transport process across the endothelium of capillaries in the villus processes of the choroid plexus). Each villus is lined with a single layer of cuboidal epithelium and has a central stromal core. The apical tight junctions represent the blood-CSF barrier. Na-K ATP are located in the microvilli extrudes sodium ion into the ventricle which osmotically draws water along with itself. Na^+ transport is balanced by counter transport of K^+ and / or H^+ ion. Carbonic anhydrase catalyses formation of bicarbonate inside the cell, with the H^+ ion being fed back to the Na^+ transporter as a counter ion in exchange of K^+.

2. **Ependymal surface:** The ependymal surface is also believed to be a site of CSF production and may contribute up to 15-30% of the total CSF production.

3. **Brain parenchyma:** Intracerebral injection studies suggest bulk flow of brain interstitial fluid in white matter which is an important source of non-choroidal CSF production.

   Clinical studies have shown that the CSF formation rate is around 20 ml/hour in adults and the total CSF volume in the ventricles and subarachnoid space is approximately 150 ml.

CSF absorption

The rate of CSF absorption is pressure dependent and relatively linear over a wide physiologic range. CSF formation is independent of pressure whereas CSF absorption increases linearly after 68 mm H_2O pressure. Below 68 mm H_2O pressure there is no CSF absorption. The formation and absorption rates become equal beyond 112 mm H_2O pressure.

Site of CSF Absorption

1. Arachnoid villus
2. Brain capillaries
3. Choroid plexus
4. Lymphatic system
5. Nerve root sleeves

   With the single exception of choroid plexus papilloma that results in CSF overproduction, hydrocephalus results basically secondary to impaired absorption.

Classification and Aetiology

In the past, depending on the site of obstruction hydrocephalus was classified as (i) Non-communicating - Blockage of CSF pathway at or proximal to the outlet foramina of the fourth ventricle.
(ii) Communicating - Obstruction located in the basal subarachnoid cisterns, subarachnoid sulci or the arachnoid villi.

Anatomic Aetiologic Classification of Hydrocephalus

A. Obstruction of CSF pathways

Non-communicating	*Communicating*
1. Congenital	**1. Congenital**
• Acqueductal obstruction	• Arnold-Chiari malformation
• Atresia of foramen of Monro	• Dandy Walker malformation
• Dandy Walker malformation	• Encephalocoele
• Benign intracranial cysts	• Incompetent arachnoid villi
• Arnold-Chiari malformation	• Benign cysts
• Skull base anomalies	
• X-linked acqueductal stenosis in males	
2. Neoplastic	**2. Neoplastic**
• Choroid plexus papilloma	
• Medulloblastomas, ependymomas, craniopharyngiomas, astrocytomas	
3. Inflammatory	**3. Inflammatory**
• Infectious ventriculitis	• Infectious meningitis
• Chemical ventriculitis	• Subarachnoid hemorrhage
• Intraventricular haemorrhage	• Chemical arachnoiditis
B. Overproduction of CSF Choroid plexus papilloma	

Pathophysiology

The subarachnoid channels adjacent to the arachnoid villi represent the first CSF compartment to dilate and reduce CSF pressure. Subsequently with progressive dilatation of the subarachnoid channels, the increase in CSF pressure is transmitted to the venticular system resulting in ventriculomegaly. Ventricular enlargement causes displacement of primary cerebral arteries and a reduction in the calibre and number of the secondary and tertiary vessels causing diminished blood flow and ischaemia.

The effects of raised ICP on the developing brain include:
1. White matter atrophy.
2. Stretching and damage of ependymal epithelium with formation of ventricular diverticulae.
3. Spongy edema of the brain parenchyma.
4. Fenestration of the septum pellucidum and thinning of the interhemispheric commisure.

The atrophy involves primarily the axons, and neurons of the grey matter are selectively spared because of better blood supply. The previous view of using cerebral mantle thickness as a prognostic criterion in hydrocephalus is therefore losing favour.

Clinical Presentation

The signs and symptoms related to hydrocephalus depend on the age of the patient, causative factor, associated malformations or cerebral insult and the severity and progression of the disease.

Newborn and Infant

The infant with hydrocephalus presents with macrocrania, a bulging anterior fontanelle, poor feeding and lethargy. The infant may have sutural diastasis particularly the squamo-parietal suture. The other signs of hydrocephalus include scalp vein distention, Parinauds phenomenon (sun set sign caused by pressure on the tectal plate) and Macewen's sign (cracked pot resonance). The infant will have delayed milestones and difficulty in head control. Apneic bouts and bradycardia are usually associated with posterior fossa anomalies and are rarely seen in other causes of progressive hydrocephalus. During the first three months of life, normal head growth velocity is 2 cm/month. Head circumference more than 97th percentile for gestation age is suggestive of hydrocephalus. Transillumination can be appreciated in cases of hydranencephaly and in infants less than 9 months of age with cerebral mantle less than 1 cm. Cranial nerve palsies and stridor may also be seen in infants. The discrepancy between head and chest circumference may suggest hydrocephalus. Normally the head measures about 1 cm more than the chest circumference until late in the first year when it reverses.

Older Child

The inability of the fused cranium to expand means that older children usually have a more acute presentation and the triad of severe headache, vomiting and lethargy is commonly seen. Papilloedema is commonly seen in children unlike infants. Delayed motor and cognitive development and subtle behavioural changes are noted. A mild spastic diplegia with positive Babinski sign can also be elicited. The other indicators of hydrocephalus include decreased active leg motion, poor placing and positive support reflexes.

Differential Diagnosis of Macrocrania

1. Hydrocephalus
2. Subdural fluid — Hygroma / Hematoma / Effusion
3. Brain oedema
   • Toxic - Lead encephalopathy
   • Endocrine - Galactosaemia
4. Familial or constitutional macrocrania
5. Gigantism
6. Achondroplastic dwarfism
7. Leukodystrophy e.g. Alexander's disease
8. Lysozymal disorders
9. Aminoaciduria
10. Thickened skull e.g. Thalassemia, cranioskeletal dysplasias
11. Hydranencephaly

Imaging

The goals of imaging in hydrocephalus are:
1. Confirm the presence of hydrocephalus.
2. Evaluate etiology of hydrocephalus
3. Assess result of treatment and prognosticate in terms of long-term intellectual development.

Ultrasonography

Ultrasound is used in the presence of an open anterior fontanelle the relative ease and noninvasive nature makes ultrasonography particularly useful in evaluating the premature infant. It is also useful for follow-up screening.

Computed Tomography

CT scanning is the most commonly used imaging modality to evaluate macrocrania or signs of raised intracranial pressure. The cause and site of obstruction can usually be defined and with contrast enhancement tumours as well as vascular lesions can be visualized. Dilatation of the temporal horns is a sensitive indicator of raised intracranial pressure. The presence of periventricular edema or ooze suggests high intracranial pressure.

Magnetic Resonance Imaging

The axial, coronal and sagittal images available with MRI provide a more exact position and extent of the lesion. MRI can also locate small tumours in the upper cord and brainstem, which may be missed on a CT scan.

Ventriculography and Cisternography

Ventriculography is used for evaluating patients with suspected ventricular loculation and for mass lesions extrinsically compressing the ventricular system. The role of these investigations has diminished following the advent of MRI.

Other Diagnostic Studies

CSF evaluation: CSF examination for protein and cell content is important prior to shunt placement in post-meningitic hydrocephalus. Fat laden cells are indicative of brain damage in post infection states and can also be evaluated by CSF examination.

ICP monitoring: In infants the role of ICP monitoring is not clear and it has little predictive value regarding the progression of hydrocephalus.

Neuropsychologic evaluation: The child with hydrocephalus can exhibit problems with learning and development. Subtle changes in school performance or MPQ assessment may indicate progression of hydrocephalus or shunt dysfunction.

Cerebral blood flow and Doppler studies: Transcranial doppler flow studies and PET scanning have also been used for diagnosing and follow-up of hydrocephalous.

Trans systolic time (TST) is a new Doppler index used to evaluate intracranial pressure.

Fundus evaluation to assess severity of raised intracranial pressure.

Post-meningitic Hydrocephalus

Meningitis of bacterial (including tubercular) and nonbacterial origin is the most common cause of acquired hydrocephalus, which produces obstruction to CSF flow usually at the subarachnoid level. The incidence of hydrocephalus following meningitis ranges between 1-5%. Intrauterine viral infection with cytomegalovirus, rubella, mumps, varicella and parainfluenza are also responsible for congenital obstructive hydrocephalus of the non-communicating variety.

Post TBM Hydrocephalus

Neurotuberculosis constitutes almost half of the cases of childhood tuberculosis and TB meningitis is the commonest manifestation of CNS tuberculosis. The causes of hydrocephalus following TB meningitis include:
- Communicating hydrocephalus due to blockage of basal cisterns by the tuberculous exudate in the acute stage and adhesive leptomeningitis in the chronic stage.
- Non-communicating hydrocephalus caused by blockage of the aqueduct or outlet foramina of the fourth ventricle.

Post-haemorrhagic Hydrocephalus in the Premature Infant

Hemorrhage into the germinal matrix of the immature brain and extension into the ventricular system remains a major problem in premature neonates. Post haemorrhagic hydrocephalus is secondary to a fibrous thickening of the meninges with an obliterative arachnoiditis and obstruction of CSF flow through the normal subarachnoid pathways.

Diagnosis

Diagnosis is confirmed on ultrasonography or documentation of raised intracranial pressure. Post haemorrhagic hydrocephalus presents with - increasing occipito-frontal head circumference, tense anterior fontanelle, lethargy, feeding difficulty, bradycardia and ventilator dependency. The other manifestations include SIADH, persistent metabolic acidosis, abnormal eye movements and hypertonia.

Treatment

The communicating hydrocephalus resulting secondary to intraventricular hemorrhage can be managed by:
1. Serial lumbar punctures - Repeated lumbar punctures are done to relieve intracranial pressure as necessitated

by clinical or ultrasonological examination. Serial lumbar punctures have been reported to resolve post haemorrhagic hydrocephalus in selected cases in 1-6 weeks.

2. Acetazolamide (50-100 mg/kg/day) and furosemide (2 mg/kg/day) with careful electrolyte and acid base status monitoring.

3. Ventriculostomy/Valveless shunts

The recent use of flexible ventriculoscopes for irrigation, evacuation of blood or to lyse intraventricular septations may decrease the need for shunting.

Management of Antenatally Detected Hydrocephalus

The treatment of antenatally detected hydrocephalus has been tempered over the last decade because of various adverse factors:

1. The incidence of associated anomalies with antenatally detected hydrocephalus is reported to be as high as 81%. Moreover 20-40% of these anomalies can be missed on antenatal sonography.

2. The high rate of complications associated with the ventriculo-amniotic shunt and need for multiple revisions secondary to dislodgement and blockage.

3. Serial cephalocentesis requires multiple punctures and does not allow consistent reduction of intra cerebral pressure.

Recent studies have dampened the enthusiasm of treating antenatally detected hydrocephalus in view of the poor prognosis and ill-defined natural history of the disorder. It is now accepted that the overall mortality in foetuses with antenatally detected ventriculomegaly is around 70% while only 50% of the survivors show normal intellectual development.

Congenital CSF Anomalies of the Posterior Fossa

The restricted area of the posterior fossa with its vital contents and frequent aberrant anatomy poses a diagnostic and therapeutic challenge. The various anomalies seen are:

(i) Arachnoid and neuroepithelial cysts
(ii) Dandy-Walker malformation
(iii) Isolated fourth ventricle
(iv) Pulsion diverticulum
(v) Mega cisterna magna and ex-vacuo states.

Treatment

The goals in the treatment of hydrocephalus include:
• Decrease the intracerebral pressure to safe levels.
• Increase the volume of brain parenchyma to maximize the child's neurological development.
• Minimize the likelihood of complications, detect and aggressively treat any complications.

• Maintain the integrity of CSF pathways to prevent ventricular coaptation and preserve the potential for life without shunt dependency.

Medical Treatment

The medical treatment of hydrocephalus is not an alternative for shunt surgery but has a definite role in some clinical situations. The potential for spontaneous arrest of hydrocephalus exists in infants because of the linear increase in CSF absorption seen with increase in ICP. The four modalities of medical treatment of hydrocephalus are:

1. Removal of CSF

The rate of CSF production is around 0.02 ml/min in neonates and the total ventricular CSF volume varies between 5-15 ml. Serial lumbar puncture for CSF removal is indicated in (a) Hydrocephalus secondary to intraventricular haemorrhage in infants (b) Treatment of normal pressure hydrocephalus in adults. Meninigitis, vertebral osteomyelitis and hypernatremia are the potential complications of the procedure.

2. Decrease CSF production

(a) Carbonic anhydrase inhibitors - Acetazolamide is a potent inhibitor of carbonic anhydrase Furosemide is another agent used in inhibiting choroidal CSF production. Both the drugs can reduce CSF flow by 50-60% at sufficient doses. Acetazolamide is given in the dose of 50-100 mg/kg and furosemide at 1 mg/kg. Nearly all infants receiving acetazolamide at these doses will develop metabolic acidosis. Furosemide on the other hand causes metabolic alkalosis and nephrocalcinosis.

3. Decrease brain water content

Osmotic diuretics increase the outflow of water from the interstitial space into the capillaries. Osmotic diuretics are effective temporarily in reducing ICP but prolonged use can lead to a rebound effect with an increase in interstitial water. Isosorbide, mannitol, urea and glycerol are the common agents, which have been used.

4. Increase CSF absorption

Hyaluronidase, urokinase, streptokinase and tissue plasminogen activator have been used experimentally to lyse fibrin blocking the subarachnoid villi following haemorrhage.

Surgical Treatment

The decision to perform a CSF shunting procedure has to be taken with care. The risks involved in performing the procedure are low but the nature of complications associated with shunting are serious. There is a very variable course and progression of hydrocephalus and its effect on intellectual development. Studies have demonstrated that a cerebral mantle of 2.8 cm is adequate to achieve normal MPQ status in follow-up. It is believed that the goal for treating a child with hydrocephalus is to achieve a cerebral mantle of 3.5 cm by the age of 5 months. The indications for shunt surgery are:

1. Cortical mantle < 1 cm on initial radiological investigation or thinning of the cortical mantle on follow up.
2. Evidence of falling MPQ values on follow-up.
3. Evidence of papilledema and features of raised ICP like periventricular ooze on CT scan.
4. Head size > 2SD above normal at initial presentation.

Ventricular catheters are usually made of Silastic (silicone polymer) and have radio-opaque markings or barium impregnation for visualisation.

The proximal catheter is placed in the lateral ventricle ideally anterior to the foramen of Monro. Presently the peritoneum is the preferred receptacle for the distal catheter.

Four types of valves are currently available: Slit valve, Ball in cone valve, Diaphragm valve and Miter valve.

Ventricular shunt complications include:

(A) Common to all types of shunt
  1. Malfunction
     - Obstruction
     - Disconnection or fracture
     - Shunt migration
  2. Shunt infection
  3. Overdrainage
     - Slit ventricle syndrome
     - Subdural/Extracerebral CSF collections
     - Craniosynostosis
  4. Seizures
  5. Pneumocephalus
  6. Isolated ventricle syndromes
(B) Complications unique to vascular shunts
  1. Cardiac complications:
     - Mural thrombosis
     - Endocarditis
     - Cardiac arrhythmias

  - Cardiac tamponade secondary to right atrial perforation
  - Distal shunt migration and pulmonary embolization
  - Superior vena cava obstruction
  2. Pulmonary complications
     - Pulmonary thromboembolism
     - Pulmonary hypertension and cor pulmonale
  3. Shunt nephritis
(C) Complications unique to peritoneal shunts
  1. Inguinal hernia and hydrocele
  2. Ascites
  3. Cyst formation
  4. Intestinal volvulus and obstruction
  5. Bowel perforation, bladder perforation
  6. Intraperitoneal spread of infection and malignancy.

Long-term Follow-up Results

Mortality in hydrocephalus patients is usually related to the aetiology and associated conditions. Most published series report long-term survival rates of 50-90% in surgically treated patients. The natural history of untreated hydrocephalus is dismal and only 20% of patients survive till adulthood.

The best functional results after shunt surgery are obtained in infants below 5 months of age. The care of children with hydrocephalus requires a multimodality approach. Early treatment and regular follow-up can insure a favourable outcome in these children.

Acknowledgement

Some photographs in this chapter have been taken from Textbook of Neonatal Surgery Ed DK Gupta, MBD publishers, New Delhi 2000 with prior permission from the publishers.

BIBLIOGRAPHY

1. Newborn surgery. Ed. Prem puri. Arnold Publishers, London, 2003.
2. Pediatric surgery Eds. Prem puri and Michael hoellwarth, springer, germany 2006.
3. Textbook of Neonatal surgery, Ed. DK Gupta MBD publishers, New Delhi 2000.

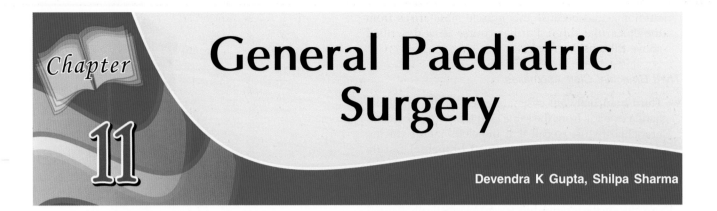

Devendra K Gupta, Shilpa Sharma

BRANCHIAL ARCH ANOMALIES

Phylogenetically the branchial apparatus is related to gill slits of fish and amphibians; hence the name 'branchial' derived from Greek for gills. Rathke in 1828 described the development of the pharyngeal arches in the human fetus.

Embryology

At the fourth week of embryonic life, the development of the branchial or pharyngeal arches contributes to the formation of various structures between the developing head and the heart (i.e. the face, neck, oropharynx, and the larynx). There are six branchial arches; the last two are rudimentary. Each arch has a bar of mesoderm. Caudal to each of the four arches is an internal pouch lined with endoderm. Externally is branchial cleft, lined with ectoderm. Between each bar, a branchial plate, composed of endoderm and ectoderm, separates the branchial cleft from the branchial pouch. The second arch grows caudally to join with fifth arch and, ultimately, covers the third and fourth arches. The buried clefts become ectoderm-lined cavities, which normally involute around week 7 of development. If a portion of the cleft fails to involute completely, the entrapped remnant forms an epithelium-lined cyst with or without a sinus tract to the overlying skin.

Pathophysiology

Branchial clefts 2, 3, and 4 fuse into one structure referred to as the cervical sinus of his created by downward growth of the overlapping second arch's ventral pole, which normally involutes completely. If a portion of the cleft fails to involute completely, the entrapped remnant forms an epithelium-lined cyst with or without a sinus tract to the overlying skin.

There are also few older theories to explain the origin of the branchial sinus. The "Inclusion Theory" suggests that the cystic alteration of cervical lymph nodes is stimulated by trapped epithelium derived from epithelial inclusions, brachial cleft, pharyngeal pouch and parotid gland. Another explanation is that it is as a result of recurrent tonsillitis and pharyngitis, leading to spread of squamous epithelium of pharynx via the lymphatic system to regional lymph nodes. Subsequent growth of this epithelium and cystic degeneration of the node forms the cyst.

Types and Features

First Branchial Cleft Anomalies

First branchial cleft cysts are divided into two types : I and II. Type I cysts are located near the external auditory canal. Most commonly, they are inferior and posterior to the tragus (base of the ear), but they may also be in the parotid gland or at the angle of the mandible. They may be difficult to distinguish from a solid parotid mass on clinical examination. Type II cysts are associated with the submandibular gland or found in the anterior triangle of the neck.

Second Branchial Cleft Anomalies

- The second branchial cleft accounts for 95% of branchial anomalies. Second branchial cleft remnants account for the majority of branchial cleft abnormalities. Anomalies can occur anywhere along an embryologically defined tract that extends from the external opening, the anterior border of the junction of the middle and lower thirds of the sternocleidomastoid muscle, passes between the internal and external carotid arteries superficial to cranial nerves IX and XII, and enters the oropharyngeal tonsillar fossa. However, these cysts may present anywhere along the course of a second branchial fistula, which proceeds from the skin of the lateral neck, between the internal and external carotid arteries, and into the palatine tonsil.
- Fistulas of the second arch would have an external opening at the anterior border of the lower third of

sternomastoid because this muscle mass arises from the epicardial ridge. Further course is as described above till tonsillar fossa.

Third Branchial Cleft Anomalies

- Third branchial cleft cysts are rare. A third branchial fistula extends from the same skin location as a second branchial fistula (recall that the clefts merge during development); however, a third branchial fistula courses posterior to the carotid arteries and pierces the thyrohyoid membrane to enter the larynx. Third branchial cleft cysts occur anywhere along that course (e.g., inside the larynx), but are characteristically located deep to the sternocleidomastoid muscle.
- A fistula formed from the third branchial arch has its external opening in the same area as the second branchial fistula. The tract passes deep to the platysma, ascending along the common carotid sheath, but this time passing behind the internal carotid artery. The tract crosses the hypoglossal nerve but will not ascend above the glossopharyngeal nerve or the stylo-pharyngeus muscle, which are third branchial bar derivatives. The tract is superficial to the superior laryngeal nerve that supplies fourth branchial bar derivatives. The internal opening is in the pyriform sinus, the area formed from the third branchial cleft.

Fourth Branchial Cleft Anomalies

- Fourth branchial cleft cysts are extremely rare. A fourth branchial fistula arises from the lateral neck and parallels the course of the recurrent laryngeal nerve (around the aorta on the left and around the subclavian artery on the right), terminating in the pyriform sinus; therefore, fourth branchial cleft cysts arise in various locations, including the mediastinum.
- Fourth pouch sinuses also arise from the pyriform sinus but in contrast they course inferior to the superior laryngeal nerve. Complete fourth branchial apparatus anomalies have never been conclusively demonstrated. Theoretically, because of their site of origin, fistulas or sinus tracts originating in this branchial region would loop around the right subclavian artery on the right or the aortic arch on the left, and course superiorly to the upper esophagus (Fig. 11.1).

Incidence

The exact incidence in the population is unknown. There is no recognised ethnic predilection or sexual predilection recognised. Branchial cleft cysts are the most common congenital cause of a neck mass. In 2-3% of cases it is bilateral. 75% arise from the second cleft, 20% from the first, and a few remaining from the third and fourth clefts.

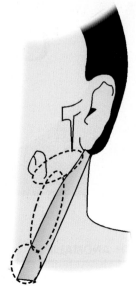

Fig. 11.1: Diagram showing the characteristic location for the outer opening and internal drainage for each of the first and second branchial cleft sinuses and fistulae

Presentation

Branchial cleft cysts are congenital in nature, but they may not present clinically until later in life, usually by early adulthood. Many branchial cleft cysts are asymptomatic. It commonly presents as a solitary, painless mass in the neck of a child or a young adult. A history of intermittent swelling and tenderness of the lesion during upper respiratory tract infection may exist, due to the lymphoid tissue located beneath the epithelium. Spontaneous rupture of an abscessed branchial cleft cyst may occur, resulting in a purulent draining sinus to the skin or the pharynx. Discharge may be reported if the lesion is associated with a sinus tract. Depending on the size and the anatomical extension of the mass, local compressive symptoms, such as dysphagia, dysphonia, dyspnea, and stridor, may occur.

Differential Diagnosis

- Lymphadenopathy - reactive, infective, neoplastic
- Vascular malformations
- Neoplasm
- Lymphatic malformation -cystic hygroma (Fig. 11.2)
- Ectopic thyroid tissue
- Ectopic salivary tissue.

Investigations

No investigations need to be obtained in the work up of a branchial cleft cyst but if there is doubt about the diagnosis radiological investigations are required.

- In cases of sinus or fistula, especially in third and fourth branchial anomalies, sinogram or barium

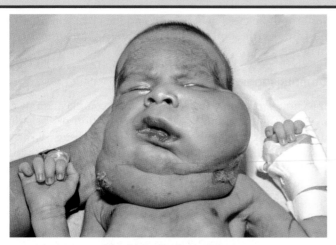

Fig. 11.2: Cystic hygroma

contrast study can delineate the course of the anomaly. Barium swallow should be performed after the resolution of acute inflammation in order to decrease the chance of false-negative results.

- Ultrasonography helps to delineate the cystic nature of these lesions.
- A contrast-enhanced CT-scan shows a cystic and enhancing mass in the neck. It may aid preoperative planning and identify compromise of local structures.
- MRI allows for finer resolution during preoperative planning. The wall may be enhancing on gadolinium scans.
- FNAC of the lesion can be done if there is doubt about diagnosis or high suspicion of neoplastic condition is present.

Histologic Findings

Most branchial cleft cysts are lined with stratified squamous epithelium with keratinous debris in 90% of cases, 8 % of them are composed of ciliated columnar epithelium; and 2% show both types of epithelium. Usually the lumen is filled with viscid yellow fluid character-istically containing large amounts of glittering cholesterol crystals. In a small number, the cyst is lined with respiratory (ciliated columnar) epithelium. Lymphoid tissue is often present outside the epithelial lining. Germinal center formation may be seen in the lymphoid component, but true lymph node architecture is not seen. In infected or ruptured lesions, inflammatory cells are seen within the cyst cavity or the surrounding stroma.

Treatment

Medical treatment: Antibiotics are required to treat infections or abscesses.

Surgical treatment: Surgery is indicated for branchial anomalies because there is a lack of spontaneous

regression, a high rate of recurrent infection, the possibility of other diagnoses, and rare malignant degeneration.
- Surgical excision is definitive treatment for this condition.
- A series of horizontal incisions, known as stepladder incision, is made to fully dissect out the occasionally tortuous path of the cyst.
- Surgery is best delayed until the patient is at least age 3 months.
- Definitive surgery should not be attempted during an episode of acute infection or if an abscess is present.
- Surgical incision and drainage of abscesses is indicated if present, usually along with concurrent antimicrobial therapy.

First branchial remnants are often closely associated with the facial nerve and external auditory canal. Identification and dissection of the facial nerve is a necessary step. Visualisation of the tract at operation may be aided by injecting into the fistula methylene blue dye or quick-hardening polymers. The dissection may be facilitated by prior catheterisation of the fistula.

Complications of Branchial Cyst

- Untreated lesions are prone to recurrent infection and abscess formation with resultant scar formation and possible compromise to local structures. Rarely squamous cell carcinoma arising in a branchial cleft cyst in adults is described.
- Complications of surgical excision result from damage to nearby vascular or neural structures, which include carotid vessels and the facial, hypoglossal, vagus, and lingual nerves.

Prognosis

- Following surgical excision, recurrence is uncommon, with a risk estimated at 3%, unless previous surgery or recurrent infection has occurred, in which case, it may be as high as 20%.

THYROGLOSSAL CYST

The thyroglossal cyst is a benign midline neck mass arising from the remnant of thyroglossal duct. The cyst is usually located at the midline of the neck. It is the most common congenital neck mass. It is found in 7% population. Majority of patients are less than 10 years old. There is an equal gender distribution. They are usually asymptomatic and the majority of them occur in close proximity to the hyoid bone. Over 60% of them lie just inferior to the hyoid bone at about the level of the thyroid cartilage.

Thyroglossal cysts result from the dilatation of a remnant or failure of closure and obliteration of thyro-glossal tract, which is formed during primitive thyroid descended from its origin at the base of the tongue the foramen caecum to its permanent location, low in the neck. This duct usually atrophies by about 10 weeks of development. The cysts are usually found between the isthmus of the thyroid gland and the hyoid cartilage, or just above the hyoid cartilage. Of interest, about 50% of the population has a pyramidal lobe of the thyroid, and the pyramidal lobe of the thyroid is the most common remnant of the thyroglossal tract.

Location

Thyroglossal cyst present in 5 different locations
1   Infrahyoid type accounts for 65% and is mostly found in the paramedian position.
2   Suprahyoid type accounts for nearly 20% and is positioned in the midline.
3   Juxtahyoid cysts make up 15% of cases.
4   Intralingual location occurs in approximately 2% of cases.
5   Suprasternal variety occurs in approximately 10% of cases.

Symptoms of Thyroglossal Duct Cyst

Thyroglossal duct cysts most often present with a palpable asymptomatic midline neck mass at or below the level of the hyoid bone. Some patients will have neck or throat pain, or dysphagia. Often, it presents with infection requiring drainage prior to excision or as a fistula following incomplete surgery.

On examination, the cyst rises as the patient swallows or protrudes tongue, which is the pathagnomonic sign of a thyroglossal duct cyst because of its attachment to the tongue via the tract of thyroid descent and attachment to laryngeal apparatus via suspensory ligament of Berry. Often, it presents with infection requiring drainage prior to excision.

Differential Diagnosis

The most common condition to be thought in the differential diagnosis is going to be the dermoid cyst, and next being the pretracheal lymphadenopathy, sebaceous cysts, lymphatic malformations and uncommon cysts or masses of the neck, like schwannomas and cysticercosis etc.

Histology

Histologically it is a well-defined cyst with an epithelial lining consisting either squamous or respiratory epithelium. Sometimes islands of thyroid tissue lying in the walls of these cysts may be seen and the cysts will usually be filled with some sort of mucous or mucopurulent material.

Complications

Infection is probably the most common complication. It is managed with antibiotics, needle aspiration or incision drainage. If incision and drainage is done it may complicate future management by generating thyroglossal fistula with scarring and creating abnormal tissue planes, making future dissection difficult.

Carcinoma is probably the most dreaded complication of a thyroglossal duct cyst. It is extremely rare and there is excellent long-term survival. Most of these are papillary carcinoma (80% to 85%). About 6% of them are follicular. There have been few cases of squamous cell carcinoma in thyroglossal cysts reported in literature.

Thyroid ectopia is found in about 10% of cases and usually it is going to be in the lingual area. Patient with a thyroglossal duct cyst with the ectopic thyroid tissue it may be their only source of functioning thyroid tissue. If a Sistrunk were done on this patient without knowing it the patient would then end up in hypothyroidism, leading to myxoedema coma.

Diagnosis of Thyroglossal Duct Cyst

Diagnosis is usually made clinically. Laboratory analysis includes a haemogram with total leucocyte count to rule out infection. Ultrasound is the gold standard for imaging and is done in almost every patient with this condition for diagnosis and to identify normal thyroid. FNAC is useful in diagnosis and to rule out other condition. Thyroid isotope scans and thyroid function studies are ordered preoperatively to demonstrate that normally functioning thyroid tissue is in its usual location.

Treatment for Thyroglossal Duct Cyst

Treatment options
•   The definitive treatment of a non-infected thyroglossal cyst is an elective Sistrunk operation
•   A thyroglossal cyst abscess requires drainage
•   An infected thyroglossal cyst without abscess should be treated with antibiotics and subsequently a Sistrunk operation is done.

Sistrunk's operation consists of excision not only of the cyst but also of the path's tract and branches. The intimate association of the tract with hyoid bone mandates simultaneous removal of the central portion of the hyoid bone to ensure complete removal of the tract.

The Sistrunk's procedure does have its fair share of major complications; although uncommon, they can be fairly morbid. Recurrence is by far the most common complication of doing a Sistrunk's procedure. Hypothyroidism can also occur, as already mentioned. Also fistulas can occur and can be quite morbid and difficult to deal with when they do occur. The other major complications are abscess, airway injury, tracheotomy, and nerve paralysis.

Prognosis

Recurrence occurs in approximately 3-5% of the cases and is increased by previous incomplete excision and a history of recurrent infections.

CLEFT LIP AND PALATE

Introduction

Cleft lip and palate is a congenital anomaly, presenting in a wide variety of forms and combinations. Cleft lip and palate are among the most common of congenital deformities. Cleft lip ranges from notching of the lip to a complete cleft, involving the floor of the nose, and may be associated with a cleft of the primary palate (alveolus/premaxilla), and with clefts of the secondary palate (hard and soft palate). Chinese physicians were the first to describe the technique of repairing cleft lip. Currently Millard technique of rotating the medial segment and advancing the lateral flap; thus, preserving the Cupid's bow with the philtrum is widely done.

Embryology

During the early stages of pregnancy, the upper lip and palate develop due to insufficient mesenchymal migration during primary palate formation in the fourth through seventh week of intrauterine life normally, as the face and skull are formed; these tissues grow towards each other and join up in the middle. When the tissues that form the upper lip fail to join up in the middle of the face, a gap occurs in the lip. Usually, a single gap occurs below one or other nostril (unilateral cleft lip). Sometimes there are two gaps in the upper lip, each below a nostril (bilateral cleft lip).

Etiology

What causes clefts is not known exactly, but most believe they are caused by one or more of three main factors: an inherited gene defect from one or both parents, environment exposure to any teratogenic agent like anticonvulsant drugs e.g. phenytoin, and sodium valproate, during pregnancy is associated with a 10-fold increase and is twice more in infants whose mothers smoke or consume alcohol during pregnancy (poor early pregnancy health or exposure to toxins such as alcohol or cocaine) and genetic syndromes like Vander Woude syndrome, Pierre

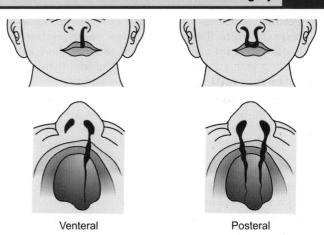

Venteral　　　　　　Posteral

Fig. 11.3: Cleft lip and cleft palate, facial clefts clefts drawing indicating the possibilities of oral and facial clefts

Robin and Down syndrome are associated with clefts of the lip and palate.

Classification

Veau Wardill categorised clefts into 4 major types (Fig. 11.3).
1. Clefts of the soft palate alone
2. Clefts of the soft and hard palate
3. Complete unilateral clefts of the lip and palate
4. Complete bilateral clefts of the lip and palate.

This classification does not provide a means of classifying clefts of the lip alone and ignores incomplete clefts. Kernohan stripped–Y classification describes the cleft of the lip, the alveolus, and the palate. In this classification, the incisive foramen defines the boundary between clefts of the primary palate (lip and premaxilla) and those of the secondary palate.

Incidence

The incidence of cleft lip is approximately 1 in 1000 live births. The incidence in the Asian population is twice as great but in the black population it is less than half. Male children are affected more than female children. Isolated unilateral clefts occur twice as frequently on the left side as on the right and are 10 times more common than bilateral clefts. Combined cleft lip and palate is the most common presentation (50%), followed by isolated cleft palate (30%), and isolated cleft lip or cleft lip and alveolus (20%). In 10% of cases clefts are bilateral.

Complications of Clefts

The complications of cleft lip and cleft palate can vary greatly depending on the degree and location of the cleft. They can include all or some or all of the following:

- **Feeding:** Problems with feeding are more common in cleft children; there can be nasal regurgitation or aspiration into airway. Special feeding devices or feeding with ink filler is advised. Children with a cleft palate may need to wear palate prosthesis.
- **Ear infections and hearing loss:** Cleft palate can affect the function of the Eustachian tube and increase ascending infection of middle ear which is a primary cause of repeated ear infections. Hearing loss can be a consequence of repeated otitis media.
- **Breathing:** When the palate and jaw are malformed, breathing becomes difficult especially when associated with Pierre Robin syndrome.
- **Speech problem:** Normal development of the lips and palate are essential to speak clearly. The causes of speech problem are incorrect lip pressures, tongue malposition, velopharyngeal incompetence, abnormal neuromuscular function, abnormal jaw relationships, abnormal dentition and secondary hearing loss due to otitis media. Speech therapy helps with language development after surgical repair.
- **Dental problems:** Cleft involving the gums and jaw can affect the growth of teeth and alignment of the jaw. Orthodontic appliance or bone graft surgery helps this problem. A defect in the alveolus can (1) displace, tip, or rotate permanent teeth, (2) prevent permanent teeth from appearing, and (3) prevent the alveolar ridge from forming.

Investigation

No investigation is needed for confirmation of diagnosis, as it is a clinical diagnosis. Hoemogram for anaesthesia purpose and throat swab is done for excluding beta haemolytic streptococci carrier state, which can cause disruption of postoperative palate wound by producing fibrinolysin. Cardiac evaluation, including echocardiography, if cleft is associated with cardiac anomalies.

Treatment

Aims of Treatment

Therapeutic goals to be achieved by primary surgery are restoration of normal anatomy, restoration of normal/near normal function, promotion of normal development resulting in satisfactory facial appearance, speech, hearing, and skeletal jaw relationships.

Timing of Surgery

- Cleft lip repair - between birth and 3 months
- Cleft palate repair - by one year of age
- Follow-up surgeries - between age 2 and late teen years.

Operative Procedures

For lip: (unilateral/bilateral, complete/incomplete) procedures including Millard, Delaire, Le Mesurier, Pfeiffer

and others are available. Millard introduced the rotation-advancement technique, which is the most commonly used method today for the repair of unilateral clefts. The technique preserves the Cupid's bow and the philtral dimple and improves nasal tip symmetry. The rotation-advancement lengthens the lip by means of a rotation incision that releases the medial lip element, allowing the Cupid's bow to rotate downwards into normal position. The lateral lip element is advanced into the gap created by rotation of the medial element, thus completing reconstruction of the upper lip (Figs 11.4A to D).

For cleft palate: One-stage or two-stage, methods of closure include Von Langenbeck, Veau, Kilner- Wardill, Delaire, Malek, Furlow and others. Cleft palate repair requires more extensive surgery and is usually done when the child is 10 to 15 months old. The principle of cleft palate surgery is an incision made on both sides of the separation, moving tissue from each side of the cleft to the centre or midline of the roof of the mouth. This rebuilds the palate, joining muscle together and providing additional length in the palate so the child can eat and learn to speak properly (Figs 11.5A and B).

Secondary Surgery: Secondary surgery should result in an improvement of the above, where the outcomes of primary surgery have been shown not to meet accepted standards. Secondary procedures like bone grafting, gingivo-periosteoplasty is done later for good cosmetics and function. Dental Care and Orthodontia help align the teeth and take care of any gaps that exist because of the

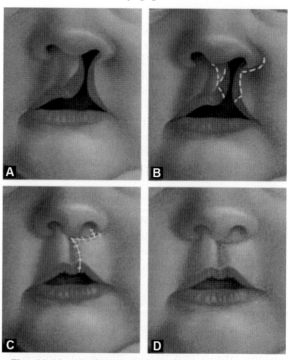

Figs 11.4A to D: Showing cleft lip repair before and after operation A, B, C and D

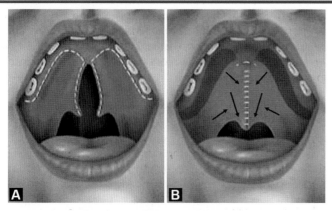

Fig. 11.5: Showing cleft palate surgery. Pre and postoperation moving tissue from each side of A and B the cleft to the centre or middle of the roof of the mouth

cleft. A child with cleft palate may have trouble speaking and can make the voice nasal and difficult to understand. Some will find that surgery fixes the problem completely. In children with velopharyngeal anomalies, surgical management includes revision of palatoplasty, pharyngoplasty, pharyngeal wall implant, palatal pushback, and Tonsillectomy/adenoidectomy in association with other programmed procedures. Shortly after the initial surgery is completed, the speech therapist will do complete assessment about speech and developing communication skills from 15 months of age. Emotional and social issues are to be considered and psychiatrist advice should be sought if needed.

Postoperative Care and Follow-Up

In the immediate postoperative period, feeding care, complete pain control, wound care is essential. Subsequently during follow-up in cleft clinics, assessment of outcome and consideration for secondary procedure should be made. Speech assessment and dental alignment are an essential part of programmed follow-up.

Complications of Cleft Surgery

Early complications

- Airway obstruction
- Bleeding/haematoma
- Wound breakdown
- Necrosis of tissues
- Nerve injury
- Damage to teeth
- Infection
- Formation of excess scar.

Late complications

- Abnormal dental occlusion
- Abnormal palatal morphology

- Oro-nasal fistulae
- Development of abnormal jaw relationships
- Poor acceptable function
- Abnormal facial balance
- Psychological and social problem.

Prognosis

The outcome is good for improved facial development, improved appearance, good psychological and social acceptance and favorable speech and dental alignment.

Prevention

Since little known about the cause of cleft lip and palate, the most sensible approach is simply to ensure a healthy pregnancy by avoiding teratogenic drugs, alcohol and smoking during pregnancy.

INGUINAL HERNIA AND HYDROCELE

It is the protrusion of the abdominal viscous into a peritoneal sac (the processus vaginalis) in the inguinal canal (Fig. 11.6). The contents of the sac are usually intestine but may be omentum, Meckel's diverticulum, and ovary and fallopian tube in girls. The incidence of paediatric inguinal hernia is between 0.8-4.4% [1]. The male : female ratio is 6 : 1. The patent processus vaginalis (without a hernia) is present in 80% of boys at birth, in 40% at 2 years and in 20% of adult men [2].

Conditions that may predispose to the development of congenital inguinal hernia include undescended testis, bladder exstrophy, ascites, ventricular peritoneal shunt, peritoneal dialysis, repair of exomphalos or gastroschisis, meconium peritonitis, cystic fibrosis and connective tissue disorders [3].

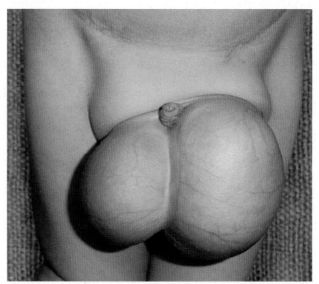

Fig. 11.6: Bilateral inguinal hernia

In children it is almost always an indirect inguinal hernia (hernial sac originating lateral to the deep epigastric vessels) unlike the direct one (medial to the same vessels) seen in adults. Most of the inguinal hernias are apparent and present before 6 months of age. However, many a times there is only a history provided by the parents of the swelling that appears in the inguinal region, especially when the child cries. The swelling disappears when the child is either calm or goes to sleep. A reliable history is usually enough to establish the diagnosis, though there is no evidence of such an anomaly when the baby is presented for examination.

Diagnosis

On physical examination, cough or cry impulse is the most important sign. A soft bulge that is reducible on digital pressure is also a diagnostic feature. Hernia in neonates may be transilluminant so it is not a very reliable test to differentiate it from hydrocele.

The spermatic cord may feel thickened or "rustle" on palpation, as the contiguous folds of the peritoneum slide over one another ("silk glove" sign). Confusion may occur if there is an undescended testis in the inguinal region. A hydrocele shows brilliant transillumination, is irreducible and its upper limit is identifiable distal to the external ring. On eliciting history, a hydrocele fills from below upwards while an inguinal hernia appears from above downwards. An encysted hydrocele of the cord may mimic as an irreducible indirect inguinal hernia, but can be distinguished by traction on the testis: the encysted hydrocele will move up and down while an incarcerated hernia is immobile at the external inguinal ring. Hydroceles have a light blue colour through the skin, while meconium peritonitis with meconium or blood in the processus will look black or dark blue. Neonatal hydroceles are rarely very tense, and the testis within can be felt or at least transilluminated, to confirm its normalcy. Other differential diagnoses include testicular torsion, lymphadenitis and torsion of the testicular appendices in which the blue dot sign is apparent at the upper pole of the testis. Needle aspiration is contraindicated in inguinal swelling for the fear of perforating the intestines.

Treatment

Once confirmed, inguinal hernias never regress and all inguinal hernias would need surgical repair as and when diagnosed. In the Western world, the premature infants with hernia are not discharged unless the hernia has been repaired, as the chances of incarceration are very high. For this, an expert Paediatric anaesthetist is required, as anaesthesia risks may be higher. Postoperative apnea is also, common in premature babies and at times may even require ventilatory support. In the developing countries, as the facilities for anaesthesia and the postoperative support for the premature babies and the newborns are very limited, hence all such babies should either be referred to a higher centre or the surgery be deferred till the risk of anaesthesia is low.

There should not be any undue delay in deciding in favour of surgery as the spontaneous disappearance of inguinal hernia does not occur, risk of incarceration is greater in infants, and the operation is simple with almost 100% success. However, the surgery is technically more difficult and the risk of injury to the vas and testicular vessels is greater in long-standing and incarcerated hernias.

Herniotomy

Herniotomy is performed through an incision in the lower most transverse inguinal skin crease. In neonates, the inguinal canal is not developed and the external inguinal ring lies over the internal inguinal ring so the incision is limited to the medial portion of the skin crease. The sac is identified after splitting the cremasteric muscles, the contents are reduced and the sac is transfixed high at the level of the internal inguinal ring. Herniorapphy (repair of the inguinal canal) is not required in children as the posterior wall is normal and strong enough. Bilateral repair can easily be done at the same time and should ideally be done in all patients presenting with bilateral hernias.

In infants under the age of one year, the contra-lateral sac is present in about 50% of cases. The issue of contralateral exploration in an ipsilateral hernia is debatable and the opinion varies from centre to centre. Direct inguinal hernia and femoral hernia require Cooper's ligament repair in addition to the ligation of the sac.

Irreducible Hernia

If not treated surgically, inguinal hernias are known to get complicated with obstruction and even strangulation. It occurs when the intestine gets struck at the internal inguinal ring. If it is prolonged, the blood supply may also get hampered to cause strangulation. There is a sudden increase in the size of the hernia with severe pain and the symptoms of bowel obstruction appear (vomiting and abdominal distension). On examination, a hard, tender and a fixed mass in the groin is palpable with increased bowel sounds on auscultation. It may be confused with the torsion of testis, acute inguinal lymphadenitis and tense infected hydrocele. The treatment for the obstructed (without vascular compromise) inguinal hernias includes:- an adequate sedation and administration of the analgesics to calm the baby, cold fomentation (to reduce the oedema and a gentle pressure is applied to reduce the hernial contents. It is contraindicated if the signs of peritonitis are present.

After reduction of the hernia the child should be admitted to the hospital and checked hourly to be sure that the damage to the intestine or testis has not occurred and also to reduce a recurrent incarceration promptly if it occurs. Herniotomy is performed preferably after 48 hours when the tissue oedema has subsided. In cases of irreducible and strangulated hernias, an urgent surgical exploration is mandatory.

Postoperative Complications

1. Scrotal swelling. Fluid accumulation may occur but it resolves spontaneously.
2. Ascending testis – iatrogenic undescended testis.
3. Recurrence rate upto 20% has been reported in incarcerated hernias.
4. Injury to the Vas deferens. This may be avoided by not holding the vas directly with the forceps and assuring its position during ligation of the sac.
5. Testicular atrophy. It may occur in incarcerated hernia.
6. Intestinal injury has been reported in association with incarcerated hernia.
7. Mortality may be related to prematurity and cardiac disease.

Hydrocele

It is formed due to the accumulation of fluid in the scrotum due to persistent communication *via* a patent processus vaginalis from the peritoneal cavity (Fig. 11.7). Rarely, it is secondary to epididymo-orchitis, tumour or torsion of testis. It is usually asymptomatic, but large sized hydroceles cause not only dragging pain but also likely to get infected. Trauma may also occur to the sac with formation of haematocele. In all such cases, the testis is not palpable separately. The upper pole of the swelling is easily reachable. It reduces gradually on lying down for long

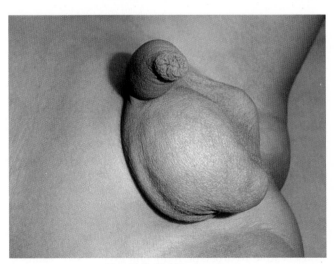

Fig. 11.7: Right hydrocele

and is transilluminant (hernia is a neonate may also be Transilluminant). There is no cough impulse present. Left sided hydroceles are more common as it takes longer for the left processus vaginalis to close down and thus it remains patent with the peritoneal cavity.

The condition needs to be differentiated from inguinal hernia and the underlying pathologies like tumours and torsion of the testis should not be missed. Spermatocele and varicocele are non-transilluminant, have worm like feeling on palpation and is separate from the testes.

Surgical treatment is rarely indicated as most cases would have spontaneous resolution as the child grows and the processus vaginalis closes. However, surgery is always indicated in all those cases of hydroceles that do not disappear by the age of 2 years, hydroceles that appear de-novo i.e. those which appear afresh in infancy and also those which are larger and symptomatic. The surgical procedure is a simple herniotomy (closure of the communication from the peritoneal cavity) as is done for inguinal hernia, with no attempt to excise the sac completely.

Bibliography

1. Gupta DK. Common Surgical Problems in Children. In. Text Book of Neonatal Surgery (Ed. D.K.Gupta) Modern Publishers, New Delhi. 2001, chapter 18, pp 109-117.
2. Gupta DK, Rohatgi M. Inguinal Hernia in Children: An Indian Experience. Pediatr Surg Int. 1993; 8:466-468.
3. Gupta DK, Sharma Shilpa. Common Inguinoscrotal problems in Children, in Recent Advances in Surgery, Vol 10, Ed. Roshal Lal Gupta, 2006 Chapter 8:147-161.

UMBILICAL HERNIA

An umbilical hernia is a abnormal protrusion of the abdominal lining, or abdominal viscera, usually the bowel loops through a congenital weakness in the area around the navel part of the intestine, and/or fluid from the abdomen.

The defect is caused by incomplete closure of the muscle of the abdominal wall at the umbilical ring, through which the umbilical blood vessels passed to provide nourishment to the developing fetus.

Incidence

The exact incidence is unknown, but may be as high as 1 in 6 infants. Low birth weight and premature infants are also more likely to have an umbilical hernia. Boys and girls are equally affected. Umbilical hernias occur slightly more frequently in infants of African American descent. The vast majority of umbilical hernias are not related to any disease condition. However, umbilical hernias can be associated with rare diseases, such as mucopolysaccharide storage diseases, Beckwith-Wiedemann syndrome, Down syndrome, and others.

Clinical Features

A physical examination reveals the hernia. Although often appearing at or just after birth, these hernias can also occur at any time during later life. The hernia generally appears as a soft swelling beneath the skin that often protrudes when the infant is upright, crying, or straining. Depending on the severity of the hernia, the area of the defect can vary in size, from less than 1 to more than 5 centimeters in diameter. Small (less than 1 cm) hernias usually close spontaneously without treatment by age 3 to 4 years. Those that do not close may require surgery.

During examination, the contents are reduced in a calm child and the defect is assessed by passing the finger tips into the umbilical ring. This is noted so that on follow-up the reduction in size of the defect can be appreciated.

In extremely rare instances, bowel or other tissue can protrude and become strangulated due to hampering of blood flow to a section of bowel and require emergency surgery.

Treatment

Strapping the umbilical hernia with a small tape over a suitable coin during the early months of life will cause the hernia to shrink and also disappear in 60% cases. Many umbilical hernias close spontaneously by ages 3 to 4. If closure does not occur by this time, surgical repair is usually advised. In younger children, only if the hernia is causing problems, enlarging, if there is an episode of incarceration or if the hernia is very large, surgical repair may be recommended. The decision for surgery should only be made after a comprehensive examination by a Paediatric Surgeon.

Surgery to repair the hernia is performed under general anaesthesia.

A small incision is made at the base of the belly button. If any intestine is present in the hernia, it is placed back into the abdominal cavity. The opening in the muscle is then repaired with multiple layers of stitches to prevent another hernia. A dressing is placed to keep the belly button flat.

While premature infants and children with certain medical conditions may require overnight observation in the hospital, most children are able to return home within a few hours after surgery.

Paraumbilical Hernia

A paraumbilical hernia is one that develops around the area of the umbilicus. After birth, although the umbilical cord disappears, the weakness or gap in the muscle may persist. Hernias can occur in this area of weakness at any time from birth through late adulthood, as the weakness progressively bulges and opens, allowing abdominal contents to protrude through. In addition to navel deformity and an associated bulge, the signs and symptoms include pain at or near the navel area.

Follow-Up

Once the hernia is closed, it is unlikely that it will reoccur. However, the risk of recurrence is increased in patients who have wound infections following surgery or associated connective tissue disorders.

INTUSSUSCEPTION

The disorder is characterised by telescoping of one of the portions of the intestine into a more distal portion, leading to impairment of the blood supply and necrosis of the involved segment. Of the three forms (ileocolic, ileoileal and colocolic), ileocolic is the most common. It is the most frequent cause of intestinal obstruction during the first 2 years of life.

Aetiologic considerations: The most common form is idiopathic and occurs classically between 4 and 7 months of age. A pathologic lead point may be found in only 2-8% of the cases, especially after 2 years of age. The predisposing factors include Henoch-Schoenlein purpura, Meckel diverticulum, parasites, constipation, inspissated fecal matter in cystic fibrosis, foreign body, lymphoma and infection with rotavirus or adenovirus.

Clinical Features

These include episodic abdominal pain, vomiting and rectal passage of bloody mucus. Fever and prostration are usually appearing 24 hours after the onset of intussusception and signify transmural migration across congested serosa. A sausage-shaped lump may be palpable in the upper abdomen in early stages. Rectal examination may show a cervix-Like mass and blood on the examining finger.

Diagnosis

Plain X-ray abdomen may reveal absence of bowel gas in the right lower quadrant and dilated loops of small bowel.

Ultrasound will show a target sign in upper abdomen or in left iliac fossa due to presence of intussuscetum within the bowel.

Barium enema may show the intussusception as an inverted cap or a claw sign may be seen. There is an obstruction to the retrograde progression of barium into ascending colon and cecum. In the area of intussusception, there may be a ceiling-spring appearance to the column of barium.

Treatment

Conservative hydrostatic reduction gives good results in a large majority of the cases, provided that there is no evidence of strangulation, perforation or severe toxicity. It is performed by insertion of an unlubricated balloon catheter into the rectum. The balloon is then inflated and pulled down against the levator ani muscles. Thereafter, buttocks are strapped together. From a height of 90 cm, barium is allowed to flow into the rectum. Under fluoroscopy, the progress of barium is noticed. Total reduction is judged from:

- Free flow of barium into the cecum and reflux into the terminal ileum.
- Disappearance of the lump,
- Passage of flatus and/or stools per rectum,
- Improvement in the patient's general condition
- Passage of charcoal, placed in child's stomach by the nasogastric tube, per rectum.

Surgical/ reduction is indicated in patients who are unfit for hydrostatic reduction or who fail to respond to hydrostatic reduction after 2 attempts.

Prognosis

Left unreduced, intussusception is invariably fatal. Spontaneous reduction with recurrent episodes is known in older children.

SURGICAL JAUNDICE IN CHILDREN

Yellow discoloration of the skin and the sclera of the eyes and body fluids due to increased level of bilirubin is called as jaundice. Jaundice is a common problem in paediatric age group. The common clinical problems are neonatal jaundice and viral hepatitis. Neonatal jaundice affects 60% of full-term infants and 80% of preterm infants in the first 3 days after birth. Although transient and self-limiting in most of the cases but some cases may be due to pathological reason. This section mainly aims to provide a bird eye view about the physiology of bilirubin metabolism, causes of jaundice in children and emphasis on the common neonatal surgical jaundice e.g. biliary atresia and its management.

Bilirubin Metabolism

Bilirubin, a by-product of the breakdown of haemoglobin (the oxygen-carrying substance in red blood cells), is produced when the body breaks down old red blood cells. Bilirubin is a by-product of heme catabolism. In the neonate, destruction of senescent erythrocytes accounts for 75% of the bilirubin produced. Almost completely insoluble in water, bilirubin must be bound to albumin for transport in the plasma. Bound bilirubin coexists with a small-unbound fraction determined by both the molar ratio of albumin to bilirubin and the binding affinity of albumin. Bilirubin is conjugated to glucuronic acid in the liver in a reaction catalysed by uridine diphosphate glucuronyl transferase (UDPGT). The bilirubin glucuronide, which is water-soluble, is secreted by active transport into the bile canaliculi and becomes concentrated in the gallbladder before excretion into the intestinal tract. In the intestine, some of the bilirubin glucuronide can be deconjugated to water-insoluble unbound bilirubin, which readily enters the entero- hepatic circulation. Deconjugation and resorption of bilirubin is minimal in adults, because of the action of intestinal bacteria, which progressively convert the bilirubin glucuronide into water-soluble stercobilins and urobilins that are excreted in the stool.

Physiologic Jaundice

Jaundice in healthy, full-term newborns has been termed physiologic because hyper- bilirubinemia occurs universally in neonates. Before birth, an infant gets rid of bilirubin through the mother's blood and liver systems. After birth, the baby's liver has to take over processing bilirubin on its own. Almost all newborns have higher than normal levels of bilirubin. In most cases, the baby's systems continue to develop and can soon process bilirubin. However, some infants may need medical treatment to prevent serious complications, which can occur due to the accumulation of bilirubin.

Total serum bilirubin concentration usually peaks at 5 to 12 mg/dL on the second or third day after birth. In newborns, the activity of UDPGT is limited because of immaturity of the liver enzyme system. At birth, the UDPGT activity level is only 0.1% to 1% that of the adult. Activity increases over time but does not reach adult levels until 6 to 14 weeks after birth. As a result, bilirubin accumulates. Infants lack intestinal bacterial flora, very little bilirubin glucuronide is converted to stercobilins and urobilins, with the result that both conjugated and unconjugated bilirubin are excreted as the golden-yellow pigment characteristic of the stools of the newborn. Jaundice should be considered non physiologic, or pathologic, if it occurs less than 24 hours after birth, if bilirubin levels rise at a rate of greater than 0.5 mg/dL per hour or 5 mg/dL per day, if total bilirubin levels exceed 15 mg/dL in a full-term infant or 10 mg/dL in a preterm infant, if evidence of acute haemolysis exists, or if hyper bilirubinemia persists beyond 10 days in a full-term infant or 21 days in a preterm infant. (However, mild breast-milk jaundice may persist for up to 2 weeks in breast-fed infants).

Kernicterus

Severe hyperbilirubinemia could result in kernicterus. This condition is characterised by bilirubin staining of the basal ganglia and involves diffuse neuronal damage, which results in severe neurologic sequelae. Kernicterus rarely occurs with unconjugated bilirubin levels lower than 20 mg/dL (340 μmol/litre) but typically occurs when levels exceed 30 mg/dL. When levels are between 20 and

Table 11.1: Guidelines for treatment of neonatal jaundice				
Age (hr) Total serum bilirubin level (mg/dL)	Consider phototherapy	Initiate phototherapy	Initiate exchange transfusion intense phototherapy fails	Initiate exchange transfusion
24-48	≥ 12 mg%	≥ 15 mg%	≥ 20 mg%	≥ 25 mg%
49-72	≥ 15 mg%	≥ 18 mg%	≥ 25 mg%	≥ 30 mg%
> 72	≥ 17 mg%	≥ 20 mg%	≥ 25 mg%	≥ 30 mg%

30 mg/dL, concomitant conditions such as prematurity and haemolytic disease may increase the risk of kernicterus.

Clinically, bilirubin encephalopathy progresses through three phases. In the first 2 to 3 days the infant is lethargic and hypotonic and sucks weakly. Progression is marked by hypertonia (especially of the extensor muscles), arching, opisthotonic posturing, fever, seizures, and high-pitched crying. In the final phase, the patient is hypotonic for several days and then gradually becomes hypertonic. Affected children have marked developmental and motor delays in the form of choreoathetoid cerebral palsy. Mental retardation may also be present. Other sequelae include extrapyramidal disturbances, auditory abnormalities, gaze palsies, and dental dysplasia.

Diagnosis

The initial diagnosis of hyperbilirubinemia is based on the appearance of jaundice at physical examination. The child is often placed by an open window so he/she may be checked in natural light. Blood samples may be taken to determine the bilirubin level in the blood.

Treatment

Most cases of newborn jaundice resolve without medical treatment within two to three weeks, because most often it is due to physiologic jaundice. It is important that the infant is feeding regularly and having normal bowel movements. If bilirubin levels are high, the infant may be treated with phototherapy exposure of the baby's skin to fluorescent light. The bilirubin in the baby's skin absorbs the light and is changed to a substance that can be excreted in the urine. This treatment can be done in the hospital and is often done at home with special lights, which parents can rent for the treatment. Treatment may be needed for several days before bilirubin levels in the blood return to normal. The baby's eyes are shielded to prevent the optic nerves from absorbing too much light. Another type of treatment used is a special fiberoptic blanket. There is no need to shield the baby's eyes with this treatment, and it can be done at home. Light emitted at a wavelength of 425 to 475 nm converts bilirubin to a water-soluble form that can be excreted in the bile or urine without glucuronidation.

Multiple factors can influence the effectiveness of phototherapy, including the type and intensity of the light and the extent of skin surface exposure. "Special blue" fluorescent light has been shown to be most effective, although many nurseries use a combination of daylight, white, and blue lamps. Recently, fiberoptic blankets have been developed that emit light in the blue-green spectrum. These are effective, convenient forms of phototherapy. The intensity of light delivered is inversely related to the distance between the light source and the skin surface.

Phototherapy acts by altering the bilirubin that is deposited in the subcutaneous tissue. Therefore, the area of the skin exposed to phototherapy should be maximised. This has been made more practical with the development of fiberoptic phototherapy blankets that can be wrapped around an infant. Double phototherapy can reduce bilirubin levels twice as fast as single phototherapy and can be accomplished by using the combination of a blanket and a bank of lights or by using two banks of lights. In rare cases, where bilirubin levels are extremely high, the baby may need to receive an exchange blood transfusion (Table 11.1).

Biliary Atresia

Biliary atresia (BA) is a rare disease characterised by a biliary obstruction of unknown origin that presents in the neonatal period. It is the most important surgical cause of cholestatic jaundice in this age group. The common histopathological picture is one of inflammatory damage to the intra- and extrahepatic bile ducts with sclerosis and narrowing or even obliteration of the biliary tree. Untreated, this condition leads to cirrhosis and death within the first year of life. Surgical treatment usually involves an initial attempt to restore bile flow: the Kasai portoenterostomy, which is performed as soon after diagnosis as possible. Later, liver transplantation may be needed for failure of the Kasai operation or because of complications of cirrhosis. BA remains the commonest indication for paediatric liver transplantation throughout the world. The reported incidence of BA varies from 5/100,000 live births.

Aetiology

The aetiology of BA remains unknown. Some cases seem to be related to abnormal morphogenesis of bile ducts occurring early in gestation, while others appear to arise as a result of later perinatal damage to normal developed bile ducts. The role of viruses has been extensively studied. An association of BA with cytomegalovirus respiratory syncytial virus, Epstein-Barr virus, and human papilloma virus has been reported, and alternatively, no association has been found with hepatitis A, B and C viruses. Reovirus type 3 can cause cholangitis resembling BA in mice and may be associated with spontaneous BA in the rhesus monkey. In human neonates, the association of reovirus type 3 and BA has been suggested in several studies but not supported in others. A strictly genetic cause is unlikely although familial cases of BA have been reported. Biliary atresia is associated with various congenital anomalies such as polysplenia, asplenia, cardiac or intra abdominal defects (situs inversus, pre-duodenal portal vein, absence of retro-hepatic inferior vena cava, intestinal malrotation).

Types of Biliary Atresia

- Type 1 Atresia limited to common bile duct (3%)
- Type 2 Gallbladder, cystic duct and common bile duct patent (25 %)
- Type 3 Complete extrahepatic biliary atresia porta hepatic (75%).

Clinical Features

The clinical triad of biliary atresia is jaundice (conjugated, and beyond two weeks of life), acholic (white) stools and dark urine and hepatomegaly. The general condition of the child is usually good and at least initially there is no failure to thrive. Later signs include splenomegaly (suggesting portal hypertension), ascites and haemorrhage (which can be intracranial, gastrointestinal or from the umbilical stump and is due to impaired absorption of vitamin K).

Investigations

Ultrasonography

On ultrasonography biliary atresia is suspected if the gallbladder is shrunken despite fasting, if the liver hilum appears hyper-echogenic ("triangular cord sign"), or if there is a cyst at the liver hilum. There should be no evidence of bile duct dilatation. Syndromic biliary atresia infants may show other features such as multiple spleens, a preduodenal portal vein, absence of the retro hepatic vena cava etc.

Hepatobiliary Scintigraphy (HIDA scans)

It demonstrates failure of excretion of the radioisotope into the intestine. Hepatobiliary scintigraphy using imino-diacetic (IDA) radiopharmaceuticals provides clinically useful information on the function of the biliary tract. Phenobarbital premedication (5 mg/kg per day for a minimum of 5 days in divided doses) is used in infants who are being examined for neonatal jaundice to increase the accuracy of 99 mTc-IDA scintigraphy in differentiating extrahepatic biliary atresia from neonatal hepatitis. Biliary atresia can be ruled out in an infant if a patent biliary tree is shown with passage of activity into the bowel. If no radiopharmaceutical is noted in the bowel on imaging up to 24 hours but with good hepatocyte function it is suggestive of obstruction of biliary tree. HIDA scan can rule out biliary atresia if there is excretion.

Magnetic Resonance Cholangiopancreatogram (MRCP)

MRI of the hepatobiliary tree gives idea about the anatomy of the biliary tree and identifies a choledochal cyst. It is non- invasive but availability and need for sedation for newborn is an issue.

Cholangiography

In the cases where the gallbladder seems normal on US scans, cholangiography is needed to assess the morphology and patency of the biliary tree. The cholangiogram can be performed by open operative technique.

Liver Biopsy

The main features suggesting BA are bile plugs, ductular proliferation, portal oedema and/or fibrosis. As in any other cause of neonatal cholestasis, giant cell transformation may be observed.

Other Tests

Biochemical liver function tests show cholestasis (with elevated liver enzymes and gamma glutamyl transferase).

Management

The current management of BA patients involves Kasai's operation, which aims to restore bile flow by excising the atretic extrahepatic biliary tree and anastomosing small bowel to the portal hilum to maintain bile flow. The important steps of the operation are after section of the falciform, left and right triangular ligaments; the liver is exteriorized out of the abdominal cavity. The entire extrahepatic biliary tree is excised together with the fibrous tissue situated inside the bifurcation of the portal vein at the level of the porta hepatis. A 45 cm Roux- en -Y loop is prepared and passed through the mesocolon to the liver hilum. An anastomosis is fashioned between the cut edge of the transected tissue in the porta hepatis and the antimesenteric side of the Roux- loop. A liver biopsy is performed. The following are the complications of biliary atresia as such and Kasai's operation.

Postoperative Complications

Early Postoperative

1. Fluid and electrolyte imbalance.
2. Bleeding diathesis.
3. Hepatorenal syndrome.
4. Absence of bile drainage.
5. Anastomotic leak.
6. Burst abdomen.
7. Persisting ascitic leak.
8. Hepatic encephalopathy.

Late Complications

1. Diet and nutrition problem.
2. Physical, mental and sexual dysfunction.
3. Pruritus.
4. Ascites.
5. Adhesive obstruction.
6. Anastamotic stricture.
7. Recurrent cholangitis.
8. Progressive cirrhosis.
9. Portal hypertension.
10. Hepatopulmonary syndrome and pulmonary hypertension.
11. Malignancies.
12. Progressive disease needing transplantation of liver.

Patients who present late with failing liver function or those who develop progressive liver damage after Kasai's operation need liver transplantation to save the life. Biliary atresia is the commonest indication for liver transplantation in children.

BIBLIOGRAPHY

1. Gastroenterology series of monographs and text books-extahepatic biliary atresia, Fredric Daum 1983.
2. Manual of neonatal care, fifth edition, year 2003, Lippincott Williams Company. Author: John P. Cloherty, Eric C. Eichenwald and Ann R. Stark.
3. Paediatric surgery third edition, year 2000 W.B. Saunders Company. Ed.Keith W.Ashcraft.
4. Text book of neonatal surgery, first edition, year 2000, Modern Publisher's: Ed. D.K. Gupta.

CHOLEDOCHAL CYST

Introduction

The term choledochal cyst is derived from chole - relating to bile, dochal - containing or receiving or duct, cyst - fluid collection. Choledochal cyst is considered as congenital problem of the bile ducts characterised by abnormal permanent cystic dilatations of the extrahepatic biliary tree, intrahepatic biliary radicles, or both.

The first script about choledochal cyst was published by Vater and Ezler in 1723. Douglas made first clinical report in a 17-years-old girl who presented with classical symptoms. Alonso-Lej et al. made detailed description of choledochal cysts in 1959. The classification system for choledochal cysts was further refined by Todani et al. in 1977 and currently includes 5 major types and it is followed till now.

Types of Choledochal Cysts

Depending on the location and type of choledochal cysts they can be classified into 5 types by Todani classification, which is described below.

- **Type I choledochal cysts**
  Constitute 80-90% of the lesions. It is characterised by dilatations of the entire common hepatic and common bile ducts or segments of each. They can be saccular or fusiform in configuration. In this form of abnormality, the gallbladder usually enters the choledochal cyst itself, which is really a dilated common bile duct. The right and left bile ducts and the ducts within the liver are usually normal in size in these instances.

- **Type II choledochal cysts**
  It is characterised by isolated protrusions or diverticulum (outpouching) that project from the common bile duct wall although the common bile duct itself is normal. They may be sessile or may be connected to the common bile duct by a narrow stalk.

- **Type III choledochal cysts**
  It is characterised by cystic dilatation of the intra-duodenal portion of the common bile duct. There is some degree of narrowing or blockage in the distal end of common bile duct (CBD). Another term used for these cysts is choledochocele.

- **Type IV choledochal cysts**
  It is characterised by dilation of biliary ducts within the liver and also outside the liver. There are two types of type IV choledochal cysts. Type IVA cysts are characterised by multiple dilatations of the intrahepatic and extra hepatic biliary tree. Most frequently, multiple cysts of the intrahepatic ducts accompany a large solitary cyst of the extrahepatic duct. Type IVB choledochal cysts consist of multiple dilatations that involve only the extrahepatic bile duct.

- **Type V choledochal cysts**
  This type is characterised by dilatation of the intrahepatic biliary radicals only with normal bile duct system outside the liver. Often, numerous cysts are present with interposed strictures that predispose the patient to intrahepatic stone formation, obstruction, and cholangitis. The cysts are typically found in both hepatic lobes. Occasionally, unilobar disease is found and most frequently involves the left lobe.

Aetiology

The aetiology of choledochal cyst in its various forms of presentation is not precisely known. However, the so-called "common channel theory" stands out as the most likely explanation. In almost all instances of choledochal cyst there is an abnormal arrangement of the pancreatic and bile duct junction in which the junction is high above the level of the muscle in the wall of the duodenum, which controls the direction of flow within these ducts. With an abnormal pancreaticobiliary duct junction, there is free-flow of pancreatic juice into the common bile duct extending up to the level of the liver. In the fetus, some of the digestive enzymes in pancreatic juice may damage the wall of the forming common bile duct resulting in duct dilation (enlargement) and a downstream blockage. The reason for the abnormal pancreaticobiliary junction seen in patients with choledochal cyst is likely to be based on genetic or hereditary factors. Additionally, choledochal cysts and bile duct abnormalities are much more common in oriental than in other populations, another suggestion that hereditary factors are involved. On the other hand, these abnormalities do not tend to run in families from one child to the next, so multiple factors must be involved. The large number of females is suggestive of a sex-linked genetic problem.

Clinical Presentation

It is common in persons of Asian ancestry, especially those of Japanese origin. Choledochal cysts are more prevalent in females. The female-to-male ratio is approximately 3-4:1.

Approximately 70% of paediatric patients with choledochal cysts have signs or symptoms related to the cyst before they are aged 10 years. A choledochal cyst may not become clinically apparent until the patient is an adult. In many adult patients, sub clinical bile duct inflammation and biliary stasis have been ongoing for years. Adults with choledochal cysts can present with hepatic abscesses, cirrhosis, recurrent pancreatitis, cholelithiasis, and portal hypertension.

The clinical history and presentation of a patient with a choledochal cyst varies with the patient's age. Overt dramatic signs and symptoms are more common in infancy, whereas manifestations are more subtle and protean in adulthood.

Infants frequently come to clinical attention with jaundice and the passage of acholic stools. These infants present with a clinical picture of complete bile duct blockage and jaundice. Numerous infants have been noted to have a choledochal cyst in utero on prenatal ultrasound, but following birth it appears that jaundice takes one to three weeks to become evident if this presentation occurs in early infancy, a work up to exclude biliary atresia may

be initiated. Infants with choledochal cysts can have a palpable mass in the right upper abdominal quadrant; this may be accompanied by hepatomegaly.

Children in whom the condition is diagnosed after infancy present with a different clinical constellation, which includes intermittent bouts of biliary obstructive symptoms or recurrent episodes of acute pancreatitis. Children in whom biliary obstruction is present may also have jaundice and a palpable mass in the right upper quadrant. The correct diagnosis is occasionally more difficult in children with pancreatitis. Often, the only clinical symptoms are intermittent attacks of colicky abdominal pain. Biochemical laboratory values reveals elevations in amylase and lipase levels. This leads to the proper diagnostic imaging work up.

The so-called adult form of choledochal cyst presents with frequent complaints of vague epigastric or right upper quadrant abdominal pain, jaundice, and occasionally a soft mass can be felt in the right upper area of the abdomen. Indeed, the most common symptom in adults is abdominal pain. A classic clinical triad of abdominal pain, jaundice, and a palpable right upper quadrant abdominal mass has been described in adults with choledochal cysts, although this is found in only 10-20% of patients. Cholangitis can be part of the clinical presentation in adult patients with biliary obstruction.

Complications

Choledochal cysts not appearing until adulthood can be associated with a number of serious complications resulting from long-standing biliary obstruction and recurrent bouts of cholangitis. Other complications include cholelithiasis, severe pancreatitis, hepatic abscesses, cirrhosis, and portal hypertension. The poor drainage causes infections in the bile duct in many patients. Some patients develop repeated attacks of pancreatitis since the pancreatic duct may enter into the bile duct with abnormal junction. If the cyst is not removed at the time of surgery then this exposes the patient to future development of bile duct cancer in the wall of the cyst. The most worrisome complication of choledochal cysts is cholangiocarcinoma. The reported rate of this malignancy in patients with choledochal cysts is 10-30%. The incidence of cancer in a choledochal cyst is twenty times greater than in the general population. 20% of the adult population with a choledochal cyst will develop cancer in a cyst if the cyst is not removed. By the age of 50 years up to 50% of patients will have cancer in the cyst.

Diagnosis

Blood Tests

No blood test is specific for the diagnosis of choledochal cyst; further studies indicate the status of the patient and any possible complications. Since the most common sign of a choledochal cyst is jaundice, the main finding is an increase in bilirubin in the blood. At times, in cases of severe cholangitis or long-standing biliary blockage, patients may show signs of a decrease in blood clotting.

Radiological Imaging

The only sure way to diagnose a choledochal cyst is some form of radiological study. As mentioned previously, prenatal ultrasound frequently identifies a choledochal cyst that may be present in the fetus. Immediately following birth, the most helpful initial screening study is abdominal ultrasound since this study is capable of showing the entire bile duct system within and outside the liver, the gallbladder, and the pancreas.

Most people feel that in the newborn with jaundice and an enlarged biliary tree outside the liver shown on ultrasound, no further diagnostic studies are required preoperatively. In addition to ultrasound examination in the newborn, some physicians also like to obtain a nuclear medicine scan or a CT-scan.

Because of the subtle clinical presentation of most older children, this age group may require additional studies, particularly because of the intermittent nature of jaundice seen in this age group. In older patients, injections of the bile duct system with dye (contrast) either through the skin or by means of a scope placed in the duodenum while performing X-rays or special MRI techniques may be needed.

In addition to demonstrating the common channel frequently seen in these patients, these studies are particularly useful for defining the precise anatomy so that planning an appropriate operation can be undertaken. At the time of an operation, X-rays using a contrast injection directly into the bile duct system (operative cholangiogram) are usually performed in order to confirm all of the preoperative findings. It usually does not take very long to obtain all of the preoperative information necessary to plan operative correction. While diagnostic studies are being accumulated, measures are undertaken to make sure the patient is in the best possible preoperative condition. Antibiotics are usually a part of this preparation.

Ultrasound is noninvasive, it involves no radiation exposure, and its findings are sensitive and specific for the diagnosis. Patients with choledochal cysts most often have symptoms referable to the hepatobiliary system, and most US operators are familiar with the anatomy of this area.

Abdominal US findings can help in detecting associated conditions and complications of choledochal cysts, such as choledocholithiasis, intrahepatic biliary dilatation, portal vein thrombosis, gallbladder or biliary neoplasms, pancreatitis, and hepatic abscesses; other supportive studies may be ordered, including abdominal CT, magnetic resonance imaging (MRI), or magnetic resonance cholangiopancreatographic (MRCP) examinations. These studies demonstrate the cyst with more precise anatomic detail. In addition, important anatomic relationships to surrounding structures are better defined than with other modalities (Fig. 11.8).

CT-scans of a choledochal cyst demonstrate a dilatated cystic mass with clearly defined walls, which is separate from the gallbladder. The fact that this mass arises from or actually is the extrahepatic bile duct usually is clear from its location and its relationships to surrounding structures. The cyst is typically filled with bile, which produces water-like attenuation. Depending on the patient's age and clinical history, the wall of the cyst can appear thickened, especially if multiple episodes of inflammation and cholangitis have occurred.

Use of MRI and MRCP techniques is increasing dramatically for the noninvasive diagnosis of biliary and pancreatic diseases. Choledochal cysts are no exception. These cysts appear as large fusiform or saccular masses that may be extrahepatic, intrahepatic, or both, depending on the type of cyst. They produce a particularly strong signal on T2-weighted images. Associated anomalies of the pancreatic duct, its junction with the common bile duct, and the long common channel formed by the 2 are usually well demonstrated on MRI/MRCP images.

Hepatobiliary scintigraphic modalities are used commonly in the setting of acute cholecystitis and in the investigation of neonatal jaundice. In addition, these techniques are useful in the diagnosis of choledochal cysts (Fig. 11.9).

Nonvisualization of the gallbladder in children is not necessarily indicative of acute cholecystitis and that

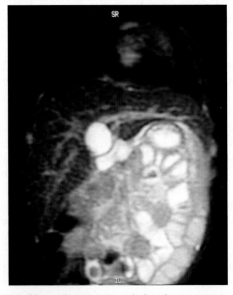

Fig. 11.8: Magnetic resonance cholangiopancreatographic (MRCP) showing choledochal cyst

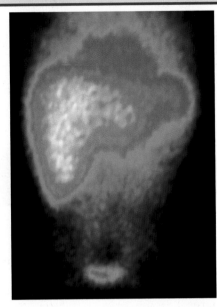

Fig. 11.9: HIDA scan showing filling defect due to choledochal cyst

large choledochal cysts may compress the gallbladder, leading to nonvisualisation.

Treatment

The only effective treatment is surgical correction other measures only serve the purpose to maximise the patient's condition before operation.

The treatment for choledochal cysts is surgical. The preferred procedure today is to completely remove (excise) the dilated duct system outside the liver and to drain the common bile duct as it exits the liver into a loop of intestine designed to prevent backflow of intestinal contents into the liver, thus protecting the patient from cholangitis. As long as no blockage occurs at the level of the suture line between the bile duct system and the intestine, these patients do very well long-term.

The treatment of choice for a type I choledochal cyst is complete excision of the cyst with construction of a Roux-en-Y biliary-enteric anastamosis to restore biliary continuity with the gastrointestinal tract.

Type II choledochal cysts can usually be excised entirely, and the defect in the common bile duct can be closed primarily over a T-tube. This approach can be used because, typically, type II choledochal cysts are lateral diverticulum of the bile duct.

Therapy for type III choledochal cysts, or choledo-choceles, depends on the size of the lesion. Choledo-choceles with a diameter of 3 cm or smaller may be approached endoscopically and effectively treated by means of sphincterotomy. Choledochoceles larger than 3 cm in diameter are often associated with some degree of duodenal obstruction. These cysts can be excised surgically if fearible.

For type IV choledochal cysts, the dilatated extrahepatic duct is completely excised, and a Roux-en-Y biliary-enteric anastomosis procedure is performed. No therapy is specifically directed at the intrahepatic ductal disease, except if intrahepatic ductal strictures, hepatolithiasis, or hepatic abscesses are present. In these patients, interventional radiological techniques can be performed. If the disease is limited to specific hepatic segments or a lobe, these may be resected.

A type V choledochal cyst, or Caroli disease, is defined only by the dilatation of the intrahepatic ducts. If dilatation is limited to a single hepatic lobe, usually the left, the affected lobe is resected. Patients who have bilobar disease and signs of biliary cirrhosis, portal hypertension, or liver failure may be candidates for liver transplantation.

BIBLIOGRAPHY

1. Paediatric surgery - Diagnosis and Management, Eds. DK Gupta, Shilpa Sharma and Richard Azizkhan, Jaypee Bros., New Delhi - 2008.

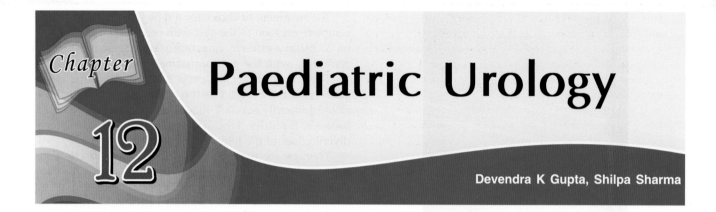

Paediatric Urology

Devendra K Gupta, Shilpa Sharma

HYDRONEPHROSIS

Hydronephrosis reflects an aseptic dilatation of the pelvicalyceal system as a result of a functional or mechanical obstruction at Pelviureteric junction (PUJ) or somewhere distally. PUJ obstruction is the most common cause of hydronephrosis, discovered antenatally on ultrasound or presenting later in childhood. If left untreated, complications may set in and lead to progressive renal insufficiency.

Hydrodynamics

Urine passes from renal pelvis into ureter by anatomical continuity at the pelviureteric junction and peristaltic contractions from pelvis to ureter. Normal basal pressure in the renal pelvis varies from 5-25 cm of water. An obstruction causes initial rise in pressure leading to dilatation. This results in fall of renal pressure and the equilibrium is maintained for long without symptoms and the renal damage is slow.

Aetiology

1. Idiopathic obstruction. Intrinsic abnormality – commonest cause due to muscle defect (only longitudinal fibers, excess of collagen, may be due developmental arrest).
2. Angulation and adhesions at PUJ.
3. Aberrant vessels (20%).
4. Ureteral stenosis/hypoplasia.
5. Polyp, papilloma, valve in the ureter at PUJ.
6. Persistent fetal ureteral folds.
7. Secondary PUJ due to Vesicoureteric reflux (5-10%): Reflux increases urine load on ureter and pelvis leading to dilatation, onset of infection leads to periureteritis – fibrosis- true obstruction.

Clinical Presentation

Patients with congenital hydronephrosis due to PUJ may remain asymptomatic throughout their life. However, they may develop symptoms at any stage depending on the degree and duration of obstruction.

- Renal lump – unilateral bilateral, tense cystic/soft, small/large
- Pain – high pressure, acute obstruction, infection, stone
- Infection, stone – rare and requires to rule out VUR/obstruction
- Acute presentation – intermittent lump, nausea, vomiting (Dietl's)
- Hematuria – rare, usually after trauma
- Renal failure – usually in single kidney with PUJ
- General features – failure to thrive, anaemia
- Chance finding – antenatal, postnatal on ultrasound/Intravenous urogram (IVU).

Investigation

1. Routine haemogram, renal biochemistry.
2. Urine examination – Microscopy and culture.
3. **Ultrasonography** – First modality for anatomical dilatation. It is mainly operator dependent. It is a good screening modality of first choice, non-invasive and can detect ureteric dilatation/bladder/urethra pathology also. It is also helpful to assesses the other kidney and differentiate hydronephrosis from other lumps – tumours, multicystic kidney, multilocular cysts. It is useful for diagnosis of antenatal hydronephrosis.
4. **Nuclear imaging** – Diureteric renogram (DTPA) for function, clearance and Glomerular filteration rate (GFR). Diureteric renogram is useful for differentiating the obstructed from non obstructed system and provides individual renal function. It is now the ideal investigation for screening and for follow-up evaluation. The grading on the diureteric scan is normal function: if function is 40% or more, Moderate function between 10-40% and Poor function less than 10%.
5. Antegrade pyelography, if there is doubt in the diagnosis of PUJ or in suspected cases of vesicoureteric junction obstruction.

6. Intravenous urogram (IVU) is now replaced by ultrasound and renogram. IVU is indicated in presence of duplex system, horseshoe kidney or ectopic ureteric opening. It is the traditional investigation for precise anatomy and function. Crescent sign due to contrast medium in the stretched collecting ducts is diagnostic. IVU is a reliable indicator of recoverable renal function.

7. Micturating cystourethrogram is indicated if the ureter is dilated, there is bilateral hydronephrosis or in presence of urinary tract infection.

8. Pressure flow studies – Whitaker's tests is done in equivocal cases. It is now rarely needed after the advent of nuclear imaging.

In all neonates with antenatally detected hydronephrosis, an ultrasound examination is performed first at birth within a week and then repeated at 4-6 weeks of age to confirm persistence of hydronephrosis. The renal scintigraphy is performed at 4-6 weeks when the renal maturity has better developed. Only 4-10% cases of hydronephrosis due to PUJ may have associated vesico-ureteric reflux, unilaterally or bilaterally, requiring evaluation for that. Micturating cystourethrogram (MCU) is not recommended in all cases with PUJ. It is recommended in selected cases who present with the followings; (a) poor urinary stream, (b) history suggestive of urinary tract infection (UTI), (c) bilateral PUJ obstruction and (d). if the ultrasound had suggested dilated ureter and/or bladder and posterior urethral changes indicating obstruction distal to PUJ.

If the renal scan shows an enlarged renal pelvis, with significant delay in excretion and a persistent rising curve, with or without decrease in split renal function, the diagnosis of PUJ obstruction is essentially confirmed.

Over 50-70% cases with hydronephrosis detected before birth, may completely resolve with the passage of time, without any risk of loss of renal functions. Function may remain stable in 20-30% cases despite presence of hydronephrosis. However, in 10% cases the function would deteriorate. Hence, a close follow up is required in most of these especially during the first 2 years, to identify the subgroup of children who would demonstrate obstruction and require surgery.

Preoperative percutaneous nephrostomy (PCN) drainage is warranted in patients with infected hydronephrosis, a giant hydronephrosis, bilateral gross hydronephrosis and in a solitary functioning hydronephrotic kidney presenting with uremia. Preoperative drainage restores the deranged renal parameters, provided there is no inherent dysplasia. PCN drainage may be kept for 3-4 weeks in all children who present with poorly functioning kidneys due to hydronephrosis.

Indications for Surgery

1. All children presenting with symptoms- lump, pain and infection.

2. PUJ associated with horse shoe, pelvic and crossed fused kidney.

3. If the split renal function is less than 40 % in the affected side, supported by delayed excretion and an obstructive renogram curve.

4. Deterioration in split renal function from normal to less than 40 % function.

5. A fall of more than 10% of the original value on the affected side at follow-up.

6. Postnatal anteroposterior diameter of the pelvis is more than 20 mm on USG.

Surgical Procedures Include

1. Excision of PUJ.
2. Formation of a funnel shaped renal pelvis.
3. Dependent drainage.
4. Watertight and tension free anastomosis.
5. Excision of the redundant pelvis.
6. A straight pelvi-ureteric anastomosis, without any redundancy around PUJ.

The surgical exposure to the kidney is a critical factor in achieving the above said goals. Appropriate access to the kidney may be achieved through lumbar, lumbotomy or the subcostal incisions. The classical Anderson Hynes or a variation thereof is the commonest procedure performed using the open technique. It is applicable to most variants of the anomalous anatomy and is particularly useful in cases of high insertion of the ureter and presence of lower polar crossing vessels. The technique allows a complete excision of the abnormal segment of the upper ureter, excision of the redundant pelvis, a dependent drainage and a wide pelvi-ureteric anastomosis.

Choice of Drains

Following PUJ repair, the need for postoperative urinary drainage and the choice of placing a nephrostomy tube, double "J" stent or a single transanastomotic stent (TAS) has always been controversial. Whereas the use of internal "J" stents or the nephrostomy drainage needs to be carefully individualised, the perirenal area is always drained with a corrugated drain or a closed suction drain. This prevents any collection around the anastomosis, sepsis and scarring. It is brought out either through the lateral part of the main wound or a separate stab skin incision.

Complications

Bleeding: Bleeding is common after nephrostomy drainage. Bleeding can jeopardize the repair by formation of clots. Slight haematuria settles down gradually in next few days. A frank bleeding requires an immediate exploration. Irrigation of the nephrostomy tube should be avoided, as it introduces infection and can disrupt the suture line.

Urine leak: Urine leak may occur within the first 24 hours. Drainage lasting over a week is of concern, because subsequent peripelvic and periureteral fibrosis harms the anastomosis and can cause secondary obstruction. Prolonged leakage can be managed by placing a double J stent endoscopically across the anastomosis and also keeping the bladder empty with a Folley's catheter. A percutaneous nephrostomy may be required if the infection has set in.

Obstruction: If obstruction develops at the PUJ it can be managed by leaving the stent or the nephrostomy tube in place for long, until the infection clears and the PUJ opens up on a nephrostogram. For obstruction which persists, attempt should be made to place a double J stent from below. If these measures fail, allow the area to heal for 10-12 weeks before contemplating a redo pyeloplasty. With the availability of endourologic intervention procedures, many cases of obstruction are now amenable to endoscopic retrograde stenting, balloon dilatations or percutneous incisions of strictures at PUJ.

Redo cases: For a case of redo pyeloplasty, emphasis is on gaining an adequate surgical access for a wide variety of surgical options. If the procedure is being done within first week or so of the initial pyeloplasty, same incision is reopened. A transperitoneal anterior approach may be preferred for all difficult redo cases and so also for the PUJs associated with Giant hydronephrosis, horse shoe kidney, duplex hydronehrotic moiety, cross fused renal ectopia and the pelvic kidney. It offers a direct and wide access to the complicated and an anatomically abnormal PUJ. The possible redo procedures include repeat pyeloplasty, ureterocalicostomy, ureteric replacement by appendix or an ileum, auto transplantation or even nephrectomy.

Ureterocalicostomy

Anastomosis of the proximal ureter directly to the lower pole calyceal system is best suited as a salvage procedure for cases with the difficult re-do pyeloplasty. Also in the patients on prolonged nephrostomy drainage, the identification of the renal pelvis becomes very difficult due to shrinkage and scarring. In such situations, the choice is to anastomose the lower pole calyx with the available ureter after excising the overlying renal parenchyma. This procedure is therefore best suited for kidneys with a large, dilated lower pole calyx with overlying thinned out parenchyma. Sufficient cortex must be removed to protect the proximal ureter from entrapment. The calyx must also be partly mobilized to create a tension free anastomosis.

In cases of horse shoe kidney with hydronephrosis, though, an extraperitoneal flank approach is enough for the unilateral cases. For those requiring bilateral procedures, a transperitoneal approach is preferred. The vascular supply to the horse shoe kidney is quite variable, with the isthmus and lower pole frequently receiving blood from the common iliac. The gonadal vessels pass over these lower renal vessels. The ureters lie nearer the midline than normal. Division of the isthmus which was once thought to be the cause of obstruction must not be done.

Endoscopic Procedures

The benefits of endourologic management of PUJ obstruction are less well established and in some cases offer no advantage over open pyeloplasty especially in younger children. It can be performed retrograde or antegrade. Several factors like the age of patient, the presence of primary or secondary PUJ, the degree of obstruction, the presence of crossing vessel and the overall differential function determine the success of the endoscopic procedure. However, the procedure is not suitable for the neonates and the infants with primary PUJ obstruction due to the technical. In the older children, the ureter caliber is more or less like that of adults, thus these patients may benefit from the endourologic procedures. Children with secondary PUJ obstruction respond better to the endourologic interventions. The success rate is less (77%) in case of massive hydronephrosis as compared to those with moderate disease (95%).

Laparoscopic pyeloplasty was developed in an attempt to duplicate the high success rates achieved with open pyeloplasty while offering advantages of minimally invasive techniques. Laparoscopic pyeloplasty can be performed in most patients with PUJ, however, an expertise in laparoscopy is required for an effective and purposeful procedure. The indications for laparoscopic pyeloplasty include a failed retrograde or antegrade pecutaneous endopyelotomy, patients with anatomic abnormalities such as horse shoe or pelvic kidney, patients with crossing vessels crossing at PUJ and the extremely dilated pelvis. The contraindications of laparoscopic pyeloplasty are small intrarenal pelvis, kidneys with poor function following the prolonged obstruction and the failed open pyeloplasty.

BIBLIOGRAPHY

1. Gupta DK, Chandrasekharam VV, Srinivas M, Bajpai M. Percutaneous nephrostomy in children with ureteropelvic junction obstruction and poor renal function. Urology. 2001 Mar;57(3):547-50.
2. Josephson S, Dhillon HK, Ransley PG. Post-natal management of antenatally detected, bilateral hydronephrosis. Urol Int. 1993;51(2):79-84.
3. Koff SA, Campbell KD. The nonoperative management of unilateral neonatal hydronephrosis: natural history of poorly functioning kidneys. J Urol. 1994 Aug;152(2 Pt 2):593-5.
4. Koff SA. The beneficial and protective effects of hydronephrosis. APMIS Suppl. 2003;(109):7-12.
5. Morin L, Cendron M, Crombleholme TM, Garmel SH, Klauber GT, D'Alton ME. Minimal hydronephrosis in the fetus: clinical significance and implications for management. J Urol. 1996 Jun;155(6):2047-9.

6. Onen A, Jayanthi VR, Koff SA. Long-term follow-up of prenatally detected severe bilateral newborn hydronephrosis initially managed nonoperatively. J Urol. 2002 Sep;168(3): 1118-20.
7. Perez LM, Friedman RM, King LR. The case for relief of ureteropelvic junction obstruction in neonates and young children at time of diagnosis. Urology. 1991 Sep;38(3):195-201.
8. Ransley PG, Dhillon HK, Gordon I, Duffy PG, Dillon MJ, Barratt TM. The postnatal management of hydronephrosis diagnosed by prenatal ultrasound. J Urol. 1990 Aug;144(2 Pt 2):584-7.
9. Ulman I, Jayanthi VR, Koff SA. The long-term follow-up of newborns with severe unilateral hydronephrosis initially treated nonoperatively. J Urol. 2000 Sep;164(3 Pt 2):1101-5.

EXSTROPHY OF BLADDER

Bladder exstrophy is a congenital defect that is characterised by malformation of the bladder and urethra, in which the bladder is essentially inside out and exposed on the outside of the abdomen through the defect below the umbilicus. Because the bladder is exposed to the outside of the body, urine constantly dribbles out and the child develops local infection and ammoniacal dermatitis. Boys will have a short penis, which is bent towards the dorsal aspect of penis called chordee. In the female, the clitoris is bifid. The urethral opening is on the dorsal aspect (epispadias) and the anus and vagina are anteriorly displaced. Additionally, the pelvis pubic ramus is widely separated (Pubic diastasis), outwardly rotated legs and feet, and there is displacement of the umbilicus upwards.

Embryology

Many believe that it is caused abnormal persistence of the cloacal membrane. If this membrane does not disappear at proper time during fetal development, anterior aspect of the bladder and the soft tissue covering the lower abdomen are never formed correctly. As a result, neither the bladder nor the skin and the muscle of lower abdominal wall close leading to exstrophy of bladder.

Incidence

This disorder occurs one in every 30,000 live births. It is two to three times more common in boys than girls. If a child has bladder exstrophy the chance of his sibling having bladder exstrophy is increased to about 1 in 100.

Issues in Exstrophy of Bladder

1. **Epispadias:** The urethra is not formed completely and the urethral meatus is on the dorsal aspect of penis. In boys, the penis is flattened and is bent towards the abdomen called as dorsal chordee. In girls, the urethral opening is located between a divided clitoris and labia minora. After reconstruction of urethra it increases the resistance to urinary flow and helps in the bladder growth. Cantwell Ransley's epispadias repair is the commonly done operation and carried out when the child around 2-3 years.

2. **Vesicoureteric Reflux:** Reflux is a condition where urine goes back up from the bladder into the kidneys. Reflux becomes serious when infected urine in the bladder travels to the kidneys, which can lead to scarring of kidney leading to loss of kidney function. All patients after bladder closure are put on antibiotic prophylaxis to prevent urinary tract infection and scarring of kidney. Reimplantation of ureter is done during bladder neck repair or augmentation surgery.

3. **Pubic Diastasis:** Separation of the pubic bones, which does not allow the bladder to remain inside the body and can cause waddling gait.

4. **Small Bladder Capacity:** All exstrophy of bladders are small at birth, some smaller than others. The extent to which the bladder will grow cannot be definitely determined. Successful bladder closure and epispadias repair increase urethral resistance and help the bladder to grow. If the balder capacity does not improve and the intravesical pressure remains high the patient will need to increase the size of the bladder by augmentation surgery using a patch of colon, stomach or ileum. After augmentation few complications may be encountered. The spectrum of complication observed is electrolyte imbalance, acid base imbalance, impaired sensorium, altered hepatic metabolism, abnormal drug metabolism, growth retardation, bone disorder and malignant changes.

5. **Incontinence of Urine:** The bladder neck and sphincter complex are not well formed in these patients and hence they have incontinence of urine. After bladder closure and epispadias repair the continence slowly improves with time. If it does not improve, then bladder neck repair surgery has to be done around 3- 5 years. Some children may require clean intermittent catheterisation to adequately empty their bladders. Use of agents like collagen, silicone and other substances, which can now be injected at the neck of the bladder may help to increase resistance and to improve the continence.

6. **Bladder Stones:** The incidence of stone formation varies incidence range from 10 to 25% and up to 52% after augmentation cystoplasty. The predisposing factors are chronic bacteriuria, urinary stasis, immobility, and mucus production, and metabolic abnormality, foreign body like sutures, catheters and staples.

7. **Urinary Tract Infections:** They are prone for urinary infection due to VUR, repeated catheterisation or mucus production after augmentation with bowel.

8. **Inguinal Hernias and Undescended Testes:** There can be bilateral inguinal hernia and undescended testes due to abnormal muscle development of anterior

abdominal wall. These need correction later. Undescended testis is thought to be due to unclosed bladder creating reduced abdominal muscle.

9. **Genital and Reproduction Problem:** The fertility in males is questionable though they are not impotent and is due to retrograde ejaculation or scarred or damaged vas deference. Almost all females are able to have children but will need caesarean section for delivery due to adherent uterus abnormal utero vaginal angle.

Investigation

1. **X- ray of the pelvis**
   To know the degree of pubic diastasis.
2. **Ultrasonogram**
   It diagnoses renal anomaly, hydroureteronephrosis, and renal damage due to reflux, bladder capacity and post void residue after the bladder closure.
3. **Renal isotope scan**
   Nuclear imaging include DTPA for drainage pattern and differential renal function, DMSA for renal scars due to reflux and GFR for global renal function.
4. **Micturating cystourethrogram (MCU)**
   Done after the bladder closure to know the bladder contour, capacity, VUR, urethral profile and post void residue.
5. **Urodynamic study**
   To know the bladder capacity, bladder pressure, compliance, detrusor sphincter coordination, uroflometry, post void residue, etc.

Treatment

The treatment is only surgical. The primary goals of reconstruction are:
- Closure of the bladder and urethra
- Closure of the abdominal wall
- Preservation of kidney
- Good urinary continence
- Sexual function
- Improved appearance of genitalia.

A. **Staged repair:** There are usually three stages of reconstruction. The goal of this staged reconstruction is to have patients with a normal urinary tract, satisfactory external genitalia, and adequate dry intervals.
   1st Stage - Closure of bladder and abdomen (24-48 hours of life).
   2nd Stage - Epispadias repair (2-3 yrs).
   3rd Stage - Achieve urinary continence by bladder neck repair and augmentation (4-5 yrs).
   The first stage involves internalisation of the bladder and closing the abdomen and should be performed, ideally, within the first 48 hours of life, if at all possible.

Within this time frame, the bones are pliable, the changes in the bladder lining have not occurred yet and the bladder and abdominal wall can usually be closed without disrupting the bony pelvis (iliac osteotomies) .

The second stage consists of reconstruction of external genitalia in male child epispadias repair with reconstruction of phallus and in females clitoral repair is done at 2-3 years of age. Later if bladder is too small to cope with urinary volume and it will lead to incontinence of urine, high pressure within the bladder leading to kidney damage due to poor drainage and vesico ureteric reflux. In this case, a bladder enlargement (augmentation) by using stomach, ileum or colon can be done which will increase the bladder size, reduce the bladder pressure and improve the continence. This is usually done at 4-5 years of age, and often coincides with a reconstruction of the bladder neck. If the patient does not improve with regards to urinary continence closure of bladder neck and creation of continent catheterisable channel from the bladder onto the abdominal wall namely the Mitrofanoff operation can be carried out (Figs 12.1A and B).

B. **Single stage total reconstruction of exstrophy bladder** Because of improvement in surgical technique, good postoperative care and safe anaesthesia total reconstruction of the exstrophy can be under taken in single stage. The outcome following single stage reconstruction is found to be better than staged repair.

BIBLIOGRAPHY

1. Adult and paediatric urology, third edition, year 1991, Mosby publication, author Jay Y. Gillenwater, John T. Gray hack.
2. Paediatric surgery third edition, year 2000 W.B. Saunders Company. Author Keith W.Ashcraft.

UNDESCENDED TESTIS (UDT) CRYPTORCHIDISM

An undescended testis (UDT) is one, which cannot be made to reach the bottom of the scrotum and remains high along its line of descent (Fig. 12.2). The incidence of undescended testis is 2.7 to 3% at birth in the full term infants. The incidence decreases to around 1 % after 1 year of age and thereafter remains the same. It is much more common in premature infants approaching 100% at gestational age of 32 weeks or less.

An ectopic testis is one that has strayed from the inguinal canal, usually to the thigh, perineum, base of penis, femoral or even to the other side of the scrotum. The superficial inguinal pouch is the most common site for the ectopic testis. Ascending testis is one that has descended once and was there in the scrotum at birth, but as the spermatic cord fails to elongate at the same rate as the

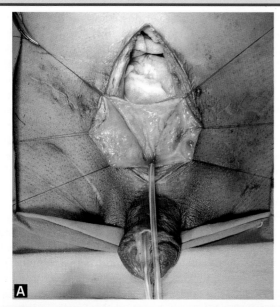

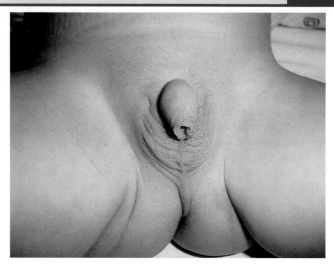

Fig. 12.2: Bilateral undescended testes with underdeveloped scrotum

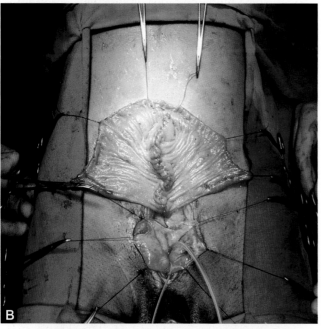

Figs 12.1A and B: Showing the exstrophy of bladder being opened up for augmentation

body growth, the testis ascends up progressively, and becomes high in inguinal canal by the childhood. An impalpable testis is quite uncommon (less than 10%) and agenesis is rare (2% of all cases of UDT and about 20% of all impalpable testis). A fully descended but grossly hypoplastic testis may be impalpable and identified only on exploration.

The retractile testis is a testicle having completed the descent process but is not in its normal scrotal position secondary to a hyperactive cremasteric reflex. Strong contraction of the cremaster muscle may pull the testis

from the scrotum into the superficial inguinal pouch. Abnormally highly located gubernacular attachment may cause the testis to migrate high during a cremasteric reflex. The cremasteric reflex becomes most active at ages 5 to 9 years. Ascent of the testis at this time may prevent the prepubertal testis from growing normally, as commonly seen with gliding and severe retractile testis. The testis and scrotum are usually well developed. It is possible to bring the testis into the scrotum by dragging the testis and it remains there for sometime. The Chair test (Orr) may be helpful to bring down the retractile testis in difficult cases. The child is asked to sit on a chair keeping both feet on the seat with extreme flexion of the knees towards the chest. Testicular function and fertility are normal. It is now believed that there is no role of hormonal therapy.

Embryology

During the 5-6th week of gestation, the gubernaculum forms from a band of mesenchyme and extends from the genital ridges through a gap in the abdominal wall musculature to the genital swellings which will develop into the scrotum. Primordial germ cells from yolk sac migrate along the dorsal mesentry of the hind gut to reach the genital ridges.

During the 7th week, under the influence of H-Y antigen, the indifferent gonads differentiates into fetal testes.

Fetal testis becomes normally active by the 8th week, secreting testosterone and mullerian inhibiting substance (MIS). MIS is secreted by fetal sertoli cells stimulated by FSH from pitutary and causes regression of the mullerian ducts.

During the10-15th week, testosterone produced by leydig cells stimulate differentiation of wolffian duct to form the epididymis, vas deferens and seminal vesicle.

Leydig cells are stimulated by placental choronic gonadotropin and pituitary LH. Differentiation of external genitalia depends on the presence of 5-a-reductase, which converts testosterone to dihydrotestosterone. The processus vaginalis forms as a hernial sac through the weakness in the abdominal wall adjacent to the gubernaculum and gradually extends into the scrotum. The process of testicular descent remains dormant until the seventh month of gestation.

At the seventh month, the gubernaculum increases in size, distending the inguinal canal and scrotum. The testis then descends through the inguinal canal into the scrotum. Epididymis, attached to gubernaculums, precedes the testis in its descent into the scrotum.

Thus the normal descent of testes occurs at about the seventh month of fetal life when the gubernaculum swells and shortens, drawing the testis through the inguinal canal into the scrotum.

After the descent, gubernaculum persists as fibrous band, the gubernacular ligament. Processus vaginalis is completely obliterated prior to birth.

Factors Responsible for Testicular Descent

1. Traction of the testis by the gubernaculum or cremaster muscle or both.
2. Differential body growth.
3. Increase in intraabdominal pressure.
4. Development and maturation of the epididymis.
5. Changes resulting from androgen environment- milieu, directly or indirectly mediated through the spinal nucleus of genitofemoral nerve innervating the gubernaculum which stimulates the release of calcitonin gene related peptide (CGRP).
6. Role of oestrogen and MIS.

Failure of the descent may occur because of the hormonal failure (inadequate gonadotropins and testosterone), dysgenetic testis or an anatomic abnormality such as abnormal or malplaced gubernaculum, obstruction of inguinal canal or scrotum or the shortened vas and/or vessels.

Sequelae of Non-Descent

1. Infertility: The higher temperature of the extrascrotal testis causes testicular dysplasia with interstitial fibrosis and poor development of seminiferous tubules thus hampering the spermatogenesis. Testosterone production is unaffected by the testicular position, thus a male with bilateral undescended testes will develop secondary sexual characters yet may be sterile.
2. Trauma: The testis in inguinal region is also more prone to direct trauma.
3. Torsion: The chances are greatest in the postpubertal period when testis usually increases in size.

4. Neoplasia: The most serious complication due to the associated dysplasia existing in the testis is a higher chance of malignancy if left untreated (10-20 times on the affected side and about 7 times on the contralateral side). The risk of malignant degeneration is though, not altered by doing an orchiopexy, yet, few workers now have indicated that an early orchiopexy before one year of age or so may actually decrease the incidence of malignancy. Malignancy, usually a seminoma, develops only in the second or third decade of life.
5. Hernia due to patent processus vaginalis.
6. Atrophy results in untreated cases.
7. Feeling of incompleteness psychologically.

On examination, always look for a hernia. The position and the size of the testis should be noted, if impalpable, ectopic locations of the testis should be examined. There are many associated anomalies that are quite common with UDT: intersex disorders, prune belly syndromes, exstrophy bladder, spina bifida posterior urethral valves and prune belly syndrome (Fig. 12.3). Any child with unilateral or bilateral UDT associated with hypospadias, needs to be investigated for intersexuality by performing chromosomal analysis, hormones assessment, genitogram and the tests to confirm the presence or the absence of the Mullerian structures.

Histological Changes

Pathological changes may occur as early as 6 months. Impaired Leydig cell development has been shown as early

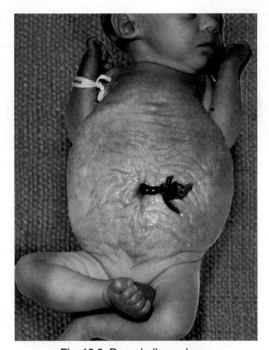

Fig. 12.3: Prune belly syndrome

as 2-6 months, whereas sertoli and germ cells appeared normal. There could be delayed germ cell maturation, reduced germ cell number and hyalinisation of seminiferous tubules. These changes are reversible upto 2 years of age. Histologic changes in crytorchid testis include degeneration of mitochondria, loss of ribosomes, increase in the collagen fibres in the spermatogonia and sertoli cells.

Treatment

The histological changes in the testes occur as early as six months of postnatal life and therefore, a child who has an undescended testis should be operated at the earliest to prevent them. The best time for orchiopexy is about 1 year of age, but where facilities of surgical expertise and paediatric anaesthesia are available, it may be considered even before 9 months of age. A still early surgical procedure is usually associated with higher complication rate with injury to the vessels and the vas (2-3%). Figure 12.4 outlines the algorithm for management of impalpable undescended testes.

Methods of Orchiopexy

1. **Extra-dartos pouch- Conventional Orchiopexy**
   An inguinal incision is made, the hernial sac is dissected from the cord structures and a high ligation of the sac is done. The testis is placed in an extra-dartos

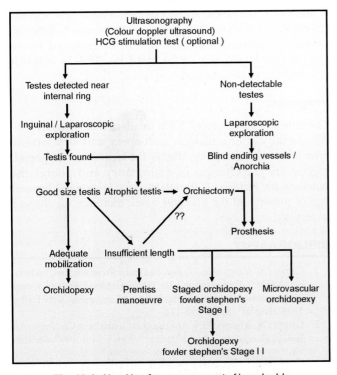

Fig. 12.4: Algorithm for management of impalpable undescended testes

pouch in the scrotum; an adequate dissection should be done to avoid tension on the pedicle while placing the testis in scrotum. Any torsion of the pedicle should be avoided. Retroperitoneal dissection and careful snipping off of lateral peritoneal bands will give an adequate length to the cord.
   If the testis does not reach the scrotum easily then the inferior epigastric artery and vein can be ligated and the testis brought directly through the transversalis fascial floor (Prentiss maneuver).

2. **Transcrotal orchiopexy**
   It is performed through a skin crease incision in the neck of the scrotum. High ligation of processus vaginalis, dissection of the spermatic cord and placement of the testis in an ipsilateral subdartos pouch constructed through the same incision is done. Advantage includes minimal dissection through a single incision and avoidance of disruption of the inguinal canal.

3. **Fowler Stephen's Technique**
   It comprises of division of the main testicular vessels and relies on delicate vasal and cremasteric collaterals for testicular survival and growth. It is associated with 50-100% atrophy rate.

4. **Staged Fowler Stephen's Technique**
   It is a 2 stage procedure. Ligation of the spermatic vessels to gain length is done as stage I operation by open or laparoscopic method to allow the collateral blood supply to develop without mobilizing the testes. After about 6 months waiting, at second stage, the testis can be brought into scrotum by inguinal exploration. The testicular blood supply is supported by the artery to the vas.

5. **Multistage Orchiopexy**
   The testis is mobilised and brought into the inguinal canal as far as possible. The testis and spermatic cord are wrapped with a silicone sheath to prevent adhesions. After 1 year waiting, at second stage, the testis is brought down to the scrotum.

6. **Microvascular orchiopexy (Testicular auto transplantation)**
   Microvascular transfer of testes is the best procedure to avoid atrophy of the testis but it needs great surgical expertise and the equipment. This procedure involves high mobilisation of the testicular vascular pedicle and also carefully safeguards the vas and vasal collaterals. Following division of the blood supply, the testis is transferred to the scrotum and immediately revascularised by one arterial and one or two venous anastomosis to the inferior epigastric vessels. In expert hands, a success rate of over 80-90% is now possible.

7. **Refluo Technique**
   It consists of full venous drainage by microvascular anastomosis of the testicular vein to the inferior

epigastric vein, but relies on the arterial input from the vasal collaterals.

8. **Ombredanne's Procedure**

The testis is put into the contralateral scrotal sac through the scrotal septum.

In cases of impalpable testis, in about 50% a useful testis can be brought down and in the other 50% there is either possibly a testicular agenesis or atrophy due to the intra-uterine torsion resulting in the vanishing testis. A useless and potentially neoplastic testis must be removed. If the testis is difficult to be brought to the root of the scrotum, it should be brought down as much as possible but without any tension and fixed, possibly to the pubic tubercle to make it easily palpable for detection of enlargement, if any.

Role of Hormones

Hormones, human chorionic gonadotrophins (HCG) and Gonadotrophin releasing hormones (GnRH) therapy play multiple roles. Hormones, mainly the HCG, have been used for the detection of anorchia in cases of impalpable testis. In cases of bilateral UDT, an HCG test (1000 IU on alternate days for 3 injections) is performed to see change in level of testosterone. A less than 20-fold rise is indicative of anorchism and surgery is not indicated in these patients. These days laparoscopy is a much better modality for this purpose.

HCG is also used to achieve partial or complete descent of undescended testis and the secondary benefits for redo cases, i.e for the enlargement of the testicular volume, the vessels and the scrotum. Under the HCG effect, the spermatic vessels become more pliable and the length of the cord is also increased. The scrotum becomes more capacious. The results following the hormonal therapy are known to be better if the testis is low-lying (inguinal or high scrotal), retractile, unilateral, good in volume and in boys above 8 years of age. Since the therapy is effective in only 20-30 % cases, it is not widely used.

Laparoscopy

Paediatric laparoscopy has evolved as an important tool in the search for the impalpable testis. Laparoscopy has 95% sensitivity for locating a testis or proving it absent. It seems to offer a safe and reliable diagnostic and therapeutic option to patients with impalpable testis.

Intraabdominal detection allows more testes to be brought down to the scrotum. Laparoscopy obviates the need for groin exploration in many cases.

Technically a first stage Fowler-Stephens' procedure can be performed easily and effectively with the help of a laparoscope.

If the testicular vessels are seen to end blindly this signifies that the testis is absent on that side and that no surgical exploration is necessary. If the vessels are seen to enter the internal inguinal ring, an inguinal exploration or laparoscopic assisted orchiectomy or orchiopexy is required.

If the testis is seen in the abdomen a decision may be made either to perform an extraabdominal exploration and attempt to place the testis in scrotum or to clip the testicular vessels and perform an orchiopexy at a later date.

Complications of Orchiopexy

1. Failed orchiopexy.
2. Recurrence of undescent due to inappropriate choice of surgical technique.
3. Testicular reascent. Testis becomes tethered to the operative scar and retracts out of the scrotum over time with increasing body growth.
4. Testicular atrophy.
5. Vas and vessel injury.

Indications for Orchiectomy

1. Malignancy.
2. Testicular atrophy.
3. High intra-abdominal testis that cannot be brought down.

Prosthesis

If orchiectomy has been done, for psychological reasons - a prosthetic placement should be performed, firstly in the childhood as it allows the growth of the scrotum. Later on around puberty, the prosthesis can be replaced by an appropriate sized one if the need be. This is only for psychological satisfaction.

Prognosis

There is 2% recurrence, 2-5% incidence of atrophy, 70-80% fertility after unilateral orchiopexy and 40% fertility after bilateral orchiopexy. Higher the location of the gonad, higher are the chances of malignancy and poorer the outcome for fertility. If the orchiopexy is delayed beyond age of puberty in the bilateral cases, there are no chances of fertility.

BIBLIOGRAPHY

1. Gupta DK. Indigenized Teflon Testicular Prosthesis in Children- an AIIMS Experience. In Ambiguous Genitalia and Hypospadias (Ed DK Gupta) Printext Publishers, New Delhi. 1999 chapter 18, pp 113-114.
2. Gupta DK, Menon PSN. Ambiguous Genitalia in Children . An Indian Perspective. Ind J Pediatr. : Ind. J. Ped. 1997; 64: 189-94.
3. Gupta DK. Paediatric Intersex Disorders. In. Ambiguous Genitalia and Hypospadias (ed. DK Gupta) Printext Publishers, Delhi. 1999 chapter 7, pp57-62.

4. Gupta DK, Sharma Shilpa. Common Inguinoscrotal problems in Children, in Recent Advances in Surgery, Vol 10, Ed. Roshal Lal Gupta, 2006 Chapter 8:147-161.

5. Gupta DK. Use of hormones for testicular descent in Recent Advances in Paediatrics Ed. Suraj Gupta, Jaypee brothers. New Delhi 1991, p 113-115.

4. Rohatgi M, Gupta DK, Menon PSN, Verma IC, Rao PS and Rajalaxmi M. Hormonal Therapy in Undescended testis. Ind. J. Pediatr. 1991; 58: 79-83.

PHIMOSIS

Phimosis is defined as the excessive tightness of the foreskin, preventing retraction behind the glans. At birth, if the meatus is visible at the glans (even without any prepucial retraction), there is no phimosis. The separation of prepuce from the glans surface continues and is completed by the age of about 2 years. At this age, if the prepuce can not be retracted fully or balloons out on micturition, there is phimosis. It occurs in only 1-2% males. Usually, it is mild and a simple separation and retraction is all that is required in most cases. An epithelial debris is usually present at the coronal sulcus and forms the source of constant irritation and infection. A forced retraction may worsen the phimosis by producing tears in the foreskin, which heals with scarring and contraction. If there is pooling of urine and repeated attacks of balanoposthitis, then simple dilatation of the foreskin can be done with due care regarding the local hygiene.

After the age of 2 years, adhesinolysis can be done as a outpatient procedure (stretching and forcibly separating the glans from the inner layer of prepuce). Daily retraction and cleansing of the glans is very important and must be continued for at least for 10-15 days. This will prevent recurrence of the phimosis. An antibiotic cream may be used as a lubricant to prevent readhesion formation. Few centres promote the use of steroid creams for this purpose. It is not our practice to use any steroids for this. It must be emphasized that after retraction of the prepuce, the same must be reposited back on to the glans, to avoid any risk of paraphimosis. A dorsal slit in the prepuce may be needed if the prepuce is too tight. Circumcism is the last resort and indicated only if the prepucial skin is scarred and fibrotic and dilatation and adhesinolysis have not been successful.

Circumcism is a tradition in some religions and performed as a routine in all male babies even without phimosis. It is interesting to know that female circumcism is also practiced in some areas of Saudi Arabia on religious grounds.

Chapter 13

Paediatric Oncology

Devendra K Gupta, Shilpa Sharma, Robert Carachi

WILMS TUMOUR

Introduction

Wilms tumour (WT) or nephroblastoma is the most common type of renal malignancy that affects children. It is an embryonal tumour that develops from remnants cells of immature kidney. The condition is named for Carl Max Wilhelm Wilms, a 19th-century German surgeon, who wrote one of the first medical articles about the disease in 1899.

Epidemiology

The overall annual incidence is approximately 8 per million children less than 15 yrs of age. It accounts for 6-7% of all childhood cancers. The mean age of presentation for unilateral disease is 3.5 yrs and for bilateral disease, 2.5 yrs. The tumour presents at an earlier age among boys. The disease occurs with equal frequency in girls and boys worldwide. Wilms' tumour has been linked to various genetic syndromes and birth defects such as:

- WAGR (Wilms tumour, aniridia, ambiguous genitalia, and mental retardation) syndrome.
- Beckwith-Wiedemann syndrome (macroglossia, gigantism, and umbilical hernia)
- Denys-Drash syndrome (WT, pseudohermaphroditism, and glomerulopathy)

Children with these genetic syndromes should be screened for Wilms tumour every three months until age 8 years. An ultrasound test may be used for screening

Wilms tumour has also been linked to various birth defects such as:

- Hemihypertrophy.
- Cryptorchidism
- Congenital aniridia
- Hypospadias

Pathogenesis

Nephrogenic rests are thought to be precursor lesions to Wilms tumour. Nephrogenic rests have been defined as a focus of abnormally persistent nephrogenic cells. These rests are found in 1% of unselected paediatric autopsies, 35% of kidneys with unilateral Wilms tumour and nearly all kidneys with bilateral Wilms tumour.

It has been postulated that in most people these rests resolve but in some, can give rise to Wilms tumour.

Molecular Genetics

Wilms tumour appears to primarily result from loss of certain tumour suppressor genes as opposed to activation of oncogenes. Knudsen and Strong proposed that WT results from two mutational events based on loss of function of tumour suppressor genes.

The first mutation, the inactivation of the first allele of the specific tumour suppressor gene, involves prezygotic and postzygotic aspects. Prezygotic (constitutional or germline) mutations are inherited or they result from a *de novo* germline mutation. This mutation is present in all body cells and predisposes the patient to familial and/or multiple WT. Postzygotic mutations occur only in specific cells, and they predispose patients to single tumours and sporadic cases of WT.

The second mutation is inactivation of the second allele of the specific tumour suppressor gene.

Several chromosomal regions have been implicated with development of Wilms tumour:

- Band 11p13—**WT1**, Wilms tumour suppressor gene, may explain associations with WAGR and Denys-Drash syndromes
- Band 11p15—**WT2**, may explain associations with Beckwith-Wiedeman syndrome
- 17q—harbors familial locus **FWT1**
- 19q—harbors familial locus **FWT2**

Several chromosomal regions have been associated with phenotype of Wilms tumour:

- **16q**
- **1p**
- **17p**
- **7p**

Pathology

Wilms tumours are mostly solitary lesions but can be multifocal in 12% cases.

Gross Appearance

Uniform pale gray or tan colour on section, but can give a variegated appearance due to hemorrhage and necrosis. They are usually sharply demarcated and are surrounded by a distinct intrarenal pseudocapsule composed of compressed atrophic renal tissue. Cysts are also commonly encountered.

Histology

Wilms tumour is composed of three cell types
- Blastemal—Undifferentiated small blue cells
- Epithelial—Usually seen as abortive glomeruli and tubules
- Stromal—usually as immature spindled cells or can manifest as cartilage, osteoid or fat.

Depending on presence of different types of cell types Wilms can be termed as triphasic or monophasic.

Wilms tumour can be separated into two prognostic groups on the basis of histopathology:
- **(FH) Favourable histology:** Absence of anaplasia in the tumour in considered as favourable histology.
- **(UFH) Unfavourable/Anaplastic histology:** Presence of markedly enlarged polypoid nuclei within tumour samples. Anaplasia is associated with resistance to chemotherapy and may still be detected after preoperative chemotherapy. Anaplasia is found in 5% of tumours.

Clinical Presentation

Most children are brought to medical attention because of an abdominal mass (Fig. 13.1). Other frequent symptoms at diagnosis are abdominal pain, fever, and hematuria. Hypertension may also be present in 25 % of children with Wilms tumour.

The child may also present with acute abdomen due to rupture of the tumour in the peritoneal cavity.

On examination the mass is examined with serious efforts to recognise signs suggestive of associated syndromes. Varicocele may be present due to obstruction of spermatic veins due to tumour thrombus in the renal vein or inferior vena cava, on left side.

Investigations

Laboratory Studies

- Complete blood count
- Basic metabolic profile
- Coagulation assay (acquired Von Willebrand's disease in 8% patients)
- Urinalysis

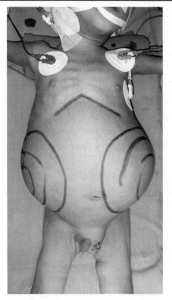

Fig. 13.1: Synchronous bilateral Wilms tumour in a child presenting with abdominal masses

Imaging Studies

- Ultrasound
  - Initial diagnosis of a renal or abdominal mass, possible renal vein or inferior vena cava (IVC) thrombus, information regarding liver and other kidney
- Computed tomography scan
  - Differential diagnosis of a kidney tumour versus adrenal tumour (neuroblastoma)
  - Liver metastases
  - Status of opposite kidney (7% patients have bilateral Wilms' tumour)
  - Lymph node assessment
  - Status of chest with respect to metastases
  - Renal vein or IVC thrombus (6 % of cases have IVC thrombus).
- Chest X-ray—As a baseline for pulmonary metastases
- Bone scan/ skeletal survey—Routinely not done in all cases of Wilms tumour. Indicated in cases with pulmonary or hepatic metastases and in patients with symptoms suggestive of bone involvement.

Histology

In National Wilms Tumour Study Group (NWTSG) protocol patient is explored at presentation if resectable, then nephrectomy specimen or if unresectable, a biopsy is submitted for histopathological examination for assessing the FH and UFH.

Staging

National Wilms Tumour Study Group (NWTSG) staging for renal tumours:

- **Stage I:** The tumour is limited to the kidney and has been completely excised. The renal capsule and the tumour were not ruptured. The vessels of the renal sinus are not involved and there is no residual tumour after surgical resection.
- **Stage II:** The tumour extends beyond the kidney but was completely resected. There is regional extension of the tumour (i.e., penetration of the renal capsule, extensive invasion of the renal sinus). Blood vessels outside the renal sinus may contain tumour (tumour thrombus or infiltration). The tumour may have been biopsied, or there was local spillage of tumour confined to the flank. There is no evidence of tumour at or beyond the margins of resection. Free floating inferior vena caval thrombus.
- **Stage III:** Residual nonhematogenous tumour confined to the abdomen or any of the following: Lymph node involvement in the hilum or pelvis, diffuse peritoneal spillage either before or during surgery, peritoneal implants, tumour beyond the surgical margin either grossly or microscopically tumour not completely resected because of local infiltration into vital structures, IVC thrombus that is adherent to the venaoucaval wall, tumour infilterating a cuff of bladder.
- **Stage IV:** Hematogenous or lymph node metastasis has occurred outside the abdomen or pelvis.
- **Stage V:** Synchronous bilateral involvement has occurred. Each side is assigned a stage from I to III, and histology is based on biopsy findings.

The most common sites of metastases are lung, regional lymph nodes, and liver.

Treatment

Multidisciplinary Treatment planning by a team of cancer specialists (paediatric surgeon or paediatric urologist, paediatric radiation oncologist, and paediatric oncologist) with experience in treating Wilms' tumour is required to determine and implement optimum treatment.

There are basically two important treatment protocols:
- **NWTS** (National Wilms' Tumour Study group): Surgery (and staging) are done at presentation and treatment is decided according to the staging
- **SIOP** (Société Internationale d'Oncologie Paediatrique): Upfront chemotherapy is given at presentation. After few cycles of chemotherapy staging is done and future treatment is decided.
- **UKCCLG** (UK Cancer Children's and Leukemia Group): Diagnostic biopsy is done then chemotherapy is given.

Surgical Principles

According to the NWTSG protocol, the first step in the treatment of WT is surgical staging followed by radical nephrectomy via transabdominal route. Following points are to be remembered while operating on Wilms' tumour:

- Accurate assessment of the extent of disease for staging and to assess resectability
- Complete tumour removal without rupture
- Contralateral kidney must be palpated and inspected
- Lymph node sampling is mandatory
- Margins of resection and residual tumour should be marked with titanium clips.

Nephrectomy is not done (only staging and biopsy done) in following circumstances:
- Solitary kidney
- Bilateral Wilms' tumour
- Unresectable tumour
- Poor general condition of patient (high operative morbidity and mortality)
- IVC thrombus extending above the level of hepatic veins.

Chemotherapy is given for 5 wks, after which patient is reassessed for resectability. In the author's experience, Fine needle aspiration cytology (FNAC) has been practiced routinely over decades without any untoward effects. The diagnostic accuracy in expert hands is high. Supplementation with immunocytochemistry helps to rule out other round cell tumours in cases with diagnostic dilemmas. An open, biopsy for histopathological confirmation, in cases appearing unresectable clinically, may not be needed if facitilies for FNAC are available.

Chemotherapy

Depending upon the stage and histopathology, the chemotherapy regime is charted:
- **Regimen EE4A**—18 week course of Actinomycin D and Vincristine
  - All Stage I and Stage II FH (Favourable histology) tumours
- **Regimen DD4A**—24 week course of actinomycin D, vincristine, doxorubicin
  - Stage III—IV FH WT and Stage II - IV Focal anaplasia
- **Regimen I**—24 week course of vincristine, doxorubicin, cyclophosphamide, etoposide
  - Stage II - IV diffuse anaplasia

The dose in infancy should be decreased by 50%.

Radiotherapy

Wilms' tumour is a highly radiosensitive tumour. Higher doses were used in the past, but documentation of radiation related side effects has led to decreases in radiation doses. Indications of radiotherapy are:
- Stage II, III, IV with unfavourable histology
- Stage III and IV with favourable histology
- Metastatic disease (to metastatic site)
  Abdominal irradiation 1080cGy in six fractions
  Lung irradiation 1200 cGy in nine fractions (> 18 mts)

Patients in age < 18 month are given radiation only if there is no response to chemotherapy, 900cGy in six fractions with 150cGy supplementation to the metastases.

Prognostic Factors

The most important adverse prognostic factor is the presence of anaplasia. Other prognostic factors are regional lymph node involvement and presence of metastases.

Follow Up

All patients are reviewed every 3 months for the first year, and then every 6 months for another 2 years. During each of the follow-ups in the first three years it is recommended to get a radiological evaluation. This may be an ultrasound or CECT scan in addition to a chest X-ray. The likelihood of recurrence after the first 3 years is less however, these patients should be followed up every year for various long-term complications.

Complications

Surgical Complications

- Small bowel obstruction (7%)
- Hemorrhage (6%)
- Wound infection, hernia (4%)
- Vascular complications (2%)
- Splenic and intestinal injury (1.5%)

Long-term Complications

- **Renal function**: The rate of chronic renal failure (CRF) is 1% overall. Of these cases, 70% are children with bilateral WT. In unilateral WT, the rate is 0.25%. The most common cause of CRF is the treatment-related causes such as surgery or radiation. Unrecognized renal disease, such as Denys-Drash syndrome, is rare. The damage produced by radiation is dose-dependent, and the rate of impaired creatinine clearance is approximately 20% with total abdomen irradiation with less than 1200 rads.
- **Cardiac function**: The fact that anthracyclines such as doxorubicin produce cardiac muscle impairment in 5% of those receiving a cumulative of 400 mg/m2 is well known. The overall incidence rate of some form of cardiac damage is 25% in those treated with anthracycline. Overall incidence of cardiac failure is 1.7%. The mean time to the onset of cardiac failure is 8 years.
- **Pulmonary function**: Radiation pneumonitis is encountered in 20% of the cases receiving total pulmonary radiation. The rate of diffuse interstitial pneumonitis with varicella and Pneumocystis infection is 13%.
- **Hepatic function**: Actinomycin D and radiation may damage the liver. Hepatic venoocclusive disease (VOD) is a clinical syndrome of hepatotoxicity and consists of jaundice, ascites, hepatomegaly and weight gain.
- **Gonadal function**: Chemotherapy may affect gonadal function in boys but rarely affects the function of ovaries. Abdominal irradiation may induce ovarian failure if ovaries were in the target field.
- **Musculoskeletal function**: Clinical rickets is possible due to renal tubular Fanconi's syndrome caused by drugs that are too cytotoxic. Skeletal sequelae of radiation, including scoliosis or kyphosis, result from uneven growth when the radiation was unilaterally targeted to the vertebral bodies and the dose was higher than 2000 rads.
- **Second malignant neoplasm**: These may result from inherited disposition and treatment, bone tumours, breast cancer, and thyroid cancer. The rate after a medium follow-up of 15 years is 1.6%, which is 5 times the expected rate. Limiting the intensive chemotherapy and radiotherapy and reserving the intensive treatment regimens only for the high stages and the cases with unfavourable histology possibly can limit second malignant neoplasm.

Prognosis

The outcome of 202 cases seen in last 17 years, the survival rate was 95% for Stage I and II tumours, 75% for Stage III tumours, 62% for Stage IV tumours and 40% for Stage V tumours. The number of cases Stagewise was Stage I–19.3%, Stage II–15.8%, Stage III–43.0% Stage IV–15.3% and Stage V–6.4%.

NEUROBLASTOMA

Introduction

Neuroblastoma is the most common extracranial solid tumour in children, accounting for 8% to 10% of all childhood cancers. Neuroblastoma is exclusively a paediatric neoplasm and is the most common cancer diagnosed during infancy. It is a malignancy of the sympathetic nervous system arising from neuroblasts (pluripotent sympathetic cells).

Epidemiology

Incidence of neuroblastoma is approximately 8 to 10 per million children younger than 15 yrs. It is marginally more common in boys than in girls, with a male to female ratio of 1.1:1.0.The mean age at diagnosis is 17.3 months.

Etiology

Neuroblatoma develops from postganglionic sympathetic neuroblasts. Microscopic neuroblastic nodules are usually present in adrenal gland of all fetuses. These nodules peak at 17 to 20 weeks of gestation and regress by the perinatal period. Although these nodules probably represent remnants of normal adrenal development, nevertheless they represent cells from which neuroblastoma develops.

These tumours frequently have features of neuronal differentiation. Neuroblastomas may occasionally show spontaneous differentiation to ganglioneuroblastoma or ganglioneuroma.

Genetics

The most important genetic abnormality of prognostic significance is gene amplification of MYCN proto-oncogene present on short arm of chromosome 2. More than 10 copies of MYCN are associated with poor prognosis. Approximately 25% of patients with neuro-blastoma exhibit MYCN amplification.

Deletion of the short arm of chromosome 1 is the most common chromosomal abnormality present in neuro-blastomas, and it confers a poor prognosis. The 1p chromosome region likely harbours tumour suppressor genes or genes that control neuroblast differentiation. Neuroblastomas also exhibit deletions of 11q, 14q, and unbalanced gain of 17q.

Total content of DNA in cell as measured by flow cytometry is also of prognostic significance in infants. Hyperdiploid tumours (DNA index >1) have better prognosis as compared to diploid tumours.

Three neurotrophin receptor gene products, TrkA, TrkB, and TrkC, are tyrosine kinases that code for a receptor of members of the nerve growth factor (NGF) family. It has been demonstrated that TRKA expression is inversely correlated with MYCN amplification.

Pathology

Neuroblastoma falls into the broader category of small round blue cell neoplasms of childhood. The three classic histopathologic patterns of neuroblastoma, ganglioneuro-blastoma and ganglioneuroma reflect a spectrum of maturation and differentiation.

Neuroblastoma is composed of small uniform cells with scant cytoplasm and hyperchromatic nuclei. The presence of neuropil and Homer-Wright pseudorosette are diagnostic of neuroblastoma. These pseudorosettes, observed in 15-50% of tumour samples can be described as neuroblasts surrounding eosinophilic neuritic processes.

Ganglioneuroma on the other hand is composed of mature ganglion cells, neuropil and Schwannian cells.

Ganglioneuroblastoma comprises of tumours with histology spanning the extremes of ganglioneuroma on one hand and neuroblastoma on other.

Light microscopy is frequently unable to differentiate neuroblastoma from other small blue round cell tumours. Inmmunohistochemistry with NSE, chromogranin, synaptophysin, and S-100 stains usually are positive. Electron microscopy can be useful because ultrastructural features like presence of microfilaments, microtubules and dense core granules are diagnostic for neuroblastoma.

Earlier Shimada and Joshi pathological classification was in use but now International Neuroblastoma Pathology Classification that combines the best features of these two systems has been developed. The tumours are divided into those with favourable and unfavourable histopathology depending upon histology, age and mitosis-karyorrhexis index (MKI). MKI is defined as total number of necrotic tumour, mitotic cells and cells with lobulated, pyknotic or malformed cells per 5000 cells examined.

Favourable Histopathology
- Any age; ganglioneuroma maturing or mature
- Any age; ganglioneuroblastoma, intermixed
- Less than 1.5 years old; neuroblastoma; poorly differentiated or differentiating and low or intermediate MKI
- 1.5 years up to less than 5 years old; neuroblastoma; differentiating and low MKI.

Unfavourable Histopathology
- Any age; ganglioneuroblastoma, nodular
- Any age neuroblastoma; undifferentiated and any MKI, or high MKI
- 1.5 years up to less than 5 years old; neuroblastoma; poorly differentiated tumour and any MKI, or inter-mediate MKI
- Equal to or greater than 5 years old; neuroblastoma; any subtype and any MKI.

Clinical Features

Because neuroblastoma can arise from any site along the sympathetic nervous system explains the multiple anatomic sites where these tumours occur; location of tumours appears to vary with age. Tumours can occur in the abdominal cavity (40% adrenal, 25% paraspinal ganglia) or involve other sites (15% thoracic, 5% pelvic, 3% cervical tumours, 12% miscellaneous). The signs and symptoms in neuroblastoma reflect the location of primary, regional and metastatic disease.

Most with neuroblastoma have abdominal primaries and present with an asymptomatic abdominal mass that usually is discovered by the parents or a caregiver (Fig. 13.2). Symptoms produced by the presence of the mass depend on its proximity to vital structures and usually progress over time:
- Tumours arising from the paraspinal sympathetic ganglia can grow through the spinal foramina into the spinal canal and compress the spinal cord. This may result in the presence of neurologic symptoms, including motor, sensory deficits and even bladder and bowel dysfunction.
- Tumours may compress the lymphatic or venous drainage resulting in scrotal or lower extremity oedema.

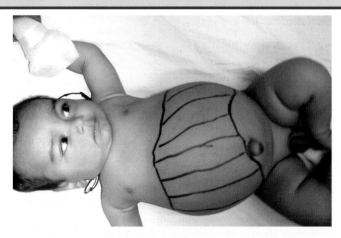

Fig. 13.2: A baby with neuroblastoma IV S presenting with hepatomegaly

- Sudden enlargement of abdominal mass may be due to haemorrhage into the tumour.
- Thoracic neuroblastomas (posterior mediastinum) may be asymptomatic and usually are diagnosed by imaging studies obtained for other reasons. Presenting signs or symptoms may be insignificant and involve mild airway obstruction or chronic cough, leading to a chest radiograph. Occasionally they may result in superior vena cava syndrome.
- Thoracic tumours extending to the neck can produce Horner's syndrome. Primary cervical neuroblastoma is rare but should be considered in the differential diagnosis of masses of the neck, especially in infants younger than 1 year with feeding or respiratory difficulties.

Metastatic extension of neuroblastoma occurs by both haematogenous and lymphatic routes. Haematogenous spread occurs most often to bone, bone marrow, liver, and skin.

- Extensive metastases to liver may result in respiratory compromise.
- Metastases to bone may cause bone pain and limping. Periorbital ecchymosis and proptosis secondary to metastatic disease to the orbits may be the presenting complaint. The presence of bone metastases can lead to pathologic fractures.
- Skin involvement especially in infants with stage 4S is characterized by variable number of nontender bluish subcutaneous nodules. Blueberry muffin baby is the term sometimes to describe extensive involvement of skin.
- Symptoms of bone marrow failure (anaemia, bleeding and infection) may be present if there is extensive involvement of bone marrow.

Minority of patients may present with paraneoplastic syndromes

- Opsomyoclonus: Child presents with myoclonic jerking and random eyeball movements. Antineural antibodies against the tumour may cross react with neurons in cerebellum and may cause opsomyoclonus.
- Secretory diarrhoea and hypokalaemia may be the manifestation of tumour secretion of VIP (vasoactive intestinal peptide).

Constitutional symptoms like fever and failure to thrive may be the presenting complaint.

Investigations

Laboratory Investigations

- Complete blood counts
- Basic metabolic panel
- Urinary catecholamines: Increased levels are detected in 90% to 95% of neuroblastomas patients. Urinary homovanillic acid (HVA), metabolite of DOPA and dopamine, and vanillylmandelic acid (VMA), metabolite of epinephrine and epinephrine are measures. 24-hour measurements are preferred as compared to spot samples. Higher HVA/ VMA is associated with less differentiated tumour.

Other investigations

Imaging is required to know the origin and extent of disease. CT or MRI is done to determine the extent of primary.

Metastases are common in neuroblastoma; therefore, possible sites of metastases are investigated to rule out involvement:

- Bone: Skeletal survey and bone scan (technetium 99)
- Bone marrow: Bilateral bone marrow aspiration and biopsy from posterior superior iliac spine. Single positive study is enough to diagnose bone marrow metastases.
- Abdominal imaging with CT or MRI
- Chest radiograph AP and lateral. Chest CT is only done if chest radiograph is abnormal or abdominal tumour extends into the chest.

MIBG (methyliodobenzylguanadine) scintigraphy: MIBG accumulates in catecholaminergic cells including most neuroblastomas and provides a specific way of identifying primary and metastatic disease if present.

Diagnostic criteria

Diagnosis of neuroblastoma is established if:

- An equivocal pathological diagnosis is made from tumour tissue by light microscopy, with or without immunohistology, electron microscopy, or increased urine catecholamines or metabolites; or
- Bone marrow aspirate or biopsy containing unequivocal tumour cells, and increased urine catecholamines or metabolites.

Staging

Earlier multiple staging systems were in use. International Neuroblastoma Staging System (INSS) was developed to make the staging of neuroblastomas around the world.

- **Stage 1:** Localized tumour with complete gross excision, with or without microscopic residual disease; representative ipsilateral lymph nodes negative for tumour microscopically (i.e., nodes attached to and removed with the primary tumour may be positive).
- **Stage 2A:** Localized tumour with incomplete gross excision; representative ipsilateral nonadherent lymph nodes negative for tumour microscopically.
- **Stage 2B:** Localized tumour with or without complete gross excision, with ipsilateral nonadherent lymph nodes positive for tumour. Enlarged contralateral lymph nodes must be negative microscopically.
- **Stage 3:** Unresectable unilateral tumour infiltrating across the midline, with or without regional lymph node involvement; or localized unilateral tumour with contralateral regional lymph node involvement; or midline tumour with bilateral extension by infiltration (unresectable) or by lymph node involvement. The midline is defined as the vertebral column. Tumours originating on one side and crossing the midline must infiltrate to or beyond the opposite side of the vertebral column.
- **Stage 4:** Any primary tumour with dissemination to distant lymph nodes, bone, bone marrow, liver, skin, and/or other organs, except as defined for stage 4S.
- **Stage 4S:** Localized primary tumour, as defined for Stage 1, 2A, or 2B, with dissemination limited to skin, liver, and/or bone marrow (limited to infants younger than 1 year). Marrow involvement should be minimal, i.e., <10% of total nucleated cells identified as malignant by bone biopsy or by bone marrow aspirate. More extensive bone marrow involvement would be considered to be Stage 4 disease.

Prognostic factors

- **Age:** Infants have better prognosis than older children
- Early Stage of disease (I and II) is better
- **Tumour site:** Cervical neuroblastomas have better prognosis, maybe due to their early detection. Pelvic and thoracic tumours carry a better prognosis than abdominal tumours.
- Cortical bone involvement is associated with poor prognosis.
- **Tumour pathology:** Favourable or unfavourable as determined by International Neuroblastoma Pathology Classification

Genetic markers

- MYCN amplification
- Hyperdiploid karyotype
- 1p loss of heterozygosity
- TrkA

Treatment

Principles of Surgery

Surgery plays an important role in the diagnosis and management of neuroblastoma.

Advances in chemotherapy have made sacrifice of vital structures during resection, unnecessary. Gross complete resection should be attempted if possible. Non-adherent, intracavitary lymph nodes should be sampled. Role of random liver biopsy to rule out hepatic metastases is controversial. Liver biopsy is still indicated in infants as imaging studies may miss diffuse involvement of liver.

Principles of Radiotherapy

Neuroblastoma is a radiosensitive tumour. Role of radiotherapy in management of neuroblastoma is clearly defined in following setting:

- Infants with Stage 4S disease who present with respiratory distress secondary to hepatomegaly and have not responded to chemotherapy.
- Total body irradiation is used as a part of many preparative regimens for autologous bone marrow transplant.
- To decrease spinal cord compression in patients with intraspinal extension of tumour, who present with neurological symptoms.
- Treating problematic metastatic disease at diagnosis
- Palliative management of pain in end-stage disease.

Role of radiotherapy in patients with locoregional disease is not well defined. Use of more dose intensive chemotherapy has made routine use of radiotherapy questionable. Radiotherapy may still be of benefit in patients whose tumour has responded incompletely to both chemotherapy and attempted resection and also has unfavourable biologic characteristics.

Principles of Chemotherapy

In patients of intermediate or high-risk neuroblastoma chemotherapy is the predominant modality of treatment. Drugs used in treatment of neuroblastoma are cyclophosphamide, cisplatin, doxorubicin and etoposide. Other drugs useful or under investigation are ifosfamide, carboplatin, irinotecan and topotecan.

Risk-related Treatment

Prognostic factors may determine the clinical behaviour of the tumour. Thus, most oncology study groups now divide the patients according to their risk groups. The COG Risk Stratification System has been developed from more than two decades of experience with clinical trials in Children's Cancer Group (CCG) and Paediatric Oncology Group (POG).

Treatment of Low-risk Disease

Surgery alone is effective as initial therapy in Stage 1 and 2 neuroblastoma. Recurrences are often salvageable with surgery.

Treatment for rare subset of these patients with MYCN amplification needs further evaluation, as relapses are frequent after surgery.

In patients with Stage 4S neuroblastoma, resection of primary tumour does not affect the outcome. Patient with respiratory distress secondary to hepatomegaly are treated initially with chemotherapy.

Treatment of Intermediate Risk Disease

Chemotherapy is the predominant modality for treatment of neuroblastoma. Cyclophosphamide, cisplatin, doxorubicin and etoposide are given for 12 to 24 weeks. Surgical resection of residual disease is done. Radiotherapy is reserved for patients with progression despite surgery and chemotherapy or for patients with unfavourable features and unresectable primary tumour after chemotherapy.

Treatment of High-risk Disease

Neuroblastoma is typically sensitive to initial chemotherapy so patients are given induction chemotherapy consisting of very high doses of cyclophosphamide, cisplatin, doxorubicin and etoposide with the goal of causing maximum reduction in tumour bulk. After a response to chemotherapy, resection of the primary tumour should be attempted, followed by myeloablative chemotherapy, sometimes total-body radiation, and autologous stem cell transplantation. Because of significant improvements in time to recovery and a lower risk of tumour cell contamination, most centres now recommend the use of peripheral blood stem cell support over bone marrow for consolidation therapy. Finally therapy against minimal residual disease is started with the goal of eradicating this chemoresistant residual disease by using agents, which are not typically cytotoxic.

Patients are treated with oral 13-cis-retinoic acid for 6 months. Retinoids are helpful by promoting cellular differentiation with decrease in proliferation of neuroblastoma cells.

Prognosis and Survival

The 5 year survival rates are approximately 80% for infants, 50% for children 1-5 years and 40% for children

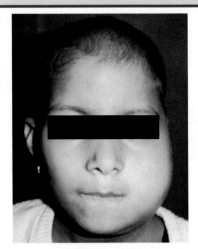

Fig. 13.3: Submandibular rhabdomyosarcoma

older than 5 years. Children with disseminated disease have a high mortality rate. The 3 year event free survival for high-risk patients treated with conventional chemotherapy, radiotherapy and surgery is less than 20%. Bone marrow transplantation has been found to improve survival.

RHABDOMYOSARCOMA

Introduction

Rhabdomyosarcoma (RMS) is the most common soft tissue tumour in children. It is a ubiquitous tumour occurring almost everywhere but most commonly in the head and neck, testis and the genitourinary (GU) areas (Fig. 13.3). RMS is the third most common neoplasm after neuroblastoma and Wilms tumour, comprising 15% of all extracranial paediatric solid tumours. Multimodal treatment approach, risk-adapted therapy, refinements in tumour grouping and better supportive care have resulted in good survival rates with 73 % children having failure free survival for more than 3 yrs.

Epidemiology

Annual incidence of RMS in children less than 20 yrs of age is 4-5 cases per million children. Almost two-thirds of cases of RMS are diagnosed in children <6 years of age although there is another mid-adolescence peak. It is slightly more common in males than in females (1.3-1.4: 1).

Etiology

Majority of cases of RMS occur sporadically, but few cases have also been associated with some familial syndromes like Li-Fraumeni syndrome and neurofibromatosis.

Molecular biology

In the last decade specific genetic alterations associated with the development of this tumour have been uncovered.

The two major histologic subtypes of RMS, i.e. embryonal RMS (ERMS) and alveolar RMS (ARMS) are associated with characteristic but distinct genetic alterations.

ARMS have a translocation between long arms of chromosome 2 and 13; t (2; 13)(q35; q14) or between chromosomes 1 and 13 which generate PAX3-FKHR and PAX7-FKHR fusion proteins respectively. ERMS have allelic loss at chromosome 11p15.5.

The most common oncogene abnormalities observed in RMS are RAS mutations.

Pathology

Gross Appearance

Rhabdomyosarcomas are grossly firm, nodular and of variable size and consistency. They are well circumscribed but not encapsulated and often tend to infiltrate extensively into adjacent tissues. Sarcoma botryoides subtype has characteristic grape-like appearance with its grape-like clusters of tumours arising from a mucosa-lined area.

Histology

RMS falls into the broader category of small round blue cell neoplasms of childhood. The characteristic feature that helps in characterizing the tumour, as RMS is identification of skeletal myogenic lineage, which can be done in following ways:
- **Light Microscopy:** Presence of cross-striations or characteristic rhabdomyoblast.
- **Immunohistochemistry:** Muscle-specific proteins, like desmin, muscle-specific actin, and myosin, myoglobin, Z band protein and Myo D can be identified by immunohistochemical staining.
- **Electron microscopy:** Identification of actin-myosin bundles or Z band.
  RMS was traditionally classified by Horn and Enterline in 1958. Due to lack of consensus between pathologists led to development of a new International Classification of Rhabdomyosarcoma, which was reproducible and prognostically useful. RMS was classified as:
1. Superior prognosis
   - Botryoid
   - Spindle cell
   Both uncommon variants of ERMS
2. Intermediate prognosis
   - Embryonal
3. Poor prognosis
   - Alveolar
   - Undifferentiated

Embryonal RMS: Stroma rich, spindle cell appearance, less dense and no evidence of alveolar pattern. *Botryoid type* has characteristic appearance of tumour layer under the epithelium. *Spindle cell* type has characteristic spindle shaped cells with abundant collagen in between them. Approximately two-thirds of newly diagnosed RMS belongs to the embryonal type.

Alveolar RMS: Presence of any alveolar pattern. Small round cells, densely packed.

Clinical Features

Site of Primary

- Head and neck- 35%
  1. Parameningeal-16%
  2. Orbit- 9%
  3. Other head and neck- 10%
- Genitourinary- 22%
- Extremity- 18%
- Others (trunk, intrathoracic, perineal, biliary tract)- 25%

Presentation

Some typical presentations by location of nonmetastatic disease are as follows:
- Orbit—Proptosis or dysconjugate gaze
- Paratesticular—Painless scrotal mass
- Prostate—Bladder or bowel difficulties
- Uterus, cervix, bladder—Menorrhagia or metrorrhagia
- Vagina—Protruding polypoid mass (botryoid, meaning a grape-like cluster)
- Extremity—Painless mass
- Parameningeal (ear, mastoid, nasal cavity, paranasal sinuses, infratemporal fossa, pterygopalatine fossa) - Upper respiratory symptoms or pain

Pattern of Spread

Nearly 25% of newly diagnosed cases have distant metastases with most of them having a single site involvement. The lung is the most common site of metastases (50%). Other sites of involvement are bone marrow, bone, and lymph node.

Investigations

Laboratory Studies

- Complete blood count
- Basic metabolic profile

Imaging Studies

- Plain X-ray films of affected part
- Skeletal survey
- Bone scan
- Computed tomography scan
- Magnetic resonance (especially for head and neck and extremity tumours)

Histology

Incisional or excisional biopsy is taken and submitted for histopathological examination.

Bilateral bone marrow aspiration and biopsy

Staging

Following two staging systems are currently employed in combination:
- **Clinical group staging system**
  - Group I—Tumour completely removed
  - Group II—Microscopic residual tumour, involved regional nodes, or both
  - Group III—Gross residual tumour
  - Group IV—Distant metastatic disease
- **TNM staging system**
  - Tumour—Confined to the site of origin (T1); extends beyond the site of origin (T2)
  - Node—No regional node involvement (N0); regional node involvement (N1); nodes unknown (NX)
  - Metastasis—No metastasis (M0); metastases present at diagnosis (M1)
  - Stage 1—Orbit, head/neck (not parameningeal), and GU tract (not bladder/prostate)
  - Stage 2—Other locations, N0, or NX
  - Stage 3—Other locations, N1 if tumour less than 5 cm, N0 or NX (if tumour >5 cm)
  - Stage 4—Any site with distant metastases

Treatment

Multimodal approach for treating RMS has resulted in better survival rates.

Various treatment protocols are in use for treatment of RMS:
- Intergroup RMS Study (IRS): First study in 1972. Treat cases with aggressive surgery, routine RT, prolonged chemotherapy for up to 2 yrs.
- Malignant Mesenchymal Tumour Study (MMTS): Non Radical surgery/biopsy followed by chemotherapy. RT omitted if complete remission

Surgery

Complete surgical excision has been the cornerstone of treatment. Now with multimodal (chemo+RT+ surgery) therapy local control rates of 95%. Surgery has evolved with avoidance of mutilating procedures and stress on organ preservation. There is no role of tumour debulking. Lymph node sampling is only necessary in extremity RMS.

Surgical Principles: Head and Neck

Non-surgical treatment for orbital RMS is standard. Biopsy followed by chemotherapy and radiotherapy achieves more than 90% survival. Eventration is reserved for recurrent or residual disease.

Other head and neck lesions are usually treated by biopsy followed by chemotherapy and radiotherapy with resection of the residual disease and reconstruction. Some superficial lesions can be excised primarily.

Surgical Principles Bladder and Prostate

Partial cystectomy is done for lesions at the dome of bladder, sarcoma botryoides that is pedunculated and excision of residual nodule. Bladder can usually be preserved without compromising survival rates. Cystectomy must be resorted to when adjuvant therapy fails.

Intracavitary radiotherapy has revolutionised treatment of these cases.

Surgical Principles: Paratesticular RMS

Radical inguinal orchidectomy is done and if scrotal violation is also there then hemiscrotectomy is also done. Retroperitoneal lymph node dissection is unnecessary in less than 10 yr old in which excellent cure rate can be achieved with chemotherapy. In children older than 10 yrs modified retroperitoneal lymph node dissection is done.

Surgical Principles: Vagina/ Uterus/ Vulva

Biopsy followed by chemotherapy and radiotherapy with limited resection or partial vaginectomy for the residual disease. Hysterectomy is only rarely required.

Surgical Principles: Extremities

Limb sparing wide local excision (2 cm margins) and regional LN biopsy is done. Amputation is rarely done and reserved for:
- Neurovascular bundle involvement
- Local recurrence
- Skeletally immature child
- Pain control in weight bearing limbs.

Chemotherapy

VAC (Vincristine, Actinomycin-D and Cyclophosphamide) is the gold standard for combination chemotherapy. Chemotherapy is usually given for 52 wks.

Low risk cases (Clinical group 1/2 orbit or eyelid and clinical group I paratesticular RMS) only VA (Vincristine and Actinomycin-D) given for 32 wks is sufficient.

In infants the dose is decreased by half.

Radiotherapy

RMS is a radiosensitive tumour therefore radiotherapy is important in achieving local control. In clinical group II and stage 3 clinical group I cumulative dose of 41.4 – 45.0 Gy and in clinical group III, 50.4 – 54.0 Gy is given. This is given in daily fractions of 180 – 200 cGy. Treatment field comprises of initial pretreatment tumour volume with a 2 cm margin. Actinomycin D is stopped during radiotherapy.

With some exceptions radiotherapy is started after 9-12 wks of chemotherapy.

Prognostic factors

Presence of metastases is the most important prognostic factor. Other prognostic factors are site (orbit having best prognosis), histology, surgical resectability and age of the child. Overall in non-metastatic disease a 3 yr failure free survival rate of 76% can be achieved.

HEPATOBLASTOMA

Introduction

Hepatoblastoma is a form of liver cancer that usually occurs in infants. In contrast to hepatocellular carcinoma, it arises in an otherwise normal liver. Of all liver masses in children, approximately two-thirds are malignant and of these two-thirds are due to hepatoblastoma.

Epidemiology

Most cases of hepatoblastoma occur in infancy or very young childhood. The incidence of malignant liver tumours in infancy is 11.2 per million and decrease throughout childhood with incidence of 1.5 per million in children less than 15 yrs.

The mean age of diagnosis is around 19 months with the tumour being more common in boys, ratio of 1.4:1.0 to 2.0:1.0.

Aetiology

The aetiology of hepatoblastoma is unknown. Hepatoblastoma is linked to a number of genetic syndromes, the most important being Beckwith-Wiedemann syndrome and familial polyposis coli. Other syndromes associated with hepatoblastoma are Li-Fraumeni syndrome, trisomy 18 and glycogen storage disease type I.

There is increased incidence of hepatoblastoma in premature infants, therefore, there is need to determine specific factors related to prematurity which contribute to tumourigenesis as well as need for surveillance of the survivors of extreme prematurity.

Molecular Biology

The most common karyotype changes are extra copies of entire chromosomes most commonly 2 and 20.

Pathology

Gross

About 80% of hepatoblastoma are solitary with 60% involving the right lobe. They are lobulated tan yellow color with areas of haemorrhage and necrosis.

Histology

Broadly hepatoblastoma can be classified as Epithelial type or Mixed epithelial and mesenchymal type.

Epithelial type (56%)
- Foetal (31%): cords of neoplastic hepatocytes smaller than normal cells of foetal liver with nuclear to cytoplasmic ratio.
- Embryonal (19%): Primitive tubules formed by small epithelial cells with minimal cytoplasm.
- Macrotrabecular (3%): Cells grow in trabeculae of 20 to 40 cells in a repetitive pattern within the tumour
- Small cell undifferentiated (3%): Uniform population of cells lacking evidence of stromal or epithelial differentiation.

Mixed epithelial and mesenchymal type (44%)
- With teratoid features (10%)
- Without teratoid features (34%)

Clinical features

Most patients are asymptomatic at presentation. Asymptomatic mass palpated by either parent or pediatrician is the presenting complaint in 68% of patients. Other presentations are abdominal distention, anorexia, weight loss, abdominal pain and vomiting. Jaundice is rare (Fig. 13.4).

Pattern of spread

Majority of metastases occur in the lungs. Bone lesions have been reported but it is unclear whether these represent true metastases or are areas of demineralization. Metastases to brain or bone marrow are rare.

Investigations

Laboratory Investigations

- Complete blood counts: Anaemia and thrombocytosis are commonly observed.
- Basic metabolic panel: Liver enzymes are usually normal but may be raised.
- AFP (alpha-fetoprotein): Levels are increased in more than 80% of cases of hepatoblastoma. AFP is a major

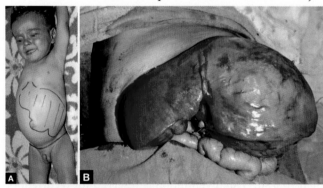

Figs 13.4A and B: Hepatoblastoma of the left lobe of liver (A) clinical appearance (B) operative findings

serum protein synthesised by fetal liver cells, yolk sacs, and the GI tract. Although elevated AFP levels are not specific for hepatoblastoma, they provide an excellent marker for response to therapy, disease progression, and detection of recurrent disease. The half-life of AFP is 5 to 7 days and levels fall to reference levels 4 to 6 weeks after complete resection. Interpretation of AFP levels can be difficult because hepatoblastoma tends to occur within the first 2 years of life. Reference range AFP levels are comparatively high at birth and even higher in premature infants, which can complicate interpretation of this value. By age 1 year, adult levels of less than 10 ng/ml have been reached. Hepatoblastomas with very low or very high levels of AFP are associated with poor prognosis.

Imaging Studies

- Plain abdominal radiograph: may reveal right upper quadrant mass and calcification.
- Ultrasound: Homogenous, encapsulated tumour that may be associated with portal venous or caval invasion
- CT scan of abdomen: Predominantly hypodense lesion with pathological areas of arterialization. Calcification may be present in 40% cases.
- MRI can also be done instead of CT scan: Low signal on T1 weighted sequences and heterogenous signal on T 2 weighted sequences.
- CT scan of chest: To exclude pulmonary metastases.

Histology

According to SIOPEL (Society of Paediatric Oncology Epithelial Liver Group) diagnosis is usually established on the basis of clinical setting, radiological findings and AFP values, biopsy is recommended in children less than 6 months of age or more than 3 yrs of age to differentiate from other tumours (hemangiothelioma and hepatic cell carcinoma).

- High Risk Case
- Low Risk Case

Staging

Paediatric oncology group staging of hepatoblastoma.

- Stage I (favourable histology): Complete resection with pure foetal histology
- Stage I (unfavourable histology): Complete resection with histology other than pure foetal type.
- Stage II: Microscopic residual disease, preoperative or intraoperative spill
- Stage III: Unresectable or partially resected tumours, positive lymph nodes
- Stage IV: Metastatic disease.
  PRETEXT (Pretreatment classification scheme) alternative staging system developed by International

Society of Paediatric Oncology based upon number of liver segments involved as determined by preoperative imaging studies. The liver is divided into four sectors. An anterior and a posterior sector on the right and a medial and a lateral sector on the left. Staging is done according to tumour extension with in the liver as well as involvement of hepatic vein (v), portal vein (p), regional lymph nodes or distant metastases (m).

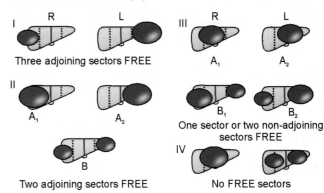

Treatment

Cooperative group trials have enabled development of treatment protocols for treatment of hepatoblastoma. From various studies it is clear that only chance for cure from hepatoblastoma is if sometime during treatment there is grossly complete resection. Most hepatoblastomas on other hand show good response to drugs, which shrinks the tumour thereby increasing the chances of resectability. Therefore, there are two principal strategies in treatment of hepatoblastoma:

- SIOPEL recommends no attempt for primary resection and giving the patient preoperative chemotherapy routinely.
- POG (Paediatric Oncology Group) promotes primary resection of tumour at presentation reserving chemotherapy for obviously unresectable tumours.
- German group: Because of concern that resistance may develop after 3 to 6 courses of chemotherapy and tumour may rapidly develop, primary resection of small localized tumour is advocated therefore a low resection rate (20%) is observed.

Surgery

Goal of hepatic tumour resection in general is to completely excise the tumour with at least a 1 cm margin. Anatomical resection is undertaken as they are associated with less intraoperative and postoperative morbidity and mortality. Lymph nodes at porta and hepatoduodenal ligaments are also removed and sampled. There is no significant difference in local tumour recurrence with microscopic positive as against negative margins.

Presence of microscopic residual disease does not necessarily mean a poor prognosis with respect to local tumour recurrence, nor does it imply the need for heroic chemotherapy or surgical salvage procedures. Extrahepatic disease is a more important predictor or outcome than surgical margins.

Orthotopic liver transplantation (OLT) is now accepted as a treatment modality for patients with unresectable tumours. Liver cancers now account for approximately 2% of all liver transplants in children. Early referral to a transplant surgeon should be considered in following situations:

- Multifocal PRETEXT 4 Hepatoblastoma
- Large, solitary PRETEXT 4 Hepatoblastoma, involving all four sectors of the liver
- Centrally located tumours involving main hilar structures or main hepatic veins

Chemotherapy

Cisplatin (CDDP) is accepted as the single most useful agent in treatment of hepatoblastoma. Other drugs which are used Doxorubicin (DOX), 5 Flurouracil (5FU), Vincristine (VCR) and Carboplatin. Use of Irinotecan is under investigation.

Radiotherapy

Radiotherapy does not play a major role in treatment of hepatoblastoma.

Prognostic Factors

The most important prognostic factor is complete tumour resection. Other prognostic factors are degree of mitotic activity in tumour cells (more than 2/hpf associated with poor prognosis), pure foetal histology (only if tumour completely resected) and AFP levels at presentation and a fall in response to chemotherapy, is good for prognosis.

HEPATOCELLULAR CARCINOMA (HCC)

This tumour occurs in older children, usually adolescent. It may present with a papable hepatic mass, abdominal pain and rarely jaundice. The serum Alpha feto protein is raised. In children, HCC can complicate viral hepatitis or metabolic liver disease. It is an aggressive tumour with poor pregnosis. It is chemoresistant and is usually advanced at diagnosis. Survival at 3 years is less than 25%.

GERM CELL TUMOURS

Germ cell tumours account for 2–4% of all malignant diseases in children. They occur in both male and female gonads and occur in a wide variety of paraxial sites. They can be benign or malignant. The importance of these tumours lies in the clearer definition of the role of surgery in treatment. Most malignant tumours are sensitive to chemotherapy and the accuracy of tumour marker measurement is an indicator of the success of treatment. Thus, correct surgical management of testicular tumours results in over 60% cure by orchiectomy alone, saving those patients the risks of permanent effects of the toxicity of chemotherapy. It is also likely that careful attention to surgical detail in the excision of benign sacro coccygeal teratomas in infants may prevent some malignant germ cell tumours.

The age distribution of malignant germ cell tumours as a group reflects the relative frequency of the tumours mentioned above. There is an early peak representing malignant recurrence after excision of sacrococcygeal teratoma in infants, and a later one for the cluster of testicular tumours in males in early puberty.

Embryology and pathology

In the normal embryo, germ cells are first identified at 4 weeks in the caudal aspect of the yolk sac wall, having arisen from the endoderm at the neck of the yolk sac (the endodermal sinus). Migration of these cells cephalad to the gonadal ridges is complete by 6 weeks. At this stage, the gonadal ridges extend along side the vertebral column from cervical to lower lumbar levels. Germ cells which aberrantly migrate further (e.g. to pineal and sacro-coccygeal sites) or remain outside the coalescence of gonadal tissue near the developing kidney, may be presumed to lose appropriate growth-regulating influences.

The steps leading to production of benign teratomas and malignant tumours are unknown, but a general explanation in terms of the stage and pathway of differentiation of the germ cell is possible. If it is unipotential, and committed to form gonadal precursors of the gametes, malignant transformation results in the undifferentiated germinoma. The multipotential cell, whether intra- or extragonadal, differentiates in a benign form to teratoma and under oncogenic influences to a range of malignant types (Fig. 13.5). It is noted that teratomas predominate in females between birth and 15 years, with a female: male ratio of 7:1 for sacrococcygeal teratomas. This increased susceptibility may be related to pathology in the steps leading to embryonic meiotic activity of germ cells in females.

Further clues to pathogenesis may be found in some well documented risks of malignancy in gonads. Family studies of phenotypic females with 46XY genotype show a high risk of gonadal malignant dysgerminoma, so-called 'gonadoblastoma'. In the undescended testis, the increased risk of malignancy is well documented. Premalignant intratubular germ cell neoplasia in an undescended testis has been documented as leading to invasive germ cell malignancy, as well as being found in tubules adjacent to established malignant disease. This appearance is not found in yolk sac tumours in the descended testis of early infancy, including those associated with teratoma. This

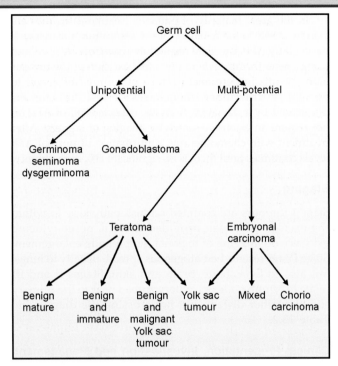

Fig. 13.5: Scheme of relationship in germ cell tumours

Table 13.1: Histopathology classification of germ cell tumours	
Germinoma	(a) Intratubular germ cell neoplasia
	(b) Invasive (dysgerminoma, seminoma)
Teratoma	(a) Mature/benign
	(b) Immature
	(c) Malignant (teratoma plus one or more malignant elements)
Embryonal carcinoma (adult type)	
Endodermal sinus tumour (yolk sac tumour)	
Choriocarcinoma	
Gonadoblastoma	

From Ref. 23, with permission from Wiley-Liss, Inc, New York

suggests that maldescent may be associated with an oncogenic influence on the germ cells and a different mechanism operates in the origin of malignant germ cell tumours associated with benign teratoma.

The overlap of histopathological appearances of tumours arising in different sites has led in the past to a confusion of different nomenclatures and ascriptions of the embryological origin of the tissues. Further confusion has arisen from the finding of immature elements in benign teratomas, especially those of the ovary.

Benign teratomas contain mature representation of all three embryonic germ layers. In some ovarian lesions, however, immature neuroectodermal tissue resembling neuroglia may invade outside the teratoma and across the peritoneum. Metastatic tissue appears nevertheless on microscopy as benign neuroglia.

Of the four main histological types of malignancy, yolk sac tumours (also known as endodermal sinus tumours) are the commonest in early infancy and may occur as malignant foci within an otherwise benign teratoma. Embryonal carcinoma is found in older children and in mixed histology types it co-exists with yolk sac tumours. Mixed tumours account for up to a quarter of cases (Table 13.1). Germinomas (testicular seminoma and ovarian dysgerminoma) are relatively rare in children. Choriocarcinoma is very rare, and presents in two forms: the gestational form in a sexually active teenager; and the non-gestational form which occurs in gonads or in males in extragonadal axial sites.

Though some patterns of chromosomal abnormalities have been identified in germ cell tumours, none so far has formed the basis of a prognostic test, except that aneuploidy is an unfavourable sign.

Malignant germ cell tumours are aggressive neoplasms with local invasive spread occurring early in instances of ovarian and mediastinal primaries. Testicular tumours in contrast often present clinically while still localized to their organ of origin. Metastatic spread is found in 20% of patients at presentation, in either regional lymph nodes or via hematogeneous spread to the lungs or occasionally the liver.

Tumour Markers

Alpha-fetoprotein (AFP), first identified as a serum marker of liver tumours, is in clinical practice almost invariably secreted to high levels by malignant germ cell tumours, a serum level greater than 100000 ng/ml being common. AFP is a glycoprotein with a serum half-life of about 5.5 days. The foetal and neonatal liver secretes AFP in large quantities and newborn levels of 50000 ng/ml are normal with still higher levels noted in premature infants. Marked variability of the rates of fall in the first 4 months of life make interpretation of changes of serum AFP difficult in this era. After the 8th month of life, levels remain low at less than 20 ng/ml. After infancy, the expected fall after total removal of a secreting tumour (Fig. 13.6) is easily plotted on a logarithmic chart, and any deviation from this line is considered evidence of residual or recurrent disease. Similarly, any elevation of the serum AFP level after removal of a benign teratoma is evidence of growth of a malignant yolk sac tumour.

Beta-human chorionic gonadotrophin (b-HCG) is secreted by some embryonal carcinomas and germinomas, and is presumed to arise from cells simulating syncytiotrophoblast. b-HCG is not associated with yolk sac tumours, but may be positive in instances of mixed tumour, from the embryonal carcinoma element. It is invariably present in patients with choriocarcinoma. Logarithmic graph with an even steeper slope than AFP can be constructed for

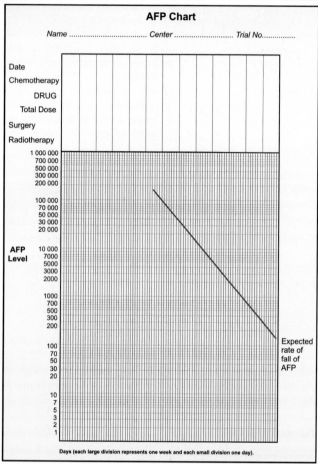

AFP Chart

Name .... Center .... Trial No................

Date
Chemotherapy
DRUG
Total Dose
Surgery
Radiotherapy

AFP
Level

Expected
rate of
fall of
AFP

Days (each large division represents one week and each small division one day).

Fig. 13.6: Logarithmic chart for plotting the fall of AFP during treatment

monitoring the progress of patients with tumours secreting this tumour marker.

Some central nervous system germ cell tumours secrete markers, either AFP or b-HCG. An international study showed that there was correlation between tumour markers and histology in only 48% of patients. Elevation of cerebrospinal fluid (CSF) levels of markers over a simultaneous serum sample give a good indication of the nature of a tumour seen on imaging, or of recurrence of known tumour within the central nervous system (CNS) after initial treatment.

In the great majority of patients, treatment regimes are closely linked to the behavior of the serum tumour markers, particularly AFP. Excellent results have been reported without using chemotherapy where operative excision of the tumour alone results in permanent return of serum AFP levels to normal. Furthermore, metastases or residual tumour discovered by a deviation from the expected fall of AFP do not require an extensive search by imaging or surgery. After treatment with chemotherapy, confirmation of normal AFP levels continues until there is no significant risk of recurrence.

Staging

Stage I tumours are confined on histopathology to within the excised specimen provided there is no convincing evidence on imaging of regional lymph node enlargement. Stage IV represents hematogenous spread, usually to lungs, but also to liver, bone, brain and skin. Stages II and III relate to lymph node or cavitary spread near to the primary site or further distant, but not crossing the diaphragm, Table 13.2.

Clinical Presentation, Investigation and Management

Testis

The finding of a painless and hard enlargement of a previously normal testis is the commonest presentation. In most cases the obvious change in testicular size and consistency leads to medical intervention before local invasion or distant metastases have occurred. In the absence of pain, the differential diagnosis includes other malignancies, particularly paratesticular rhabdomyosarcoma and testicular involvement in leukemia. Serum AFP levels should be measured urgently and a chest radiograph should be obtained to exclude metastases.

Ultrasound examination of the retroperitoneal tissues, both iliac and at the level of the renal vessels, will detect significant enlargement of lymph nodes. An abdominal CT study is more accurate in assessing the lymph node presence and status. Except for a complete blood count, other investigations are not justified, since removal of the tumour and histological examination of the whole testis and inguinal cord should be carried out promptly.

	Table 13.2: Staging	
		Site of original tumour
Stage	Uterine, vaginal, prostatic or sacrococcygeal	Abdominal, retroperitoneal, thoracic or other
I	Tumour confined to organ/site of origin	Tumour confined to the site of origin and respectable
II	Tumour spread limited to the pelvis	Local spread
III	Tumour spread limited to the abdomen (excluding liver)	Extensive spread confined to one side of the diaphragm (excluding liver)
IV	Tumour spread to the liver or beyond the abdominal cavity	Tumour spread to the liver, to both sides of the diaphragm, and/or to bones, bone marrow or brain

From Ref 24, with permission from Wiley-Liss, Inc, New York

Trans-scrotal biopsy or any scrotal incisions are contraindicated. A groin incision is made which should be wider than for herniotomy. The inguinal canal is opened and the cord mobilized at the internal ring. A double throw of a silicone vascular loop is placed around the cord to act as a vascular clamp. The scrotal tumour is then mobilized through the scrotal neck and delivered into the groin wound (Figs 13.7A to C). If tumour is confirmed, following high ligation of the cord at the internal ring, orchidectomy is performed. If the scrotal skin has followed the testicular mass upwards, careful dissection is undertaken to ensure that no tumour is left behind. Biopsy must be performed at this stage if it is feared that invasion of scrotal tissue has occurred. This is rarely required. Hemiscrotectomy may be necessary if the scrotal skin is involved. There is no case for retroperitoneal node sampling or dissection. Postoperatively, AFP should be measured regularly and the results charted. Particular note is taken of any histological evidence of tumour extension to the cut end of the cord, or any breaching of the capsule of the tumour in the scrotum.

Stage I testicular germ cell tumours should carry a virtually 100% survival rate.

Ovary

In contrast to testicular tumours, ovarian malignant germ cell tumours usually present after the first decade of life and with widespread pelvic or intra-abdominal tumour spread. In advanced cases, ascites and cachexia are found. In the majority of girls abdominal pain leads to the finding of a lower abdominal mass (Figs 13.8A and B) and its nature is established by the results of aquiring serum AFP or b-HCG levels. Abdominal radiographs may show a mass teratoma containing bone or teeth (Fig.13.9) and a mixed echogenicity appearance on ultrasound exami-nation suggests the presence of solid and cystic components. The presence of these findings while compatible with a benign teratoma, do not exclude malignant germ cell tumour. Clues to malignancy will come from CT or MRI evidence of invasion of pelvic wall tissues or other viscera, or evidence of obstruction of ureters. Chest radiograph and ultrasound examination of lymph nodes are called for in all suspected cases of malignant germ cell tumour.

If investigations suggest that surgical excision is possible, this should be undertaken. Rarely when a benign teratoma is being removed, evidence of peritoneal deposits of neuroglial tissue may be found and biopsy is required. The prognosis is good and chemotherapy not required. A needle biopsy serves to make a histological diagnosis. Laparoscopy may be a highly suitable instrument to control the acquisition of several samples of an invasive tumour.

Following chemotherapy, and re-evaluation on scanning, an additional role for the surgeon may be at second-look

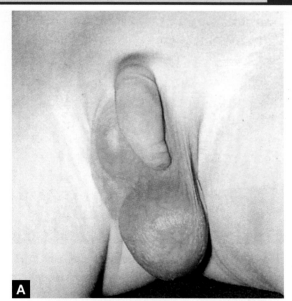

Fig. 13.7A: Clinical photograph of a testicular tumour (orchioblastoma)

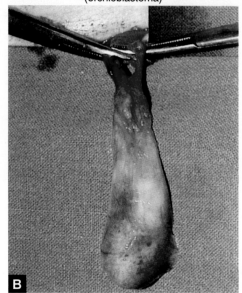

Fig. 13.7B: Operative photograph showing groin incision cord clamping and removal of tumour

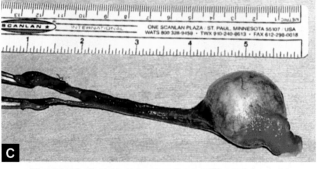

Fig. 13.7C: Orchidectomy specimen with cord clamped

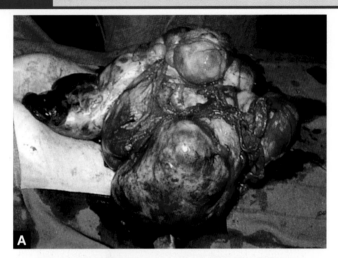

Fig. 13.8A: Malignant ovarian tumour filling the abdomen

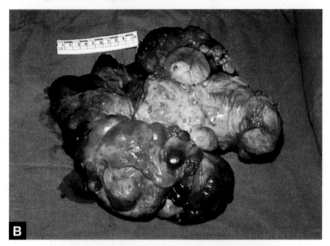

Fig. 13.8B: Tumour excised

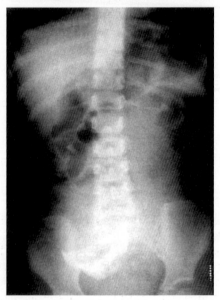

Fig. 13.9: Iliac crest bone in an ovarian tumour (desmoid)

laparotomy or laparoscopy to check for any residual malignancy and of course to excise any benign teratoma.

Sacrococcygeal

Teratomas in the newborn are most common in girls, are almost always benign and 40% of them are sacrococcygeal. Altman et al noted and classified the varying anatomical presentation with Type I virtually all external and without presacral extension, and Type IV, entirely presacral and without external component. Type IV teratomas tended to present late and are more difficult to detect. Some teratomas, however, are now found on prenatal ultrasound studies sometimes causing obstructive uropathy. These tumours may be inherently more associated with malignant germ cell tumours, but in any case, a neglected tumour acquires a high risk of malignancy after 6 months of age.

It is likely, therefore, that prompt and correct surgical management will prevent the occurrence of some malignancies. The teratoma should be excised with a margin of surrounding subcutaneous tissue. It must be detached carefully from pelvic floor muscles, and any intrapelvic extension protruding through them requires very exact attention to surgical detail to minimize long-term sequelae in the urinary tract and rectum/anal canal. The pelvic floor muscles will need careful repair in relation to the repositioned anal canal (which in Altman Types I and II is often found tilted to face forwards). Teratomas of Types III and IV, mainly or entirely intrapelvic, require a combined abdominal and perineal approach. On occasions, these tumours may so fill the pelvis that risks of damage to the rectum during surgery are very high; and a colostomy may rarely be warranted until the integrity of the rectum has been checked by contrast imaging some weeks after the excision of the teratoma. Rarely a pubic symphysiotomy may afford some vital extra dissection space during removal of a difficult intrapelvic teratoma.

In all cases, the coccyx itself must be excised with the tumour to minimize the risk of either benign or malignant recurrence which can occur in 30% of cases in which the coccyx is left in place at the original procedure.

After excision of the teratoma, follow-up evaluation using serum AFP levels as a guide to an event-free postoperative status must take normal infant levels of AFP into account. Until 8 months of age, regular rectal examination is justified, after which serum AFP levels will yield accurate evidence, not only of pelvic, but of any possible metastatic yolk sac tumour. Malignant recurrence in the site of excision of a sacrococcygeal teratoma (or malignancy associated with a neglected tumour) is very unlikely to be surgically excised (Figs 13.10A and B). Symptoms usually include constipation or obstruction of the urinary tract or both. A primary pelvic tumour will need to be distinguished by scanning from some benign

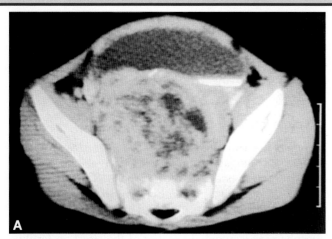

Fig. 13.10A: CT scan showing mixed density pelvic recurrence of a malignant yolk sac tumour in a patient aged 16 months

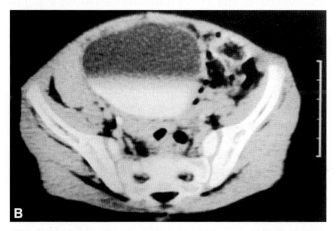

Fig. 13.10B: Pelvic CT scan after chemotherapy showing complete disappearance of the yolk sac tumour recurrence

lesions, including anterior lipomeningocele, presacral neuroblastoma and pelvic rhabdomyosarcoma. The serum AFP will almost certainly confirm the diagnosis. In a primary tumour, biopsy is obligatory, but this may be omitted where a sacrococcygeal teratoma has previously been excised. After chemotherapy, surgical excision of any residual teratoma is required. Frequently no malignant tissue is found in the specimen after chemotherapy.

Other Extracranial Sites

Wherever benign teratomas are found, malignant germ cell tumours may occur in relation to them. Teratomas are found in association with almost all intraperitoneal organs and also occur in the retroperitoneum. The most common mode of presentation is with abdominal pain leading to the discovery of a mass, although a mass may have been noted on antenatal ultrasound. In any case, retroperitoneal lesions tend to present in very small children.

In contrast, mediastinal teratoma occurs in older children and adolescents. Mediastinal tumours are mainly found in the anterior superior compartment apparently arising from the thymus. They may reach considerable size before compression of the major airways produces cough, wheezing and breathlessness. Hemoptysis has been reported and may be related to extension of teratoma into a bronchus. Occasionally these tumours may be hormonally active and induce precocious puberty. Plain radiographs of the chest may show features of teratoma (calcification) and CT scanning will elucidate the involvement of airways and other major structures. After obtaining serum AFP and b-HCG levels, biopsies should be planned. If the serum AFP level is normal, the lesion is probably benign and should be excised. In cases of malignancy chemotherapy is likely to be successful and primary surgery is only indicated if a very well defined tumour can be removed without damage to vital structures. 'Debulking' surgery is contraindicated. After chemotherapy, excision of any residual teratoma and tumour is planned using further scans and serum AFP levels as a guide to response.

Extracranial teratomas in the head and neck tend to occur in early life and often present in the newborn. Cervical teratoma is often detected on prenatal ultrasound examination. Delivery of these infants should be performed at a high-risk delivery centre with paediatric surgeons available at delivery, as prompt organization of an adequate airway (including possible tracheostomy) may be life-saving. Excision of a benign teratoma in this region may be surgically demanding. A malignant yolk sac tumour occurring in the teratoma site is easily dealt with by chemotherapy. Most patients can be managed on the basis of serum AFP estimations without the need for repeated scanning.

Intracranial Tumours

Only 2–3% of intracranial tumours are of germ cell origin, but the majority of pineal tumours are of this group. Suprasellar tumours also occur, with girls more likely to be affected. The chief presenting symptom in suprasellar tumours is diabetes insipidus, and in pineal tumours, raised intracranial pressure. Abnormal eye movements, oculomotor palsies and visual field disturbances may be observed and hormonally active tumours may induce precocious puberty.

The discovery of a pineal tumour on CT or MRI scanning is highly indicative of a malignant germ cell tumour. MRI is most likely to detect a small suprasellar lesion, and often shows the characteristic mixed density of these tumours. CT scanning with contrast shows the bright enhancement corresponding to the increased vascularity that often accompanies these lesions.

The next move in investigation is to measure levels of tumour markers silmultaneously in serum and CSF samples. In addition, the cytology of the CSF is important since positive findings of malignant cells indicate CNS metastatic spread.

The largest current treatment study, successfully piloted for over 3 years, runs under the auspices of the Société Internationale d'Oncologie Paediatrique (now the International Society of Pediatric Oncology) (SIOP). The protocols avoid surgery where possible, in marked contrast to the surgical emphasis in some North American centres.

Yolk sac tumours, embryonal carcinoma (including mixed tumours) and choriocarcinoma accounts for just over one-third of intracranial germ cell tumours. In the presence of characteristic scanning features and positive tumour markers, the tumour should not be biopsied, thus sparing the patient the risks of intruding into a highly vascular intracranial lesion. To date, though results in secreting CNS tumours are not good, biopsy confers no known added value to management. In the absence of cytological evidence of CNS spread, chemotherapy (see below) is instituted. Following regression, radiotherapy is given focally to the lesion, with a surrounding margin. With positive cytology, or if CNS metastases were found on scanning at presentation, complete craniospinal axis radiotherapy is required.

In a few cases, during chemotherapy, tumour markers may disappear without full regression of the tumour on imaging. This occurs most commonly in a mixed malignant tumour where b-HCG secreting choriocarcinoma disappears leaving embryonal elements of poor chemosensitivity. Alternatively, a benign teratoma may constitute the residue. Under these circumstances, surgical excision is essential.

Germinomas do not secrete markers, and biopsy is essential to differentiate them from other CNS tumours, including all the more common types. Mediastinal germ cell tumours in boys with b-HCG positive tumour markers have been reported in patients with Klinefelter's syndrome. Germinomas, like their gonadal counterparts, are highly radiosensitive, and survival of over 90% is achievable. The two possible approaches include craniospinal axis irradiation with a boost to the primary tumour site and chemotherapy with focal radiotherapy to the primary site. To date, no trial of these two methods has been evaluated. Since good results are obtained, very large numbers and wide international collaboration would be required to show a difference in survival, or in morbidity. Most germinomas occur in teenagers, and radiotherapy does not result in the cognitive disorders seen, for instance, after treatment of CNS leukaemia in the young.

Where early and urgent surgical management of hydrocephalus with increased intracranial pressure has been required, the risks of tumour dissemination via the ventriculoperitoneal shunt must be borne in mind. Chemotherapy has shown as much success in treating systemic dissemination from ventriculoperitoneal shunting as in treating CNS metastases from extracranial tumours.

Chemotherapy

Advances in chemotherapy have led to: a) a clearer role for surgery and biopsy; b) improved survival; and c) lower levels of toxicity and long-term sequelae. Thus, because of toxicity or late effects, some highly effective regimes are now reserved for relapsed or incompletely responding patients. For instance, the alkylating agent cyclophosphamide is avoided because of the effect on fertility, except with Adriamycin® (doxorubicin), vincristine, actinomycin-D and cyclophosphamide (Adria-VAC) in relapsed patients. The lung toxicity observed with use of bleomycin has led to careful modification of the dose and method of administration of this highly effective agent. Finally, for extracranial tumours, carboplatin has been substituted for the more ototoxic and nephrotoxic cisplatin. The formula for the administration of carboplatin has been refined.

Results are now available from the UKCCSG's second germ cell tumour trial (GCII) showing that carboplatin, etoposide and bleomycin (JEB) are effective and less toxic than previous regimens in the treatment of extracranial non-gonadal malignant germ cell tumours. In this trial, which ran from 1989 to 1995, courses of JEB were given every 3 weeks until remission was achieved (assessed by normal serum AFP and/or b-HCG levels and radiological findings), followed by two further courses. In each course, etoposide 120 mg/m was given intravenously over 1 hour on each of days 1–3, carboplatin 600 mg/m2 intravenously over 1 hour on day 2 and bleomycin 15 mg/m2 intravenously over 15 minutes on day 3.

Among the 44 survivors of chemotherapy in GCII, 43 are evaluable and none has renal impairment; four children have deafness. This contrasts with renal impairment in six of 30 evaluable children in the previous trial (CGI) and deafness in 11. In GCII, toxicity appears to be among the lowest yet, while still comparing favourably for survival with all previous trials worldwide (Fig. 13.11).

For intracranial germ cell tumours, mostly those secreting tumour markers, the current SIOP study uses cisplatin, etoposide, and ifosfamide (PEI), in four courses before further evaluation with a view to subsequent radiotherapy or surgery.

Radiotherapy

The high chemosensitivity of most malignant germ cell tumours excludes radiotherapy from treatment programs.

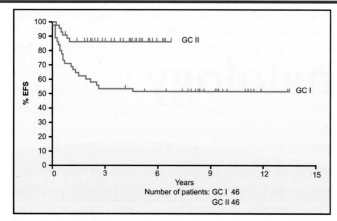

Fig. 13.11: Event-free survival for 46 cases treated in GCI (the six low dose VAC cases were excluded) and all 46 cases treated in GCII

Rarely a focal metastasis in a resistant tumour may be treated to relieve symptoms. The chief exception is germinoma. Few gonadal germinomas occur in childhood, but they are highly radiosensitive, and good results are obtained. Similarly, the intracranial germinoma has been successfully treated by radiotherapy for more than two decades. In adolescents, the dose required is unlikely to produce the cognitive effects seen in the irradiated brain of the young child. However, some suprasellar germ cell tumours present with an effect on the pituitary, and irradiation may extend the damage. Lack of growth hormone in adults may be harmful and lead to obesity and other symptoms, and endocrine surveillance is required after therapy in all such patients.

Prognosis

The correct combination of surgery and chemotherapy has recently resulted in excellent outcomes, building on the fine results for testicular tumours which have been achieved over the last decade. Many testicular tumours are cured by correct surgical management alone. Though up to 25% of these are either metastatic at presentation or relapse after appearing to be Stage I, survival at or near 100% is reported. Two patients died out of 74 in UKCCSG GCI, after a low dose of VAC (vincristine/actinomycin-D/cyclophosphamide) was given for metastases. All patients receiving full dose VAC survived. It is expected that patients in the later trial GCII will have at least as good results with fewer toxic effects.

Ovarian tumours prove more difficult to manage, and 25% relapse after initial chemotherapy or fail to respond to first line treatment. Of the extragonadal tumours, the rare primary sites including vagina, uterus and prostate carry the best prognosis. A quarter of malignant tumours recurring in the site of a sacrococcygeal teratoma may show relapsing or persistent disease, and mediastinal primary tumours carry a similar poor prognosis. However, a number of relapsing patients are salvaged by Adriavac or other more toxic chemotherapy regimes.

The advance in chemotherapy can be judged by the difference in 5-year event-free survival in GC1 (46%) and GCII (87%).

BIBLIOGRAPHY

1. Gupta DK, Carachi R (Eds) Pediatric Oncology. Jaypee Brothers, New Delhi, 2007.

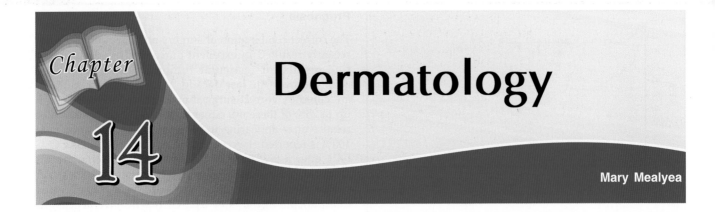

Dermatology

Mary Mealyea

INTRODUCTION

The function of the skin is to provide a barrier between the outside world (i.e. the environment) and our internal organs. This barrier provides, physical, mechanical, chemical and immunological protection from the external environment. It also has important sensory, endocrine and thermoregulatory functions.

The skin is a complex organ consisting of three layers: Epidermis, dermis and subcutaneous fat. Within the three layers there are many types of cells (Fig. 14.1).

The epidermis is the outside layer of skin that is a continually regenerating living barrier. More than 90% of its cells are keratinocytes. The keratinocytes mature and move up to form an outer layer of dead cells. These form a waterproof protective layer.

Melanocytes are found in the basal layer of the epidermis. These cells produce melanin, which absorbs and scatters ultraviolet light, visible light and near infrared radiation. Thus providing a physical barrier protecting against damage from sunlight. Melanosomes (packets of melanin) protect the nucleus from the harmful effects of ultraviolet radiation. Without this protection skin cancer may develop.

Diseases affecting the epidermis usually result in abnormal scale, change in pigmentation or loss of surface integrity resulting in an erosion or the production of an exudate.

The dermis contains collagen and elastic fibres, which provide an elastic tough supportive layer under the epidermis. Specialised structures within this layer include hair follicles and sweat glands. It also contains mast cells, macrophages and lymphocytes.

The subcutaneous layer provides some added protection in the form of shock absorption.

It is also an energy store and helps to maintain body heat. This layer is made up of adipocytes that form lobules and are separated by fibrous septae. The blood supply is carried in this septae.

COMMON TERMS USED

Erythema	– A patch of redness caused by capillary dilatation or hyperaemia
Macule	– A small circumscribed flat area of altered skin colour
Papule	– A small (< 5 mm) solid elevated skin lesion
Plaque	– A large (> 5 mm) solid elevated skin lesion
Nodule	– A circumscribed elevated solid skin lesion
Vesicle	– A small (< 5 mm) fluid-filled elevated skin lesion
Bulla	– A large (> 5 mm) fluid-filled elevated skin lesion
Pustule	– A small (< 5 mm) pus containing, elevated skin lesion

Fig. 14.1: Diagram of structure of normal skin

Epidermis

Dermis

Sebaceous gland

Fat

Collagen

Sweat gland

Hair follicle

Wheal	– A transient skin lesion consisting of an elevated pale centre with a surrounding flare of erythema. Often described by patients as 'blisters'. It is characteristic of urticaria and can be produced by the release of histamine in the dermis.
Scale	– A sheet of adherent corneocytes in the process of being shed
Crust	– Dried exudate consisting of a mixture of serum and scale, sometimes with erythrocytes and leucocytes
Ulcer	– A discontinuity in the skin surface involving the complete loss of epidermis.
Erosion	– A superficial ulcer
Excoriation	– A scratch mark
Lichenification	– A patch or plaque in which the epidermis appears to be thickened and the normal skin creases are more prominent
Scar	– A patch or plaque in which the skin surface has lost the normal surface crease, contour and skin appendages

History

As in any other branch of medicine a careful history is important. The history, not only about the rash or lesion, but also about general health and relevant family history is fundamental to making a correct diagnosis. In children obviously this information will be obtained from a parent or carer but it should be from the person who is most involved with the care of the child and who can give an accurate history.

Important questions about the rash or lesion

- When and where and how did it begin?
- Has it changed and if so how?
- Does it come and go?
- Does anything make it better or worse?
- Is it itchy, painful or tender?
- Does anyone else in the family have a similar rash or lesion?
- How is their general health, are they otherwise well and thriving?

The examination

The close examination of the whole skin under good light is important. There are three aspects to the examination.
1. The distribution of the rash or lesion. Is it limited to one particular area or areas or widespread, in other words where is its location? Is it symmetrical or segmental?

2. The morphology of the primary lesion. In other words what does a lesion look like when it first appears? What shape, colour and size is it? Is it scaly or smooth or does it form blisters?
3. The configuration of the rash. Are lesions separate or in groups? Is it discrete or confluent? Is it annular or linear?

Diagnosis

The history and examination will often be enough to make a diagnosis. If there is still doubt then some further investigations may be required such as skin scrapings or hair sent to mycology if fungal infection is suspected. Swabs to check if there is bacterial or viral infection. Blood tests may be required and occasionally a biopsy.

VASCULAR ANOMALIES

Vascular birthmarks are classified according to that suggested by Mulliken and Glowacki in 1982. This classification was slightly modified and accepted in 1996 by the International Society for the Study of Vascular Anomalies. Essentially vascular birthmarks fall into one of two categories: Vascular tumours or vascular malformations. Tumours are vascular lesions in which there is hyperplasia of the vessels while malformations are lesions in which there is dysplasia of the vessels.

Vascular Tumours

The most common vascular tumour is the infantile haemangioma, sometimes known as a strawberry naevus or birthmark. About 10% of infants will be diagnosed with one. They are more common in girls and in premature infants. Chorionic villous sampling during pregnancy also increases the risk.

This benign proliferation of endothelial cells has a very distinctive history. The lesion is not usually present at birth; if present it is in the form of a faint bruise like mark. It normally becomes evident within the first few weeks of life and has a period of rapid growth. It can increase in size considerably and continue to grow for up to 12 months (Fig. 14.2). It is then followed by a period of slow involution over a number of years (Fig. 14.3).

Infantile haemangioma can be superficial where all the growth is above the skin or deep where the growth is below the skin surface. Often there is a combination of superficial and deep (Fig. 14.4).

The appearance is often of a rapidly expanding bright red plaque, this is the superficial component. The deeper component can be more difficult to diagnose and usually takes longer to involute than the superficial one. This is a fast flow lesion and so is warmer than surrounding skin. If there is doubt about the diagnosis Doppler ultrasound can be helpful.

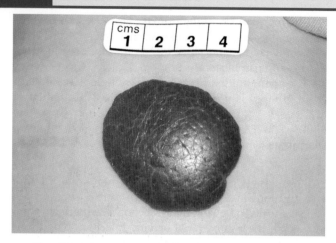

Fig. 14.2: Infantile haemangioma before signs of involution

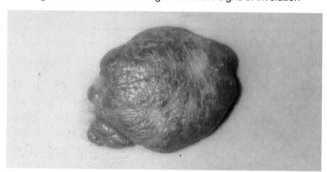

Fig. 14.3: Infantile haemangioma showing the first signs of involution

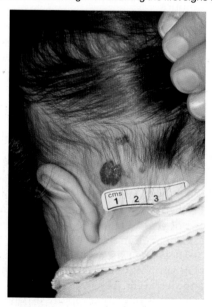

Fig. 14.4: Infantile haemangioma of neck mainly deep type with small superficial component

Most haemangioma do not require any treatment. After the growing phase they begin to pale or whiten on the surface and then slowly shrink down. A small number of the large ones do not completely involute and require some

cosmetic tidying up in the form of laser treatment or surgery.

There can be significant and serious complications of some haemangioma and this largely depends on their site, these are listed below (Figs 14.5 and 14.6).

Site	Complication
Around the eye causing restricted vision	May result in permanent eye sight problems e.g. amblyopia
Lip and perineum	ulceration bleeding and infection
Beard area	pressure on larynx and trachea
Nose	cartilage damage
Ear canal	hearing problems
Large facial ones	PHACE syndrome
Midline lumboscaral	Spinal dysraphism

Treatment if required is usually with corticosteroids, either topical, intralesional or systemic which will usually halt the growing phase. They have to be started early during the growing phase and will have to continue throughout until the growing phase has stopped which can be several months.

Embarking on a fairly long course of oral steroids has to be given careful consideration as to whether the benefits outweigh the risks. The dose has to be reasonably high between 2-4 mg/kg/day to be effective in halting the growing phase and this will need to continue probably for several months. These children obviously need careful monitoring to check height and weight, urine for sugar and BP.

PHACE SYNDROME

This is a rare syndrome where there is an association of posterior fossa brain malformations, haemangiomas, arterial anomalies, coarctation of the aorta, cardiac defects and eye abnormalities. It is usually associated with large segmental facial haemangioma.

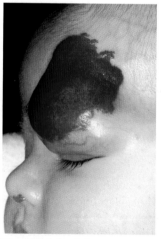

Fig. 14.5: Infantile haemangioma on eyelid

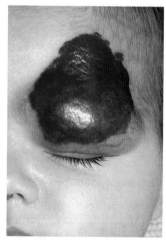

Fig. 14.6: Infantile haemangioma on eyelid closing the eye and requiring treatment with oral steroids

Other Less Common Types of Haemangioma/ Vascular Tumour

Two other types of vascular tumours can sometimes be confused with infantile haemangiomas. These are the tufted angioma and the Kaposiform Haemangio-endothelioma. The history and behaviour of these two vascular tumours will give a clue to the diagnosis but usually a biopsy is required to confirm the diagnosis.

They may look like Infantile haemangiomas but do not give the classic history. They may or may not be present at birth.

The main concern with these two tumours is that they may be associated with Kassabach-Merritt phenomenon. Rapid swelling of the tumour occurs with bruising and purpura. There is a severe thrombocytopaenia with platelet trapping and some consumption of fibrinogen and coagulation factors. This condition is always life threatening and requires urgent treatment.

Congenital Haemangioma: These haemangioma look like infantile haemangioma but are present and fully formed at birth. They do not have a growing phase and either involute quite rapidly or do not change at all.

Diffuse Neonatal Haemangiomas: Numerous small cutaneous and visceral haemangioma. Hepatic lesions can lead to high output cardiac failure. Gastrointestinal ones can present with bleeding.

Multiple Neonatal Haemangiomas: Multiple small cutaneous haemangiomas without visceral lesions.

VASCULAR MALFORMATIONS

Vascular malformations are composed of dysplastic vessels and can be made up of capillary, venous, arterial, arteriovenous, lymphatic or a combination of vessels.

Capillary Malformation

The most common type of capillary malformation is the Salmon patch. This is a red patch, often in the shape of a V, on the forehead. It sometimes involves the upper eyelids, nose, and upper lip. It can also form a patch at the nape of the neck (Fig. 14.7). These patches are present in about 50% of infants and usually disappear by the age of 2 years although the ones on the nape of the neck often persist. They are of no consequence.

The next most common type of capillary malformation is often referred to as a **Port-Wine Stain** (Fig. 14.8). It is a flat red mark that can occur anywhere on the body and is present at birth. It can sometimes fade a little in the first year but then darkens again. Eventually, it becomes quite purple in colour. It does not resolve on its own but requires treatment with laser. These are slow flow lesions and so is the same temperature as surrounding skin.

If the capillary malformation is within the ophthalmic division of the trigeminal nerve segment on the face there is a risk of Sturge-Weber syndrome. This is a triad of— capillary malformation in ophthalmic division of the trigeminal nerve, eye and brain abnormalities.

Venous malformations are also slow flow vascular malformations so the skin temperature is normal. They often appear as bluish compressible birthmarks. They can be quite extensive and radiological imaging may be necessary to determine the extent. Craniofacial lesions can cause bony deformities resulting in functional impairment. Treatment is aimed at preventing this. Treatment is difficult but surgical excision and percutaneous sclerotherpy may be helpful.

Arteriovenous Malformations are more serious lesions, which can worsen over time especially around the time of puberty or because of some kind of trauma to it either accidental or ill advised surgery.

They are fast flow lesions so warmer to the touch than surrounding skin. They can look like other vascular birthmarks. They are warm like haemangiomas but do not have the classic history of rapid growth and then slow involution. They may appear like Port-Wine stains but are warm to touch unlike Port-Wine stains, which have normal skin temperature. If there is any doubt about the diagnosis Doppler ultrasound should confirm the diagnosis and MRI scan will show the extent of the lesion.

DISORDERS OF PIGMENTATION

Either too much pigment or too little can pose quite a distressing cosmetic problem. This is particularly so in darker skinned individuals as the pale or white patches standout more.

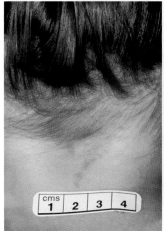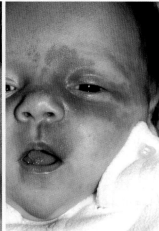

Fig. 14.7: Salmon patch on the nape of the neck

Fig. 14.8: Capillary malformation Port-Wine stain on the face

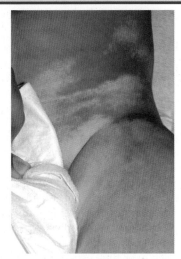

Fig. 14.9: Hypomelanosis—congenital hypopigmented area in groin area, upper thigh and lower trunk

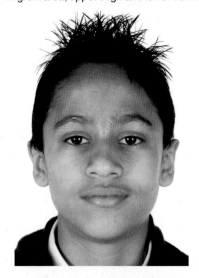

Fig. 14.10: Pityriasis Alba

Post-inflammatory Hypo and Hyper-pigmentation

Any kind of inflammation in the skin can result in changes in the pigment, either hypo-pigmentation or hyper-pigmentation. Even when all the inflammation is settled the change in pigment remains for sometime before completely resolving (Fig. 14.9).

This is particularly seen in atopic eczema. In darker skinned individuals the inflammation instead of appearing red as in white skin may only appear as darker areas of skin along with a palpable rash.

PITYRIASIS ALBA

This is a form of post-inflammatory hypo-pigmentation where pale patches appear mostly on the face (Fig. 14.10). These are more evident in the summer time when the sun

has darkened the rest of the skin. They usually fade over the winter but may return again the following summer. Many parents and even doctors get very concerned about this because they confuse it with vitiligo. However Pityriasis Alba, which is a benign condition and eventually clears even without treatment, is a form of hypopigmentation while vitiligo is complete depigmentation. If the skin is dry an emollient can be prescribed and if any inflammation is evident, and mostly it is not, a mild topical steroid can be used for a week or two.

VITILIGO

This usually presents with symmetrical white patches that can occur anywhere. The white patches occur because of depigmentation caused by the destruction of melanocytes. This can be a major cosmetic problem depending on where the white patches are. It is obviously more noticeable on dark-skinned individuals. The areas of skin appear as chalk white but developing vitiligo in dark-skinned individuals may show various shades between normal skin and totally depigmented skin (Fig. 14.11).

About 25% of those with vitiligo develop it before the age of 10. The vitiligo is most commonly generalised but can be segmental. Patches of vitiligo can also affect the hair and mucous membranes.

Vitiligo is thought to be a type of autoimmune disease in which there is a complete loss of melanocytes. There is often a family history of vitiligo or of other autoimmune diseases. Children themselves with vitiligo rarely show signs of other autoimmune diseases and routine screening is not required.

Treatment with potent topical steroids may stimulate repigmentation. Parents, however, should be warned that the white patches, because there is no pigment, are more susceptible to sun damage and should therefore be

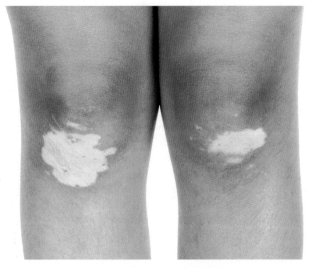

Fig. 14.11: Vitiligo showing the symmetrical depigmented patches

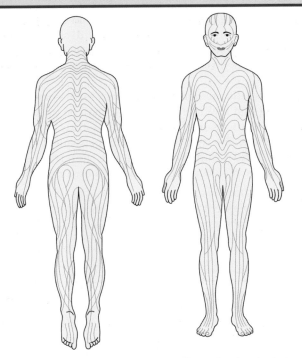

Fig. 14.12: Blaschko lines-represent lines of embryological neuroectodermal migration

protected with either clothing or sunscreen. More recently topical tacrolimus has also been found in some cases to be effective.

PIEBALDISM

This is another condition in which there are white patches because of lack of melanocytes in the skin. However this is an inherited condition in which there is a defect in the proliferation and migration of melanocytes during embryogenesis. It can be differentiated from vitiligo by the fact that it is present at birth and is not progressive.

HYPOMELANOSIS OF ITO

This condition is characterised by hypo-pigmented patches or streaks, which often follow the lines of blaschko (Fig. 14.12). They are usually present at birth, but may develop in the first two years of life. Thereafter they usually remain stable. This is usually a benign condition but may be associated with other abnormalities.

TUBEROUS SCLEROSIS

This inherited condition has manifestations in the skin, central nervous system, the eye and viscera. It may initially present with a number of hypo-pigmented macules usually called ash leaf macules. These macules can be a variety of shapes—oval, lance shaped, ash leaf or small confetti like shapes.

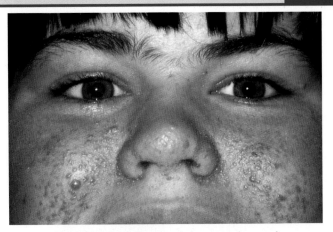

Fig. 14.13: Angiofibromas (adenoma sebaceum)

Other cutaneous features include angiofibromas of the face, connective tissue naevi (forehead plaques and shagreen patches), and periungual fibromas (Fig. 14.13). Any child who presents with hypo-pigmented patches should be carefully followed up and monitored for other signs of tuberous sclerosis.

Other conditions, which may present with hypo-pigmentation, are pityriasis versicolor, lichen sclerosus and leprosy.

CAFÉ AU LAIT MACULES

These are light brown, flat, round or oval lesions, which may have an irregular border. They can occur anywhere on the body. They may be present at birth or develop in the first few months. They can however increase in number and size throughout childhood.

When there are only a few lesions (less than 5) it is usually insignificant and not associated with any other abnormalities. However, they may be a marker for neurofibromatosis especially when there are more than 5.

Neurofibromatosis is an inherited condition with manifestations in the skin, eye, bone, soft tissues and central nervous system. There should be at least 5-6 café au lait macules greater than 5 mm present to warrant suspicion and other signs should be looked for such as axillary and inguinal freckling, lisch nodules in the eyes, and a family history (Figs 14.14 and 14.15). These children should be followed up and carefully monitored for any changes in their skin. Regular checks on BP, height, weight and examination of the spine should be carried out. They should be referred to ophthalmology for regular eye examinations.

One very large café au lait macule, particularly if it has a jagged margin may be a marker for McCune-Albright syndrome. This syndrome is a triad of café au lait macules, polyostotic fibrous dysplasia and endocrine disorders.

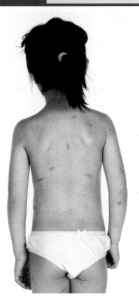

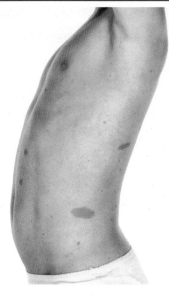

Fig. 14.14: Neurofibromatosis showing café au lait macules

Fig. 14.15: Neurofibromatosis showing café au lait macules and axillary freckling

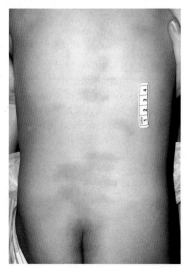

Fig. 14.16: Dermal melanocytosis—Mongolian blue spots

DERMAL MELANOCYTOSIS

Mongolian spots: 80% of Asian and African-American babies are born with or develop in the first few months of life a Mongolian blue spot. This is a patch of blue-grey or darker pigmentation usually located over the sacrum and lower back (Fig. 14.16). It can however be more extensive and involve the trunk, buttocks and lower limbs. They are completely benign and the majority fade and clear before adulthood. If seen in combination with a capillary malformation (Port-Wine stain) it may be part of a syndrome called Phakomatosis pigmentovascularis.

Naevus of Ota: Blue-grey pigmentation in the periorbital region in ophthalmic and maxillary divisions of the trigeminal nerve distribution on the face is known as a naevus of ota. It is common in Asian babies and also more common in girls.

It is usually present at birth but may not become evident until the first few months of life. It may be mistaken for bruising but its unchanging and lasting appearance differentiates the two. It is generally permanent and may in fact darken and increase in size. Referral for ophthalmologic review should be made to exclude glaucoma.

Naevus of Ito: This is similar to the naevus of Ota but the blue-grey pigment colour is on the shoulder area, neck, upper arms and upper trunk area. It does not resolve but is generally a benign condition.

EPIDERMAL NAEVI

Epidermal Naevus

These lesions often present at birth or shortly after. They are usually initially light brown in colour and may be slightly raised or papillomatous. Later, they often become warty and are sometimes mistaken for viral warts. They are usually linear although they can be oval (Fig. 14.17).

Sebaceous Naevus

This naevus is typically found on the scalp but may also be found on the face or neck (Fig. 14.18). It is present at birth but is not always recognised as at this stage it is often flat and the changes are subtle. Later, it is noticed as a round, oval or linear patch of alopecia. However, on close examination it will be noticed that the patch of skin on the scalp in a different colour from the rest of the scalp. It is usually a slightly pink/yellow/orange colour. It remains hairless and in adolescence becomes slightly raised and warty.

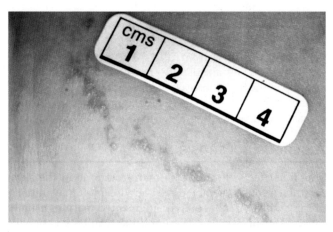

Fig. 14.17: Linear epidermal naevus—following the lines of Blaschko

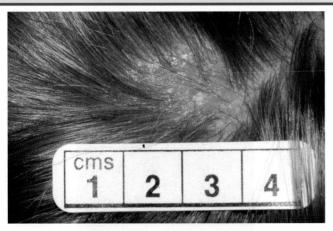

Fig. 14.18: Sebaceous naevus on the scalp

The sebaceous naevus is thought to be a variant of the epidermal naevus and is derived from the adnexial structures especially apocrine and sebaceous.

There is a very small risk of development of benign and malignant tumours but usually later in life. Therefore treatment is usually excision in late childhood or adolescence.

BLISTERING DISORDERS

Epidermolysis Bullosa (EB)

Epidermolysis bullosa is a group of rare inherited diseases characterised by blistering due to friction or trauma to the skin. There are defects in the complex network of proteins in the layers of the skin, which in effect hold the skin together.

This means that even the slightest pressure on the skin can cause blister formation. The skin then lifts off leaving raw eroded areas, which are painful.

There are a number of subtypes, which are determined by the inheritance pattern and the level in the skin where the defect and therefore the split (blister) occur. A biopsy is needed to make the diagnosis. The subtypes range from severe with a poor prognosis to fairly mild. The main types are EB simplex, junctional EB and **dystrophic EB.**

There is no cure for this condition and the child is subject to daily dressings and care of their skin. Great care needs to be exercised when handling these babies and children to prevent further blistering. The mucous membranes may be involved and when the gastro-intestinal tract is affected problems with nutrition occur. The teeth and eyes may need special care and mobility is often a problem.

The main job of the dermatologist is to make the diagnosis and then co-ordinate care for these children. They will need special nursing care and may need referral to numerous other specialities.

Staphylococcal Scalded Skin Syndrome (SSSS)

This condition is caused by Staphylococcus aureus, which produce an exotoxin resulting in an acute illness with blister formation. The initial symptom is often tender erythema of the skin, which is often worse in the flexural and periorificial areas. The mucous membranes are not generally involved. At this stage, the child may be generally unwell with fever, irritability, conjunctivitis or rhinitis. This is followed quickly by the development of large flaccid bullae (blisters), which are fragile with a thin roof comprised only of the upper layer of the epidermis. These quickly peel away to leave large moist glistening denuded areas, which are extremely painful. These bullae are in fact sterile (Fig. 14.19).

The source of the infection is not always clear but may be from the, nasopharynx, the umbilicus in a neonate, urinary tract infection, conjunctiva, or a cutaneous wound.

This condition usually affects young children. It is potentially life threatening and prompt treatment with appropriate IV antibiotics is required. Semi-occlusive dressings with petrolatum will ease the pain and analgesics as required. Recovery is usually rapid and healing occurs without scarring.

The diagnosis is usually made based on the typical clinical picture but if there is any doubt biopsy will confirm the split in the skin to be in the upper epidermis.

If this condition occurs in the neonate it may be confused with epidermolysis bullosa, and in the older child with toxic epidermal necrolysis (TEN). Biopsy will differentiate. In TEN the split in the skin is lower and the mucous membranes are often involved. TEN is a more serious illness with a potentially poorer prognosis so

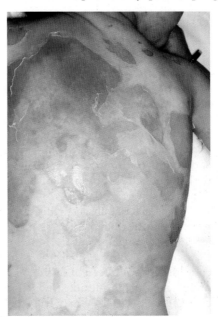

Fig. 14.19: Staphylococcal scalded skin syndrome

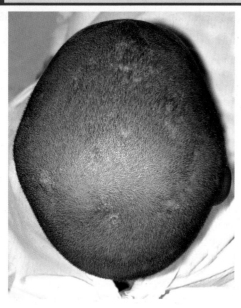

Fig. 14.20: Tinea capitis showing widespread involvement of the scalp

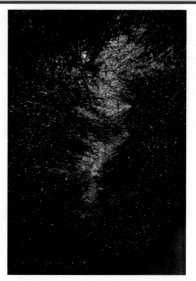

Fig. 14.21: Tinea capitis showing small area of scaling and hair loss

making the correct diagnosis is important and starting the correct treatment is essential. Drug reactions are the commonest cause of TEN and therefore the offending one needs to be withdrawn. Supportive measures such as correcting any electrolyte and fluid imbalance as well as care for the skin, which may need to be done in a specialised burns unit, are needed.

Fungal Infection

Fungal infection (dermatophytes) can affect any part of the body, affecting hair skin or nails, and are named after the part of the body affected.

Tinea capitis is fungal infection of the scalp. It can be quite discrete affecting only a small patch of scalp causing scaling and hair loss or it can be more widespread, with scaling, hair loss and sometimes pustules, affecting most of the scalp (Figs 14.20 and 14.21). Many types of fungi cause this and among them are *Trichophyton tonsurans, T. rubrum, T. soudanese, T. violeceum* and *Microsporum canis.*

A kerion may develop. This consists of pustules and painful tender nodules, which may coalesce and expand. There is marked inflammation with pain and tenderness and an underlying bogginess of the scalp from which there may be oozing, crusting and hair loss. This is frequently misdiagnosed as a bacterial abscess. Treatment however is not surgery but anti-fungals such as griseofulvin or terbinafine. If not treated promptly hair loss may be permanent. A common source of infection is from cattle.

Tinea corporis (fungal infection of the body) appears as round annular expanding lesions, which are slightly scaly especially at the edge. They may be slightly red and inflamed and have tiny pustules (Figs 14.22 to 14.24). These lesions are often mistaken for eczema and treated with topical steroids, which masks the appearance and is then called tinea incognito.

Tinea corporis can usually be treated successfully with topical anti-fungals but if it is very widespread may need systemic treatment.

Tinea of the nails (tinea unguium) results in the nails becoming thickened, yellowish and crumbly. In adults and older children treatment generally needs to be systemic and for a long course, about three-six months or more. One would be reticent to embark on such a long course of systemic treatment in young children particularly if the tinea unguium is not bothering them. Topical treatment or just observation may be the most appropriate treatment for them. Fortunately tinea unguium is uncommon in children.

Diagnosis of fungal infection is made by plucking hair samples, taking skin scrapings or nail cuttings for culture and examination. It is important to identify the source of the infection, which may be human, animal or soil. If it is

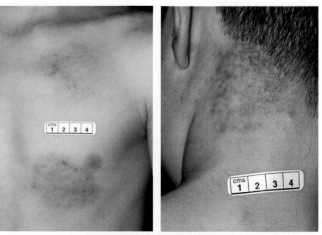

Figs 14.22 and 14.23: Tinea corporis

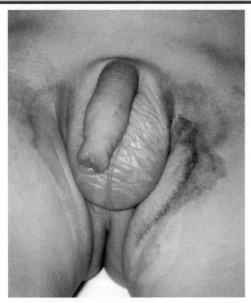

Fig. 14.24: Tinea cruris—fungal infection of groin area

from a family pet or other animal known to the family it needs to be examined and treated by a vet.

Scabies

Human scabies is caused by *Sarcoptes scabiei ssp*. Hominis. Infants even as young as 4-5 weeks old can be affected. Babies are unable to scratch so the symptoms are often irritability, poor sleeping and feeding. A generalised erythematous vesiculopapular rash is seen and the papules are commonly found on the palms and soles of babies (Fig. 14.25).

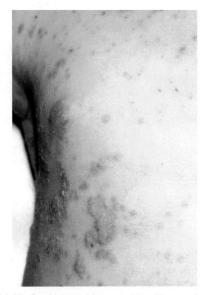

Fig. 14.25: Scabies—widespread pruritic papules seen over the trunk and axilla

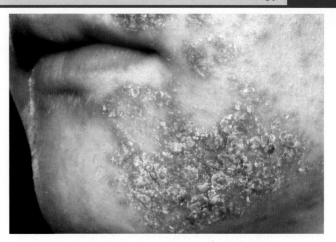

Fig. 14.26: Impetigenised atopic eczema

In older children, itch is the predominant feature especially at night. Scabies should be considered part of the differential diagnosis in any slightly atypical itchy rash especially if other family members are itchy. In children with eczema it can be the cause of a sudden flare of their eczema. The presence of burrows confirms the diagnosis but are not always evident.

Treatment is usually with topical permethrin 5% cream and all family members and regular contacts should be treated at the same time.

Impetigo

Impetigo is a superficial skin infection mostly caused by *Staphylococcus aureus* but occasionally by *Streptococcus pyogenes*. Impetigo normally develops on skin which is already affected by a primary skin disease such as atopic eczema or an area of skin which has been traumatised by either an insect bite, laceration, burn or other condition resulting in a break in the normal skin barrier (Fig. 14.26). It tends to occur more frequently in hot humid climates.

Impetigo is generally recognised by its honey colour crusted plaques. It can be localised to a small area of skin or become more generalised especially when it is secondarily infecting previously diseased skin. Most children with impetigo remain well although they may have some localised adenopathy. In children with eczema the infection may be quite subtle and appear only as a flare of the eczema with some yellow crusting.

If only a small area is affected a topical antibiotic such as mupirocin may be sufficient otherwise swabs should be done for sensitivities and the appropriate antibiotic started. Flucloxacillin is usually the antibiotic of choice.

Atopic Eczema

This is one of the most frequently seen conditions in paediatric dermatology. It commonly presents after the first few weeks of life as a red rash on the face and scalp. It then becomes more widespread especially on the extensor aspects of the limbs but usually spares the nappy area. As the child becomes older the flexures of the limbs become the main site with excoriations, lichenification, and exudates. In severe cases, it can be extensive and widespread (Figs 14.27 to 14.30).

Eczema is always itchy but it is not always apparent in neonates, young infants or children with any degree of physical weakness. It may manifest itself in these children as irritability and poor sleeping.

This is a chronic relapsing condition and is associated with a family history of atopy (atopic eczema, asthma, hay fever or allergic rhinitis). It is distressing to the child because of the constant itch but also to the whole family who become very stressed because of an irritable child who sleeps poorly. Parents are particularly distressed because of lack of sleep and a feeling of failure because they do not seem able to comfort or help their child.

There is no cure for eczema but the majority of children can have their symptoms controlled and most of them grow out of it before adulthood.

The principal features of eczema are, dry skin, red itchy inflammation and frequent bouts of secondary infection. Treatment is therefore aimed at controlling these symptoms.

The skin is very sensitive and many things such as woollen or nylon clothing, perfumes, soap, animal dander and house dust mite will all cause a flare of the eczema. Excessive heat and sweating may also irritate the skin. Avoidance of such irritants is therefore important.

Moisturisers should be applied to the skin frequently and regularly to prevent the skin drying out. These also, especially the greasier ones, form a barrier on the skin to help prevent irritants and infection getting in. Moisturisers should continue to be applied even when the skin is not red and itchy. Bath oil and a moisturising soap substitute should also be used. Once, it is under control many

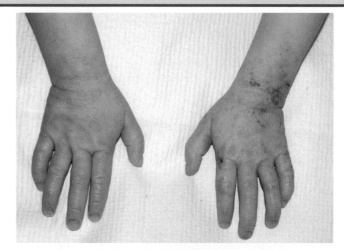

Fig. 14.28: Flared eczema of the hands showing lichenification and an area of crusted infection

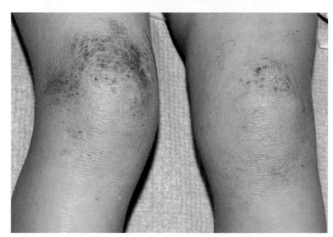

Fig. 14.29: Flared eczema of knees showing lichenification and infection

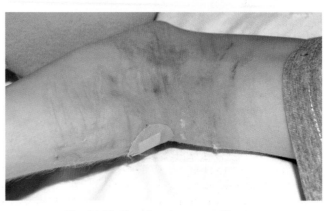

Fig. 14.30: Excoriated eczema of the arm

children can keep their eczema settled with moisturisers alone and very occasional topical steroid.

The itch and inflammation of eczema is best controlled with topical steroids. Weak steroids are used for the face, folds and napkin area. Stronger steroids may be required

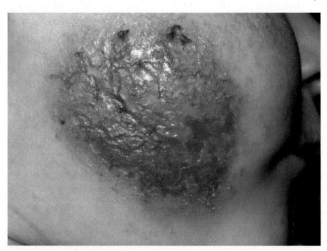

Fig. 14.27: Excoriated eczema of face

intermittently for severe flares but should only be given under close supervision. Moderate to potent steroids are usually required for intermittent use on the limbs and trunk.

Topical tacrolimus is proving a useful alternative to topical steroids particularly on the face. This is especially so around the eyes where strong steroids are usually contraindicated. However, the long-term safety of tacrolimus has not been well-established yet, so a degree of caution should be used and sun protection is advised when using it.

Infection with *Staphylococcus aureus* is a problem for many individuals with eczema and it is often the cause of a sudden severe flare, which does not respond to their normal treatment. Swabs for culture and then appropriate oral antibiotics may be necessary. Regular use of a soap substitute, which has an antiseptic as one of its ingredients, can be helpful in reducing infection.

Treatment for atopic eczema is quite complex with different creams and ointments to be used at different times. It can be quite confusing for parents; therefore time spent writing out a treatment plan and then going over it with the parents is very worthwhile. Follow up care to ensure that treatment is being applied properly and appropriately and the skin is settling and coming under control is important.

Restriction of diet is usually unnecessary and should only be done when there is clear evidence of a reaction to a particular food. It should then be done under the supervision of a paediatric dietician.

Fortunately most children respond to these measures but for the ones with more severe eczema wet wrap bandaging for limited periods may be helpful. Children who are still unresponsive and whose eczema is making them miserable may require systemic treatment such as azathioprine.

Eczema Herpeticum

Children with atopic eczema do not handle the herpes simplex virus normally and when infected with it the infection can become widespread and the child systemically unwell. Admission to hospital is often necessary for IV acyclovir. The infection is recognised by numerous small discrete erosions. Swabs should be taken for confirmation of the diagnosis. If possible children with eczema should avoid contact with people who have cold sores (Herpes simplex). In particular, family members with a cold sore should not kiss children especially those with eczema. The herpes simplex virus cannot be eradicated and the child will suffer recurring episodes of localised colds sores or even widespread eczema herpeticum.

Seborroheic Eczema

This is a condition generally affecting children in the first year of life. Characteristically there is a greasy, yellowish, thick scale on the scalp, usually known as cradle cap (Fig. 14.31). When more extensive the face, especially the eyebrows, nasolabial folds and malar eminences, the ears, and the chest can also be affected with erythema and yellow greasy scale (Fig. 14.32). Unlike atopic eczema where the napkin area is spared in seborrhoeic eczema the napkin area is often affected especially the folds (Fig. 14.33). The axillary area can also be similarly affected.

This condition is often confused with atopic eczema but the classic clinical picture and distribution of the rash along with the fact that the rash is not itchy and therefore

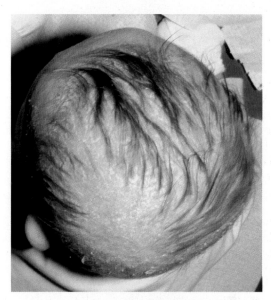

Fig. 14.31: Seborrhoea of the scalp—cradle cap

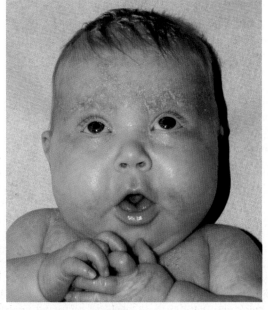

Fig. 14.32: Seborrhoeic dermatitis showing yellow scaling of eyebrows, forehead and scalp

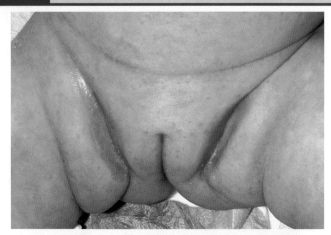

Fig. 14.33: Seborrhoeic dermatitis showing involvement of the folds in napkin area

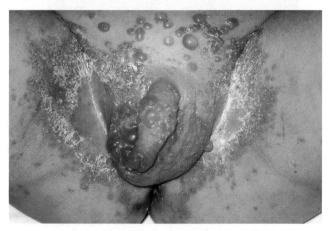

Fig. 14.34: Napkin dermatitis

the child is usually happy and content differentiates the two. In young babies, there can be an overlap and they can in fact have both atopic and seborrhoeic eczema.

Candida albicans often invades the affected areas and therefore treatment, which is with a mild to moderate steroid, may be combined with an anticandidal preparation.

Napkin Dermatitis

The most common type of napkin rash is irritant contact dermatitis due to the contact of urine and faeces with the skin. The rash is initially red and scaly but quickly becomes deeply erythematous with a typical glistening or glazed appearance (Fig. 14.34). It typically spares the folds of the napkin area. It is very painful and the child is miserable especially at each nappy change. If left untreated punched out ulcers and erosions develop.

Nappies should be changed as soon as they are soiled and a thick emollient such as zinc and castor oil cream or petrolatum jelly should be used to act as a barrier to urine and faeces.

When napkin dermatitis occurs a mild potency steroid may be applied two to three times a day and thick emollients should be applied at each nappy change. If candida or bacterial infection is also suspected an antibiotic or anticandidal agent should be added.

Psoriasis

Psoriasis is uncommon in children under 10 years but when it does occur it can have a similar distribution to seborrhoeic eczema affecting mainly the scalp, ears and napkin area especially in young children. In fact, in some children only the napkin area is involved and the diagnosis is difficult and may be confused with irritant napkin dermatitis or seborrhoeic eczema.

In older children, it can have the same distribution as in adults, i.e. the scalp, ears, elbows, knees and peri-umbilical area (Figs 14.35 to 14.37). Occasionally only the scalp is affected. It may or may not be itchy and there is often a family history of the condition.

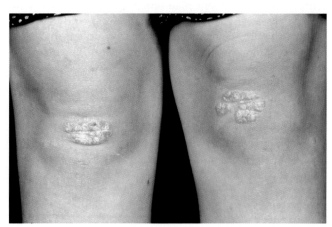

Fig. 14.35: Psoriasis—plaque located over the pressure point of the knee

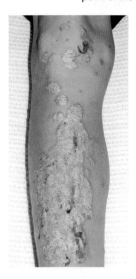

Fig. 14.36: Psoriasis—typical plaques with silvery scales

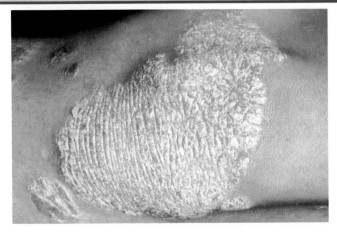

Fig. 14.37: Psoriasis

Psoriasis occurs as large well-demarcated scaly plaques with a red or pink base or as guttate lesions, which consist of numerous small round red scaly lesions usually beginning on the trunk but becoming more widespread. Nail changes including nail pitting, onycholysis and subungual hyperkeratosis may be present.

Children are more prone to guttate psoriasis, which often occurs after a throat infection. This type may clear completely and stay clear but normally psoriasis is a chronic relapsing condition.

Treatment is with emollients and mild steroids for face, nappy area and folds and tar preparations for elsewhere. Dithranol and calcipotriol can be used in slightly older children.

MELANOCYTIC NAEVI

These are localised proliferations of melanocytes and they are often classified according to where the naevus cells lie in the dermis or epidermis and whether or not they are present at birth or acquired throughout childhood.

Acquired naevi are generally small brown lesions < 5 mm in size and evenly pigmented with a regular shape and border. Malignant melanomas are rare before puberty but may be suspected, if the edge becomes irregular, the colour becomes uneven or there is rapid growth. Children with a family history of malignant melanoma are at slightly increased risk.

Congenital Melanocytic Naevus (CMN) is present at birth or within the first few months of life. They are usually categorised by their size. Small are 1-1.5 cm, intermediate are 1.5-20 cm and greater than that are called large or giant. The margin of these congenital naevi is often irregular as is the colour and surface (Figs 14.38 and 14.39). They are often hairy and grow in size in proportion to the child's growth.

Small CMNs occur in 0.01 of the population, intermediate CMNs occur in 0.1 of the population and large or giant CMNs occur in 0.001% of the population (Fig. 14.40).

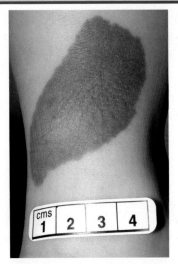

Fig. 14.38: Congenital melanocytic naevus

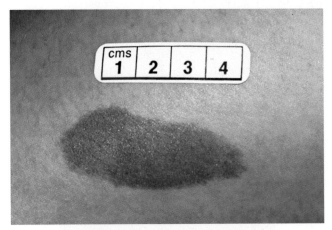

Fig. 14.39: Melanocytic naevus

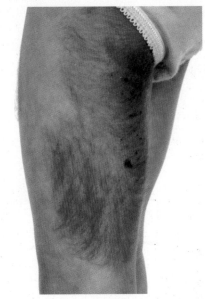

Fig. 14.40: Giant congenital hairy-pigmented naevus

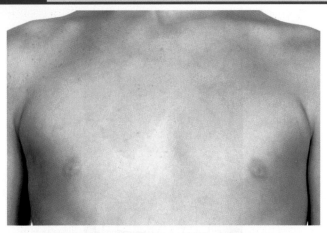

Fig. 14.41: Naevus spilus-speckled lentiginous naevus

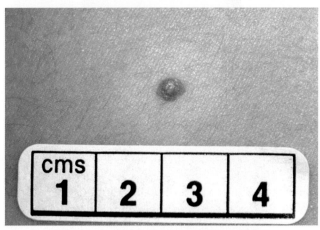

Fig. 14.42: Halo naevus

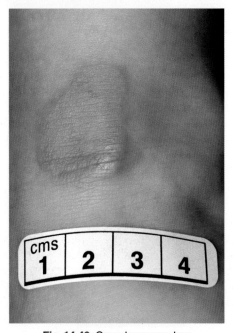

Fig. 14.43: Granuloma annulare

Small and intermediate CMN do not seem to be at increased risk of developing malignant melanoma but if so the risk is quite small. However, those with the large or giant type have an increased risk of between 6-8%.

However, in children with darker skins these lesions are less common as is malignant change.

Naevus spilus or speckled lentiginous naevus occurs as a light tan patch, which gradually develops small dark spots within it (Fig. 14.41).

Halo Naevus

Occasionally, a white patch occurs around a pigmented naevus (Fig. 14.42). This reaction is mostly seen in children and is benign. Sometimes the naevus in the centre also depigments. This reaction is thought to be an immunological one and the patient may also have vitiligo or a family history of it.

Granuloma Annulare

The cause of these lesions is unknown but they occur in children and adults. They are mostly to be found over bony prominences on the back of the hands or dorsum of the feet but they can occur anywhere. They begin as an expanding ring of pink papules. As it expands the central area clears leaving a roughly annular-shaped lesion with a beaded edge (Fig. 14.43). It is entirely asymptomatic but in adults can be associated with diabetes. These lesions are sometimes diagnosed as fungal infection but the differentiating feature is that granuloma annulare is not scaly.

These lesions can also appear as more flat purplish lesions and can be found as single or multiple lesions. They spontaneously involute and require no treatment. Intralesional steroid can sometimes hasten the resolution process but is very painful.

Pyoderma Gangrenosum

Pyoderma gangrenosum is an uncommon condition in children but can occur in association with ulcerative colitis or Crohn's disease. It starts off as a small nodule or pustule, which quickly expands to form an ulcer. The edge has a characteristic undermined bluish appearance (Fig. 14.44). As well as treating the underlying disease topical and or oral steroids are the treatment of choice although recently topical tacrolimus has been found helpful.

Urticaria

This is a common condition at any stage in life although rarely seen before the age of 6 months. It starts acutely with transient red raised blotches, which expand and move around with each individual lesion clearing completely within 24 hours leaving normal skin behind.

The acute form lasts for up to 6 weeks but it may go on to become chronic and last several months or even years.

In children, this condition is often triggered by a viral infection although often no cause is found and investigations are unhelpful and unnecessary. However, a careful history should be taken of events leading up to the onset of the rash to exclude drugs or foods.

Angioedema may or may not accompany an episode of urticaria. Angioedema can be quite frightening for the individual and their family as they associate it with anaphylaxis. There is deep swelling of the eyelids, lips and sometimes the hands and feet. However, it is usually mild and transient and there are no breathing difficulties or hypotension.

Treatment is with non-sedating anti-histamines, which should be given on a regular basis until the episode is over.

Angioedema of a more serious nature does occur with anaphylaxis and hereditary angioedema. Anaphylaxis is a medical emergency as along with the urticaria and angioedema there is dyspnoea and hypotension. However, for the majority who have urticaria this does not happen and the prognosis is good. If laryngeal oedema has not occurred during the first few hours it is unlikely to occur thereafter.

Hereditary angioedema is due to either deficiency of or loss of function of C1 esterase inhibitor. The diagnosis is made on the basis of the symptoms of, abdominal pain, vomiting and massive oedema and a family history but is confirmed by doing a functional assay of C1 esterase inhibitor.

Erythema Multiforme

Erythema multiforme develops as a reaction most often to an infection like herpes simplex or a drug. It is an acute self-limiting condition with typical target lesions mainly affecting the peripheral limbs. It can also affect the mucous membranes when it can be much more serious requiring hospital admission. However, it is usually a mild condition lasting several days or 1-2 weeks. Treatment is of the underlying infection or cessation of the offending drug.

Erythema Nodosum

This condition presents as tender, red nodules often on the shins of the legs but can occur anywhere (Fig. 14.46). It is due to inflammation of the subcutaneous fat.

It is a reactive process usually caused by infections such as Streptococcus, tuberculosis, brucellosis and leprosy. Drugs such as sulphonamides, and oral contraceptive can also be responsible in older children. Erythema nodosum can also be associated with sarcoidosis, ulcerative colitis, Crohn's disease and Behcet's disease.

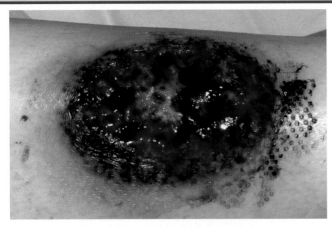
Fig. 14.44: Pyoderma gangrenosum

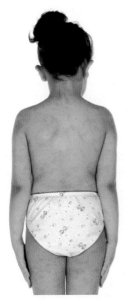
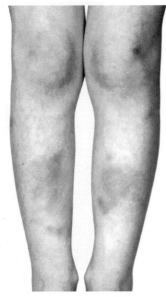
Fig. 14.45: Widespread urticaria
Fig. 14.46: Erythema nodosum

The appearance of the lesions can be quite dramatic, sometimes forming giant urticarial plaques with irregular borders, which move about in a bizarre fashion (Fig. 14.45). These giant lesions do not signify a more serious form of the disease. Often as they clear they do so from the centre leaving rings, which can mimic erythema multiforme. The lesions are described as very itchy but excoriations are rarely seen. The patient or parent often describes them as blisters because of the wheal like appearance of them. It is therefore important to ask if fluid comes out of them to which the answer is no.

In fact, most often when the patient arrives at the clinic the skin is completely normal indicating the transient nature of the condition. It is therefore important to try to get an accurate description of the lesion. Episodes may occur daily to begin with but generally as the condition improves episodes become less frequent.

Viral Warts

Warts are a common occurrence in children. They are caused by the human papilloma virus of which there are several types. They most commonly appear on the hands and feet but can occur anywhere on the body surface. They initially appear as smooth skin coloured papules but slowly enlarge and develop an irregular hyperkeratotic surface. They may appear as a slender stalk in which case they are called filiform warts and are commonly found on the face especially the nostrils of the nose and the lips. Viral warts usually spontaneously resolve once the immune system recognises and overcomes the virus but it may take many months.

If treatment is desired wart paints containing salicylic acid are usually effective. Cryotherapy with liquid nitrogen is also usually effective but is painful and not advised in young children.

Genital warts are less common and when they occur, especially in the older child, may be caused by sexual abuse. However, they can be caused by autoinoculation from warts elsewhere on the same individual or from a carer who has hand warts. In the young child (under age 4), they may also be caused by vertical spread from the mother *in utero* or during delivery. The virus may lie dormant and not manifest itself for some months or even years. It is often best to leave these warts to spontaneously resolve, as treatment with cryotherapy is inevitably painful.

Molluscum Contagiosum

This is a viral infection, which produces crops of pearly dome shaped papules with an umbilicated centre (Fig. 14.47). The condition is self-limiting and clears once the individual has developed his or her own immunity

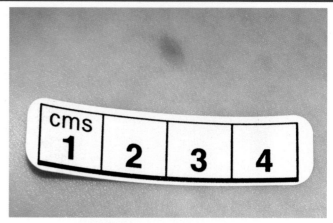

Fig. 14.48: Juvenile xanthogranuloma

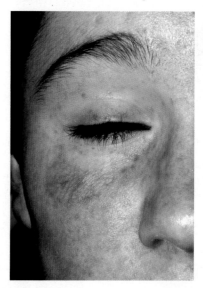

Fig. 14.49: Juvenile xanthogranuloma—plaque type

but it can take several months. This is mainly an infection affecting children and is quickly spread by contact with infected individuals often through shared baths, towels or swimming pools. The lesions are asymptomatic until they are beginning to clear when they develop an area of erythema around them, which is itchy. At this stage, children often scratch them and they can be susceptible to secondary infection. An antiseptic paint should be applied to prevent this.

Treatment is usually not necessary. Cryotherapy is effective but painful and not advised in young children.

Juvenile Xanthogranuloma

These lesions have a very characteristic yellow/orange colour. They can occur as single or multiple lesions and are usually restricted to the skin but can occur in other organs. They usually present as nodules in the skin but can occur as plaques (Figs 14.48 and 14.49).

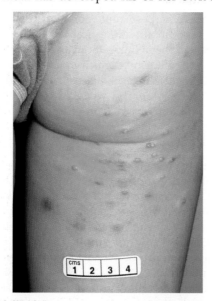

Fig. 14.47: Molluscum contagiosum—umblicated papules

A common site for them is the lateral eyebrow area and these lesions do not have a central nervous system connection and are therefore of less concern (Fig. 14.50).

KELOID SCAR

Keloid scars are caused by an exaggerated response to skin injury. Darker skinned individuals seem to be more at risk of these and there is sometimes a familial tendency.

The scarring grows out beyond the original site of injury (Fig. 14.51). The chest and shoulder area seem to be most vulnerable to this type of scarring but the face scalp and back of neck can also be quite badly affected often as a result of acne.

Treatment with intralesional steroid can sometimes flatten the scar and silicone gel can be applied topically but it is not always successful.

MASTOCYTOSIS

Brown, reddish brown or yellow brown lesions can present either as individual lesions (mastocytomas) or as multiple lesions (urticaria pigmentosa) (Fig. 14.52). These lesions usually present during the first two years of life but can be congenital. In the early stages they urticate and blister with any kind of friction. These lesions are full of mast cells, which release histamine to produce the typical wheal and flare reaction or blister.

The prognosis is generally good. The blistering usually stops by about the age of two and the lesions themselves often eventually spontaneously clear. Affected children should avoid histamine-releasing agents such as aspirin, opiates and cholinergic medications.

A small number of children, especially those with numerous lesions, may develop systemic symptoms such as flushing, headache, diarrhoea, and tachycardia. An antihistamine with or without the addition of H_2 blockers can help. Cromolyn sodium is usually effective for patients with gastrointestinal symptoms.

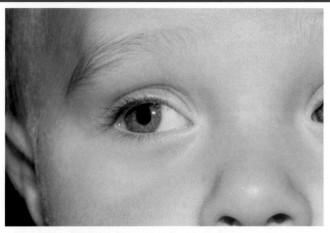

Fig. 14.50: Dermoid cyst at the lateral eyebrow area

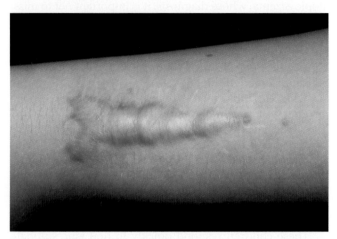

Fig. 14.51: Keloid scar—an abnormal reparative reaction to skin injury. Keloids are characterised by proliferation of fibroblasts and collagen

They are usually benign and self-limiting affecting infants and young children. Lesions may be present at birth but most occur in the first year of life. Rarely there can be an association with neurofibromatosis, juvenile myeloid leukaemia or urticaria pigmentosa, particularly when multiple lesions are present.

Dermoid Cyst

These present as asymptomatic skin-coloured or slightly bluish nodules and occur anywhere on the face, scalp or spinal axis. Although these are congenital lesions, caused by faulty development of the embryonic fusion lines, they are not always noticed until early childhood when they begin to enlarge.

Midline or nasal dermoid cysts can have an intracranial connection and have the potential to become infected resulting in meningitis. These cysts should be surgically excised after radiological imaging.

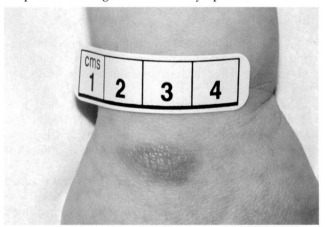

Fig. 14.52: Mastocytoma—these lesions urticate if rubbed

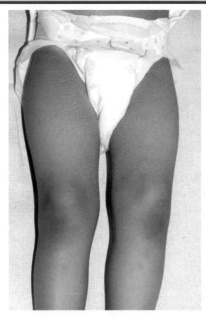

Fig. 14.53: X-linked ichthyosis

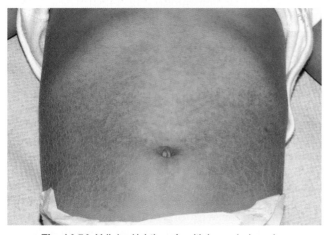

Fig. 14.54: X-linked ichthyosis with large dark scales

Ichthyosis

This is a group, if inherited disorders where the process of keratinisation is abnormal resulting in marked scaling and dryness of the skin, which ranges from mild to severe and incapacitating.

The commonest type is ichthyosis vulgaris, which may appear no more than a very dry skin. A light-coloured fine scale, which is most obvious on the limbs and tends to spare the flexures, is evident. It is inherited as autosomal dominant.

X-linked recessive ichthyosis affects boys and is much rarer than ichthyosis vulgaris affecting 1 : 2000. It can initially present as a collodion baby at birth with a shiny adherent film encasing the whole body. This shiny film is shed in the first few days leaving behind either normal

skin, X-linked or more frequently lamellar ichthyosis (Figs 14.53 and 14.54).

X-linked ichthyosis is due to deficiency of the enzyme steroid sulphatase, the activity of which can be measured in the blood to give the diagnosis. It is characterised by large brown scales especially seen on the legs and trunk and affects the flexures. There is a small risk of affected boys having hypogonadism and undescended testes.

The treatment for all the ichthyoses is emollients, which will not cure the condition but can make the individual more comfortable. For more severely affected individuals topical or systemic retinoids may help.

Acrodermatitis Enteropathica

There are some other conditions, which may present like atopic eczema, whose diagnosis, it is important not to miss. Children with atopic eczema are otherwise well so when a child with eczema like rash has other symptoms such as failure to thrive, diarrhoea, an odd distribution of rash or a purpuric element to it, it is important to consider some other less common diagnoses.

Acrodermatitis enteropathica is an autosomal recessive disorder, which causes zinc malabsorption and deficiency. Zinc deficiency can of course also result from poor intake of zinc.

Babies affected by this have a typical eruption affecting mainly the cheeks and chin, the hands and feet and the nappy area (Fig. 14.55). They usually have diarrhoea, failure to thrive and irritability. Measuring the zinc plasma level points to the right diagnosis.

These children respond quickly to oral zinc sulphate but treatment may have to be long-term.

Wiskott-Aldrich Syndrome

Wiskott-Aldrich syndrome is another condition, which can present like atopic eczema but again the rash is atypical. There is usually a haemorrhagic component with

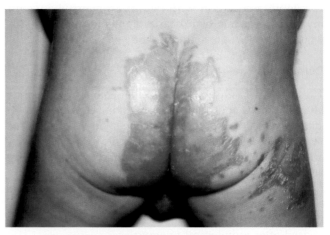

Fig. 14.55: Acrodermatitis enteropathica—buttocks

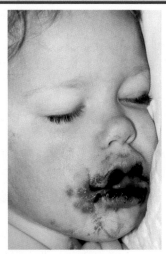

Fig. 14.56: Herpes simplex of mouth

purpura and patchier and the child is unwell with bloody diarrhoea, frequent infections and failure to thrive. Many of the immunodeficiency disorders can also present with an eczematous rash but again there are other features, which should lead to the correct diagnosis.

Herpes Simplex Infections

Cutaneous infections with herpes simplex virus are not uncommon in children. Primary herpes gingivostomatitis is the most common clinically apparent herpes infection. It is characterised by fever, malaise, headache and small eroded vesicles on the lips and oral mucosa (Fig. 14.56). Herpetic infections of the fingers and thumb may occur during the course of herpetic gingivostomatitis if children put them in their mouths. Herpetic genital infections are much less common in children than they are in adults. Sexual abuse should be considered a possibility in children with herpes genitalis.

No effective therapy is available for herpetic gingivostomatitis though oral acyclovir can be used. In children with gingivostomatitis healing usually occurs in 7-10 days.

BIBLIOGRAPHY

1. Lawrence A. Schachner and Ronald C Hansen. Paediatric Dermatology, 2003 Mosby.
2. Lawrence F Eichenfield, Ilona J Freiden, Nancy Esterly. The Textbook of Neonatal Dermatology. WB Saunders Company, Philadelphia, 2001.

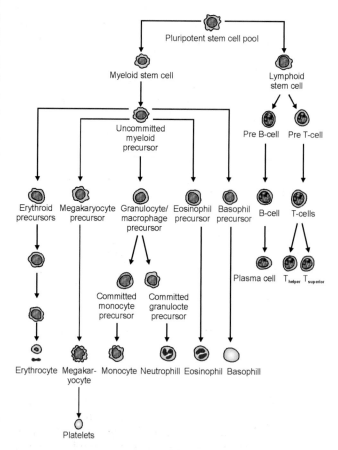

Haematological Disorders

Chapter 15

Krishna M Goel

HAEMATOPOIESIS

Within a few days of embryonic implantation "blood islands" develop in the human yolk sac. Cells from these islands develop into vascular endothelium and primitive blood cells. These pluripotent stem cells known as progenitor or CFU-GEMM (colony forming unit, granulocyte—erythroid/megakaryocyte—macrophage) cells produce red cells, white cells except lymphocytes and platelets (Fig. 15.1). Most haematopoiesis in the foetus takes place from progenitor cells seeded to the liver. Bone marrow haematopoiesis is present from about 10 weeks' gestation and by term has taken over almost all of the foetal haemopoietic function. Control of erythropoiesis in the foetus is through hepatic erythropoietin mediated by foetal tissue oxygen concentration. There is a switch to renal erythropoietin a few weeks after birth.

All of the white cell series and platelets are identifiable in foetal blood by about 14 weeks' gestation and the granulocyte series is controlled by the hormone GSF and platelets by thrombopoietin.

Modern haematology embraces many complicated techniques which have added greatly to our understanding of the nature of some of the less common disorders, e.g. haemolytic anaemias, haemoglobinopathies, megaloblastic anaemias, etc. None the less, the blood disorders commonly encountered in paediatric practice can most often be dealt with by use of relatively simple standard techniques.

THE NORMAL BLOOD PICTURE IN INFANCY

Considerable variations in normal values during the early days of life have been recorded by different workers. There are several reasons for this. Blood samples obtained by venipuncture in early infancy have lower values for haemoglobin and red cell counts than those obtained by heel prick and individual infants show a wide variation in values. In routine clinical practice only fairly large

departures from normal ranges are likely to prove significant.

Haemoglobin

The Hb concentration in blood from the umbilical cord is high with a mean of 17 g/dl (17 g/100ml). Values up to 20 g/dl may be recorded. A venous sample of the infant's

Fig. 15.1: Haematopoiesis in the embryo and foetus

blood some hours after birth may reveal an even higher Hb level with a mean of 19 g/dl, and a skin-prick sample is likely to be still higher with a mean of 21 g/dl. This rise in Hb values just after birth is probably due to haemo-concentration due to diminutioin in the plasma volume, in addition to the infusion of red cells which may occur when late clamping of the umbilical cord is practised.

The oxygen-carrying capacity of the blood is related to the total circulating red cell mass (RCM) which can vary in normal infants between 30 and 50 ml/kg depending on whether the cord is clamped early or late. Haemoglobin concentration and haematocrit can correlate poorly with the RCM especially in pre-term infants. The RCM can vary between 12 and 24 ml/kg in infants with a haematocrit of 0.3 (30%) due to compensatory reductions of plasma volume.

The Hb value falls to 10-11 g/dl by the age of 8-12 weeks but rises again to between 11 and 13 g/dl between the ages of 6 months and a year. Thereafter, the Hb level increases to 11.5-15 g/dl by the age of 10-12 years, and reaches normal adult values (men = 13.5-18 g/dl; women = 11.5-16.5 g/dl by the age of 15 years. The explanation for the fall in Hb level during the early weeks of life is that, although erythropoiesis continues at a high level found in the foetus for about 3 days after birth, an abrupt decline in erythropoiesis then occurs and the marrow erythroid count falls from 40 000 to 6000 per mm^3. This is reflected in a fall in the reticulocyte count from 3 or 4% just after birth to under 1% one week later.

At birth 50-65% of the Hb is of the foetal type (Hb-F) which resists denaturation with alkalis. It has a slightly different electrophoretic mobility and a quite different oxygen dissociation curve from adult type haemoglobin (Hb-A). After birth Hb-F is slowly replaced by Hb-A so that after a year of age only small amounts of Hb-F are still present. In certain diseases, such as thalssaemia and sickle-cell anaemia, Hb-F is produced in excessive quantity. The value to the foetus of Hb-F appears to be that of a greater affinity for oxygen at low tensions than Hb-A and an ability to release CO_2 more readily.

Since the discovery in 1949 of the first abnormal haemoglobin molecule (Hb-S) a great deal of information has accumulated about the molecular structure of haemoglobin. Over 100 variant forms of human haemo-globin have now been recognised. Some of these are associated with serious disease in various parts of the world.

Red Cells

The red cell count at birth varies between 5.5 and 7.5 million per mm^3. The count falls to about 5-5.5 millions after 2 weeks and thereafter runs parallel to the Hb level. Scanty eosinophilic normoblasts are found in the peripheral blood at birth. Erythrocytes at birth have a larger diameter (about 8.4 µm) than in the adult. The mean adult value of 7.2 µm is reached after 1 year.

White Cells

The total white cell count at birth is about 18,000 per mm^3 The adult value of 6,000 - 7,000 per mm^3 is not reached for 7-10 years. At birth about 60 per cent of the white cells are polymorphonuclear (11,000 per mm^3) and 30 per cent are lymphocytes (5,400 per mm^3). During the ensuing two weeks the polymorphonuclear count falls to within the normal adult range (3,500-4,500 per mm^3) where they remain during the rest of childhood. On the other hand, the lymphocytes, predominantly of the large type in infancy, rise rapidly to about 9,500 per mm^3 at two weeks and only slowly fall during the next 12 years to the adult level of about 1,500-2,000 per mm^3. It is important to remember the comparatively high lymphocyte count in normal children if mistaken diagnoses such as glandular fever or leukaemia are to be avoided. The monocyte ratio in children tends to be somewhat higher than in adults. Eosinophils and basophils show no special characteristics.

The normal blood volume in infancy is 85 ml/kg.

Key Learning Point
Normal values It is essential to remember age-related haematology reference ranges for diagnostic purposes.

IRON DEFICIENCY OR NUTRITIONAL ANAEMIA OF INFANCY

This is the only deficiency disease seen commonly among infants and children in the UK at the present time. The highest incidence of anaemia is found in the lower socio-economic groups.

Aetiology

Several factors, singly or in combination, can result in this deficiency state. Breast milk and cow's milk are low in iron. Therefore unduly prolonged milk feeding (human or cow's) or feeding whole cow's milk in early infancy results in iron deficiency. This is perhaps the most commonly found factor. Another important factor is the influence of birth weight. It is well-known that pre-term infants and others of low birth weight (such as twins or triplets) are particularly likely to develop iron-deficiency anaemia. Infants, whatever their maturity, have a body iron content of about 75 mg per kg fat free body weight. The bulk of the infant's iron endowment (66 to 75%) is represented by haemoglobin iron. One gram of haemoglobin contains 3.4 mg of iron. Complications of pregnancy or the perinatal period that result in blood loss will compromise the infants' iron endowment. The smaller infant grows more rapidly in proportion to his birth weight than the larger with a corresponding need for a larger increase in his red cells and haemoglobin. As the amount of iron absorbed is very low during the first four months of life the small infant more rapidly exhausts his storage iron (in liver and spleen) and develops overt signs of iron deficiency. Unless extreme, the presence of maternal iron deficiency does not appear to compromise the iron endowment of the foetus. Infections, to which the iron deficient infant is prone, further aggravate the anaemia. Finally, the possibility of chronic blood loss from e.g. oesophagitis, a Meckel's diverticulum or hook worm infestation, or of iron malabsorption must always be considered in cases of iron deficiency anaemia. Occult gastrointestinal bleeding can occur in infants who have been started on whole cow's milk early in life. Convenience foods are often low in iron. Red meat, eggs and green vegetables are sources of iron.

Key Learning Points
• Nutritional iron deficiency anaemia is seen commonly among infants and children during their 1st year. • Breast milk and cow's milk are low in iron. • Also convenience foods are often low in iron.

Clinical Features

A mild degree of nutritional anaemia probably affects over 25 per cent of infants during their first year. The onset is rarely before the fifth month of life. When the anaemia is severe there is obvious pallor of skin and mucous membranes. Splenomegaly may be present and there may be cardiomegaly and a haemic systolic murmur. The anaemia is microcytic and hypochromic (Fig. 15.2). Serum iron is markedly reduced (normal mean = 18 µmol/l; 100 mg per 100 ml), and the saturation of the iron binding protein of the serum is reduced from 33 per cent to 10 per cent or less. The serum ferritin concentration is reduced (less than 10 mg/ml). Bone marrow shows normoblastic hyperplasia and an absence of stainable iron. Ferritin is an acute phase protein and it is increased in inflammatory disease. Thus serum ferritin could be normal even in the absence of iron stores.

Key Learning Point
Ferritin is an acute phase protein and it is increased in inflammatory disease. Thus serum ferritin could be normal even in the absence of iron stores.

Prevention

In the term infant, iron deficiency is best prevented by the avoidance of whole cow's milk as a drink until 12 months and by the introduction of mixed feeding with foods rich in iron at the age of 4 months. In the pre-term infant iron should be given orally from the age of four weeks. The term infant should receive 1 mg of iron per kg per day and the pre-term infant 3 mg/kg/day.

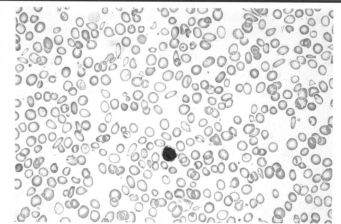

Fig. 15.2: Peripheral blood smear of a child with iron deficiency anaemia. Lymphocyte represents a normal size red cell, hence microcytic hypochromic red cells with some red cells

Treatment

In most cases the anaemia can be rapidly corrected with oral iron unless there are good reasons for using another route. Among the ferrous salts such as sulphate, fumarate, succinate, glutamate, gluconate and lactate the sulphate salt is considered to be the salt of choice. Ferrous salts show only marginal differences between one another in efficiency of absorption of iron. Ferric salts are much less well-absorbed. The oral dose of iron in an average child is 3 to 6 mg of elemental iron per kg daily administered two to three times daily between meals. The therapeutic response to iron therapy may be verified by any one of the following methods. A reticulocytosis may be noted 2 to 3 days after the start of therapy with a peak rise at 7 to 10 days. The haemoglobin concentration should rise by about 1-2 g/l per day or 2 g/100 ml over 3-4 weeks. Once normal haematological values have been attained iron should be continued for an additional three months to reconstitute depleted iron stores. The most common reason for lack of response in children is poor compliance; poor absorption is rare in children. Parenteral administration of iron as iron dextran or iron sucrose is indicated only if it is not possible to achieve compliance with use of oral iron or under the unusual circumstances in which iron malabsorption occurs.

CASE STUDY
A two year old Asian girl presented with poor appetite and pallor. Mother's main concern was that her daughter looked pale as compared to her siblings. There was no history of bleeding from any orifice of her body. On examination, she was anaemic and had haemic murmur. Otherwise no positive finding. Hb 6 g/dl. Blood film: Hypochromic and microcytic red cells and no target cells seen. Serum ferritin < 5 µg/ml. Stools negative for intestinal parasites. ***Diagnosis:*** Nutritional iron deficiency anaemia.

THE MEGOBLASTIC ANAEMIAS (FOLATE DEFICIENCY, VITAMIN B$_{12}$ DEFICIENCY)

Folate Deficiency

True megoblastic erythropoiesis is rare in paediatric practice. Folate is absorbed unchanged in the duodenum and jejunum. It is provided by most foods including meat and vegetables. The most common cause is malabsorption of folic acid in the older child with inadequately treated coeliac disease. However, folate deficiency may also be caused by inadequate intake, increased requirements (haemolytic anaemia), disorders of folate metabolism (congenital and acquired) drugs, and increased excretion in children on special diets. The symptoms of folate deficiency anaemia are similar to vitamin B$_{12}$ deficiency except that neuropathy is not a feature of folate deficiency. Also the peripheral blood and bone marrow changes in folate deficiency are indentical to those found in vitamin B$_{12}$ deficiency.

Hyper-segmentation of the neutrophils in the peripheral blood is the single most useful laboratory aid to early diagnosis (Fig. 15.3). The red cell or serum folate assay is a sensitive, reliable guide to the presence of folate deficiency and remains the best way of confirming early folate deficiency. Successful treatment of patients with folate deficiency involves correction of the folate deficiency as well as amelioration of the underlying disorder and improvement of the diet to increase folate intake. It is usual to treat folate deficient patients with 1 to 5 mg folic acid orally daily.

Key Learning Points
• Megaloblastic anaemia is rare in children.
• There is no justification for prescribing multiple-ingredient vitamin preparations containing vitamin B$_{12}$ or folic acid.

Vitamin B$_{12}$ Deficiency

Vitamin B$_{12}$ deficiency in children is exceedingly rare. If it occurs it is caused either by a specific malabsorption of vitamin B$_{12}$ or as part of a generalised malabsorption syndrome. Vitamin B$_{12}$ is provided by foods of animal origin, fish, meat, eggs and milk. After resection of the terminal ileum there is a risk of a megaloblastic anaemia developing 2-3 years later once the liver stores are depleted. Those most vulnerable are children who lose terminal ileum as a result of tumour (lymphoma), NEC, Crohn's disease or trauma. Most cases of vitamin B$_{12}$ deficiency occur during the first 2 years of life and others manifest later in childhood until puberty.

The clinical signs and symptoms of vitamin B$_{12}$ deficiency are related primarily to the anaemia but can also be complicated by subacute combined degeneration of the spinal cord. Glossitis with papillary atrophy may also be seen.

The haematological findings are indistinguishable from those of folic acid deficiency. The peripheral blood and bone marrow findings can be identical but the serum vitamin B$_{12}$ level is low. A Schilling test may be necessary to diagnose vitamin B$_{12}$ malabsorption.

Most patients with vitamin B$_{12}$ deficiency require treatment throughout life. Vitamin B$_{12}$ therapy results in reticulocytosis that peaks in 6-8 days and falls gradually to normal by 12th day. Bone marrow returns completely from megaloblastic to normoblastic in 72 hours.

THE HAEMOLYTIC ANAEMIAS

The causes of haemolytic anaemia, which may be defined as one in which the life span of the red cells is shortened. The red cell life span in children is 120 days, 60-80 days in neonates and even shorter in premature babies. The classification of haemolytic disorders is as shown in Table 15.1.

Table 15.1: Classification of haemolytic disorders
(i) *Inherited haemolytic disorders*
(a) Defects in the structure of the red cell membrane
Hereditary spherocytosis
Hereditary elliptocytosis
(b) Quantitative haemoglobin disorder
Thalassaemias
(c) Qualitative haemoglobin disorder
Sickle cell disease
(d) Defects of red blood cell metabolism
G6PD deficiency
Pyruvate kinase deficiency
Other enzyme disorders
(ii) *Acquired haemolytic disorders*
• Immune
– Autoimmune haemolytic anaemia
– Alloimmune haemolytic disease of the newborn

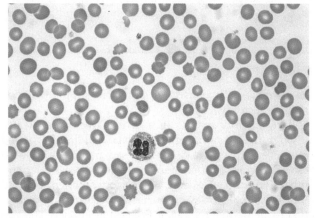

Fig. 15.3: Megaloblastic blood picture with oval macrocytic red cells

HEREDITARY SPHEROCYTOSIS (CONGENITAL HAEMOLYTIC JAUNDICE)

Aetiology

Hereditary spherocytosis is one of the most common inherited haemolytic anaemias encountered in paediatrics. This disease is inherited in an autosomal dominant fashion but in 25% of the cases neither parent appears to be affected. This is most likely the result of spontaneous mutation. At present it seems likely that the physiologically important abnormality is an inherent instability of the red cell membrane. It is certain that the major part of the haemolysis of the abnormal red cells takes place in the spleen.

Key Learning Point
Hereditary spherocytosis is one of most common inherited haemolytic anaemias encountered in paediatrics.

Clinical Features

The disease is quite variable in its severity. However, most affected children will, at sometime, manifest one or more of the cardinal features of the disease: Anaemia, jaundice (unconjugated bilirubin) and splenomegaly. It can cause haemolytic icterus in the neonatal period and kernicterus has been described. It is, however, rare for the disease to appear in infancy. More commonly it presents during later childhood with pallor and lassitude; less often with jaundice and highly coloured urine. Children may present with an acute abdomen from splenic infarcts. It may remain symptomless until adult life when biliary colic due to gall-stones is not uncommon. Acute haemolytic crises with severe anaemia and icterus require emergency treatment but they are, in fact, uncommon. Splenomegaly is usually present whatever the degree of haemolysis in hereditary spherocytosis. The red cells are unable to sustain a normal biconcave shape because of their metabolic defect. They are spheroidal with a smaller diameter than normal. It is usually easy to differentiate microspherocytes in well-stained blood films (Figs 15.4A and B). They appear unduly dark in colour and small in diameter than normal biconcave erythrocytes. A significant reticulocytosis is usually found. High figures may be reached during a crisis but the absence of a reticulocytosis does not exclude the diagnosis. Increased osmotic fragility of the red cells is an important diagnostic feature. The test is much more reliable when performed on a quantitative basis but is not pathognomonic of hereditary spherocytosis, being sometimes abnormal in acquired haemolytic anaemia, and infrequently it may be normal in the neonatal period. In hereditary spherocytosis Coombs' test is negative. Routine ultrasound of the gallbladder should be done to determine whether biliary pigment stones have developed. These should be removed at the time of splenectomy.

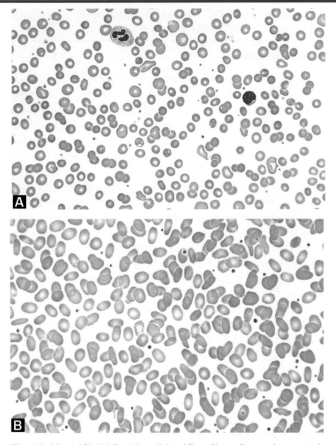

Figs 15.4A and B: (A) Peripheral blood film of hereditary spherocytosis showing microspherocytes and polychromasia: (B) Blood film of a child with elliptocytosis

CASE STUDY

A four year old Caucasian boy presented with pallor and lassitude. On examination, he was anaemic and had slight scleral icterus. He had no lymphadenopathy or hepatomegaly but had 7 cm splenomegaly. His mother had splenectomy at 8 years of age. Hb 6.2 g/dl, WBC 6.6 x 10^9/l, platelet count 300 x 10^9/l, reticulocyte count 40 x 10^9/l. Blood film revealed numerous microspherocytes. Total bilirubin was elevated at 160 µg/l with an unconjugated bilirubin of 150 µg/l. AST /ALT normal. Ultrasound examination of gallbladder negative for gallstones.
Diagnosis: Hereditary spherocytosis

Treatment

Treatment usually consists of folic acid supplimentation and splenectomy.

Splenectomy results in a return to normal health although it does not alter the metabolic defect in the red cells. It should always be advised in the child with hereditary spherocytosis since even mild disease interferes with growth and well-being. Splenectomy renders the child more susceptible to severe bacterial infections and there is good evidence that the risk is greatest in infancy. This can be reduced by immunisation with polyvalent. pneumo-coccal vaccine At present re-immunisation is recommended every five years. Also *Haephilus influenzae type b*, and Neisseria meningitides (menigococcus) may cause infection. In addition the child should receive life long oral prophylactic phenoxymethyl penicillin and for those allergic to penicillin erythromycin should be used. If the child has not been previously immunised against *H. influenzas* it would be worthwhile giving *Hib.vaccine*. In our opinion splenectomy should be postponed until the child is about 5 years old. Children should carry a card with information about their lack of spleen. They should be educated on the potential risk of infection. There is no evidence that further delay is useful, and it may be harmful, since the risk of cholelithiasis increases in children after the age of 10 years. Control of the anaemia can meantime be achieved by blood transfusion. Rarely, in the neonatal period a rising serum bilirubin level may necessitate an exchange transfusion to eliminate the risk of kernicterus. Box 15.1 shows the indications for splenectomy in children.

BOX 15.1: Indications for splenectomy

- *Medical*
  — Hereditary spherocytosis
  — Hereditary elliptocytosis
  — Severe pyruvate kinase deficiency
  — Autoimmune haemolytic anaemia—warm IgG antibody type
  — Chronic immune thrombocytopenic purpura
  — Hypersplenism—who develop significant anaemia or thrombocytopenia
  — Sickle cell anaemia—acute splenic sequestration crisis
  — Thalassemia major—increasing transfusion requirements caused by hypersplenism
- *Surgical*
  — Splenic trauma, splenic cysts, tumours, Gaucher's disease
  — Thalassemia major—massive splenomegaly—for relief from mechanical stress

---

THE THALASSAEMIAS

The thalassaemia syndromes are characterised by deficiencies in the rate of production of specific globin chains. A microcytic hypochromic anaemia results.

Developmental Changes in Haemoglobin Synthesis

Normal adult and foetal haemoglobin contains four globin chains (Table 15.2). The thalassaemia syndromes are a heterogeneous group of disorders of haemoglobin (Hb) synthesis resulting from a genetically determined reduced rate of production of one or more of the four globin chains of haemoglobin—α (alpha), β (beta), δ (delta) and γ (gamma). This results in an excess of the partner chains which continue to be synthesised at a normal rate. The alpha chain types are carried on chromosome 16 and the beta, delta and gamma on chromosome 11. Each type of

Table 15.2: Globin chains of normal haemoglobins			
Adult	-	Hb A	$\alpha_2 + \beta_2$
	-	Hb A$_2$	$\alpha_2 + \delta_2$
Fetal	-	Hb F	$\alpha_2 + \gamma_2$
		H Bart's	γ_4
		Hb H	β_4

thalassaemia can exist in a heterozygous or a homozygous state. The most common is beta thalassaemia (Cooley's anaemia) which involves suppression of beta-chain formation. In homozygotes, there is a severe anaemia with a high level of Hb-F (alpha 2, gamma 2), some Hb-A2 (alpha 2, delta 2) and a complete absence of, or greatly reduced (normal) Hb-A (alpha 2, beta 2). Heterozygotes on the other hand suffer from only mild anaemia with reasonable levels of Hb-A, somewhat raised Hb-A2, but Hb-F levels rarely in excess of 3 per cent. Children of the mating of two such heterozygotes have a 1 in 4 chance of suffering from the homozygous state for beta thalassaemia. They will not present clinically, however, until later infancy when the effects of beta-chain suppression develop because Hb-A formation fails to take over from the production of Hb-F in the normal way. The other main type of thalassaemia involves suppression of alpha-chain production and as alpha chains are shared by Hb-A, Hb-A2 and Hb-F it is to be expected that alpha thalassaemia would become clinically manifest in foetal life.

Tetramers of gamma chains may be produced (Hb-Bart's) which result in a clinical picture very similar to that in hydrops foetalis with massive hepatosplenomegaly and generalised oedema, with stillbirth or early neonatal death. In haemoglobin, H disease, on the other hand, tetramers of gamma chains (Hb-H) are present in excess and there is considerable clinical variability: From a picture indistinguishable from Cooley's anaemia to an absence of specific signs. Heterozygotes for alpha thalassaemia cannot be detected with certainty. The thalassaemias are uncommon in persons of British stock but they are commonly seen in children of Mediterranean, Middle Eastern, Indian, Pakistani origin as well as in South-East Asia where they constitute a major and distressing public-health problem. The distribution parallels with that of falciparum malaria for which the trait appears to have a selective advantage.The clinical account which follows refers only to the most common variety of beta thalassaemia in the homozygous state (beta thalassaemia major—Cooley's anaemia).

Key Learning Point

The clinical severity of beta thalassaemia ranges from thalassaemia minor (usually symptomless), thalassaemia intermedia (with anaemia plus splenomegaly but not transfusion dependent) to thalassaemia major (transfusion dependent).

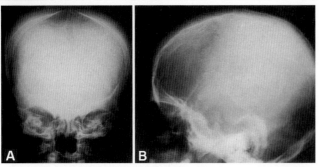

Figs 15.5A and B: Lateral view of the skull showing expansion of the diploic space and a hair on end appearance of the skull vault

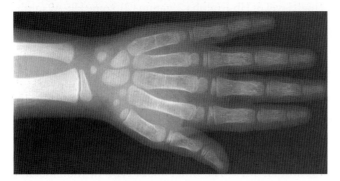

Fig. 15.6: AP view of the hand showing mild generalised osteopenia, coarsening of the trabecular pattern, medullary widening and cortical thining

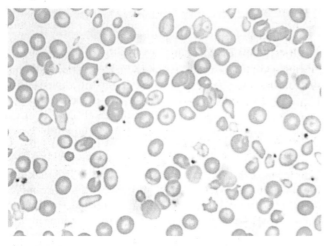

Fig. 15.7: Peripheral blood smear of a child with homozygous beta-thalassaemia showing a target cell

branous bones of the skull are thickened and lateral views of the skull show the "hair on end" appearance (Fig. 15.5). The facies has a Mongoloid appearance due to thickening of the facial bones. The hands may become broadened and thickened due to changes in the metacarpals and phalanges. These bone changes are due to the hyperplasia of the bone marrow (Fig. 15.6). Blood examination shows a severe hypochromic anaemia with marked anisocytosis and poikilocytosis. Many microcytic red cells lie side-by-side with large (12-18 mm), bizarrely shaped cells. In some of the latter cells and abnormal central mass of haemoglobin gives to them the appearance of "target cells" (Fig. 15.7). Reticulocytosis is marked and Howell-Jolly bodies may be numerous. Serum unconjugated bilirubin concentration is increased. There is increased serum iron while the iron-binding capacity is fully saturated and lower than in normal children. The haemoglobin pattern in beta thalassaemia major consists mainly of Hb-F, which may amount to 90 per cent of the total and of Hb-A2; Hb-A is totally absent or greatly reduced. Most children affected by beta thalassaemia major can be kept in reasonable health, if they are maintained on a high blood transfusion regimen which prevents the Hb level from falling 11 g/dl. Other laboratory abnormalities commonly found in homozygous beta thalassaemia are mostly due to complications of transfusional haemosiderosis. However, even with the best available treatment, growth failure becomes apparent before puberty. In boys, there is usually a complete or partial failure of pubertal growth and sexual maturation. In girls the failure tends to be less severe with irregular or scanty menstrual periods. However, secondary amenorrhoea may develop from iron overload. Other effects may include endocrine, hepatic or renal failure and overt diabetes mellitus.

CASE STUDY

A one year old Asian boy presented with pallor, poor feeding, failure to thrive and recurrent upper respiratory infection. On examination he was anaemic and had a massive hepatosplenomegaly.
Hb 5.2 g/dl, WBC and platelet counts were normal. Peripheral blood film showed markedly hypochromic, microcytic red cells, anisocytosis and target cells and some basophilic stippling. Reticulocyte count 10%. He had mildly raised unconjugated bilirubin, otherwise ALT and AST were normal.
The most likely diagnosis was beta thalassaemia major.

Clinical Features

This condition is characterised by a chronic haemolytic anaemia which becomes manifest later in infancy but not in the newborn. Pallor is constant and icterus not uncommon. Splenomegaly increases throughout childhood. Hepatomegaly is also present, largely due to extramedullary erythropoiesis. Pathognomonic skeletal changes can be demonstrated radiographically. Mem-

Treatment

The prognosis in beta thalassaemia has improved in recent years and could improve still further if the best available management were to be everywhere pursued. This has been well-described under three major categories: choice of transfusion scheme; hypersplenism and splenectomy; iron chelation therapy. The objective of the transfusion scheme should be to maintain haemoglobin between

10 and 14 g/dl with a pre-transfusion haemoglobin of 10 - 11 g/dl. Patients should have their red cells genotyped to reduce the risk of sensitisation due to repeated blood transfusions. This regimen will reduce the stimulus to unlimited bone marrow expansion and so prevent such undesirable manifestations as cardiomegaly, stunting of growth and the disfiguring, Cooley's facies. This regimen has become standard therapy for β thalassaemia major. On the other hand, the degree of hypersplenism has not always been appreciated and it may be marked even in the absence of thrombocytopenia or leucopenia. Its presence greatly increases the blood requirements. The rate of splenic enlargement is variable even in well-transfused patients and the massive size of the spleen may lead to abdominal discomfort. Often the transfusion requirement increases as the spleen enlarges. Eventually most patients undergo splenectomy which usually leads to improved physical well-being and a reduction in the transfusion requirement. Splenectomy should be delayed if possible until the child is 5 years of age because of the risk of post-splenectomy infection. Splenectomised children should receive lifelong oral penicillin prophylaxis and polyvalent pneumococcal and hib vaccine.

Desferrioxamine is the only effective agent available for chronic iron chelation. This should be commenced to prevent iron overload before the third birthday and when the infant is dry at night. Desferrioxamine can be administered subcutaneously overnight with a small infusion pump. There is also general agreement that ascorbic acid 100-200 mg daily by mouth enhances the effectiveness of desferrioxamine therapy.Ferritin levels should be used to monitor iron load.

Iron overload is responsible for cardiac, hepatic and endocrine problems which are reduced by chelation therapy. Because of the hypothalamic-pitutary dys-function testosterone or oestrogen supplements may be indicated for hypogonadism. Growth hormone may also be required. Insulin for those who develop diabetes. Children will require folic acid supplements due to increased demands of increased erythropoiesis. Bone marrow transplantation is the only curable option for those with fully matched HLA compatible sibling donors.

The only rational approach to thalassaemia on a world scale must lie in programmes developed towards prevention. These have been based on prospective detection of heterozygotes followed by genetic counselling.

Beta Thalassaemia Minor and Thalassaemia Intermedia

The beta thalassaemia heterozygotes are asymptomatic. The haemoglobin is slightly reduced to 9-12 g/dl and the red cell count is high. On the contrary, patients with thalassaemia intermedia are symptomatic. They have a milder clinical course than those with thalassaemia major

and are not blood transfusion dependent and should not be subjected to transfusion inappropriately.

SICKLE CELL DISEASE

Aetiology

This disease is almost confined to the black African races.It is one of the most prevalent autosomal recessive haemoglobinopathies. Homozygotes suffer from sickle cell anaemia in which all of their haemoglobin is of the Hb-S variety (homozygous SS disease).The other sickling syndromes are the double heterozygous states such as Hb SC disease (HbSC) and sickle beta thalassaemia (Hb S Beta thal). The abnormality in Hb-S lies in the beta peptide chains, the alpha chains being normal. The aberration in the beta chains is due to the substitution of valine for glutamic acid in the No.6 position. Heterozygotes reveal the sickle cell trait (AS) and their haemoglobin is composed of about 60 per cent Hb-A and 40 per cent Hb-S. The trait is found in about 7-9 per cent of American black people but it is much more prevalent in some African tribes. It provides increased resistance to malignant tertian malaria. Hb-S has a distinctive electrophoretic pattern which is due to its abnormal molecular structure. This type of haemoglobin forms crescent-shaped crystals under reduced oxygen tension, and it is this property which is responsible for the sickled shape of the erythrocytes in people who possess the gene. Haemolysis in sickle-cell anaemia appears to be due mainly to impaction of the sickled cells in the capillaries, especially in organs where the oxygen tension is low. Capillary obstruction leads to infarcts in various organs, e.g. spleen, intestine, bones, kidneys, heart, lungs and brain.

Key Learning Point
Most infants with sickle cell disease (SS) are functionally asplenic by one year of age because of repeated splenic infarction.

Clinical Features

The sickle cell trait (AS) is symptomless unless it is associated with another haemoglobinopathy or with thalassaemia. Sickle cell anaemia (SS) often presents during the first year with pallor, listlessness and mild jaundice, but not before 6 months of age. The onset of symptoms is, however, delayed for six months or longer until the Hb-F of the infant has been replaced by Hb-S. In some cases, there are recurrent haemolytic crises with acute symptoms such as severe abdominal pain and rigidity, pain in the loins, limb pains, localised paralyses, convulsions or meningism. Cerebrovascular occlusion can lead to hemi-plegia and cranial nerve palsies.

The lung is also one of the major organs involved in sickle cell disease. Clinical lung involvement commonly

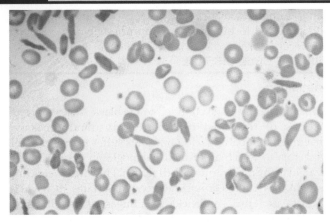

Fig. 15.8: Pereipheral blood smear of a child with sickle cell disease showing sickled red cell.

takes two major forms: The acute chest syndrome and sickle cell chronic lung disease. Acute chest problem is manifested by fever, chest pain and infiltrates in the chest radiograph. Chronic lung disease is due to repeated episodes of infection and infarction.

Symmetrical painful swellings of the fingers and feet (hand foot syndrome-dactylitis) may develop due to infarction of the metacarpals and metatarsals. X-rays show severe bone destruction and periosteal reaction. They may also reveal radial striations in the skull. Chronic haemolytic anaemia interferes with growth and nutrition so that the child is often stunted in later years. Spleno-megaly may be marked, but sometimes disappears in later childhood. Cholelithiasis may develop as in other haemolytic anaemias. In adults the large joints may become swollen and painful with serious crippling. The peripheral blood shows a normochromic anaemia, reticulcytosis and polymorphonuclear leucocytosis. In addition there is an increase in the serum unconjugated bilirubin and a decrease in red cell osmotic fragility. In a crisis excess urobilinogenuria is marked. Sickled cells may be seen in ordinary blood films (Fig. 15.8). The diagnosis can be confirmed by demonstration of the characteristic mobility of Hb-S on starch gel electrophoresis. Children affected with sickle-cell anaemia also have some Hb-F in their circulation.

CASE STUDY

A three year old Nigerian boy presented with pallor and a painful swollen right index finger. On abdominal examination he had splenomegaly 4 cm below the left costal margin. Most likely diagnosis is sickle cell disease with dactylitis.

Treatment

There is no cure for sickle cell disease but blood trans-fusions are frequently required for anaemia. Because of the high incidence of serious bacterial infections in patients

with sickle cell anaemia, the index of suspicion for infection should be high. Antibiotic choice should include agents effective against *pneumococcus, Haemophilus influenzae*, salmonella and *Staphylococcus aureus*. The risk of pneumococcal infection in particular is high in the first two years of life. Therefore penicillin prophylaxis should be started by the age of 4 months. In vaso-occlusive crises, rest in bed and relief of pain are essential. Dehydration and acidosis should be quickly corrected. With careful supervision and the use of blood transfusion many children with sickle cell anaemia (SS) reach adult life. Splenectomy is indicated when there is evidence of hypersplenism. Folate deficiency is particularly common in sickle-cell disease and 5 mg of folic acid should be given daily. Death can occur suddenly from cardiac failure, renal failure or cerebral infarction and patients of black African extraction should always be tested for sickling before anaesthesia. Sickle cell testing is an important considera-tion in any child from geographical areas where sickle cell disease is prevelant before any elective surgery is carried out. Post-operative preparation may require blood transfusion, and hypoxia and acidosis should be avoided during the operation. Antenatal diagnosis can be made on chorionic villous biopsy in the first trimester of pregnancy. At present the role of bone marrow trans-plantation is limited. Some patients benefit clinically from hydroxyurea.

OTHER HAEMOGLOBINOPATHIES

It has already been noted that there are three normal haemoglobins each of two identical pairs of globin polypeptide chains with an iron-containing haem group inserted into each chain. In the healthy adult 98 per cent of the Hb-A is composed of two alpha and two beta chains ($\alpha_2\beta_2$). About 2 per cent of adult Hb is Hb-A composed of two alpha and two delta chains ($\alpha_2\delta_2$). Foetal Hb or Hb-F is composed of two alpha and two gamma chains ($\alpha_2\gamma_2$). However, over 100 abnormal haemoglobins have now been recognised in which the aberration generally consists of a single amino acid substitution in one pair of the peptide chains due to gene mutation. That is to say, they are determined by alleles of the genes for normal Hb-A, Hb-A_2 or Hb-F. The different haemoglobins carry different electrical charges so causing them to move at different speeds in an electrical field and they can usually best be identified by electrophoresis. The different haemo-globinopathies vary widely in their effects, from no apparent effect on health to a fatal disease (e.g. Hb-S). The homozygote for the gene will, of course always be much more severely affected than the heterozygote, as in sickle-cell disease.

The homozygote for Hb-C presents with manifestations similar to those in sickle-cell disease but sickling and bone changes do not occur. The heterozygote is usually symptomless but blood films show target cells and there is increased osmotic resistance. The homozygote for Hb-E on the other hand, suffers only from a mild normochromic anaemia with numerous target cells and increase in osmotic resistance, while the heterozygote is asymptomatic. Haemoglobin M disease is very different in that it causes methaemoglobinaemia.

Having now considered thalassaemia and a few of the haemoglobinopathies in both the homozygous and heterozygous forms, it remains to point out that some anaemic children are found to have inherited the genes for two abnormal haemoglobins, one from each heterozygous parent, or more commonly for beta thalassaemia and one abnormal haemoglobin. They are, in fact, mixed or double heterozygotes. Thus there has been described beta thalassaemia with haemoglobin S (or C, D or E) as well as S/C, S/D combinations, etc. The effects produced by these states depend upon the peptide chains involved. Thus, if both abnormal genes affect the same type of chain the effects are much more severe than if they affect different chains, i.e. the mixed heterozygous state is more crippling than the double heterozygous state. For example, in both S/C disease and Hb-S/beta thalassaemia the beta chains are involved. This means that no Hb-A can be formed because no normal beta chains can be produced, a state called "interaction" and the resulting clinical manifestations are very similar in severity to the homozygous S/S state (sickle cell anaemia). On the other hand, when both an alpha and a beta chain abnormality are inherited (e.g. as in alpha thalassaemia with beta chain haemoglobins S, C or E) the effect is usually no more severe than when only one of the abnormalities is present because no "interaction" has taken place. Some of these abnormal haemoglobin states can only be accurately identified by family studies, employing sophisticated techniques. The matter is of practical importance because of the differences in prognosis.

GLUCOSE 6 PHOSPHATE DEHYDROGENASE DEFICIENCY

Glucose 6 phosphate dehydrogenase deficiency is the most common red blood cell enzyme abnormality associated with haemolysis. It affects people throughout the world with the highest incidence in individuals originating from most parts of Africa, from most parts of Asia, from Oceania, and from Southern Europe.

G-6-PD A is the commonest variant associated with haemolysis and is found in 10-15% of African-Americans. G-6-PD Mediterranean is the commonest variant in white people of Mediterranean origin and G-6-PD Canton is the commonest in Asia. It is X-linked and haemolysis is mainly confined to males. The magnitude of haemolysis is variable and is dependent on the degree of oxidant stress. Most variants of G-6PD deficiency cause acute haemolysis and

not chronic haemolysis on taking a number of common drugs. They are also susceptible to developing acute haemolytic anaemia upon ingestion of fava beans (broad beans, Vicia faba); this is termed favism and can be more severe in children or when the fresh fava beans are eaten raw.

The diagnosis of G-6-PD deficiency is suggested by Coomb's negative haemolytic anaemia associated with drugs or infection. The specific diagnosis of G-6-PD deficiency can be made by spectrophotometric enzyme measurements. Special stains of the peripheral blood may reveal Heinz bodies during haemolytic episodes.

Treatment

There is no specific treatment for haemolysis due to G-6-PD. Patients should be educated about which drugs to avoid. The risk and severity of haemolysis is almost always dose related. The most common drugs implicated are the sulphonamide antibiotics and antimalarial drugs and other potential sources of oxidant stress (See Box 15.2). G-6-PD deficiency may protect against malaria.

BOX 15.2: Drugs commonly associated with acute haemolysis in most G-6-PD deficiency

- Primaquine
- Pamaquine
- Sulphanilamide
- Sulphapyridine
- Sulphamethoxazole
- Salazopyrin
- Septrin
- Dapsone
- Thiazolesulphone
- Nitrofurantoin
- Nalidix acid
- Naphthalene in mothballs

Pyruvate Kinase Deficiency

Pyruvate kinase deficiency is the commonest red cell enzyme deficiency in north Europeans. It presents in the neonatal period with anaemia and jaundice. Diagnosis requires measurement of pyruvate kinase in the red blood cells. The degree of haemolysis varies greatly and is sometimes severe enough to require frequent red blood cell transfusions. There is a beneficial response to splenectomy.

AUTOIMMUNE HAEMOLYTIC ANAEMIA (AIHA)

Aetiology

This is not a common problem in paediatric practice but it may present as an acute emergency. There are two major classes of antibodies against red cells that produce haemolysis in man: IgG and IgM. Autoimmune haemolytic anaemia can be warm or cold antibody type. The IgM antibody is generally restricted to the clinical entity of cold haemagglutinin disease because it has a particular affinity for its red cell antigen in the cold (0° to 100°C). IgM induced immune haemolytic anaemia is most commonly associated with an underlying mycoplasma infection or cyto-megalovirus, mumps and infectious mononucleosis infections.

The IgG antibody usually has its maximal activity at 37°C and, thus, this entity has been termed warm antibody induced haemolytic anaemia. IgG induced immune haemolytic anaemia may occur without an apparent underlying disease (idiopathic disease); however it may also occur with SLE, rheumatoid arthritis and certain drugs. Warm type AIHA can be severe and life-threatening.

Clinical Features

In some children the disease has an alarmingly acute onset with fever, backache, limb pains, abdominal pain, vomiting and diarrhoea. Haemoglobinuria and oliguria may be present. Pallor develops rapidly and icterus is common. Frequently, the pallor, listlessness and mild icterus develop more insidiously. Splenomegaly is common. The urine may be dark in colour due to the presence of excess urobilinogen. Reticulocytosis is often marked and there may be many erythroblasts in the peripheral blood. Spherocytosis with an increased fragility of the red cells may simulate congenital spherocytosis. However, in acquired haemolytic anaemia Coombs' test is positive and serum unconjugated bilirubin concentration is increased.

Treatment

In many patients with IgG or IgM induced immune haemolytic anaemia no therapeutic intervention is necessary, since the haemolysis may be mild. However, in some children with significant anaemia complete recovery follows emergency blood transfusion. In less acute cases the haemolytic process continues after transfusion. Corticosteroids are of great value in the treatment of AIHA. Oral prednisolone 2 mg/kg/d should be given until the haemolysis is brought under control. Thereafter, the dosage is progressively reduced to achieve the smallest main-tenance dose compatible with a reasonable haemoglobin value (10 - 12 g/dl). When long-term steroid therapy proves necessary a careful watch must be kept for undesirable side-effects such as osteoporosis, diabetes mellitus, etc. When haemolysis cannot be controlled with a reasonable dosage of steroid, the question of splenectomy arises.

In children who do not respond to steroids immuno-suppresion has been used, e.g. ciclosporin, cyclo-phosphamide and high dose intravenous immuno-globulin. Blood transfusion may be required. The least incompatible blood should be used if clinically indicated.

APLASTIC AND HYPOPLASTIC ANAEMIA

This group of anaemias is poorly understood and clearly contains a considerable number of quite separate diseases which present clinically in somewhat similar ways. The defect in erythropoiesis may affect all elements of the marrow or only one, such as the erythropoietic tissue. There may be virtually no formation at all of the precursors or red cells, leucocytes or platelets. Fortunately, these conditions are not common, but those to be considered here occur sufficiently frequently in paediatric practice to merit the attention of all who have to handle sick children.

CONGENITAL HYPOPLASTIC ANAEMIA (BLACKFAN DIAMOND ANAEMIA)

Aetiology

This disease presents in early infancy as an apparent aplasia of the red cells. Granulocytes and platelets are unaffected. In most cases, the bone marrow shows a gross deficiency or erythroblasts but shows normal maturation of myeloid and megakaryocyte cells. The incidence is the same in boys as in girls but the disease tends to be milder in its effects on boys. Its occurence in siblings has been reported in several families and family studies have suggested an autosomal recessive mode of inheritance.

Clinical Features

The presenting feature is pallor, which becomes apparent in the early weeks or months of life. Irritability becomes obvious only when the anaemia is severe in degree. Short stature is common and characteristic facial features are described of a snub nose, wide-set eyes and a thick upper lip. There are no haemorrhagic manifestations. Hepatic or splenic enlargement is unusual but may develop as a consequence of cardiac failure. Haemic systolic murmurs are common. The anaemia, often severe, is normocytic and normochromic. Reticulocytes are absent or scanty. White blood cells and platelets show no abnormalities (Fig. 15.9).

Course and Prognosis

This is greatly influenced by treatment. Repeated blood transfusions lead to haemosiderosis which causes a typical muddy bronze skin pigmentation. Cirrhosis of the liver ultimately develops with failure of sexual maturation. Portal hypertension and hypersplenism occasionally develop. The long bones often show marked growth-arrest lines. Osteoporosis and delayed bone age are common. Affected children are frequently dwarfed but mental development proceeds normally. The prognosis is not good in the long term; on the other hand, spontaneous remissions have frequently been reported, even after puberty and several hundred transfusions.

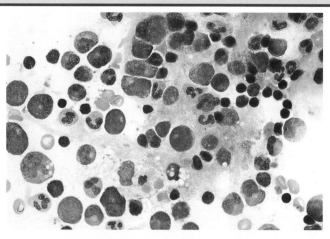

Fig. 15.9: Marrow film of a child with Blackfan Diamond anaemia – virtually no red cell precursors on the film.

Treatment

Repeated transfusions of packed red cells, always after careful cross-matching, are frequently required over periods of many years. In some cases there is a marrow response to prednisolone in an initial dose of 2 mg/kg/d in four divided doses, but only if treatment is started before three months of age. The dosage should thereafter be reduced to the smallest which will maintain a reasonable haemoglobin level and normal reticulocyte count and is given on alternate days. When repeated transfusions are necessary the development of haemosiderosis can be delayed with the iron chelating agent desferrioxamine to treat iron overload. In these children, bone marrow transplantation may be considered.

FANCONI-TYPE FAMILIAL APLASTIC ANAEMIA

Aetiology

This autosomal recessive disorder affects all three elements of the bone marrow (pancytopenia). Chromosomal studies in some cases have revealed an abnormally high number of chromatid breaks, endoreduplications and other minor abnormalities.

Clinical Features

Pallor may become obvious in early infancy, but more often the onset is delayed until between the ages of 3 and 10 years. Purpura and ecchymoses are not uncommon and there may be bleeding from mucous membranes. Defects in the radius and/or thumb or accessory thumbs are common. Mild hyperpigmentation, hypogonadism and short stature have frequently been reported, and endocrine studies have revealed growth hormone deficiency, isolated or combined with deficiencies of gonadotrophins and ACTH. Other congenital abnormalities seen less frequently include microcephaly, squints and anomalies of the heart or renal tract. The blood shows a normocytic, normochromic anaemic, leucopenia, granulocytopenia and thrombocytopenia. Reticulocytes are scanty or absent. Leukaemia not infrequently appears in relatives and occasionally in the patient. The diagnosis is readily overlooked in patients who lack the characteristic congenital abnormalities but useful diagnostic pointers are the presence of Hb-F, 1-2 g/dl in the blood and of chromosomal abnormalities in the lymphocytes.

Treatment

Repeated blood transfusions may be necessary in spite of the risks of transfusion haemosiderosis. Death is common during childhood but a sustained remission can sometimes be obtained with a combination of prednisolone 0.4 mg/kg on alternate days and oxymetholone 2 to 5 mg/kg daily. The latter drug can give rise to hepatoblastoma. Therapy with human growth hormone may cause an increase in growth velocity if a deficiency of GH has been confirmed. Also successful bone marrow transplantation has been reported in patients with Fanconi's anaemia.

ACQUIRED HYPOPLASTIC ANAEMIA

This is a rare disease in childhood and most cases are "idiopathic". The bone marrow is rarely completely aplastic in such patients. Some cases are secondary to the toxic effects of drugs such as chloramphenicol, phenylethylacetylurea, carbimazole, thiouracil, phenybutazone and gold salts.

Clinical Features

The onset may be acute or insidious with increasing pallor, listlessness, malaise, bruises, purpura and sometimes bleeding from mucous membranes. Death is due to haemorrhage into internal organs or to intercurrent infection. The blood shows a normocytic, normochromic anaemia, thrombocytopenia, leucopenia and granulocytopenia. Bone marrow must always be examined by needle biopsy or trephine. Marrow examination is, furthermore, the only way in which hypoplastic anaemia can be distinguished from aleukaemia leukaemia. The prognosis is grave when the marrow examination reveals gross hypoplasia of all the blood forming elements, but in less severe cases there is always hope of a spontaneous or induced remission.

Treatment

Life can be prolonged by repeated transfusions of packed red cells. Platelet transfusions can also help to prolong life. Remissions can sometimes be obtained with a combination of prednisolone and oxymetholone as described for the treatment of Fanconi's anaemia. However, the treatment of choice is bone marrow transplantation from histocompatible sibling or family donor. Bone marrow transplantation is more likely to be successful if blood transfusions have been irradiated and kept to a minimum to avoid sensitisation to donor transplantation antigens.

ALBERS-SCHÖNBERG DISEASE (OSTEOPETROSIS, MARBLE BONES)

Aetiology

This is a genetic disorder of bone, usually autosomal recessive. The cortex and trabeculae of the bones are thickened and the marrow is crowded out. Extramedullary erythropoiesis in the liver and spleen may prevent anaemia for a variable period. It is now recognised that the cause of osteopetrosis is a defect or deficiency of osteoclasts or their precursors which are derived from the pluripotent haemopoietic stem cells. Bone resorption is inhibited.

Clinical Features

The disease may present in infancy with progressive lose of vision due to optic atrophy, with cranial nerve palsies or with deafness. In later childhood the mode of presentation is a pathological fracture or increasing pallor. The anaemia is leuco-erythroblastic in type. There is progressive hepatosplenomegaly. The most characteristic diagnostic signs are to be found in radiographs of the skeleton (Figs 15.10A to C). The bones, including the base of the skull, ribs, vertebrae, scapulae and pelvis show increased density. Typical zones of decreased density can be seen at the metaphyses and running parallel to the borders of scapulae and ilia; these still contain marrow. This disease should be differentiated from pykno-dysostosis. This is an autosomal recessive disease that resembles osteopetrosis except that the clinical manifestations are mild and not associated with haematologic or neurologic abnormalities.

Treatment

It is now possible to cure some infants with the severe form of the disease by bone marrow transplantation from a histocompatible sibling. Infants with compatible donors should be transplanted as early as possible to avoid irreversible damage from bone encroachment on cranial nerves.

THE THROMBOCYTOPENIC PURPURAS

Purpura is an extremely common clinical phenomenon in childhood and has many causes. The principal pathogenic factors are capillary defects and thrombocytopenia, sometimes both being present. In most cases the purpura

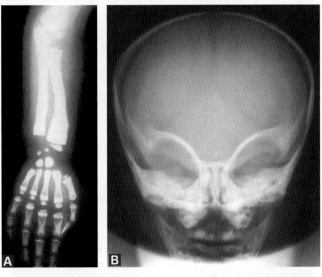
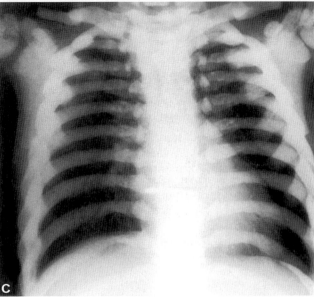

Figs 15.10A to C: (A) Osteopetrosis showing zones of increased density at metaphyseal ends of long bones, (B) Face spectacles or showing "White spectacle sign" (C) Showing increased density in ribs.

is symptomatic of another disease. It occurs due to decreased capillary resistance or bacterial micro-emboli in acute infections such as meningococcal (and other) septicaemia, bacterial endocarditis, typhus and typhoid fever, scarlet fever, etc. It may arise in scurvy, uraemia and snake-bite. Severe intrapartum hypoxia sometimes causes petechiae, especially over the head, neck and shoulders of the newborn. A similar mechanical effect is sometimes seen in the child who has had a severe and prolonged convulsion and in whooping cough. Symptomatic thrombocytopenic purpura occurs in leukaemia, hypoplastic anaemia and in states of hypersplenism.

Table 15.3: Thrombocytopenia in childhood		
Disorders of production	*Disorders of destruction*	*Abnormal distribution*
Leukaemia	DIC	Giant haemangioma
Solid tumour	HUS	
Aplastic anaemia	Acute ITP	
TARS	Chronic ITP	
Drug induced	Autoimmune diseases (SLE)	
e.g. cytotoxic therapy,	TTP	
sodium valproate,	Intravascular prosthetic	
phenytoin, carbamezepine	devices	
	INTP	

DIC = Disseminated intravascular coagulation
HUS = Haemolytic uraemic syndrome
ITP = Idiopathic thrombocytopenic purpura
TTP = Throbotic thrombocytopenic purpura
TARS = Thrombocytopenia with absent radius syndrome, Giant
         haemangioma
      = Kasabach-Merritt syndrome
INTP = Isoimmune neonatal thrombocytopenic purpura

Fragmentation of platelets as well as red cells, with thrombocytopenia and haemolytic anaemia may occur in cases of giant haemangioma and after cardiac surgery. Congenital defects in the capillaries are ssen in such rare conditions as hereditary haemorrhagic telangiectasia (Osler's disease) and cutis hyperelastica (Ehler's-Danlos syndrome). It will be clear, therefore, that purpura reflects a blood disorder in only a minority of cases. Nonetheless, the more important primary diseases in which purpura is a prominent feature are conveniently discussed in this chapter.

IDIOPATHIC THROMBOCYTOPENIC PURPURA (ITP)

Idiopathic thrombocytopenic purpura (ITP) accounts for the majority of cases of childhood thrombocytopenia and has been classified into acute and chronic forms. It is a clinical diagnosis reached by exclusion of other causes of thrombocytopenia (Table 15.3).

Clinical Features

Most cases in childhood have an acute onset. The peak age is 2-4 years with a male : female ratio of 1 : 1. There has frequently been a recently preceding, non-specific upper respiratory infection or other common childhood illness and immunisations have been associated. The first manifestation may be bleeding from mucous membranes such as epistaxis, bleeding gums or haematuria. Generalised purpura and/or ecchymoses are characteristic and often profuse. The spleen may be palpable but never becomes very large. Life may be endangered in severe cases by blood loss or by subarachnoid haemorrhage. The differentiating characteristic of this acute form is the spontaneous and permanent recovery within 6 months of onset.

Key Learning Points
Meningococcal septicaemia comes into differential diagnosis of a widespread petechial rash but is unlikely in a well child. Non-accidental injury with bruises is unlikely because of the abnormal platelet count.

Chronic cases are also seen in which crops of purpura and ecchymoses persist beyond 6 months and occur more frequently in girls. Children who have the chronic form of idiopathic thrombocytopenic purpura may present at any age, although children over 10 years of age are at a greater risk than those in the younger age group. The blood shows a diminished platelet count. Spontaneous bleeding can occur when the count will be low and often is less than $10 \times 10^9/l$. The WBC and haemoglobin are normal. Blood film shows no abnormality other than the absence of platelets.

A bone marrow examination is needed only when there is an atypical presentation or abnormalities other than absent platelets on the blood film or if steroids are going to be used as treatment (Fig. 15.11).

CASE STUDY

A 6 year old girl presented with a 48 hour history of bruises on her legs and numerous petechiae over face and chest. She had epistaxis a few hours prior to hospitalisation. She had no previous history of easy bruising or being on any medication. In fact she had been previously healthy. On examination she had widespread petechiae. She had no other positive finding and in particular had no lymphadenopathy or hepatosplenomegaly. Hb 12.5 g / dl, WBC 10.6 x $10^9/l$, neutrophil count $5.6 \times 10^9/l$ and platelet count $1.5 \times 10^9/l$. The blood film except for the absence of platelets was normal. Immunoglobulins normal. Blood urea, creatinine and U and Es normal.

The most likely diagnosis in this girl with isolated thrombocytopenia is idiopathic thrombocytopenic purpura (ITP).

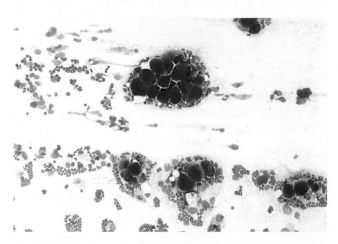

Fig. 15.11: Bone marrow of a child with idiopathic thrombocytopenic purpura—showing excess megakaryocytes

Treatment

Unfortunately the clinician cannot predict whether a given child will have the more common acute self-limiting form, develop a chronic course, or be in the 1% of children who have their course complicated by a sudden spontaneous life-threatening gastrointestinal or central nervous system haemorrhage. However, in most children the acute attack of thrombocytopenic purpura undergoes spontaneous remission within six months and does not again appear. There is rarely any need for a quick decision about some form of specific treatment. Despite very low platelet counts of even less than $10\times10^9/l$, major haemorrhage is rare and only symptoms are usually bruising. The patient should be treated and not the platelet count. Life-threatening intracranial haemorrhage is a very rare event. When bleeding is severe and persistent, blood transfusion combined with steroid therapy is usually successful in initiating a remission. This may be permanent or temporary. Platelet transfusions should be used only when life-threatening bleeding episodes occurs, since they achieve only a transient haemostatic response. Intravenous administration of very large doeses of human immuno-globulins also can lead to a rapid but usually transient rise in platelet count. Therefore intravenous immuno-globulin does not seem to be indicated as the therapy of choice in the acute phase of ITP. Elective splenectomy is followed by permanent return of the platelets to normal levels in only about 80 per cent of cases. For this reason, we have been reluctant to recommend it unless the disease is persistent or there are repeated acute attacks.

NEONATAL THROMBOCYTOPENIC PURPURA

It is well-recognised that the infant of a mother who is suffering from idiopathic thrombocytopenic purpura or thrombocytopenia secondary to systemic lupus erythematosus may be born with severe thrombocytopenia. The infant usually exhibits generalised purpura, and during the first few days of life there is a risk of severe haemorrhage into organs such as the brain, adrenals or pericardium. The pathogenesis has been shown to be the transplacental passage of antibodies which are directed against antigens common to all platelets. If the infant's platelet count falls below $10\times10^9/l$, prednisolone 2 mg/kg/day should be prescribed for 2-3 weeks with later reduction of the dosage. This type of neonatal thrombocytopenia has to be differentiated from neonatal, isoimmune thrombo-cytopenia in which there is foeto-maternal incompatibility for a platelet antigen absent in the mother and expressed on the foetal platelet membranes(INTP).The mother is platelet antigen (PLA-1) negative and anti-platelet antibodies pass to the foetus and destroy the foetal platelets. The situation is analogous to Rh or ABO incompatibility, but there are as yet no reliable tests to predict the birth of an affectedd baby during pregnancy. In contrast to Rh sensitisation, first born infants may be affected and the risk of recurrence in future pregnancies is high. The diagnosis can be confirmed by the demons-tration of antiplatelet antibodies in the maternal serum. These tests, together with a normal maternal platelet count and the exclusion of other known causes of neonatal thrombocytopenia (e.g. neonatal infection—including TORCH infections—toxoplasmosis, rubella, CMV, herpes simplex, syphilis, disseminated intravascular coagulation, drug induced or autoimmune thrombocytopenia) often establish the diagnosis of neonatal isoimmune thrombo-cytopenia. The best form of treatment is probably transfusion of platelets lacking the offending antigen, i.e only the mother's platelets, which can be obtained by plateletpheresis. Exchange transfusion, steroids and intravenous immunoglobulins have also been used but the more effective treatment remains the transfusion of compatible platelets.

WISKOTT-ALDRICH SYNDROME

This is a rare X-linked recessive disorder affecting only males. It is characterised by the triad of severe thrombo-cytopenia, eczema and immunodeficiency. The majority of children die from overwhelming infection at an early age. Those who survive may develop reticulo-endothelial malignancies such as lymphoma and myeloid leukaemia. The usual mode of presentation is during infancy with typical atopic eczema which may later be superceded by asthma. The bleeding tendency results in purpura or oozing from mucous membranes. Infections such as otitis media, pneumonia, septicaemia, meningitis and virus diseases constitute the major threat to life. Recent studies have revealed a immunological deficiency in this disease involving both humoral and cellular immunity. There is absence or reduction in isoagglutinins, progressive lymphopenia and failure to produce antibodies to some antigens after an appropriate challenge.

Treatment

Apart from blood and platelet transfusions little could be done for children with this disease until recently.There is a good response to splenectomy. Therefore in spite of the risks of splenectomy in an immunocompromised child, splenec-tomy may be justified. Otherwise bone marrow transplantation is the only curative treatment for this disease.

HENOCH SCHÖNLEIN PURPURA

See chapter 16 on Rheumatology.

BLOOD CLOTTING DEFECTS

The mechanism of blood clotting is extremely complex and modern tests used to define the various congenital and

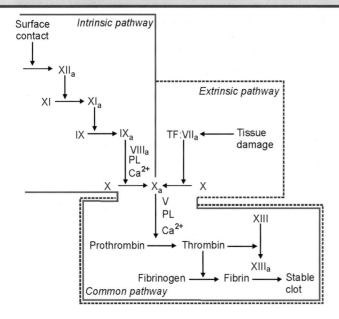

Fig. 15.12: Diagrammatic representation of the coagulation cascade.

acquired defects in this mechanism are only for the expert haematologist. The paediatrician must, however, have sufficient knowledge of the clinical types of clotting deficiency to use rationally the help which the haematologist has to offer.

The Blood Coagulation Cascade and Screening Tests of Homeostasis

The classical blood coagulation cascade involves the intrinsic pathway and the extrinsic pathway. Although the mechanism of blood clotting is extremely complex it is easier to understand it under these two headings. Intrinsic blood coagulation is initiated by contact of the flowing blood with a foreign surface while the extrinsic pathway is thought to be primarily responsible for initiating haemostasis as shown in Figure 15.12.

Screening Tests

Screening tests of haemostasis include platelet count, the bleeding time-measures platelet function and interaction with vessel wall, and clotting factors such as fibrinogen and factor viii. The precise diagnosis of each coagulation disorder may require very sophisticated coagulation tests.

The prothrombin time (PT) measures the extrinsic pathway (factors VII, X, V, II, and fibrinogen) and the activated partial thromboplastin time (APTT) measures the intrinsic pathway (measures the coagulation activity of factors XII, HMWK, PK, XI, IX, VIII, X, V, II and fibrinogen). The thrombin clotting time (TCT) measures the conversion of fibrinogen to fibrin. It is prolonged when fibrinogen is low from consumption, in hypo/dys-fibrinogenaemia, in the presence of heparin and fibrin

degradation products (FDPs)/D-dimers. Direct estimation of fibrinogen is included since PT, APTT, TCT are insensitive to levels of fibrinogen over 100 mg/dl.

HAEMOPHILIA A

Aetiology

Haemophilia A is the second most common inherited haemorrhagic disorder occuring in all ethnic groups. Deficiency of functionally active factor VIII is inherited as an X-linked recessive trait affecting males. Affected females are extremely rare.

Clinical Features

It is rare for haemophilia to become manifest during the first year of life. The outstanding feature is bleeding. The clinical severity of the condition is highly variable. It is classified according to the plasma concentration of factor VIII: Severe <1 IU/dl, moderate 1-5 IU/dl and mild > 5 IU/dl. This may take the form of prolonged oozing from a minor injury such as a cut lip or finger, from an erupting tooth, after the loss of a deciduous tooth or from the nose. There may be dangerous and persistent bleeding from circumcision or tonsillectomy if haemophilia has not been discovered. A common event is severe haemarthrosis, especially in a knee-joint after quite minor strain. A blow may result in a massive haematoma on any part of the body. A deeply situated haematoma may threaten life by pressure on vital structures such as the trachea or a large artery. In some children who are severely affected repeated haemarthroses may lead to fibrous ankylosis and crippling (Fig. 15.13). Bleeding from gastro-intestinal or renal tracts

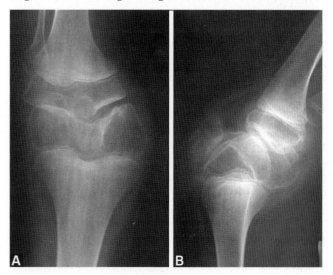

Figs 15.13A and B: AP and lateral view of the knee showing marked enlargement of the epiphyses around the knee, narrowing of the joint space, mild periarticular osteopenia, widening of the intercondylar notch, and mild increase in the soft tissue density within the joint itself, corresponding to haemosiderin deposition.

is not rare. Cases vary considerably in severity but run true to type within each individual family. There is a fairly high mutation rate, and the absence of a family history of "bleeders" does not exclude the diagnosis.

HAEMOPHILIA B (CHRISTMAS DISEASE)

Aetiology

Deficiency of factor IX is inherited as an X-linked recessive trait. It accounts for about 15% of all "bleeders", being much less common than true haemophilia A.

Clinical Features

The disease cannot be distinguished from haemophilia A on clinical grounds.

Diagnosis of Haemophilia A and B

Both in haemophilia A and B activated partial thromboplastin time (APTT) is prolonged because of the low levels of either Factor VIII or Factor IX. But estimating factor VIII or factor IX levels will help in confirming the diagnosis and classifying the severity. In haemophilia A the vWF:Ag and ristocetin co-factor activity (measurement of vWF activity) are normal. In both haemophilia A and B the bleeding time and prothrombin time (PT) are normal.

VON WILLEBRAND DISEASE

Aetiology

Von Willebrand disease (vWD) is caused by a deficiency or defect of vWF, which is responsible for the adherence of platelets to damaged endothelium. This bleeding disorder has been recognised with increasing frequency in children in recent years. It is inherited as an autosomal dominant characteristic and thus affects both sexes equally. The gene is situated on chromosome 12.

Clinical Features

The haemorrhage is of the "capillary" type rather than the "clotting deficiency" type as seen in haemophilia. Common presenting features include epistaxis, prolonged bleeding from cuts or dental extractions and excessive bruising. Gastro-intestinal bleeding can occasionally be alarming and menorrhagia may be a problem in the adult.

Diagnosis

The bleeding time is prolonged because of abnormal platelet adhesion. The APTT is prolonged relative to the reduction in factor VIII. The vWF:Ag and ristocetin co-factor activities (vWF activity) are reduced. The prothrombin time (PT) is normal.

Management of Haemophilia A, Haemophilia B and Von Willebrand disease

(i) All children who are likely to require blood products on a regular basis should be vaccinated against hepatitis A and B.

(ii) Alternatives to blood products should be used if appropriate and, when not, recombinant products should be used to avoid the risk of viral transmission.

(iii) Most children with severe haemophilia A will need Factor VIII concentrate and this should be recombinant. Factor VIII 1 U/kg will raise the Factor VIII:C level by 2 IU/dl and has a half-life of 8-12 hours. For mild haemorrhage a level of 30 IU/dl is required, for established haemarthrosis a level of around 50 IU/dl and for surgery 80-100 IU/dl are recommended.

(iv) Haemophilia B replacement therapy will need Factor IX concentrate. Factor IX concentrate 1 U/kg will raise the FIX:C level by approximately 1 IU/dl and the half-life is about 24 hours. Minimum level of FIX:C of 20 IU/dl is necessary for early bleeding episodes, 40 IU/dl for more advanced muscle or joint bleeding and an initial level of 60 IU/dl for surgery.

(v) Treatment of mild vWD is with desmopressin if this has been shown to raise the vWF and FVIII:C into a haemostatic range. If not, treatment is with vWF concentrates or FVIII concentrates, which contain adequate amounts of vWF. By definition, these will not be FVIII recombinant products and should be viricidally treated.

(vi) Boys with severe haemophilia A and B generally receive prophylactic treatment thrice and twice weekly, respectively. This will greatly reduce the frequency of bleeds and thus chances of reduced arthropathy.

(vii) About 10% of boys with haemophilia A may develop antibodies to FVIII:C when FVIII replacement fails to stop bleeding. Recombinant FVIII is now used to bypass the inhibitor. A smaller percentage (6%) of boys with haemophilia B develop inhibitors.

(viii) The problems seen in haemophilia are changing as the treatment advances. Recombinant products will hopefully stop the transmission of viral infection and consequently the liver disease. Prophylaxis will reduce damage to joints with less painful chronic arthropathy and the need for replacement later in life. Home treatment allows a more normal life with less dependency on the haemophilia centre.

DISSEMINATED INTRAVASCULAR COAGULATION (DIC)CONSUMPTION COAGULOPATHY

Disseminated intravascular coagulation is the commonest acquired haemostatic defect that occurs when there is *in vivo* activation of the coagulation mechanism resulting

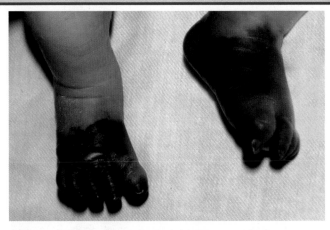

Fig. 15.14: A child with purpura fulminans who developed gangrene of both feet.

in an accelerated rate of conversion of fibrinogen to fibrin. Fibrin may or may not be deposited within blood vessels but resulting in disseminated microthrombi. It is always caused by some underlying disease process. Infection is the most common cause of disseminated intravascular coagulation. Within this category bacterial septicaemia (gram negative bacterial infections) with associated septic shock is the most frequent infectious casue of DIC. Haemolytic uraemic syndrome, meningococcal septicaemia, falciparum malaria, haemolytic transfusion reactions and some snake venoms can induce a consumption coagulopathy. Virus induced DIC occurs predominantly in immunocompromised patients. In children one of the most fulminant of DICs follows meningococcal septicaemia. Fungal infections are rarely a cause of DIC. Regardless of the underlying primary disease in the majority of patients the main clinical finding is bleeding and only a small number of patients will show thrombosis or thromboembolic episodes. Microthrombi formation can lead to the syndrome of *Purpura fulminans*, which is characterised by perpheral gangrene of fingers and toes (Fig. 15.14).

Diagnosis

The laboratory findings consist of thrombocytopenia, anaemia with red cell fragmentation on the blood film, prolonged PT, APTT, and TCT, low fibrinogen and elevated FDPs or D-dimers.

Treatment

The aim of treatment of DIC is to control bleeding and to eliminate the threat of fibrin deposition. The management objectives include control or removal of the underlying disease, replacement of depleted pro-coagulants with fresh frozen plasma, cryoprecipitate and platelets and in selected cases medical interruption of the consumptive process

with anticoagulants and platelet inhibitor drugs. Virus-inactivated FFP and cryoprecipitate are now available. In the presence of peripheral gangrene protein-C concentrate may be beneficial. Also, the use of exchange transfusion in newborns and plasma exchange in older children has been reported to be beneficial in some cases.

> **CASE STUDY**
>
> A six month old comatosed infant presented with fever, convulsions, and numerous petechiae and purpura covering nearly all his skin. The echymotic patches on his feet became necrotic and gangrenous. He had meningococcaemia and disseminated intravascular coagulation. He had purpura fulminans.

ACUTE LEUKAEMIAS

In childhood, leukaemia is nearly always of the acute variety. On the basis of morphologic classifications, they are divided into lymphoblastic (ALL) and non-lymphocytic (ANLL) or acute myeloid leukaemia (AML) types.

Approximately 80 to 85% of acute leukaemias in children are lymphoblastic and 15 to 20% are due to acute myeloid leukaemia (AML). Chronic myeloid leukaemia and myelodysplasia are rare. The exact cause of leukaemia remains unknown although the list of risk factors associated with chilhood ALL is substantial.

Clinical Features

The most common symptoms and clinical findings reflect the underlying anaemia, thrombocytopenia and neutropenia that result from the failure of normal haematopoiesis. Therefore, the most common presenting features are rapidly progressive pallor and spontaneous haemorrhagic manifestations such as purpura, epistaxis and bleeding from the gums. These are associated with increasing weakness, breathlessness on exertion, malaise, anorexia and fever. In some cases, the onset takes the form of a severe oropharyngeal inflammation and enlargement of the cervical lymph nodes which does not respond to antibiotics. In two-thirds of children with ALL the onset is with bone pains and half of these will have radiological bone changes. Arthralgia, secondary to leukaemic infiltration of joints may be difficult to differentiate from other non-malignant disorders such as juvenile idiopathic arthritis or osteomyelitis. Extramedullary leukaemic spread causes lymphadenopathy, hepatomegaly and splenomegaly. In some patients, however, the signs are confined to pallor and haemorrhage of variable severity and distribution. Infrequently jaundice may develop or there may be early evidence of involvement of the central nervous system. Ophthalmoscopy frequently reveals retinal haemorrhages.

However, clinicians should be aware of the fact that ALL may mimic a number of non-malignant conditions.

Blood Picture and Bone Marrow Findings

In addition to severe anaemia the peripheral blood films will show immature cells. These are most often lymphoblasts, less commonly myeloblasts and other granulocytic precursors, rarely monoblasts or neoplastic megaloblastic erythroid cells. The total white cell count is often raised to between 20,000 and 30,000 per mm³; only rarely to a very high figure. Thrombocytopenia is almost invariably found. Reticulocytes are usually scanty. It is, however, rarely justifiable to base the diagnosis of leukaemia on the peripheral blood picture alone. Bone-marrow biopsy will nearly always confirm the diagnosis beyond doubt, the films and sections showing gross leukaemic infiltration by immature or abnormal white cell precursors, diminution in erythropoietic activity and disappearance of megakaryocytes.

The majority of children presenting with ALL will have more than 80% of their marrow cells consisting of lymphoblasts, whereas it is not uncommon to see the presence of only 30 to 50% blasts in the bone marrow in acute non-lymphocytic leukaemia. The majority of childhood acute leukaemias (85 to 90%) can be readily separated into lymphoid or myeloid (Figs 15.15 and 15.16) subtypes on the basis of morphology alone. Thus, although in most cases the diagnosis is apparent from the morphology, the final diagnosis of ALL rests on confirmatory cytochemical staining patterns, immunophenotype and cytogenetic studies. These studies are of therapeutic significance in lymphatic leukaemias.

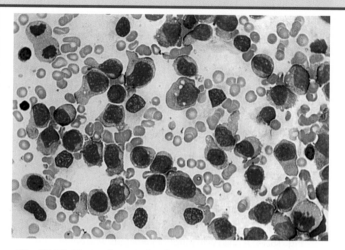

Fig. 15.16: Photomicrograph of bone marrow of a child with acute myeloid leukaemia showing myeloblasts.

MENINGEAL AND TESTICULAR LEUKAEMIA

Meningeal and testicular leukaemia became a major problem when the duration of life for children with acute leukaemia progressively lengthened as the result of treatment with modern anti-leukaemic drugs. This manifestation commonly develops in patients who are in complete haematological remission and the incidence has exceeded 50% in some series. Not infrequently the meningeal relapse coincides with a systemic relapse. It is probable that a few nests of leukaemic cells are already present when the patient first presents, and as the cytotoxic drugs do not readily cross the blood-brain barrier these neoplastic cells are able to multiply in the largely protected environment of the brain and meninges. The child, who has been in systemic remission for months or even some years, develops headache, vomiting and meningism. A rapid increase in weight due to the increased appetite of hypothalamic damage is not uncommon. There may be neurological signs such as squint, ataxia, or visual disturbance, but more often the only signs are of increased intracranial pressure including papilloedema. Cerebrospinal fluid will show a pleiocytosis due to leukaemic blast cells with increased protein and reduced glucose. The recent introduction of cranial or craniospinal radiation combined with intrathecal methotrexate has drastically reduced the incidence of meningeal relapses.

Testicular

The testes are a major site of extramedullary relapse in boys with ALL. Clinically, overt testicular relapse presents as painless testicular enlargement that is usually unilateral.

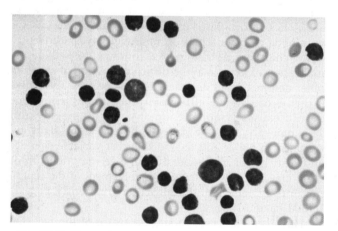

Fig. 15.15: Photomicrograph of bone marrow of a child with ALL.

Prognostic Factors

Prognostic factors may be influenced by the treatment given.

(i) WBC and age are important prognostic indicators and are used to stratify treatment. Children with a WBC greater than $50 \times 10^9/l$ and those more than 10 years of age have a less favourable outcome than those who are younger with a lower WBC. Infants less than 1 year of age have a particularly poor outlook.

(ii) Girls have a more favourable prognosis than boys.

(iii) *Immunophenotype:* Common ALL or B-lineage disease does better than T-cell ALL. Mature B-cell ALL is more characteristic of a Burkitt type lymphpma than a leukaemia and is treated as such.

(iv) *Cytogenetics:* Hyperdiploidy and t(12,21) are favourable; near haplodiploid, t(9,22) and t(4,11) are poor prognostic indicators. AML 1 amplification also appears to be associated with a poor outlook.

Management

Supportive care: children should receive adequate intravenous hydration and allopurinol prior to commencing therapy. They may require red cell and platelet support to correct anaemia and thrombocytopenia and antibiotics for febrile neutropenia.

Chemotherapy

The outlook for standard-risk ALL is now at least 70-80% and this is achieved with combination intensive chemotherapy. The rate of cell kill is a vital prognostic indicator (the faster the disease clears the better the outcome).

Treatment of ALL is arbitrarily divided into the following:

Induction Therapy: This refers to the initial weeks of treatment, which aims to eradicate disease from the bone marrow and allow it to repopulate with normal cells. Children are stratified by their age (<10 years) and by WBC ($< 50 \times 10^9/l$) to the intensity of their induction therapy. The combination of dexamethasone (superior to prednisolone because of better control of CNS disease), vincristine and asparaginase ± daunorubicin, depending on the child's age and WBC results in remission in at least 95 % of children.

Intensification/consolidation: The intensity is tailored to the prognostic group. Combination chemotherapy is used to prevent drug resistance developing.

CNS –directed treatment: CNS-directed therapy is important in reducing the risk of CNS relapse, although dexamethasone and intensive chemotherapy contribute. Intrathecal methtrexate, high-dose systemic methotrexate and cranial radiation have been employed. Cranial radiation is now reserved for the treatment of CNS leukaemia because of its associated neuropsychological impairment and learning difficulties. Intrathecal methotrexate is currently used in the UK.

Maintenance/continuing Chemotherapy: This involves daily 6-mercaptopurine, weekly methotrexate and four weekly vincristine and dexamethasone. Currently in the UK, boys receive treatment for three years and girls for two years.

Co-trimoxazole (Septrin) is given throughout as prophylaxis against *Pneumocystis carinii pneumonia* (PCP).

Acute Myeloid Leukaemia (AML)

The presenting signs and symptoms in this type of leukaemia are similar to those seen in children with ALL. FAB M4-M5 subtype manifest with extramedullary disease, including infiltration of gum and skin, lymphadenitis and CNS involvement. Sometimes, there are rare features such as chloromas, which are solid masses of myeloblasts which can develop around the orbits, spinal cord or cranium.

Investigations are similar to those for ALL. The myeloblasts usually contain Auer rodes and these are seen only in AML.

Treatment

About 90% of children with AML achieve remission with one or two courses of intensive combination chemotherapy. Usually a total of four blocks of treatment are required. Allogenic bone marrow transplantation is reserved for those children in whom response to chemotherapy is slow. The disease free survival is now in the region of 60%.

Stem Cell Transplantation

Stem cells are primal undifferentiated cells which retain the ability to differentiate into other cell types. This unique ability allows the stem cells to act as a repair system for the body and replenishing other cells as long as the organism is alive thus change the face of human disease.

The sources of stem cells are bone marrow, blood from placenta and umbilical cord. Stem cell transplantation may be defined as autologous (recipients own stem cells), syngeneic (twins stem cells) or allogenic (stem cells from sibling, non-sibling related or unrelated donor).

Allogenic treatment stem cell transplantation is generally employed in leukaemia and primary bone marrow disorders. Stem cell transplantation has also been used in Hunter syndrome, Hurler syndrome, thalassaemia major, sickle cell disease, immunodeficiency/inborn errors of metabolism.

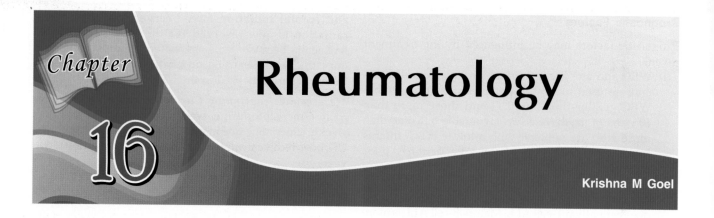

Chapter 16

Rheumatology

Krishna M Goel

RHEUMATOLOGY

In view of the voluminous information available on the structure and biosynthesis of collagen it has become possible to explain a number of genetic diseases on the basis of molecular defects in collagen biosynthesis. Acquired diseases involving collagen are clearly important in medicine but knowledge of how acquired diseases alter collagen synthesis or metabolism is still fragmentary. In this chapter only the rheumatic diseases of significance will be dealt with in order of clinical importance (Table 16.1).

JUVENILE IDIOPATHIC ARTHRITIS (JIA)

The well known clinical picture of chronic polyarthritis with lymphadenopathy, splenomegaly, a rash and pericarditis was first described in Britain by George Frederick Still in 1896. Since then the term "Still's disease"had been used to encompass the whole spectrum of rheumatoid arthritis in children. Recently the problem of nomenclature and classification was reviewed and the term juvenile idiopathic arthritis (JIA) has been accepted. It is an autoimmune disease. Rarely there is a family history of juvenile idiopathic arthritis (JIA), only a few sibling pairs of juvenile idiopathic arthritis have been reported. However, there is high prevalence of rheumatoid arthritis among first and second degree relatives.

The term juvenile idiopathic arthritis (JIA) indicates a chronic inflammatory arthritis of childhood onset that begins before 16 years and persisting for at least 6 weeks with no known cause. It would be appropriate to recognise these clinical variations by separating juvenile idiopathic arthritis (JIA) into three subtypes.

Subtypes of juvenile idiopathic arthritis

1. Systemic JIA
2. Polyarticular JIA: rheumatoid factor (RF negative, rheumatoid factor (RF) positive

3. Oligoarticular JIA
   (a) Persistent oligoarticular JIA: confined to 4 or fewer joints during the first 6 months of disease
   (b) Extended oligoarticular JIA: involvement of more than 4 joints after the first 6 months of disease

Systemic JIA

The major signs and symptoms of this subtype of juvenile idiopathic arthritis (JIA) are systemic. The most common

---

Table 16.1: Differential diagnosis of arthritis in children

Acute rheumatic fever (ARF)
Juvenile idiopathic arthritis (JIA)
    Systemic - onset JIA
    Polyarticular - onset JIA
        Rheumatoid factor positive
        Rheumatoid factor negative
    Oligoarticular - onset JIA
Infection
    Viral arthritis, septic arthritis, Lyme disease, osteomyelitis, discitis, gonococcal arthritis, tuberculous arthritis
Juvenile dermatomyositis
Vasculitic syndromes
    Henoch Schönlein purpura (anaphylactoid purpura)
    Kawasaki disease
    Polyarteritis
Paediatric systemic lupus erythematosus, Neonatal lupus
Juvenile scleroderma: systemic and localised
Juvenile ankylosing spondylitis (JAS)
Juvenile psoriatic arthritis
Reactive arthritis:
Reiter syndrome, post-streptococcal arthritis, post-enteric arthritis, arthritis in ulcerative colitis and Crohn's disease
Behcet disease
Sarcoidosis
Malignancy: leukaemia, neuroblastoma
Trauma : accidental, non - accidental
Enthesitis related arthritia (ERA)
Non - organic limb pains (Idiopathic limb pains)
Undefined or unclassified arthritis

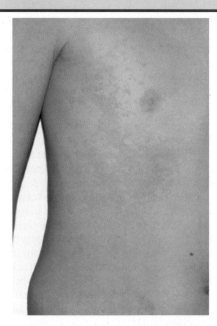

Fig. 16.1: Rheumatoid rash—characterised by salmon pink macules, usually coming and going with the fever spikes.

age of onset of the disease is under 5 years but it can occur throughout childhood. Boys are affected as frequently as girls. Characteristic features are high remittent fever, generalised lymphadenopathy, splenomegaly, poly-morphonuclear leucocytosis and a rash. The rash has an irregular outline and is coppery red in colour. It is rarely pruritic and never purpuric (Fig. 16.1). The best time to look for the rash is just after the child has had a hot bath or at the height of the temperature elevation. The fever shows diurnal swings as large as 2 or 3°C which are rarely seen in acute rheumatic fever (ARF). Acute pericarditis is not very rare in this form of juvenile idiopathic arthritis but endocardial involvement is exteremely rare. Joint mani-festations are usually present at an early stage although they may initially amount to arthralgia without visible swelling.

When the joints are involved they are frequently large ones e.g. knees, hips, ankles, elbows and wrists. The cervical spine is another commonly affected site, presenting with pain, limitation of movement and torticollis. Also peripheral joints may be involved. Uveitis probably never occurs in children with systemic JIA. However all children with juvenile idiopathic arthritis should be screened for uveitis by slit-lamp microscopy at the diagnosis of juvenile idiopathic arthritis.

Laboratory findings include anaemia, leucocytosis, an elevated ESR and CRP. The ANA is rarely positive. For investigations in a child with acute arthritis see BOX 16.1. The systemic JIA frequently runs a course of remission and relapses. Macrophage activation syndrome is a rare but life-threatening complication of systemic JIA.

Key Learning Points
ARTHRITIS versus ARTHRALGIA Arthritis: objective inflammation of a joint: redness, swelling, heat and pain Arthralgia: pain in a joint without objective findings on clinical examination

Polyarticular JIA (rheumatoid factor negative, rheumatoid factor positive)

Children with polyarticular JIA are divided into two groups: those with a negative rheumatoid factor and a small group with a positive rheumatoid factor. This subtype involves five or more joints but is not accompanied by the severe systemic manifestations such as high fever and rash of systemic JIA. Girls are much more frequently affected than boys and although this subtype of juvenile idiopathic arthritis can occur at any age it is more often seen in children over the age of 5 years. Those with a positive rheumatoid factor are usually over 10 years of age and are more likely to develop destructive joint disease.

BOX 16.1: Laboratory Tests Investigations in a child with acute arthritis
Full blood count and blood film
Erythrocyte sedimentation rate (ESR) in mm in 1st hour and C-reactive protein (CRP) in mg/l
Throat swab
Urinalysis (Urine dipstix)
Antinuclear antibody (ANA) test
Antistreptolysin titre (serial titres)
Viral titres (Parvovirus, rubella, Epstein-Barr, CMV)
Blood culture(s) (if indicated)
Arthrocentesis (if septic arthritis suspected)
Plain X-ray (to exclude trauma, tumour and infection)
Magnetic resonance imaging (MRI) of the joint (when plain X-rays are normal)
Chest X-ray (for cardiomegaly, pericardial effusion, infection)
ECG (for prolonged PR interval)
Echocardiography

Oligoarticular JIA

Oligoarticular JIA is the most frequent type of arthritis in children in North America and Europe. On the contrary, systemic JIA and polyarticular JIA predominate in most parts of Asia including Japan, China and India. Oligoarticular JIA occurs predominantly in young girls less than 4 years old. It is defined persistent oligoarthritis affecting 4 or fewer joints during the first six months of disease.

It is essential to remember that children with oligo-arthritis do not have constitutional symptoms and signs of a systemic or chronic illness. If oligoarthritis is considered as a single entity the knee and then the ankle

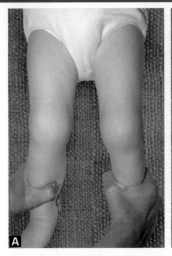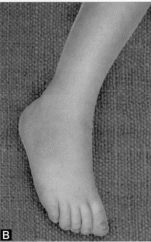

Figs 16.2A and B: Oligoarticular JIA - (A) Swelling of both knees (B) Swelling of right ankle

are the most commonly involved joints (Figs 16.2 A and B) but other large joints and small joints may be involved. The hip joint is almost never affected. While the risk of chronic anterior uveitis exists in all forms of juvenile idiopathic arthritis it is particularly common in oligo-articular type, especially in those with a positive antinuclear antibody (ANA) test. It occurs in 10-30% of children usually within 4 years of the onset of arthritis (Fig. 16.3). Rheumatoid factor is almost universally absent.

The prognosis of oligoartcular JIA is good although the course may be prolonged and may evolve into an extended oligoarthritis i.e. addition of newly affected joints to a total of more than 4 joints after 6 months of disease.

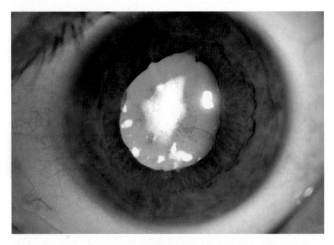

Fig. 16.3: Oligoarticular JIA—Showing synechiae, irregular pupil and complicated cataract as a result of prolonged chronic iridocyclitis

Key Learning Points

Laboratory tests are of limited value for making a diagnosis of JIA. Tests for rheumatoid factor are not useful for diagnosis, because they are usually negative. But they are important for making the appropriate diagnosis of a child with rheumatoid factor positive polyarticular JIA.

CASE STUDY

A 2-year-old girl presented with a swollen, hot and painful right knee for 8 weeks. There was a vague history of being fallen from a chair. At no time she had fever or constitutional symptoms. On examination she had active synovitis of right knee. Patellar tap was positive. Full blood count, U and Es, LFTs were normal. ESR 40 mm in one hour and CRP 60 mg/l. Urine dipstix negative. Rheumatoid factor negative. ANA positive in a titre of 1/256. Slit-lamp microscopy normal. She was treated with one intra-articular injection of triamcinolone hexacetonide and oral naproxen. She responded to this treatment satisfactorily. She was followed up for 2 years. During this time her arthritis did not spread to any other joint. Also she did not develop uveitis. So by definition she had persistent oligoarticular JIA.

MANAGEMENT OF JIA

The treatment of juvenile idiopathic arthritis has changed dramatically in the last 15 years. It is vital to diagnose the disease and treat it early, before soft-tissue deformities and joint damage become irreversible. The assumption that juvenile idiopathic arthritis will usually resolve by adulthood is incorrect.

Initial treatment for most children with JIA consists of intra-articular corticosteroid injections and non-steroidal anti-inflammatory drugs (NSAIDs). Since NSAIDs are not disease modifying drugs they are mainly used to treat pain, stiffness and fever. Differences in anti-inflammatory activity between different NSAIDs are small, but there is considerable variation in individual patient tolerance and response. A large proportion of children will respond to any NSAID; of the others, those who do not respond to one may well respond to another. The possible association of Reye syndrome with salicylates have resulted in other NSAIDs replacing aspirin.

In juvenile idiopathic arthritis, NSAIDs may take 4-12 weeks to be effective. If appropriate responses are not obtained within these times another NSAID should be tried. Therefore the choice of NSAID will mainly depend on the convinience of dosing regimen. The naproxen is very popular in the dosage of 15-20 mg/Kg/d, given in two divided dosed. Other NSAIDs for use in JIA include ibuprofen, diclofenac, indomethacin, mefenamic acid and piroxicam. In children serious gastrointestinal side effects are rare although gastritis and/or duodenitis, gastro-duodenal ulcer, perforation and bleeding have been reported (Figs 16.4 A and B). As children appear to tolerate

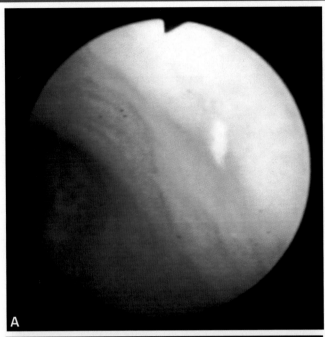

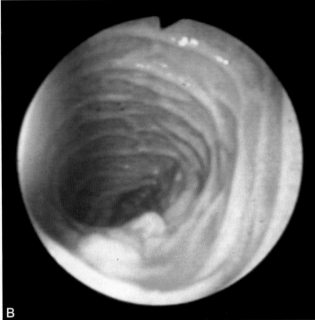

Figs 16.4A and B: Upper GI endoscopy (A) Showing antral erosion secondary to NSAIDs (B) Duodenitis secondary to NSAIDs

NSAIDs better than adults the use of gastroprotective drugs such as ranitidine and omeprazole may not be necessary.

Corticosteroids are the mainstay of treatment for controlling serious systemic manifestations of systemic JIA. However there is no evidence that systemic steroids are disease modifying. In those children who do not respond to oral steroids the use of periodic intravenous pulses of methylprednisolone (30 mg/Kg/per dose, maximum of 1g) is very useful.

Key Learning Points

Malignancy
Occasionally a child in whom a diagnosis of JIA has been made turns out to have malignancy e.g. leukaemia or neuroblastoma. This rare occurrence, should be kept in mind when examining any child with bone pain.

Corticosteroid injections especially in patients with oligoarthritis is an effective way to treat active arthritis. They are injected locally for an anti-inflammatory effect. They should be used at the onset of disease rather than later. The long-acting (depot effect) triamcinolone hexacetonide 1mg/Kg/joint (total of 40 mg) is more effective than other forms of injectable corticosteroids. On the whole it is safe, although in some cases patients have become Cushingoid but this side effect is transient. Triamcinolone acetonide and methylprednisolone may also be considered for intra-articular injection into larger joints, whilst hydrocortisone acetate should be reserved for smaller joints.

Key Learning Points

Administration of corticosteroids may result in suppression of growth and may affect the development of puberty. The risk of corticosteroid - induced osteoporosis should be considered in those on long-term corticosteroid treatment.

Disease modifying drugs (DMRDs) found to be effective in juvenile idiopathic arthritis are sulphasalazine, methotrexate and biologic agents e.g. etanercept. Anti-rheumatic drugs such as hydroxychloroquine, oral gold, or D-penicillamine are not significantly effective in the treatment of juvenile idiopathic arthritis.

Methotrexate is the most commonly used drug and is effective particularly in children with extended oligo-arthritis and polyarthritis and relatively less effective in systemic juvenile idiopathic arthritis. Methotrexate is tolerated well in children with doses commencing at 0.3 mg/Kg/week and increased to a maximum of 1 mg/Kg/dose/week (no more than 25 mg/week). Subcutaneous methotrexate may be more effective than oral route. It is not clear when a patient should stop taking methotrexate because the disease will flare up in as many as 60% of patients but most of these patients respond when methotrexate is recommenced. Supplementation with folic acid 1 mg daily or 5 mg weekly, usually at least 24 hours after the dose of methotrexate has shown to lessen the side effects without affecting the efficacy of methotrexate. Patients on methotrexate should be carefully monitored by checking liver function tests, full blood counts (including differential white cell count and platelet count) and renal function tests.

Etanercept a biologic agent is a soluble tumour necrosis factor (TNF) receptor. It is given subcutaneously twice weekly and is highly recommended in children aged 4-17 years with active extended oligoarticular and polyarticular JIA who have not responded adequately to methotrexate or who are intolerant of it. It is essential that children should be screened for tuberculosis, prior to anti-TNF therapy. Adverse effects of etanercept are generally mild, mainly injection site reactions, upper respiratory tract infections and headaches. Recently infliximab another biologic agent has been used in children with juvenile idiopathic arthritis.

Autologous stem cell transplantation (ASCT) has been used in refractory cases of systemic JIA. However, it carries a significant mortality risk. Therefore ASCT should only be carried out when all other treatment options have failed.

In addition patients with JIA should receive influenza vaccine, pneumococcal vaccine and varicella-zoster vaccine. Preferably children should receive varicella - zoster vaccine prior to starting methotrexate. No serious side effects due to these vaccines have been encountered even in immunosuppressed patients.

PHYSIOTHERAPY AND OCCUPATIONAL THERAPY

Physiotherapy and occupational therapy are important adjuncts to medication because they help maintain and improve range of motion of joints, muscle strength and skills for activities of daily living. Exercises may be performed in the warm water of the hydrotherapy pool.

A physiotherapist should plan an exercise programme tailored to the child's needs. The role of an occupational therapist is to keep the child as independent as possible. The occupational therapist will assess any difficulties the child with arthritis may have and will teach the child techniques to make problem activities easier, e.g. by using specially designed cutlery.

SURGICAL TREATMENT

Most cases of juvenile idiopathic arthritis do not require surgery. However, some children may need total hip replcement or knee arthroplasty. Every attempt should be made to delay surgery until skeletal maturity if possible.

ENTHESITIS RELATED ARTHRITIS (ERA)

Enthesitis related arthritis is a chronic arthritis with enthesitis i.e. inflammation at points where tendons, fascia, and capsule insert to bone (Fig. 16.5). The disease is common in boys who are more than 8 years old. The main features consist of pain, stiffness and finally loss of mobility of the spine. It should be suspected in a child with chronic arthritis of the axial and peripheral skeleton plus enthesitis. Both ANA and rheumatoid factor tests are negative but most patients will have HLA-B27 positive. In

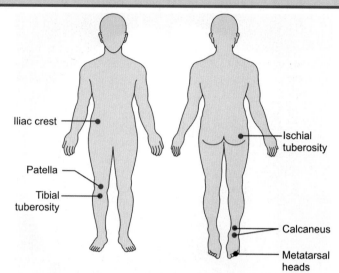

Fig. 16.5: Enthesopathic sites in children with enthesitis related arthritis

enthesitis related arthritis the uveitis is symptomatic as compared to uveitis in children with oligoarthritis where it is painless. Treatment requires NSAIDs and sometimes corticosteroids or sulphasalazine. Some patients respond to methotrexate. It has been found that anti-TNF medications are highly effective.

JUVENILE PSORIATIC ARTHRITIS

Psoriatic arthritis is rare in childhood. It is more common in girls than in boys. The mean age of onset of arthritis is about 10 years but children of any age can be affected. Asymmetrical polyarthritis, frequently involving the distal interphalangeal joints is the most frequent pattern, but can involve both large and small joints (Fig. 16.6). The major difference between JIA and psoriatic arthritis is the paucity of systemic manifestations. It is interesting that nearly 50% of children with psoriatic arthritis will have either minimal skin disease or no skin involvement at all for several years and therefore may initially diagnosed as cases of juvenile idiopathic arthritis. The diagnosis is suggested by the presence of arthritis and psoriasis or by arthritis and two of the following:
1. Nail pitting or onycholysis (loosening or separation of a nail from its bed)
2. Dactylitis
3. A family history of psoriasis in a first degree relative

All children with psoriatic arthritis should have a slit-lamp examination every 6 months because of the occurrence of asymptomatic anterior uveitis. In some children ANA may be positive.

Most children with psoriatic arthritis can be treated satisfactorily with non-steroidal anti-inflammatory drugs

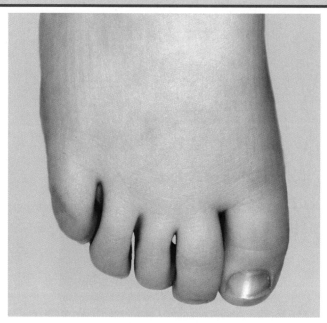

Fig. 16.6: Psoriatic arthritis—Dactylitis of the second toe

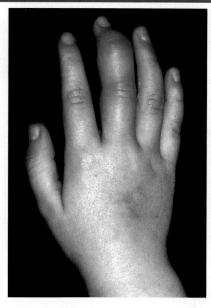

Fig. 16.7: Reiter syndrome - Dactylitis of 3rd right finger

(NSAIDs) but some may require disease modifying anti-rheumatic drugs (DMRDs) such as sulphasalazine.

JUVENILE REACTIVE ARTHRITIS

(a) Post-enteric reactive arthritis

Post-enteric reactive arthritis should be considered in any child with gastroenteritis and arthritis of the large joints of the lower extremity. It is immune mediated arthritis. The synovial fluid is sterile on culture. The various bacteria implicated in reactive arthritis are Salmonella species, Shigella flexneri, Yersinia enterocolitica and Chlamydia trachomatis.

(b) Post-streptococcal reactive arthritis

Children with sustained fever, arthritis and a preceding streptococcal infection who do not fulfill Jones criteria of acute rheumatic fever may be diagnosed as having post-streptococcal reactive arthritis.

(c) Arthropathy in inflammatory bowel disease

Arthritis is the commonest extraintestinal mani-festation of inflammatory bowel disease. It seems that the incidence is generally somewhat higher in ulcerative colitis than in Crohn's disease. It predo-minantly affects large joints, especially the knees and ankles but involvement of the spine (spondylitis) has been reported.

The onset of arthritis usually follows bowel symptoms by months or years but in some children arthritic symptoms develop at the same time, while occasionally the arthritis is the first manifestation. In general, the episodes of active arthritis occur when the underlying bowel disease is active. The prognosis for ultimate joint function is excellent.

(d) Juvenile Reiter syndrome

Reiter syndrome with the typical triad of urethritis, arthritis and conjunctivitis is rare in children. The most common cause of this syndrome in childhood is an infective diarrhoea, due to Shigella or Salmonella or other enteric pathogens. The knee is the most commonly involved joint but ankles and single toes or fingers can be affected (Fig. 16.7). Diagnosis of Reiter syndrome is primarily clinical. The prognosis is usually good with gradual amelioration of signs and symptoms.

JUVENILE DERMATOMYOSITIS (JDM)

Juvenile dermatomyosis is a multisystem, autoimmune connective tissue disorder in children. The onset is usually insidious with facial erythema, proximal muscle weakness and general constitutional upset but occasionally the onset is acute. It may occur at any age from the second year into adolescence. A heliotrope - violaceous colouration of the eyelids and periorbital skin is quite characteristic of this disorder and periorbital oedema is also common. (Figs 16.8A and B). There may be erythematous rash over the knuckles also known as Gottron's papules (Fig. 16.9). Calcification is common in children affecting more than 50% cases. It primarily involves the muscles and the subcutaneous tissues (Fig. 16.10). Calcinotic nodules can be a serious long-term problem (Fig. 16.11).

The diagnosis of juvenile dermatomyositis is based mainly on the combination of the clinical features of

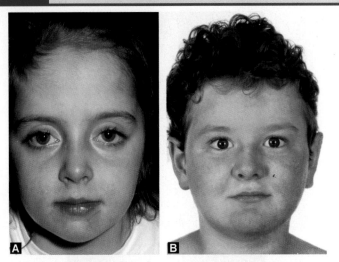

Figs 16.8A and B: Two different patients at diagnosis of juvenile dermatomyositis showing malar and forehead rash and heliotrope disclouration of the upper eyelids

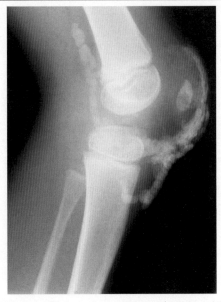

Fig. 16.10: Juvenile dermatomyositis—lateral view of the knee showing subcutaneous and interfascial calcification

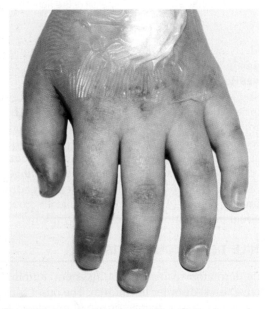

Fig. 16.9: Juvenile dermatomyositis—Gottron's papules - erythematous papules over MCP and PIP joints

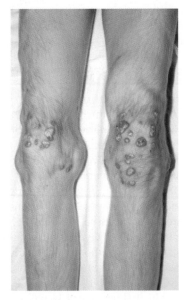

Fig. 16.11: Juvenile dermatomyositis—Calcinotic nodules

symmetrical muscle weakness and the typical cutaneous manifestations. It may be confirmed by finding of an elevation in serum muscle enzymes (creatine kinase). If the clinical diagnosis is clear cut, then there is no need to perform muscle biopsy or any other tests. Also an ultrasound of muscle(s) and a positive magnetic resonance imaging (MRI) of muscle(s) are very useful tools in supporting the diagnosis of juvenile demamtomyositis. EMG is not done these days.

Treatment

Various therapeutic measures have been employed at one time or another but corticosteroids have received considerable attention. A high dosage of steroid such as oral prednisolone is recommended, beginning with 1.5 - 2 mg/Kg/d as a single morning dose or in three divided doses. Once the acute phase is controlled, usually by 4 weeks of therapy, it is desirable to reduce the dose to an alternate day regimen. Patients who are very ill at diagnosis would

CASE STUDY

A 4-year-old girl presented with a 3 month history that she was unable to climb stairs and had morning stiffness of large joints. On examination she had an erythematous rash on face, axillae and back and heliotrope discolouration of eyelids. She had Gottron's papules on her hands. There was proximal muscle weakness and weakness of neck flexors. Hb, ESR, CRP, and white blood cell counts were normal. creatine kinase was high at 600 iu/l (reference range 10 - 180 iu/l). She did not require muscle biopsy or any other tests. She responded well to oral prednisolone 2 mg/Kg/d, which was gradually tapered and stopped one year later.

Diagnosis: Juvenile dermatomyositis

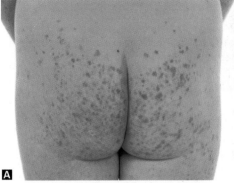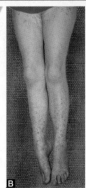

Figs 16.12A and B: Henoch-Schönlein purpura - (A) Purpuric rash on buttocks (B) rash on legs

benefit from intravenous methylprednisolone pulse therapy (30 mg/Kg/dose-up to 1g).

VASCULITIC SYNDROMES

There are four common vasculitic syndromes of children - Henoch-Schönlein purpura, Kawasaki disease, polyarteritis nodosa and Takayasu's disease. This section will deliberately concentrate on the vasculitic diseases of significance to a paediatrician.

Henoch-Schönlein Purpura (Anaphylactoid Purpura)

Henoch - Schönlein purpura (HSP) is a systemic vasculitis, involving skin, joints and the kidney. Other organs less frequently affected include the central nervous system, gonads and the lungs. Certain vaccines and drugs may precede the development of Henoch-Schönlein purpura, but a definite evidence to support these theories is lacking. Also a few reports in the past implicated B-haemolytic streptococcus as a significant specific cause but subsequently publications have failed to support this.

The disease has a wide variety of manifestations but the diagnosis is rarely difficult and is based essentialy on the rash which is characteristic in appearance and distribution. The most prominent symptoms may arise from swollen painful joints, or from areas of angio-oedema elsewhere. Whilst in other children the onset is with severe abdominal pain with or without melaena. It is in such cases that a mistaken diagnosis of intussusception has sometimes led to an unnecessary laparotomy. Another mode of presentation in boys is with an acute scrotal swelling which can be mistaken for a torsion of the testis. In the majority of cases the rash is the most striking feature and causes the parents to seek medical advice but sometimes it may appear after the abdominal pain. Characteristically the rash appears first as small separate urticarial lesions, both visible and palpable. These soon become dusky red or frankly purpuric. In the typical case the rash is most profuse over the extensor surfaces of the knees, ankles, dorsum of the feet, arms, elbows and forearms (Figs 16.12 A and B). The face, abdomen and chest are completely spared. On the contrary the purpuric/petechial rash in meningococcal disease may appear on any part of the body. Central nervous system involvement may present as headache, seizure or hemiparesis. Lung involvement presents as pulmonary haemorrhage.

Renal involvement is more common than is usually recognised and may occur in 20% of children. The clinical presentation can vary from microscopic haematuria to a typical acute glomerulonephritis or to a nephrotic syndrome. While the majority of children with renal involvement make a complete recovery a few may go on to develop persistent proteinuria, hypertension and deteriorating renal function. It is suggested that urinalysis should be carried out for 2 months after resolution of the rash, to ensure that renal involvement is not missed.

There are no specific laboratory tests which would help with the diagnosis of Henoch Schönlein purpura. The platelet count is within the normal range. Coagulation studies are normal.

Treatment

There is no specific treatment for Henoch-Schönlein purpura, and a large majority of children will require no treatment. The supporting treatment is aimed at symptomatic relief of arthritis and abdominal pain. Non - steroidal anti- inflammatory drugs (NSAIDs) seem to be effective in most cases and there is no evidence that they induce gastrointestinal haemorrhage in these children. Prednisolone at a dose of 2 mg/Kg/d seems to relieve symptoms rapidly in most cases. Immunosuppresive drugs such as cyclophosphamide or azathioprine are used in children with biopsy proven crescentic glomerulonephritis.

Kawasaki Disease

Kawasaki disease is an acute vasculitis affecting infants and children. It is characterised by prolonged fever, mucosal inflammation, skin changes and cervical lymphadenopathy (Figs 16.13A to C). The disorder is a systemic vasculitis with predilection for the coronary arteries. It was described by Dr Tamasaku Kawasaki in the Japanese literature in 1967 and in the English literature in 1974. Since then it has been recognised in children of every ethnic origin although Asian children are affected 5 to 10 times as often as Caucasian children. It is a disease of young children and 80% of cases are younger than 5 years. The peak age of onset is one year and the disorder is more common in boys.

The generally accepted diagnostic criteria are outlined in Table 16.2. A definite diagnosis of Kawasaki disease can be made when at least five of the six principal signs are present. In the absence of pathognomonic clinical or laboratory signs it is extremely difficult to diagnose mild or incomplete cases. Therefore it is essential sometimes to keep an open mind and occasionally follow a child as a "possible case" with repeated clinical and cardiac evaluations. However in most cases the diagnostic criteria are clearly identifiable and a definite diagnosis of Kawasaki disease can be made.

Coronary artery aneurysms develop approximately in 15-20% of untreated children with Kawasaki disease, within 4 to 6 weeks of disease onset. Two-dimensional echocardiography will detect nearly all patients with acute coronary artery disease.

Table 16.2: Diagnostic guidelines for Kawasaki disease

Principal signs
1. Fever persisting for 5 days or more
2. Polymorphous rash
3. Bilateral conjunctival congestion
4. Changes of lips and oral cavity, reddening of lips, fissured lips, strawberry tongue, diffuse hyperaemia or oral and pharyngeal mucosa
5. Acute non-purulent cervical lymphadenopathy
6. Changes of peripheral extremities: reddening of palms and soles, indurated oedema of hands and feet, membranous desquamation from finger tips

Five of these six symptoms are required for a diagnosis of Kawasaki disease to be made, though four will suffice if there is evidence of coronary artery aneurysm. As with all diagnostic criteria, these are not 100% sensitive and specific. Children who do not have the requisite number of criteria may have incomplete or atypical Kawasaki disease.

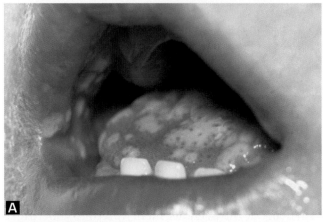

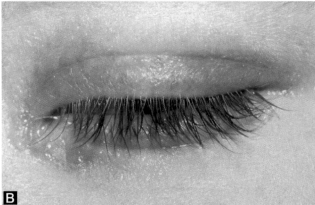

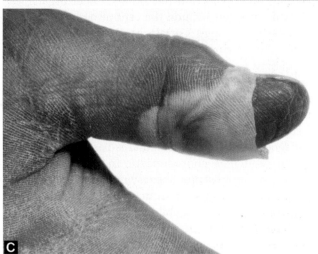

Figs 16.13A to C: Kawasaki disease (A) Strawberry tongue and sloughing of filiform papilla (B) Non-purulent conjunctivitis (C) Desquamation of thumb

Other less frequent features include arthritis, arthralgia, urethritis, diarrhoea, aseptic meningitis, sterile pyuria, myocarditis, pericarditis, alopecia, jaundice, uveitis and hydrops of the gall bladder. Blood tests show leucocytosis, a raised ESR/CRP and during the second week of illness there may be thrombocytosis.

Treatment

Early initiation of aspirin therapy and intravenous normal immunoglobulin (IVIG) remains the mainstay of treatment to prevent thrombus formation and ischaemic heart disease. Aspirin is used for its anti-inflammatory and anti-thrombotic effects. Initially aspirin is given to obtain anti-inflammatory effect by giving doses of 30 - 80 mg/Kg/d in 4 divided doses, in the acute phase of illness. Thereafter it is reduced to 3-5 mg/Kg/d for its anti-platelet effect. Aspirin should be continued until ESR and platelet count return to normal, unless coronary artery abnormalities are detected by echocardiography.

Treatment with intravenous normal immunoglobulin (IVIG) for all children diagnosed within the first 10 days of illness reduces the incidence of coronary artery aneurysms by 70%. The recommended dose of normal immunoglobulin (IVIG) is 2g/Kg and it should be administered as a single dose over 8-12 hours. However, children with a delayed diagnosis of Kawasaki disease may also benefit from IVIG.

> **CASE STUDY**
>
> A 2-year-old boy presented with a 5 day history of fever, cough, runny nose and a macular rash on his trunk. On examination he had suffusion of ocular conjunctivae, bilateral cervical lymphadenitis, an inflamed throat, strawberry tongue, induration of palms and soles and a temperature of 40^{0}C. He had no hepatosplenomegaly, arthritis and no peeling of skin and no neck stiffness. Hb 10g/dl, WBC 20 × 10^9/l with preponderance of polymorphs. Platelet count 600 × 10^9/l. ESR 80 mm in 1st hour. C-reactive protein 60 mg/l. 2-D echocardiography showed dilatation of right coronary artery. Urine clear both biochemically, microscopically and bacteriologically. Viral serology negative.
> The most likely working diagnosis was Kawasaki disease. He was treated with aspirin and IVIG. He recovered unscathed and did not develop any problems.

Juvenile Polyarteritis Nodosa

Polyarteritis nodosa (PAN) is one of the least common types of vasculitis seen in children. It is a necrotising vasculitis of medium sized muscular arteries with associated aneurysmal formation.

Clinically the symptoms are due to involvement of the vessels of the kidney, central nervous system, muscle and viscera. Coronary artery involvement and myocardial infarction may occur.

No specific serlogical markers are available for the diagnosis of PAN although some patients may have circulating anti-neutrophil cytoplasmic antibody (ANCA). Skin or muscle may be biopsied to detect histological changes of fibrinoid necrosis of small and medium sized arterial walls. Renal biopsy is generally avoided as there is a significant risk of bleeding.

Juvenile Takayasu Arteritis (TA)

This is another form of vasculitis in children. The cause remains unknown. There is a preponderance of female patients in children with Takayasu arteritis. It presents with cardiomegaly, hypertension, fever, nodules, abdominal pain, arthralgia, weight loss and chest pain. Early diagnosis and aggressive therapy with corticosteroids and immunosuppresive agents have shown variable efficacy in Takayasu arteritis.

PAEDIATRIC SYSTEMIC LUPUS ERYTHEMATOSUS (SLE)

Systemic lupus erythematosus is a multisystem auto-immune disease and the literature continually expands our knowledge of the varied and seemingly infinite manifestations and course of this complex disorder. Only a few children develop SLE in the early school years. Most cases occur between 11 and 15 years of age and it is more common in girls.

Drug-related lupus is clinically identical with paediatric SLE. In children the most common cause of drug - related lupus is the administration of anticonvulsant drugs.

> **LEARNING TIP**
>
> Earlier diagnosis of paediatric SLE and rapid introduction of aggressive immunosuppressive therapy would lead to an improved outcome.

Clinical Manifestations

In the childhood form of SLE, as in the adult, the clinical symptomatology may be variable and unpredictable with any number of organ systems eventually becoming involved. The children frequently present with constitutional symptoms and the characteristic erythematous "butterfly" rash on cheeks and bridge of nose. In one third of patients, the rash is photosensitive (Figs 16.14A and B). In addition, various skin manifestations may occur such as non-specific erythemata, purpura, telangiectasia, urticaria, alopecia and abnormal pigmentation. Raynaud phenomenon is less common in paediatric SLE. Anaemia in which there may be evidence of haemolysis (autoimmune haemolytic anaemia), thrombocytopenia and leucopenia may occur.

Renal involvement—the lupus nephritis is a grave manifestation, being the most commonly identifiable cause of death in SLE. Lupus nephritis is relatively more common and severe in children in China, and in East Asian countries.

Joint involvement is not uncommon and varies from arthralgia to arthritis closely resembling that of juvenile

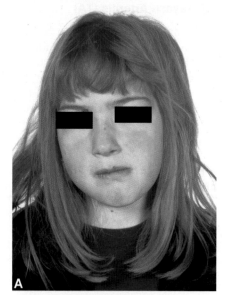

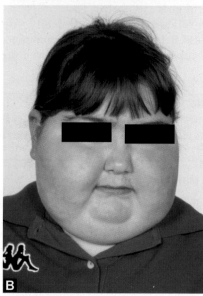

Figs 16.14A and B: Systemic lupus erythematosus (A) Malar - butterfly rash (B) Same patient with extreme iatrogenic hypercorticism Cushingoid syndrome)

idiopathic arthritis. Heart involvement may occur in this disease in the form of myocarditis, endocarditis and pericarditis. Manifestations of central nervous system involvement include convulsions and mental confusion and various localising manifestations due to focal vascular lesions. Enlargement of the liver and spleen may be found. Lymphadenopathy with generalised lymph gland enlargement is yet another clinical manifestation. There may be a rapidly progressive retinopathy and extensive retinal haemorrhages, exudates and papilloedema.

Laboratory Findings

The diagnosis of systemic lupus erythematosus is associated with a large assortment of autoantibodies. Presence or absence of particular autoantibodies influences the confidence with which this diagnosis is made. Antinuclear autoantibodies are present in up to 100% of patients. Anti- double stranded DNA (dsDNA) is the most specific antibody for lupus, while anti-single stranded DNA (ssDNA) is relatively non-specific and commonly found in other connective tissue disorders. For a detailed autoantibody profile in connective tissue disorders in children see BOX 16.2.

BOX 16.2: Autoantibodies in connective tissue disorders in children

Autoantibody	Disease
Antinuclear antibody	SLE, JIA,JDM, scleroderma
Antibodies to extractable nuclear antigen	SLE, mixed connective tissue disease
C1q antibody	SLE (particularly lupus nephritis)
Anti - cardiolipin antibodies	SLE, anti - phospholipid syndrome
Double - stranded DNA antibodies	SLE
Histone antibodies	Drug - induced lupus
Lupus anticoagulant	SLE, anti - phospholipid syndrome
Rheumatoid factor	Juvenile idiopathic arthritis
Ro/SS –A	SLE, neonatal lupus
SCL – 70	Scleroderma
Anti - Sm antibodies	SLE
U1RNP	Lupus nephritis
Centromere antibodies	CREST syndrome

SLE: systemic lupus erythematosus; JDM: juvenile dermato-myositis; JIA: juvenile idiopathic arthritis; CREST: calcinosis, Raynaud's, oesophageal dysmotility, sclerodactyly, telangiectasia.

Treatment and Prognosis

Prior to the availability of modern therapeutic measures, the majority of children with SLE died either from lupus affecting multiple organs or from infections. Children without renal involvement may do well with a combination of corticosteroids and methotrexate or azathioprine. The controlled trials have shown clear cut benefit of pulsed intravenous cyclophosphamide over steroids alone in reducing clinical and serological activity of lupus, histological damage, and end - stage renal failure. Prior to the use of cyclophosphamide the prognosis for children with continuing active renal disease following cortico-steroid therapy alone was poor.

NEONATAL LUPUS

Infants born to mothers with active SLE may present with transient manifestations of SLE such as skin rash, complete heart block, thrombocytopenia, leukopenia and haemolytic anaemia. Mothers of these babies are SS-A/Ro positive. Most manifestations of neonatal lupus resolve with the clearance of transplacentally transferred maternal antibodies and rarely require any treatment.

However, infants with marked thrombocytopenia may benefit from a short course of corticosteroid therapy. In very extreme cases exchange transfusion is useful. Heart block is lifelong and babies usually need pacing.

CASE STUDY

An 8-year-old girl presented with a 3 month history of feeling very tired, unable to walk, ulcers in her mouth, painful knees, wrists, elbows and fingers and a facial rash. She had been off school for 2 months. On examination she had a typical butterfly facial rash and active synovitis of knees, wrists and elbows. Blood pressure 100/60 mm Hg. No other positive finding was detected. The following investigations were carried out: Hb 8.5 g/dl, WBC $3.3 \times 10^9/l$, neutrophils $2.4 \times 10^9/l$, platelet count $391 \times 10^9/l$, ESR 75 mm in 1st hour, clotting profile normal, AST 40 iu/l, ALT 30 iu/l, albumin 31g/l, protein 80 g/l. creatinine 36 umol/l, Urea 5.2 mmol/l, creatine kinase 42 iu/l, Complement C3 0.26 g/l ($\downarrow$), Complement C4 0.06g/l($\downarrow$) Urine clear (Dipstix) Direct Coomb's test positive, ANA titre 1:256, Double stranded DNA more than 1000 iu/ml, Crithidia test positive, Anti-Ro positive, Anti-Sm negative, Anti-RNP negative, Anti-Scl 70 positive, Anti Jo1 positive, IgG cardiolipin antibody less than 10 iu/ml(N) IgM cardiolipin antibody less than 10 iu/ml(N).

She was initially treated with pulse methylprednisolone and a course of oral prednisolone. She responded to this treatment and did not develop lupus nephritis or any other complication.

Diagnosis: Active paediatric systemic lupus erythematosus.

JUVENILE SCLERODERMA

Scleroderma is an autoimmune connective tissue disease. There are two main categories of scleroderma
- Systemic disease
- Localised disease

JUVENILE SYSTEMIC SCLEROSIS

The systemic sclerosis is exceptionally rare in childhood, and its course unpredictable. The patches of skin with scleroderma become oedematous and the atrophic and inelastic, becoming adherent to the underlying tissues. The consequent atrophy and tightening of the skin gives a characteristic appearance of pinched nose and pursed lips. The hands become shiny with tapered finger ends and restricted movement, producing claw - like deformities which may also affect the feet. Raynaud phenomenon is common. The well known gasrointestinal system involvement with oesophageal fibrosis and dysphagia is much less common in the childhood form of the disease. Pulmonary fibrosis and renal involvement may occur. Sjögren syndrome (sicca syndrome of dry mouth and eyes) is not uncommon in this condition. An apparently slowly developing form of scleroderma, described largely in adults

and called CREST syndrome, may be found in children. CREST is an acronym for calcinosis, Raynaud phenomenon, oesophageal dysfunction, sclerodactyly and telangiectasia.

There are no specific laboratory tests diagnostic of scleroderma. Antinuclear antibodies (ANA) are frequently found in sera of children with juvenile systemic sclerosis.

Treatment

No treatment at the present time is of any certain value. Thus the treatment of juvenile systemic sclerosis poses one of the frustrating challenges in paediatric rheumatology.

JUVENILE LOCALISED SCLERODERMA (MORPHEA, LINEAR SCLERODERMA)

Morphea

Localised scleroderma is a rare disease. It differs from systemic sclerosis in that it is usually limited to the skin and subcutaneous tissues and is very rarely associated with systemic manifestations (Fig. 16.15A).

Linear Scleroderma

Linear scleroderma is characterised by scleroatrophic lesions affecting an upper or lower extremity (Fig. 16.15B). ANA can be present in any of the localised scleroderma.

Treatment

Physiotherapy and occupational therapy have a major role in the management of juvenile localised scleroderma, especially when joint structures are involved. Since these

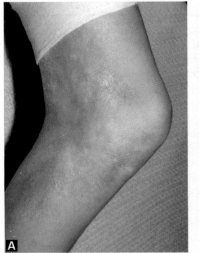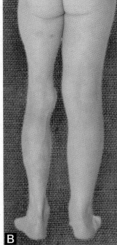

Figs 16.15A and B: Morphea (A) localised morphea on knee (B) linear scleroderma affecting left lower limb showing growth failure of the limb

disorders are benign in many patients and often spontaneously go into remission after a few years, any medication, (if not of proven value in children), should be used with caution.

JUVENILE ANKYLOSING SPONDYLITIS (JAS)

Juvenile ankylosing spondylitis is a rare condition in childhood which may present as asymmetrical polyarthritis of hips and knees rather than the classical lumbo-sacral manifestations. Iritis and scleritis may precede the joint involvement and it may take several months or years before a definite diagnosis can be made.

Laboratory findings are not particularly helpful in this disorder as rheumatoid factor and antinuclear antibody tests are negative. The presence of HLA B -27 positivity will support the diagnosis provided other clinical features of JAS are present. Plain X-ray examination is unhelpful because the typical changes in the sacroiliac joints described are rarely seen. However, in these patients MRI of sacroiliac joints will show changes of sacroiliatis. The treatment of JAS consists of the use of NSAIDs, DMRDs and a physical therapy programme.

BEHCET SYNDROME

This syndrome is rare in children and is seen more commonly in children from the Middle East and Japan. It is characterised by recurrent oral and genital ulceration and eye inflammation. Additional associated clinical features are arthritis, fever and less commonly there can be involvement of gastrointestinal, cardiovascular and nervous systems. Laboratory findings are not diagnostic. Colchicine is relatively safe and effective medication in children with Behcet syndrome.

LYME DISEASE

In 1977 Steer and his colleagues announced the discovery of a new disease called Lyme disease which they proved was transmitted by the deer tick Ixodes dammini. In 1982 it was discovered that infectious agent is a spirochaete (Borrelia burgdorferi). The clinical syndrome consists of a febrile illness with a characteristic rash, erythema chronicum migrans. Arthritis may be the initial manifestation of Lyme disease. It is oligoarticular type of joint involvement. The diagnosis should be confirmed with Lyme serology (ELISA and immunoblot assays). Lyme disease should generally be treated with doxycycline in children over 12 years of age. Also intravenous administration of cefotaxime, ceftriaxone or benzylpenicillin is recommended for 2-4 weeks.

SARCOIDOSIS

Sarcoidosis is a multisystem condition characterised by chronic noncaseating granulomas. It is uncommon in children. The disease is charasterised by fever, arthritis, uveitis, erythema nodosum and pulmonary disease. The uveitis either anterior or posterior is granulomatous with formation of course keratic precipitates. Serum levels of angiotensin - converting enzyme (ACE) are raised. Biopsy of appropriate tissue demonstrates typical granulomas.

In some cases no specific treatment is necessary since spontaneous resolution occurs. Mild general symptoms and arthralgia may be treated with NSAIDs. When more specific treatment is needed steroids are the usual choice.

TUBERCULOUS ARTHRITIS

Tuberculosis remains a major cause of skeletal tuberculosis in many developing countries. Tuberculous arthritis in children is a chronic, insidious arthritis affecting spine and synovium of knee, hip and wrist being the most common sites. Dactylitis has also been noted as the presenting sign in children. The most frequent presenting symptom is pain, swelling, tenderness, muscle wasting and decreased range of movement. There may be general detrioration in health with loss of weight, poor appetite and low grade fever.

The ESR and C-reactive protein are usually raised and Mantoux test is positive. However, a normal ESR and a negative Mantoux test do not exclude the diagnosis of tuberculosis. Confirmation of diagnosis is made by the identification of Mycobacterium tuberculosis in the synovial fluid or by histology of the synovium.

Early diagnosis is important to prevent spread to a contaguous joint. The treatment of tuberculous arthritis is medical.

BENIGN JOINT HYPERMOBILITY SYNDROME (BJHS)

Generalised joint laxity is a feature of the hereditary connective tissue disorders such as Marfan's syndrome, Ehlers - Danlos syndrome and osteogenesis imperfecta. A subject is considred hypermobile if he can perform two of the following three maneuvers: passive opposition of both thumbs to the volar aspect of the forearms, passive hyperextension of the fingers so that they lie parallel to the extensor aspect of both forearms; and active hyperextension of both elbows beyond 180 degrees.

Hypermobility is relatively common in the general population. The term benign joint hypermobility syndrome has been coined to clinical situation in which there is generalized joint laxity associated with musculoskeletal complaints without cutaneous or internal signs of connective tissue disease in otherwise normal subjects. In young children this syndrome is observed equally in both sexes but towards puberty it predominates in girls. The knees are the most frequent sites of complaint but occasionally the ankles may also be affected. The discomfort usually comes after exercise and the whole clinical picture is consistent with an episode of traumatic synovitis. There is a strong familial tendency to this syndrome and the diagnosis is therefore essentially clinical combined with an awareness of family history. The management is mainly reassurance as to the absence of serious disease and activity which precipitates symptoms should be avoided if possible. Most young subjects will grow out of their complaints altogether.

Key Learning Points
Hypermobility:
• Consider hypermobility if child is able to:
• Passively oppose the thumb to the volar aspect of the forearms
• Passively hyperextend fingers so they are parallel to the extensor aspect of forearms
• Active hyperextension of both elbows beyond 180 degrees

LIMB PAINS OF CHILDHOOD WITH NO ORGANIC DISEASE (IDIOPATHIC LIMB PAINS)

So - called 'limb pains' or 'growing pains' are more common in childhood than all the other rheumatic diseases put together. Growth in children involves two phases - 'shooting up' and 'filling out'. A limb may show bony growth followed by (not accompanied) by muscle growth. It may be that in such a shooting up phase, extra strain is put upon the muscle, which tires easily and gives pain towards the end of the day or during the night when relaxation is incomplete. They can also start after a minor accident such as falling over, or they may be triggered by being upset or stress for example having exams at school. These factors make the muscles in arms and legs tense up and feel tight thus the pain. A history of rheumatic disorders is common in the families of children with idiopathic limb pains than in controls. Therefore parents often become worried and feel their child suffers from rheumatic disease. In two-thirds of affected children limb pains occur during the daytime or evening. In the remainder the pains are predominantly nocturnal, and can wake the child and may be severe enough to cause crying. The age group mainly affected is 9-12 years, and girls more than boys. The children site pain between joints, suggesting that the pain is muscular. Most children like to have the area gently rubbed by a parent, which effectively excludes juvenile rheumatoid arthritis. With reassurance based on discussions, it should be possible to convince parents that their child does not suffer from a rheumatic disorder. Occasionally, children have psychosomatic musculo-skeletal pain and these should have a full psychological evaluation. They should respond well to treatment directed toward decreasing pain and restoring function.

CASE STUDY
A-10-year-old girl presented with nocturnal lower limb pains for six months. At no time she had swelling or tenderness of any of her joints. She had no other symptoms but she had been worried about her exams. Her maternal grandmother had osteoarthritis and maternal aunt was crippled with rheumatoid arthritis. On her clinical examination no positive finding was detected. In particular she had no evidence of active synovitis.
Full blood count, urea and electrolytes, liver function tests, rheumatoid factor, ANA, ESR and CRP were normal. She was diagnosed as having non-organic nocturnal lower limb pains. Parents and the child were reassured that she did not have rheumatoid arthritis. With firm reassurance within a few weeks her symptoms settled and she was discharged from follow up.
Diagnosis: Idiopathic nocturnal lower limb pains.

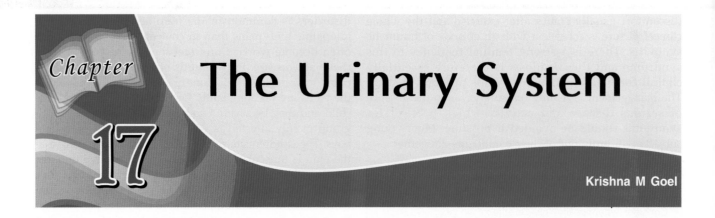

Over the past four decades progress has been achieved in the classification of renal disease and this has been particularly in the realm of glomerular disorders. This has been possible because of electron microscopy and immunofluorescence in the identification within renal tissue of immunoglobulins and complement components. On the basis of experimental work it has been shown that there are mainly two types of immunologically mediated glomerular diseases:

1. Due to deposition of antigen antibody complexes (immune complex glomerulonephritis); and
2. Due to the action of autoantibodies against constituents of glomerular basement membrane (anti-GBM disease).

Classification at present is based on a combination of factors, e.g. aetiological agents, association with systemic disease, identification of basic immunopathogenic mechanisms and correlation with clinical findings (Table 17.1).

Interestingly the spectrum of paediatric renal diseases in Asian countries is similar to that seen in the Western countries although certain conditions are more common such as post-dysenteric haemolytic uraemic syndrome, malarial nephropathy, hepatitis-B nephropathy and nephropathy associated with leptospirosis, snake-bite and other envenomations. In this chapter only common glomerulonephritides in relation to paediatric practice will be discussed.

ACUTE POST-STREPTOCOCCAL GLOMERULONEPHRITIS (APSGN)

Acute post-streptococcal glomerulonephritis (APSGN) is a syndrome consisting of frank haematuria, proteinuria with accompanying oliguria, volume overload and usually, a mild increase in plasma creatinine. In the Indian sub-continent, China, Thailand, Nigeria, South Africa, acute post-streptococcal glomerulonephritis is common as compared to its incidence in the Western countries. In most cases there is a history of a preceding infection 7-21 days before the onset of renal manifestations. In the majority this infection is due to one of the group A beta haemolytic streptococci, most often nephritogenic types 4,12,25 and 49. It has been presumed that during the latent period of 7-21 days an antigen-antibody reaction takes place between the streptococcal endotoxin and the cells of the glomerulus. The underlying renal histology is typically an acute proliferative glomerulonephritis.

Apart from the cases due to streptococcal pharyngitis, some cases may occur following skin infection (pyoderma) or rarely middle ear infection. In developing countries the outbreaks of APSGN are often due to pyoderma while in developed countries they are associated with pharyngeal infection. The simultaneous occurrence of acute rheumatic fever and APSGN has been reported but is extremely rare.

Table 17.1: Classification of glomerulonephritis
Primary glomerulonephritis
Acute post-streptococcal glomerulonephritis
IgA nephropathy
Anti-glomerular basement membrane antibody disease
Goodpasture syndrome
Glomerulonephritis of uncertain aetiology
Minimal change nephrotic syndrome (MCNS)
Focal segmental glomerulosclerosis (FSGS)
Membranous nephropathy
Glomerulonephritis associated with systemic disease and infections
Henoch Schönlein purpura, systemic lupus erythematosus, scleroderma, polyarteritis nodosa, Wegener granulomatosis, infective endocarditis, shunt nephritis, hepatitis B and C, malaria, syphilis, toxoplasmosis, parvovirus B19, cytomegalovirus, filaria, HIV associated renal disease, Epstein-Barr virus infection.
Hereditary disorders
Congenital nephrotic syndrome
Familial nephritis-Alport syndrome, Sickle-cell disease
Other conditions
Diabetes mellitus, amyloidosis, heavy metal poisoning - mercury

Clinical Features

Usually the child is of school age and the onset is abrupt with fever, malaise, headache, vomiting and the passage of red, or smoky or brown coloured urine. The preceding tonsillitis or other cutaneous infection has usually resolved by this time. Examination reveals mild oedema, most obvious in the face and hypertension of moderate severity. Urinary output is reduced. There is proteinuria but it is usually in the non-nephrotic range (<2 g/l). Microscopy of urine shows red blood cell casts and hyaline or granular casts are less frequent during the acute phase. Causes of dark or discoloured urine are shown in Box 17.1.

BOX 17.1: Causes of dark or discoloured urine in children

Rifampicin
Nitrofurantoin
Metronidazole
Dexferrioxamine
Beetroot
Black-berries
Urate crystals
Myoglobinuria
Haemoglobinuria
Alkaptonuria, porphyria
Food colourings

Key Learning Point

It is essential to establish that red urine is due to haematuria by looking for red blood cells on urine microscopy.

Haemolytic streptococci are frequently isolated from the throat swab and in most cases the antistreptolysin-O (ASO) titre is raised within 10-14 days following a streptococcal infection and anti-DNAse B will be positive. The blood urea and serum creatinine concentrations are frequently raised but a normal level need not invalidate the diagnosis. During the first week or two of acute post-streptococcal glomerulonephritis (APSGN) very low levels of serum complement are found which rise as recovery takes place. For investigations of APSGN see Box 17.2.

BOX 17.2: Investigations of APSGN
FBC
U and E's
LFT's
Immunoglobulins
ASO titre (anti-DNAse B)
Complement screen
ANF
Urine protein creatinine ratio
Urine culture
Renal ultrasound

Course and Prognosis

The prognosis of acute post-streptococcal glomerulonephritis in childhood is excellent. Complete recovery can be expected in about 90% of children without significant alteration in renal function. Resolution of the oliguria usually occurs within a week and this is associated with blood pressure normalisation and a fall in -plasma creatinine. Frank haematuria may remain for 2-3 weeks but in the longer-term, proteinuria is usually gone by 3-6 months and microscopic haematuria by 1-2 years.

Treatment

The treatment of acute post-streptococcal glomerulonephritis is symptomatic. It includes fluid and salt restriction and management of the associated hypertension with nefedipine and frusemide. Also atenolol and enalapril can be used for lowering the blood pressure. Penicillin should be prescribed at the start of treatment to eradicate any surviving haemolytic streptococci, e.g. oral penicillin-V 250 mg four times daily for children aged 6-12 years and 125 mg four times daily for children aged 1-6 years daily for 7 days or erythromycin 50 mg/kg/d in four divided doses orally for 10 days as an alternative to penicillin in hypersensitive patients.

Since immunity to nephritogenic streptococci is type specific and long-lasting, recurrent attacks of APSGN are rare. Therefore penicillin prophylaxis as in acute rheumatic fever is not indicated.

CASE STUDY

A five-year-old girl presented with an acute onset of periorbital puffiness and tea coloured urine. Three weeks previously she had a sore throat from which she had recovered. She also complained of headache, nausea and vomiting and abdominal pain. She had oliguria.

On examination she had periorbital puffiness and minimal ankle oedema. Blood pressure was 90/60 mmHg (normal for her age). Urine revealed 4+blood and 2+ protein and red blood cell casts. Blood urea 10 mmol/L and creatinine 140 mmol/L. Complement C3 was 0.6 g/L(low) but C4 was normal. ASO titre 1200 Todd units/ml. Hb 10g/l, WBC and platelet counts normal. Her haematuria and proteinuria resolved by 6 weeks. Complement C3 returned to normal range at 8 weeks. She recovered unscathed.
Diagnosis: APSGN

PRIMARY IgA NEPHROPATHY(IgAN)

Primary IgA nephropathy occurs at all ages but is commom during the second or third decades of life and affects boys more often than girls. It seems to be uncommon in India but it is probably the most common chronic glomerulonephritis in other parts of the world, e.g. Japan, France, Italy and Australia.

The most common clinical presentation of IgA nephropathy is recurrent episodes of painless haematuria following an upper respiratory infection. The interval between the appearance of haematuria ranges from 1-2 days compared to 1-2 weeks in APSGN. Serum IgA levels are increased in this condition but serum complement concentrations are usually normal. The normal level of complement concentration differentiates it from post-infectious glomerulonephritis. A proven form of therapy for IgA nephropathy does not exist.

NEPHROTIC SYNDROME

This is the commonest clinical syndrome in the world. It is characterised by gross proteinuria ($>1g/m^2/24hr$) and hypercholesterolaemia are always present. Oedema resulting from build up of salt and water is usually severe. Other abnormalities such as raised plasma aldosterone and anti-diuretic hormone levels are prominent in childen with massive proteinuria and oedema. Hypertension, azotaemia and haematuria either microscopic or frank rarely occur in childhood. The cause of idiopathic nephrotic syndrome remains unknown, but evidence suggests it may be a primary T-cell disorder—the most common form that leads to glomerular podocyte dysfunction.

Idiopathic nephrotic syndrome has a reported incidence of two to seven cases per 100,000 children. However, in the Indian sub-continent the incidence is estimated at 90-100 per million population. There are three distinct histological variants of primary idiopathic nephrotic syndrome:
  (i) Minimal-change nephritic syndrome (MCNS)
 (ii) Focal segmental glomerulosclerosis (FSGS)
(iii) Membranous nephropathy.

Minimal change nephrotic syndrome (MCNS) and focal segmental glomerulosclerosis (FSGS) may represent opposite ends of one pathophysiological process or distinct disease entities. By contrast, membranous nephropathy is a distinct disease and is rare in children.

Clinical Features

Although the idiopathic nephrotic syndrome is seen at all ages the majority of cases occur between 1½ and 5 years. It seems to affect boys more often than girls. Its occurrence in siblings is rare. The first manifestation is oedema which causes swelling of the face, legs and abdomen, often starting after a viral upper respiratory tract infection. Gross ascites is the rule; indeed in some children peripheral oedema may be relatively slight while ascites is massive in amounts. Hypertension is typically absent. Proteinuria is also very heavy; at least 10 g may be lost each day. Haematuria is uncommon. Appropriate laboratory studies establish the correct diagnosis—see Box 17.3.

BOX 17.3: Investigation in a child with nephrotic syndrome
FBC, U and E's, creatinine, LFT's, ASO, C3/C4
Urine culture, urinary protein/creatinine ratio
Blood culture
Urinary sodium concentration in those children at risk of hypovolaemia
Varicella status prior to steroid therapy

Complications of Nephrotic Syndrome

The main complications are infection, thrombosis and hypovolaemia.

Infectious complications

Many children with nephrotic syndrome died of inter-current pyogenic infections in the pre-antibiotic era. This susceptibility is presumably due to the decreased level of factor B, transferrin and immunoglobulins lost in urine. The most typical infection is primary pneumococcal peritonitis although pneumonia and cellulitis, empyema, bone and joint infections, sepsis and tuberculosis are also common. In the Indian subcontinent tuberculosis is a problem. Therefore every child with nephrotic syndrome should be screened for the presence of tubrculosis before starting steroid therapy and to exclude it during the subsequent management. Pneumococal vaccination is recommended for children who have nephrotic syndrome.

Thromboembolic complications

Thromboembolism is the most severe and fatal complication of nephrotic syndrome.

Hypovolaemia

Children with nephrotic syndrome while very oedematous could be intravascularly depleted. A urinary sodium of <10 mmol/L is a good marker of hypovolaemia.

Management

Before the introduction of corticosteroids there was no satisfactory form of therapy. Fortunately it is now possible in the majority of nephrotic children to induce diuresis and complete or partial remission of proteinuria with steroids. Bed rest is rarely indicated.

A well balanced and healthy diet containing the recommended dietary reference value for protein is recommended with a "no added salt" regimen. If the child's appetite remains poor, a complete nutritional and energy supplement is necessary. Fluid restriction may also be helpful. These restrictions are lifted once the child goes into remission.

Treatment of Initial Presentation of Idiopathic Nephrotic Syndrome

On the basis of randomised controlled trials involving children with a first episode of steroid-responsive nephotic syndrome it is recommended that a 12 weeks initial course of prednisolone significantly decreases the risk of relapses. The dose of prednisolone is based on surface area and the recommended 12 weeks programme is as follows:

- Prednisolone 60 mg/m² daily for 4 weeks followed by
- Prednisolone 40 mg/m² on alternate days for 4 weeks followed by
- Prednisolone 5-10 mg/m² each week for another 4 weeks then stop.

Traditionally patients receive divided doses but once daily treatment also seems to be effective.

If the patient is very oedematous, oliguric, showing evidence of hypovolaemia, intravenous 20% salt poor albumin, 1g /kg given over 4-6 hours is very effective, particularly if supplemented by intravenous frusemide 2 mg /kg. A low serum albumin alone is not an indication for intravenous albumin.

Key Learning Points
Steroid responsive nephrotic syndrome
Roughly 95% of children with nephrotic syndrome (MCNS) will respond to steroid therapy within 2-4 weeks. A remission is defined when urine is free of protein (or trace only) for 3 or more days. If proteinuria persists beyond the first 4 weeks of steroid therapy, the child should have a renal biopsy.

Frequently Relapsing and Steroid Dependent Idiopathic Nephrotic Syndrome

Up to 60% of steroid responsive patients with nephrotic syndrome may have one or more relapses. Some of these children can be managed with low-dose prednisolone given daily or on alternate days, but many will still relapse, especially if they have intercurrent infections. Steroid induced side-effects develop in a large number of these children.

Frequent relapses are diagnosed if there is:

2 or more relapses within 6 months of initial response 4 or more relapses in any 12 months period and steroid dependent nephrotic syndrome if : 2 consecutive relapses during steroid tapering or within 14 days of cessation of steroids. Treatment with cyclophosphamide, chlorambucil, ciclosporin and levamisole to reduce the risk of relapses is supported. Ciclosporin is an important steroid spairing agent in the treatment of steroid-responsive nephrotic syndrome. The proportion of children with frequent relapses and steroid dependence in the Indian sub-continent is high but the final outcome is satisfactory.

Steroid-resistant Idiopathic Nephrotic Syndrome

The management of children with steroid-resistant nephrotic syndrome is difficult, most children failing to achieve remission show progressive renal damage.

A few children around 20-25% with idiopathic FSGS respond to an 8 week course of high dose corticosteroids. However, immunosuppressive drugs such as cyclophosphamide, levamisole, chlorambucil and ciclosporin have provided an alternative line of treatment for these children. Also, newer immunosuppressive agents such as mycophenolate mofetil and sirolimus have a place in the treatment of idiopathic primary FSGS.

Key Learning Point
Steroid toxicity
Cushingoid facies, obesity, hirsutism, striae, hypertension, impaired glucose tolerance, posterior subcapsular cataracts, emotional problems and growth retardation.

Course and Prognosis

The main prognostic indicator in nephrotic syndrome is responsiveness to steroids. On the whole as many as 60-80% of steroid responsive nephrotic children will relapse and about 60% of those will have 5 or more relapses. If the child is more than 4 years of age at presentation and remission occurs within 7-9 days of the start of treatment without haematuria are predictive of fewer relapses. Finally, steroid resistant FSGS children with the current treatment modalities available a few will achieve a sustained remission. For children with refractory nephrotic syndrome progress to end-stage renal disease is inevitable.

CONGENITAL NEPHROTIC SYNDROME

Congenital nephrosis is a rare disorder in which inheritance is probably autosomal recessive. It appears to have a peculiarly high and familial incidence in Finland (Finnish type). The hallmarks of the disease are an abnormally large placenta associated with heavy proteinuria, oedema and ascites. It is unresponsive to steroid therapy and cytotoxic drugs. The affected infants die from intercurrent infections or progressive renal failure.

Another condition that causes nephrotic syndrome in the first months of life is diffuse mesangial sclerosis. The pattern of inheritance is not yet clear although it appears to be genetic.

URINARY TRACT INFECTIONS

Urinary tract infection is one of the common diseases of paediatric practice. The most common infecting organism is *E.coli* and the highest incidence of disease is in the first 2 to 3 years. Less frequently, the organisms are the

Streptococcus, *Pseudomonas aeruginosa* and rarely the *Salmonella* group. There has long been controversy as to the route by which the organisms reach the kidney. Haematogenous spread undoubtedly occurs, especially in the newborn, but the present tendency is to attach more importance to ascending infection via the urethral lumen or the lymphatics. Urinary stasis due to congenital anomalies of the renal tract or to acquired causes of obstruction such as calculi predisposes to infection.

Clinical features

Urinary tract infections occur four times more frequently in girls than in boys, with the exception of the first 6 months of life. The higher female incidence after the early months of life has been attributed to the short female urethra and ascending infections.

The onset of the acute stage is usually sudden with fever, pallor, anorexia, vomiting and tachycardia. Urinary tract infection is one of the few causes of rigor in young children. However, in children symptoms pointing to the renal tract are often absent. In some cases, however, the mother may have observed that there is frequency of micturition or that the infant screams during the act of urination.

In older children frequency and dysuria make diagnosis easier although their absence does not exclude the diagnosis. Some children may present with new or increase enuresis.

Key Learning Points
Indications for examining urine: Abdominal pain and unexplained vomiting Frequency of micturition, dysuria or enuresis Failure to thrive Prolonged jaundice in the newborn Non specific illness Haematuria

Key Learning Points
Urine analysis should be part of routine investigation of every ill infant or child. A pure growth of more than 10^5 colony forming units or any growth on suprapubic tap urine is significant.

Diagnosis

The diagnosis must be based upon examination of the urine including microscopy and culture. If there is any delay, storage at 4°C will permit accurate diagnosiss certainly for 24 hours. Urine microscopy can make a useful contribution to diagnosis, especially when urgent treatment need to be initiated without culture results. Significant pyuria is defined as >10 WBC per cu mm. Pyuria however, is not diagnostic of UTI. Also the absence

of pyuria, particularly in children with recurrent UTI does not exclude significant bacteriuria.

However, an active infection can be present in the child upon the presence of a clean catch or suprapubic bladder urine (SPA) in an infant or a mid stream (MSSU) urine specimen in an older child of a growth of more than 100,000 (10^5) colony forming units of pathogenic organisms per ml or any growth on SPA sample is significant.

Course and Prognosis

In the majority of cases of acute urinary tract infections complete recovery occurs with adequate treatment. A proven urinary tract infection in any child is an indication for further investigation. They may include plain radiograph, ultrasonography, intravenous urography, micturating cystography and gamma camera renography, ^{99}TcDTPA and DMSA renal scans. Their use should be tailored to the clinical situation in each case. See Box 17.4 for basic learning points.

BOX 17.4: Basic learning points
Ultrasound is the most sensitive method for detection of renal parenchymal damage and for evaluation of differential renal function **DMSA** scan is very sensitive for the detection of renal scarring damage, the evaluation of divided renal function (normal if it lies between 45 and 55%), assessment of ectopic renal tissue, assessment of suspected horse-shoe kidney and investigation of a child with hypertension. **MCUG** is the definite method for detecting the bladder and urethral anatomy **DTPA** is the indirect radionuclide cystography but the child should be toilet trained (3-3½ years of age) Uses are : assessment of reflux, assessment of obstruction. $^{99-m}$**Tc-MAG3** is non-invasive technique for the follow-up of vesico-ureteric reflux (VUR) previously assessed by MCUG

Management

General nursing measures include a large fluid intake, antipyretic agents when there is high fever and a laxative if the patient is constipated. If at all possible antibiotic therapy should not be commenced until the diagnosis has been fully established or at least appropriate urine cultures have been obtained so that the organism and its antibiotic sensitivity can be determined. However, in any unwell child especially in infants and children under the age of 2 years, it would be unwise to withhold antibiotic once urine cultures have been taken and treatment should be started with the "best guess" antibacterial agent in full dosage. Full dose antibacterial therapy is given for 7-10 days. However, if there is no clinical response within 24-48 hours, the antibiotic should be changed. At present the following drugs are suitable for oral administration for short full dose courses.

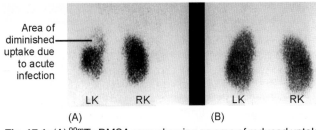

Area of diminished uptake due to acute infection

LK   RK   LK   RK

(A)   (B)

Fig. 17.1: (A) ^{99m}Tc DMSA scan showing an area of reduced uptake of the scanning agent in the upper part of the left kidney at the time of an acute urinary tract infection. The function in the kidney was also reduced. (B) The appearance had returned to normal on a follow-up scan.

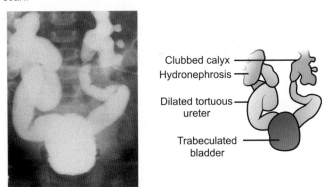

Clubbed calyx
Hydronephrosis
Dilated tortuous ureter
Trabeculated bladder

Fig. 17.2: Cystogram showing bilateral vesico-ureteric reflux

- Trimethoprim
- Augmentin
- Nitrofurantoin
- Cephradine.

The use of intravenous therapy should be considred in the infant and young child and in all children who are sufficiently ill to need hospitalisation. A third generation cephalosporin, e.g. cefotaxime or ceftazidime or a combination of aminoglycoside and augmentin would be appropriate. There is no consensus over the duration of intravenous therapy, however it seems reasonable to give it for a minimum of 5 days.

A prophylactic dose of a suitable antibiotic should be continued at least until investigation of the urinary tract has been completed. The drug dosage should be adjusted to the child's age and weight and antibiotics presently suitable for prophylaxis are:

Trimethoprim: 1-2 mg/kg/d
Nitrofurantoin: 1 mg/kg/d
Augmentin: 0-1 year 125/31 – 2.5 ml/d
              1-6 years 125/31 – 5 ml/d
              6 – 12 years 250/62 – 5-10 ml/d

To reduce the risk of dental decay, liquid preparations should be sugar free and must not be diluted with sugar containing diluents.

The long-term management of infants and children with a history of recurrent UTI, renal scarring (Fig. 17.1) or other imaging abnormalities, e.g. vesico-ureteric reflux (Fig. 17.2) should be tailored to the individual patient. However, it would seem appropriate to maintain patients with definite risk factors on some form of antibiotic prophylaxis until the age of 5 years.

Urinary Tract Imaging

A significant number of urinary tract anomalies will be detected in children of both sexes who present with UTI. Therefore all children should have some urinary tract imaging after a first UTI (see Box 17.5).

BOX 17.5: Urinary tract imaging
Initial
0-1 years
Urinary tract ultrasound, ^{99m}Tc DMSA scan, MCUG. MCUG scan should be carried out when the urine is sterile and should be carried out if there is gross dilatation of the collecting system and/or obstructive uropathy is suspected.
1-5 years
Urinary tract ultrasound, ^{99m}Tc scan: if there is a history of recurrent UTI, or a family history of VUR/reflux nephropathy. If an abnormality on either of these two imaging studies is found, a reflux study should be done. (a) in a pre-continent child – MCUG or a direct isotope cystography (b) in a continent and cooperative child: ^{99m}Tc DTPA or MAG3 scan.
>5 years
Urinary tract ultrasound alone unless there is a history of recurrent UTI or a family history of VUR/reflux nephropathy, a ^{99m}Tc DMSA scan should be done. If an abnormality is detected on either of these two imaging studies then a ^{99m}Tc DTPA or MAG3 indirect radionuclide cystogram should be considered.
Follow-up
Subsequent imaging should be individualised, depending upon the age of the child and the presence or absence of abnormalities on initial imaging.

CASE STUDY

A six-month-old girl presented with fever (38°C), irritability, listlessness, vomiting and not finishing her feeds. On examination she looked ill and pale. Otherwise she had no positive finding. Hb 8.6 g/dl, WBC 16×10^9/L (neutrophils 12×10^9/L), platelet count normal, CRP 98 mg/L. Urine : blood 2+ and protein 2+, pus cells 200/ mm^3. CSF sterile on culture. Blood and urine cultures yielded a heavy growth of *E.coli*. Urinary tract ultrasound normal. She responded to a course of intravenous cefotaxime 100 mg/kg for 7 days satisfactorily.
Diagnosis: *E. coli* septicaemia with UTI.

Haematuria

Unless there is an obvious lesion of the prepuce or meatus, haematuria is always of serious significance. Table 17.2 shows the differential diagnosis of haematuria in children. Fear on the part of the parents usually leads to early

Table 17.2: Differential diagnosis of paediatric haematuria

1. Glomerular
   a. Acute streptococcal glomerulonephritis
   b. Henoch-Schönlein purpura
   c. IgA nephropathy
   d. Systemic lupus erythematosus
   e. Haemolytic uraemic syndrome
   f. Shunt nephritis
2. Urinary tract
   a. Urinary tract infection
   b. Haemorrhagic cystitis
   c. Renal calculi
3. Vascular
   a. Sickle cell disease
   b. Renal vein thrombosis
   c. Thrombocytopenia
4. Interstitial
   a. Renal tuberculosis
   b. Cystic disease
   c. Hydronephrosis
   d. Wilms' tumour
   e. Acute tubular necrosis
   f. Drugs, e.g. NSAIDs, etc

Table 17.3: Causes of hypertension in infants and children

1. Renovascular disease
   – Renal artery stenosis
   – Renal artery aneurysm
   – Renal artery thrombosis
   – Polyarteritis nodosa
2. Renal parenchymal disease
   – Chronic glomerulonephritis
   – Polycystic disease of kidneys
   – Haemolytic uraemic syndrome
   – Reflux nephropathy
   – Obstructive uropathy
   – Renal failure
3. Renal tumours
   – Nephroblastoma
   – Phaeochromocytoma
   – Neuroblastoma
4. Congenital adrenal hyperplasia
5. Conn and Cushing syndrome
6. Essential hypertension
7. Drugs: Corticosteroid therapy
8. Coarctation of aorta

investigation of haematuria. Haematuria may also be accompanied by pain when there passage of a blood clot. Painless haematuria may be a presenting feature in many children with glomerulonephritis and in rare instances of Wilms tumour. In the newborn haematuria may be the presenting sign of renal vein thrombosis. Trauma may produce frank blood in the urine and minor trauma which causes haematuria suggests an underlying lesion such as hydronephrosis. Also haematuria can occur in general diseases such as thrombocytopenic purpura and leukaemia. In a few children with haematuria no firm diagnosis is made. There are certain substances including medications which can alter the colour of urine and thus simulate gross haematuria (See Box 17.1).

Key Learning Point
Urinary tract infection is the common cause of macroscopic (frank) haematuria.

RENAL TUBERCULOSIS

Symptomatic tuberculosis of the kidney and urinary tract is uncommon in children. Most cases of renal tuberculosis have evidence of concomitant, usually pulmonary tuberculosis, which is frequently inactive. The interval between primary tuberculosis and development of active renal tuberculosis could take a very long-time, e.g. 5-15 years.

Clinical presentation consists of dysuria, frequency of micturition, flank pain and occasionally gross haematuria. Sterile pyuria is typical of renal tuberculosis. Tuberculin

test is positive. Positive culture of three morning urine specimens for mycobacteria will establish the diagnosis. Standard anti-tuberculous therapy is recommended.

HYPERTENSION IN CHILDREN

The incidence of hypertension in children is thought to be somewhere between 1 and 3%. In children most cases of hypertension are of secondary aetiology. Also in the younger hypertensive patient it is more likely that the hypertension is due to a correctable disorder. About 80-90% of cases of severe or sustained hypertension in children are due to some form of renal disease. Causes of hypertension in children are as outlined in Table 17.3. A diagnosis of essential hypertension can be made only after exclusion of all other known causes of hypertension. It is commonly found in obese children.

As shown in Figure 17.3, normal blood pressure readings vary according to the age of the child. The most reliable definition is a systolic or diastolic blood pressure above the 95th centile of the expected blood pressure for the child's age, which is confirmed on at least two measurements. Blood pressure levels below the 90th centile are normal. The "gold standard" for blood pressure measurement is mercury sphygmomanometry and this should be used to confirm hypertension found using automated devices.

Clinical Features

Children with quite severe hypertension may be asymptomatic and hypertension is usually detected on routine physical examination. The most common symptoms are

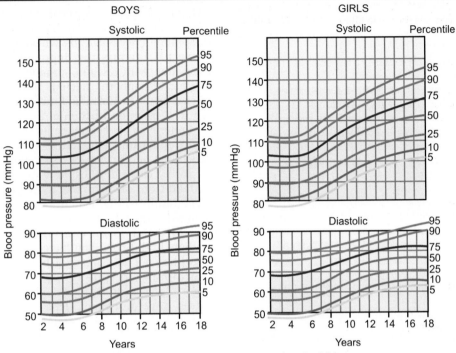

Fig. 17.3: Normal blood pressure values in children

headache, nausea, vomiting, polyuria, polydipsia and abdominal pain. Needless to say, blood pressure measurement is essential in a child with headache, in spite of the fact that there is a strong family history of migraine. Some children may present with convulsions, epistaxis, visual disturbances and facial palsy. Symptoms related to catecholamine excess, such as palpitations, sweating and weight loss may suggest the presence of a phaeochromocytoma.

Physical examination should include careful inspection of optic fundi for evidence of hypertensive retinopathy. Other important findings that suggest renovascular hypertension are cardiomegaly and the presence of an upper abdominal bruit. Physical examination should also include a neurological evaluation, palpation of the abdomen for a mass and inspection of skin for café-au-lait spots, neuromas and neurofibromas. Cushingoid features or evidence of virilisation suggest disturbances of adrenocortical function. Upper limb hypertension associated with delayed or absent femoral pulses suggest the diagnosis of coarctation of aorta.

Investigation of Hypertension

It is vital to remember that single high blood pressure values are not reliable. All children with persistent hypertension should have some evaluation but the question arises how intensive it should be; laboratory investigations should include full blood count, CRP, U and E's, creatinine, LFT's, routine urinalysis, urine culture, chest X-ray, ECG, and echocardiography. If renal aetiology is suspected: renal imaging such as renal ultrasound with Doppler, DMSA and DTPA renal scans, intravenous urography, renal angiography and renal biopsy. If catecholamine excess suspected : CT/MRI imaging of abdomen, abdominal angiography with selective venous sampling.

If corticosteroid excess suspected: urinary steroid profile, steroid suppression tests, adrenal CT/MRI and selective adrenal venous steroid sampling.

Management of Hypertension

Children with severe hypertension should be treated because of the high incidence of morbidity and mortality. Most children with hypertension will require general advice regarding diet, exercise and lifestyle.

In children with retinopathy, encephalopathy, seizure or pulmonary oedema immediate steps should be taken to lower the blood pressure. Therefore they may need intravenous anti-hypertensive therapy initially. Drugs that can be used belong to five categories, which are most suitable for the first line treatment of children with hypertension. These are diuretics, adrenorecepter blockers, ACE inhibitors, calcium antagonists, and vasoilators. Other classes of drugs may be used in certain situations (See Box 17.6).

BOX 17.6: Antihypertensive drugs in children aged 1 month – 12 years
1. Diuretics
   Frusemide: 0.5 mg/kg orally 2-3 times a day or 0.5 to 1 mg/kg IV repeated every 8 hours as necessary
   Spironolactone: 1-3 mg/kg/d orally in 1-2 divided doses
2. Angiotensin converting enzyme (ACE) inhibitors
   Captopril: 0.3 mg/kg/d orally in three divided doses
   Enalapril: 0.1 mg/kg/d orally in 1-2 divided doses
3. Calcium channel blockers
   Nifedipine: 0.25 mg/kg/d orally in 1-2 divided doses
   Amlodipine: 0.05 mg/kg/d once daily
4. Adrenergic blockers
   Labetalol: 1-3 mg/kg/hour intravenously(infusion only)
   Atenolol: 1 mg/kg/d orally in one dose
5. Vasodilators
   Hydralazine: 0.15-0.25 mg/kg/dose IV repeated every 4-6 hours as necessary
   Minoxidil: 0.2 mg/kg/d in 1-2 divided doses

Mild hypertension (use one of the following)
   Nifedipine, Amlodipine, Atenolol
Moderate hypertension (use one of the following)
   Nifedipine, Amlodipine, Atenolol, Enalapril
Severe hypertension (use one of the following)
   Nifedipine, Amlodipine, Atenolol, Enalapril

Key Learning Points

Blood pressure check
Blood pressure should be routinely measured in a child at least on the first paediatric consultation
Children who are at risk of developing hypertension, e.g. with known renal disease, must have their blood pressure checked routinely.

RENAL VEIN THROMBOSIS

Renal vein thrombosis is a microvascular angiopathy which used to occur more frequently in dehydrated and seriously ill infants. The intravascular coagulation spreads from within the intrarenal vessels into the larger veins and ultimately to the renal vein. In an ill infant the appearance of gross proteinuria, haematuria and an enlarged kidney suggest the diagnosis. The baby may also have significantly raised blood pressure. The colour Doppler ultrasound will be useful in making the diagnosis of renal venous thrombosis. Supportive therapy with re-establishment of an adequate circulating volume is most important and treatment of any primary underlying disorder is indicated.

RENAL CALCULI (UROLITHIASIS)

Aetiology

There are three main types of renal calculi in children, i.e.
• Endemic
• Infective
• Metabolic.

The great majority of renal calculi found in children are secondary to infection of the renal tract, especially by urea-splitting *Proteus vulgaris*, which by maintaining a high urinary pH favours the deposition of phosphate in combination with calcium, ammonium and magnesium. The typical "staghorn" calculus fills the renal pelvis and calyces (Fig. 17.4). Calculus formation is especially likely when there is an obstruction in the renal tract, e.g. at the pelvi-ureteric or vesicoureteric junction. Nephrocalcinosis is the deposition of calcium salts within the renal parenchyma and it may be associated with urolithiasis. Very rarely calcium phosphate or oxalate stones are a manifestation of primary hyperparathyroidism or hypervitaminosis D. Calculi may also develop after prolonged immobilisation. Cystinuria, one of the inborn errors of metabolism, is a rare cause of renal stone formation. In this condition there is a defect in the tubular reabsorption not only of cystine but also of lysine, arginine and ornithine. In spite of the passage of the typical hexagonal crystals in the urine only a minority of affected children develop calculi. This condition must not be confused with the quite separate metabolic disorder called cystinosis in which cystine is deposited in body tissues. Another exceedingly rare cause of renal lithiasis, also an inborn error of metabolism is primary hyperoxaluria. Other inherited metabolic diseases which increase the excretion of very insoluble substances and thus formation of renal stones are Lesch-Nyhan syndrome, 2,8-dihydroxy adeninuria, xanthinuria and the orotic acidurias.

In certain parts of the world, e.g. India and other developing countries, endemic urolithiasis leads to the formation of vesical calculi, which are composed of ammonium acid urate (Fig. 17.5). There is evidence

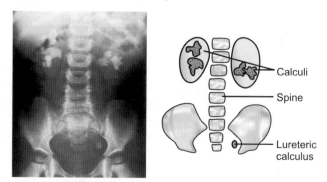

Fig. 17.4: Staghorn calculus

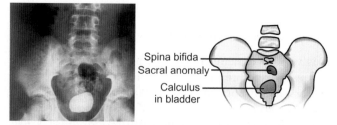

Fig. 17.5: Calculus in bladder

implicating dietary factors in their pathogenesis, where the major source of dietary protein are cereals instead of meat.

Clinical Features

The majority of children present as cases of urinary tract infection with pyuria. Classical renal colic with haematuria is relatively uncommon in childhood.

Diagnosis

Calculi cause acoustic shadows and have a characteristic ultrasound appearance, therefore renal calculi can be diagnosed by renal ultrasound examination. However, the presence of a renal calculus may be overlooked by ultrasound examination. Therefore it can be confirmed by an abdominal X-ray and an IVP may be necessary to establish calyceal anatomy prior to lithotripsy. Spiral computed tomography is the most sensitive method for diagnosing renal calculus. In confirmed cases it is wise to determine the urinary output of calcium, cystine and oxalate so that metabolic disorders are not overlooked.

Treatment

This consists of sterilisation of urine by appropriate antibiotic therapy and removal of the calculus either by lithotripsy or by an operation. Also percutaneous nephrolithotomy in children before school age is a safe and effective procedure for treating renal stones.

HYPOPHOSPHATAEMIC RICKETS (PHOSPHATURIC RICKETS)

In this disease rickets develops at a later age, than is usual in infantile rickets, and it is resistant to vitamin D in ordinary doses. It appears to be casually related to a deficiency in the tubular reabsorption of phosphate. The disease is usually transmitted by a dominant gene on the X chromosome; affected males have only affected daughters, whereas affected females have equal numbers of affected and healthy children irrespective of sex. The condition is therefore, more common in girls, but because they have one normal X chromosome the severity of the disorder is less than in affected males. In a few cases an autosomal recessive pattern of inheritance has been reported.

Clinical, Biochemical and Radiological Features

The child develops the classical features of rickets modified from the vitamin D deficient infantile variety only by the patient's age. These include enlargement of epiphyses, rachitic rosary, and deformities of the limbs. Bilateral coxa vara frequently results in a characteristic waddling "penguin" gait. Short stature with disproportionate shor-

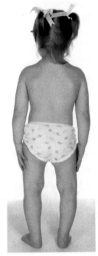

Fig. 17.6: A girl with hypophosphataemic rickets showing short stature and bow legs

tening of the lower limbs is the most important clinical manifestation (Fig.17.6).

Urinary excretion of calcium is small whereas the output of phosphate is exces-sive. The phosphate reabsorption percentage is less than 85% in spite of low plasma phosphate and parathyroid hormone (PTH) values. The plasma biochemical findings in the blood are the same as those usually found in infantile vitamin D deficiency rickets, namely a normal plasma calcium, reduced plasma phosphate and increased alkaline phosphatase. The plasma concentration of 25-OHD$_3$ is usually normal and that of 1, 25 (OH)$_2$ D$_3$ is slightly low or normal. Aminoaciduria which is commonly found in vitamin D deficiency rickets is not a feature of hypophosphataemic rickets. Radiological features are those of rickets, e.g. cupped, frayed and broadened metaphyses, broadened epiphyses, osteoporosis, deformities and pathological fractures (Fig. 17.7).

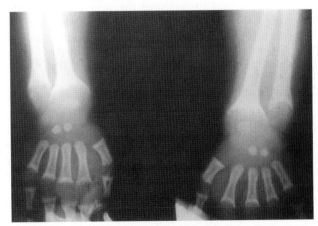

Fig. 17.7: X-rays of wrists and hands showing changes caused by rickets

Treatment

The most effective treatment appears to be a combination of 1-4 g of oral elemental phosphate per day with either oral 1, 25 $(OH)_2$ D_3 initially 15 nanograms per kg once daily, increased if necessary in steps of 5 nanograms/kg daily every 2-4 weeks (maximum 250 nanograms) or 1 a -OHD$_3$ 25-50 nanograms/kg once daily, adjusted as necessary (maximum 1 microgram). Initially phosphate supplementation may cause diarrhoea but tolerance to the regimen usually develops within 1-2 weeks. Frequent estimations of plasma calcium are necessary to detect hypercalcaemia due to overdosage. Vitamin D therapy alone rarely corrects dwarfism and even if started in early infancy may fail to prevent its development. Patients with residual skeletal deformities may need surgical correction with bilateral tibial and femoral osteotomies, usually after growth has ceased.

CASE STUDY

A 5-year-old boy presented to the paediatric clinic with bilateral bowing of the legs. The child was of Scottish origin, had a normal diet and no gasrointestinal symptoms. On examination he had short stature, reduced dental enamel and bilateral varus deformity of the knees. He did not have any wrist swelling.
Investigations performed:
    Ca 2.31 mmol/L (reference range 2.2 - 2.7 mmol/L)
    Po$_4$ 0.56 mmol/L (reference range 0.9 - 1.8 mmo;/L)
    PTH 8.5 pmol/L (reference range 0.9 - 55 pmol/L)
    25HCC 74 nmol/L (reference range 15 - 85 nmol/L)
    Phosphate excretion index high
    Tubular reabsorption rate of phosphate low: <85% (normal 85 - 95%)
Diagnosis: Hypophosphataemic rickets

RENAL FANCONI SYNDROME (CYSTINOSIS)

This syndrome embraces a group of biochemical disorders resulting from multiple renal tubular defects: glycosuria, aminoaciduria, tubular acidosis, phosphaturia, potassium loss and occasionally sodium loss and uricosuria. Cystine crystals are found throughout the reticuloendothelial system but there is no gross excretion of cystine in the urine as in cystinuria which is a quite separate inborn error of metabolism. The disease is inherited as an autosomal recessive trait.

Clinical Features

The physical features usually appear in early infancy and resemble those of hyperchloraemic acidosis. The features, failure to thrive, anorexia, vomiting and severe constipation are constantly present. Thirst and polyuria may also have been noted by the mother. A feature characteristic of cystinosis is photophobia. This is due to the presence of cystine crystals in the cornea but it is not always present. Rickets makes its appearance after some months of illness. Its appearance in a wasted infant is in contrast to infantile rickets which is more commonly found in well grown infants (Fig. 17.8).

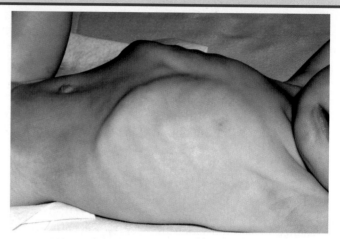

Fig. 17.8: Rachitic rosary and generalised wasting

Diagnosis

This is based initially on the presence of glycosuria and aminoaciduria. Radiological changes are typical of rickets. Cystinosis can be confirmed by the detection of cystine crystals in the cornea with a slit-lamp, or by finding them in bone marrow or lymph node biopsy material. White cell cystine levels are raised and this is now used in diagnosis and monitoring treatment.

Treatment

The rickets requires large doses of calciferol for healing (50,000 - 300,000 units daily). Alternatively 1 alpha OHD may be used in the dosage of 25-50 nanograms/kg once daily orally. The metabolic acidosis can be corrected with oral sodium bicarbonate 1-3 mmol/kg/d. If hypokalaemia is present some of the sodium salt should be replaced by potassium citrate or potassium bicarbonate. The daily intake of potassium salt may need to be as much as 5 g. Renal transplantation has been successful in children with cystinosis who develop end-stage renal disease.

CASE STUDY

A 2-year-old Asian boy presented with a history of "not growing" and polydipsia. Parents were first cousins. His height was between the 0.4th -2nd centile and weight between the 2nd-9th centile. He had widening of both wrists. No other positive finding.
Investigations performed:
Hb 10.4 g/dl, WBC 7.2x10^9/L, platelets 315x10^9/L, plasma sodium 130 mmol/L, potassium 2.9 mmol/L, chloride 94 mmol/L, bicarbonate 28 mmol/L, urea 5.6 mmol/L. creatinine 115 micromol/L, calcium 2.26 mmol/L, phosphate 0.87 mmol/L, alkaline phosphatase 315 u/L, parathormone (PTH) 9.3 pmol/L (reference range 0.9 - 5.5 pmol/L), 25HCC 64 nmol/L (normal), leucocyte cystine 4.26 nmol of ½ cystine per mg of protein (normal <0.3 nmol of ½cystine per mg of protein).
Diagnosis: Nephropathic cystinosis

NEPHROGENIC DIABETES INSIPIDUS (NDI)

This is a rare condition which must be differentiated from central-neurogenic or pituitary diabetes insipidus (CDI) due to failure of production by the posterior pituitary of antidiuretic hormone (ADH). In NDI the renal tubules fail to respond to vasopressin and reabsorb water normally. The condition has been transmitted as an X-linked trait in most of the reported families, only males being affected. The concentrating defect can be partial or complete.

Clinical Features

Excessive thirst, and polyuria start soon after birth. Failure to thrive, anorexia, constipation and vomiting are common. Deprivation of fluids or a high environmental temperature leads to fever, prostration and hypernatraemic dehydration because these children cannot produce urine of high specific gravity. There is a particular risk during infancy when the patient is unable to determine his/her own fluid intake. Usually the child is non-selective in his choice of fluids, and they wake from sleep to drink and may drink from inappropriate sources e.g. toilet cistern and bath water or any other source of fluid available. Another clinical feature is that growth may also be retarded.

Diagnosis

Diagnosis can be confirmed by the failure to respond to vasopressin (vasopressin test) and by the marked inability to concentrate the urine during water deprivation (a urine osmolality estimated four hours later-normal response is a urine osmolality of over 800 mOsm/kg).

In NDI benefit may be gained from the paradoxical anti-diuretic effect of thiazides, e.g. chlorothiazide 10-20 mg/kg twice daily (maximum 500 mg).

Key Learning Points

Vasopressin test
In NDI there is little change in pre and post-vasopressin urine osmolality.
In CDI the pre-vasopressin test osmolality is < 300 mOs/kg, but post-vasopressin urine osmolality is makedly increased i.e. > 800 mOs/kg.

CASE STUDY

A 3-month-old boy was born at 38 weeks gestation with a birth weight of 3kg. Neonatal period uneventful. He was bottle-fed. He was irritable, took his bottle feeds satisfactorily. Milk offered to him was never enough and was always thirsty—so he was offered flavoured water which he took eagerly. His weight gain was poor. On examination he was well hydrated. In fact he had no positive finding. Urine dipstix and culture negative. Urinary tract ultrasound normal. Plasma urea 12 mmol/L, sodium 164 mmol/L, creatinine 60 μmol/l. He was given DDAVP 0.5 μgram intranasal and urine osmolality 4 hours later was 200 mOs/kg.
Diagnosis: Nephrogenic diabetes insipidus (NDI)

RENAL TUBULAR ACIDOSIS (RTA)

Two main mechanisms are recognised in renal tubular acidosis. In one mechanism in the presence of systemic acidosis the kidney is unable to excrete sufficient hydrgen ions to lower the urinary pH below 6. This mechanism is responsible for the classical or distal RTA (type 1). In this type giving an ammonium chloride load fails to depress urinary pH below 6.0 and the excretion rates of ammonium and titratable acid are reduced. In the other mechanism, operative in proximal renal tubular acidosis (type 2) the proximal tubule is unable to conserve filtered bicarbonate adequately or in other words there is bicarbonate wastage. In this type 2 RTA the response to ammonium chloride loading test is normal. Type 3 is a mixture of distal and proximal RTA and type 4 is associated with a deficiency of aldosterone production or resistance to its action (pseudohypoaldosteronism).

Distal Renal Tubular Acidosis (Type 1 RTA)

Primary distal renal tubular acidosis is usually sporadic but can be inherited as an autosomal dominant trait.

The classical disorder occurs more frequently in girls and usually presents after the age of 2 years with polyuria and polydipsia. Muscular weakness and flaccid paralysis may result from hypokalaemia. Often the initial manifestation of the disease is growth failure.

Laboratory findings consist of hyperchloraemic metabolic acidosis, failure of urinary pH to fall below 6 even in the presence of severe metabolic acidosis. Renal potassium loss is reflected in the persistent hypokalaemia.

Secondary distal renal tubular acidosis can occur in children with vitamin D intoxication, obstructive uropathy, medullary sponge kidney, Marfan syndrome and after renal transplantation.

Treatment

Treatment is aimed at correcting the metabolic acidosis by using sodium bicarbonate 1-3 mmol/kg/d. Potassium supplementation may also be required to correct the hypokalaemia.Striking improvement in growth can be expected with this regimen.

Proximal Renal Tubular Acidosis (Type 2)

The primary and secondary forms of proximal renal tubular acidosis are rare, therefore they will not be discussed in this chapter.

ENURESIS

Enuresis refers to the persistent involuntary or inappropriate voiding of urine. This can occur while the child is asleep (nocturnal) or in the daytime (diurnal). The disorder may have been - primary or come on at a later stage - secondary. Primary (continuous) enuresis is the sleep wetter who has never been dry for extended periods. Whilst secondary enuresis is the onset of wetting after a continuous dry period of at least 6 months.

Nocturnal enuresis is a commonly occurring disorder which affects approximately 10% of children at the age of 5 and 5% at the age of 10 years with 1 or 2% continuing to wet throughout the teens. Enuresis is seen world-wide in all cultures and races. It is crucial that parents understand that the child is not wetting the bed on purpose and that the enuresis is not voluntary.

Nocturnal enuresis is not primarily a child psychiatric problem and it occurs with similar prevalence as all the rest of the psychiatric disorders put together. There is frequently a family history and it is usually a mono-symptom with family discord and emotional factors being secondary to the inconvenient and undesirable symptom. There is an increased incidence of wetting amongst populations of children with child psychiatric problems, but the correlation is not with any specific disorder. While it is assumed enuresis is associated with anxiety, it more often occurs in children in poor social circumstances where early training has not been established. Some children have had disturbing life events at the time when night-time bladder control should be acquired and the symptom is more frequent in children with other developmental delays and with encopresis, one mechanism being that the faecal impaction fills the space occupying the pelvis and presses on the bladder neck, giving rise to incomplete voiding of urine.

Associated urinary tract problems and other medical problems are unusual but should be kept in mind when a new case is seen. Structural anomalies such as reflux into mega-ureters are associated with incomplete bladder emptying and a reduction in the amount of urine voided at any time. Although it is easy to test for urinary tract infections, most children with urinary tract infections do not bed-wet and most bed-wetters are not infected. Children with mono-symptomatic nocturnal enuresis are unlikely to have an organic cause. The physical examination results in almost all children with nocturnal enuresis are completely normal. However urine should be tested both biochemically and bacteriologically.

Key Learning Point

Children with mono-symptomatic nocturnal enuresis are unlikely to have an organic cause.

Treatment

Treating enuresis can be frustrating for the parents, the child and the paediatrician. Parents should be firmly reassured that the problem of bed-wetting may resolve with time and that these children are not at fault for wet episodes. Treatment is not appropriate in children under 5 years and it is usually not needed in those aged 7 years and in cases where the child and parents are not anxious about the bed wetting. Drug therapy is not usually appropriate for children under 7 years of age. However it can be used on a short-term basis, for example, to cover periods away from home.

Tricyclic anti-depressants such as imipramine, amitiptyline and less often nortriptyline are used but behaviour disturbances may occur and relapse is common after withdrawal. Treatment should not normally exceed 3 months and toxicity following overdosage with tricyclics is of particular concern.

Antidiuretic hormone, in the form of desmopressin is available as a nasal spray or it may be given by mouth as tablets. The initial recommended dose of the nasal spray is 20 µg, one 10 µg spray per nostril. The starting dose for the tablet is one 0.2 mg tablet by mouth before bedtime. Particular care is needed to avoid fluid overload and treatment should not be continued for longer than 3 months without stopping it for a week for full reassessment.

The most effective treatment is the pad and buzzer—an enuresis bell, for well motivated children aged over 7 years. Great care is needed in securing the cooperation of the child, the parents and the siblings. The alarm initially acts as a stimulus that awakens the child when micturition occurs. Ideally the child then awakens, inhibits voiding, gets out of bed, and goes to toilet to complete voiding. With time the alarm creates a conditional response in which the physiologic stimuli that cause micturition cause inhibition of voiding and awakening. Attention to detail is important so that false alarms caused by inadequate cleaning of the pad, excess sweating or the pad folding over on itself should be avoided. If there is no response after 3 months, it is better to withdraw the enuresis bell. It has been reported that between 40-70% children respond to this device. Also use of an alarm may be combined with drug therapy if either method alone is unsuccessful.

The simple technique of "lifting" a child when the parents go to bed sometimes solves the problem at a practical level. The use of star charts should be reserved for those children who wish to fill them in. All too often there is an expectation that the star chart will work and if it does not there is loss of face for the child, the parent or the doctor.

Therefore a set treatment package for enuretic children should be avoided. It is essential to check out the feelings, attitudes and family relationships before deciding whether a family therapy or psychodynamic approach is needed before using the pad and bell technique.

CASE STUDY

An 8-year-old boy presented with a history of bed-wetting for 2 years. There was no.history of daytime wetting. His father used to wet his bed but stopped wetting at the age of 12 years. On examination no positive finding was detected, in particular examination of lumbo-sacral spine, lower limbs and perineum was normal.

Urine was clear both biochemically and bacteriologically. Urine concentrating ability normal.

He did not respond to oral desmopressin 200 micrograms at bedtime daily for 3 months. However, he responded to an enuresis alarm after being on it for 2 months. His wetting did not return when seen for review 6 months later.

Diagnosis: Secondary nocturnal enuresis.

HAEMOLYTIC URAEMIC SYNDROME (D+HUS, D-HUS)

Haemolytic uraemic syndrome is much commoner in infants and children than in adults. Also this condition accounts for most children with primary acute renal failure requiring specialist renal care. The cascade leading from gastrointestinal infection to renal impairment is complex. It is characterised by the triad of microangiopathic haemolytic anaemia, thrombocytopenia and acute renal failure. There are two subtypes of HUS. The first is associated with diarrhoeal prodrome (D+HUS) and the second is not associated with antecedent diarrhoea (D-HUS).

The association between haemolytic uraemic syndrome (D+HUS) and enteric *E.coli* type 0157:H7 shows that this is the type responsible for HUS. It produces cytotoxin active or vero-cells called "vertoxin". It is usually transmitted by ingestion of contaminated food or water and by person to person contact. Also the association of shigellosis with HUS is well established. However, the incidence of HUS in India has declined with the decline in the virulent form of shigella dysentery.

The D-HUS is much rarer in childhood. The D-HUS is atypical, seen in older children and can be familial, drug induced or recurrent.

Clinical Features

It is characterised by abdominal cramps, watery diarrhoea changing to bloody diarrhoea, vomiting, pallor and is frequently accompanied by convulsions. Oliguria is constantly present but not always appreciated. Hypertension may be severe. The blood shows a severe anaemia, thrombocytopenia and reticulocytosis. Some of the red cells are characteristically misshapen—acanthocytes—burr cells—triangular cells and others with a "broken eggshell" shape are common. The blood urea is greatly elevated. The urine shows protein, red cells and granular casts. Proteinuria is in the non-nephrotic range (1-2 g/d). It has been recognised that in many of these cases sequential studies of the circulating clotting factors will show evidence of a consumptive coagulopathy due to disseminated intravascular coagulation (DIC).

Prognosis of HUS

In children with HUS the complete recovery rate is about 70%, but a small number die in the acute stage of the illness; some die without recovering renal function after weeks on dialysis and other children left with hypertension and chronic renal failure. In children who develop end-stage renal disease successful renal transplantation has been reported.

Treatment

In D+HUS, no specific therapy has been beneficial. There is no benefit from anticoagulant or throbolytic therapy nor from IV prostacyclin, steroids or gammaglobulins. The mainstay of treatment for children with HUS is the management of acute renal failure (ARF).

Prevention

The only way to prevent HUS is to prevent primary infection by developing efficient human and animal reservoir strategies, i.e. control and improvement of food safety procedures.

ACUTE RENAL FAILURE

Acute renal failure is defined to describe a precipitous deterioration in renal function. The hallmark of acute renal failure is progressive rise in plasma creatinine and urea due to accumulation of nitrogenous waste products of metabolism. The metabolic derangements include metabolic acidosis and hyperkalaemia, and disturbances of body fluid balance, especially volume overload and variety of effects on almost every organ of the body. Oliguria or anuria is the cardinal feature (see Box 17.7).

BOX 17.7: Definition of ARF

Oliguria-urine output: $<300/m^2/day$ or 0.5 ml/kg/hr

Anuria – urine output: < 1 ml/kg/day

Hypekalaemia – potassium > 6.0 mmol/L

Clinical fluid overload

Oedema

Hypertension

Aetiology

The causes of acute renal failure may be divided into three sub-groups as outlined in Table 17.4.
1. Pre-renal
2. Intrinsic renal
3. Post-renal

The causes of ARF in developing countries differ from those in developed countries and there are also other regional variations. Post-dysenteric HUS used to be the most common cause of ARF in the Indian sub-continent

Table 17.4: Causes of acute renal failure

1. Pre-renal
   Gastroenteritis, blood loss, insensible losses, burns, sepsis, anaphylaxis, diabetic ketoacidosis
2. Intrinsic renal failure
   a. Vascular: renal vein thrombosis, HUS, HSP, SLE
   b. Glomerular: post-streptococcal glomerulonephritis
   c. Acute tubular necrosis: intravascular haemolysis in G6PD deficiency, sepsis, snake-bite, falciparum malaria, leptospirosis
3. Post-renal
   a. Renal calculi
   b. Neurogenic bladder
   c. Posterior urethral valves
   d. Ureterocele

during the 1970s to 1980s, but its incidence has now decreased. Also stings by poisonous scorpions, wasps and bees may occasionally lead to ARF.

Clinical Evaluation of a Child with ARF

In evaluating a child with acute renal failure the clinical history, physical examination and laboratory tests should give some clues to the cause of ARF. It is essential to exclude both pre-renal and post-renal causes before considering the intrinsic renal causes.

Pre-renal ARF should be suspected when there is a history of diarrhoea, vomiting, fluid or blood loss. Acute gastroenteritis with dehydration and shock is the most common cause of pre-renal failure. It is typically associated with high plasma urea to creatinine ratio, increased urine osmolality (>500 mOsm/kg), urinary sodium concentration < 20 mEq/l and fractional excretion of sodium less than 1%. The intrinsic renal parenchymal disorder can often be diagnosed by microscopic urinalysis and extrarenal manifestations of multisystem disease. Also in intrinsic ARF the urinary sodium is high (>40 mEq/L), urinary osmolality is low (< 300 mOs/kg) and fractional excretion of sodium is more than 1%. Ultrasonography is the ideal imaging tool in renal failure because of its non-dependence on renal function. It allows visualisation of structural anomalies, pelvicalyceal system, assessment of renal size and calculi, thus help to ascertain as to whether ARF is post-renal.

Key Learning Point

Acute renal failure
Falciparum malaria, leptospirosis and snake-bite are important causes of ARF in India and in some other Asian countries.

MANAGEMENT OF ACUTE RENAL FAILURE

Fluid Therapy

As a rule of thumb fluid therapy should equal insensible fluid losses plus output (urine, vomiting, diarrhoea, etc.). Potassium containing fluids should not be given.

Hyponatraemia

Hyponatraemia is the common finding in children with ARF, and is most frequently secondary to water excess rather than sodium loss. If doubt exists, it is safer to restrict water intake until the cause becomes clear. Profound hyponatraemia (plasma sodium < 120 mmol/L) may cause neurological problems. Therefore correction of hypo-natraemia to a sodium level of around 125 mmol/L should be considered. Also consider Dialysis.

Hyperkalaemia

Hyperkalaemia is the most serious problem associated with ARF and causes cardiac dysfunction which may lead to death of the patient. Hyperkalaemia arises from the inability to excrete potassium in the urine and is worse in the presence of an acidosis. Potassium intake must be minimised and correction of acidosis undertaken. If ECG changes are present, or if serum potassium rises above 7 mmol/L then emergency treatment is indicated i.e. 10% calcium gluconate 0.5-1 ml/kg by slow IV infusion over 5-10 minutes to reduce the toxic effect of high potassium on the heart.

The choice of potassium lowering agent remains a matter of personal choice. Many favour the use of nebulised salbutamol as it acts by moving potassium from the extracellular into the intracellular space. Also calcium resonium 1 g/kg can be given orally or rectally to expedite the elimination of potassium from the body. However, the onset of action is relatively slow and has a very limited role in the management of hyperkalaemia associated with ARF. Also consider Dialysis.

Hypocalcaemia

Hypocalcaemia is quite common in ARF but it rarely causes symptoms. If symptomatic then calcium can be given by slow intravenous infusion of 10% calcium gluconate 0.5 ml/kg/hr. The infusion rate being titrated according to the blood calcium level. If resistant check Mg.

Hyperphosphataemia

Phosphate restriction and phosphate binders, e.g. calcium carbonate should help to deal with this problem.

Metabolic Acidosis

Metabolic acidosis is a uniform and early accompaniment in this condition because of the important role of the kidneys in regulating and maintaining normal body homeostasis. When acidosis is present it should be treated with sodium bicarbonate. Intravenous 8.4% sodium bicarbonate 1-2 ml/kg equivalent to 1-2 mmol/kg should be administered where blood pH values are less than 7.25. Adequacy of pH correction should be monitored by regular measurement of blood gases. Rapid correction of acidosis may cause hypocalcaemia and tetany or seizures. Therefore rapid correction should be avoided.

Anaemia in ARF

Mild to moderate anaemia is often present in ARF. Anaemia, when present to a significant degree, may potentiate the complications, especially cardiac failure, and may be beneficial to correct by small transfusions of recently collected packed red cells.

Hypertension

Severe symptomatic hypertension can occur in association with salt and water overload. Treatment of hypertension mainly consists of restriction of fluid and sodium intake and anti-hypertensive therapy. It is vital that it is adequately controlled.

Infection in ARF

Infection is a most serious complication and every effort must be made to prevent it and to treat it if it develops.

Nutrition in ARF

Acute renal failure is a hypercatabolic state and requires aggressive nutritional support. The aim of dietary treatment is:
- Control of dietary potassium
- Control of dietary sodium
- Control of dietary phosphate
- To tailor fluid intake to maintain fluid balance
- Vitamin and micronutrient supplements

Peritoneal Dialysis or Haemodialysis

Acute peritoneal dialysis (PD) is frequently indicated and may be life saving. Although acute PD is the preferred choice for children, but if complications occur with PD, then haemodialysis may be necessary. In patients with multi-organ failure, haemofiltration may be required.

CHRONIC RENAL FAILURE (CRF)

Chronic renal failure (CRF) is defined, if the glomerular filtration rate (GFR) is less than 50 ml/minute/1.73 m² surface area. This means that there is moderate to severe renal impairment leading to metabolic abnormalities i.e. secondary hyperparathyroidism and growth impairment. In course of time there will be further deterioration of renal function. However, renal replacement therapy either by dialysis or renal transplantation will not be needed until the GFR falls below 10 ml/minute/1.73 m² surface area. The initiation of renal replacement therapy marks the onset of end-stage renal disease. The causes of CRF are shown in Table 17.5.

Table 17.5: Causes of chronic renal failure in children

1. Congenital abnormalities
   - Aplasia, hypoplasia, obstructive uropathy, reflux nephropathy, Prune belly syndrome
2. Hereditary conditions
   - Juvenile polycystic kidney disease, cystinosis, congenital nephrotic syndrome, hereditary nephritis
3. Glomerulonephritis
   - Multisystem disease: SLE, HSP, HUS
4. Miscellaneous
   - Renal vascular disease

Clinical Presentation

Children with CRF present in a variety of ways. It could be related to the primary renal disease or as a result of impaired renal function. The history and clinical examination may provide useful information to the underlying cause of CRF, but in some children the cause will only be revealed by specific investigations.

Management

Nutrition

Poor growth and nutritional status are common in children with CRF. Children with CRF tend to be anorexic and may have their energy intakes below the estimated average requirement for age. Therefore nutritional therapy should be instituted to promote improved well being and growth.

Fluid and Electrolyte Balance

Water intake is determined by the child and should therefore be offered freely to satisfy thirst. Some children may need sodium chloride intake of 4-6 mmol/kg/d for their normal physical and intellectual development while others may need their sodium intake reduced. Most children with CRF are able to maintain potassium homeostasis satisfactorily despite fluctuations in intake.

Acid-base Status

Sodium bicarbonate supplement in a dose of 2 mmol/kg/d is frequently required to correct metabolic acidosis. Treatment should be monitored and dosage adjusted according to blood gas measurements of pH and bicarbonate concentration.

Renal Osteodystrophy or Renal Bone Disease

Vitamin D requires hydroxylation, by the kidney and liver to its active form therefore the hydroxylated derivative alfacalcidol or calcitriol should be prescribed for children with CRF. Alfacalcidol is generally preferred in children as there is more experience of its use and appropriate formulations are available.

Hypertension

If the child's systolic or diastolic blood pressure is repeatedly in excess of the 90th centile for age, it should be treated with anti-hypertensive therapy.

Infection

Urinary tract infection or any other bacterial infection should be treated appropriately.

Anaemia

CRF is associated with normochromic normocytic anaemia due to inadequate erythropoietin production. Recombinant human erythropoietin is available, is safe and is effective in treating anaemia in children with CRF. The clinical efficacy of epoetin alfa and epoetin beta is similar.

Growth

Growth retardation is a common problem in children with CRF. If, despite optimal management, growth remains poor i.e. the child's height velocity is below minus 2SD, a trial of.synthetic human growth hormone, somatropin, produced using recombinant DNA technology should be considered.

Management of end-Stage Renal Failure

Successful renal transplantation is the treatment of choice, for all children with end-stage renal failure. There is a choice between living-related kidney donation and cadaveric transplantation. Living donor transplantation avoids an unpredictable long wait for a suitable cadaveric graft and facilitates pre-emptive transplantation. Dialysis should be seen as a complement to transplantation which may be needed before or between transplants but not an alternative to transplantation. However, dialysis is the only active treatment available for infants with end-stage renal failure, since transplantation is not usually undertaken in children weighing less than 10 kg.

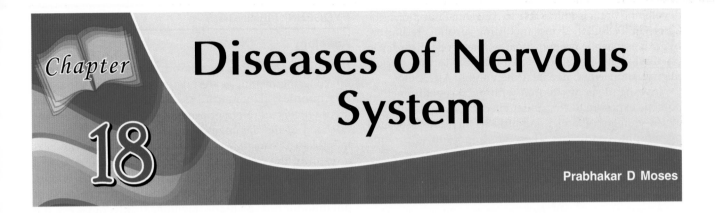

Chapter 18

Diseases of Nervous System

Prabhakar D Moses

Diseases of the nervous system contribute to a significant proportion of childhood morbidity and mortality and consequently considerable parental anxiety. Precise and prompt diagnosis helps in cure, limiting disability and proper counselling. This chapter focuses on the common neurological disorders seen in childhood and comprises the following sections.

- Congenital malformations of CNS
- CNS infections
- Acute hemiplegia in childhood
- Acute cerebellar ataxia
- Acute flaccid paralysis
- Neurocutaneous syndrome
- Neurodegenerative disease
- Neuromuscular disorders
- Autonomic nervous system
- Convulsions in infancy and childhood
- Cerebral palsy
- Learning disorders.

CONGENITAL MALFORMATIONS OF CNS

The common congenital anomalies of the central nervous system are neural tube closure defects, hydrocephalus, failure of development of part of brain (aplasia or hyperplasic) and neuronal migration defects.

(Section on neural tube closure defects and hydro-cephalus: See chapter 10 on Neonatal Surgery).

MICROCEPHALY

Microcephaly is due to failure of normal brain growth and is defined as a head circumference that is more than three standard deviations below the mean for age and gender. Microcephaly can be divided into primary and secondary types.

Primary Microcephaly

Primary microcephaly is frequently genetically determined (autosomal recessive) and may be familial. Apart from its smallness the head has a characteristic shape with narrow forehead, slanting frontoparietal areas, pointed vertex and flat occiput. The ears are often large and abnormally formed. Generalised muscular hyper tonicity is a common feature. Convulsions frequently develop. These children have profound learning disorder (Fig. 18.1).

Primary microcephaly is also associated with recognisable malformation syndromes in particular chromosomal anomalies like trisomy 21, 18 and 13, and non-chromosomal syndromes such as Cornelia de Lange syndrome.

Secondary Microcephaly

Secondary microcephaly results from severe brain damage during pregnancy or the first 2 years of postnatal life. The

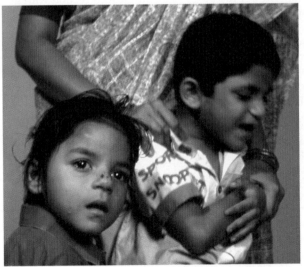

Fig. 18.1: Familial microcephaly with mental retardation.

developing brain is vulnerable to congenital infections (the acronym TORCH), drugs including alcohol, radiation, hypoxic-ischaemic encephalopathy, metabolic disorder in particular maternal diabetes and maternal hyper-phenylalaninaemia, neonatal meningitis, AIDS, etc.

Investigations of children with microcephaly include possible exposure to congenital infection, drugs, radiation, etc, assessment of family and birth history and associated dysmorphic conditions. These are important to provide genetic and family counselling.

CRANIOSYNOSTOSIS

Craniosynostosis results from premature fusion of single or multiple cranial sutures leading to deformity of skull and face. The cause of craniosynostosis is unknown but is due to abnormality of skull development. Craniosynostosis can occur isolated or as part of genetic syndromes like Crouzon's disease, Apert's syndrome and Carpenter's syndrome. Mutations of the fibroblast growth factor receptor gene family have been shown to be associated with craniosynostosis. Clinical features include abnormal asymmetric craniofacial appearance, sutural ridging and premature closure of fontanelles. In sagittal synostosis lateral growth of skull is restricted, resulting in a long narrow head (scaphocephaly). In coronal synostosis expansion occurs in a superior and lateral direction (brachycephaly). This produces shallow orbits and hypertelorism. Involvement of several sutures results in skull expansion towards the vertex (oxycephaly). Frontal plagiocephaly is characterized by unilateral flattering of forehead. Neurological complications include raised intracranial pressure, hydrocephalus, proptosis, optic atrophy and deafness. The diagnosis can be confirmed by plain skull X-ray or CT scan. Surgical correction with good outcome is possible.

INFECTION OF THE NERVOUS SYSTEM

Infections of the nervous systems particularly meningitis form a significant proportion of serious infection in childhood.

Acute bacterial meningitis
Aseptic meningitis
Tuberculous meningitis
Viral encephalitis.
Brain abscess
Neurocysticercosis

The common types of meningitis are pyogenic, tuberculous and aseptic. Rare forms are mycotic (torulosis, nocardiosis, cryptococcal, histoplasmosis), syphilitic and protozoal (malaria and toxoplasmosis).

PYOGENIC MENINGITIS

Aetiology

Excluding the neonatal period the common bacteria infecting the meninges are pneumococcus (Streptococcus pneumonia), Haemophilus influenza type b and meningococcus (Neisseria meningitidis). Haemophilus infection of the meninges is most common in children 2 months to 3 years of age. The incidence has come down as a result of the conjugated *H.influenzae* vaccine. The next most common meningeal infection is due to pneumococcus; this may be secondary to upper respiratory infection or pneumonia but 'primary' meningeal infections are not uncommon. In infants and children meningococcal meningitis is usually sporadic but epidemics can occur. The disease is seen most commonly in the late winter and early spring. In infants both staphylococcal and streptococcal meningitis are occasionally seen, most often secondary to infection elsewhere, e.g. bone, skin, middle ear or lungs. A meningomyelocoele, congenital or acquired CSF leak across cribriform plate, middle and inner ear and compound fractures of the skull may also act as portals of entry. In immunosuppressed children and in patients undergoing neurosurgical procedures, including ventri-culoperitoneal shunts, meningitis can be caused by a variety of bacteria such as Staphylococcus, Enterococcus and *Pseudomonas aeruginosa*.

Clinical Features

Symptomatology is common to all types of bacterial meningitis and the causal organism is most often determined by examination of the cerebrospinal fluid. There are a few characteristic signs peculiar to meningo-coccal infections. The important one from the diagnostic point of view is a generalised purpuric rash although this is seen only in a minority of cases. It is also characteristic of meningococcal meningitis to develop suddenly and unheralded, whereas there is usually a preceding history of respiratory infection in cases due to Heamophilus or Penumococcus.

The onset of bacterial meningitis is usually sudden with high fever, irritability, refusal of feeds, vomiting, headache in older children and general malaise. Convulsions are common. Young infants show a tense bulging anterior fontanelle, indicative of increased intracranial pressure, and head retraction is common. The older the child the more likely is there to be nuchal rigidity, but its absence in the baby by no means excludes the diagnosis. Kernig's sign is useful in older children and may not be observed in infants. Blurring of consciousness of varying degree is the rule and increases in severity as the disease progresses. Hypertonia and decerebrate posturing may be seen in late cases. Focal neurological abnormalities such as paralytic squints, facial palsy or haemiplegia sometimes develop. Deafness due to damage to the auditory nerve may be permanent. Papilloedema is infrequently found.

In infants the disease sometimes has a more insidious onset with diarrhoea and vomiting, irritability and "bogginess" of the anterior fontanelle. The diagnosis is easily missed unless a high index of suspicion is maintained.

Diagnosis

Lumbar puncture is indicated whenever the possibility of meningitis has crossed the physician's mind and normally treatment should not be started before CSF has been obtained. However, it is reasonable to give intramuscular benzylpenicillin 250,000 units before transfer to hospital or lumbar puncture in a child suspected to have meningococcal meningitis by virtue of the characteristic purpuric or petechial rash seen in meningococcal infection. In pyogenic meningitis the cerebrospinal fluid will be turbid or frankly purulent. The white cell count may be in thousands/mm^3, the majority being polymorphs. The protein content of the fluid is raised (above 0.4g/l; 40 mg/100 ml) and the glucose is greatly reduced (below 2.5 mmol/L; 45 mg/100 ml). Gram stain films of the centrifuged deposit may reveal Gram-positive diplococci, often very numerous, in pneumococcal infection, Gram-negative pleomorphic coccobacilli in haemophilus infection and Gram-negative intra and extracellular diplococci in meningococcal infection. Rapid identification of bacterial antigen in CSF can be obtained by use of latex agglutination test. The final cause is determined by CSF culture but this may be sterile if prior antibiotic had been administered.

Complication and Sequelae

In the acute stage, raised intracranial pressure due to cerebral oedema, subdural effusion or hydrocephalus may develop. Electrolyte imbalances particularly hyponatraemia may occur as also anaemia. Recurrent convulsions including status epilepticus can further damage the brain. Permanent brain damage with motor and learning deficits are more common in infants, in part due to the greater difficulty and delay in diagnosis. Symptomatic epilepsy is less common. Nerve deafness can develop early in the illness and unpredictably.

Treatment

Bacterial meningitis ought rarely to be fatal today. Management of bacterial meningitis encompasses many aspects of treatment including antibiotics, correction of fluid and electrolyte imbalances, anticonvulsant medi-

Table18.1: Antibiotic therapy in children with bacterial meningitis		
Age Group	*Drug (IV)*	*Dose Per Day*
Infants 1-3 months	Ampicillin and Cefotaxime	200 mg/kg/day in 4 doses 200 mg/kg/day in 4 doses
Older infants and children	1 Cefotaxime or Ceftriaxone	200 mg/kg/day in 4 doses 100 mg/kg/day in single dose
	2 Ampicillin and Chloramphenicol	200 mg/kg/day in 4 doses 75-100 mg/kg/day in 4 doses
	3 Benzylpenicillin	400,000 units/kg/day in 4-6 doses

cation, anti-cerebral oedema measures and possibly dexamethasone therapy.

The major factor in selecting antibiotic therapy for children with bacterial meningitis is the continually changing pattern of antibiotic resistance. Therefore knowledge of local susceptibility patterns is essential. Antibiotic therapy should eventually be aimed against the specific organism causing the meningitis but initial therapy is directed against all usual bacterial pathogens for the age group of the patient. The recommended antibiotics schedule for initial treatment of bacterial meningitis in different age groups is as shown in Table 18.1.

Currently a minimum of 10 days of antibiotic treatment or for 5 afebrile days whichever is longer is recommended. It has been demonstrated that intravenous dexamethasone used as an adjunctive therapeutic agent in dosage of 0.6 mg/kg/day in 4 doses for 4 days is responsible for a significantly lower incidence of neurological sequelae including hearing impairment.

Anti-cerebral oedema measures include restriction of fluid intake to two-thirds of the normal requirement, use of isotonic intravenous solution and at times intravenous mannitol. Convulsions are best controlled with intravenous midazolam, lorazepam or diazepam. Recurrence of seizures is prevented by IV phenytoin.

When treatment is adequate a prompt improvement can usually be expected with a subsidence of fever within 48-96 hours. If fever persists with continuing irritability, bulging of the fontanelle, focal seizures and at times focal deficits, the presence of a subdural effusion should be suspected. This is most commonly encountered in infants with meningitis due to Haemophilus. Cranial ultrasound examination will be helpful to confirm the diagnosis. Subdural taps should be done through the coronal sutures on both sides. The subdural fluid is xanthochromic and protein rich. Repeated subdural taps may be required before the accumulation stops. Routine lumbar puncture at the completion of antibiotic therapy is not advised. Anaemia may have to be corrected by blood transfusion. The child with meningitis requires a high standard of professional nursing.

THE WATERHOUSE-FRIDERICHSEN SYNDROME

This is due to acute bilateral adrenal haemorrhage seen most commonly in fulminating cases of meningococcal septicaemia. Death occurs usually before the meningitis has had time to develop, and may, in fact, take place after an illness of only a few hours' duration. The characteristic clinical picture is seen in an infant who suddenly becomes ill with irritability, vomiting and diarrhoea and tachypnoea or Cheyne-Stokes breathing. The heart rate is very rapid. The infant becomes rapidly drowsy/unconscious. Peripheral cyanosis is associated frequently with a patchy purple mottling of the skin, which resembles post-mortem lividity. The child may die at this stage, about 6-8 hours from the onset of the illness. In less fulminating cases a diffuse purpuric and ecchymotic eruption appears which is very characteristic of meningococcal septicaemia. The blood pressure may be so low as to be unrecordable. In the toddler the course of the illness tends on the whole to be less rapid than in the infant. The meningococcus is not always successfully isolated in blood cultures but can sometimes be cultured from the fluid contents of purpuric blebs on the skin. Disseminated intravascular coagulation may also develop in fulminating cases of meningococcal septicaemia and should always be sought by appropriate laboratory tests. Full blood count with platelet count, blood film for fragmentation of red cells, clotting screen including fibrinogen levels, FDPs or D dimers.

Treatment

In cases where the adrenal cortex has been destroyed by haemorrhage, recovery is impossible. In some cases of fulminating meningococcal septicaemia, however, there is intense congestion of the adrenal glands without much haemorrhage. It is in these cases, which are clinically indistinguishable from the fully developed Waterhouse-Friderichsen syndrome, that energetic treatment can save life and lead to complete recovery. A continuous intravenous infusion of 5% dextrose in 0.18% saline should be commenced. Penicillin should be given by direct injection in the dosage mentioned above. Hydrocortisone hemisuccinate 100 mg should be injected intravenously via the infusion at the start of treatment, to be followed by 50 mg 6-hourly for 24-48 hours; thereafter-decreasing doses of prednisolone are given orally for another few days.

Prevention of Bacterial Meningitis

Routine immunisation of infants with conjugated Haemophilus influenzae type b vaccine is recommended. For close contacts of children with Haemophilus influenzae and meningococcal meningitis, chemoprophylaxis with rifampicin at a dosage of 20 mg/kg/day for 2-4 days is advised.

ASEPTIC MENINGITIS

Definition

Aseptic meningitis refers to mostly viral meningitis as well as other forms of meningitis where Gram stain and routine bacterial culture reveal no organisms.

Sporadic cases occur throughout the year, and from time to time sizeable epidemics occur. Hospital based studies looking at the different aetiologies of childhood meningitis have found that aseptic meningitis is 2-3 times more common than bacterial meningitis; also pyogenic meningitis is more common in younger children whereas aseptic meningitis is seen across all age groups.

Aetiology

Many viruses can cause aseptic meningitis. These include enteroviruses (particularly Coxsackie and ECHO viruses), viruses of mumps, measles, Herpes simplex and Herpes zoster, the mouse virus of lymphocytic choriomeningitis and Epstein-Barr virus. Mumps virus can cause aseptic meningitis without any of the other manifestations of this disease. Coxsackie virus can cause meningitis and paralysis, which is indistinguishable clinically from classical poliomyelitis. Non-viral agents, which can cause aseptic meningitis, include Leptospira (icterohaemorrhagiae and canicola), Treponema pallidum, Toxoplasma gondii and Trichinella spiralis.

Clinical Features

The onset is usually sudden with fever, headache, neck pain, vomiting, malaise, diarrhoea or constipation. In some cases, especially of poliomyelitis there is a preceding illness about 1 week earlier with fever, headache, malaise, sore throat and abdominal pain. The temperature chart in such cases shows two "humps", sometimes called "the dromedary chart". The child may be drowsy, apathetic and irritable when disturbed, but marked blurring of consciousness is uncommon. Slight nuchal rigidity is usually found. In the infant the anterior fontanalle may be tense and full. Compared to bacterial meningitis, meningeal signs and focal seizures are less common in aseptic meningitis. Exanthem may precede or accompany the CNS signs.

Diagnosis

The cerebrospinal fluid is clear or only slightly hazy. The cell count varies from 50 to 1000/ mm^3 (may be higher in lymphocytic choriomeningitis) with lymphocytic predominance. The glucose content is normal but the protein content is moderately elevated (50-200mg/100ml). The culture remains sterile. The main differential diagnosis is partially treated pyogenic meningitis. CSF bacterial antigen detection test can be helpful. The causative virus can be identified in the stools. The serum (at least two specimens taken within a 10-day interval) may be tested for neutralizing antibody or complement fixation in rising titre. Identification of the viral DNA after PCR amplification in CSF is now possible but may give false positive result.

Treatment

In the great majority spontaneous recovery occurs. Symptomatic measures to relieve fever, headache or muscle pain are required. Specific treatment is available only for Herpes simplex infection (Acyclovir).

ACUTE ENCEPHALITIS AND ENCEPHALOPATHY

The term encephalitis denotes infection affecting the brain substance. The term encephalopathy is used to describe functional disturbances of the brain without actual infection of the brain.

Aetiology

All of the viruses mentioned in connection with the aseptic meningitis can cause acute encephalitis. Others include arbo viruses like Japanese encephalitis virus, influenza virus, cytomegalic inclusion disease in infancy, and the viruses of rabies, HIV, encephalitis lethargica and the zymotic diseases such as measles and varicella. Special mention must be made of Herpes simplex virus (HSV). In the newborn infant HSV type 2 can cause a disseminated infection involving many tissues with a grave prognosis. In the older children Herpes simplex virus type 1 infection of the brain causes acute necrotising encephalitis affecting particularly the temporal lobe.

In the Indian subcontinent, Japanese encephalitis transmitted by Culex mosquito is common, often in epidemic form, during the monsoon season.

Clinical Features

These are extremely protean. The onset of the illness is usually acute and a prodromal stage with general malaise, fever, headache and vomiting often precedes signs of CNS involvement. The acute encephalitic stage may show varying disturbances of cerebration from the gradual onset of stupor or coma to the sudden onset of violent convulsions. Headache, fever, irritability, mental confusion, abnormal behaviour, and seizures may be marked. Focal neurological signs of many kinds are encountered such as cranial nerve palsies, speech disturbances, spastic palsies, cerebellar disturbances and abnormalities in the various reflexes. In cases of acute necrotising encephalitis caused by herpes virus type 1, in addition to the clinical manifestation described above, some cases have had neurological signs suggestive of an expanding lesion in the brain, particularly in the temporal lobe.

The outcome is always doubtful in every case of encephalitis and especially grave in acute necrotising encephalitis. Death is not uncommon. The case fatality rate in Japanese encephalitis has varied between 25 and 45 percent. Although complete recovery is possible, many are left with permanent disability such as mental deterioration, hemiplegia or paraplegia, and epilepsy. In some children an apparently good recovery is followed later by learning difficulties or behaviour problems.

Diagnosis

The diagnosis is usually made on clinical grounds supported by CSF analysis, which shows a mild pleocytosis and increase in protein. EEG typically shows diffuse slow-wave abnormalities. Focal findings and Periodic Lateralised Epileptiform Discharges (PLEDS) on EEG or CT or MRI, especially involving the temporal lobes, suggest HSV encephalitis. Virological studies are often successful in determining the causal agent.

Treatment

With the exception of herpes encephalitis, treatment of other viral encephalitis is essentially supportive and consists of control of hyperpyrexia and convulsion, reduction of raised intracranial pressure, and expert nursing, the latter being of utmost importance. Convulsions must be controlled with intravenous midazolam or diazepam or phenytoin. A clear airway must be ensured by proper positioning and frequent pharyngeal suction. Rarely, tracheal intubation and mechanical ventilation may be required. Frequently, tube feeding or intravenous fluids are indicated. Patients should be monitored for signs of raised intracranial pressure and managed appropriately. Fluid and electrolyte balance must be maintained. Distension of the bladder must be anticipated and controlled by an in-dwelling catheter.

For HSV encephalitis, intravenous acyclovir is given in a dose of 10 mg/kg every 8 hours for 10 days. During the convalescent stage physiotherapy, occupational therapy and rehabilitation treatment are important.

In addition to the viral encephalitis, which may occur, early in the infectious fever such as measles, rubella and chickenpox, an encephalitic illness of later onset may occur during the period of recovery. This is characterised histologically by extensive demyelination in the brain substance and the pathogenesis is probably a vasculopathy mediated by immune complexes with lesions occurring in central nervous tissue myelin. This is known as post-infectious or acute disseminated encephalomyelitis (ADEM).

Sclerosing Panencephalitis

There is yet another type of encephalitis produced by measles virus which develops some years after apparent recovery from the measles illness itself. The disease is called subacute sclerosing panencephalitis (SSPE). Histologically the disease is characterized by intranuclear inclusions, and under the electron microscopy these are seen to contain tubular structures typical of the nucleocapsids of paramyxoviruses. Measles antigen has also been demonstrated in the brain by fluorescent antibody techniques and measles virus itself has been isolated from brain tissue of patients with SSPE. The initial attack of measles usually antedates the onset of encephalitic manifestation by several years. Infection with measles during infancy seems to increase the risk of SSPE. The disease has also been reported to follow immunisation with live measles virus vaccine but the risk is very much less than with wild measles virus infection. Viral mutation, abnormal immune response to measles virus or subtle predisposing immune deficiency has been proposed to explain the persistent measles virus infection of the CNS.

Clinical Features

The onset is insidious over a period of months and occurs mostly from 5 to 15 years of age with preponderance among boys. There is insidious deterioration of behaviour and school performance progressing to a state of dementia. Major epileptic seizures may occur. A somewhat characteristic form of myoclonic jerk is commonly seen in which the child makes repetitive stereotyped movements with rhythmic regularity (2-6 per minute); each begins with shock-like abruptness typical of the myoclonic jerk, but then the elevated limb remains "frozen" for a second or two before, and unlike the usual myoclonic jerk, it gradually melts away. Pyramidal and extra-pyramidal signs are common. The final stage of decerebrate rigidity, severe dementia and coma is reached about 1 year or more from onset and death occurs usually 1-3 years after diagnosis. Rarely, clinical arrest has been reported.

The CSF cell count is usually normal. Although the total protein content of the CSF may be normal or only slightly elevated, the gamma globulin fraction is greatly elevated resulting in a paretic type of colloidal gold curve. On CSF electrophoresis, oligoclonal bands of Ig are often observed. High levels of antibody in CSF in dilutions of 1 equal 8 or more to measles are found. The EEG at the start of the illness may show only some excess slow-wave activity. Later in the illness bilateral periodic complexes typical of the disease appear. The EEG then shows high-amplitude slow-wave complexes, frequently having the same rhythmicality as the myoclonic jerk, sometimes with a frequency of 6-10 seconds (burst–suppression episodes). Finally the EEG becomes increasingly disorganized with random dysrhythmic slowing and lower amplitudes.

Treatment is mainly supportive. Administration of inosiplex (100 mg/kg/24 hr) may prolong survival and produce some clinical improvement. Measles vaccination is the most affective measure to prevent SSPE.

Acute Encephalopathy

The term acute encephalopathy refers to acute cerebral disorder associated with convulsions, stupor, coma and abnormalities of muscle tone. There is no actual infection of the brain substance. In some cases there has been a recent preceding virus infection. Rarely it may be related to the administration of a vaccine. Occasionally the child may have an underlying inherited metabolic defect such as maple syrup urine disease, organic aciduria or fatty acid, peroxisomal or mitochondrial metabolic defect. The cerebrospinal fluid is usually normal and apart from oedema the findings in the brain are remarkably inconspicuous. One distinct clinicopathological entity is Reye syndrome. Here an acute encephalopathy with fatty degeneration of the viscera in a young child is associated with hypoglycaemia, hyperammonaemia, greatly elevated aminotransferases, metabolic acidosis and respiratory alkalosis with prolongation of the prothrombin time. The CSF generally is clear and acellular with a normal protein concentration and reduced glucose level. At autopsy the liver is enlarged and shows gross fatty change, being greasy and pale yellow in colour. The brain shows only oedema. However, electron microscopy reveals distinctive mitochondrial changes in both hepatocytes and neurons. The syndrome follows viral infection with influenza B and varicella. The evidence to support a possible association between Reye syndrome and aspirin ingestion is not absolute but sufficient to discourage the use of aspirin for children. Treatment remains nonspecific in this syndrome because the precise aetiology and pathogenesis remain obscure. None the less the correction of hypoglycaemia, electrolyte imbalance, bleeding diathesis, metabolic disturbances and control of intracranial pressure may suffice in the early cases. The mortality and morbidity are high in late cases.

TUBERCULOSIS OF THE CENTRAL NERVOUS SYSTEM

Tuberculosis of the central nervous system is the most serious complication of primary tuberculosis in children. The clinical presentation commonly takes the form of meningitis. Less commonly, single or multiple tuberculomata enlarge and present as intracranial tumours. Tuberculous disease may also be confined to the spinal cord.

Tuberculous Meningitis

This develops following the rupture of a caseous subcortical focus (Rich focus) into the subarachnoid space and is commonest in children between 6 months to 5 years of age. Sometimes it is preceded by a head injury or an intercurrent infection such as measles, mumps or pertussis. Human immunodeficiency viral (HIV) infection predisposes children to tuberculous infection including TB meningitis. The onset of symptoms is insidious and progress gradually over some weeks and may be grouped into stages, which give a guide to prognosis. In infants the disease may run a more rapid course. Initially, the symptoms are non-specific and include lethargy, irritability, anorexia, headache, vomiting, abdominal pain, constipation and low-grade fever. The child's consciousness is unimpaired and neurological signs are absent. Unless there is a high index of suspicion and a positive contact history, the diagnosis is easily missed at this stage. About 2 weeks later the intermediate stage develops with obvious blurring of consciousness, nuchal rigidity, positive Kernig's sign and focal neurological signs such as cranial nerve paralysis (ophthalmoplegia and facial paralysis) and hemiplegia. Seizures may develop. Raised intracranial pressure may manifest as full "boggy" fontanelle in an infant and "cracked pot resonance" in the older child. Funduscopy may reveal choroidal tubercles indicating an associated miliary tuberculosis, papilloedema or the development of optic atrophy.

The third and final stage is characterized by coma, decerebrate rigidity, paralytic squints, unequal or dilated pupils, other neurological signs, and marked wasting. Convulsions are common. Vasomotor instability and terminal hyperpyraexia may occur. The combination of cerebral vasculitis, infarction, cerebral oedema and communicating hydrocephalus due to obstruction to CSF flow at the level of basal cisterns, leads to severe brain damage with little hope of recovery and the incidence of permanent brain damage such as hydrocephalus, blindness, deafness, mental retardation and learning impairment are high.

Diagnosis

The diagnosis is based on a positive contact history, clinical examination, positive Mantoux test, chest radiograph and CSF analysis. Mantoux test may be negative in advanced stages and in severe malnutrition. The CSF is often under pressure and may be clear or opalescent depending on the cell count. The CSF cell count varies between 50-500/mm^3 with lymphocyte predominance. The protein content is raised above 40 mg/100 ml and may be even in gms/100 ml. The glucose content is low between 20-40 mg/dl. The final proof is the detection of tubercle bacilli by acid-fast stain of the CSF sediment or cobweb clot, and mycobacterial culture. Identification of specific DNA sequences of Mycobacterium tuberculosis after polymerase chain reaction (PCR) amplification in the CSF is possible but there are risks of contamination and false positive results. Cultures of other fluids, such as gastric aspirate or urine may help confirm the diagnosis. CT or MRI scan of the brain will show basal exudate, communicating hydrocephalus, cerebral oedema and focal ischaemia.

Tuberculous meningitis is most likely to be mistaken for partially treated pyogenic meningitis or aseptic meningitis due to viruses. In these cases the onset is usually much more acute than in tuberculosis cases, with brisk fever and obvious early rigidity of the neck and spine. The cerebrospinal fluid may show a lymphocytic pleocytosis but in viral aseptic meningitis there is no fall in sugar content, the protein content is less markedly raised and a spider-web clot rarely, if ever, forms. There will be no other indications of tuberculosis in these cases. Detection of bacterial antigen in CSF by latex agglutination test and a positive bacterial CSF and blood culture will help to differentiate pyogenic meningitis. In older children tuberculous meningitis can simulate brain tumour, but the cerebrospinal fluid and CT or MRI scan of the brain will reveal the true state of affairs. Tuberculomas in children are often infratentorial in location, and may be single or multiple.

Treatment

In tuberculous meningitis the results depend upon the stage at which treatment is started. The prognosis for young infants is generally worse than for older children. The optimal chemotherapy is the use of a combination of antituberculous drugs with good penetration into the CSF and low toxicity, for sufficient duration. A suggested regimen is isoniazid (5-10 mg/kg), rifampicin (10 mg/kg), pyrazinamide (25-30 mg/kg) and ethambutol (20 mg/kg) given in single daily dose on an empty stomach for the first 2 months followed by isoniazid, rifampicin and ethambutol for another 10 months. Rifampicin may cause gastric upset, red coloured urine and a rise in liver transaminases but these side effects are rarely severe. Isoniazid may cause convulsions in young infants and peripheral neuropathy in older patients. Although children taking isoniazid may have transient elevation of serum transaminase, clinically significant hepatoxicity is rare. Corticosteroids are normally administered during the first few weeks of treatment to reduce cerebral oedema and prevent formation of adhesions and hydrocephalus. Initially dexamethasone 0.6 mg/kg/day in 3-4 divided doses is given, followed by prednisolone (1-2 mg/kg/day) for 2-4 weeks and gradually tapered off.

Good nursing care and adequate nutrition are important. Anticonvulsant therapy may be required to control seizures. Close family contacts should be screened for tuberculosis.

Complication

During treatment neurological complications may arise due to obstructive hydrocephalus, thrombosis of cerebral vessels and the involvement of cranial nerves in basal exudate. Serial cranial CT scans should be performed on all patients to detect the presence or development of hydrocephalus. Ventriculoperitoneal shunt surgery may be necessary.

BRAIN ABSCESS

Pus accumulation in brain parenchyma may occur as a complication of meningitis, due to haematogenous spread of septic emboli from infective endocarditis and congenital cyanotic heart disease (especially tetralogy of Fallot), extension of infection from chronic otitis media and mastoiditis, and penetrating head injuries. The site of abscess depends on the source, e.g. chronic otitis media and mastoiditis lead to abscess formation in temporal lobe and cerebellum. The usual organisms are streptococcus (especially Streptococcus viridans), anaerobic organisms, Staphylococcus aureus and gram-negative organisms particularly citrobacter. In immune compromised children fungal organisms may be responsible.

The symptoms and signs usually develop over 2-3 weeks and initially are non-specific with low-grade fever and headache. Later signs of raised intracranial pressure, seizures and focal neurological signs develop. Cerebellar signs may be obvious. The diagnosis is confirmed by contrast CT scan which shows a central area of low density with marked 'ring' enhancement and surrounding area of low density due to oedema. There may be shift of the midline. Lumbar puncture should not be performed in a child suspected to have brain abscess. The treatment consists of appropriate antibiotics and aspiration of the pus. The usual antibiotic combination is a third-generation cephalosporin, metronidazole and benzyl penicillin. Associated infection such as mastoiditis should be treated.

BRAIN TUMOUR IN CHILDREN

Brain tumours are the second most common tumour in children. Although the aetiology of most brain tumours are unknown, certain neurocutaneous syndromes like neurofibroma and tuberous sclerosis predispose to development of brain tumours. Infants and young children have higher risk of developing brain tumours. The commomn histological the tumour types are – Medulloblastoma/primitive neuroectodermal tumour. Astrocytoma, ependymoma and craniopharyngioma.

Most brain tumours in children are malignant and are situated usually in the posterior cranial fossa. The children usually present with signs of raised intracranial pressure which can be mistaken for meningitis. Gait disturbances and ataxia are common with cerebellar tumours.

Supratentorial tumours may present with focal seizures and deficits. Craniopharyngioma occurring in the suprasellar region is minimally invasive and may present with visual disturbances and neuroendocrine deficiencies.

Diagnosis of brain tumour is confirmed by neuro-imaging studies (MRI/CT scan). When brain tumour is suspected lumbar puncture should not be done as it might produce coning and sudden death. Surgery is the preferred mode of treatment. Radiation and chemotherapy have also contributed to improved prognosis.

NEUROCYSTICERCOSIS

Neurocysticercosis is the most common parasitic infestation of the central nervous system, and is caused by pork tapeworm Taenia solium in its larval stage. Human cysticercosis usually results when humans ingest vegetables contaminated with the eggs of Taenia solium. The cysticerci develop almost anywhere but particularly in the skin, muscle, brain and eye. Neurocysticercosis has been reported even in young children. It manifests commonly with seizures, but can also cause signs of increased intracranial pressure, meningitis, behavioural disorders, paresis and hydrocephalus. The seizures are mostly focal in nature. A phenomenon peculiar to patients in the Indian subcontinent is the solitary cysticercus granuloma which shows up as a single, small, enhancing lesion on the contrast enhanced computerised tomography (CT) scan, with significant surrounding oedema located superficially near the cortex (Fig. 18.2). The usual

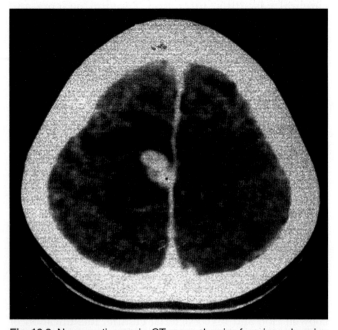

Fig. 18.2: Neurocysticercosis. CT scans showing four ring enhancing lesions close to the midline in the left fronto-parietal region with surrounding oedema

presentation is a simple partial seizure often with post-ictal deficit in the form of monoparesis or hemiparesis. The deficit is usually temporary and the CT lesion resolves spontaneously over a period of time. Serologic tests like enzyme-linked immunosorbent assay (ELISA) and enzyme-linked immuno electrotransfer blots (EITB) can be useful to confirm the diagnosis. Since active solitary parenchymal lesions resolve spontaneously, only anti-epileptic drug is advised usually for a six-month period. However persistent, enlarging or multiple lesions need anticysticercal drugs. Albendazole is preferred at a dosage of 15 mg/kg/day in 2 divided doses for 28 days. A worsening of symptoms may follow the use of Albenda-zole due to host inflammatory response to dying parasite. A short course of steroids for about 5 days can ameliorate these effects.

ACUTE HEMIPLEGIA IN CHILDHOOD (ACUTE INFANTILE HEMIPLEGIA)

This is a characteristic clinical syndrome seen in both infants and children. Most cases are associated with a preceding pyrexial illness such as tonsillitis, cervical adenitis, tooth infection or sometimes tonsillectomy. The presence of abnormalities in the internal carotid and first part of the middle cerebral arteries has been clearly demonstrated in cases investigated within a few days of the onset. These have ranged from complete occlusion to very marked narrowing of the lumen of the carotid and its branches. A good case is made that this arterial obstruction is the consequence of an inflammatory arteritis of the carotid following throat or neck gland infection.

Clinical Features

The disease may present in one of two ways. In the more common, the child suddenly goes into status epilepticus with high fever and deep coma. The convulsions may be generalised or unilateral. After some hours or days of critical illness, the fits cease and consciousness slowly returns. Hemiplegia is then found to be present, with dysphasia in right-sided cases. The upper motor neuron weakness and spasticity affect principally the face and arm, and recovery in the leg precedes and exceeds that of the arm.

In the second mode of presentation the child, after a recent febrile illness, suddenly develops a hemiplegia, with or without dysphasia; convulsions do not occur and if there is loss of consciousness it is of short duration.

In either type of case signs of recovery are obvious after a week or two, although the hemiplegia rarely completely disappears. Intelligence may be unimpaired, although in some cases serious mental retardation or epilepsy persists permanently. If the hemiplegia remains severe, defective growth and shortening of the arm and leg result.

The cerebrospinal fluid shows no abnormality at the inception of the illness but some days later a slight rise in cells and protein may develop; later, ventricular enlarge-ment occurs on the affected side of the brain with displacement of the ventricular system to that side with enlargement of the sulci. This atrophic change is, in fact, most marked in the territory supplied by the middle cerebral artery, but sometimes it is also seen in the territory of the anterior cerebral artery. The posterior part of the hemi-sphere is rarely affected. MRI and CT would demonstrate these changes.

Diagnosis

Other causes of acute hemiplegia in childhood should be excluded. Thrombosis of the internal carotid artery may result from trauma caused by falls on objects, e.g. a pencil in the mouth, which penetrates the tonsillar fossa. Acute hemiplegia may be the presenting feature of haemophilus influenzae meningitis and is also seen as a complication in tuberculous meningitis and encephalitis (particularly herpes). Abscess from middle ear infection or congenital heart disease can also present with hemiplegia. Infla-mmatory arteritis due to autoimmune disorders like systemic lupus erythematosus, polyarteritis nodosa and Takayasu arteritis can also cause hemiplegia in children. Prolonged seizure can cause a temporary paralysis – Todd's paralysis – that recovers within 48-72 hours. Hemiplegia can occur due to thrombosis in an otherwise normal vessel in hypercoagulable states, examples of which are polycythaemia in congenital cyanotic heart disease, leukaemia, protein C and protein S deficiency, sickle cell disease and post-splenectomy. Metabolic disorders associated with hemiplegia include homo-cystinuria, Fabry disease and mitochondrial disorders (MELAS). Additional causes of hemiplegia include Sturge-Weber syndrome, brain tumour and familial hyper-lipidaemia.

Treatment

Other causes of hemiplegia such as meningitis and encephalitis should be excluded by early lumbar puncture. Investigations should be directed towards identifying an underlying disease process. Status epilepticus is best treated with intravenous midazolam, lorazepam or diazepam followed by maintenance anticonvulsant therapy. Persisting tonsillar or dental sepsis should be treated with an appropriate antibiotic. Routine use of anticoagulant therapy or aspirin is not recommended.

ACUTE CEREBELLAR ATAXIA

This condition refers to sudden onset of ataxia, often following a viral infection, such as varicella, coxsackie virus or echovirus infection, by 2-3 weeks. It is most common in children aged 2-5 years and is thought to be due to an immune response to the viral agent affecting the cerebellum. It is a diagnosis by exclusion. Other clearly defined causes, e.g. infratentorial tumours, otogenic cerebellar abscess, anticonvulsant drugs like phenytoin, alcohol ingestion, glue-sniffing, lead encephalopathy and the various leucodystrophies and hereditary types of ataxia have to be excluded.

Clinical Features

In the typical case the onset of cerebellar signs in a child aged 2-5 years is sudden. There may have been a preceding viral infection. The principal feature is the typical reeling ataxia. Truncal ataxia may cause difficulty in sitting. There may be a tremor or wobble of the head. Hypotonia is common and the deep reflexes may be diminished. The child may be irritable or abnormal in personality but there is no blurring of consciousness. Other cerebellar signs may be elicited, e.g. nystagmus, intention tremor, dysmetria or jerky explosive speech (dysarthria). The optic fundi are normal. Vomiting may occur but there are no other indications of an increase in intracranial pressure. The cerebrospinal fluid is usually normal.

The differential diagnosis from the other causes of cerebellar ataxia is essential and usually possible on careful assessment of the history and physical findings. Computerised axial tomography (CT scanning) should be arranged if there is any suspicion of tumour.

In most instances complete recovery can be expected within a period of weeks. A few cases have long-term sequelae.

Treatment

Symptomatic measures only are possible.

ACUTE FLACCID PARALYSIS

Acute flaccid paralysis is defined as onset of weakness and floppiness within 2 weeks in any part of the body in a child less than 15 years of age. The common causes of acute flaccid paralysis are acute paralytic poliomyelitis, Guillian-Barre' syndrome, traumatic neuritis and transverse myelitis. Other causes include non-polio enterovirus infections, encephalitis, meningitis, toxins, etc.

ACUTE POLIOMYELITIS

This is caused by poliovirus, which comprises three serotypes: Types 1, 2 and 3 of which type 1 is the commonest cause for poliomyelitis. Transmission is primarily person-to-person via the faecal-oral route. Unimmunised children 6 months to 3 years of age are most susceptible. In 90-95% of infected individuals, poliovirus infection is inapparent. In the remaining infected individuals, one of the three syndromes may occur.

(i) Abortive polio is characterized by a minor illness with low-grade fever, sore throat, vomiting, abdominal pain and malaise. Recovery is rapid and there is no paralysis.

(ii) Non-paralytic aseptic meningitis is characterized by headache, neck, back and leg stiffness preceded about a week earlier by a prodrome similar to abortive polio. The child may be drowsy and irritable; spinal stiffness is manifested by the tripod sign. There is no paralysis.

(iii) Paralytic poliomyelitis occurs in about 1% of infected individuals. Symptoms often occur in two phases with a symptom free interval: The minor consisting of the symptoms of abortive poliomyelitis and the major illness characterized by high grade fever, muscle pain and stiffness followed by rapid onset of flaccid paralyses that is usually complete within 72 hours (Fig. 18.3).

There are three types of paralytic poliomyelitis:

(a) Spinal poliomyelitis: This accounts for newly 80% of paralytic poliomyelitis. It results from a lower motor neuron lesion of the anterior horn cells of the spinal cord and affects the muscles of the legs, arms and/or trunk. Paralysis is asymmetrical and the sensory system is intact. The affected muscles are tender; floppy and tendon reflexes are lost or diminished.

(b) Bulbar poliomyelitis results from involvement of lower cranial nerves and can cause facial paralysis, difficulty in swallowing, eating or speech and respiratory insufficiency.

(c) Bulbospinal poliomyelitis involves both bulbar cranial nerves and spinal cord.

Life is endangered in case of bulbar involvement with inability to swallow and obstruction of the airway and when the muscles of respiration are involved.

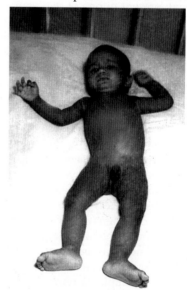

Fig. 18.3: Acute flaccid paralysis due to poliomyelitis.

As the acute phase of paralytic poliomyelitis subsides over 4 weeks, recovery begins in paralysed muscles. The extent of recovery is variable depending upon the extent of damage caused to the neurones by the virus. Maximum recovery takes place in the first six months after the illness but slow recovery can continue up to two years. After two years, no more recovery is expected and the child is said to have post-polio residual paralysis. Affected muscles atrophy and deformities such as pes cavus, talipes or scoliosis and ultimate shortening of the affected limb may develop.

Poliovirus can be isolated from the stool specimen. Paired serum may be tested for neutralising antibody in rising titre. The cerebrospinal fluid is clear or only slightly hazy. The cell count varies from 50 to a few hundreds per cubic millimeter with lymphocytic predominance. The sugar level is normal but the protein content is elevated leading at times to 'cyto-albumino dissociation'.

Treatment is mainly supportive with complete bed rest, proper positioning of the affected limb and passive range of movement at the joints. Massage and intramuscular injection should be avoided during the acute phase of illness. Children with bulbar involvement and respiratory paralysis would need hospitalisation and close monitoring. Moist heat and analgesics can be given to relieve pain and fever. Physiotherapy plays an important role during recovery. Orthosis may be required for ambulation and children with fixed deformities and contractures may require orthopaedic surgery.

Poliomyelitis can be prevented by active immunization with trivalent oral polio vaccine. Besides in endemic countries, national immunisation days (or Pulse Polio Immunisation) are conducted in which 2 doses of oral polio vaccine are administered at an interval of 6 weeks to all children aged 0-5 years regardless of previous vaccination history. Ongoing surveillance of all acute flaccid paralysis (AFP) cases is an important aspect of polio eradication. This involves AFP case reporting, investigation, stool collection and laboratory confirmation. After the AFP case investigation and stool specimen collection, outbreak response immunisation is organized in the community and children aged 0-5 years are given one dose of trivalent oral polio virus vaccine regardless of their prior immunisation status.

ACUTE POSTINFECTIOUS POLYNEUROPATHY (GUILLAIN-BARRE' SYNDROME)

It is an acute inflammatory demyelinating polyneuropathy affecting the spinal nerve roots, peripheral nerves and cranial nerves. It involves primarily the motor but sometimes also sensory and autonomic nerves. It typically occurs after recovery from a viral infection or in rare cases, following immunisation. The commonly identified triggering agents are *Helicobacter jejuni*, cytomegalovirus, Epstein-Barr virus and Mycoplasma pneumoniae. It is believed to be due to a "cross-reactive" immune attack by host antibodies and T-lymphocytes on nerve components. Guillain-Barre` syndrome is now appreciated as a heterogeneous spectrum of disorders with distinct subtypes. Some patients have mainly loss of myelin while others have predominantly axonal damage, which tend to be more severe. Another subtype, the Miller-Fisher syndrome, consists of acute onset of ataxia, areflexia and ophthalmoplegia.

Clinical Features

After an upper respiratory febrile illness or acute gastroenteritis, the child develops increasing muscle weakness and tenderness with loss of deep tendon reflexes. The lower limbs are the first to be affected followed by involvement of the trunk, upper limbs and finally the bulbar muscles (Landry's ascending paralysis). Proximal and distal muscles are involved relatively symmetrically. Sensory changes tend to be minimal. Intercostal and diaphragmatic paralysis may endanger life. Bilateral facial paralysis is common. Autonomic nervous system involvement may manifest with tachycardia and hypertension. In the typical Guillain-Barre' syndrome the cerebrospinal fluid shows a high protein content with little or no pleiocytosis, but these changes are inconstant and may be late in appearing. Motor nerve conduction velocities are greatly reduced. Electromyogram shows evidence of acute denervation of muscle.

Treatment

Most cases recover spontaneously over a period of weeks to months with supportive treatment with good nursing care and physiotherapy. Respiratory paralysis may necessitate tracheostomy and assisted ventilation. Rapidly progressive paralysis is treated with intravenous immunoglobulin therapy (0.4 gm/kg/day) administered for 5 days. Plasmapheresis, steroids and/or immuno-suppressive drugs are alternatives.

NEUROCUTANEOUS SYNDROME

Neurocutaneous syndrome (The Phakomatoses) are disorders with manifestation in skin and central nervous system. Most are autosomally inherited and have a high rate of tumour formation. The common phakomatoses are neurofibromatosis, tuberous sclerosis, Sturge-Weber syndrome, von Hippel-Lindau disease and ataxia telengiectasia.

NEUROFIBROMATOSIS (VON RECKLINGHAUSEN'S DISEASE)

This is the commonest neurocutaneous syndrome and is transmitted as an autosomal dominant characteristic.

There is abnormality of neural crest migration. Two gene defects have been identified; one on chromosome 17 which leads NF-I with mainly cutaneous features and peripheral nerve abnormalities, and the other on chromosome 22 with mainly central nervous system involvement and acoustic neuroma formation after the age of 20.

The earliest and pathognomonic signs of neuro-fibromatosis are the café-au-lait spots or patches which are irregularly shaped hyperpigmented brownish macules often present at or shortly after birth and may vary in size and number with age. Presence of six or more café-au-lait spots greater than 0.5 cm in diameter in prepubertal children is considered diagnostic of neurofibromatosis. Other cutaneous manifestations are axillary or inguinal freckling and presence of pedunculated neurofibromas. Palpable neurofibromata are to be detected along the course of subcutaneous nerves. The brain may be the site of formation of hamartomatous nodules, and various types of tumours (glioma, ependymoma, meningioma) may occur in the brain, optic nerve, spinal cord or spinal nerve roots. Approximately 10-20% of patients manifest with seizures, intellectual deficit and speech and motor delay. Lisch nodules are seen in the iris with increasing age. Osseous lesions include progressive kyphoscoliosis in childhood, sphenoidial dysplasia and cortical thickening of long bones with or without pseudoarthrosis.

Treatment

There is no specific treatment and therapy is symptomatic and includes genetic counselling and early detection of treatable complication. Neurosurgical intervention is often necessary to remove symptomatic tumours of the central and peripheral nervous system.

TUBEROUS SCLEROSIS (EPILOIA)

Tuberous sclerosis is one of the phakomatoses with manifestations in the skin, central nervous system, and eye as well as hamartomata of internal organs such as kidney, heart, lung and bone. The disease is transmitted as an autosomal dominant trait with gene defects identified on chromosomes 9 and 16. Seizures are the commonest presenting symptom and may present in infancy with infantile spasms or partial seizures. Hypopigmented areas of skin, sometimes assuming an ash-leaf shape, are the earliest skin manifestation (Fig. 18.4). The characteristic rash of butterfly distribution and papular character on the face and nose known as adenoma sebaceum appears later (Fig. 18.5). Other skin lesions include shagreen patch – a leathery plaque – usually in the lumbosacral area and café-au-lait spots.

The characteristic brain lesion consists of tubers typically present in the subependymal region made of abnormal giant cells and sclerosis due to overgrowth of

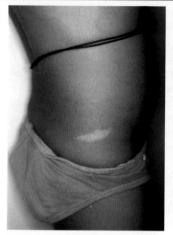
Fig. 18.4: Tuberous sclerosis. Hypopigmented macule.

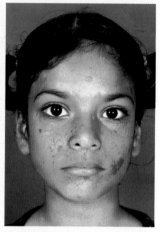
Fig. 18.5: Tuberous sclerosis. Adenoma sebaceum in a characteristic malar distribution and chin lesions as well.

astrocytic fibrils. These tubers undergo calcification and also at times malignant transformation. Mental retardation is a common feature. Ophthalmoscopy may show characteristic yellowish-white phakomata on the retina. The heart may be the seat of a rhabdomyoma or tubers. In some cases there are teratomata or hamartomata of the kidneys, liver, bone and lung.

The diagnosis of tuberous sclerosis is based on the combination of characteristic cutaneous lesions, seizures, intellectual deficit and visceral tumours. Neuroimaging studies demonstrate subependymal-calcified nodules adjacent to lateral ventricles. The white matter in cerebral lesions is either calcified or hypodense. There is no specific treatment for tuberous sclerosis. Management consists mainly of seizure control and genetic counselling. Infantile spasm associated with tuberous sclerosis is best treated with vigabatrin.

STURGE-WEBER SYNDROME
(Encephalofacial angiomatosis)

This disease consists of cutaneous port-wine haemangioma of the upper face and scalp, which is predominantly limited by the midline, and a similar vascular anomaly of the underlying leptomeninges on the same side (Fig. 18.6). The brain beneath becomes atrophic and calcified particularly in the occipital and parietal regions (Fig. 18.7). The mode of inheritance of this disease is not clear.

The port-wine stain is present at birth. Convulsions confined to the contralateral side of the body develop in infancy. In time a spastic hemiparesis and hemiatrophy may develop on the contralateral side. Mental deterioration ultimately appears and progresses. Glaucoma may also develop in the ipsilateral eye and require surgical

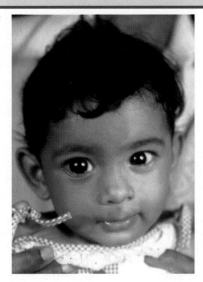

Fig. 18.6: Sturge-Weber syndrome. Port-wine nonelevated cutaneous haemangioma in a trigeminal distribution, including the ophthalmic division.

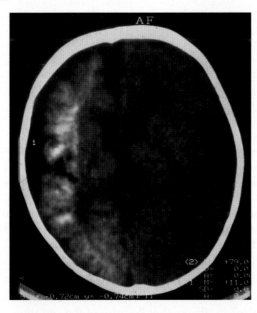

Fig. 18.7: Sturge-Weber syndrome. CT scan showing intracranial calcification.

intervention. Radiographs of the skull in later childhood show a characteristic double contour or "tramline" type of calcification.

Treatment is symptomatic and directed at control of seizures and glaucoma. If seizures are refractory to drug therapy surgical resection of the affected lobe or hemispherectomy may be indicated. In some cases the facial naevus can be corrected by cosmetic laser surgery.

ATAXIA – TELENGIECTASIA (LOUIS-BAR SYNDROME)

Ataxia telengiectasia is characterized by progressive cerebellar ataxia, oculocutaneous telengiectasia, choreo-athetosis, recurrent sinopulmonary infections, and immunological dysfunction. It is an autosomal recessive condition with the abnormal gene located to chromosome 11. The first symptom to appear is a progressive cerebellar ataxia beginning in the second or third year of life. There may be, in addition, choreo-athetotic movements and a tendency to turn the eyes upwards when focussing. Telengiectases appear between the ages of 3 and 7 years. They are found on the bulbar conjunctiva, malar-eminences, ears and antecubital fossae. These children suffer severely from infections of the sinuses and lungs; indeed bronchiectasis is a frequent cause of death. They have a much higher risk of developing lymphoreticular malignancy. These are explained by abnormalities of immunologic function resulting in reduction of serum and secretory IgA, IgE, IgG2 and IgG4. There is hypoplasia of the thymus and cellular immunity is also impaired. Alpha-feto protein level is elevated. There is no specific treatment. Infection should be controlled with suitable antibiotics. In malignant change, steroids may give temporary relief.

VON HIPPEL-LINDAU DISEASE

This is a rare autosomal dominant inherited disorder characterized by haemangiomatous cystic lesions in the retina and cerebellum, sometime also in spinal cord, kidney, liver and pancreas. It may present with the signs of a cerebellar tumour (progressive ataxia and raised intracranial pressure) or with loss of vision due to retinal detachment. Renal carcinoma and phaeochromocytoma are frequently associated. Surgical treatment is indicated for the cerebellar and visceral tumours and photo-coagulation and cryocoagulation for the retinal angiomas.

NEURODEGENERATIVE DISORDERS

These are rare progressive degenerative disorders that usually result from specific genetic and biochemical defects. The characteristic features are loss of developmental milestones, intellect, speech and vision often associated with seizures. They may affect primarily the grey matter, i.e. cortical neurones resulting in early symptoms of seizures and intellectual deterioration, or the white matter with early pyramidal tract involvement.

Neuronal ceroid lipofuscinoses: These are autosomal recessive disorders characterised by accumulation of autofluorescent intracellular lipopigment. There are three clinical types namely infantile type, late infantile type and juvenile type. In the types with onset in infancy, myoclonic seizures are a prominent feature with progressive loss of vision and developmental milestones.

The white matter degenerative diseases (leucodystrophies) include metachromatic leucodystrophy, Krabbe's globoid body leucodystrophy, adrenoleucodystrophy and Schilder's disease.

Metachromatic leucodystrophy: This autosomal recessive disorder is characterized by accumulation of cerebroside sulphate in the white matter of the brain, the peripheral nerves, the dentate nucleus, basal ganglia and in other organs such as the kidneys due to deficiency of the enzyme arylsulphatase A. There is widespread demyelination with neuronal and axonal loss. The sulphatide stains metachromatially with basic polychrome dyes. Three clinical forms of the disease have been described.

1. *Late infantile form:* This the most common type with its onset between 6 and 24 months. Deterioration in walking due to progressive and mixed pyramidal and cerebellar damage is soon followed by deterioration in speech and social development, loss of the ability to sit or feed without help, fits, misery and withdrawal, finally a decorticate posture leading to death some 5 months or longer from the onset.

2. *Juvenile type:* This has an onset between 6 and 10 years. The first signs are educational and behavioural deterioration, followed after some months or years by disorders of gait mostly extrapyramidal with some pyramidal signs. Progress towards dementia and death may take more than 5 years.

3. *Adult type:* Onset 16 years to adulthood. Psychiatric changes predominate.

Krabbe's globoid body leucodystrophy: Krabbe's globoid body leucodystrophy is characterized by accumulation of globular bodies in white matter due to deficiency of the enzyme galactocerebroside β-galactosidase. The onset is in early infancy with incessant crying followed by apathy. Generalised rigidity, seizures, head retraction, blindness, inability to swallow and death may ensue in a year or so. Peripheral nerve involvement may cause absent deep tendon reflexes.

Adrenoleucodystrophy: This is an X-linked recessive disorder with onset usually between 5 and 15 years of age with progressive psychomotor deterioration, ataxia, dementia, loss of vision and hearing. There is evidence of adrenocortical insufficiency with skin pigmentation. The blood level of very long chain fatty acid is increased. Death occurs within 10 years of the onset. Bone marrow transplant at an early stage is helpful.

Heredo degenerative ataxias: These are inherited progressive ataxias. The commonest type is Friedrich ataxia, which is an autosomal recessive disorder with the abnormal gene located in chromosome 9. The onset of symptoms is in childhood and before puberty with pes cavus, kyphoscoliosis and ataxia. There is nystagmus and intention tremor. Involvement of dorsal columns leads to loss of vibration and position sense. There is absent deep tendon reflexes particularly ankle jerk and the plantar response is extensor. Optic atrophy and dysarthria may appear late in the course of the disease. Cardiac involvement can lead to intractable congestive cardiac failure. Death may be delayed for 10-15 years, but it may occur earlier from cardiac failure.

Hereditary motor – sensory neuropathies: This group of progressive degenerative disorders of the peripheral nerves affects predominantly the motor nerves, and sensory and autonomic involvement appears later.

Charcot-Marie-Tooth peroneal muscular atrophy: This disease starts in late childhood with progressive weakness and lower motor neurone type of flaccid atrophy of the peroneal and tibial muscles and of the small muscles of the feet resulting in parlaytic talipes equinovarus. Later, wasting of the calf muscles gives the legs an inverted wine-bottle appearance. At a late stage, weakness and wasting affect the hands and forearms. The ankle jerks are lost but the knee jerks remain brisk. Sensory involvement is manifested by some loss of vibration and positional sensation. Most cases are transmitted as autosomal dominant.

NEUROMUSCULAR DISORDERS

SPINAL MUSCULAR ATROPHY (SMA)

The principal feature of this disease is progressive degeneration and loss of motor neurones in the anterior horns of the spinal cord. It is a relatively common disease of infancy inherited as a recessive trait. The genetic locus is on chromosome 5. There are 3 clinical types differentiated by age of onset and severity of weakness.

SMA type 1 (WERDNIG-HOFFMANN DISEASE): This is the most severe form and may be present at birth or appear within a few weeks. Its onset in utero may be recognized by the mother because of the cessation of fetal movements. There is severe flaccidity and weakness of the muscles of the trunk and limbs. The proximal muscles tend to be more severely paralysed than the distal. The deep tendon reflexes are absent. Fasciculation in the muscles of the tongue may be seen. The infant has an alert expression. When the intercostals and other accessory muscles of respiration become affected dyspnoea, intercostal recession and paradoxical respiration develop. Eventually the diaphragm is involved rendering the infant prone for chest infection and respiratory failure. The loss of power to suck further aggravates the terminal stages of the illness. Death usually occurs before 2 years of age. There is no specific treatment.

SMA type 2: This type has a later onset and is obvious by the end of the first year. There is progressive weakness with severe wasting leading to deformities particularly scoliosis. They rarely learn to walk and are confined to wheelchair. Deaths occur before 10 years of age.

SMA type 3 (KUGELBERG-WELANDER SYNDROME): This is a milder type of paralysis with onset after the age of 2 years and is compatible with a prolonged course. There is proximal muscle weakness involving the pelvic and shoulder girdle muscles. Skeletal deformities readily develop. In some cases, the bulbar muscles become involved. These children may learn to walk, but ultimately become confined to a wheel chair. They may live up to middle age.

Electromyography shows a denervation pattern and muscle biopsy can also help to confirm the diagnosis. Spinal muscular atrophy has to be differentiated from other causes of "floppy infant syndrome". In benign congenital hypotonia, hypotonia dates from or soon after birth. The deep tendon reflexes although sluggish can usually be elicited and muscle fibrillation is not seen. The true diagnosis of benign congenital hypotonia becomes clear with the passage of time (5-9 years), when slow but not always complete recovery takes place. Muscle biopsy is normal in benign congenital hypotonia.

MYASTHENIA GRAVIS

This is an immune-mediated disorder of neuromuscular function caused by a reduction of available acetylcholinie (Ach) receptors at the neuromuscular junction due to circulating Ach receptor-binding antibodies. It is an autoimmune disorder and patients with myasthenia gravis have higher incidence of other autoimmune diseases particularly thyroiditis.

Clinical Features

Most cases are in girls and the ocular muscles are usually first affected; the child presents with ptosis or complaints of diplopia; the muscle weakness tends to be more severe as the day goes on. The pupillary reflexes are normal. The bulbar muscles are often next affected. The voice is then weak, swallowing and chewing become difficult, and there may be asphyxial episodes due to the aspiration of upper respiratory secretions and saliva. When the facial muscles are affected a lack of expression is a striking feature. Easy fatiguability of muscles is a characteristic feature but muscle atrophy and fibrillary twitchings do not occur. The deep tendon reflexes are usually present. In the worst cases the muscles of the limbs and those responsible for respiration are affected. As in the adult, the myasthenic child may run a prolonged course of remissions and relapses, but there is a tendency for the disease to reach a static phase some 5 years from the onset. There is always a risk of death from aspiration of food into the respiratory passages, from respiratory failure due to involvement of respiratory muscles or from intercurrent respiratory infection.

Neonatal myasthenia gravis occurs in newborn infants born to myasthenic mother and is due to the placental transfer of antibodies to acetylcholine receptors from mother to baby. The manifestations include a weak cry, generalized severe hypotonia, feeble sucking reflex and attacks of choking and cyanosis. They are temporary and disappear within a few weeks.

Diagnosis

Myasthenia gravis should be suspected in the presence of ptosis, strabismus, bulbar palsy or severe muscular hypotonia during infancy or childhood. The diagnosis is confirmed by the immediate response to intravenous injection of edrophonium – a short acting cholinesterase inhibitor. Atropine sulphate should be available during the edrophonium test to block acute muscarinic effects. Electromyogram demonstrates decremental response to repetitive nerve stimulation. Anti acetyl choline receptor antibodies may be measured in the plasma. Although the thymus gland is hyperplastic this is not radiologically obvious unless there is an actual thymoma, which is extremely rare in childhood.

Treatment

This should be medical in the first instance and consists of a cholinesterase inhibitor. The most useful drug for continuous treatment is pyridostigmine bromide given orally with a starting dosage of 1.5 mg /kg every 3-8 hours according to the clinical response. The other drug that can be given is neostigmine. Over dosage of cholinesterase's results in prolonged depolarisation of muscle end plates and muscle paralysis (cholinergic crisis). The short-acting edrophonium may be used to differentiate between cholinergic crisis and myasthenic crisis. Edrophonium injection will aggravate cholinergic crisis and transiently improve myasthenic crisis.

Apart from anticholinesterase drugs, immuno-suppressive drugs (corticosteroids and azathioprine) may be used to reduce antibodies to acetylcholine receptors. Plasmapheresis is effective in some myasthenic children as also intravenous immunoglobulin therapy. The position of thymectomy in the treatment of myasthenia gravis in childhood is not yet clear. The indications for thymectomy are inadequate control of the muscular weakness with drugs and duration of the disease of less than 2 years.

MUSCULAR DYSTROPHY

Muscular dystrophies are a group of inherited disorders characterized by progressive degeneration of muscle fibres.

Duchenne Muscular Dystrophy

This is the commonest type of muscular dystrophy. It is inherited as a X-linked recessive trait with a high new mutation rate. The abnormal gene is located at Xp21 locus on the X-chromosome, which leads to deficiency of dystrophin protein in the muscle fibre. The onset is usually before the third or fourth years of life. There may be a history of delay in walking. The child may fall unduly often, or has great difficulty in climbing stairs. Weakness begins in the pelvic girdle and the gait assumes a characteristic waddle so that the feet are placed too widely apart and there is an exaggerated lumbar lordosis. A quite characteristic phenomenon – Gower's sign – is seen when the child, lying on his back on the floor, is asked to stand up. He will roll to one side, flex his knees and hips so that he is "on all fours" with both knees and both hands on the ground; he then extends his knees and reaches the erect posture by "climbing up his own legs", using his hands to get higher up each leg in alternate steps. Weakness of the shoulder muscles may render the child unable to raise his hands above his head. Pseudohypertrophy of the calf muscles with wasting of thigh muscle is characteristic. Tendon reflexes become progressively diminished and finally cannot be elicited. By the age of 10 years the child is usually confined to a wheel chair. Skeletal and postural deformities particularly scoliosis may later become severe. Heart may fail from involvement of the myocardium. Mental retardation occurs in about 30% of cases. Death is usual during adolescence from intercurrent respiratory infection, respiratory or cardiac failure.

The serum creatine kinase is greatly elevated and is often above 10,000 IU/L (normal up to 150 IU/L). Electromyography (EMG) shows myophathic changes and muscle biopsy with immunohistochemical staining for dystrophin is confirmatory. Periodic cardiac assessment is necessary.

Treatment

There is no effective treatment for this disease. Physiotherapy is important to prevent or delay contracture. Lightweight calipers and later bracing of the spine may prolong ambulation. Steroids such as deflazacort may give short-term benefit. Psychological support is needed for the child and the family. Healthy female carriers often have elevated serum levels of creatine kinase. Antenatal diagnosis is possible using DNA analysis.

BECKER MUSCULAR DYSTROPHY

This sex-linked recessive disorder is similar but milder than Duchenne muscular dystrophy. The progress is slower and affected boys remain ambulatory until late adolescence or early adult life.

The other less common muscular dystrophies include Facioscapulohumeral muscular dystrophy, Limb-girdle muscular dystrophy and Dystrophia myotonica.

Facioscapulohumeral Muscular Dystrophy

This form of dystrophy is transmitted as an autosomal dominant trait and can affect both sexes. The onset may be in early childhood or early adult life, most often with weakness and lack of expression in the facial muscles. In time the child cannot close his eyes, wrinkle his forehead or purse his mouth. The lips project forwards due to weakness of the orbicularis oris to give the appearance of "tapir mouth". Weakness of the shoulder girdle muscles, especially the pectoralis major, serratus magnus, trapezius, spinati, deltoid, triceps and biceps results in winging of the scapulae, inability to raise the arms above the head and looseness of the shoulders. Then the pelvic girdle becomes affected, glutei, quadriceps, hamstrings and iliopsoas, so that there is lumbar lordosis and a broad-based gait. This form of muscular dystrophy usually runs a prolonged and relatively benign course well into adult life. Indeed, the face only may be affected during most of childhood and severe crippling may be long delayed. The diagnosis can be confirmed by muscle biopsy. Elevated levels of serum creatine kinase are found only in some cases.

Treatment

None is available at the present time.

Limb-girdle Muscular Dystrophy

This form of dystrophy affects mainly the muscles of hip and shoulder girdles. It is usually inherited as an autosomal recessive characteristic. Males and females are equally affected.

This rarely appears during the first decade. Weakness first becomes obvious in the muscles of the shoulder girdle with winging of the scapulae and difficulty in raising the arms. Later the muscles of the pelvis girdle become affected. The facial muscles are never affected. The disease runs a slow course but usually leads to death before the normal age. Serum creatine kinase levels may be normal or moderately raised. Muscle biopsy reveals myopathic changes.

This type of muscular dystrophy is extremely rare in paediatric practice.

Dystrophia Myotonica (Myotonic Dystrophy)

This disorder is inherited as an autosomal dominant with the locus being on the long arm of chromosome 19. Affected children nearly always have affected mothers (rather than fathers). It has been regarded as a disease of adult life, characterised by delayed muscle relaxation and atrophy (especially of the hands, masseters and sternomastoids), baldness, cataract and testicular atrophy. Clinical manifestations in childhood differ from the adult picture.

The clinical features in the neonate or older infant include hypotonia, facial diplegia and jaw weakness, delayed motor development and speech, talipes and respiratory problems. Mental retardation is relatively common. Clinical evidence of myotonia is absent (although it may be demonstrated by electromyography). Cataracts do not occur. Electromyography is the most helpful investigation. Muscle biopsy with special staining techniques and electron microscopy will confirm the diagnosis. DNA analysis will demonstrate the abnormal DM gene on chromosome 19. There is no effective treatment. If myotonia is significant, then phenytoin may be helpful.

AUTONOMIC NERVOUS SYSTEM

FAMILIAL DYSAUTONOMIA (RILEY-DAY SYNDROME)

This is a rare familial, autosomal recessive disorder, characterised by autonomic neuropathy and peripheral sensory neuropathy. The striking features are severe hypotonia, muscle weakness with areflexia, relative indifference to pain, excessive salivation and sweating, absent tears and recurrent pneumonia. The corneal reflex is usually absent. Difficulty in swallowing is common. There may be delayed psychomotor development and generalised seizures. Recurrent pyrexial episodes are common. In older children, attacks of cyclical vomiting with associated hypertension, excessive sweating and blotching of skin are not infrequent. Urinary frequency has also been noted in some patients.

Treatment

No specific treatment is available. Prompt treatment of respiratory infection, adequate fluid and electrolyte therapy for cyclical vomiting, topical ocular lubricants to prevent corneal ulcer and psychiatric treatment where indicated are advocated. Most affected children die in childhood.

MOVEMENT DISORDERS

The control of voluntary movement is affected by the interaction of the pyramidal, extra-pyramidal and cerebellar systems. The effects of disease of the extra-pyramidal system on movement are bradykinesia, rigidity, postural disturbance and involuntary movements namely chorea, athetosis, tremor and dystonia. Chorea is a jerky, semi-purposive, non-repetitive involuntary movement affecting the limbs, face and trunk. Causes of chorea in childhood include rheumatic chorea, extra-pyramidal

cerebral palsy, Wilson's disease and post-encephalitic sequalae.

WILSON'S DISEASE

This disease, inherited as an autosomal recessive trait, is an inborn error of copper metabolism resulting in an excessive accumulation of copper in the liver, brain, cornea and other tissues. The gene for Wilson's disease has been mapped to chromosome 13.

Clinical Features

Hepatic presentation in the form of jaundice, hepato-megaly, cirrhosis or portal hypertension, is predominant in children younger than 10 years of age. Neurological presentation is predominantly in older children with basal ganglia lesion, e.g. coarse tremors of the extremities (wing-beating tremor), dystonia, dysarthria, dysphasia, drooling, emotional instability, deterioration in school performance and dementia (Fig. 18.8). A characteristic finding is the Kayser-Fleischer ring, a golden brown discoloration due to deposition of copper at the corneal limbus.

Diagnosis

The serum ceruloplasmin level is decreased and urine copper excretion is increased particularly after a 1gm D-penicillamine challenge test. Liver function is usually deranged and slit-lamp examination of the eyes reveals K-F ring. Liver biopsy may reveal cirrhosis and excessive copper content.

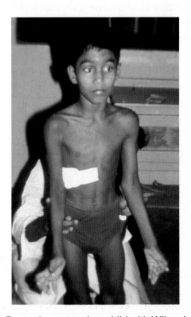

Fig. 18.8: Dystonic posture in a child with Wilson's disease.

Treatment

Early treatment with chelating agent can show marked improvement. Oral D-penicillamine is given in doses of 500 mg to 2 gm per day; the drug should be continued for life. Zinc reduces copper absorption and 100-150 mg/day can be given as an adjuvant therapy. A low-copper diet (excluding cocoa, nuts, liver, shellfish, mushrooms and spinach) is also advised. It is essential to screen siblings of patients with Wilson's disease.

Rheumatic Chorea (Sydenham's Chorea, St. Vitus Dance)

This major manifestation of rheumatic fever may occur in association with other manifestations such as polyarthritis and carditis but it frequently appears as a solitary and rather odd phenomenon. It is, in fact, the only major rheumatic manifestation which can affect the same child more than once, and sometimes several times, without the development of any of the other manifestations of acute rheumatic fever. For these reasons and also because the ESR and ASO titre remain normal in uncomplicated chorea, the precise relationship of this disease to rheumatic fever has been the subject of an unresolved controversy. It is more common in girls. The clinical features fall into four main groups.

a. Involuntary purposeless, non-repetitive movements of the limbs, face and trunk, e.g. grimacing, wriggling and writhing. The movements can be brought under voluntary control temporarily. They are aggravated by excitement and they disappear during sleep. The first indication may be that the child begins to drop things or her handwriting suddenly deteriorates or she gets into trouble with her elders for making faces. Sometimes the movements are confined to one side of the body (hemichorea).

b. Hypotonia may result in muscular weakness. It also causes the characteristic posture of the outstretched hands in which the wrist is slightly flexed, whereas there is hyperextension of the metacarpophalangeal joints. Occasionally the child is unable to stand or even to sit up (chorea paralytica).

c. Inco-ordination may be marked or only obvious when the child is asked to pick a coin off the floor.

d. Mental upset is often an early sign. Emotional lability is almost constant. School work usually deteriorates. Infrequently the child becomes confused or even maniacal (chorea insaniens).

As regards the management of rheumatic chorea carbamazepine, haloperidol, sodium valproate and prednisolone have been tried. Prophylactic chemotherapy with penicillin is required as for rheumatic fever.

CONVULSIONS IN INFANCY AND CHILDHOOD

Convulsion is a common acute and potentially life threatening event encountered in infants and children. About 5% of children would have had one or more convulsion by the time they reach maturity.

Aetiology

Seizures may be either provoked or unprovoked. The common provoking factors include high fever, perinatal damage, hypoglycaemia, hypocalcaemia, intracranial infections, head injury, tumours, inherited metabolic disorders and developmental anomalies of the brain. In some infants repeated seizures are due to an inborn error of brain metabolism, whereby the daily requirements of pyridoxine greatly exceed that in a normal diet. This state is known as pyridoxine dependency and it is rapidly amenable to treatment. Various other metabolic disturbances, in addition to hypoglycaemia already mentioned, can cause convulsions. These include hyponatraemia from water intoxication or from retention of water, acute infections of the brain tissues, hypernatraemia from severe hypertonic dehydration, inappropriate use of oral rehydration solution, disease of the hypothalamus or frontal lobe, and lead poisoning. Finally, hypertensive encephalopathy as a cause of convulsions in childhood is not excessively rare.

Unprovoked seizures are the result of a brain disorder producing recurrent spontaneous paroxysmal discharges of cerebral neurones. The term epilepsy is used when two or more unprovoked seizures occur at an interval of greater than 24 hour apart. However the close inter-relationship between the provoked and unprovoked groups, which overlap each other, must not be forgotten. It should be stressed further that in a high proportion of epileptic children and in a similar proportion with provoked seizures a family history of epileptic seizures or of infantile convulsions is obtainable.

Whereas there is a 1 in 200 risk of any child or adolescent experiencing an epileptic seizure, approximately one-third of children and adolescents with learning disabilities, cerebral palsy and autistic disorders will develop epileptic seizures.

Classification

Epileptic seizures are generally classified based on the clinical features of the attack and the accompanying EEG. The International classification of epilepsy is shown in Table 18.2. The electroencephalographic changes are frequently characteristic in the different clinical types but this correlation is by no means firm and a good deal of overerlap and mixing of types occur. A normal EEG does

Table 18.2: International classification of epileptic seizures

1. Partial seizures (attacks begin focally)
   i.   Simple partial (consciousness retained)
   ii. Complex partial (consciousness impaired)
   iii. Partial seizure with secondary generalisation
2. Generalised seizures
   i.   Tonic-clonic (grand mal)
   ii. Absences (petit mal)
   iii. Myoclonic seizures
   iv. Atonic seizures
3. Unclassified seizures

not preclude the diagnosis of epilepsy especially the interictal recording.

Epilepsy in children is also classified by syndrome. Epileptic syndrome is a complex of signs and symptoms that define a unique epilepsy condition. The uses of syndromic classification are better management with appropriate medication, identification of candidates for epileptic surgery and prediction of prognosis. The important epilepsy syndromes are infantile spasms (West syndrome), febrile convulsions, Lennox-Gastaut syndrome, benign myoclonic epilepsy of infancy, benign childhood epilepsy with centrotemporal spikes (Rolandic epilepsy), Ohtahara syndrome, juvenile myoclonic epilepsy (Janz syndrome) and progressive myoclonic epilepsy (Lafora disease). Some epileptic children remain unclassifiable.

A patient is said to be in status epilepticus when seizure lasts or occurs in succession for more than 30 minutes without intervening periods of recovery. It is a true medical emergency and can end fatally or with permanent sequelae of hypoxic brain damage. Secondary metabolic complications appear when convulsive status is prolonged. Lactic acidosis becomes prominent and cerebrospinal fluid pressure rises. Initial hyperglycaemia is followed by hypoglycaemia and autonomic dysfunctions appear consisting of hyperthermia, excessive sweating, dehydration, hypotension and eventually shock. Cardiovascular, respiratory and renal failure may result.

Generalised Seizures

Tonic-clonic Seizure (Grand Mal)

This is the commonest clinical manifestation of epilepsy. Its features include sudden loss of consciousness, possible injury from falling, tonic followed by clonic spasms, tongue biting, possible urinary or faecal incontinence, and frothing at the month. It is followed by post-ictal sleep, or a period of confusion or automatism. A careful examination is essential to exclude a provoking cause, which requires specific treatment. In febrile convulsion the convulsion is short, solitary and occurs at the onset of the illness. A prolonged or recurrent convulsion in a febrile child may

well herald idiopathic epilepsy and the physician should be guarded in his prognosis in these circumstances. In grand mal epilepsy the EEG shows most often frequent high-voltage spikes, but there may instead, or in addition, be spike-and-wave or slow-wave patterns. Even a normal EEG is not uncommon in major epilepsy and in no sense excludes such a diagnosis when the history is typical. Evaluation with cranial CT or MRI scan for children with generalised tonic-clonic seizures is not routinely required.

Absences (Petit Mal)

This diagnosis should be reserved for those children, usually girls above the age of 4 years, who show brief, often frequent, lapses of consciousness unassociated with twitching or loss of balance in which the EEG shows a characteristic 3 per second spike-and-wave pattern. Consciousness and activity are resumed suddenly after a few seconds. There is no post-ictal confusion or drowsiness. Activation, particularly hyperventilation, often can precipitate electrical and clinical seizures. Having the patient take about 60 deep breaths per minute for 3-4 minutes often precipitates a typical attack. Petit mal seizures are differentiated from complex partial seizures by their increased frequency, shorter duration, absence of loss of body tone, balance or post-ictal phenomenon. The distinction is important in treatment. Petit mal attacks show a tendency to disappear towards puberty (pyknolepsy). Unfortunately they are not infrequently replaced by grand mal.

Myoclonic Epilepsy

These attacks consist of brief, sudden, often symmetric muscular contractions of the head and neck, or of limbs. They may occur as the sole manifestation of epilepsy or in children who also have grand mal seizures. The muscular contractions may be sufficiently violent to throw the child to the ground, and repeated soft tissue injuries may occur. This type of epilepsy occurs due to multiple causes particularly degenerative and metabolic disease. The EEG frequently shows atypical slow spike-and-wave or polyspike discharges, which are more or less asymmetrical.

Infantile Spasms

These attacks, often extremely numerous each day, consist of a series of sudden jerks of the whole body, head and limbs. Most often the head and trunk flex suddenly forward while the arms jump forwards (salaam seizures) or up alongside the head, but the spasms may also be opisthotonic (extensor) in nature. Mixed flexor-extensor spasms are the most common type followed by flexor spasms; extensor spasms are the least common. The onset is usually between the ages of 3 and 9 months. In about half of the infants developmental retardation has been present before the onset of the fits and attributable to such perinatal insults as hypoxia, hypoglycaemia and intracranial haemorrhage, or to prenatal causes such as developmental malformations, toxoplasmosis and tuberous sclerosis, or to an inborn metabolic error such as phenylketonuria. Other infants have appeared to develop quite normally until the onset of the attacks. In some of these the aetiology is known, e.g. encephalitis. Others are "cryptogenic". The fits often become less frequent with the passage of time and may cease spontaneously. The EEG always shows gross abnormalities; the most severe and characteristic has been termed "hypsarrhythmia". This amounts to total chaos with asynchrony, high amplitude irregular spike-and-wave activity, no recognized discharges and no formal background activity. The triad of infantile spasms, retardation and hypsarrhythmia has become known as the West syndrome. The seizures usually are refractory to standard anticonvulsants. Long-term mental and developmental outcome of patients with infantile spasms is poor.

Atonic Seizures

In these attacks the child suddenly loses muscle tone and drops to the floor with transient unconsciousness. This type of seizure is usually seen in children with severe learning difficulty.

Partial Seizures

Partial seizures are those in which there is clinical or EEG evidence of focal onset. They are subdivided into (i) simple, i.e. without alteration of consciousness and (ii) complex, with impairment of consciousness. A partial seizure may progress to a generalised seizure.

(i) *Simple partial seizure:* These may be either motor or sensory in nature. In typical simple motor seizures, twitching or jerking starts in one area, arms or limb, and spreads in an orderly fashion until one half of the body is affected. This may be followed by a transient hemiparesis – Todd paralysis. In simple sensory seizures the patient complaints of paraesthesia or tingling in an extremity or face. Simple partial seizures often indicate structural brain disease, the focal onset localizing the organic lesion. Conjugate deviation of the head and eyes to one side may indicate a lesion in the opposite frontal lobe. Tingling in a foot incriminates the opposite postcentral sensory cortex.

(ii) *Complex partial seizure (Psychomotor seizure or temporal lobe epilepsy):* These attacks generally consist of an aura followed by impaired consciousness and automatism. The aura may take many forms, e.g. sudden fear, unpleasant smells or tastes, abdominal pain or tinnitus. Impaired consciousness may be brief and difficult to appreciate. The automatic behaviour

frequently consists of abnormal repetitive movements, e.g. jaw movements, smaking the lips, eye fluttering or blinking, or staring, clasping or fumbling with the hands. Sudden difficulty in speaking or incoherence is common. The most distressing features involve mental disturbances, e.g. violent tantrums, dream-like states or the déjà vu phenomenon (the mental impression that a new experience has happened before). Various types of visual, auditory or olfactory hallucinations may occur. There may be post-ictal confusion or sleepiness. This type of epilepsy is often difficult to diagnose in childhood because the young child is unable to describe the emotional or sensory elements of the seizures. It may take various forms, each rather bizarre and their epileptic basis should be indicated by their continued recurrence without obvious cause. The EEG typically shows a focal discharge from the temporal lobe, slow wave or spike-and-wave. Some children show spikes originating from other lobes. Various lesions have been noted in the temporal lobe by MRI scans and during surgery. The most common is mesotemporal sclerosis in the region of Ammon's horn. This may be a sequel to perinatal hypoxia but status epilepticus itself, as in prolonged febrile convulsion, may be the asphyxial incident, which is followed by temporal lobe seizures. Other pathologies identified include hamartoma, vascular malformation, post-encephalitic gliosis and low-grade tumours.

Febrile Seizures

Febrile seizures are convulsions precipitated by fever, not due to an intracranial infection or other definable CNS cause. Febrile seizures are the most common type of seizures during childhood with an incidence of 3-4%. They are age dependent and occur between 6 months and 5 years of age and are precipitated by a rapid rise of temperature to 39°C or greater due to viral fever, URI, acute otitis media, etc, in the early course of the fever. There may be a family history of febrile seizure in parents or siblings.

Clinical Features

Febrile seizures are classified as simple (85%) or atypical/complex (15%). The majority (simple) seizures are typically brief generalized tonic-clonic seizure lasting a few seconds to a few minutes followed by full recovery. Febrile seizures are considered as atypical/complex when the duration of seizure is longer than 15 minutes, repeated convulsions occur within the same day, when the seizure is focal or post-ictal focal deficit is noted. Febrile seizure lasting more than 30 minutes may be called febrile status and may leave a sequel, if untreated; particularly temporal lobe epilepsy due to mesial temporal sclerosis.

The risk of recurrence of febrile seizure is 30%. Most recurrences occur within the first year of the first febrile seizure. The future risk of epilepsy is 1% in simple febrile seizure and 9% when 2 or more risk factors are present. The risk factors are atypical febrile seizure, a positive family history of epilepsy, an initial febrile seizure before 9 months of age, delayed developmental milestones or a pre-existing neurological disorder. Intermittent prophylaxis with clobazam in a dose of 0.5 mg /kg/dose q12h × 2 days at the onset of fever has been found to decrease the chance of recurrence of febrile seizures. High-risk cases with several risk factors may be given sodium valproate (20-40 mg/kg/day) or phenobarbitone (3-5 mg/kg/day) for 1½-2 years.

Diagnosis

The first step is to make sure the child actually had a seizure. This depends on a careful history from a witness of the event, a thorough neurological examination and an EEG. The conditions that mimic seizures include breath-holding spells, reflex anoxic seizures, syncope, tics and movement disorders, migraine, benign paroxysmal vertigo, narcolepsy, night terrors and pseudo-seizures.

Breath-holding attacks: These occur not infrequently in infants or toddlers and they are usually precipitated by pain, indignation or frustration. There are two types of breath-holding attacks, the more common cyanotic form and the less common pallid form also called as reflex anoxic seizures.

Cyanotic breath-holding attack: Shortly after the onset of a fit of loud crying, the infant or toddler suddenly stops breathing in expiration and becomes cyanosed. If inspiration does not quickly follow the infant loses consciousness and goes rigid with back arched and extended limbs. He may have a few convulsive twitches. Respiration always starts again with rapid recovery and there is no danger to life. These attacks cease spontaneously as the child matures usually before 5 years of age. EEG shows no abnormality. The parents need to be reassured about its harmless nature and natural course. No specific treatment is necessary apart from correction of anaemia if present.

Pallid breath-holding attacks (reflex anoxic seizure): These occur in infants and children who have exaggerated vagal cardiac reflexes. Attacks may be precipitated by pain, which causes reflex cardiac asystole with sudden onset of extreme pallor, loss of posture and muscular hypotonia, and at times a tonic seizure. Recovery takes place as quickly as the onset with the resumption of ventricular contractions. No treatment is usually necessary. However if attacks are very frequent, oral atropine sulphate may be given.

The second step is to exclude a provoking factor for the seizure. Blood glucose and calcium measurement should be performed. Seizures in the first year of life or if associated with developmental delay will warrant a wider metabolic screen. Routine lumbar puncture is not indicated unless there is a reasonable suspicion of a CNS infection. When convulsions recur, EEG is essential. Computerised tomography and MRI scans may be required in some cases particularly in partial seizures.

Treatment

General: Most seizures are often self-limited and would have subsided by the time the child reaches a health care facility. If the child is still convulsing, airway, respiration and circulation are first assessed and maintained. This is followed by prompt termination of seizure activity by administration of 0.1mg/kg IV Lorazepam or 0.2 mg/kg IV of Diazepam. If vascular access is not possible, rectal diazepam at 0.5 mg/kg or intranasal midazolam may be administered. Cessation of seizure is followed by the determination of the underlying cause and treatment of this where possible.

Anticonvulsants: The majority of children with a first unprovoked seizure will not have a recurrence. Hence anti-epileptic drug treatment should not be commenced routinely after a first unprovoked tonic-clonic seizure. Risk factors for recurrence include remote symptomatic aetiology, abnormal EEG, a history of prior febrile convulsions and age less than three years. In newly diagnosed epilepsy, the aims of treatment are to control, or prevent if possible, the recurring seizures of the epileptic, and to achieve this with one drug. The choice of the antiepileptic drug should be determined where possible by the syndromic diagnosis and potential adverse effects. Generalised tonic clonic epilepsy can be treated with sodium valproate, carbamazepine, phenytoin or pheno-barbitone. Ethosuximide and sodium valproate are both effective in controlling childhood absence epilepsy. Myoclonic epilepsy is usually treated with sodium valproate or clonazepam. The first line drug in partial seizure is carbamazepine. However sodium valproate, phenytoin, lamotrigine, clobazam, oxcarbazepine and vigabatrin are all effective as monotherapy in the treatment of focal seizures. In drug resistant generalised epilepsy, clobazam, clonazepam and lamotrigine are effective as add-on treatments. Lamotrigine, gabapentin, topiramate and oxcarbazepine are effective as add-on therapies for focal seizures.

The treatment of infantile spasms (West's syndrome) is unsatisfactory; they are resistant to most conventional anticonvulsant drugs, although they sometimes cease spontaneously with time. At present, corticotrophin (ACTH) or corticosteroids is recommended as first line treatment. The therapeutic efficacy of these two drugs is relatively equal and one may be effective if the other drug fails. ACTH is given intramuscularly in doses of 40 units/

day and prednisolone is given orally in doses of 20-30 mg/day. A 21-day course of treatment is usually sufficient; although in some cases prolonged but reduced dosage is necessary. In West's syndrome secondary to tuberous sclerosis, vigabatrin is superior. Benzodiazepines, clonazepam and nitrazepam are the alternative drugs for the treatment of infantile spasms.

Adverse effects from antiepileptic drugs are common and are a major cause of discontinuing drug treatment. Many adverse effects are dose related and predictable. These can be minimised by gradual escalation of the dose, regular monitoring of the serum concentration of the drug and appropriate dose reduction. Idiosyncratic drug reactions usually arise early in treatment. Rash is a common adverse effect in children and is associated with carbamazepine, phenytoin and lamotrigine. Rarely, a severe hypersensitivity syndrome may occur which may be life threatening. Sodium valproate has very little sedative action. The dosage is 20-30 mg/kg/day given in a twice-daily dose. Adverse reactions include mild nausea, vomiting and transient alopecia. Significant weight gain can occur. In a few children it has caused acute liver failure and pancreatitis. The value of estimating the serum concentration of valproate is less than for other drugs as it seems to have a longer action than its half-life (4-14 hours) would suggest. Tremor and thrombocytopaenia are dose related side effects. Carbamazepine rarely causes drowsiness and has considerable advantage for children and adolescents, in whom learning ability is very important. It may cause ataxia if started in full doses too abruptly. The usual dose is 10-20 mg/kg/day given in 2-3 divided doses started at a lower dose and increased gradually. Phenytoin is given in a dose of 5-10 mg/kg/day in 2 divided doses. There are very many interactions between phenytoin and other drugs. Over dosage results in ataxia and it is helpful to monitor serum concentration. An unwelcome although reversible side effect is hypertrophy of the gums, seen in a sizeable proportion of patients. Prolonged medication can result in hirsutism, coarsening of the facies towards an acromegaloid appearance and acne. Very rarely in children it causes megaloblastic anaemia responding to folic acid. The major side effects of benzodiazepines are behavioural with clobazam and clonazepam causing over activity, aggression, sleep disturbance and poor concentration. In some children excessive sedation and hypotonia occur. Development of tolerance to their antiepileptic effects is another problem. Clonazepam is started with a single evening dose of 250-500 micrograms gradually increasing to a daily dose of 0.1-0.2 mg/kg/day in three divided doses. Phenobarbitone causes impairment of cognitive function, drowsiness, restlessness and behaviour disturbances in a fair proportion of patients. Antiepileptic drugs have teratogenic side effects.

Overall, 60-70% of children who have been seizure free on drugs for two years or more will remain seizure free when the drugs are withdrawn. Sudden discontinuation of antiepileptic drugs, particularly phenobarbitone and benzodiazepines should be avoided.

Social management: The epileptic child whose convulsion can be prevented or rendered infrequent should attend an ordinary school and live as normal a life as possible. The physician must by explanation and advice bring the parents to accept the need for an unrestricted existence and even to accept a few risks. Certain restrictions such as riding a bicycle in the city streets or swimming unsupervised are clearly unavoidable, but they should be reduced to the minimum. For many children and their families, social and psychological factors far outweigh those problems associated with the prevention and control of seizures. Families who have a child with epilepsy should be given clear, accurate and appropriate information about the condition, its treatment and the implication for everyday living. A multidisciplinary approach provided within a specialist clinic, with support and advice from a clinical nurse specialist, with help from relevant voluntary support organizations and occasionally from psychologists and psychiatrists has proved helpful to some families. Special schooling may be necessary for the learning-impaired epileptic. Schools should be given written information on epilepsy and its management.

CEREBRAL PALSY

Cerebral Palsy (CP) is defined as a central motor dysfunction affecting muscle tone, posture and movement resulting from a permanent, non-progressive defect or lesion of the immature brain. It is one of the common chronic neurological disorders in children.

The incidence of cerebral palsy is in the region of 2.5 per 1000 in childhood. Figures have always varied from one country to another. The problem is, therefore, a large one. It is essential to stress, also, that children who suffer from cerebral palsy frequently have other severe handicaps. The associated co-morbid conditions result mostly from damage to other parts of the brain by the same damaging event. Approximately 50% of cerebral palsied children have an intelligence quotient (IQ) below 70, as compared with 3% of the general population. Epileptic seizures are common in cerebral palsied children and speech defects occur in about 50%. Deafness, frequently unexpected, is common particularly high-tone deafness. Squints occur in almost one-half of all affected children. Refractive errors are common. Dental problems are also common, such as gingivitis due to defective chewing, tooth grinding and malocclusion.

Aetiology

The causes of cerebral palsy can be generally classified as prenatal, perinatal and postnatal causes. However, sometimes, it is impossible to determine the precise cause of cerebral palsy in the individual patient. The prenatal causes include genetic factors, intrauterine infection during pregnancy, radiation, cerebral infarction, metabolic and toxic factors and hypoxia. Approximately half of all cases of cerebral palsy are associated with preterm delivery and low birth weight. The precise nature of this relationship is not clear although hypoxia and hypotension are important factors. Although the perinatal risk factor of birth asphyxia is a well-recognized cause of cerebral palsy particularly in the term baby, the incidence of birth asphyxia among cases of cerebral palsy is not high. The main pathological lesions found in preterm infants who later develop cerebral palsy are periventricular leucomalacia and intracerebral haemorrhage. Lesions in the full term infants who develop cerebral palsy are mainly due to hypoxic ischaemic encephalopathy and are seen in thalami and basal ganglia or in the cortex and sub-cortical white matter. Postnatal causes of cerebral palsy include hypoglycaemia, hyper-bilirubinaemia, meningitis, subdural haematoma, acute infantile haemiplegia and trauma.

Classification of cerebral palsy: Cerebral palsy may be classified in terms of physiologic, topographic, aetiologic and functional categories Table 18.3.

Clinical Features

(1) Spastic cerebral palsy: This group shows the features of upper motor neurone type of pyramidal tract lesion such as spastic hypertonicity, exaggerated deep tendon reflexes, ankle clonus and extensor plantar response. It may be symmetric or asymmetric and may involve one or more extremities. In spastic diplegia the lower limbs are affected more than the upper limbs. In spastic quadriplegia there is marked involvement of all four limbs. Involvement of one side of the body is termed spastic haemiplegia.

Spastic diplegia: This type of cerebral palsy also called Little's disease, affects particularly the preterm babies. Term babies with perinatal asphyxia are also prone. The most common neuropathologic finding is periventricular leucomalacia and/or haemorrhage. These babies, often evolve through a dystonic phase when at the age of 2-3 months they may be stiff with extensor hypertonia which may last until 7 or 8 months of age when it is replaced by spasticity. Spasticity is of two types. The flexor muscles are mainly affected in tonic spasticity and extensor muscles such as triceps and quadriceps in phasic spasticity. The phasically spastic muscles show brisk tendon reflexes and often the clasp-knife phenomenon. Tonically spastic muscles show decreased lengthening reaction and rapidly develop contractures. The hip flexors, hamstrings and calf muscles together with adductors of hip form the main tonic groups in the lower limbs, causing the child to be flexed at hip, knee and in equinus at the ankle with the legs usually internally rotated and the characteristic scissoring posture (Fig. 18.9). The upper limbs are flexed at elbow and wrist, and the fingers are flexed across the adducted thumb with marked spasticity of the pronators. Atrophy below the waist occurs in many patients. In spastic diplegia of low birth weight babies epilepsy is uncommon and intelligence is only moderately reduced whereas in diplegia of term asphyxiated babies, epilepsy, mental retardation, micro-cephaly, speech and behaviour disorders are more common.

Table 18.3: Classification of cerebral palsy: Cerebral palsy may be classified in terms of physiologic, topographic and functional categories		
Physiologic	*Topographic*	*Functional*
Spastic	Diplegia	Class I – No limitation of activity
Athetoid	Hemiplegia	
Rigid	Quadriplegia	Class II – Slight to moderate limitation
Ataxic	Double hemiplegia	
Tremor	Triplegia	Class III – Moderate to severe limitation
Atonic	Paraplegia	
Mixed	Monoplegia	Class IV – No useful physical activity

Adapted from Minear WL A classification of cerebral palsy Pediatrics 18:841; 1956

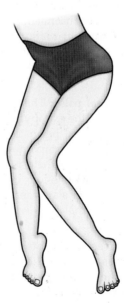

Fig. 18.9: Drawing from Little's monograph illustrating one of his cases of spastic diplegia. (Little Deformities of the human frame, 1953)

Spastic quadriplegia: This is the most severe form of cerebral palsy often the result of intrauterine disease, usually malformation and in some due to hypoxic ischaemic encephalopathy in term newborns. There is marked motor impairment of all four extremities. Feeding is difficult because of pseudobulbar palsy with increased incidence of gastro-oesophageal reflux and aspiration syndrome. There is a high association with mental retardation and seizures. Speech and visual abnormalities are common. Neuropathologic findings include severe periventricular leucomalacia, multicystic encephalo-malacia and cerebral dysgenesis. Positional deformities are common resulting in windswept posture of lower limbs, dislocation of hip, pelvic tilt, scoliosis and rib deformities.

Spastic haemiplegia: This type of cerebral palsy affects one side of body. The majority are congenital and the result of maldevelopment, prenatal circulatory disturbances or perinatal stroke in the distribution of middle cerebral artery. Postnatal causes include acute CNS infection, acute infantile haemiplegia, cerebral thrombosis particularly in congenital cyanotic heart disease and subdural haematoma. The right side is more often affected than the left, and the arm more severely than the leg. The condition may be missed during the neonatal period. Later reduced movement and abnormal posturing on one side and rarely hand preference may be observed. There is delay in walking and hand manipulation skills on the affected side. The upper limb assumes a flexed posture at the elbow and wrist with adduction at the shoulder and forearm pronated. In the lower limb the hip is partially flexed and adducted, the knee flexed and the foot in equinus position. The child walks with a circumducting gait. There is growth arrest of the affected extremities, particularly the hand. Cortical sensory loss and haemianopia are not infrequent. Convulsions and mental retardation are seen in about one fourth of these children. Neuropathologic findings show an atrophic cerebral haemisphere with a dilated lateral ventricle.

(2) Dyskinetic cerebral palsy: This type of cerebral palsy results from damage to the extrapyramidal system usually the result of jaundice and perinatal asphyxia. There is defect of posture and involuntary movement. It could take the form of athetosis, choreoathetosis, rigidity or dystonia. Pathologic findings include lesions in the globus pallidus, subthalamic nucleus and status marmoratus (lesions in the basal ganglia and thalamus with a marbled appea-rance).

Athetosis: The affected infants go through an early hypotonic phase characterized by lethargy, poor head control and feeding difficulty. This is followed after 4 months of age by the dystonic phase associated with extensor hypertonia, arching attacks and abnormal persistence of primitive reflexes. The stage of involuntary movement is obvious after 2 years consisting of slow writhing distal movements. When athetosis is caused by kernicterus there is often a high-tone deafness. The child is dysarthritic and drooling may be prominent. Seizures are uncommon and intelligence may be well preserved.

Choreoathetosis: In this type the writhing athetotic movements have in addition jerky, irregular, rapid movements involving the face and proximal extremities. Stress and excitement may exacerbate the chorea.

Dystonia: This type affects the trunk and proximal muscles of the limbs and consists of abnormal twisting and sustained movements, which may be either slow or rapid. These children tend to be more severely affected.

(3) Ataxic cerebral palsy: In a small proportion of children with cerebral palsy, the clinical manifestation indicate a cerebellar defect, e.g. ataxic reeling gait, intention tremor and past pointing, dysdiadokokinesia, hypotonia and diminished deep tendon reflexes. Most of these cases are congenital in origin and due to malformations of the cerebellum and may have an autosomal inheritance. A few cases are due to perinatal asphyxia and hydro-cephalus, and meningitis. Most patients have congenital hypotonia. Motor milestones and language skills are typically delayed.

(4) Tremor: This type of cerebral palsy is rare and characterised by a constant, severe coarse tremor. Spasticity and athetosis are rare but true extrapyramidal rigidity is not infrequently also present.

(5) Hypotonic cerebral palsy: In a few children cerebral palsy takes the form of a hypotonic quadriplegia without any spasticity. Many infants destined to develop typical spastic diplegia pass through a hypotonic phase. The true situation is usually revealed by adductor muscle spasm, but in some cases differentiation from hypotonic cerebral palsy depends upon continued observation. In benign congenital hypotonia there has usually been a normal birth and later normal development, whereas in hypotonic cerebral palsy there has often been perinatal asphyxia and is associated with severe learning difficulties.

(6) Mixed cerebral palsy: Mixed cerebral palsy includes manifestations of both spastic and extrapyramidal types; often an ataxic component is present. These patterns of motor impairment are the result of involvement of large areas of brain affecting the cortex, subcortical areas and basal ganglia.

The Early Diagnosis of Cerebral Palsy

The diagnosis of CP depends upon a combination of motor delay, neurologic signs, persistence of primitive reflexes and abnormal postural reactions. Infants with an abnormal obstetric or perinatal history are at increased risk to develop cerebral palsy and should be monitored closely. Clues to an early diagnosis include abnormal behaviour, psychomotor delay and abnormal oromotor or oculomotor patterns.

Neurobehavioural signs suspicious of cerebral palsy are excessive docility or irritability. A typical history includes poor feeding in the neonatal period. The baby often is irritable, sleeps poorly, vomits frequently, is difficult to handle and cuddle, and has poor visual attention.

Motor tone in the extremities may be normal or increased. Persistent or asymmetric fisting may be present. Poor head control and excessive head lag may be early motor signs. However, increased neck extensor and axial tone may make head control appear early in cerebral palsy. In many cases spasticity may not be identified until six or seven months of age. Dyskinetic patterns are not typically apparent until approximately 18 months. Ataxia may not become obvious until even later.

Primitive reflexes in cerebral palsy may be asymmetric or persistent. In normal infants, most primitive reflexes related to posture (tonic labyrinthine, tonic neck and neck-righting and body righting reflexes) disappear when the infants are between three and six months of age. These reflexes often are not appropriately integrated or inhibited in children with cerebral palsy. Thus, delay in the disappearance or exaggeration of a primitive reflex may be an early indicator of cerebral palsy. Other abnormal signs can be elicited when the infant is held in vertical suspension. During the first few months, the appropriate response is for the baby to assume a sitting position ("sit in the air"). An abnormal response is persistent extension of the legs and crossing (scissoring), which is due to adductor spasm.

The practice parameter from the American Academy of Neurology and the Child Neurology Society recommends the following approach to the evaluation of the child with cerebral palsy. All children with cerebral palsy should undergo a detailed history and physical examination. It is particularly important to determine that the condition is static rather than progressive or degenerative. It is also important to classify the type of cerebral palsy. Screening for mental retardation, ophthalmologic abnormalities, hearing impairment, speech and language disorders, and disorders of oro-motor functions are warranted as part of the initial assessment. An EEG is recommended when there are features suggestive of epilepsy. Neuroimaging is recommended to both establish an aetiology and for prognostic purposes. MRI is preferred to CT scan. Metabolic and genetic testing is considered if the clinical history or findings on neuroimaging do not determine a specific structural abnormality or if there are additional atypical features in the history or clinical examination.

Management

The management of children with cerebral palsy has many facets such as physiotherapy, play therapy, orthoptic care, pharmacotherapy, hearing aids, speech therapy, correction of refractive error, orthopaedic surgery, special education, etc. It is the responsibility of the paediatrician to coordinate the whole management. Parents are an integral part of the management team.

The objectives of the treatment programs are to improve function, prevent deformity and to encourage independence. A proper assessment of the child noting his capabilities and disabilities (motor, mental, speech, vision, hearing and psychologic) is made. The earlier in the child's life treatment can be begun the better will be the result. An early infant stimulation programme during the first 2 years of life with emphasis on more than just improving motor deficits is emphasized. Physiotherapy combined with orthotics with occasional plaster immobilisation and orthopaedic surgery remains the mainstay of treatment. Drugs have a limited role in cerebral palsy. Pharmacotherapy to decrease spasticity includes benzodiazepine, baclofen, botulinum toxin and dantrolene. Selective dorsal rhizotomy has to be occasionally resorted to, to decrease spasticity. It has been claimed that levodopa will occasionally produce dramatic results in children with athetoid cerebral palsy. Anticonvulsant drugs are indicated in epilepsy. In a few older children with congenital haemiplegia complicated by frequent and uncontrollable epileptic seizures, the operation of haemispherectomy has abolished the seizures. Some cerebral palsied children of normal intelligence, specially those with haemiplegia and diplegia, may manage well in a normal school. On the other hand, the spastic or athetotic child who is severely crippled but educable is best educated in a special school (day or residential) for cerebral palsied children. The family of the cerebral palsy child needs regular counselling and the benefits of community services to cope with the stress of bringing up a child with cerebral palsy.

LEARNING DISORDERS (Developmental Retardation)

Words used to describe individuals with learning disorders such as the terms mental deficiency, mental retardation or mental handicap are taken to mean a failure of development of the mind. This is in contrast to dementia, which means a disintegration of the fully developed mind. As a group these children have in common learning difficulty. The severely affected have difficulty learning to walk, feed, dress and communicate. The more mildly affected have difficulty, in acquiring social and physical skills to enable them to earn a living and cope with the demands of society. Words used to describe the severity of the learning difficulty, e.g. idiot, imbecile; feeble-minded, moron have become terms of abuse and even the terms mental retardation and handicap are being abandoned. The WHO classifies mental handicap into profound IQ 0-20; severe IQ 20-34; moderate IQ 35-49 and mild IQ 50-70. Although IQ measurement is a rather too broad assessment on which to base specialised education input for the child, a rough educational classification is that children with an IQ of less than 50 are severely educationally subnormal (ESN) and those between 50 and 70 have moderate ESN. There are, of course, varying degrees of severity of learning difficulty. Those with an IQ below 50 are likely always to need care and attention and unlikely to be educable in any formal sense. Those with an IQ between 70 and 90 are not included within the group of learning disordered children, but they are likely to be educationally backward and to be placed in the lower educational stream of a normal school. Some, in fact, require the facilities and specially trained staff of a special school.

Aetiology

The vast majority of cases of learning disorder can be placed in one of two broad aetiological groups, primary amentia which is due to inheritance or defects in the child's genetic material; and secondary in which the brain, derived from a normal germ plasm, has been damaged by environmental influences which may be operative prenatally, perinatally or postnatally. In some cases both genetic and environmental factors combine to result in brain damage. It must be stressed, however, that in individual patients it is quite often impossible to determine the precise cause of the mental retardation. For example, in the case of a severely retarded child, apnoeic and cyanotic attacks in the first week of life could indicate brain damage resulting from anoxia or respiratory difficulties due to malfunctioning of an abnormally formed brain.

Inheritance

A large number of single gene defects have been uncovered as causes of learning disorder. Many of these fall into the category of inborn errors of metabolism. They are now numerous and include phenylketonuria, maple syrup urine disease, the organic acidurias, homocystinuria, argininosuccinic aciduria, Hartnup's disease, galactosaemia, pyridoxine dependency, Niemann-Pick disease, Gaucher's disease, Tay-Sach's disease, mucopolysaccharidoses and others such as Sturge-Weber syndrome, tuberous sclerosis and neurofibromatosis. Some cases of sporadic cretinism and all cases of non-endemic familial goitrous cretinism are also due to single gene defects. Another rare example is familial dysautonomia (Riley-Day syndrome). While the single gene defects cited above are each relatively rare, it has been recognized that X-linked genes are quite frequently responsible for non-specific mental retardation. In many of the affected males a marker X-chromosome has been identified. The marker in this "fragile X syndrome" is a "fragile site" occurring at band q27 or q28 (i.e. towards the end of the long arm) of the X-chromosome. However, not all males with X-linked non-specific mental retardation have this fragile site on the X-chromosome. At least three distinct forms of X-linked mental retardation have been described which seem to breed true within families. The most clearly definable is found in males with the marker X-chromosome and macro-orchidism. The enlarged testes become obvious after puberty and are only occasionally noticeable at birth. The degree of learning difficulty is usually severe but may be mild. Specific speech delay is common and is associated with a characteristic rhythmic quality of "litany speech". Epilepsy may be a feature in some severely affected boys. In another group of families both the marker X chromosome and macro-orchidism are absent but the other clinical features are indistinguishable from those described above. In the third type of X-linked mental retardation there is no marker chromosome but the affected boys show microcephaly, severe retardation and small testes. The female carriers of the marker X-chromosome are generally of normal intelligence although some have been mildly retarded, possibly related to non-random X-inactivation in the central nervous system. Chromosome analysis of boys with non-specific learning disorder is essential for genetic counselling. When the characteristic clinical features described above are present in a boy with no family history the recurrence risk seems to be about 10%.

Some types of mental retardation have been clearly related to gross chromosomal abnormalities. The most severe degrees are usually produced by non-dysjunction during gametogenesis in the mother, leading to trisomy for one of the small acrocentric autosomes. In these conditions the long-recognised correlation with advancing maternal age has been explained on the assumption that the aging ovum is more prone to favour non-dysjunction. Down's syndrome is the most common of the trisomies (about 1.8 per 1000 live births) and is a major cause of profound and severe learning disorder. Only a rare case falls into the moderate category.

The next most common autosomal trisomies in live-born children are trisomy 13 (Patau's syndrome) and trisomy 18 (Edward's syndrome) with frequencies of about 0.5 and 0.1per 1000 live births respectively. Each causes such severe and multiple abnormalities including profound learning disorders that those affected rarely survive infancy.

A variety of structural chromosome anomalies have also been found associated with severe learning disability. The best defined of these is the cri-du-chat syndrome, which is due to partial deletion of the short arm of chromosome 5. About two-thirds of the patients have been females and its frequency at birth is 1/50,000 to 1/100,000 or less. The name of this syndrome derives from the characteristic mewing-like cry, which is present from the neonatal period. The birth weight is low. Both physical and mental development is markedly retarded. In Wolf syndrome many similar features to the cri-du-chat syndrome occur, although the cat-like cry is often absent. It is due to partial deletion of the short arm of chromosome 4.

Rett's Syndrome

In 1966 Rett described 22 mentally handicapped children, all of them girls, who had a history of regression in development and displayed striking repetitive hand movements. It is now evident that this clinical disorder affects between 1 in 10,000 to 1 in 30,000 female infants, with signs of developmental regression appearing during the first year of life and accelerating during the second year of life. At the onset of the regression in locomotion, manipulation and speech, screaming attacks are common. Rhythmic hand movements with fingers usually adducted and partly extended are characteristic with patting or lightly clapping them, banging the mouth or wringing and squeezing intertwined fingers. In some girls there are choreiform trunk and limb movements and dystonia. As they grow older the girls become more placid, their lower limbs progressively stiff with wasting, scoliosis and respiratory dysrhythmias, hyperventilation and apnoeic episodes. The cause is unknown although a defective gene on the X chromosome has been proposed.

Most of the genetically determined types of disordered mental function discussed so far have been of severe to moderate degree. On the other hand, rather more than 75% of all learning disordered fall into the mild learning difficulty category (IQ 50-70) and cannot be attributed to single gene or gross chromosomal abnormalities. Although, it is accepted that genetic influences play a major part in determining the child's intelligence, there is good evidence that environmental influences also affect intelligence.

Environment

In some cases learning disorder has resulted from damage to a normally developing brain by some noxious environmental influence. They may operate at various periods in the stage of development. Microbial causes of brain damage account for about 10% of all cases of learning disorder associated with microcephaly.

Prenatal

Rubella during the first 12 weeks of pregnancy can certainly damage the foetal brain. Toxoplasmosis may also be associated with mental retardation. Cytomegalovirus is the commonest known viral cause of mental retardation. About 40% of women enter pregnancy without antibodies, about twice the number who are susceptible to rubella. It has been estimated that about 1% of pregnant women in London undergo primary infection and that half of their infants are infected in utero. While most of these congenital infections are asymptomatic and only a few exhibit the severe illness, proportions are subsequently found to have learning disorders or to suffer other neurological deficits. Human immunodeficiency virus infection is a well-known cause of mental retardation. Maternal irradiation has been shown to result in mental retardation with microcephaly, and sometimes microphthalmia as in the survivors of the Hiroshima and Nagasaki atomic attacks. The effect upon a child's intelligence of adverse environmental factors during the mother's pregnancy, such as poverty, malnutrituion, excessive smoking and emotional stress are difficult to assess. They might increase the risk of learning disorder by their association with intrauterine fetal malnutrition.

Perinatal

There is a well-documented association between some of the complications of pregnancy and abnormalities of the brain including mental retardation. These complications such as antepartum haemorrhage, pre-eclampsia, breech presentation and complicated or instrumental delivery are frequently associated with intrapartum fetal anoxia. It is, however, extremely difficult to assess the importance of intrapartum or neonatal anoxia as a cause of later neurological disability.

Postnatal

Postnatal causes of mental retardation include meningitis, encephalitis, hypoglycaemia, bilirubin encephalopathy, subdural haematoma, hypernatraemia and head injury. Lead encephalopathy is a rare but undoubted cause of permanent brain damage. It remains uncertain whether low-level lead exposures; with blood levels below 1.9 μmol/l (40μg/100ml) may cause some cognitive impairment and possibly behavioural abnormalities.

Diagnosis

In most cases the diagnosis of disordered learning ability can be made in the first year of life, provided the physician is familiar with the stages of development in the normal baby and that he realises the variations, which may occur in perfectly normal babies. It is essential that a thoughtful history be obtained from the parents, to be followed by a detailed physical examination of the child. Frequently the child must be seen on several occasions before a final conclusion is possible. There may be factors which indicate that the child is "at risk" and more likely to be retarded than others. These include prematurity, complications of pregnancy or labour, a history of asphyxia neonatorum, intra or periventricular haemorrhage, jaundice in the newborn period, convulsions or cyanotic attacks, maternal rubella or a family history of learning disorder. The basis of the diagnosis of learning disorder may be conveniently discussed under four headings.

Physical Abnormalities

Certain physical features are undoubted evidence of associated mental defect. These include the characteristic signs of Down syndrome, microcephaly, cretinism and gargoylism. Other physical abnormalities are often, although not invariably, associated with learning disorder. In this group are cerebral palsy, the bilateral macular choroidoretinitis of toxoplasmosis, Turner syndrome and hydrocephalus. Certain other physical "stigmata" are seen more commonly in learning disordered than in normal people, but in themselves they can do no more than direct the physician's attention towards a more careful assessment of the child's intellectual development. Such peculiarities are a high narrow (saddle-shaped) palate, abnormally simple ears, hypertelorism, marked epicanthic folds and short, curved fifth fingers. A distinctive pattern of altered growth and morphogenesis can be recognised in the children of mothers who consume large quantities of alcohol during pregnancy. They exhibit both pre- and postnatal growth failure involving weight, length and head circumference. Neurological abnormalities include hypotonia, irritability and jitteriness, poor co-ordination, hyperkinesis, and learning difficulties, which may vary from severe to mild. Dysmorphic features include short palpebral fissures (canthus to canthus), epicanthic folds, and hypoplastic or absent philtrum, thin upper lip, broad nasal bridge with upturned nose and mid-facial hypoplasia. Other congenital anomalies may involve the heart, genitourinary system, eyes, ears, mouth or skeleton. Haemangiomata and herniae are not uncommon. Abnormal palmar creases and hirsutism have also been recorded.

Delayed Psychomotor Development

It is characteristic of the learning disordered child that his development is delayed in all its parameters. He is slow in showing an interest in his surroundings, slow in attempting to handle or play with objects, slow to sit or stand unsupported or to walk on his own, late in speaking, late in acquiring bladder or bowel control. A lack of concentration or sustained interest is also obvious. Thus, after handling a new toy or object for a minute or two he loses interest and throws it down. His lack of interest in things around him may raise the suspicion of defective vision, just as his lack of response to sounds is apt to lead to a mistaken impression of deafness. Infantile practices tend to persist beyond the normal period, e.g. putting

objects into his mouth, excessive and prolonged posturing of his hands and fingers before his eyes, drooling and slobbering. The physician must obviously be familiar with the various developmental stages of normal infants and children before he is in a position to make a judicious assessment of an individual patient. A brief outline of the more positive developmental steps is shown in Table 18.4. The best assessment is to be expected from the doctor who has had long and intimate contact with normal children in the Child Health Clinic or in their family practice, provided that during their undergraduate period they have developed the capacity to observe, and to appreciate the significance of their observations.

Abnormal Behaviour and Gestures

Learning disordered children frequently engage in types of behaviour and mannerisms, which are obviously abnormal for their age. Thus, in early infancy the retarded baby may be excessively "good" in that he will lie in his bed for long periods without crying or showing restlessness, interest in surroundings, or boredom. In other cases there is constant or prolonged and apparently purposeless crying. Teeth grinding when awake is a common and distressing habit of many with profound learning disorders. The older child may exhaust his mother by his aimless over activity, which may at times endanger his life. Certain rhythmic movements although by no means confined to learning disordered children are more commonly indulged in by them and for more prolonged periods. These include head banging, body-rocking to-and-fro, and head rolling. Profoundly disordered children frequently lack the normal capacity for affection, they may be prone to sudden rages, and they may assault other younger children.

Convulsions

Most epileptics are of normal intelligence. None the less, epileptic seizures occur more frequently among mentally retarded children than those who are normal. Frequently repeated generalised seizures lead to slowly progressive intellectual deterioration. The association of infantile spasms (hypsarrhythmia) with severe learning difficulties has been described previously.

Differential Diagnosis

The diagnosis of learning disorder is obviously one in which the physician must not be wrong or he will cause the parents unjustifiable and unnecessary grief and anxiety. Some infants have a "slow start" but catch up later, and in the absence of manifest physical signs, such as microcephaly or Down syndrome, a firm diagnosis of learning disorder should only be made after a period of observation during which the rate of development is

	Table 18.4: Developmental steps in the normal child		
Age	*Development*	*Age*	*Development*
4 weeks	Head flops back when lifted from supine to sitting position Sits with rounded back while supported Grasp reflex elicited by placing object in palm Responds to sudden noise		Discusses a picture Asks frequent questions Listens to and demands stories Likes to help mother in house, father in garden Eats with fork and spoon Can dress and undress
8 weeks	Sucks vigorously Almost no head lag when pulled into sitting position Sits with almost straight back and head only nods occasionally Grasp reflex slight or absent Smiles readily: Vocalizes when talked to	4 years	Asks incessant questions Climbs ladders and trees Engages in imitative play, e.g. doctor or nurse Uses proper sentences to describe recent experiences
12 weeks	Follows objects with head and eyes No head lag when pulled into sitting position Sits supported with straight back: Head almost steady No grasp reflex: Holds objects in hand for short time Watches own hand movements Turns head towards sounds		Can give name, age and address Draws man with features and extremities Matches four primary colours correctly Plays with other children Alternately cooperative and aggressive with adults or other children
6 months	Lifts head from pillow Sits unsupported when placed in position Rolls from supine to prone position Grasps objects when offered Drinks from cup Transfers objects from one hand to the other Responds to name Held standing can bear weight on legs and bounces up and down No more hand regard: Finds feet interesting	18 months	Can walk upstairs holding on to hand or rail Can carry or pull toy when walking Can throw ball without falling Points to three or four parts of body on request Indicates need for toilet Lifts and controls drinking cup Points to three to five objects or animals in picture book Runs safely on whole foot: Can avoid obstacles
12 months	Understands simple sentences and commands Can rise to sitting from supine position Pulls to standing position by holding on to cot side Walks holding hand or furniture Speaks a few recognisable words Points to objects which are desired Throws objects out of pram in play		Can kick a ball without losing balance Can walk upstairs: Holding rail coming downstairs Turns door handles Forms short sentences: Vocabulary of 50 words Can put on shoes and pants Demands constant adult attention Dry most nights if "lifted" at 11 p.m.
15 months	Walks unsteadily with feet wide apart; falls at corners Can get into standing position alone Tries untidily to feed himself with spoon Plays with cubes: Places one on top of another Indicates wet pants Now seldom puts toys in mouth Shows curiosity and requires protection from dangers	5 years	Runs quickly on toes: Skips on alternate feet Can tie shoelaces Can name common coins Draws recognisable complete man Names four primary colours; matches 10-12 colours
3 years	Walks upstairs with alternating feet Washes and dries hands with supervision Rides tricycle Draws a man on request – head, trunk and one or two other parts Can count up to ten		Cooperates more with friends: Accepts rules in games Protective towards younger children and pets May know letters of alphabet and read simple words

assessed. There are now available developmental screening protocols in which a child's development can be charted in a longitudinal fashion, making it easier for the less experienced doctor to detect early departures from the normal. It is easy to confuse learning disorder with cerebral palsy. Indeed the two frequently coexist. Careful neurological examination, repeated on several occasions, will reveal the motor handicaps of cerebral palsy. The deaf child has frequently been diagnosed as mentally retarded, sometimes with tragic results. This mistake should not occur when the physician takes a detailed history and follows it with a careful physical examination. The deaf child will, of course, show a lively visual interest and his motor skills will develop normally. A difficult if not very common problem is the child who fails to develop speech (developmental dysphasia). He is readily confused with the learning disordered child although here too a careful history and period of observation will reveal that in other respects his psychomotor development is proceeding normally. Particular caution is required in the intellectual assessment of the child who has been emotionally deprived by the break-up of his home, death of his mother, or who has been otherwise bereft of normal security. It may require a long period outside an institution before he can be assessed.

Until recently many autistic children were wrongly labeled mentally defective. In a sense such children are defective because they cannot be normally educated and the prognosis is not good. None the less, the autistic child has often a revealing intelligent expression, and in his reactions to objects and various test materials shows considerable innate ability to the careful observer. The most characteristic features of infantile autism are a complete lack of interest in personal relationships which contrasts with an interest in inanimate objects; frequently a preoccupation with parts of the body; a tendency to react violently and unhappily to changes in environment; loss of speech or failure to acquire it, or the meaningless use of words or phrases; grossly abnormal mannerisms such as rocking, spinning or immobility (catatonia). The most outstanding feature of the autistic child is the way he rejects social contacts. None the less, although he is aloof, does not respond to a greeting with a smile, does not wave goodbye and so forth, he is yet aware of social contact. Thus, he may engage furiously in one of his more irritating mannerisms when someone enters his presence and cease whenever he is left alone. There is an odd high incidence of professional and educated people among the parents of autistic children. Such children, of course, are wrongly placed in institutions for profound and severe learning disorders. Some have responded considerably to psychotherapy as outpatients or inpatients in departments of child psychiatry. None probably becomes a normal child.

Intelligence Tests

Psychological testing and evaluations are of considerable although limited value in providing an estimate of a child's probable potential ability. They cannot, naturally, take into account the influence of such variables as zeal, ambition, interest, encouragement or the lack of it, good or bad teaching so forth. There are many aspects of intelligence and personality and the various tests assess these in different degrees. It is not proposed here to describe these tests in detail; they are reliable only in the hands of the expert. The most commonly used are: the Gesell tests for infants and the modifications of Cattell and Griffiths; for older children the Stanford-Binet scale and the revised test of Terman and Merrill, also the Wechsler Intelligence Scale for Children; for adolescents and adults the Wechsler Adult Intelligence Scale and Raven's Progressive Matrices. There are also several useful personality tests of which the

best for the mentally retarded are the Rorschach test and the Good enough "Draw-a-Man" test. In the case of the school child it is also important to enquire as to educational progress. An evaluation of the results of various tests competently performed is of great value in planning suitable education or training for the mentally handicapped child.

Investigations: Depending on the history and physical examination the following investigations may be done. Thyroid function test, metabolic screening for inborn error of metabolism, cranial CT or MRI scan, EEG, karyotyping including examination for fragile-X syndrome, TORCH infection screen, etc.

The Prevention of Learning Disorders

The prevention of neurological disorder has become increasingly possible in recent years. Indeed, the more efficient application of knowledge, which has been available to us for some years, would considerably reduce the present incidence of brain damage from such disturbances as perinatal hypoxia, hypoglycaemia, kernicterus and hypernatraemia and the prevalence of maternal rubella by the institution of anti-rubella vaccination. Screening programmes during the neonatal period for several of the treatable inborn errors of metabolism such as phenylketonuria, homocystinuria, maple syrup urine disease, galactosaemia as well as congenital hypothyroidism are making some impact upon the number of learning impaired children.

A most common development in the field of prevention is to be found in prenatal diagnosis. This is most often based upon examination of the amniotic fluid obtained by transabdominal amniocentesis between the 14th and 16th weeks of pregnancy and supported by ultrasonography. Sampling of chorionic villi or fetal blood or tissue may also be employed in selected cases. Chromosome analysis of amniotic cell cultures may reveal abnormalities such as trisomies 21, 13 and 18, or trisomy affecting the sex chromosomes (XXX and XXY). It may, on the other hand, lead to a diagnosis of 21/14 translocation in the fetus when one of the parents is known to be a translocation carrier and other more complex translocations have also been demonstrated. The sex of the fetus can also be determined when there is a known sex-linked inherited disease in a family, and where the risk to male progeny is 50:50. While most of the X-linked disorders are not associated with learning disorder (e.g. haemophilia) a few, such as Hunter syndrome do lead to progressive mental deficiency.

Recent years have seen a rapid increase in the number of inborn errors of metabolism, which are capable of prenatal diagnosis. A considerable number of these are associated with progressive neurological deterioration. Most are autosomal recessives although a few are X-linked. The laboratory techniques involved include enzyme assays on cultured amniotic fluid cells, measurement of metabolites, and biochemical analysis of the liquor.

Analysis of fetal blood obtained at fetoscopy has also been applied in the prenatal diagnosis of the haemoglobinopathies. Molecular genetic techniques allow earlier diagnosis and intervention.

When severe and irreversible disorders of the fetus are recognised prenatally therapeutic abortion may be considered. This is a complex problem with ethical, legal and religious implications. Occasionally, prenatal testing will reveal a treatable disease, as when congenital adrenal hyperplasia due to 21-hydroxylase deficiency is confirmed by a high level of 17-hydroxyprogesterone in the amniotic fluid, when no delay should arise in instituting appropriate treatment from the time of the infant's birth. In practice it has been found that in the majority of cases involving prenatal diagnosis the extreme parental anxiety, which is common in this situation, is relieved because in most instances the fetus is found not to be carrying the chromosomal or enzyme abnormality.

Prenatal diagnosis demands careful selection of patients as the techniques are not entirely devoid of risk and there can be no absolute guarantee of success. Not only must there be full discussion and investigation of the family problems, but there must also be close liaison between the clinicians, geneticists and the laboratories. This should preferably be undertaken before and not after the female partner has become pregnant. Suitable indications for prenatal diagnosis include:

1. Advancing maternal age, where the risk of chromosome abnormalities, particularly trisomy, is increased.
2. When either parent is a translocation carrier or has chromosomal mosaicism with a high risk of an abnormal fetus.
3. When there has previously been a child with a chromosomal abnormality such as Down syndrome.
4. In families with X-linked and certain autosomal recessive diseases.

Management of Children with Learning Impairment

The concept of management rather than treatment is central to the care of the learning disordered child. Treatment involves measures aimed at curing or improving a disorder or disability. Management is the continuing totality of all treatments of all the patient's dimensions – somatic, intellectual, emotional and social.

It must first be stated that with the exception of cretinism, phenylketonuria, galactosaemia, and a few other rare inborn errors of metabolism there is at the present time no specific treatment for the learning disordered. The only drugs of value are anticonvulsants for children who also have epileptic seizures, and sedatives for restless hyperkinetic children.

Secondly, once the physician has reached a definite diagnosis of developmental delay in a child, but not before, he must impart this information to the parents. This task requires time, tact, abundant sympathy and understanding, but it must be discharged in simple unambiguous phrases. In the case of the very young child, the doctor would be wise not to commit himself too firmly or too soon to an assessment of degree or to a forecast as to educability. These matters can be resolved with time, and it is the physician's duty to see the child and his parents regularly, and to be prepared to give of his time to answer their many questions. In particular, the irrational feelings of guilt, which many parents have on hearing that their child has a significant learning disorder, must be assuaged by quiet discussion and explanation. Some parents will refuse to accept the situation at first. They may "go the rounds" of the specialists seeking a happier diagnosis. This is completely understandable. At the end of the day they will still require and merit all the help, which their personal physician can offer. This is often particularly necessary when the child is at home with normal brothers and sisters where many different stresses and strains can arise. Genetic counselling will frequently be indicated, and the physician should also consider discussing contraception with the parents. They may well need guidance as to where these services can be obtained. Many professionals including teachers, therapists, social workers, and psychologists are involved in the management of these children.

Integration in regular schools is frequently an appropriate option. Otherwise the child is educated at a special school (day or boarding). His progress there will depend not only upon his innate ability but also on the support and training he receives, and has earlier received, from his parents. The child, who proves unable to benefit from formal education at a special school, can be placed in an occupation or training centre. Here he is taught social behaviour and simple manual skills. While the child whose IQ is around 50 is never likely to be educable to the extent that he can be self-supporting, it is a considerable advantage to him to become socially acceptable. It is undesirable that a mentally retarded child should be sent to an ordinary school if he is intellectually quite unable to benefit from such education. Suitable placement at the beginning will frequently avoid the behaviour problems and frustrations from which the retarded child must suffer if he is kept for long in an ordinary school competing with children of normal intelligence. The ability of a child to benefit from education at a special school or his suitability only for a training centre is not solely dependent on his IQ. Some children who do well at special schools have lower IQs than others who have to be transferred to training centres. Important factors are the child's personality and behaviour patterns, his home environment, and his willingness to learn. In preparation for school or training centre it is an advantage if the retarded child can be admitted to a suitable day nursery from the age of 2-3 years. This helps him to make social contact with other children while also relieving the mother of some of her load.

Children with profound learning disorder may require placement in long-term residential units specially adapted to their needs. As a general rule the earlier this category of child is placed the better, because a prolonged stay at home may cause the parents to neglect their normal children or the parents of a first-born learning disordered child to deny themselves further children. However, each case must be assessed on its merits with due regard for the parents' wishes, the home and financial circumstances, the ages and reactions of the other children in the family, and the behaviour and general condition of the child. The Down syndrome child is more often kept at home, because he is happy and good-natured. The child with aggressive or destructive tendencies is likely to be placed in an institution at an earlier age. Some retarded child find their way into institutions because they break the law and prove to be out of control, although they may be less severely retarded than other children who remain happily at home. The paediatrician often has to play an advocacy role for the learning impaired child and family.

Chapter 19

Accidental Poisoning in Childhood

Krishna M Goel

INTRODUCTION

In spite of the many educational programmes aimed at prevention and exposure to a poison, it remains the most common childhood accident. Paediatric poisonings involve three distinct groups. Poisoning in children is quite different from that in adults. Children have their special physiology and react differently to medicament as well as to poisoning.

The first group involves children between the ages of 1 and 4 years. Certain children with strong oral tendencies can be identified as especially likely to poison themselves by ingesting tablets or liquids, particularly if these have a pleasing colour or are held in an attractively labelled bottle or container. Poisoning can also occur by absorption through the skin and infiltration of the eyes i.e. ocular instillation. Patterns of accidental poisoning have been changing in recent years and while the number of children poisoned remains high, the incidence has shown a fall. There has also been a steady decline in the number of childhood deaths from poisonings. This is related to a number of factors including changes in prescribing practices, educational programmes directed towards prevention, safer packaging of dangerous drugs and safe storage of household products. Child-resistant containers have been particularly effective in reducing the incidence of death from the ingestion of prescription drugs by children. In a recent survey the rank order of poisons, drugs and chemicals, which have most often led to hospital admission, were: petroleum distillates; antihistamines; benzodiazepines; bleach and detergents; and aspirin. However, when the ratios of fatalities to ingestion were analysed to give an index of the practical danger of the substances to which children are exposed, the rank order became cardiotoxic drugs, tricyclic antidepressants, sympathomimetic drugs, caustic soda, and aspirin. While noxious plants such as laburnum, foxglove and deadly nightshade continue to be ingested, a fatal outcome is exceedingly rare. Ingestions of petroleum distillates,

insecticides such as chlorinated hydrocarbons and organic phosphates, and weed killers, particularly paraquat, are commoner in rural areas. Lead poisoning is in a different category as it usually involves ingestion over a fairly prolonged period.

The second distinct population involved in paediatric poisoning is the young 12-17 years old adolescent who ingests medications in a suicide attempt or gesture. They may require full psychiatric and social assessment. Also on the increase is "glue sniffing" i.e. inhalation of various solvent vapours and ingestion of "ecstasy" and alcohol used by teenagers as recreational drugs.

The third group is the result of parents deliberately giving drugs to their children as a manifestation of Munchausen Syndrome by Proxy. The commonest poison given by parents is table salt, anticonvulsants and opiates. In certain situations identifying poisoning can be difficult even when the doctor is alert to the possibility.

This chapter proposes to describe the general therapeutic measures applicable to acute poisoning and then to consider some of the more common individual poisonings. The possibility of poisoning should always be entertained in acute illness of sudden onset if no cause is immediately discoverable, particularly if it is associated with vomiting and diarrhoea or if there are marked disturbances of consciousness or behaviour.

ASSESSMENT OF THE CHILD AND MANAGEMENT

The primary assessment of the child with acute poisoning is essential for management. This should be done under the following acronym: **"ABCDE"**.

ASSESSMENT OF AIRWAY

If at first it is found that the child can speak or cry, this means that the airway is patent and breathing is taking place and the circulation is satisfactory. Otherwise, due to the effects of poisoning there could be loss of consciousness and this would lead to a complete or partial closure of airway. However, if the airway is not patent it should be made patent and intubation may be needed.

ASSESSMENT OF BREATHING

The child's respiratory rate should be checked. Tissue oxygen saturation must also be measured by pulse oximeter and arterial blood gas estimation should be done. There are a number of ingested substances such as opiates, which can induce respiratory depression. In such cases, oxygen should be given if there is respiratory depression, cyanosis or shock. However, if the child is breathing inadequately, support should be given by bag-valve mask with oxygen or by intermittent positive pressure ventilation in an intubated patient.

VENTILATORY SUPPORT IS INDICATED IF

- Respiratory rate is < 10 per minute
- There is poor air entry despite airway being fully open
- There is arterial blood gas measurements showing falling pO_2 and rising pCO_2

ASSESSMENT OF CONSCIOUS LEVEL

A rapid assessment of conscious level should be made by assigning AVPU method (alert, responds to voice, responds to pain, unresponsive) See Box 19.1. A detailed assessment can be made by using the Glasgow Coma Scale and Children's Coma Scale (See Box 19.2).

Box 19.1: AVPU assessment

A = Awake/alert
V = Responds to verbal stimuli (voice)
P = Responds only to pain
U = Unresponsive to all stimuli - sternal pressure, supra-orbital ridge pressure or pulling hair
Children in categories P and U will require careful assessment of their airways and ventilation. Intubation should be considered before carrying out gastric lavage or instilling activated charcoal in categories P and U.

ASSESSMENT OF CIRCULATION

It is important to assess the adequacy of the child's circulation by the following:
Heart rate, rhythm and pulse volume
Blood pressure
Peripheral perfusion: signs of poor end organ perfusion (shock) are:
- Poor peripheral pulses
- Capillary refill longer than 2 seconds
- Blood pressure may be normal in compensated shock
- Low blood pressure indicates decompensated shock

Box 19.2: Glasgow coma scale and children's coma scale

Glasgow Coma Scale (4-15 years)
Child's Glasgow Coma Scale (<4 years)

Response	Score	Response	Score
Eye opening		**Eye opening**	
Spontaneously	4	Spontaneously	4
To verbal stimuli	3	To verbal stimuli	3
To pain	2	To pain	2
No response to pain	1	No response to pain	1
Best motor response		**Best motor response**	
Obeys verbal command	6	Spontaneous, obeys verbal command	6
Localises pain	5	Localises to pain or withdraws to touch	5
Withdraws from pain	4	Withdraws from pain	4
Abnormal flexion to pain (decorticate)	3	Abnormal flexion to pain (decorticate)	3
Abnormal extension to pain (decerebrate)	2	Abnormal extension to pain (decerebrate)	2
No response to pain	1	No response to pain	1
Best verbal response		**Best verbal response**	
Oriented and converses	5	Alert, babbles, coos words to usual ability	5
Disoriented and converses	4	Less than usual words, spontaneous irritable cry	4
Inappropriate words	3	Cries only to pain	3
Incomprehensible sounds	2	Moans to pain	2
No response to pain	1	No response to pain	1

NORMAL AGGREGATE SCORE = 15

DISABILITY: ASSESSMENT OF NEUROLOGICAL FUNCTION

It is assessed by assessing the level of consciousness, posture, pupillary size and reaction to light.

Exposure

Exposure is essential for external evidence of drug abuse and drug induced rashes (e.g. purpura, swelling of lips/tongue, urticaria, angio-oedema). Record child's core and toe temperatures, because a number of drugs can cause hypo/hyperthermia.

Key Learning Points

Base line monitoring in a child with poisoning.
ECG
Pulse oximetry
Core temperature
Blood glucose level
U and E's and LFT's
Blood gases

POISON IDENTIFICATION AND ASSESSMENT OF THE SEVERITY OF OVERDOSE

Subsequent to the primary assessment of the child, it is important to evaluate the severity of the overdose. To assess this properly, obtain the identity of the substance ingested, the amount taken and the length of time the child has been in contact with poison. Sometimes it may not be easy to gather this vital information.

However, some clues about the substance taken may be obvious from the clinical signs noted during full clinical examination. An essential part of substance identification is to match the collection of signs and associated toxic effects and the offending substance as shown in Table 19.1.

Key Learning Point
Amount of poison ingested Some idea of the maximum amount of substance that could have been ingested can be obtained from counting the number of remaining tablets or volume of liquid left in the bottle and details on packaging.

Key Learning Point
Poison identification: routine toxicology screen on urine sample Substances identifiable: benzodiazepines, cocaine metabolites, methadone, opiates and amphetamines.

Treatment

Most children will be asymptomatic because they have taken only a minute non-lethal overdose or have ingested a substance which is harmless. Therefore a short period of observation in a short-stay ward or in an emergency department is often all that is needed. It is better to be safe than sorry.

On the contrary, those children who have taken a potentially lethal dose of a drug or the exact nature of the substance is unknown, then measures to minimize blood concentration of the drug should be implemented. There is an urgent need to remove the poison or to inactivate or neutralize it before it reaches the circulation. Now there is no place for the use of emetics. The routine use of gastric lavage or activated charcoal is inappropriate.

Emesis

This was the routine approach for decades. There is no evidence from clinical studies that ipecac improves the outcome of poisoned patients and thus its routine use should be abandoned.

Gastric Lavage

Gastric lavage should not be carried out routinely in the treatment of poisoned patients. Gastric lavage should not be considered unless a child has ingested a potentially life threatening amount of a poison and the procedure can be undertaken within 60 minutes of ingestion. The lavage fluid can be water or isotonic saline. After lavage, the lavage tube can be used for administering the specific antidote or activated charcoal. For those children who cannot protect their airway, intubation under general anaesthesia will be necessary. Fluid from the stomach should be collected for analysis, if necessary.

LEARNING TIP

Gastric Lavage

Gastric lavage is contraindicated if a corrosive substance e.g. acid or alkali or volatile hydrocarbon e.g. kerosene, lamp oil, lighter fluid, turpentine, paint thinners, furniture polishes and cleansing agents have been ingested.

MEDICINAL CHARCOAL

Activated charcoal is capable of binding a number of poisonous substances without being systemically absorbed (See Box 19.3). However, there are substances which it will not absorb (See Box 19.4). The effectiveness of activated charcoal decreases with time, the greatest benefit is within one hour of ingestion. Multidoses of activated charcoal to remove toxins undergoing entero-hepatic circulation are one of the simplest, active elimination techniques. The charcoal can be given via a nasogastric tube or lavage tube. The dose of activated charcoal is 1g/Kg and repeated every 2-4 hours for the first 24 hours. The complications from charcoal are negligible.

Table 19.1: Drugs and associated toxic effects	
Associated signs	*Possible toxin*
Tachypnoea	Salicylates, carbon monoxide, theophylline
Bradypnoea	Opiates, barbiturates, sedatives
Convulsions	Phenothiazines, aminophylline, salicylates, tricyclic antidepressants, insecticides, organophosphate
Hyperpyrexia	Salicylates, aminophylline, amphetamine, cocaine
Hypothermia	Aminophylline, barbiturates, phenothiazines
Hypertension	Aminophylline, amphetamines, cocaine
Hypotension	Tricyclic antidepressants, aminophylline, barbiturates, benzodiazepines, opiates, iron, phenytoin
Large pupils	Atropine, cannabis, carbamazepine, tricyclic antidepressants
Small pupils	Opiates, phenothiazines, organophosphate, insecticide
Tachycardia	Aminophylline, antidepressants, amphetamine, cocaine
Bradycardia	Tricyclic antidepressants, digoxin
Metabolic acidosis	Salicylates, ethanol, carbon monoxide

Box 19.3: List of poisons for which activated charcoal is effective

Acetaminophen	Nicotine	Barbiturates
Amphetamine	Paraquat	Phenothiazines
Atropine	Phenols	Benzodiazepines
Quinine	Camphor	Salicylates
Digitalis derivatives	Strychnine	Sulphonamides
Indomethacin	Theophylline	Tricyclic antidepressants
N-acetylcysteine		

Box 19.4: Substances not bound to charcoal

Boric acid	Lithium
Cyanide	Malathion
Ethanol	Methanol
Ethylene glycol	Petroleum distillates
Iron	Strong acids and alkalis

OTHER ELIMINATION MEASURES

- Urinary alkalinisation can be used to expedite the excretion of acidic drugs e.g. salicylate, isoniazid and phenobarbitone
- Haemoperfusion, haemofiltration and dialysis are effective in certain poisonings (See Box 19.5).

Box 19.5: Dialysis, haemoperfusion, and haemofiltration are effective in the following poisonings

Dialysis: salicylate, methanol, ethylene glycol, vancomycin, isopropanol
Haemoperfusion: carbamazepine, barbiturates, theophylline
Haemofiltration: aminoglycoside, theophylline, iron, lithium

WHOLE BOWEL IRRIGATION (WBI)

Whole bowel irrigation should not be used routinely in the management of the poisoned patient. However, it can be used to physically eliminate highly toxic substances especially those not absorbed by activated charcoal and have a long gastrointestinal transit time e.g. iron, sustained release or enteric-coated preparations. This is done by giving orally a large quantity of osmotically balanced polyethylene glycol electrolyte solution.

ANTIDOTES

A wide range of antidotes exists as shown in Box 19.6.

Box 19.6: Poisons with antidotes

Indication	Antidote
Beta-blockers	Glucagon
Benzodiazepines	Flumazenil
Carbon monoxide	Oxygen
Chloroquine	Diazepam in high doses

Contd...

Contd...

Digoxin	Digoxin specific antibodies
Hypoglycaemic agents	Glucose
Iron salts	Desferrioxamine
Isoniazid	Vitamin B_6
Lead	Calcium EDTA, BAL
Methanol	Ethanol
Methaemoglobin producing agents	Methylene blue
Morphine derivatives (opiates)	Naloxone
Organophosphates	Atropine
Paracetamol	N-acetylcysteine
Ethylene glycol and methanol	Fomepizole (Antizol)

SALICYLATE POISONING

Accidental poisoning in children due to salicylate has recently declined in incidence following the packaging of salicylates in child resistant containers and also because aspirin is being superseded by paracetamol and ibuprofen as the standard domestic analgesic. Salicylate is usually ingested in the form of aspirin (acetyl salicylate). This is often accidental but sometimes it has been given with therapeutic intent by the parents and even by the doctor. On occasion, oil of wintergreen (methyl salicylate) a source of the salicylate, has been swallowed, one teaspoonful of which contains the equivalent of 4 g aspirin. Salicylate poisoning can also occur due to local application of ointments containing salicylic acid.

Prognosis in the individual case is determined much more by the interval of time, which has elapsed between the ingestion of the poison and the start of treatment than, by the level of the serum salicylate. Indeed, the toddler can show signs of severe poisoning with a salicylate level as low as 2.9 mol/l (40 mg/100ml). With the exception of rheumatic fever, juvenile idiopathic arthritis (JIA) and Kawasaki disease, aspirin should not be prescribed for infants or children.

Clinical Features

Rapid, deep, regular, acyanotic breathing or air hunger is almost diagnostic of salicylate poisoning. Cases may be misdiagnosed as "pneumonia" but the hyperpnoea of salicylate poisoning is quite different from the short, grunting respirations of pneumonia. Other early manifestations of salicylate poisoning such as nausea and vomiting are difficult to evaluate in infants and toddlers and they cannot often describe tinnitus.

The hyperpnoea has a double aetiology. It is due initially to direct stimulation by salicylate of the respiratory center of the brain. The resultant over breathing washes out CO_2 from the lungs and causes a respiratory alkalosis with a blood pH (>7.42) and lowered PCO_2 (<33mmHg). This alkalotic phase is commonly seen in adults with salicylate poisoning, but in young children, an accelerated fatty-acid catabolism with excess production of ketones results in the early establishment of a metabolic acidosis. By the time the poisoned toddler reaches hospital the blood pH is usually reduced (<7.35). The compensatory hyperventilation of metabolic acidosis adds to the stimulant effect of salicylate on the respiratory centre so that the over breathing of the poisoned child is often extreme. A side effect of salicylate overdosage is fever. There is also a disturbance of carbohydrate metabolism and the blood glucose may rise above 11.1 mmol/l (200 mg/100 ml) although not above 16.7 mmol/l (300 mg/ 100 ml). Hypoglycaemia has been recorded but it is uncommon.

The child with salicylate poisoning shows peripheral vasodilatation until near to death. Death is preceded by cyanosis, twitching, rigidity and coma.

CASE STUDY

A 12-year-old boy presented with severe icthyosis. He was treated with topical 2% salicylic acid in simple cream applied to the whole body twice daily. The salicylate concentration was increased to 5% on day 3 of treatment and 10% on day 5. On day 8 he developed symptoms of salicylate toxicity. His blood salicylate level was 3.3 mmol/l. Topical salicylate treatment was stopped. Intravenous fluids and bicarbonate were given and complete clinical and biochemical recovery was achieved after two days.

This case illustrates that significant percutaneous salicylate absorption can occur especially when salicylate preparations of increasing strength are used.

Diagnosis: salicylate poisoning in dermatological treatment.

Treatment

The immediate treatment is gastric emptying. So gastric lavage can be undertaken up to 4 hours after ingestion. Also activated charcoal should be given to those patients who have ingested sustained release salicylate preparations.

On arrival at hospital blood is taken for estimation of the plasma salicylate level, electrolytes, renal function, blood glucose, clotting profile and acid base status. However, repeated salicylate measurements are necessary and reliance should not be placed on a single salicylate level. The salicylate levels will usually rise over the first 6 hours if enteric-coated preparation is ingested.

Urinary alkalinisation enhances excretion of salicylates, sodium bicarbonate should be infused over 4 hours. Patients with unresponsive acidosis, convulsions, coma, renal failure or continuing deterioration should be considered for haemodialysis. Haemoperfusion is not recommended. Forced diuresis is no longer used.

PARACETAMOL POISONING

While paracetamol accounts for a large number of attempted suicides in adults (either alone or in combination with dextroproxyphene as "Co-proxamol", cases of serious poisoning are rare in children. Paediatric paracetamol elixir preparations ingested by the toddler very rarely cause toxicity. Nonetheless, as it can lead to irreversible liver and renal failure, any child who may have ingested in excess of 150 mg/kg should be admitted to hospital without delay. However, children are more resistant to paracetamol-induced hepatotoxicity than adults. Doses of less than 150 mg/Kg will not cause toxicity except in a child with hepatic or renal disease.

Clinical Features

The first symptoms are nausea, vomiting and abdominal pain. Evidence of severe liver damage may be revealed by elevated levels of aspartate aminotransferase (AST) and alanine aminotransferase (ALT) over 1000IU/l and of renal impairment by a plasma creatinine concentration over 300 µmol/l (3.4 mg/100ml). The child may become comatose and die from respiratory arrest.

Treatment

Correct treatment of paracetamol poisoning includes oral activated charcoal and a paracetamol blood level to be taken 4 hours following ingestion. Plasma concentrations measured in less than 4 hours cannot be interpreted. Specific treatment is with intravenous infusion of N-acetylcysteine. Nomogram shows the level of blood paracetamol at which acetylcysteine should be given intravenously (Fig. 19.1). Those whose plasma-paracetamol concentration is above the normal treatment line are treated with acetylcysteine by intravenous infusion (or, if acetylcysteine is not available, with methionine by mouth, provided the overdose has been taken within 10-12 hours and the child is not vomiting). If the treatment was started within 8 hours of ingesting the overdose, the risk of liver or renal damage is insignificant.

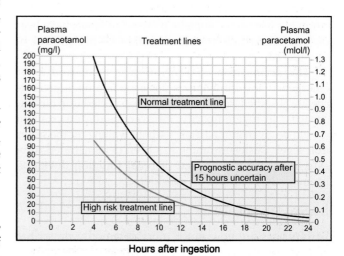

Hours after ingestion

Fig. 19.1: Nomogram for use in paracetamol ingestion

ACUTE IRON POISONING

Iron poisoning is most common in childhood and is usually accidental. The most common source of acute iron poisoning is ferrous sulphate tablets, which the young child mistakes for sweets. Other ferrous salts such as gluconate or succinate are less dangerous. If over 20 mg/Kg of elemental iron has been taken, toxicity is likely. Over 150 mg/Kg may be fatal.

Clinical Features

The symptoms are vomiting, diarrhoea, haematemesis, melaena, pallor, and metabolic acidosis. Hypotension, coma and hepatocellular necrosis occur later. Coma and shock indicate severe poisoning.

CASE STUDY

A 2½-year-old Asian boy was found with an empty bottle of ferrous sulphate tablets (ferrous sulphate 200 mg containing 65 mg of ferrous iron). His mouth was full of crushed pieces of tablets. His mother took him to a nearby paediatric A and E unit. On examination he had a temperature of 98.4°C, pulse 120 per minute, respiratory rate 40 per minute and blood pressure 90/55 mmHg. He was drowsy; otherwise clinical examination was unremarkable. Hb 12.6 g/dl, WBC and platelet count normal, U and E's and LFT's normal, HCO_3 16 mmol/l. Serum iron 60 µmol/l.

He was gastric lavaged with normal saline. He was treated with desferrioxamine 15 mg/Kg per hour intravenously for 24 hours. He did not develop any complications and recovered unscathed. He was discharged home, well, 2 days later.

Treatment

On arrival in hospital gastric lavage should be performed with 1% solution of sodium bicarbonate. Activated charcoal is not helpful. X-ray of the abdomen may help substantiate the number of tablets ingested and a repeat X-ray will demonstrate whether or not gastric emptying has been complete. If large quantities have been consumed, whole bowel irrigation (WBI) should be considered.

The serum iron concentration is measured as an emergency and intravenous desferrioxamine is given to chelate absorbed iron in excess of the expected iron binding capacity. In severe toxicity, intravenous desferrioxamine should be given immediately without waiting for the serum iron level. Desferrioxamine has been demonstrated to be safe. If severe impairment of renal function develops, haemodialysis should be considered.

Barbiturate Poisoning

Barbiturates are now much more commonly prescribed and are rarely encountered as a cause of poisoning in children.

Clinical Features

In most cases the child is only extremely drowsy. Infrequently, the child may be flushed, excited, restless and may vomit. In severe cases the child is comatose, unresponsive to stimuli and may show respiratory depression with cyanosis, absence of deep reflexes and circulatory failure with hypotension. Skin blisters mainly over bony prominences, peripheral nerve pressure lesions may develop.

Treatment

For those who have ingested more than 25 mg/kg within one hour give activated charcoal 1g/kg by mouth or via nasogastric tube. Forced diuresis is ineffective and potentially dangerous. Haemodialysis is of no value.

POISONING BY ANTIHISTAMINES

The common prescribing of antihistamines of many kinds has, unfortunately, increased the opportunity for young children to ingest them accidentally. There is sometimes a fairly long period between ingestion and the appearance of symptoms. These include anorexia, progressive drowsiness, stupor and signs such as inco-ordinated movements, rigidity and tremor. Poisoning by two of the newer non-sedating antihistamines, terfenadine and astemizole may predispose to the development of ventricular tachyarrhythmias.

Treatment

Activated charcoal should be considered up to four hours post-ingestion, as gut motility is impaired. Treatment is otherwise largely supportive.

POISONING BY TRICYCLIC ANTIDEPRESSANTS

The frequent use of antidepressants for adults has resulted in a rapidly increasing incidence of their accidental ingestion by children. Moreover, these drugs are prescribed for enuresis in children and the fact that overdosage can produce dangerous toxic effects in a young child is not sufficiently stressed to the parents.

Clinical Features

Mildly affected children develop drowsiness, ataxia, abnormal postures, agitation when stimulated, dilated pupils and tachycardia. Thirst and nystagmus have been present in some cases. In severely affected children convulsions may be followed by coma and severe respiratory depression. Cardiac arrhythmias such as ventricular tachycardia and various degrees of heart block with profound hypotension in children are prominent and dangerous.

Treatment

As there is no known antidote, the management of poisoning with the tricyclics is mainly symptomatic. Activated charcoal should be administered. In addition, alkalinisation up to an arterial pH of at least 7.5 has been shown to reduce cardiac toxicity. This can be achieved by hyperventilation and by infusing sodium bicarbonate in a dose of 1 kg/kg.

The cardiac rhythm should be continuously monitored by electrocardiography. If cardiac arrhythmias develop they can be treated with anti-arrhythmic measures. Life threatening arrhythmias may respond to cardioversion.

ATROPINE POISONING

This type of poisoning may arise from ingestion of the plant Deadly Nightshade. It may also occur when drugs such as tincture of belladonna, atropine or hyoscine are taken accidentally or prescribed in excessive doses. Antidiarrhoeal agent Lomotil that contains diphenoxylate and atropine is toxic to some children at therapeutic dosage.

Clinical Features

The onset of symptoms is soon after ingestion, with thirst, dryness of mouth, blurring of vision and photophobia. The child is markedly flushed with widely dilated pupils. Tachycardia is severe and there may be a high fever. Extreme restlessness, confusion, delirium and incoordination are characteristic. In babies there may be gross gaseous abdominal distension. In fatal cases circulatory collapse and respiratory failure precede death.

Treatment

This can only be symptomatic and supportive. Gastric lavage followed by the instillation of activated charcoal is effective.

POISONING BY DIGOXIN

The increasing number of older adults taking digitalis preparations in the community is resulting in accidental ingestion by children, of cardiac glycosides. The most commonly involved preparation is digoxin. Children require treatment if they have ingested more than 100 µg/kg body weight. The toxic effects may not become marked for some hours and it is important to treat every case as potentially dangerous.

Clinical features

The most striking presenting feature is severe and intractable vomiting which is largely due to the action of digoxin on the central nervous system. Other neurological manifestations include visual disturbances, drowsiness and convulsions, which are usually delayed for several hours in their appearance. The cardiac manifestations of digoxin intoxication in a previously healthy child are: exaggeration of normal sinus arrhythmia which is a common early finding, and sinus pauses with nodal escape beats may occur. Other findings include sinus bradycardia, nodal rhythm, coupled idio-ventricular rhythm and complete heart block.

Treatment

Treatment in the first instance is with activated charcoal. Repeated doses may be required. The electrocardiograph should be continuously monitored and the serum electrolytes frequently measured because hyperkalaemia may aggravate digoxin toxicity. Hyperkalaemia should be corrected using ion exchange resins, glucose and insulin or dialysis. Salbutamol and calcium infusions should be avoided because of their potential to destabilize the myocardium.

Bradyarrhythmias may require treatment with atropine or cardiac pacing. Tacchyarrhythmias may respond to lignocaine or phenytoin. Cardioversion should be used only as a last resort because of the possibility of inducing asystole. Digoxin-specific antibody fragments are indicated for the treatment of known or strongly suspected digoxin or digitoxin overdosage, where measures beyond the withdrawal of the cardiac glycoside and correction of any electrolyte abnormality are felt to be necessary. Exchange transfusion, peritoneal dialysis and haemodialysis are of no value because most of the drug is tissue bound and plasma concentrations are low.

POISONING BY PETROLEUM DISTILLATES, INSECTICIDES AND WEEDKILLERS

Ingestion of petroleum distillates is a common childhood problem because they are readily available in most households, including developing countries where kerosene, in particular, is used for heating, cooking and lighting. Petroleum distillates (petrol, paraffin, turpentine, turps substitute, white spirit and kerosene) cause irritation of mucous membranes, vomiting and diarrhoea, when ingested, and respiratory distress, cyanosis, tachycardia and pyrexia, when inhaled. Ingestion of more than 1 mg/kg body weight will cause drowsiness and depression of the central nervous system. Emetics and gastric lavage are contra-indicated because they increase the risk of hydrocarbon pneumonia in which there may be pulmonary oedema and haemorrhage. Children can develop symptoms up to 24 hours following ingestion. There is no evidence to support the use of steroids in the treatment of lipid aspiration pneumonitis. Antibiotics should be reserved for those who develop proven secondary bacterial infection.

Chlorinated hydrocarbon insecticides such as DDT, dieldrin, aldrin and lindane can be absorbed through the skin and respiratory tract as well as from the gastro-intestinal tract and can cause salivation, abdominal pain with vomiting and diarrhoea, and central nervous system depression with convulsions. Contaminated clothing should be removed, the child washed with soap and water and convulsions treated with diazepam.

Organophosphorus insecticides such as malathion, chlorthion, parathion, phosdrin and TEPP are cholinesterase inhibitors, which can also be absorbed from skin, lungs and intestines. The accumulation of acetylcholine in tissues causes nausea, vomiting, diarrhoea, blurred vision, miosis, headache, muscle weakness and twitching, loss of reflexes and sphincter control, and finally, loss of consciousness. Treatment is as for chlorinated hydro-carbons with, in addition, atropine sulphate 0.05 mg/kg given intramuscularly and then pralidoxime the specific cholinesterase reactivator in a dose of 25 mg/kg in 10 per cent solution by intravenous infusion at a rate not exceeding 5 mg/min. Pralidoxime is only of use if administered within 24 hours of exposure; after this the enzyme inactivation becomes increasingly irreversible. During transfer to a paediatric unit provision for intubation and assisted ventilation must be available.

Weed killers of the paraquat type may also be absorbed through skin and respiratory and intestinal tracts particularly when concentrated solutions of paraquat have been swallowed; children can experience a burning sensation in the mouth, nausea, vomiting, abdominal pain and diarrhoea, which may be bloody. Hours later, ulceration of the mouth, throat and gastrointestinal tract may occur. The absence of initial symptoms does not exclude a diagnosis of paraquat poisoning.

When low to moderate doses of paraquat have been ingested the signs of kidney and liver damage may occur after 2-3 days. Both types of damage are irreversible. After 5-10 days, or very occasionally up to 14 days after poisoning, the child may develop signs of lung damage, which is almost always irreversible. When relatively large doses of paraquat are ingested, multiorgan damage and failure occurs quickly and death usually occurs within a few hours or days. Tissue damage is probably caused by local hydrogen peroxide and this might be aggravated by giving oxygen to breathe. Paraquat absorption can be confirmed by a simple qualitative urine test.

The single most useful measure is oral administration of activated charcoal. Gastric lavage is of doubtful value.

ACUTE ALCOHOL POISONING

Episodes of acute alcohol (Ethanol) poisoning occur predominantly in infancy and preadolescence with peaks at ages 3 and 12 years and are commoner in boys. In the younger age group, ease of access to spirits and fortified wines allied with poor parental surveillance in the home are important factors. Household ethanol sources include perfumes, colognes, aftershaves, mouthwashes, and antiseptics. In the older children the episodes are more likely to occur outside the home, thus increasing the risks of physical danger from accidents and hypothermia. The younger infants are at risk of significant hypoglycaemia especially if they drink alcohol in the early morning after an obligate overnight fasting. The lethal dose of ethanol in children is only 3 g/kg, compared with the adult lethal dose of 5 to 8 g/kg.

Clinical Features

Nausea, accompanied by vomiting, ataxia and progressive loss of consciousness are the usual features. Aspiration pneumonia, hypoxic and alcoholic brain damage with cerebral oedema, hypothermia, hypoglycaemia and convulsions are not uncommon complications.

Diagnosis

This is based predominantly on history and on the finding of an elevated blood alcohol concentration. The blood glucose concentrations must be measured.

Treatment

Activated charcoal does not prevent absorption and is not indicated. Because ethanol is rapidly absorbed from the stomach, performing gastric lavage is unlikely to be of benefit.

Flumazenil and intravenous naloxone have been tried to antagonise the depressant effects of ethanol overdose. Haemodialysis has been used to treat patients with a high blood alcohol level (> 300 mg/dl).

LEAD POISONING

Lead is usually ingested in small quantities over a long period and the manifestations of poisoning develop insidiously. There are various possible sources of lead such as lead-containing paint which may be used on a child's cot, flakes or paint from plasterwork or woodwork in old Victorian houses, burnt out lead batteries or swallowed pieces of yellow crayon and lead water pipes. Pica is common in children suffering from lead poisoning and is a valuable clue to the diagnosis. It is more common in children from the poorest homes. Asian mothers, mainly for cosmetic reasons, apply Surma, which contains lead sulphide, to the eyelids and conjunctivae of infants and children. It seems that an appreciable absorption of lead in these children occurs from drainage down the tear duct or from rubbing the eyes and then licking the fingers. Other sources of environmental lead contamination are the gasoline exhaust fumes of motorcars and lead in soil. An early diagnosis is extremely important in lead poisoning because, if it is left untreated, lead encephalopathy may result in death or permanent brain damage. Lead poisoning is now defined as a blood lead level equal to or greater than 10µg per dl (0.50 µmol/l).

Clinical Features

The earliest signs such as lethargy, anorexia, vomiting and abdominal pain are too common to arouse suspicion in them, but their persistence without other discoverable cause should do so. The pallor of anaemia is a frequent and characteristic sign. Insomnia and headache frequently precede the onset of lead encephalopathy with convulsions, papilloedema and a cracked-pot sound on percussion of the skull. Radiographs of the skull may then reveal separation of the sutures. Peripheral neuropathy is uncommon in the young child but may develop with paralysis of the dorsiflexors of either the wrist or foot. Radiographs of the bones may show characteristic bands of increased density at the metaphyses (Fig. 19.2.) but this is a relatively late sign and, therefore, of limited diagnostic value. Excess aminoaciduria is a common manifestation of renal tubular damage and glycosuria may also occur. Renal hypertension has also been reported. Elevated blood lead levels are also associated with neurodevelopmental abnormalities, behavioural disturbances, learning disabilities and defects in fine and gross motor development.

The most dangerous development, both in regard to life and future mental health, is lead encephalopathy. Depending upon the amount of lead ingested, this dreaded complication may develop quite quickly or only following a long period of relatively mild ill health.

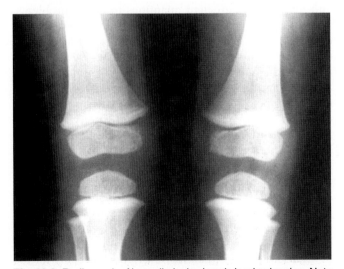

Fig. 19.2: Radiograph of lower limbs in chronic lead poisoning. Note bands of increased density "lead lines" at metaphyseal ends of the long bones

Diagnosis

The diagnosis of lead poisoning can be justified in the presence of two or more of the following findings:
  (i) Microcytic hypochromic anaemia with punctate basophilia;
 (ii) Radio-opaque foreign bodies in the bowel lumen and lines of increased density at the growing ends of the long bones;
(iii) Coproporphyrinuria;
 (iv) Renal glycosuria and aminoaciduria;
  (v) Raised intracranial pressure and protein in the cerebrospinal fluid.

Interpretation of the blood lead concentration is, unfortunately, much more difficult. While levels below 1.9 mmol/l (40 mg per 100 ml) exclude lead poisoning and levels in the region of 2.9 mmol/l (60 mg per 100 ml) are associated with clinical signs, it is possible that behaviour and learning difficulties occur at values between these levels.

Treatment

It is essential that the child be immediately removed from all sources of lead. Deposition of lead in the bones should be encouraged by giving a diet rich in calcium, phosphorus and vitamin D thereby lowering the level of lead in the blood. The most important measure is to increase the excretion of lead in the urine. In chronic lead poisoning the chelating agent of choice is probably D-penicillamine. It has the advantage of being extremely effective when given orally. A suitable dose is 20 mg/kg/day for seven days. Further courses may be required if the blood lead level rises again or if symptoms recur.

In lead encephalopathy, combination of lead with sulphydryl groups leads to inhibition of intracellular enzyme systems. The resultant cellular injury is followed by oedema, which adds further injury to the brain. The most effective and rapid method of removing lead from the brain is by the parenteral administration of sodium calcium edetate (calcium disodium versenate; CaEDTA). This therapy is combined with measures to diminish cerebral oedema. As soon as the diagnosis has been made CaEDTA 80 mg/kg/day (0.4 ml/kg/day) is given intravenously in four divided doses per 24 hours for 5 to 7 days. The CaEDTA should be given by adding each dose to 250 ml of 5 per cent dextrose solution, which is given by intravenous infusion. A second course of CaEDTA should be given some 1-10 days after the end of the first course. Subsequent courses may be required if the blood level remains elevated, or at this stage, oral D-penicillamine might be employed as described above.

The dangers of cerebral oedema are sufficiently great to demand palliative measures while CaEDTA is being used. Various measures, including surgical decompression, have been tried in this emergency. Mannitol is the safest and most effective agent. It can be given in a dosage of 2.5 g per kg by intravenous infusion of a 20 per cent solution. Dexamethasone has also been advised by the intravenous route in doses of 1 mg/kg/ day given in four equal six-hourly injections for 48 hours. Once lead encephalopathy has been allowed to develop, the risks to life and subsequent mental development are very great.

CAUSTIC INGESTION

Accidental ingestion of caustic substances by inquisitive toddlers may result in serious injury to the mouth, oropharynx, oesophagus or stomach. The most corrosive and commonly ingested caustics are the liquid form of sodium or potassium hydroxides used as drain cleaners. Other less caustic alkalis, which may be ingested, are bleach (sodium hypochlorite), laundry and dishwasher detergents and disinfectants usually kept in the kitchen.

Ingestion of these substances is most likely to result in injury to the oesophagus, but if ingested in large amounts, they can produce extensive damage to the upper gastro-intestinal tract. If the hydroxide concentration is high it may lead to perforation of the oesophagus and thus penetration into the peri-oesophageal tissues, which may cause mediastinitis. The presence of oral burns confirms that ingestion of a caustic substance has taken place but it does not suggest the degree of oesophageal damage. Dyspnoea, stridor or hoarseness suggests laryngeal injury. Products that become trapped in the oesophagus cause the most damage e.g. batteries or dishwasher tablets.

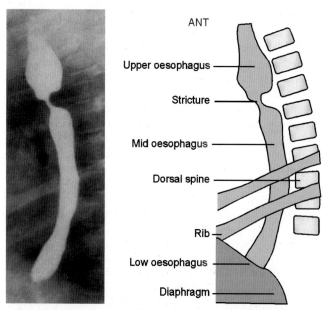

Fig. 19.3: Oesophageal stricture: barium swallow showing short smooth stricture secondary to caustic ingestion

Treatment

All children with caustic ingestion should be admitted for observation of at least 24 hours. The outcome for most children following corrosive ingestion is good. Attempts at neutralisation of corrosives or gastric decontamination should be avoided.

Persistence of drooling and dysphagia after 12-24 hours of ingestion are indications of oesophageal scar formation and warrants upper gastrointestinal endoscopy (Fig. 19.3.). It seems that steroid treatment does not minimise the formation of scar tissue and stricture. Children with oesophageal stricture usually respond to repeated dilatations but some require oesophageal replacement surgery.

SWALLOWED FOREIGN BODIES

Foreign body ingestion is common in children because they have a tendency to explore and to taste new objects and, thus, they swallow bizarre and multiple objects. Most foreign bodies swallowed pass through the alimentary tract without symptoms. However, if the foreign body is lodged in the oesophagus, it should be removed imme-diately through an endoscope to avoid serious complica-tions of oesophageal obstruction, asphyxia or media-stinitis. In the absence of symptoms, the manage-ment simply consists of an X-ray of the abdomen to confirm the presence of a radio-opaque object and a careful watch kept on the stools until the foreign body is recovered.

Disc batteries (button batteries) are often ingested in young children these days due to their widespread use in electrical products in the home. These batteries contain alkalies in sufficient concentration to cause caustic injuries and mercury in sufficient quantities to create problems. However, the highly toxic mercuric oxide is converted to essentially non-toxic elemental mercury on leakage or complete disintegration of the battery (Fig. 19.4). In addition, mercuric oxide is poorly soluble and not well absorbed and this may account for the very low incidence of mercury poisoning and, therefore, children may not need chelation therapy. The vast majority of battery ingestions is benign and can be managed without endoscopic or surgical intervention. Evaluation and treatment of the burns caused by the battery is the same as that for other alkali burns (see caustic ingestions). Batteries lodged in the oesophagus must be removed by endoscopic means. If they have recently passed into the stomach, purgation can speed their passage, if, however, they have been in the stomach for more than 3 hours their removal by endoscopy is essential. However, it is less likely for the battery to produce obstruction as it would have been disintegrated and, therefore, removal by endoscopy may not be required.

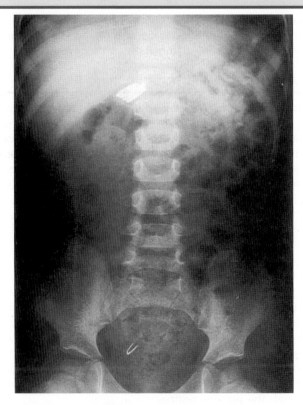

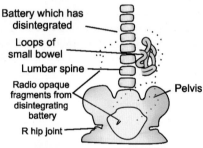

Fig. 19.4: X-ray of abdomen showing disintegrating battery

ACUTE CARBON MONOXIDE POISONING

Carbon monoxide (CO) is an odourless, colourless gas and poisoning causes hypoxia, cell damage and death.

Carbon monoxide is produced by the incomplete combustion of carbon containing fuel, such as gas (domestic or bottled), charcoal, coke, oil and wood. Gas stoves, fires, car exhaust fumes, paraffin heaters are all potential sources.

The symptoms of carbon monoxide poisoning are non-specific and include headache, fatigue, confusion, nausea, dizziness, visual disturbances, chest pain, shortness of breath, loss of consciousness and seizures. The classical signs of carbon monoxide poisoning such, as cherry-red lips, peripheral cyanosis and retinal haemorrhages are uncommon. A carboxyhaemoglobin level of 10% or more or the presence of clinical signs and symptoms after known exposure to carbon monoxide are indicative of acute carbon monoxide poisoning.

Treatment

The child should be moved to fresh air, the airway cleared and oxygen 100% administered as soon as available. High concentrations of oxygen hasten the dissociation of carboxyhaemoglobin. Patients with neurological signs or symptoms or those with evidence of cardiovascular abnormalities may need hyperbaric oxygen therapy. Unconscious patients should have early cranial imaging and may need aggressive treatment to control cerebral oedema.

SNAKE BITE

Snake bite is a major medical problem in many parts of the world. The snakes of medical importance are the vipers (e.g. carpet viper, Russell viper, adder etc) and the elapids (cobra, mamba, krait etc). In the Indian sub-continent, the most important species are cobra, common krait, Russell's viper, but in South East Asia the Malayan pit viper, green pit viper and the monocellate cobra cause most bites and deaths. In Britain, the adder or viper is the only venomous species.

Clinical Manifestations

The earliest symptoms related to the bite are local pain, bleeding from the fang puncture, followed by swelling and bruising extending up the limb and tender enlargement of regional lymphnodes. Clinical effects of systemic envenoming usually involve haemorrhage and coagulation defects resulting in incoagulable blood. Systemic elapid poisoning usually causes neurotoxic effects, which, in untreated cases, results in ptosis and life threatening paralysis of the respiratory muscles. In victims of envenoming by sea snakes and Russell's vipers in Sri Lanka and South India, muscles become tender and painful and develop myoglobinuria. In rural and coastal regions of India and Thailand, snake-bite is a frequent cause of acute renal failure.

Management of Snake-Bite

(i) First aid and resuscitation

The first aid treatment should be carried out immediately or very soon after the bite. The bitten limb should be immobilized as far as practicable with a splint or sling. Most of the traditional first aid methods are potentially harmful and should not be used. As far as the snake is concerned, do not attempt to kill it, as this may be dangerous. However, if already killed, it should be taken to hospital with the patient so that it may be identified. Cardiopulmonary resuscitation (CPR) may be needed, including administration of oxygen and establishment of intravenous access. Airway, respiratory movements (breathing) and circulation must be checked immediately.

(ii) Antivenom treatment

The most important decision in the management of a patient bitten by a snake is whether or not to give antivenom, the only specific treatment for envenoming. There is abundant evidence to suggest that with severe envenoming, the benefits of this treatment outweigh the risks of antivenom reactions.

Antivenom is indicated if there are signs of systemic envenoming, local swelling involving more than half the bitten limb, extensive blistering or bruising, bites on digits and rapid progression of swelling. Monovalent or monospecific antivenom neutralises the venom of only one species of snake. Polyvalent or polyspecific antivenom neutralises the venoms of several different species of snakes, usually the most important species from a medical point of view in a particular geographical area. The dose of antivenom should not be based on the patient's size, but on the amount required to neutralise the toxin; thus in general, children should receive the full adult dose.

Key Learning Point
Snake bite antivenom treatment Children should be given the same dose of antivenom as adults

There is no absolute contraindication to antivenom treatment, but those who have reacted to horse or sheep serum in the past and those with a strong history of allergic disease should be given antivenom only if they have signs of systemic envenoming. However, allergic reactions to antivenom may be prevented or ameliorated by premedication with subcutaneous adrenaline (epinephrine) 5-10 microgram/Kg. Additional protective agents such as hydrocortisone and an antihistamine may be indicated.

Patients who suffer a snake bite and have not been immunised against tetanus within the last 5 years should receive anti-tetanus toxoid.

INSECT STINGS

Stings from ants, wasps, hornets and bees cause local pain and swelling but seldom cause severe toxicity unless many stings are inflicted at the same time. If the sting is in the mouth or on the tongue, local swelling may threaten the upper airway. The stings from these insects are usually treated by cleaning the area. Bee stings should be removed as quickly as possible. Anaphylactic reactions require immediate treatment with intramuscular adrenaline (epinephrine), self-administered (or given by a carer). Intramuscular adrenaline (e.g. EpiPen) is the best first-aid

treatment for children with severe hypersensitivity. A short course of an oral antihistamine or a topical corticosteroid may help to reduce inflammation and relieve itching.

PLANT AND MUSHROOM POISONING

Plants found in the home, garden and field now constitute the most common source of ingested poison in children. The fruits, seeds or roots of many common plants are poisonous. Fortunately, poisonous plants are rarely ingested in quantities sufficient to cause serious illness. However, the symptoms of poisoning from plants can include:
- Vomiting
- Stomach cramps
- Irregular heart beat
- Burning to the mouth
- Convulsions.

The type and severity of symptoms will vary according to the type of plant eaten. Any amount of any wild mushroom is considered to be very dangerous (See Box 19.7 for symptoms of mushroom poisoning). Deliberate ingestion of magic mushroom is also a potential source of poisoning. Identification of the plant must be attempted early and a computerised database can be accessed through the poisons centres.

Box 19.7: Symptoms of mushroom poisoning: symptoms typically appear 6 to 8 hours after eating but the symptoms can develop as soon as 2 and as late as 12 hours after ingestion.
Bloated feeling Nausea and vomiting Watery or (bloody) diarrhoea Muscle cramps Abdominal pain **Severe cases can include:** Liver damage, high fever, convulsions and coma Death (usually 2-4 days after ingestion).

Caution should be used in accepting common names of plants or in identifying a plant from a verbal description of its fruit or foliage. If substantial doubt exists, a portion of the plant should be brought for identification. However, each plant ingestion in a child must be viewed as potentially toxic until the plant has been positively identified or sufficient time has passed for a conclusion on nontoxicity. There is no way to tell by looking at a plant if it is poisonous.

DROWNING AND NEAR DROWNING

Drowning is defined as death, if the child dies within 24 hours as a result of a submersion accident and a near drowning accident if the child survives at least 24 hours after an episode of submersion. Drowning is now the most common cause of accidental death in children for a water-oriented society. Most drownings and near-drownings occur in the age group 1-2 years.

The complications of drowning are directly related to anoxia and to the volume and composition of water that is aspirated. Both fresh and salt water damage alveoli and result in pulmonary oedema. The most important complication of near-drowning accidents in addition to pulmonary injury, is the anoxic-ischaemic cerebral damage. As soon as water has entered the mouth it causes the epiglottis to close over the airway. Without oxygen, the child will lose consciousness. Thereafter bradycardia, cardiac arrhythmias, cardiac arrest and death.

Treatment

The single most important step in the treatment is the immediate institution of cardio-respiratory resuscitative measures at the earliest possible opportunity. Oxygen at the highest concentration available should be provided as soon as possible.

A deep body temperature reading (rectal or oesophageal) should be obtained as soon as possible. External rewarming is usually sufficient if core temperature is above 32°C but active core rewarming should be implemented if the core temperature is less than 32°C.

Resuscitation should not be abandoned until core temperature is at least 32°C or cannot be raised despite active measures. The decision to stop resuscitation should be taken only after all prognostic indicators have been considered (See Box 19.8).

Box 19.8: Prognostic markers in children with drowning

Submerged in water for more than 3-8 minutes
No gasp after 40 minutes of full CPR
Persisting coma
Arterial blood pH less than 7.0 despite treatment
Arterial blood PO$_2$ less than 60 mm Hg despite treatment.

There is no evidence that osmolality specific (salt versus fresh water) drowning affects the probability of survival.

Metabolic Diseases

Krishna M Goel

INBORN ERRORS OF METABOLISM

There has been a remarkable increase in our knowledge of the inborn metabolic errors in recent years, largely brought about by the introduction of new biochemical techniques. The term "inborn errors of metabolism" was first used by Garrod in 1908 when he described albinism, alkaptonuria, cystinuria and pentosuria. Garrod, noting the frequency of consanguineous matings in the pedigrees of his patients, correctly inferred the genetic origin of these disorders. He went further and suggested that they arose through the medium of defective enzyme activities. At the present time there are over 1,500 known recessive and X-linked human genetic diseases, all of which can be expected to have an underlying specific inherited metabolic disorder. So far in only about 200 is the precise enzyme defect known, although the chromosomal location of more than 700 of these genes is now known. In this book it would clearly be impracticable to consider the whole subject, which is, indeed, now far beyond the competence of any one individual. An attempt has been made to portray a broad outline of the subject and some of the more common or important diseases in the group receive more detailed considerations. Others are considered in other chapters under the various systems of the body.

GENERAL AETIOLOGICAL CONSIDERATIONS

It is now certain that genes act through the control of complex intracellular biochemical reactions. The concept of "one gene - one enzyme" is now firmly established. It follows, therefore, that an abnormal or defective enzyme activity must be related to an abnormal or mutant gene. Our understanding of the nature of gene activity was greatly furthered by the work of Watson and Crick when they described the structure of the deoxyribonucleic acid (DNA) molecule. A gene is composed of DNA and the structure of the DNA molecule determines the specific function of the gene. This structure consists of two helical chains of phosphate-sugar each coiled round the same axis. The chains are held together by purine and pyrimidine bases, which are at right angles to the axis of the molecule. There are four such bases in the DNA molecule - adenine (a purine), thymine (a pyrimidine), guanine (a purine) and cytosine (a pyrimidine). The genetic function is coded, as it were, by the particular sequence of these alternating pairs of purine and pyrimidine bases along the length of the DNA molecule. The activity of the DNA molecules on the chromosomes transmits information to the molecules of ribonucleic acid (RNA) within the cell nucleus. There are also four nitrogen bases in the RNA molecule-adenine, guanine, cytosine and uracil (instead of thymine as in DNA). The RNA or "messenger" molecules then diffuse out into the cytoplasm and pick up individual amino acids which come together to form polypeptide chains and proteins on the ribosomes. The sequence of bases along the RNA molecule is the code, which determines the order of incorporation of amino acids into the particular polypeptide chains. A mutation, therefore, consists of an alteration in the sequence of bases in the DNA molecule and consequently in the RNA molecule. This usually results in the substitution of one amino acid for another in the polypeptide chain. For example, the haemoglobin in sickle-cell anaemia (HbS) differs from normal haemoglobin (HbA) only in that valine occupies the position in the haemoglobin peptide sequence normally occupied by glutamic acid.

In the case of a defective enzyme system it is also likely that there is formed an enzyme protein, which is structurally abnormal. Thus, a single amino acid substitution at the active centre of the protein could profoundly alter the kinetics of the catalytic process and so result in loss of activity. The same kind of thing could obviously occur in peptides and protein macromolecules other than haemoglobin and enzymes, and the inborn errors of metabolism should now be taken to include all the specific molecular abnormalities, which are genetically determined. They can for clinical purposes be divided into four types.

1. Disturbances in structure of protein molecules,
   e.g. the haemoglobinopathies.
2. Disturbances in synthesis of protein molecules,
   e.g. haemophilia, Christmas disease, congenital afibrinogenaemia, congenital hypogammaglobulinaemia, and Wilson's disease where caeruloplasmin is deficient.
3. Disturbances in function of protein molecules,
   e.g. enzyme deficiencies like phenylketonuria, galactosaemia, adrenocortical hyperplasia and many others.
4. Disturbances in transport mechanisms,
   e.g. Hartnup disease, cystinuria, nephrogenic diabetes insipidus, renal glycosuria, de Toni-Fanconi syndrome, vitamin D-resistant rickets.

In 1961 the first success was achieved in "breaking the code" which the sequences of base pairs in the DNA and RNA molecules represent. Each amino acid is specified by a set of three bases out of the possible four nitrogen bases in the DNA and RNA molecules. This is a triplet code, which gives $4^3 = 64$ different possibilities, and each base triplet has been called a "codon". Some examples of the code in relation to the RNA molecule are as follows:

Phenylalanine	=	Uracil/Uracil/Uracil
Methionine	=	Uracil/Guanine/Uracil
Tryptophan	=	Uracil/Guanine/Guanine
Leucine	=	Uracil/Uracil/Adenine

A mutation usually involves the addition or deletion of a single base and as this may occur at random anywhere along the base-pair sequence it follows that many different (alternative) genes (or alleles) may be generated by different mutations in any given gene. For example, in a typical gene with 900 nitrogen bases coding a polypeptide chain of 300 amino acids as many as 2,700 different alleles might arise from different mutations, each causing the replacement of a single base because, of course, each of the 900 bases may be altered to one of three others by different mutational events. Such a great variety of different mutant alleles are not merely theoretical. Over three hundred variants of haemoglobin A have now been identified, the great majority differing from normal HbA by only a single amino acid substitution, although only a few are associated with overt disease. In the same way an enzyme protein can be altered in many ways by different mutant alleles, although when they result in the loss of enzyme activity they will all have similar metabolic and clinical consequences. In phenylketonuria different degrees of enzyme deficiency have now been recognised which are believed to reflect the effects of different mutations of the same gene, and a similar explanation has been suggested for the fact that some patients with homocystinuria respond to pyridoxine and others do not.

As the triplet code from 4 bases gives 64 different possibilities it follows that any one of the 20 amino acids must be able to be coded by more than one base triplet or codon. It would appear that of the 64 possible triplet sequences 61 each specify one out of the 20 amino acids, and that most amino acids are coded by two or more different base triplets. The remaining 3, sometimes called "nonsense triplets" do not code for any amino acid. They are concerned with chain termination, i.e. they define the point in the synthesis of the polypeptide at which the end of the chain is reached. In the majority of mutations involving a single base change the base triplet (or codon) for one amino acid is replaced by the base triplet for another resulting in the substitution of one amino acid for another in the polypeptide chain - as in the abnormal haemoglobins. On the other hand, if this single base change were to involve one of the "nonsense triplets" which code for chain termination the result would be the synthesis of a greatly shortened polypeptide chain which would fail to add up to a viable and functional form of protein. The effect could be a complete failure to synthesise the specific enzyme protein or, alternatively, a severe reduction in the rate of its synthesis so that very little is actually present at any one time. In other rare instances complete failure to form the enzyme may arise from a deletion of parts of the DNA sequence of the gene rather than from a single base change.

The basis of many of the inborn errors of metabolism is highly complex and even now not fully worked out. There are, in fact, certain other factors still to be mentioned and which are known to be concerned with the activity of any enzyme. This activity is, of course, determined by the aminoacid sequence of its constituent polypeptide chains, which dictate its three-dimensional molecular structure. But the quantity of enzyme, which is actually present, is also clearly important, and this is the resultant of the rates at which it is being synthesized in the cells and at which it is being broken down and denatured. Enzyme activity is further influenced by the presence of particular activators, inhibitors, repressors, coenzymes, etc. It will become clear in the accounts of some of the individual inborn errors, which follow that these factors may sometimes explain the variations, which are now being demonstrated within diseases previously thought to be more or less uniform in their manifestations.

Diagnosis depends on both the clinician having a high index of suspicion and on the appropriate test(s) being carried out. The local laboratory has a key role to play by guiding these investigations so that the most appropriate preliminary "screening" tests are carried out first. Many of the more specialised tests (i.e. specific enzymes) will only be required later to confirm a diagnosis.

DISORDERS OF AMINO ACID METABOLISM

PHENYLKETONURIA

Aetiology

"Classical: phenylketonuria (persistent hyperphenyl-alaninaemia > 240 μmols/l, relative tyrosine deficiency and excretion of an excess of phenylketones) is transmitted as an autosomal recessive trait, so that in any family in which the disease has appeared the chances of future children being affected will be 1 in 4. Parents of affected children are both asymptomatic carriers. The incidence of the "classical" form of PKU in the United Kingdom is about 1 in 10,000 births. In recent years the development of sensitive screening tests based upon the estimation of blood phenylalanine has shown that hyperphenyl-alaninaemia is not necessarily associated with the presence of phenylketones in the urine. The terminology relating to these other types of hyperphenylalaninaemia is confused, as is our understanding of their aetiology and has included such names a atypical PKU, mild PKU, phenyla-laninaemia, etc. Recent genetic studies have provided an explanation for this variation. Over 150 different mutations of the phenylalanine hydroxylase gene have been identified.

Pathogenesis

In normal individuals phenylalanine, which is an essential amino acid, is converted in the liver to tyrosine by the activity of phenylalanine hydroxylase. The gene for phenylalanine hydroxylase is located on chromosome 12 and contains 13 exons and messenger RNA is not readily available. Therefore a high proportion of affected subjects are compound heterozygotes rather than homozygotes. In consequence the blood phenylalanine increases to 1815-6050 μmol/l (30 - 100 mg per 100 ml) within two or three weeks of birth, and after a phenylalanine load the blood level of tyrosine does not rise. The blood phenylalanine is then converted by phenylalanine transaminase to phenylpyruvic acid and other degradation products such as phenyllactic acid, phenylacetic acid and ortho-hydroxyphenylacetic acid. The precise chemical cause for the inevitable mental retardation in "classical" PKU is not known but is probably related to the high phenylalanine concentration and to deficiencies of the neurotransmitters noradrenaline, adrenaline and dopamine. The fair hair and blue eyes are due to the deficient availability of melanin, which is synthesised like the neurotransmitters from tyrosine (Fig. 20.1).

The pathogenesis of the other types of hyperpheny-lalaninaemia is much less clearly defined. In one group, which may be called "mild" PKU, the blood phenylalanine values remain between 1210 and 1815 μmol/l (20 and 30 mg per 100 ml). The urinary ferric chloride test for

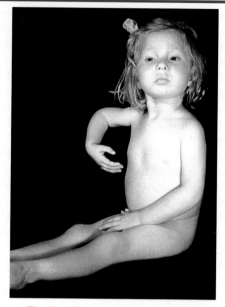

Fig. 20.1: Untreated phenylketonuria

phenylpyruvic acid is usually weakly positive, but if it is not, phenylketonuria develops if a high-protein diet or a phenylalanine-loading dose is given. Enzyme studies on some of these patients have shown complete absence of phenylalanine hydroxylase. In a third group of cases the blood phenylalanine ranges from 302 to 1210 μmol/l (5 to 20 mg per ml), and phenylpyruvic acid is not excreted in the urine because the level of blood phenylalanine is too low for transamination to occur. In a few such infants enzyme study of liver biopsy material has shown phenylalanine hydroxylase activity of less than half to one-tenth of normal. There are, however, other possible causes of hyperphenylalaninaemia. Several patients have been described with choking attacks, muscular hypotonia, developmental delay and convulsions, and mild to moderate hyperphenylalaninaemia. Liver phenylalanine hydroxylase activities have been normal and there has been continued clinical deterioration in spite of adequate dietary control. In these patients there is defective synthesis of tetrahydrobiopterin or of biopterin from dihydro-biopterin. As tetrahydrobiopterin is the cofactor for phenylalanine hydroxylase its deficiency prevents the conversion of phenylalanine to tyrosine even though the phenylalanine hydroxylase enzyme is normal. Deficien-cies of tetrahydrobiopterin will also interfere with the conversion of tyrosine to dihydroxyphenylalanine (DOPA) and noradrenaline and the conversion of tryptophan to serotonin, as tetrahydrobiopterin is also a cofactor for the enzymes involved. These tetrahydrobiopterin defects are found in about 1% of hyperphenylalaninaemic children and treatment is with tetrahydrobiopterin L-DOPA (dihydroxyphenylalanine) and L-5 hydroxytryptophan and a peripheral decarboxylase inhibitor. There is a blood spot-screening test available for total blood biopterin and this should be done in all hyperphenylalaninaemic children. The diagnosis of dihydropteridine reductase deficiency can be made prenatally on amniotic fluid cells and underlying gene defects have been identified. Other instances of hyperphenylalaninaemia may be due to deficiency of phenylalanine transaminase which converts phenylalanine to phenylpyruvic acid and in these patients neither an increased protein intake nor a phenylalanine load would result in phenylketonuria. In this group of patients, not only diagnosis but also the question of management raises considerable anxiety. Finally, in some infants there seems to be only a delayed maturation of one or more enzyme systems, especially if they are prematurely born and receiving parenteral nutrition. Such infants, in whom the biochemical findings may mimic permanent hyperphenylalaninaemia, can only be identified when after a lapse of time there is normal restoration of enzyme activity. This emphasises the need for repeated serum phenylalanine estimations during treatment with a low-phenylalanine diet.

Clinical Features

Untreated "classical" phenylketonurics have severe learning disorders (IQ 30 or lower). They are frequently blue-eyed, fair-haired and with fair skins. Eczema is often troublesome. Some have convulsions, athetosis and electroencephalographic changes. Many show psychotic features such as abnormal posturings with hands and fingers, repetitive movements such as head-banging or rocking to-and-fro and complete lack of interest in people as distinct from inaminate objects. The tendon reflexes are often accentuated. It should be noted that infants born homozygous for the phenylketonuric trait are not brain-damaged at birth. They only become so after they start to ingest phenylalanine in their milk.

MATERNAL PKU

As a consequence of defects of phenylalanine and tyrosine metabolism in the mother abnormalities have been reported among a large number of infants of phenylketonuric women. These include mental retardation, microcephaly, congenital heart disease and intrauterine growth retardation. Congenital anomalies are uncommon in the offspring of mothers with phenylalanine concentrations below 600 µmol/l at the time of conception. However, head size, birth weight and intelligence have been shown to be inversely and linearly associated with maternal phenylalanine concentrations. Phenylalanine concentrations during pregnancy and in the period prior to conception should be maintained between 60 and 250 µmol/l. Effective contraception should be continued until control has been achieved. Biochemical monitoring should be at least twice weekly and careful fetal ultrasound examinations to assess fetal growth and anatomy should be performed. Restriction of maternal dietary phenylalanine with tyrosine supplementation when necessary begun prior to conception controls the blood phenylalanine level and metabolite accumulation in the pregnant mother with PKU just as it does in the child with PKU. Dietary treatment begun after conception seems to be much less effective. It is essential therefore those women with PKU should be appropriately counselled and supported so that their children are conceived under the best possible phenylalanine control.

Diagnosis

When it became clear that a low-phenylalanine diet improved the intelligence of patients with PKU the need for early diagnosis, before intellectual impairment had occurred, was recognised. This requirement demands the "screening" of *all* newborn infants in a community. Those infants found to give a positive result with the screening test require to be submitted to more detailed confirmatory tests.

Screening tests—The presence of phenylpyruvic acid in the urine can be quickly detected by adding a few drops of 5 or 10 per cent aqueous solution of ferric chloride to 5 ml of acidified urine, when a green colour will rapidly develop. Alternatively, a wet napkin can be tested with Phenistix (Ames and Co.), which is pressed between tow layers of the napkin to be followed by a similar green colour. This technique was widely adopted as a screening test in the United Kingdom but was soon shown in practice to have real limitations in that many cases (45 per cent) were missed during the neonatal period. The neonatal screening programmes, which are now used, permit the accurate detection of infants who have raised blood phenylalanine levels from the 5th day of life. Such infants are clearly suspect for PKU and demand confirmatory investigations. As we have already noted, some of these infants will have hyperphenylalaninaemia without phenylketonuria. The most commonly used screening test for raised blood phenylalanine in the United Kingdom at the present time is the Guthrie bacterial inhibition test, which has been proved to be extremely reliable. There are, however, several other accurate methods for the detection of hyper-phenylalaninaemia such as spectrofluorimetry or one-dimensional chromatography of plasma. Both the Guthrie test and chromatography can be modified to "screen" for several other inborn errors such as galactosaemia, tyrosinaemia, homocystinuria, maple-syrup urine disease and histidinaemia. The former test is, indeed, being so used now in some areas of the United Kingdom. Blood for the test is obtained from a heel stab between the 4th and 11th day of life, either by hospital staff or the Health Visitor in the baby's home. The objective is to identify as soon after birth as possible and before the onset of recognizable clinical symptoms, specific metabolic disorders that can then be treated to ameliorate the consequences of untreated disease. The Guthrie test is now called the "Dried Blood Spot" specimen or "heel prick test".

Confirmation of the diagnosis of PKU—All infants in whom the Guthrie or other screening test has shown a blood phenylalanine of more than 240 µmol/l (4 mg per 100 ml) on two occasions should be further investigated. The urine of an affected infant may be noted to have a mousy smell caused by phenylacetic acid.

Treatment

Treatment, which should begin as soon as after birth as possible and be continued lifelong, involves restricting the intake of phenylalanine by means of a special diet.

The accepted dietary treatment of phenylketonuria consists of reducing the intake of phenylalanine to a level, which will prevent serious hyperphenylalaninaemia. A low phenylalanine diet cannot fully substitute for the phenylalanine turnover normally exerted by hepatic phenylalanine hydroxylase. As most food proteins contain phenylalanine it is obvious that a low-phenylalanine diet must be largely synthetic and consequently expensive. Such a diet is complex and depends on the use of manufactured substitutes for many natural foods. There is, however, strong evidence that phenylalanine (Phe) restriction can prevent mental retardation if treatment is started during the first three weeks of life. Infant screening programmes now instituted have resulted in the untreated older sufferer from PKU becoming a rarity.

In infancy we prefer to start treatment with a low Phe protein hydrolysate with added tyrosine, tryptophan, carbohydrate, fat, minerals and some vitamins. The bottle-fed infant's dietary phenylalanine is obtained from measured quantities of proprietary baby milk which should be sufficient to maintain the blood phenylalanine concentration between 182 and 484 µmol/l (3 and 8 mg per 100 ml). The baby milk is divided between the day's feeds and given prior to the low phe feed. The low Phe feed is fed to satiety although care must be taken to ensure that the infant's nutritional needs are met.

Breast-fed infants obtain phenylalanine from their mother's milk. Human milk contains less phenylalanine than baby milk formulae so that more mother's milk and less low Phe formula is required to control the infant's blood phenylalanine concentrations. Mothers are encouraged to continue breast-feeding on demand but prior to three or four of the breast-feeds low phe formula 15 to 20 ml/kg (i.e. 60 ml/kg/day) is given. The volumes of low Phe formula given are adjusted to maintain a blood phenylalanine concentration of 120-360 µmol/l (2 to 6 mg per 100 ml).

Mixed feeding should be introduced between four and six months. Infants who are not breast-fed should initially have solids containing negligible amounts of phenylalanine e.g. strained vegetables and fruit, or manufactured baby foods known to have a very low phenylalanine content. Breast-fed infants should be introduced to solids, which contain some phenylalanine. Initially 50 mg phenylalanine should be given, e.g. one Farley's rusk or specific quantities of baby foods known to contain 50 mg phenylalanine. Close and relatively frequent monitoring of the blood phenylalanine levels is necessary at this stage to ensure a correct balance between the amounts of phenylalanine received from solid food and the amount received from breast milk.

Between the ages of nine and twelve months a gradual change over from low phenylalanine milks to one of the amino acid mixtures can be given. We have adopted a diet which is easy to prepare and reasonably acceptable to the child. The parents of young children starting solid food are given food tables indicating the weight of individual foodstuffs, which contain 50 mg phenylalanine (1 phenylalanine exchange). The number of exchanges required will be determined by regular measurements of the child's blood phenylalanine levels. By this means the child's food preferences can best be catered for. Fruit and vegetables (except peas and beans) can be given without restriction.

On this diet a child can sit down to a meal which, apart from the lack of meat and other protein, looks very like that of the rest of the family. PKU children can be taken to hotels and holiday camps, and we have experienced no difficulty in arranging for schools to provide the special diet. Indeed, we have been told that sometimes the child's classmates envy them their special diet.

The dietary treatment of phenylketonuria has been considered in some detail because the same principles are applicable in several of the other inborn errors of metabolism, which involve the essential amino acids. It will be obvious to the reader that the adequate treatment of the inborn errors of metabolism requires that such patients attend special centres with the necessary dietetic and laboratory facilities. Children with phenylketonuria vary greatly in their tolerance to phenylalanine and the frequency of blood testing will need to be more in some than in others. In general we test blood phenylalanine concentration weekly up to the age of 4 years, every two weeks thereafter up to the age of ten years and thereafter monthly. The parents require constant guidance and support particularly from the dietitian and, indeed, the factors, which mostly determine whether a child does well intellectually, are the intelligence and sense of responsibility of the parents. It is, of course, important also to perform psychometric tests of a type suitable for age and development periodically throughout childhood. There are as yet no clear guidelines to indicate whether the special diet can be stopped. At the present time we recommend that the diet should be continued for life.

There has been a striking difference in the state of the children who attend a PKU Clinic over the past 30 years. Then, most were retarded. Some did quite well on their special diet, but others remained on the diet for only a short period before it was decided that they were too late for significant improvement. Even although treated individuals may achieve a high academic status there can be subtle global impairment determined by the degree of control in the early years of treatment. Magnetic resonance imaging (MRI) is revealing abnormal myelin structure in most adolescents and adults with phenylalanine concentrations greater than 400 µmol/L. Overt neurological deterioration is found in some. It is now evident that we must aim for very strict control in earlier life, promote a policy of lifetime treatment and ensure a strict diet pre-conception in women likely to conceive. Effective safe gene therapy may be a reality in the not too distant future.

OTHER DISTURBANCES OF AMINO ACID METABOLISM

HYPERTYROSINAEMIA

Hereditary Tyrosinaemia Type I (hepatorenal tyrosinaemia) is due to a deficiency of the enzyme fumarylacetoacetase.hydrolase. The gene defect is in chromosome 15 (q23-q25). It presents acutely in the newborn infant with failure to thrive, vomiting, diarrhoea, hepatomegaly and bleeding disorder with bruising, haematemesis, melaena and haematuria. Plasma and urinary concentrations of tyrosine and methionine are increased and death from haemorrhage and liver failure is common. Patients with a more chronic form may occur within the same family and have in addition to liver disease, renal tubular dysfunction, hypophosphataemia and rickets. In later life hepatoma develops in more than half of those surviving the first year and many develop hepatic cirrhosis and episodes of severe acute peripheral neuropathy. Treatment with a low phenylalanine, low tyrosine diet may improve the clinical state and reduce the urinary excretion of succinylacetone and tyrosine. Liver transplantation at an early stage should be considered to avoid hepatocellular carcinomas and the renal tubular problems.

Tyrosinaemia Type 2 (Oculocutaneous tyrosinaemia) is due to a deficiency of tyrosine aminotransferase. This disorder like the Type 1 defect is inherited in an autosomal recessive mode. Eyes, skin, and central nervous system are the only organs known to be affected in tyrosinaemia type 2. It is characterised by lacrimation, photophobia with tyrosine crystals in the cornea and with associated dendritic keratitis and ulcers. Keratitis also affects the skin

and mental retardation is a feature in some affected children. Early treatment with a low phenylalanine/low tyrosine diet offers a good prognosis. The gene defect is on chromosome 16 (q22-q24). The inheritance is autosomal recessive. The primary enzymatic defect is a reduced activity of fumarylacetoacetase. A variable degree of mental retardation occurs in less than 50% of patients.

There is also **Tyrosinaemia type 3** due to the primary deficiency of 4-hydroxyphenylpyruvate dioxygenase. It is very rare.

The treatment consists of dietary restriction of tyrosine and phenylalanine to a degree sufficient to achieve a resolution of eye and skin symptoms.

ALKAPTONURIA

Alkaptonuria is due to deficiency of the enzyme homogentisic acid oxidase so that homogentisic acid, instead of being converted to maleylacetoacetate, accumulates in the tissues and is excreted in the urine. The urine is noted to turn dark on standing as the homogentisic acid is oxidized to a melanin like product or it can be made to do so immediately by the addition of ammonia or sodium hydroxide. The alkaptonuric is symptomless in childhood but in adult life develops ochronosis and arthritis. This causes an ochre-like pigmentation of sclerae, ears, nasal cartilages and tendon sheaths, also kyphosis and osteoarthritis of the large joints. The disease is usually inherited as an autosomal recessive. A few families have shown dominant inheritance. The alkaptonuria gene has been mapped to a 16c M region on chromosome $3q^2$. There is no specific treatment.

TOTAL ALBINISM

Another disturbance, which also arises from defective metabolism of the aromatic amino acids, is total albinism. Consanguineous mating has been especially frequently recorded in this autosomal recessive trait. One of the various pathways of tyrosine metabolism is its conversion to 3,4-dihydroxyphenylalanine (DOPA) by the enzyme tyrosinase. This is converted to DOPA quinone, which is then converted to melanin. In albinism tyrosinase is lacking. The patients are exceedingly fair-skinned and fair-haired with red pupils and pink or bluish irises. Astigmatism and nystagmus are common. Some are mentally backward. The only available treatment is to protect the eyes and skin from bright sunshine and to correct any refractive errors. Sunscreens are very effective in protecting the skin and should be employed whenever possible. Hyperopia, myopia, and astigmatism need to be corrected to obtain the best-corrected visual acuity.

DISORDER OF BRANCHED-CHAIN AMINO ACID METABOLISM

MAPLE SYRUP URINE DISEASE

In maple syrup urine disease (MSUD) so called because the urine from affected infants has an odour (sweet, malty, caramel like) of maple syrup or burnt sugar, neurological disturbances appear soon after birth, e.g. difficulties with feeding, absence of the Moro reflex, irregular respirations, spasticity and opisthotonus. Pronounced dehydration and metabolic acidosis are not features of acute MSUD in contrast to other disorders of organic acid metabolism. Death occurs within a few months. Early diagnosis and management are essential to prevent permanent brain damage. The ferric chloride test on the urine gives a colour reaction, which could be mistaken for phenylpyruvic acid. Urine chromatography will reveal abnormally high concentrations of the branched-chain amino acids valine, leucine and isoleucine and of their corresponding keto- and hydroxy acids. The abnormal presence in the urine of the hydroxy acids, which are responsible for the characteristic smell, suggests that an abnormal pathway, due to deficiency of the branched chain 2 oxoactodehydrogenase, reduces the keto acids. The enzyme defect can be demonstrated in leucocytes and patients cultured skin fibroblasts and it is also possible to detect heterozygous carriers by this technique.

Treatment and Prognosis

Very high blood and tissue levels of branched chain amino acids in the acutely ill newborn will require urgent treatment in the form of haemodialysis, peritoneal dialysis or blood exchange transfusions to reduce plasma levels of toxic metabolites. Long-term treatment by a life long diet low in the three branched-chain amino acids has been successful in preventing the manifestations of this disease when diagnosis was made very soon after birth. Supplementation with an amino acid mixture lacking the branched chain amino acids is necessary in a protein-restricted diet. The long-term outcome depends on early diagnosis and management. Prenatal diagnosis is possible by enzyme studies on culture amniotic fluid cells and on chorionic villi. Future developments, including liver transplantation and gene therapy, may correct the underlying metabolic defect.

ORGANIC ACIDAEMIAS

There are now described more than thirty inherited conditions characterised by an excessive urinary excretion of acidic metabolites of amino acids, carbohydrates and fats. Infants with otherwise unexplained metabolic acidosis who become acutely ill should have plasma and urine levels of a specific organic acid and its by-products analysed by gas chromatography and mass spectrometry (GLC-MS) in order to detect conditions such as 3-methylcrotonyl glycinuria, isovaleric acidaemia, glutaric aciduria, propionic acidaemia and methylmalonic acidaemia. Of these propionic and methylmalonic acidaemias constitute the most commonly encountered abnormal organic acidaemias in children. There is at present an ever-increasing number of errors of intermediary metabolism being identified using these techniques and in some effective therapies are available.

Infants with isovaleric, propionic and methylmalonic acidaemias have many symptoms in common. Babies after an initial symptom free period may present with feeding difficulties, vomiting, lethargy, respiratory distress, hypotonia and generalised hypertonic episodes. Metabolic acidosis, ketonuria, hyperammonaemia, hypocarnitinaemia, neutropenia and thrombocytopenia are almost constant findings. The acute presentation is frequently precipitated by infection or some other form of stress. Treatment with protein restriction, riboflavin and L-carnitine may slow the course of the disease, particularly in patients diagnosed before the onset of symptoms. Treatment includes stopping all protein intake and maintenance with dextrose and bicarbonate to control acidosis. The emergency treatment of organic acidurias consists of removal of toxins by haemo or peritoneal dialysis and/or blood exchange transfusions. In addition glycine in isovaleric, biotin in proprionic and vitamin B12 in methymalonic acidaemias should be given in all cases. L-carnitine (125 mg/kg/day) should be given to patients with all three disorders. The long-term treatment involves reducing accumulated toxic products, maintaining normal nutritional status and preventing catabolism. Therefore in these children protein intake is largely restricted. Prenatal diagnosis can be made by enzyme studies in amniotic fluid cells and in uncultured chorionic villi as early as the 12th week of gestation.

UREA CYCLE DISORDERS

Five well-documented diseases have been described, each representing a defect in the biosynthesis of one of the normally expressed enzymes of the urea cycle.

Only an outline of those biochemical reactions responsible for the breakdown of amino acids leading to the formation of ammonia, which is then converted, into urea and CO_2 will be presented here (Fig. 20.2). This requires 5 enzymes (the ornithine-urea cycle). Carbamyl phosphate synthetase converts ammonia and bicarbonate to carbamyl phosphate, which then condenses with ornithine under the action of ornithine transcarbamylase to form citrulline. The conversion of citrulline to argininosuccinic acid is catalysed by argininosuccinate

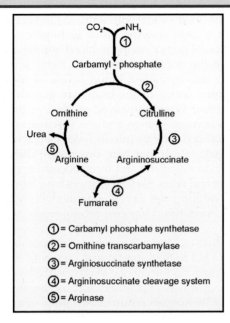

Ornithine – urea cycle diagram:

CO₂, NH₄ → ① → Carbamyl - phosphate → ② → Citrulline → ③ → Argininosuccinate → ④ → Fumarate; Argininosuccinate → Arginine → ⑤ → Urea; Ornithine

① = Carbamyl phosphate synthetase
② = Ornithine transcarbamylase
③ = Arginiosuccinate synthetase
④ = Argininosuccinate cleavage system
⑤ = Arginase

Fig. 20.2: The ornithine – urea cycle

synthetase, and argininosuccinic acid is cleaved to form arginine and fumaric acid by argininosuccinate cleavage enzyme (argininosuccinase). The enzyme arginase finally converts arginine into urea and ornithine. This synthetic process takes place in the liver and at least some of the enzymes have also been demonstrated in brain tissue, red cells and fibroblast cultures. Defects in the activity of several of these enzymes have been associated with inborn errors of metabolism in each of which mental retardation is a prominent feature due either to the toxic effects of ammonia accumulation or to the toxic effects of urea-cycle intermediates in the brain. The mechanisms leading to the toxicity of ammonia are not fully understood. The clinical manifestations of urea cycle disorders are mainly abnormalities secondary to hyperammonaemia and protein intolerance. A rapid diagnosis and institution of diet is essential for a good prognosis.

Antenatal diagnosis is available by a number of methods, particular to each disease including enzyme analysis of fibroblasts cultured from amniocytes, in utero liver biopsy, and DNA analysis.

HYPERAMMONAEMIA

Hyperammonaemia can be due to deficiency of ornithine transcarbamylase, which is inherited as an X-linked trait with variable expression in the female, and in which increased amounts of orotic acid are found in the urine; or of carbamyl phosphate synthetase. Signs usually develop in infancy with failure to thrive, vomiting, floppiness, increasing delay in milestones and episodic lethargy. A positive association between the clinical features and protein intake is a valuable diagnostic clue and episodes of coma with convulsive twitchings have been provoked

by a high protein intake. The fasting plasma ammonia level is usually greatly elevated, e.g. 205-704 µmol/l (350-1200 µg per 100 ml) as against the normal range of < 35 µmol/l (<60 µg per 100 ml). Diagnosis is confirmed by assay of the urea-cycle enzymes in liver biopsy material. In suspected cases the institution of a high-carbohydrate, protein-free diet often produces a dramatic improvement after a few days. Plasma amino acids and urinary orotate levels when measured in hyperammonaemic, non-acidotic infants provide positive identification of the specific enzyme deficiency. Long-term treatment is with a low-protein diet but the condition shows a variable clinical expression in age of onset and severity of symptoms. Even with early institution of a low protein diet and prompt treatment of metabolic crises, prognosis for normal development is guarded.

ARGINAEMIA

Argininaemia presents in childhood with hyperammonaemia, vomiting and retarded development with spastic quadriplegia, convulsions and hepatomegaly. Plasma and cerebrospinal fluid arginine concentrations are grossly elevated and the urine contains excessive quantities of cystine, lysine, ornithine, arginine and citrulline. Arginase deficiency can be demonstrated in erythrocytes.

CITRULLINAEMIA

Citrullinaemia arises from a deficiency of argininosuccinate synthetase and produces a clinical picture similar to that seen in hyperammonaemia, viz, mental retardation, episodic vomiting and coma with convulsions. The disorder is transmitted as an autosomal recessive trait. Raised levels of citrulline are found in the plasma, urine and cerebrospinal fluid and the plasma ammonia level rises sharply following a protein-rich diet and during intercurrent viral and other illnesses particularly if calorie intake is reduced so that the child becomes catabolic. Defective enzyme activity can be demonstrated in liver and skin fibroblasts. Prenatal diagnosis is possible by demonstrating enzyme deficiency in cultured amniotic cells. There is no effective treatment but a low-protein diet is worth a trial.

ARGININOSUCCINIC ACIDURIA

Argininosuccinic aciduria is due to a deficiency of the argininosuccinate cleavage enzyme. There is a severe, often fatal neonatal form and a late onset form in which there is severe mental retardation. Convulsive seizures, EEG abnormalities and ataxia may be present. In some children the hair is short and brittle (trichorrhexis nodosa). Argininosuccinic acid is normally present in very low concentrations in body fluids but in this disease high concentrations are found in the urine and cerebrospinal fluid. Deficiency of the enzyme may be demonstrated in liver, fibroblasts or erythrocytes. This disease is inherited as an autosomal recessive. The only treatment available is a restricted protein intake as the plasma ammonia level may be intermittently elevated. Prenatal diagnosis is possible either by demonstrating enzyme deficiency in cultured amniotic fluid cells or the presence of large amounts of argininosuccinic acid in amniotic fluid.

ORNITHINAEMIA

Ornithinaemia can occur in association with homo-citrullinaemia when there is deficiency of ornithine decarboxylase. There is mental retardation, ataxia and hyperammonaemia. There is a second type in which there is no hyperammonaemia or homocitrullinaemia but mental retardation, hepatic and renal disease and a generalised aminoaciduria are major features associated with a defect in hepatic ornithine keto acid transaminase. A third type presents usually with a visual defect and bizarre changes in the optic fundi due to gyrate atrophy of the choroid and retinae associated with a defect in ornithine amino-transferase. Low-ornithine diets may help.

In urea cycle disorders with hyperammonaemia the blood ammonia can be reduced with haemodialysis. In citrullinaemia and arginosuccinic aciduria, arginine infusions and a low-protein diet can help.

HISTIDINAEMIA

Histidinaemia is due to a deficiency of histidase which normally catalyses the conversion of histidine to urocanic acid. The urine contains considerable quantities of imidazolepyruvic, imidazoleacetic and imidazolelactic acids. The first of these substances reacts positively with ferric chloride solution and could lead to an erroneous diagnosis of phenylketonuria. There has always been doubt as to whether the biochemical abnormality relates to any clinical manifestations. However, prospective studies of untreated siblings with histidinaemia ascertained through probands and early detected but untreated children have indicated that the prevalence of impaired intellectual or speech development, convulsions, behavioural or learning disorders is not greater than in the non-histidinaemic population. Routine screening for early diagnosis is, therefore, probably not justifiable. Therefore treatment is rarely a consideration.

DISORDERS OF THE SULPHUR CONTAINING AMINO ACIDS

HOMOCYSTINURIA

Homocystinuria is the most common defect of the sulphur containing amino acids. Inheritance is as an autosomal recessive, and the defect is in cystathionine β-synthetase. This enzyme catalyses the condensation of homocysteine

(derived from methionine) with serine to form cystathionine. The result of this enzyme block in homocystinuria is accumulation of homocysteine in blood and tissues, and its excretion in the urine in its oxidized form, homocystine. There will also be raised blood levels of methionine; Cystathionine levels in the brain are grossly reduced. Usually the four systems involved are the eye, the skeleton, the central nervous system and the vascular system. The fully developed clinical picture includes mental retardation, seizures, malar flush, fair hair, downward dislocation of the lens, livido reticularis and thromboembolic episodes in both arteries and veins. Skeletal changes have been common, e.g. genu valgum, pes cavus, arachnodactyly, irregular epiphyses, vertebral changes, osteoporosis and pectus carinatum or excavatum. The fully developed picture resembles that of Marfan's syndrome (Marfanoid habitus of the body) but in the latter there is no mental retardation, no osteoporosis, no thrombotic tendency, the dislocation of the lens is upwards and inheritance is dominant. Some children with homocystinuria exhibit a characteristic shuffling or "Charlie Chaplin" gait; others have shown severe fatty change in the liver with little disturbance of liver function tests. Epileptic seizures may also occur. On the other hand, a considerable number of patients have a normal level of intelligence and not all cases are associated with the progressive deterioration described above. The diagnosis can be made early in infancy during screening programmes, and before clinical abnormalities have become manifest. A simple screening test when the diagnosis is suspected in the older patient is the nitroprusside/cyanide test, which does not, however, discriminate between an excess of cystine or homocystine in the urine. A positive reaction is an indication for chromatographic examination of blood and urine for increased concentrations of homosystine or methionine. When treatment is started in the neonatal period with a diet low in methionine, plus cystine supplements, normal development may be expected. Suitable amino acid mixtures with added cystine are now commercially available. Monitoring of treatment requires that the blood methionine be kept below 67 μmol/l (1 mg per 100 ml) and that there should be very low levels of homocystine in the blood and urine; it is also important to watch the blood cystine level. There are two distinct types of homocystinuria in that some cases respond completely to treatment with pyridoxine (vitamin B_6) 150-450 mg/day alone. The treatment is more successful when the diagnosis is made early. Prenatal diagnosis can be made by enzymatic assay in cultured amniotic cells and chorionic villi.

GALACTOSAEMIA

Aetiology

Classical galactosaemia (transferase deficiency) is another example of autosomal recessive inheritance and it results from the combination in one individual of two recessive genes.

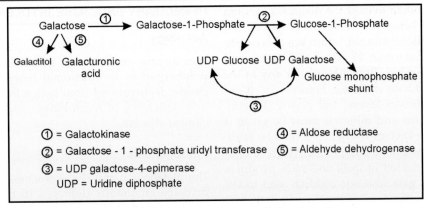

Fig. 20.3: Enzyme steps in galactose metabolism in erythrocytes

Pathogenesis

Galactose is ingested as lactose in milk, which undergoes splitting in the intestine into its component monosaccharides glucose and galactose. Milk and its products is virtually the sole source of dietary galactose in man. Galactose is then converted to glucose or energy in a series of enzyme steps (Fig. 20.3). Although the liver is the main site of this conversion, the demonstration of a similar series of enzyme reactions in red cells and the excess accumulation of galactose-1-phosphate in the erythrocytes from galactosaemic patients made it likely that the defect lay in the activity of galactose-1-phosphate uridyl transferase and in the inability to convert galactose-1-phosphate to glucose-1-phosphate (step 2 in Fig. 20.3). The accumulation in the erythrocytes of galactose-1-phosphate, believed to be the major toxic substance in galactosaemia is evidence that hexokinase activity is normal. In fact, galactosaemic red cells have been confirmed to be defective in Gal-1-P uridyl transferase and a similar deficiency has been demonstrated in liver tissue from affected patients. Gal-1-P uridyl transferase is absent in all tissues and the enzyme deficiency persists throughout life.

Clinical Features

Two main clinical types occur. The more severe develops its clinical features within two weeks of birth, after milk feeding has been started, with vomiting, disinclination to feed, diarrhoea, loss of weight, dehydration, hypoglycaemia, hepatocellular damage and renal tubular damage. The liver is enlarged with a firm, smooth edge and there may be jaundice. Splenomegaly is common. Cataracts may be seen with a slit-lamp. Finally the infant becomes severely marasmic with hepatic cirrhosis, ascites and hypoprothrombinaemia. Obvious signs and symptoms are later to appear in the less severe type although a history suggesting some early intolerance of milk may be obtained. The child may present with mental retardation, bilateral cataracts and cirrhosis of the liver. The explanation for the less severe cases may be the existence of an alternative pathway for galactose metabolism in the liver.

All the abnormalities in this disease save the mental retardation may regress rapidly on a galactose-free diet. It is, therefore, of prime importance that the diagnosis is made before irreversible brain damage has occurred. Undiagnosed cases may succumb to gram-negative sepsis.

Diagnosis

The first clue to the disease may be the finding of a reducing substance in the urine. Proteinuria may also be present. However, although Benedict's test is positive, tests based on the enzyme glucose oxidase (Clinistix) will be negative. Clinistix measures urine glucose specifically and instead a method for measuring total reducing substances (clinitest) must be used. Chromotography will then confirm that the reducing substance is galactose. There is, also, marked aminoaciduria due to renal tubular damage. Galactitol can be detected in blood and urine and may be a major factor in the toxic damage to the developing infant tissues. A valuable method of diagnosis, which can be used for umbilical-cord blood testing in the infant born into a known galactosaemic family and before milk feeds have started, is the demonstration of the absence of galactose-1-phosphate uridyl transferase activity in the red cells. An alternative test for use in the newborn is based on the excess accumulation of galactose-1-phosphate in the erythrocytes in this disease. Heterozygous carriers of the gene can be detected by quantitative estimation of Gal-1-P uridyl transferase activity in erythrocytes. It is possible to "screen" for galactosaemia during the neonatal period by a modified Guthrie test or chromatography of heel-stab blood and to start treatment before clinical features have appeared. Prenatal diagnosis by amniotic fluid cell enzyme assay is possible. In some commoner gene defects prenatal diagnosis and heterozygote testing can be performed using gene probes for the defects on chromosome 9 (p 13).

Treatment

The infant should be placed on a diet that is milk free and free from all products made with milk. When previously affected siblings are known to exist the diagnosis can and should be confirmed before the infant receives his first milk feed. Suitable milk substitutes, which are almost free from lactose, are Galactomin 17 (Cow and Gate) and Nutramigen and Pregistimil (Bristol-Myers) or any of the proprietary soya-based baby milks e.g. Formula "S" (Cow and Gate), Prosobee (Bristol-Myers) and Wysoy (Wyeth). Supplementary vitamins and minerals must be given if Galactomin 17 is used. Dietary restriction should be fairly strict during the first two years and probably there should be some lifelong restriction of milk and milk products intake. Unfortunately, galactosaemic children tend to fall below the average in mental development in spite of dietary treatment, although they remain within the educable range and have good physical health hey may also exhibit psychological disturbances, a phenomenon previously noted in phenylketonuric children also maintained on rigid dietary control. Now it is clear that the current methods of treatment, even if strictly followed, may not ameliorate the long-term sequelae, which occur regardless of when treatment was commenced. As adolescents, many develop educational difficulties, memory loss and abnormal neurological findings including ataxia, incoordination and brisk reflexes. Young women develop ovarian cysts and poor ovarian function with subfertility. Therefore a guarded prognosis should be given to parents of newly diagnosed cases. Maternal restriction of galactose is usually recommended to prevent prenatal damage in pregnancies known to be at risk of producing a galacto-saemic infant. However, it is not established that this is effective.

GALACTOKINASE DEFICIENCY

While the term "galactosaemia" has become established to denote the serious disease described above, an elevated blood galactose level may also result from a deficiency of the enzyme galactokinase by which galactose is phosphorylated to galactose-1-phosphate (Fig. 20.3). Galacto-kinase deficiency is also an autosomal recessive disorder associated with galactosuria, but the only significant pathology is the development of cataracts, which may be nuclear or zonular and is due to accumulation in the lens of galactitol. Liver, renal and brain damage do not occur. The dietary treatment as for galactosaemia prevents the development of cataracts and should be started as early in infancy as possible.

EPIMERASE DEFICIENCY

Deficiency of epimerase enzyme may produce a clinical picture similar to that of the transferase defect or may be asymptomatic. They also, if symptomatic, respond to milk free diets.

HEREDITARY FRUCTOSE INTOLERANCE

Aetiology

This disease causes severe metabolic disturbances and it is inherited as an autosomal recessive trait. It must be clearly distinguished from *benign frustosuria* which is due to a deficiency of fructokinase and which produces no clinical disease.

Pathogenesis

The metabolic pathways of fructose are complicated. The primary enzymatic defect is in fructose-1-phosphate aldolase which in the liver and intestine splits fructose-1-phosphate into two trioses, glyceraldehyde and dihydro-xyacetone phosphate. This defect results in the accu-mulation of fructose-1-phosphate, which inhibits fructo-kinase and leads to high blood levels of fructose after its ingestion in the diet. The mechanisms, which produce gastro-intestinal symptoms and hypoglucosaemia in affected infants, are not yet fully understood but the intracellular accumulation of fructose-1-phosphate probably prevents the conversion of liver glycogen to glucose.

Clinical Features

Symptoms only appear when fructose is introduced into the diet as sucrose in milk feeds, as sorbitol or as fruit juices he condition tends to be more severe the earlier the exposure to fructose. They vary in severity, partly according to the amounts of fructose ingested, and the wholly breast-fed infants remains symptomless. Common features are failure to thrive, severe marasmus, anorexia, vomiting, diarrhoea and hepatomegaly. Hypoglucosaemia may cause convulsions or losses of consciousness. Liver damage may result in jaundice, and liver function tests give abnormal results. Albuminuria, fructosuria and excess aminoaciduria may be present. Hyperfructosaemia and hypoglucosaemia develop following upon the ingestion of fructose or sucrose (glucose + fructose). Death ensues in undiagnosed infants. In milder cases in older children gastrointestinal symptoms predominate, and in some a profound distaste of anything sweet develops sponta-neously as a protective mechanism.

Diagnosis

The diagnosis is usually suspected because of its clinical presentation, by a dietary history and by a favourable response to removal of fructose from the diet. An oral fructose tolerance test (l g per kg up to a maximum of 50 g) results in a marked and prolonged fall in the true blood glucose level and a fall in the inorganic phosphorus. There will also be raised blood levels of fructose, free fatty acids and lactic acid. Fructosuria may be detected.

Treatment

Early diagnosis is important. The treatment consists simply in the life long removal of all fructose-containing foods from the diet and of sucrose from the milk feeds. Sorbitol, a fructose polymer, must not be used as a sweetening agent. An incidental benefit of the diet is that through exclusion of sucrose there is a marked reduction in the incidence of dental decay.

Hereditary Fructose 1, 6-Bisphosphatase Deficiency

Although not a defect of the specialized fructose pathway, hepatic fructose 1, 6-bisphosphatase deficiency is usually classified as an error of fructose metabolism. It manifests with spells of hyperventilation, apnoea, hypoglycaemia, ketosis and lactic acidosis and may be life-threatening in the newborn period.

HYPOPHOSPHATASIA

Aetiology

This disease is transmitted as an autosomal recessive characteristic and the heterozygous carrier state can usually be detected. Heterogyzotes may have low serum alkaline phosphatase concentrations, high urinary excretion of phosphoethanolamine, or both, without bone disease.

Pathogenesis

In some inborn errors of metabolism the absence of an enzyme activity is deduced indirectly from the demonstration that a metabolic pathway has gone wrong. In hypophosphatasia the enzyme which is defective (alkaline phosphatase) can be directly measured. Further evidence of the nature of hypophosphatasia was the demonstration by chromatography of an abnormal metabolite - phosphoethanolamine - in the plasma and urine of affected patients. Phosphoethanolamine seems to be a naturally occurring physiological substrate of alkaline phosphatase.

The consequence of this enzyme deficiency is a failure of mineralization of the skeleton, both membranous and cartilaginous. Long bones at the metaphyses show a wide irregular zone of proliferative cartilage with disorganized maturation of the cells and no evidence of calcification of the intercellular matrix. Osteoid tissue is deposited on the cartilaginous intercellular substance and on the outside of the shafts, and as it is almost completely uncalcified, fractures readily occur. There is, however, no shortage of osteoblasts, which are the normal source of alkaline phosphatase in bone.

Clinical Features

Three clinical types of hypophosphatasia have been described: (a) infantile, (b) childhood and (c) adult. In the infantile type the disease becomes obvious within a few weeks of birth. In one case, where a previous sibling had been affected, the diagnosis was established radiologically before birth. Many of the signs resemble those seen in rickets, e.g. enlarged epiphyses, "beading" of the ribs, kyphoscoliosis, bowing of the long bones which sometimes show spontaneous fractures, failure to thrive and hypocalcaemia. However, as the membranous bones are also affected the skull may be so poorly mineralized that it feels like a balloon filled with water. The anterior fontanelle and sutures may be wide and tense, but subsequently there may be premature fusion with microcephaly. In the childhood type the presenting sign may be premature loss of the deciduous teeth, increased susceptibility to infection and somatic retardation. Radiographs show an abnormal patchy calcification at the metaphyses producing an ill-defined margin distal to which there is a zone of poorly calcified osteoid. The epiphyseal lines are irregularly widened. There may also be periosteal elevation due to deposition of osteoid. The adult form may present with spontaneous fractures and radiolucent bones in the skeleton.

Diagnosis

The diagnosis should be based on a very low level of serum alkaline phosphatase for the patient's age. Biopsy of tissues normally rich in alkaline phosphatase, such as bone, will also show a greatly reduced enzyme content. The histological picture is generally indistinguishable from that of true rickets.

An inconstant but serious finding is hypercalcaemia. It may lead to renal failure. Abnormal quantities of phosphoethanolamine may be demonstrated in the urine and plasma of patients. Prenatal diagnosis of severe hypophosphatasia may be made by ultrasound evaluation of fetal skeletal calcification and reduced alkaline phosphatase activity in amniotic fluid or cells obtained from this fluid.

Treatment

Cases, which are diagnosed in early infancy, do not long survive. Treatment of children with hypophosphatasia with vitamin D has not been successful. At present there is no effective treatment for this condition.

DISORDERS OF PURINE AND PYRIMIDINE METABOLISM

Inherited disorders of purine and pyrimidine metabolism are rare disorders.

Hereditary orotic aciduria is an autosomal recessive condition in which there is failure to thrive, hypochromic anaemia with megaloblasts in the bone marrow, and increased urinary excretion of orotic acid. The underlying enzyme defect may involve one or both of the enzymes concerned in the synthesis of uridine and monophosphate, orotate phosphoribosyltransferase and orotidylate decarboxylase. Treatment with uridine, l g/day, results in correction of the anaemia and impaired growth. Prenatal diagnosis of this disorder has never been performed although theoretically this is possible.

Lesch-Nyhan syndrome is an X-linked recessive disorder in which male infants are generally normal at birth. It is characterised by central nervous system disorders of various types and excessive quantities of uric acid in blood, tissue and urine. The disorder is caused by deficiencies of the enzyme hypoxanthine-guanine phosphoribosyltransferase. Affected boys can be severely mentally retarded and have choreoathetosis, spasticity and distressing compulsive self-mutilation, or they may present with gouty arthritis and pain from ureteric colic caused by urates. A definite diagnosis of the Lesch-Nyhan syndrome can be made by the absence of hypoxanthine-guanine phosphoribosyltransferase in the peripheral circulating erythrocytes. Allopurinol and probenecid will reduce the hyperuricaemia but not correct or help the neurological problems. Prenatal diagnosis can be made by the culture of cells obtained by amniocentesis.

CONGENITAL METHAEMOGLOBINAEMIA

Aetiology

The most common form of congenital methaemoglobinaemia is inherited as an autosomal recessive trait and it is due to the absence of a normal intra-erythrocytic enzyme activity. A rare type, inherited as an autosomal dominant, has a quite different aetiology in that it is due to the formation of an abnormal haemoglobin (haemoglobin M) with a defective globulin component.

Pathogenesis

In normal haemoglobin the iron of the four-haem groups is in the reduced or ferrous state. In methaemoglobin the iron is in the oxidized or ferric state and it is incapable of combining with oxygen. In normal erythrocytes methaemoglobin is constantly being formed and in normal blood a small amount is always present. It is, however, continuously being reduced back to haemoglobin by a complex series of enzyme steps. In congenital methaemoglobinaemia there is an intra-erythrocytic defect in one of these enzyme reactions. The other form of congenital methaemoglobinaemia belongs to the haemoglobinopathies and haemoglobin M can be separated from normal haemoglobin by electrophoretic techniques.

Clinical Picture

The primary sign is a dusky slate-grey type of cyanosis, which is present from birth. It is free from respiratory or cardiac symptoms and clubbing of the fingers and toes does not develop. Some patients develop compensatory polycythaemia and some have been severely mentally retarded.

Diagnosis

The presence of excess methaemoglobin in the blood should be demonstrated by spectrophotometry.

It is important to distinguish the congenital and permanent form of methaemoglobinaemia from the temporary but dangerous acquired form, which may follow the entry into the body of certain poisons such as aniline dyes, nitrites, acetanilid and potassium chlorate. Outbreaks of acquired methaemoglobinaemia have occurred in newborn nurseries when new napkins marked by aniline dyes have been used before laundering and cases have occurred in children drinking well-water containing nitrites. Therefore assays of methaemoglobin reductase and detection of HbM are essential to confirm the specific diagnosis. It is also important to remember that cyanotic children without heart murmurs may have methaemoglobinaemia. We have seen the mistaken diagnosis of congenital heart disease made in two such cases and, in fact, one child was unnecessarily submitted to cardiac catheterisation.

Treatment

Methaemoglobinaemia due to the deficiency of enzyme methaemoglobin reductase may respond to ascorbic acid 200 - 500 mg/day or methylene blue 5 mg/kg/day, given orally or intravenously. These drugs do not, however, have any beneficial effect in haemoglobin M disease.

GLYCOGEN STORAGE DISORDERS

Glycogen is a complex high molecular weight polysaccharide composed of numerous glucosyl units linked together in the form of many branches. It is mainly found in the liver and muscle. The glucosyl units are mainly linked together through carbon atoms 1 and 4 but at the branch points the bonds are between C1 and 6. Multiple enzymes are involved in the synthesis (glycogenesis) and breakdown (glycogenolysis) of glycogen. There are still several gaps and uncertainties, which make classification of the metabolic errors of glycogen metabolism difficult. In practical paediatric practice, however, a somewhat oversimplified concept of these physiological steps will prove sufficient for the clinician's purpose. In health, human liver glycogen content varies from 0-5 per cent, while muscle glycogen is rarely as high as 1 per cent. Hepatic glycogen functions as a reserve of glucose and is utilised during fasting to maintain normoglycaemia.

Glycogenesis

Glucose reacts with ATP under the catalytic activity of hexokinase to form glucose-6-phosphate and ADP.

Glucose-6-phosphate is then converted to glucose-1-phosphate by phosphoglucomutase. The next step is the conversion of glucose-1-phosphate to glucosyl units in 1,4 linkage. While this can be achieved *in vitro* by phosphorylase, it is possible that *in vivo* it proceeds independently of phosphorylase and by means of two other steps involving UDP-glucose pyrophosphorylase and UDPG glycogen-transglucosylase. This could explain the observation of several workers that the activation of phosphorylase *in vivo* always leads to glycogen breakdown and never to glycogen synthesis. When a chain of the growing glycogen molecule reaches a critical level a branch point is established by transfer of the 1, 4 linkage to a 1, 6 linkage, this being mediated by amylo- (1, 4-1, 6)-transglucosidase (brancher enzyme).

Glycogenolysis

Glycogen can be converted back to glucose-1-phosphate by the enzymes phosphorylase, which breaks the 1,4 linkage, and amylo-1, 6-glucosidase (debrancher enzyme) which breaks the 1, 6 linkage. Glucose-1-phosphate is then converted to glucose-6-phosphate, a reversible reaction, by phosphoglucomutase. Finally, glucose-6-phosphate can be converted to free available glucose by glucose-6-phosphatase. This enzyme is found only in the liver and kidneys. Glycogen in the muscles cannot be converted to free glucose but only to pyruvate and lactate via the Embden-Meyerhof glycolytic pathway.

At least nine types of glycogenosis can now be delineated and this number is likely to increase as further enzyme deficiencies are detected by modern biochemical techniques. The investigation of such cases nowadays can only be considered complete when the chemical structure of the deposited glycogen has been determined and when the various enzymes mentioned above have been assayed. Some types have so far only been described in adults and we shall describe here only those types of glycogen storage disease, which, not infrequently, can provide diagnostic difficulties for the paediatrician.

TYPE 1 GLYCOGEN STORAGE DISEASE (VON GIERKE DISEASE - GLUCOSE-6-PHOSPHATASE DEFICIENCY

Aetiology

This was the first of the glycogenoses to be recognised. It is inherited as an autosomal recessive disorder in which consanguinity is a common feature. The heterozygous, and apparently healthy, carriers of the gene can be detected by the lowered glucose-6-phosphatase level in the intestinal mucosa.

Pathogenesis

The absence of glucose-6-phosphatase activity has been proved in this form of the disease. This enzyme normally

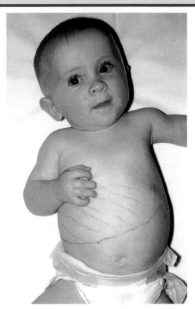

Fig. 20.4: Four-month infant with glycogen storage type 1a disease. Note rounded facies and gross hepatomegaly

liberates free glucose from glucose-6-phosphate in the liver.

Clinical Features

Gross enlargement of the liver is the most constant feature and it is often recognised in early infancy. In the severe form it may present in the neonatal period with profound hypoglycaemia and acidosis. Growth is stunted and the protuberant abdomen is often associated with an exaggerated lumbar lordosis. Genu valgum (knock knees) is common. There may be an excess deposition of fat, and xanthomatous deposits are commonly found on the knees, elbows and buttocks. Indeed, affected infants are often fat with a characteristically round face (doll like) (Fig. 20.4) There is no splenomegaly and there are no signs of cirrhosis and uric acid nephropathy may develop and there are reports of hepatic adenomata formation. The presence of fever may lead to an erroneous diagnosis of sepsis.

Type 1b has a similar clinical course with the additional findings of neutropenia and impaired neutrophil function resulting in recurrent bacterial infections. Oral and intestinal mucosa ulceration commonly occurs.

Type 1 c and type 1d have been reported in only a few patients.

Biochemical Findings

Acetonuria is common in the fasting state. Hypoglycaemia may be so severe as to precipitate convulsions and even lead to mental impairment. Hyperlipaemia and hypercholesterolaemia are marked and may even interfere with accurate measurement of plasma electrolytes. Episodes of severe metabolic acidosis develop in some cases. Plasma pyruvate and lactate concentrations are increased and the phosphate may be reduced. Renal damage from glycogenosis can cause glycosuria and aminoaciduria.

Diagnosis

Hepatomegaly with the combination of hypoglycaemia, hyperlactic-acidemia and hyperuricaemia is virtually diagnostic of Type I glycogenosis. Further evidence of von Gierke disease may be obtained from a variety of tests.

1. The glucose tolerance test (after 1.5 g glucose/kg) shows an abnormally high increase in blood sugar and a delayed fall.
2. There is a marked resistance to the hyperglycaemic response to adrenalin (0.3-0.5 ml subcutaneously) or glucagon (1 mg intravenously). In normal subjects these agents cause glycogen breakdown to glucose-1-phosphate, its subsequent conversion to glucose-6-phosphate, and liberation of free glucose there from by the action of glucose-6-phosphatase. The last step is, of course, deficient in this disease. The adrenaline or glucagon is given after an 8 hour fast and immediately after removal of a specimen of blood for estimation of the true glucose level. Thereafter the blood glucose concentrations are measured every 10 minutes for 1 hour. In healthy individuals the values increase 40-60 per cent above the fasting value. In von Gierke disease a "flat" curve is obtained.
3. Another indirect measurement of glucose-6-phosphatase activity can be obtained after an intravenous dose of galactose 1 g/kg, or fructose 0.5 g/kg. Blood glucose concentrations at 10-minute intervals are compared with the pre-injection value. In healthy persons galactose and fructose are converted via glucose-6-phosphate to free glucose, but this metabolic pathway is blocked in von Gierke disease.

Conclusive proof of the diagnosis, however, can only be obtained from a liver biopsy. The findings in this type of glycogenosis will be:
(a) A liver glycogen content over 5 per cent of wet weight.
(b) Glycogen of normal chemical structure.
(c) Absent or very low glucose-6-phosphatase activity.

Treatment

Although the enzyme failure cannot be corrected, considerable benefit can accrue from a diet in which a high intake of carbohydrate is given in frequent feeds throughout the 24 hours. Where hypoglycaemia occurs in the early hours of the morning overnight continuous intragastric feeding can produce remarkable clinical benefit. Use of slowly digested carbohydrate such as cornflour can help to maintain blood glucose concentration. Episodes of severe metabolic acidosis, often precipitated by intercurrent infections, can endanger life.

They must be promptly treated with intravenous glucose and sodium bicarbonate under careful biochemical control. Diazoxide may be of help in infants with intractable hypoglycaemia. Portocaval anastomosis, which acts by diverting glucose from the liver to the tissues, may be of help. Liver transplantation has been performed in type 1 glycogen storage disease but should be performed only after all other methods of treatment have failed or if there has been malignant transformation of adenoma. If these children can be tided over the dangerous early years their health often improves greatly during adolescence. Prenatal diagnosis of type 1 a has been possible through fetal liver biopsy.

GLYCOGEN STORAGE DISEASE OF THE HEART (CARDIOMEGALIA GLYCOGENICA: IDIOPATHIC GENERALISED GLYCOGENOSIS: POMPE DISEASE: TYPE 2)

Aetiology

Once again autosomal recessive inheritance is involved and consanguinity has been reported.

Pathogenesis

The disease may involve the central nervous system and skeletal muscles as well as the myocardium. It has been shown that the primary defect is of the lysosomal enzyme acid α-1, 4 glucosidase (acid maltase). In biopsy specimens' spontaneous glycogenolysis is rapid and the glycogen does not show the abnormal stability, which is a characteristic finding in the other types of glycogenosis.

Clinical Features

Clinically the enzyme deficiency results in two major presentations. The first, originally described by Pompe, is as follows.

The infant becomes ill in the early weeks of life with anorexia, vomiting, dyspnoea and failure to thrive. The heart is enlarged, tachycardia is present, and a systolic murmur is commonly heard. Oedema may also develop. The ECG shows a shortened P-R interval, inverted T waves and depression of the ST segments. When skeletal muscles are severely involved the degree of hypotonia may simulate Werdnig-Hoffmann disease. In some infants macroglossia has been so marked as to arouse the suspicion of cretinism. On the other hand, hepatomegaly is not prominent until cardiac failure is advanced. Glucose tolerance, adrenaline and glucagon responses are all normal. The diagnosis may be established by muscle biopsy and the demonstration of increased glycogen content. There will also be low acid maltase activity in the leucocytes. An electromyogram reveals a primary disorder of the muscles. Prenatal diagnosis is possible by determining alpha–glucosidase deficiency in cultured amniotic cells and chorionic villus biopsies.

The second presentation is more slowly progressive muscle disorder, with symptoms beginning in childhood or in adult life and manifestations limited to skeletal muscle. The muscle involvement is mainly proximal muscle weakness including impairment of respiratory function. Death results from respiratory failure.

Treatment

No effective treatment is available for this disorder.

TYPE 3 GLYCOGEN STORAGE DISEASE (LIMIT DEXTRINOSIS; DEBRANCHER ENZYME DEFICIENCY)

Aetiology

It is probable that this form of glycogen storage disease is also inherited as an autosomal recessive. It cannot be differentiated reliably from von Gierke disease by clinical examination alone.

Pathogenesis

The debrancher enzyme (amylo-1, 6-glucosidase) is absent from liver, skeletal and cardiac muscle. Glycogen deposition in the heart and skeletal muscles does not occur in von Gierke disease.

Clinical Features

Hepatomegaly is marked but hypoglycaemic problems are less troublesome and there is less interference with growth. It is common to find the same plump appearance and round face as in von Gierke disease (Fig. 20.4). In some cases, the involvement of skeletal muscles gives rise to weakness and hypotonia.

Diagnosis

Acetonuria may appear during fasting and there is a diminished hyperglycaemic response to adrenaline or glucagon. However, de-esterification of glucose-6-phosphate to glucose can proceed normally and there is, therefore, a normal hyperglycaemic response to intravenous galactose or fructose. The serum lactate level is not often raised, but there is a raised blood lipid content. The liver glycogen content is increased and it is abnormal in structure with short external chains and an increased number of 1, 6 branch points. Activity of liver amylo-1, 6 glucosidase is not detectable. It is also possible to demonstrate an elevated erythrocyte glycogen of the limit dextrin type and the enzyme deficiency can also be demonstrated in erythrocytes and leucocytes. Direct assay of the enzyme in liver and muscle tissue is confirmatory.

Treatment

Frequent feedings with a high-carbohydrate, high-protein diet and overnight nasogastric feedings can be very beneficial. Cardiac involvement is rarely clinically demonstrable but strenuous exercise should probably be avoided. No specific treatment is available for this disorder.

TYPE 4 FAMILIAL CIRRHOSIS OF THE LIVER WITH ABNORMAL GLYCOGEN (AMYLOPECTINOSIS; BRANCHER ENZYME DEFICIENCY)

This appears to be an excessively rare disease in which amylo- (1,4-1,6)-transglucosidase deficiency results in deposition of an abnormal glycogen with a molecular structure resembling the amylopectins of plants. This substance is toxic so that the patient presents with cirrhosis of the liver, splenomegaly and jaundice. Liver function tests yield grossly abnormal results and death is preceded by the development of ascites and deep jaundice. This diagnosis should be considered in all cases of familial hepatic cirrhosis. Deficiency of the branching enzyme can be demonstrated in liver and leucocytes. There is no specific treatment for type 4-glycogen storage disease.

TYPE 5 GLYCOGENOSIS (MYOPHOSPHORYLASE DEFICIENCY, MCARDLE DISEASE)

Children with myophosphorylase deficiency are asymptomatic at rest but muscle cramps occur with moderate exercise. These symptoms are usually absent or slight during the first decade. A diagnosis is made on the basis of history and the absence of elevation of lactate after exercise.

No specific treatment is available. In the absence of severe exercise the patients remain asymptomatic.

TYPE 6 GLYCOGEN STORAGE DISEASE (LIVER PHOSPHORYLASE DEFICIENCY)

In this form of glycogenosis the clinical picture simulates that described in von Gierke disease and in limit dextrinosis, although the characteristic rounded facial appearance is absent. The striking feature is hepatomegaly. Growth retardation is slight. Clinically these children have a very mild disease. Keto-acidosis is absent. Hypoglycaemia is mild and inconstant. The serum lactate level is not usually raised but there may be elevation of the serum uric acid. The blood glucose level rises after intravenous galactose. There is usually a moderate rise in the blood lipids and the red cell glycogen is elevated. Phosphorylase activity is demonstrably low in liver tissue and in the leucocytes. There is no specific therapy for this disorder. A high carbohydrate diet and frequent feedings are effective in preventing hypoglycaemia.

TYPE 7 GLYCOGEN STORAGE DISEASE (MUSCLE PHOSPHOFRUCTOKINASE DEFICIENCY, TARUI DISEASE)

The clinical features are very similar to those in type 5-glycogen storage disease. The patients experience early onset of fatigue and pain with exercise.

For diagnosis, a biochemical or histochemical demonstration of the enzyme defect in the muscle is required. There is no specific treatment available. Avoidance of strenuous exercise is advisable.

INBORN ERRORS OF LIPID METABOLISM (THE LIPIDOSES)

This group includes Gaucher disease, Niemann-Pick disease, Tay-Sachs disease and probably also metachromatic leucodystrophy and Krabbe's leucodystrophy. The chemical pathways of lipid metabolism are at present imperfectly understood. Here it will only be stated that in the lipidoses there is an abnormal intracellular deposition of sphingolipids, often widely spread throughout many organs and tissues as in Gaucher and Niemann-Pick diseases.

GAUCHER DISEASE

Aetiology

In Gaucher disease a glucocerebroside (glucosylceramide) is deposited in the tissues. The glycolipids, which go to form glucocerebroside, are derived from senescent leucocytes and erythrocytes. They are normally broken down by a series of enzymes, one of which is glucocerebrosidase. In the Type 1 form of the disease the spleen has only about 15 per cent of normal enzyme activity whereas in the Type 2 acute form glucocerebrosidase is completely absent from the spleen and other organs (including the brain).

Clinical Features

This disease appears to occur in three forms, Type 1 adult, chronic, non-neuropathic form, Type 2 infantile, acute, neuropathic form, and Type 3 juvenile subacute neuropathic form. All are inherited as autosomal recessive traits but the condition runs true to form in any single family. Gaucher Type 1 disease is particularly common in Jewish families.

Type 1 Gaucher Disease

The Type 1 chronic form is the most common. It presents at any age from a few months to late adulthood with gross splenomegaly. Hepatic enlargement may also be marked. There is also a progressive anaemia, and leucopenia and thrombocytopenia due to hypersplenism develop early in its course. Bone involvement may give rise to limb pains. Radiographs reveal a characteristic flaring outwards of the metaphyseal ends of the long bones with thinning of the cortex. This is most marked at the lower ends of the femora, which have an Erlenmeyer flask appearance. These features develop in childhood or early adult life. In older patients especially, the face, neck, hands and legs may show a characteristic brownish pigmentation, and the conjunctiva may show a wedge-shaped area of thickening with its base to the cornea (pinguecula). The serum cholesterol level is normal. The diagnosis can be confirmed by finding the lipid-filled cells, which have a typical fibrillary appearance of the cytoplasm. These should be sought in material obtained by needle puncture of the bone marrow, spleen or lymph nodes. The disease runs a slow course but death is inevitable.

Type 2 Gaucher Disease

The Type 2 infantile acute form is a rare phenomenon confined to infancy. In addition to hepatosplenomegaly there is evidence of severe cerebral involvement, which is rarely seen, in the chronic form. There may be hypertonia, catatonia, trismus, opisthotonus, dysphagia, strabismus and respiratory difficulties. Death occurs by the age of 3 years.

Type 3 Gaucher Disease

The Type 3 juvenile subacute form shares some characteristics of Types 1 and 2. Neurological features may appear early in addition to hepatosplenomegaly but the time course of progression is slower. Spasticity, ataxia, ocular palsies, mental retardation and seizures are later features. Ultimate proof of diagnosis would require tissue or white blood cell betaglucosidase assay, or liver of spleen glucocerebroside determination. Prenatal diagnosis is routine for all types of Gaucher disease.

Treatment

Treatment is now available with synthetic enzyme and bone marrow transplantation. Splenectomy is indicated when splenomegaly is massive and interferes with normal growth and development.

NIEMANN-PICK DISEASE

Aetiology

Sphingomyelin, a component of myelin and other cell membranes, accumulates within cells throughout the central nervous system and other tissues. Sphingomyelin is normally catabolized by the action of sphingomyelinase but in Niemann-Pick disease this enzyme activity is only about 7 per cent of normal.

Clinical Features

This disease also consists of a group of disorders characterised by hepatosplenomegaly and accumulation of sphingomyelin (ceramide phosphorylcholine) in organs and tissues. Three clinical forms have been identified. In Type A (acute neuropathic), which is the commonest, there is hepatosplenomegaly by 6 months of age and there are severe feeding difficulties related to central nervous system involvement. It is inherited in an autosomal recessive fashion and is more common in infants of the Jewish race. The infant's abdomen becomes greatly protuberant due to massive hepatosplenomegaly. Skin pigmentation is common and severe wasting is invariable. Deterioration in cerebral functions appears early and progresses to a state of severe incapacity with generalised muscular weakness and wasting. Pulmonary involvement is commonly found. Anaemia of severe degree is an early sign but thrombocytopenia develops late, in contrast to its early appearance in Gaucher disease. In some affected infants ophthalmoscopy reveals a cherry-red spot at the macula resembling the retinal appearance in Tay-Sachs disease and corneal opacities may be found.

Definitive proof of diagnosis would depend on demonstration of increased sphingomyelin levels in tissue specimens (usually liver or spleen) and/or identification of a specific sphingomyelinese deficiency in white blood cells, fibroblasts or visceral specimens.

In Type B (chronic non-neuropathic) there is a slightly later onset and no evidence of central nervous system impairment. Pulmonary infiltration can predispose to recurrent respiratory infections. In Type C (chronic neuropathic) there is gradual onset, usually after the age of 18 months, of neurological impairment manifest as ataxia, loss of speech with dysarthria and convulsions. Most die before the age of 15 years.

Prenatal diagnosis on cultured amniocytes is only possible for Types A and B.

Treatment

Currently there is no specific therapy for type A or B Niemann-Pick disease.

TAY-SACHS DISEASE

Aetiology

An abnormal accumulation of Gm_2 ganglioside is confined to the brain resulting in progressive cortical failure and death by 2½ to 5 years of age. These are complex lipids and their catabolism involves a succession of enzymes of which hexosaminidase is lacking in Tay-Sachs disease. There are two hexosaminidases in the body, A and B. In classical Tay-Sachs disease (Type 1) only hexosaminidase A is lacking whereas in the non-Jewish form (Type II:

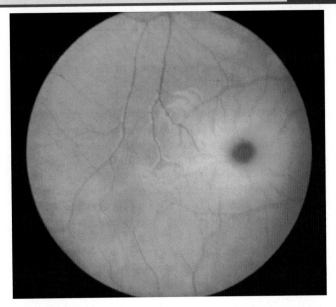

Fig. 20.5: "Cherry red spot" in the fundus of a Tay-Sachs infant

Sandhoff disease), which is clinically indistinguishable, both A and B are absent. There are also extremely rare adult and juvenile forms which have their onset after the age of 1 year and in which hexosaminidase A activity is from 10-12 per cent of normal. All types are inherited as autosomal recessive and consangunity is not uncommonly found.

Clinical Features

In this disease because the deposition of lipid is confined to the central nervous system the features are neurological in character hey appear between the ages of 4 and 6 months as delay in psychomotor development, irritability, hyperacusis for sudden noises, spasticity, generalised weakness and muscle wasting n outstanding feature is progressive loss of vision leading to complete blindness. The deep reflexes are exaggerated, at least to begin with, and the plantar responses are extensor. Ophthalmoscopy reveals primary optic atrophy and the diagnostic macular cherry-red spot on each side, surrounded by a greyish-white halo appearance (Fig. 20.5). Convulsions may occur. Ultimately there are dysphagia, dementia, blindness and a tendency to repeated respiratory infections due to accumulation of mucus. Diagnosis can be confirmed by enzyme estimations on leucocytes or in skin fibroblasts growing in tissue culture. Prenatal diagnosis is possible. Death usually occurs before the age of 3 years.

Treatment

None is available. Heterozygote screening in Ashkenazi Jewish populations, where a carrier rate of 1 in 27 is found, with appropriate genetic counselling can reduce the disease incidence.

GENERALISED GANGLIOSIDOSIS

Aetiology

The enzyme defect has been defined in this disease, which has previously been described by such names as the late infantile amaurotic family idiocy of Bielschowsky-Jansky, pseudo-Hurler and the juvenile form of Spielmeyer-Vogt. However, some cases of the last-mentioned have probably been cases of Batten's disease in which the cerebromacular degeneration is related to a lipid called ceroidlipofuscin, an unrelated disorder. There are, in fact, two biochemically distinct forms of the disease under consideration - juvenile Gm1 gangliosidosis (Type II) and generalised ganglio-sidosis (Type I). In the latter, three acid α-galactosidases (A, B and C) are absent, whereas in Type II only B and C are absent. The effect of the enzyme deficiency in Type 1 is the accumulation in the brain, viscera and bones of G_{M1} ganglioside. In Type II G_{M1} accumulates only in the neurones.

Clinical Features

In generalised G_{M1} gangliosidosis (Type I) neurological manifestations - hyperacusis, muscle weakness, inco-ordination, convulsions, loss of speech, mental retardation - develop during infancy and progress inexorably. Splenomegaly and hepatomegaly develop and in due time facial and skeletal changes resembling those of gargoylism become more obvious. Eye changes include macular degeneration, cherry-red spot, nystagmus and blindness. The full clinical picture is rarely present before the age of eighteen months can be based upon enzyme assays in leucocytes, and rectal biopsy will also reveal characteristic changes. Death occurs before the age of 5 years.

In the juvenile form (Type II) the viscera are not involved and the bones only to a slight degree. Slowly progressive neurological deterioration is the principal feature. Diagnosis is suggested by mucopolysaccharidosis - type dysmorphism (with normal urinary mucopolysaccha-rides), eye changes, multi-vacuolated foam cells in the bone marrow and vacuolization of lymphocytes in peripheral blood smear.

Treatment

None is available.

THE MUCOPOLYSACCHARIDOSES

This group of disorders, classified into 6 types, is characterised by the widespread intracellular deposition of complex substances called mucopolysaccharides (MPS) or sulphated glycosaminoglycans. They present primarily as disorders of the reticulo-endothelial system or as progressive disorders with visceral and skeletal manifestations. The mucopolysaccharides, which appear in the urine, show variations between the different clinical types and this is of help in differential diagnosis. All types of this disorder are inherited in an autosomal recessive fashion with the one exception of Hunter syndrome (MPS Type 2) in which transmission is as a sex-linked recessive. The aetiology appears to be a fault in the degradation of the mucopolysaccharides to their constituent sugars, this being related to a deficiency of one of several lysosomal enzymes, each of which normally breaks a specific bond in the mucopolysaccharide molecule. Specific enzyme deficiencies have now been identified. In Hurler syndrome (MPS Type 1-H) the missing enzyme activity is α-L-iduronidase and in Scheie syndrome (MPS Type I-S) the same enzyme is absent in spite of marked clinical differences, suggesting that Hurler and Scheie syndromes represent different mutations of the same gene with resulting but different alterations in the composition of the enzyme protein. In Hunter syndrome the missing enzyme is iduronate sulphatase he Sanfilippo syndrome, however, appears in biochemical terms to be four diseases: Sanfilippo A, due to deficiency of heparan sulphatase; Sanfilippo B, related to N-acetyl-α-glucosaminidase; Sanfilippo C, related to α-glucosaminide N-acetyl-transferase; and Sanfilippo D, related to N-acetyl-α-D-glucosaminide-6-sulphatase. There are two forms of Morquio disease, Types A and B which comprise MPS Type 4. Morquio A is related to galactosamine-6-sulphate sulphatase and Morquio B to β-galactosidase. In the Maroteaux-Lamy syndrome (MPS Type 6) the enzyme deficiency is of arylsulphatase B. A few cases of "atypical" Hurler syndrome has been described in which β-glucuronidase was the missing factor and this can be called MPS Type 7 or Sly syndrome. The number of disorders which may present with a Hurler-like phenotype and the complexities of establishing a specific diagnosis require a combined clinical and laboratory approach. Prenatal diagnosis following amniocentesis or chorionic villus biopsy is possible for all MPS.

MUCOPOLYSACCHARIDOSIS TYPE 1: HURLER'S SYNDROME

This type of mucopolysaccharidosis is associated with excessive amounts of dermatan sulphate and heparan sulphate in the urine in a ratio of about 2:1. There is deficiency of α-L-iduronidase. The superficial appearances in a typical case of "gargoylism" allow immediate diagnosis (Fig. 20.6). The head is large and scaphocephalic. The eyes are set wide apart and there are heavy supra-orbital ridges and eyebrows. The nose is broad with a flattened bridge and the lips are thick. The skin is dry and coarse. The corneae usually show a marked spotty type of opacity or cloudiness. The neck is short, there is a lumbodorsal kyphosis and the protuberant abdomen often

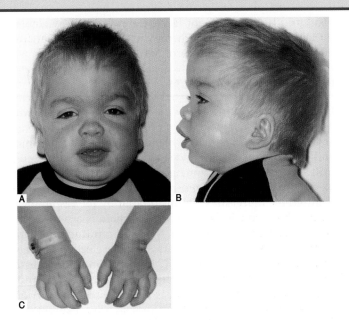

Figs 20. 6A to C: MPS 1 H: Hurler syndrome

has an umbilical hernia. The spleen and liver are considerably enlarged. The hands tend to be broader than they are long. There is characteristic limitation of extension (but not of flexion) in many joints, most marked in the fingers. The fourth and fifth fingers may be short and curved towards the thumb. Genu valgum and coxa valga are common. There are also very characteristic radiological changes in the bones. The skull shows an elongated sella turcica, widened suture lines and an unduly large fontanelle. The long bones and phalanges are broader and shorter than normal and they are often bizarre in shape. The ribs too are excessively thick. The pelvis is distorted with abnormal acetabula. The vertebral bodies have an abnormal shape with concave anterior and posterior margins and there is often a hook-like projection from the anterior border of the first or second lumber vertebra, which tends to be displaced backwards. Bone age is usually delayed. Affected children are severely mentally retarded. They show diminished physical activity. This is partly due to excessive breathlessness on exertion when the heart is involved. Cardiomegaly, precordial systolic and diastolic murmurs, and electrocardiographic evidence of left ventricular hypertrophy are commonly found. Death takes place before adult life from congestive cardiac failure or intercurrent respiratory infection.

While the child with this disorder somewhat resembles a cretin, there are very obvious clinical differences, e.g. corneal opacity, hepatosplenomegaly, limitation of extension of the interphalangeal joints, and characteristic radiological findings in the skeleton. The precise diagnosis should be based on demonstration of the specific enzyme deficiency in leucocytes or cultured fibroblasts.

MUCOPOLYSACCHARIDOSIS TYPE 2 (HUNTER'S SYNDROME)

This form of mucopolysaccharidosis is X-linked. It differs from Hurler syndrome in usually being less severe, but there is a severe form which results in death by the age of 15 years and a milder variety with survival to middle age. Clouding of the corneae does not occur but deafness is common. The urine contains large amounts of dermatan sulphate and heparan sulphate in approximately equal quantities. It reacts well with alcian blue to produce a metachromatic effect. The enzyme defect can be demonstrated in the lymphocytes. By 12 months of age radiographs show a mild but complete pattern of dysostosis multiplex.

MUCOPOLYSACCHARIDOSIS TYPE 3 (SANFILIPPO'S SYNDROME)

In this variety heparan sulphate is excreted in the urine almost exclusively. Mental deficiency is severe and there may be hyperactivity and destructive behaviour. Visceral and corneal involvement is relatively mild and the only skeletal signs may be biconvexity of the vertebral bodies and some degree of claw hand. There may also be a very thick calvarium. The enzyme deficiency can be demonstrated in cultured fibroblasts.

MUCOPOLYSACCHARIDOSIS TYPE 4 (MORQUIO'S SYNDROME)

This is probably the disease first described by Morquio in Montevideo in 1929. The urine contains large amounts of keratan sulphate, a mucopolysaccharide that is unrelated to dermatan or heparan sulphate. Mental deficiency is not a usual finding and the face and skull are only slightly affected. The neck is short, there is marked dorsal kyphosis and the sternum protrudes. The arms are relatively long for the degree of dwarfism and may extend to the knees. There is, however, no limitation of flexion of the fingers. Genu valgum with enlarged knee joints and flat feet are present. There is a waddling gait. Radiographs may reveal platybasia, fusion of cervical vertebrae and flattening of the vertebral bodies. The metaphyses of the long bones may be irregular and the epiphyses are misshapen and fragmented. Mild degrees of corneal opacity may appear at a late stage of the disorder.

MUCOPOLYSACCHARIDOSIS TYPE I-S (PREVIOUSLY TYPE 5): SCHEIE'S SYNDROME

The outstanding features are stiff joints, aortic regurgitation and clouding of the cornea (most dense peripherally). The facies shows the characteristics of gargoylism to a lesser extent than in Hurler's syndrome, intellect is but mildly impaired and survival to adulthood is common.

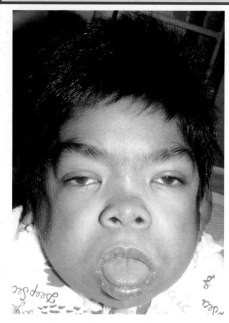

Fig. 20.7: MPS 6, Maroteaux- Lamy syndrome.

The urine shows the same distribution of mucopoly-saccharides as in Hurler's syndrome.

MUCOPOLYSACCHARIDOSIS TYPE 6 (MAROTEAUX-LAMY SYNDROME)

The principal features are severe corneal and skeletal changes as in Hurler's syndrome and valvular heart disease, but mental deficiency does not occur. Hepato-splenomegaly is usually of mild degree. The somatic features in the severe form of Maroteaux-Lamy syndrome are similar to that in Hurler syndrome (Fig. 20.7). The urine contains derma tan sulphate almost exclusively. Leucocytes or cultured fibroblasts can be tested for enzyme activity.

MUCOPOLYSACCHARIDOSIS TYPE 7 (SLY SYNDROME)

The principal features are unusual facies, protruding sternum, hepatomegaly, umbilical hernia, thoracolumbar gibbus, marked vertebral deformities, and moderate mental deficiency.

Treatment

In all types of MPS the parents must be given genetic counselling and prenatal diagnosis is also possible. Encouraging results in MPS are being obtained with bone-marrow transplantation when an appropriate well-matched donor is available. The majority of BMT in MPS have been with Hurler's syndrome, and less success has been reported in MPS 2 and MPS 3. Laronidase, an enzyme produced by recombinant DNA technology, is available for long-term replacement therapy in the treatment of non-neurological manifestations of MPS 1.

MITOCHONDRIAL DEFECTS

Energy, in the form of ATP, is generated by oxidative phosphorylation of breakdown products of metabolic fuels such as glucose, fatty acids, ketone bodies and organic and amino acids in the mitochondria. This breakdown of nutrient fuels (oxidation) generates reduced factors-NADH and reduced flavo-proteins. These must be re-oxidised for reutilisation in this process by the respiratory chain. The mitochondrial respiratory chain is a series of 5 complexes situated within the inner mitochondrial membrane. There are also two small mobile electron carriers ubiquinone and cytochrome C involved in the process. Energy substrates cross the double phospholipid mitochondrial membrane usually with a specific carrier (L-carnitine). The proton pumps of the respiratory chain components produce an electrochemical or proton gradient across the inner membrane and this charge is subsequently discharged by complex V (ATP synthesis) and the energy thus released is used to drive ATP synthesis.

Clinical Presentation

The first of the mitochondrial respiratory chain diseases were described in relation to disorders of muscle and this resulted in the term mitochondrial myopathies. It is now known that other tissues particularly the brain may be involved. Respiratory chain defects may produce isolated myopathy, eye movement disorder (ophthalmoplegia) with or without myopathy and occasionally with CNS dysfunction such as ataxia, multisystem disease, fatal lactic acidosis of infancy, and single organ dysfunction such as cardiomyopathy. The encephalopathies contain a number of recognisable syndromes such as the Kearns-Sayer syndrome characterised by progressive external ophthalmoplegia, pigmentary retinopathy and heart block, myoclonus epilepsy with ragged red fibres (MERRF) where in addition to myoclonic seizures there is weakness, ataxia, deafness and dementia. Myopathy, encephalo-pathy, lactic acidosis and stroke-like episodes (MELAS) is characterised by the recurrence of stroke-like episodes with onset usually before the age of 15 years. Cortical blindness and hemianopia usually accompany the stroke-like episodes which may be preceded by a migraine-like headache, nausea and vomiting. Dementia frequently ensues. Another syndrome known as NARP is comprised of neurogenic weakness, ataxia and retinitis pigmentosa. Unlike the other syndromes described there are no morphological changes in skeletal muscle and the mtDNA defect affects ATP synthesis.

Leigh syndrome of subacute necrotising encephalomyopathy presents with vomiting, failure to thrive, developmental delay, muscular hypotonia and respiratory problems. There may also be ophthalmoplegia, optic atrophy, nystagmus and dystonia. The disorder usually presents at around the age of 6 months but may be present from birth or may not appear until late teenage. In Leigh encephalopathy like many of the mitochondrial syndromes it is difficult to pinpoint a single biochemical abnormality. There are defects of the respiratory chain, pyruvate dehydrogenase complex and biotinidase variably present with this syndrome. Lactate and pyruvate concentrations are frequently elevated in blood and CSF and MRI scans show characteristic low density areas within the basal ganglia or less commonly the cerebellum here is occasionally an autosomal recessive pattern of inheritance in Leigh syndrome, which suggests that it may be caused by a nuclear gene rather than a mitochondrial defect. However, in some patients mutations have been found in mtDNA. There are some patients who do not fit into these clinical patterns of disease and many have been shown to have multiple defects of respiratory chain complexes due to mtDNA disorder.

Lebber hereditary optic neuropathy (LHON) is one of the commonest inherited causes of blindness in young men due to a disorder of mtDNA. Some men with the disorder have an encephalopathy with deafness and dystonia and a few develop cardiac conduction defects. There is some evidence that a gene on the X chromosome may be linked with this disorder.

There are a variety of syndromes with non-neuromuscular presentation, which involve the gastrointestinal tract with anorexia and vomiting and occasionally hepatic failure, yet others have cardiomyopathy with different degrees of heart block, renal disease with generalised aminoaciduria and haematological disorders affecting bone marrow function. In Pearson syndrome, which presents at birth or early infancy there is refractory sideroblastic anaemia, thrombocytopenia, neutropenia, metabolic acidosis, pancreatic insufficiency and hepatic dysfunction. Renal tubular disorder, diarrhoea, steatorrhoea and skin lesions with eventual liver failure have been described. Deletions of mtDNA have been identified.

Many of the respiratory chain disorders may present in the very young but there are three specific syndromes affecting the infant. The first is fatal infantile lactic acidosis. Infants present with hypotonia, vomiting and ventilatory failure and die often before the age of 6 months. A generalised aminoaciduria (de Toni Fanconi Debré syndrome), grossly increased plasma lactate concentrations, hypoglycaemia, liver dysfunction, convulsions and increased plasma calcium have been reported. The second clinical presentation is benign infantile lactic acidosis, which may present with failure to thrive, respiratory failure and hypotonia with increased plasma lactate concentrations but the condition gradually remits and by twelve to eighteen months these infants are often normal. There is a cytochrome oxidase defect, which appears to improve with age and may be related to a switch from a fetal to an adult form of complex IV. The third syndrome is the mtDNA depletion syndrome in which the infant is weak, hypotonic and has respiratory difficulties together with renal tubular disorder and convulsions. The condition is usually fatal before the age of one year.

Treatment

Children with respiratory chain defects have been treated with vitamin C (4 g per day), vitamin K (Menadione 50 mg per day) and ubiquinone (100 mg per day) in the hope that these vitamins may act as artificial electron acceptors. Some improvement in electron transfer has been suggested by NMR studies in these patients but there is some doubt as to the overall clinical benefit. Other treatments have included thiamine, biotin, L-carnitine, riboflavin and dichloracetate. As the mitochondrial respiratory chain generates free radicals, scavengers such as vitamin E might be of some clinical benefit. Unfortunately most of these conditions are progressive and result in significant disability and/or death. Considerable support of the families involved is required during the care of these infants and genetic counselling with prenatal diagnosis is available for some of these conditions.

PEROXISOMAL DISORDERS

Peroxisomes are present in every body cell except the mature erythrocyte and are particularly abundant in tissues active in lipid metabolism. They do not contain DNA and are therefore under the control of nuclear genes. A number of clinical and biochemical disorders have now been ascribed to disorders of peroxisomal metabolic functions. These functions may be catabolic and include β–oxidation of fatty acids, oxidation of ethanol and hydrogen peroxide based cellular respiration and the breakdown of purine. The anabolic functions of the peroxisomes include plasmalogen, cholesterol, and bioacid synthesis.

Table 20.1 gives a tentative classification of the peroxisomal disorders. In the Group 1 disorders there is a reduction or absence of functional peroxisomes. Zellweger syndrome is a lethal disease presenting with severe hypotonia, typical craniofacial abnormality with a high domed forehead, severe developmental delay with neurosensory defects and progressive oculo-motor dysfunction. These neurological abnormalites may be related to the neuronal migration disorders found in the brain at postmortem. There is also progressive liver dysfunction with chondrodysplasia calcificans of the

Table 20.1: Classification of peroxisomal disorders

1. **Peroxisome deficiency disorders**
   Zellweger (cerebrohepatorenal) syndrome
   Neonatal adrenoleukodystrophy
   Infantile Refsum disease
   Hyperpipecolic acidaemia
2. **Disorders with loss of multiple peroxisomal functions**
   and peroxisome structure in fibroblasts
   Rhizomelic chondrodysplasia punctata
   "Zellweger-like" syndrome
3. **Disorders with an impairment of only one peroxisomal**
   function and normal peroxisomal structure
   A. **Disorders of peroxisomal β-oxidation**
      Adrenoleukodystrophy (X-linked) and variants
      Acyl-CoA oxidase deficiency
      Bi (multi) functional protein deficiency
      Peroxisomal thiolase deficiency
   B. **Other disorders**
      Acyl-CoA: dihydroxyacetone phosphate acyltransferase
      (DHAP-AT) deficiency
      Primary hyperoxaluria Type I
      Acatalasaemia
      Glutaryl oxidase deficiency

patellae and the acetabulum. In neonatal adreno-leukodystrophy there is progressive demyelination of the cerebral hemispheres, cerebellum and brainstem with neuronal migration disturbances and perivascular lymphocytic infiltration. There is also adrenal atrophy. In infantile Refsum disease (IRD) there is developmental delay, retinitis pigmentosa, failure to thrive and hypocholesterolaemia. In the Group II disorders, Rhizomelic chondrodysplasia punctata (RCDP) is an autosomal recessive disorder characterised by short stature, a typical facial appearance, joint contractures and X-ray changes showing stippling of the epiphyses in infancy and severe symmetrical epiphyseal and extra epiphyseal calcifications in later life. Only two patients have been described as having the Zellweger-like syndrome, which is clinically indistinguishable from the classical Zellweger but shows abundant peroxisomes in the liver. In the third group of disorders with impairment of a single peroxisome function and with a normal peroxisome structure adreno-leukodystrophy, an X-linked recessively inherited disorder, usually affects males between the ages of 4 and 10 years.

Initially there may be attention deficit noticed in school followed by convulsions, visual disturbance with the later manifestations of paralysis and death. This phenotype known as childhood adrenokeukodystrophy (ALD) has been treated with long chain polyunsaturated fatty acids but there is some doubt as to the overall benefit of this form of therapy. About 25% of ALD cases present in adulthood with paraparesis whilst a few may exhibit adrenocortical insufficiency without neurological involvement. Twenty

per cent of female heterozygotes develop mild or moderate progressive paraparesis after the age of 40 years.

Pseudoneonatal ALD presents with early convulsions, muscular hypotonia, hearing loss and visual impairment due to retinopathy. **Bi-functional protein deficiency disorder** has occurred in only one patient with hypotonia and macrocephaly at birth and a single patient with **pseudo- Zellweger syndrome** had marked facial dysmorphia, muscle weakness and hypotonia at birth. The liver contained abundant microsomes but the enzyme defect was subsequently identified. The other disorders are also rare apart from primary hyperoxaluria Type I in which autosomal recessive disorder of glyoxylate metabolism there is recurrent calcium oxalate nephrolithiasis and nephrocalcinosis presenting during the first decade. There are a few, however, who present with an acute neonatal form of the disorder and early death.

Treatment

Apart from the attempt to treat X-linked ALD with fat restriction and supplementation with glycerol trioleate and glycerol trierucate, which has been shown to improve peripheral nerve function, but not as yet to effect long-term benefit there are recent reports that bone marrow transplantation may be effective in mildly affected childhood ALD patients. In more advanced X-linked ALD bone marrow transplantation worsened the clinical picture. It is hoped that gene therapy might improve the outlook for this condition. Treatment with pyridoxine may be affective in a small number of patients with primary hyperoxaluria Type I. Haemodialysis may be required during end stage renal failure in this disease and surgical removal of oxalate stones may be required. Eventually combined liver and kidney transplant becomes necessary for survival.

INHERITED DISORDERS OF INTERMEDIARY METABOLISM

Every newborn infant with unexplained neurological deterioration, ketosis, metabolic acidosis or hypoglycaemia should be suspected of having an inherited metabolic error of intermediary metabolism (Table 20.2) A high index of suspicion and rapid diagnosis can prevent death and severe neurological damage in a significant number of affected infants and will ensure adequate prenatal diagnosis in subsequent pregnancies. The newborn has a limited repertoire of responses to severe illness whether caused by overwhelming infections or metabolic defects. Most inborn errors of intermediary metabolism fall into two categories namely "intoxications" and "energy deficiencies". **Intoxications** are secondary to an accumulation of toxic compounds such as branched chain keto acids in maple syrup urine disease, most organic acidurias,

Table 20.2: Hypoglycaemia
Energy deficiencies (usually with ketonaemia)
Ketotic hypoglycaemia
Tyrosinaemia
Maple syrup urine disease
Glycogen storage diseases
Galactosaemia
Frustosaemia
Reye syndrome
Poisoning - alcohol and aspirin
Jamaican vomiting sickness
Hyperinsulinism (no ketones)
Insulinoma or nesidioblastosis
Leucine sensitivity
Poisoning - insulin

Table 20.3: Initial investigations to help categorise metabolic disorders	
Urine	Smell
	Acetone
	Reducing substances
	Keto acids (dinitrophenylhydrazine test)
	Sulphites (Sulfitest, Merck)
	pH
Blood	Blood cell count
	Electrolytes (look for anion gap)
	Calcium
	Glucose
	Blood gases (pH PCO_2, HCO_3, PO_2)
	Ammonia
	Lactic acid and pyruvic acid
	3-hydroxy butyrate, acetoacetate
	Uric acid
Store at - 20° C	Urine (as much as possible)
	Heparinized plasma, (2-5 ml)
	Do no freeze whole blood!
	CSF, 0.5 - 1.0 ml
Miscellaneous	EEG, bacteriological samples, chest X-ray, lumbar puncture, cardiac echography, cerebral ultrasound.

urea cycle defects, galactosaemia, fructosaemia and tyrosinaemia. The clinical features (vomiting, lethargy, coma, liver failure, acidosis, ketosis, hyperammonaemia) are common to most of these conditions. Treatment has to be aimed initially at removal of the toxic metabolites by peritoneal or haemodialysis, exchange transfusion and special diets, etc. **Energy deficiencies** are due in part at least to a deficiency of energy production or defect in utilization. Defects of gluconeogenesis, congenital lactic academies (pyruvate carboxylase and dehydrogenase deficiencies), fatty acid oxidation defects, disorders of mitochondrial respiratory chain and disorder of peroxisomal metabolism belong to this group. Clinical features common to this group include severe hypotonia, cardiomyopathy, failure to thrive, circulatory collapse, sudden infant death and hyperlacticacidaemia. There may also be congenital malformations such as absent corpus callosum and cerebral malformations with congenital lactic acidaemia and facial and bone anomalies with peroxisomal defects. There can be overlapping of the clinical features between the toxic and energy deficient disorders where there is accumulation of toxic compounds in addition to a deficiency of energy production. A third category of clinical presentation is **hypoglycaemia with liver dysfunction.** Convulsions and hepatomegaly with ketosis and lactic acidosis are the usual presenting features. The main diseases in that group are the glycogen storage diseases.

Table 20.3 gives a list of initial investigations, which can help categorise the metabolic disorder. More specialised investigations such as amino and organic acid analyses can then be arranged.

If the child dies it is important to have obtained urine, plasma, white blood cell DNA, fibroblast culture, and muscle and liver biopsies stored deep-frozen. Subsequent analyses may help determine the nature of the metabolic defect and allow a diagnostic and proper genetic counselling to be given to the family.

Conclusion

Although individual inherited metabolic diseases are rare and this book contains only a limited review of some of the disorders, collectively they form a major grouping of disorders causing significant mortality and an overwhelming burden of morbidity for families and the community.

Endocrine Disorders

Louis Low

HYPOPITUITARISM

Embryologically the pituitary gland is formed from the Rathke pouch, a diverticulum of the stomodeal ectoderm and the neuroectoderm of the floor of the forebrain. A number of signalling molecules and transcription factors are involved in pituitary organogenesis and the differentiation of the different cell lineages: somatotropes (growth hormone), lactotropes (prolactin), corticotropes (adrenocorticotrophic hormone), thyrotropes (thyroid stimulating hormone) and gonadotropes (luteinizing hormone, follicular stimulating hormone). Multiple pituitary hormone deficiencies can result from malformations of the hypothalamus and pituitary gland or mutations of these transcription factors. Secretion of hormones from different lineages of pituitary cells is dependent on hypothalamic releasing factors (gonadotrophin releasing hormone, thyrotrophin releasing hormone, corticotrophin releasing hormone, growth hormone releasing hormone) or suppressive hormone like somatostatin. Two hormones are secreted by the posterior pituitary gland, vasopressin and oxytocin. Vasopressin is important for the reabsorption of water by the distal renal tubules and collecting ducts. Vasopressin release is stimulated by rising plasma osmolality, fall in blood volume or blood pressure or by stress. Oxytocin release is stimulated by suckling and its role is limited to the puerperial period. Causes of hypopituitarism are shown in Table 21.1. Extent of the anterior and posterior pituitary dysfunction depends on the extent of the damage.

Clinical Features

The usual presenting features include symptoms and signs relating to the hormonal deficiencies or the underlying cause of hypopituitarism. Intracranial tumours in the suprasellar region can lead to visual field defects, neurological symptoms and symptoms and signs of raised intracranial pressure like headache and vomiting, papilloedema. Polyuria, polydipsia and dehydration may

or may not be present depending on whether there is posterior pituitary involvement. Short stature and infantile body proportions are common due to growth hormone and thyroid hormone deficiencies. Adrenal insufficiency can lead to lethargy, hypoglycaemia nausea, vomiting or even shock when the patient is under stress. In infants with hypopituitarism, the presenting features include recurrent hypoglycaemic attacks, micropenis in males (stretched penile length <2.5cm), persistent neonatal jaundice resembling the neonatal hepatitis syndrome. Microphthalmia, pendular nystagmus, optic nerve hypoplasia and signs of hypopituitarism suggest septo-optic dysplasia. Early onset of symptoms indicates a congenital or genetic cause of hypopituitarism. A proper history can usually shed light on the etiology of postnatal damage to the hypothalamus and pituitary gland.

Investigations

Assessment begins with the documentation of anthropometric data using standard techniques and the state of

Table 21.1: Causes of hypopituitarism
1 Cerebral Malformations-Holoprosencephaly, mid-line facial defects, septo-optic dysplasia, congenital hypopituitarism (transection of pituitary stalk, adenohypophysis hyperplasia, ectopic position of posterior pituitary signal on MRI scan)
2 Mutations of pituitary transcription factors genes (multiple pituitary hormone deficiency) or of pituitary hormone or pituitary hormone releasing hormone genes (isolated pituitary hormone deficiency)
3 Postnatal damage of hypothalamus or pituitary gland— traumatic or breech delivery head injury suprasellar or pituitary tumours e.g. craniopharyngioma, germ cell tumour, astrocytoma, glioma, prolactinoma-infiltrative lesions e.g. Langerhan cell histiocytosis, sarcoidosis, lymphocytic hypophysitis-pituitary apoplexy-infection, e.g. meningitis, encephalitis-autoimmune-cranial irradiation-pituitary haemosiderosis, e.g. transfusion dependent thalassaemia major

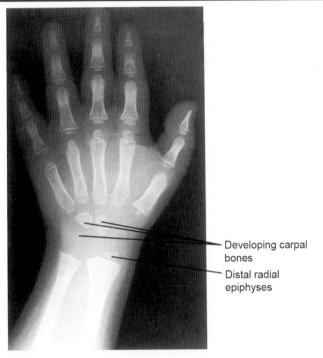

Fig. 21.1: Bone age. X-ray of the left hand and wrist of a boy aged 4 years and 3 months. The bone age using the TW II 20 bone score (Tanner and Whitehouse) is 3.8 years which is just below the 50th percentile for his age

— Developing carpal bones

— Distal radial epiphyses

the development of the genitalia and pubertal staging. An X-ray for bone age as assessed by the Greulich and Pyle and Tanner-Whitehouse Atlas will usually show retardation of skeletal maturity (Fig. 21.1) relative to the chronological age. Baseline fasting morning cortisol, thyroid hormone, thyroid stimulating hormone, prolactin, gonadotrophins and sex steroids (in pubertal age group) should be taken and one should proceed to combined pituitary hormone assessment (tests for stimulating GH and cortisol secretion together with TRH and LHRH test) if there is a strong clinical suspicion of hypopituitarism. In a patient suspected of suffering from diabetes insipidus, an accurate documentation of the daily fluid intake and urine output is required. If the patient is admitted in dehydration with serum sodium of greater than 150 mmol/L and a plasma osmolality greater than 300 mosmol/kg, a simultaneous urine osmolality less than 750 mosmol/kg is suggestive of diabetes insipidus. A water deprivation test is required for diagnosis in a patient who can compensate for the defect in urine concentration by excessive water drinking. Imaging of the hypothalamus and pituitary preferably with magnetic resonance imaging (MRI) is required after establishing a hormonal diagnosis of hypopituitarism.

Treatment

Hormonal replacement for adrenal, thyroid, gonadotrophin and growth hormone deficiency will be discussed

Table 21.2: Causes of short stature

- Genetic Short stature
- Constitutional delay in growth and puberty
- Undernutrition
- Chronic illness of all major systems, e.g. chronic renal failure, inflammatory bowel disease, congenital heart disease, inherited metabolic diseases, thalassaemia major
- Psychosocial deprivation
- Syndromal and chromosomal disorders, e.g. Turner syndrome, Noonan syndrome, Silver-Russell syndrome, Prader-Willi syndrome, William syndrome, Down syndrome
- Skeletal dysplasia, e.g. hypochondroplasia, achondroplasia, spondyloepiphyseal dysplasia
- Endocrine: hypothyroidism, multiple pituitary hormone deficiency, isolated growth hormone deficiency, genetic causes of GH deficiency and growth hormone insensitivity, pseudo-hypoparathyroidism, Cushing syndrome, Rickets
- Consequences of intrauterine growth retardation without postnatal catch-up growth

in the subsequent relevant sections of this chapter. Patients with diabetes insipidus should receive oral desmopressin (50 μg to 1000 μg/day) for control of the polyuria. Desmopression can be given by the nasal route but this preparation is being phased out.

SHORT STATURE

The factors governing human growth have already been described in the chapter on human growth and development (Chapter 2). Short stature is common but short stature due to an endocrine cause is less common. Children with a height below the 0.4th percentile (below 2.67SD) with correction for the mean parental height or growing with a subnormal growth velocity should be referred for specialist care. A genetic cause of growth hormone deficiency can be suspected if there is early onset of growth failure, a positive family history or consanguinity, extreme short stature and an extremely low GH response to GHRH, low serum IGF-1 and IGFBP-3 levels (see below). The causes of growth failure are shown in Table 21.2.

Assessment of Short Stature

The height, span, upper to lower segment ratio and previous growth record are important auxiological data. Disproportionate short stature is indicative of skeletal dysplasia. Initial investigations should include full blood count, renal and liver function tests, acid-base status, thyroid hormone, thyroid stimulating hormonal and X-ray for bone age. If the serum IGF-1 and IGFBP-3 are lower than -1SD for age in a child with significant short stature and subnormal growth velocity, then the GH/IGF-1 axis should be investigated. Growth hormone deficiency is diagnosed by an inadequate GH response of less than 20 mIU/L measured by a polyclonal radioimmunoassay or an equivalent lower value using a two-site GH assay, to two pharmacological stimuli like clonidine, L-dopa, arginine, glucagon, GHRH or insulin induced hypoglycaemia. The latter test is not favoured by some paediatric endocrinologists and should not be used in children under 5 years and of age. Assessment of the hypothalamic-pituitary adrenal axis and the gonadotrophins and TSH responses to their respective hypothalamic releasing hormone should be performed when pituitary dysfunction is suspected (glucagon and LHRH and TRH test). It is important that hypothyroidism be diagnosed and adequately treated before any investigation of the GH/IGF-1 axis. Adrenal insufficiency is diagnosed when the plasma cortisol fails to reach 500 nmol/L in response to glucagon or insulin induced hypoglycaemia. Neuro-imaging with MRI is indicated in patients diagnosed with GH deficiency or multiple pituitary hormone deficiency. Children with constitutional delay in growth and puberty (CDGP) have slow physical and pubertal maturation and a delay in bone age. The diagnosis can only be made after the other causes of short stature have been excluded.

Treatment

In children with CDGP, the final adult height although normal, is usually short of the predicted target height based on parental stature. Management includes an explanation to the parents of the natural growth pattern and the reasonable height prognosis of such children. Short courses of oxandrolone or testosterone can be used if short stature or lack of sexual development is causing significant psychosocial difficulties, but growth hormone treatment is not indicated.

Growth hormone has been approved for treatment of growth hormonal deficiency, short stature associated with chronic renal failure, Turner syndrome, Prader-Willi syndrome, small for gestational age (SGA) children who have not caught up in growth by 3-4 years of age and idiopathic short stature. The recommended growth hormone dosage is 0.7 IU/kg/week (GHD) to 1.2-1.4 IU/kg/week in divided doses daily in short SGA children. The improvement in adult height is most significant in patient with GH deficiency and early diagnosis and prompt treatment will improve the final height. A dose of GH in the range of 1 unit/kg/week in divided doses is used for the treatment of Turner syndrome, chronic renal failure and idiopathic short stature. The GH dosage can be individualized and adjusted to keep the serum IGF-1 level in the age-specific upper normal range. An improvement in the height velocity of at least 2 cm per year above the pre-treatment growth velocity is needed to justify continuation of treatment. The growth, skeletal maturation, pubertal assessment and possible side effects must be regularly monitored during GH treatment. Growth hormone treatment in childhood is relatively safe. There

was a concern that GH therapy in GH deficiency increased the risk of leukaemia and tumour recurrence but this fear has not been substantiated in recently well-conducted epidemiological studies. There is a risk of worsening of scoliosis or the development of slipped capital femoral epiphysis in the rapidly growing child treated with GH. GH therapy could be associated with insulin resistance and there is one recent report to suggest an increased risk of development of diabetes mellitus in children treated with GH. Pseudotumour cerebri can rarely occur during the early phase of GH treatment and this risk can be minimized by starting GH at a lower dose and then increase to the recommended dose gradually.

In patients with multiple pituitary hormone deficiency, growth hormone treatment may unmask hypothyroidism. It is necessary to monitor the thyroid function during GH treatment and to start thyroxine replacement if low free thyroxine level is detected. As glucocorticoid steroid in higher doses may inhibit growth, a safe low replacement dose of oral hydrocortisone of 8-10mg/m^2/day in two divided doses should be used in children with adrenal insufficiency in addition to GH deficiency. Gonadotropin deficiency can be suspected if there is micropenis since infancy in a male patient or failure to develop secondary sexual characteristics by 13 years in girls or 14 years in boys. Patients with hypogonadism can also present with arrest or delay in progress of sexual development. Puberty can be induced in boys with monthly intramuscular injections of testosterone enanthate. In females, puberty can be induced with conjugated oestrogen (premarin) or synthetic oestrogen (ethinyl estradiol) in gradual increasing dosages and cyclical oestrogen/progestagen replacement be instituted after one or two years.

TALL STATURE

The referral of children with tall stature to the endocrine service is not common and the patients are usually very tall girls who are worried about their heights. The causes of tall stature are shown in Table 21.3.

Beckwith-Wiedemann syndrome is characterized by prenatal and postnatal overgrowth, visceromegaly, omphalocoele, hemihypertrophy and neonatal hypoglycaemia. This condition is due to epigenetic errors of the imprinted gene cluster on chromosome 11p15 or mutations of cyclin-dependent kinase inhibitor gene (CDKN1C) on

Table 21. 3 Causes of Tall Stature
• Prenatal overgrowth-Beckwith Wiedemann syndrome, Sotos syndrome, Weaver syndrome
• Postnatal overgrowth-Familial tall stature, Marfan syndrome, Homocystinuria, Klinefelter syndrome
• Secondary Causes-Obesity, Precocious puberty, Growth hormone secreting tumour, Hyperthyroidism

chromosome 11p15. Patients with Sotos syndrome have macrodolichocephaly with prominent forehead and jaw and a characteristic growth pattern of rapid growth in early life followed by slowing of the growth velocity to normal by mid-childhood. Sotos syndrome is due to microdeletion of paternal chromosome 5 in the region of the nuclear receptor binding SET-domain containing gene 1 (NSD1) or intragenic mutation of NSD1. Epigenetic mutations in the imprinted gene cluster on chromosome 11p15 have been found in patients with the Sotos phenotype without NSD1 mutations. This suggests that an overlap of the molecular basis of overgrowth syndrome exists.

Skeletal features of Marfan syndrome include pectus excavatum or carinatum, scoliosis, reduced upper to lower segment ratio and a span to height ratio greater than 1.05. Other features include ectopia lentis, dilatation of the ascending aorta or pulmonary artery, mitral valve prolapse, spontaneous pneumothorax and lumbosacral dural ectasia. A positive family history (autosomal dominant inheritance) is helpful in the diagnosis. Marfan syndrome is due to mutation in the fibrillin gene (FBN1) on chromosome 15q21.1 or rarely mutation in TGF-beta receptor 2 (TGFB2) on chromosome 3p22.

Assessment of children with tall stature include identification of syndromal disorders. The pubertal status, parental stature, thyroid status and body mass index should be noted. Growth hormone excess usually resulting from a growth hormone secreting pituitary tumour, leads to growth acceleration, coarse facial features, prognathism and enlarging hands and feet. Glucose intolerance or hypertension may occur. A large pituitary tumour can cause visual field defects and headache. Growth hormone excess is occasionally associated with the McCune Albright syndrome. Further investigations include measurement of thyroid hormone, testosterone, oestradiol, LH, FSH, prolactin, IGF-1, 17α-hydroxy-progesterone. The failure of suppression of the serum growth hormone level to below 10 mIU/L during an oral glucose tolerance test (1.75G/kg to a maximum of 75G) remains the gold standard for the diagnosis of growth hormone hypersecretion. Karyotyping, X-ray for skeletal maturation and MRI scan of the brain and pituitary should be performed where indicated.

Girls may seek treatment and those with a predicted final adult height greater than +3SD could be considered for hormonal therapy (100 to 300 μg ethinyloestradiol or 7.5 mg Premarin combined with medroxyprogesterone acetate 5 to 10 mg from day 15-25 of each calendar month). Testosterone enanthate 250 to 1000 mg intramuscularly every month can be used to accelerate skeletal mutation and reduce final height in tall boys. However the use of sex hormone therapy for limiting adult height should be reserved for selected patients because knowledge in potential long-term effects and fertility is still scanty. Calf cramps and weight gain are the common side effects of high dose oestrogen in girls. In boys, acne, aggressive behaviour and hypertrichosis are the common complaints. For the other secondary causes of tall stature, treatment should be directed at the underlying condition. A pituitary growth hormone secreting tumour is managed by trans-sphenoidal surgery.

OBESITY

A 1997 World Health Organization press release declared that "Obesity's impact is so diverse and extreme that it should now be regarded as one of the greatest neglected health problems of our time with an impact on health which may well prove to be as great as that of smoking". The prevalence of obesity is on the rise in both developed and developing countries. There is currently no consistent evidence that the current epidemic of obesity is due to increased fat or caloric intake. There is an enormous range of energy intakes by children of the same age and there is little correlation between intake for age and weight for height for age. Technological advances have caused a marked reduction in the average daily energy expenditure and appears to be the key determinant of the current obesity epidemic. Television viewing and use of the computer for leisure have now been viewed as surrogate measures of physical inactivity. As much as 28% and 46% of all children and non-Hispanic black children in the United States NHANES III survey reported watching television greater than 4 hours per day. The best estimate of genetic contribution to obesity is about 25% whereas cultural transmission of life-style accounting for obesity is estimated to be about 30%. As of October 2004, 173 cases of obesity due to mutations in ten different genes have been reported and the molecular basis of at least 25 obesity syndromes is now known. There are 204 quantitative trait loci (QTLs) for obesity-related phenotypes from 50 genome-wide scans and of these 38 genomic regions harbour QTLs replicated among two to four studies. The complications of childhood obesity are show in Table 21.4.

The increase in the prevalence of obesity has been associated with a similar increase in the prevalence of type 2 diabetes in many countries. It is recommended that screening for type 2 diabetes mellitus be performed every two years in obese children and adolescents who have acanthosis nigricans and a family history of type 2 diabetes.

Obese infants and children under the age of 3 years without obese parents are at low risk of becoming obese as an adult whereas obese adolescents are at increased risk of developing adult obesity. The doctor should be able to identify obesity related syndromes and to monitor for and treat any obesity related complications developing in these obese children. Investigations to exclude a pathological cause should be undertaken if there is severe early onset of obesity or when obesity is associated with short stature or

Table 21.4: Complications of childhood obesity
1. Insulin resistance and type 2 diabetes mellitus
2. Hyperlipidaemia
3. Hypertension
4. Steatohepatitis
5. Respiratory inadequacy including obstructive sleep apnoea syndrome
6. Musculoskeletal problems including slipped capital femoral epiphysis, genu valgum
7. Tall stature and early puberty
8. Gynaecomastia or adipomastia
9. Oligomenorrhoea and hyperandrogenism
10. Psychological sequence like poor self image, disordered eating and non-specific behaviour disturbances

features suggestive of a syndromal disorder, e.g., Prader-Willi syndrome, pseudohypoparathyroidism, glucocorticoid excess, hypothalamic syndrome and Bardet-Biedl syndrome.

A preventive programme needs to have commitment from all stake-holders and be directed at the whole population. The preventive messages must be free from harm to those in the community who are not obese. Prevention should be directed towards developing a healthier lifestyle in the family and the community like increased physical activity, decreased dependence television and computer games for entertainment, and healthy eating. As children spend a significant part of the day at school, much can be done by schools to combat this epidemic by health education, providing healthy snacks, drinks and meals at school, and encouraging increased physical activity and fitness.

Once a child has developed significant obesity, measures to encourage weight loss and weight maintenance have proved disappointing in achieving these aims. Education on the nature and complications of obesity, healthy eating and life-style and psychological support on a regular basis by a team of professionals consisting of paediatricians, dietitian, exercise physiologist and psychologist have frequently been suggested but the cost effectiveness and sustainability of such programmes have been called into question. Pharmacotherapy should be restricted to treat the most severe cases of obesity associated with complications. Sibutramine, acarbose and orlistat are drugs that can be considered. Bariatric surgery employing roux-en-y gastric bypass or adjustable gastric banding has been increasingly used to treat patients with morbid obesity and severe medical complications.

THE THYROID GLAND

Disorders of the thyroid gland are, with the exception of diabetes mellitus, the most common endocrine problems of childhood. The advent of immunoassay techniques has

Table 21.5: A classification of hypothyroidism in childhood
Dysgenesis of the thyroid gland (may present as congenital hypothyroidism or juvenile myxoedema in childhood in milder cases)
Congenital atheyreosis
Maldescent
Maldevelopment
Deficiency of iodine (endemic cretinism)
Genetic basis of congenital hypothyroidism
Mutations in transcription factors resulting in thyroid dysgenesis (FOXE1, PAX8, NKX2.1)
Dyshormonogenesis
Hyporesponsiveness to TSH (TSHR or GNAS1 mutations)
Iodide transport defects (mutations in natrium-iodide symporter SLC5A5)
Thyroglobulin synthesis defects (defective TG gene)
Iodide organification defects (mutation in thyroperoxidase gene TPO or genes of oxidase proteins THOX1 and THOX2)
Pendred syndrome (SLC26A4 gene defect)
Dehalogenase defects
Thyroid hormone resistance (thyroid hormone receptor gene TRb mutation)
Ingestion of goitrogens (accidental or therapeutic)
Antenatal (iodine, thionamdies in pregnancy)
Postnatal
Primary thyroid disease, e.g. autoimmune thyroiditis, carcinoma, etc.
Pituitary hypothyroidism
Malformation of the brain e.g. holoprosencephaly
Mutations of pituitary transcription factors
Secondary to disruption of the hypothalamus-pituitary-thyroid axis, e.g. tumour, infection, irradiation, haemosiderosis

been followed by a vast increase in our knowledge of the physiology and disturbances of thyroid function and molecular mechanism of disease.

Hypothyroidism

A classification of the causes of hypothyroidism is shown in Table 21.5. It is designed upon an aetiological basis which will permit the clinician to systematically approach diagnosis and treatment. Of the various causes of hypothyroidism in childhood only endemic iodine deficiency, congenital hypothyroidism and autoimmune thyroiditis will be described in this chapter.

Endemic Iodine Deficiency

Iodine deficiency is now recognized as the commonest preventable cause of mental retardation in the world today. If the foetus and developing children in a community are not provided with sufficient quantities of iodine, the entire population will have decreased IQ, impaired motor function and hearing defect. The WHO estimates that there are still over 100 countries in our world with a significant problem with iodine deficiency. In areas of the world where iodine deficiency is found, up to 8% of the population may have deficient thyroid hormone production, TSH hypersecretion and increased iodine trapping with goitre and raised plasma $T_3 : T_4$ ratio. Neonatal serum TSH is included by WHO, UNICEF and ICCIDD in 1994 as one of the indicators for iodine deficiency disorders. If 3% to 19.9% of the neonatal TSH values exceed 10 mIU/L, mild iodine deficiency exists in that community. The prevalence of goitre in the childhood community is also an indicator of iodine nutrition status. Iodination of salt supplies can effectively reduce the prevalence of this condition.

Congenital Hypothyroidism

Apart from the rare genetic causes of thyroid dysgenesis, the causes of thyroid dysgenesis in which thyroid tissue may be absent (aplastic), deficient (hypoplastic) or abnormally sited (ectopic) are unknown but affect about 1 in 3600 of all newborns and more commonly affect female infants. Dyshormonogenesis (inborn errors of thyroid hormone biosynthesis) accounts for about 10% of all cases of congenital hypothyroidism, i.e., 1 in 40,000. These autosomal recessively inherited disorders may present with goitre.

Clinical Features

The diagnosis of severe congenital hypothyroidism should not be difficult. Indeed, the manifestations are present within a few days of birth. The presenting symptoms which are usually mild consist of feeding difficulties, skin mot-

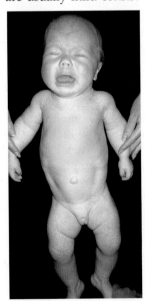

Fig. 21.2: Sporadic cretin aged 4 months. Note coarse features, large myxoedematous tongue and umbilical hernia

tling, noisy respiration and constipation. The undue prolongation of "physiological jaundice" should always arouse the suspicion of hypothyroidism. The appearance of the infants is typical if they remain undiagnosed after 3 to 4 months of age. The facial features are coarse with often a wrinkled forehead and low hairline. The hair may be dry and scanty. The large myxoedematous tongue protrudes from the mouth and interferes with feeding and breathing (Fig. 21.2). The cry has a characteristic hoarseness. The neck appears short because of the presence of myxoedematous pads of fat above the clavicles. The skin, especially over the face and extremities, feels dry, thick and cold. An umbilical hernia is common. The hands and fingers are broad and stumpy. The hypothyroid infant is frequently apathetic and uninterested in his surroundings. As times goes by, psychomotor retardation becomes obvious and partially irreversible.

However, most infants with congenital hypothyroidism are born with few symptoms or signs. None the less, the marked delay in diagnosis so commonly encountered is unnecessary and it results often in avoidable intellectual impairment. The possibility of hypothyroidism should be considered in every infant or child in whom growth is retarded. Most cases of congenital hypothyroidism are diagnosed by neonatal screening by detection of increased TSH concentrations in Guthrie card blood spots, but cases with delayed rise in TSH will be missed.

In the undetected or untreated child the body proportions remain infantile with long trunk and short legs. A tendency to stand with exaggerated lumbar lordosis and slightly flexed hips and knees is common. The anterior fontanelle is late in closing and the posterior fontanelle remains patent. The deciduous teeth are slow in erupting and radiographs may show defects in the enamel. The face and hands are frequently mildly myxoedematous and the cerebral activities are slow and sluggish. The mandible is often underdeveloped and the nasolabial configuration may be obviously that of a much younger child. The deep tendon reflexes are sometimes exaggerated with slow relaxation and there may be mild ataxia. In some cases of juvenile myxoedema, however, the only clinical indication of hypothyroidism is dwarfism with infantile proportions. In such cases sexual maturation is delayed (as in all hypothyroid children) so that the condition may be regarded as a "thyrogenic infantilism". Rarely, a hypothyroid child may present with precocious puberty.

Diagnosis

Short stature is one of the only two invariable findings in hypothyroidism. The ratio of the upper to lower (U/L) skeletal segment is also abnormal (infantile) in hypothyroid children. The lower segment is the distance from the top of the symphysis pubis to the ground; the upper segment is obtained by subtracting the lower segment from the total height. The mean body U/L ratio is about 1.7 at birth, 1.3 at 3 years and 1.1 after 7 years of age. Hypothyroid children have an unduly long upper segment because of their short age.

Delayed ossification to a more severe degree than that retardation in linear growth is the other constant finding in hypothyroidism. The assessment of bone age is based on radiographs of various epiphyseal areas, chosen according to the child's age, and their comparison with an ossification chart showing the normal ages at which the different centres should ossify (Fig. 21.3). Thus fetal hypothyroidism can be presumed in the full-term baby if

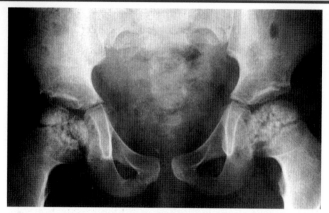

Fig. 21.3: Epiphyseal dysgenesis in femoral heads. Note stippling and fragmented appearance

the upper tibial or lower femoral epiphyses, which normally ossify at 36 fetal weeks, are absent or if they show epiphyseal dysgenesis. This appearance of dysgenesis of the epiphyses is pathognomonic of hypothyroidism. It may be florid at one area and absent at another, so that radiographs should always be taken of several areas of the skeleton. In some cases dysgenesis only appears after thyroid treatment has been started, but then only in those ossification centres which should have appeared in the normal child before that age. The presence of dysgenesis indicates that that hypothyroid state existed before the affected centre would be normally due to ossify and it permits an assessment of the age, fetal or postnatal, at which the hypothyroidism developed. The characteristic X-ray appearance is of a misshapen epiphysis with irregular or fluffy margins and a fragmented or stippled substance (Fig. 21.3). In older children, skeletal maturations is assessed with an X-ray of the non-dominant hand and wrist using the Greulich and Pyle or Tanner Whitehouse skeletal atlas. In the great majority of cases of hypothyroidism measurements of the linear height, the upper and lower segments, and a few well chosen radiographs will establish or exclude the diagnosis of hypothyroidism beyond doubt. They will also determine the age of onset of the hypothyroid state.

Investigations

A particularly sensitive biochemical test for hypothyroidism lies in measurement of the serum thyroid-stimulating hormone (TSH) using a suprasensitive assay. The TSH level (normal range < 0.5 to 5.5 mIU/L) is markedly raised (above 50 mIU/L) in primary hypothyroidism, whereas it will be low in pituitary hypothyroidism. A test of the TSH response to thyrotrophin-releasing hormone (TRH) given intravenously in a dose of 10 µg/kg to a maximum of 200 µg is rarely necessary except in a combined assessment of pituitary function.

Radioactive iodine test is never necessary to establish the diagnosis of hypothyroidism, but it can be used to provide information about the pathogenesis. For the detection and location of thyroid activity in congenital hypothyroidism, ^{123}I or ^{99m}Tc can be safely given followed by scanning of the neck for radioactivity.

Neonatal Screening for Congenital Hypothyroidism

Irreversible brain damage is a common sequel to a delayed clinical diagnosis and treatment of congenital hypothyroidism. Newborn screening for congenital hypothyroidism has been highly successful in improving the prognosis for mental development in hypothyroid neonates. The incidence of congenital hypothyroidism has been reported to be in the region of 1 in 3600. Screening is usually carried out between the 3rd and 7th days of life. In Europe and Britain, the favoured technique is by radioimmunoassay of TSH levels on dried filter paper blood spots obtained by heel stab. It involves an extremely low recall rate for repeat tests but is unable to detect the rare case of secondary (pituitary) hypothyroidism. This disadvantage does not apply to measurement of T_4 levels followed by TSH assay which is confined to specimens with low T_4 values. This latter method is favoured by many American centres. While both methods are highly reliable it is essential that infants with results in the hypothyroid range have confirmatory tests which should include clinical assessment, TSH assays, quantitative measurements of T_4 and T_3, and assessment of bone maturation by X-ray of the knee. Infants are missed despite newborn thyroid screening programmes because of human error in the infrastructure of the screening programmes. Treatment should be started as early as possible.

Treatment

The drug of choice for the treatment of hypothyroidism is L-thyroxine sodium. In infants a daily dose of 10 µg/kg up to a maximum of 50 µg daily should be given. By 5 years of age the dose should reach 75 µg daily and by 12 years the adult dose of between 100 µg and 150 µg daily, guided by clinical response, growth and skeletal maturation assessment, and measurements of plasma T_4 and TSH. The maintenance dose level is that which permits linear growth to proceed at a normal rate and does not leave the bone age retarded. The serum T_4 should be adjusted to the upper normal range. Serum TSH levels may be normal or mildly elevated in adequately treated children. It is undesirable to permit the bone age to advance beyond the chronological age. Treatment must be regularly monitored every 2 to 3 months in the first two years of life and the frequency of spaced out when the children are older.

Prognosis

The somatic response to adequate treatment before 3 months of age is invariably good but in some cases mild defects in hearing, speech and co-ordination persist despite having a normal intelligence quotient. Factors affecting outcome include the severity of congenital hypothyroidism, adequacy of thyroid hormone replacement in early life and the social economic background of the family. Reconfirmation of the diagnosis by interruption of treatment should be performed at 3 years of age especially in children who were diagnosed to have congenital hypothyroidism but with a thyroid gland in the normal location. Life-long treatment is required for patients with permanent congenital hypothyroidism.

Autoimmune Thyroiditis (Hashimoto Thyroiditis)

Autoimmune thyroiditis is the most common causes of hypothyroidism in childhood. It is one of the best examples of an organ-specific autoimmunity and the immunological phenomena are usually confined to the thyroid gland. It is caused by an interaction of multiple genetic and environmental factors like infection and dietary iodine intake. The outstanding feature is infiltration of the thyroid by lymphocytes, plasma cells and reticular cells. Hyperplasia of the epithelial cells is commonly seen. In more advanced cases the epithelial cells show degenerative changes and there may be extensive fibrosis with final destruction of the gland. Occasionally autoimmune thyroid disease may be associated with other autoimmune endocrine gland dysfunction as part of the autoimmune polyendocrine syndrome.

Clinical Features

In most children the only sign is a goitre. It rarely has the firm, rubbery consistency so typical of the adult form of the disease. Presentation is usually with a euthyroid goitre but in up to 10%, particularly in adolescence, there may be signs of thyrotoxicosis. Only a minority of affected children go on to develop hypothyroidism but it is important to monitor for signs of this state in every case as the onset of hypothyroidism is insidious and may be missed. The patient may have weight gain, slowing of growth, cold intolerance, constipation and deteriorating school performance. In adolescent patients, there may be delayed puberty or rarely precocious puberty. Hypothyroidism is diagnosed by a low total or free thyroxine level together with elevated TSH concentrating (>15 mU/L). The classical antithyroglobulin and thyroid antiimcrosomal antibodies titres are markedly elevated.

Treatment

Thyroxine should be prescribed when the child is hypothyroid to suppress the excess secretion of pituitary TSH and to diminish the size of the goitre. These children should be kept under prolonged medical supervision because some later develop other autoimmune diseases.

Hyperthyroidism

In contrast to hypothyroidism, thyrotoxicosis is a less common disorder in childhood. It usually takes the form of Graves disease with diffuse thyroid enlargement and thyrotoxic ophthalmopathy. The incidence varies from 0.1 per 100,000 in young children to 14 per 100,000 in some countries. About 35% of monozygotic twins as compared to 3% of dizygotic twins have been found to be concordant for Graves disease suggesting the importance of genetic relative to the environmental factors in disease susceptibility. The HLA-DRB1 locus and A-G polymorphism of exon 1 of the cytotoxic T-lymphocyte-associated antigen-4 (CTLA-4) have been found to be associated with Graves disease. Further chromosomal regions (5q31, 14q31, 20q11) linked to autoimmune thyroid diease have been identified by linkage analysis using the genome scan approach.

Clinical Features

The disease is more common in girls and rare before the age of 7 years. The parents may bring their child for medical advice with a variety of symptoms, such as irritability, fidgetiness, deterioration in school performance, loss of weight in spite of good appetite, excessive sweating, palpitations or nervousness. The child looks thin, and often startled because of her stare and wide palpebral fissures. There may be obvious exophthalmos (Fig. 21.4). Other eye

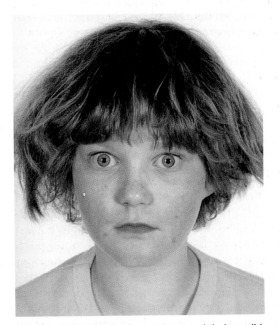

Fig. 21.4 : Thyrotoxicosis showing exophthalmos, lid retraction and goitre

signs include lid retraction, lid lag and ophthalmoplegia. There may be conjunctival injection because of exposure due to the proptosis. The skin will be flushed, warm and moist. A fine tremor of the outstretched fingers is common. The abnormal cardiovascular signs in the child include sinus tachycardia, raised systolic blood pressure and a large pulse pressure. The thyroid gland is visibly enlarged and feels soft. A bruit may be audible over the gland. Emotional lability is frequently very obvious. Menstruation may be delayed or irregular in untreated adolescent girls, and growth acceleration is commonly seen at diagnosis.

Diagnosis

This is usually obvious on simple clinical observation. The most reliable biochemical feature is an elevated total and free serum T_3 and T_4 levels with suppressed TSH documented with a suprasensitive TSH assay. Both thyroid stimulating antibody (TSAb) and thyroid blocking antibody (TBAb) epitopes are close together and are both detected in the commercially available thyroid binding inhibiting immunoglobulin (TBII) assays. TSAb bioassays are limited to specialized centres. TBIIs are disease specific and are never present in normal euthyroid individuals. TBIIs are present in 80% to 90% of children with Graves disease. The thyroglobin and thyroid antimicrosomal antibodies are present in 68% of paediatric patients.

Treatment

A trial of medical treatment should always be made with the objective of rendering the patient euthyroid for 2 years before drug therapy is withdrawn. Suitable drugs and doses are carbimazole (0.5mg/kg/day in two divided doses), and propylthiouracil (5-10mg/kg/day in 2-3 divided doses). After about 4 weeks, the dose can often be reduced according to the clinical state of the child and the T_4 and T_3 levels. An alternative approach would be the block-replace regime by maintaining the same suppressive doses of thionamides but adding a suitable replacement dose of thyroxine daily to maintain the serum T_4 in the normal range. The advantage of this regime is the lower risk of fluctuations of thyroid hormone levels and fewer blood tests in the children under treatment. With block-replace antithyroid drug treatment for two years, the remission rate is usually quoted to be 25% to 30% but frequently lower in younger children. Pubertal adolescents with a small goitre, a relatively normal body weight and not excessively high circulating thyroid hormone level at diagnosis, have a higher chance of spontaneous remission. A high iodine intake increases the risk of relapse. In patients with multiple relapses, surgery or thyroid ablation with radioactive iodine should be considered. Recent studies have not found an increased risk of thyroid and extra-thyroidal cancer after radio-iodine treatment in

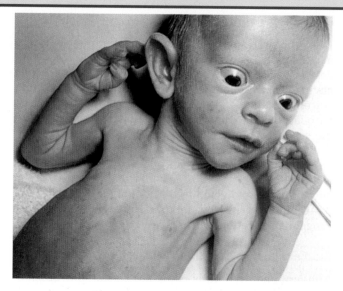

Fig. 21.5: Neonatal thyrotoxicosis

patients older than 18 years of age. At the start of antithyroid treatment, the sympathetic overstimulation can be controlled with propranolol 2 mg/kg/day in two or three divided doses. Parents must be reminded that all the antithyroid drugs can cause toxic effects, e.g. rashes, agranulocytosis and aplastic anaemia.

Transient Neonatal Thyrotoxicosis

There have been a considerable number of instances in which women who have or have had thyrotoxicosis, given birth to infants with the unmistakable signs of hyper-thyroidism in the neonatal period. The infants are restless, agitated, excessively hungry and they exhibit warm, moist flushed skin, tachycardia (190-220 per minute), tachyp-noea, exophthalmos and goitre (Fig. 21.5). The diagnosis has been made antenatally because of fetal tachycardia. Some mothers have been previously treated by partial thyroidectomy; others have received thyroid blocking drugs during pregnancy. When the mother is thyrotoxic and not on antithyroid drugs up to the time of delivery, the hyperthyroid state is present in the infant from birth. If the mother has been rendered euthyroid by drugs, the neonatal thyrotoxicosis does not develop for some days because the thyroid gland is suppressed *in utero* and during the infant's first days of life.

There is good evidence that neonatal Graves disease is caused by the transfer of maternal thyroid-stimulating immunoglobulins (TSAb or TSI) across the placenta from mother to fetus. The presence of such immunoglobulins in the mother and infant at the same time has been demonstrated both by bioassay techniques and the radioreceptor assay method. The thyroid-stimulating immunoglobulins disappear from the infant's blood after about 3 months, so that the disorder is a temporary one.

Diagnosis in the neonate is confirmed by demonstrating increased levels of total and free T_4 and T_3 and suppressed levels of TSH.

The degree of thyrotoxicosis can be alarmingly severe and prompt treatment of the newborn infant is essential. Treatment can be started with potassium iodide 2-5 mg thrice daily and propranolol 2 mg/kg/day in three divided doses. Propylthiouracil which blocks the organification of iodine, also blocks the conversion of T_4 to T_3. This drug should be started at a dose of 5-10 mg/kg/day and adjusted based on the circulating T_4 and T_3 levels. It is only necessary to continue antithyroid medication for 6 to 12 weeks. Supportive treatment with digoxin and diuretics may be required if congestive heart failure is present.

THE PARATHYROID GLANDS

Primary disorders of the parathyroid glands are exceedingly rare in paediatric practice. Much has been learned about the molecular structure and physiological activities of parathyroid hormone (PTH) in recent years and circulating PTH can be measured by RIA. PTH increases renal tubular calcium absorption and phosphate excretion, and intestinal calcium absorption. PTH also maintains serum calcium levels by stimulating osteoclastic bone resorption. It is hardly possible to consider the actions of parathyroid hormone without consideration of calcitonin. Calcitonin is also a polypeptide and is secreted from the parafollicular "C" cells of the thyroid gland. It inhibits the resorption of bone and acts as a physiological antagonist to parathyroid hormone, causing hypocalcaemia. The only disorder associated with excessive calcitonin production is medullary thyroid carcinoma which may occur as part of multiple endocrine neoplasia type IIb (MEN IIb) caused by mutations in the RET proto-oncogene.

Hypoparathyroidism

Hypoparathyroidism may occur after thyroid or parathyroid surgery or rarely radiation damage. In Asia and the Mediterranean basin, hypoparathyroidism can result from haemosiderosis in transfusion-dependent thalassaemia major patients. A rare autoimmune polyendocrine syndrome due to mutations in the autoimmune regulator gene (AIRE) can result in hypoparathyroidism which develops in childhood and is associated later with hypoadrenocorticism, and sometimes with steatorrhoea, pernicious anaemia, diabetes mellitus or elevated sweat electrolytes; moniliasis frequently precedes the endocrine manifestations. Rarely hypoparathyroidism can result from mitochondrial cytopathy. Apart from transient neonatal hypoparathyroidism due to maternal parathyroid disease, congenital hypoparathyroidism can be due to dysgenesis of the parathyroid gland, familial forms of disease (antosomal recessive, autosomal dominant, X-linked recessive), heterozygous gain-of-function

mutations of the calcium sensing receptor gene (CASR) or the DiGeorge syndrome (thymus hypoplasia, hypoparathyroidism, malformations of the outflow tracts of the heart) due to microdeletion of chromosome 22q11.

Clinical Features

The diagnosis of hypoparathyroidism is not difficult when a child presents with recurrent tetany. Other symptoms include paraesthesia ("pins and needles"), muscle cramps and carpopedal spasm. Chvostek and Trousseau signs may be elicited. More often the outstanding feature is the presence of recurrent convulsions when an erroneous diagnosis of epilepsy may easily be made. Newborn infants with hypoparathyroidism presents with jitteriness or convulsions. Some affected children have also been mentally retarded and intracerebral calcification may occur. Useful diagnostic clues are delay in the second dentition and defective enamel, ectodermal dysplasia and deformed nails, loss of hair, and moniliasis in the mouth or nails. Cataract develops later in 50% of cases. The characteristic biochemical changes are a low serum calcium (below 2.25 mmol/L) and raised serum phosphate (above 2.25 mmol/L) and normal serum alkaline phosphatase and low PTH levels by radioimmunoassay in the absence of rickets, renal disease and steatorrhoea.

Pseudohypoparathyroidism gives rise to a very similar clinical presentation, hypocalcaemia and hyperphosphataemia, but in addition, some patients have features of Albright hereditary osteodystrophy (AHO): a stocky figure with dwarfism and a rounded face, brachydactyly with shortening of the metacarpals and metatarsals of the first, fourth and fifth fingers and toes, subcutaneous calcification, mental backwardness and obesity. The serum PTH levels are markedly elevated in the presence of biochemical features of hypoparathyroidism.

Treatment

The immediate treatment for tetany is a slow intravenous injection of 10% calcium gluconate, 0.3 ml/kg after dilution over several minutes, repeated every few hours as necessary. For long-term treatment, alfacalcidol (1α-hydroxyvitamin D_3; 1α-OHD$_3$) 25-50 ng/kg or calcitriol (25-50 ng/kg) are preferred because of their shorter half-life. The dosage of the vitamin D should be adequate to maintain the serum calcium in the low normal range without inducing hypercalciuria (spot urine calcium to creatinine ratio >0.7 mmol/mmol). The patient should be monitored for the development of subcutaneous calcification, nephrocalcinosis and intracranial calcification.

Hyperparathyroidism

Hypercalcaemia due to adenoma or hyperplasia of the parathyroid glands are very rare in childhood. Neonatal primary hyperparathyroidism is caused by homozygous or compounded heterozygous mutations of the calcium sensing receptor gene (CASR) and is associated with hypotonia, anorexia, respiratory distress, dehydration and a high mortality. Urgent parathyroidectomy is required. In older children, parathyroid tumour leading to hyperparathyroidism can be associated with multiple endocrine neoplasia syndrome type I (parathyroid, pancreatic, pituitary tumours due to mutation in MEN1 gene) or multiple endocrine neoplasia type II (MTC, phaeochromocytoma, parathyroid tumour due to mutations in the RET proto-oncogene).

Clinical Features

In older children with hyperparathyroidism, bone pains and muscular weakness are the first symptoms. Peptic ulceration is unduly frequent in these patients. Anorexia, polyuria, polydipsia, vomiting, and severe constipation are common and attributable to the hypercalcaemia. The bone changes of osteitis fibrosa cystica are found. These include osteoporosis with patches of osteosclerosis. This produces a characteristic granular mottling or discrete rounded translucent areas in radiographs of the skull. Similar appearances are commonly found in the clavicles and iliac bones. Pathognomonic changes are frequently seen in the terminal phalanges of the hands where there is subperiosteal resorption of bone with a crenellated appearance. The lamina dura, a dense line of alveolar bone surrounding the roots of the teeth, disappears. A giant-cell tumour (osteoclastoma) may appear as a multilocular cyst on radiographs of the mandible or long bones. Occasionally the presenting sign is a pathological fracture at the site of such a tumour. Hypercalcaemia can lead to nephrocalcinosis and renal calculi.

The most common biochemical features are a raised serum calcium level (over 2.74 mmol) and lowered serum phosphate (below 1 mmol). These values fluctuate and several estimations in the fasting patient at intervals may be required before the diagnosis is confirmed. The plasma alkaline phosphatase is frequently but not invariably raised. There is an increased urinary output of calcium (over 10 mmol/24 hours while on an ordinary diet). This observation should be followed by estimating the 24-hour calcium output on a low-calcium diet (120 mg/day); an output in excess of 4.5 mmol/24 hours is abnormal. When the kidneys have been severely damaged by nephrocalcinosis a high serum phosphate level may simulate secondary hyperparathyroidism. In children, however, renal osteodystrophy includes the changes of rickets which are rare in primary hyperparathyroidism. Furthermore, hypocalciuria is the rule in renal failure, but hypercalciuria usually persists in primary hyperparathyroidism even when there is severe renal damage.

Treatment

Severe hypercalcaemia can be treated with intravenous fluid together with a loop diuretic and intravenous pamidronate infusion. The parathyroid tumour or hyperplastic glands should be removed surgically. Transient post-operative tetany is common and best treated with frequent intravenous doses of calcium gluconate. The results of operation are excellent provided the diagnosis has preceded irreversible damage to the kidneys.

Rickets

Rickets and osteomalacia are the consequences of decreased mineralization of the bone osteoid caused by deficiencies of calcium, phosphate or vitamin D. Rickets in childhood can be due to nutritional deficiency of vitamin D from low intake or disordered absorption of fat soluble vitamins due to diseases of the hepatobiliary and gastrointestinal systems. The condition could also result from renal tubular disorders, X-linked familial hypophosphatamic rickets or to genetic defects like loss of function mutation of the genes for vitamin D receptor or 25-hydroxyvitamin D_3 1α-hydroxylase.

Nutritional rickets has emerged again as a paediatric health issue in several parts of the world. The vitamin D intake in most adults would be 100 IU per day and pregnant and lactating women would not meet the recommended daily vitamin D intake without adequate exposure to sunlight. Dark skinned infants breastfed by vitamin D deficient mother who remain covered for cultural reasons, are particularly at risk. The clinical features of rickets are shown in Table 21.6.

The biochemical abnormalities in nutritional rickets include hypocalcaemia, hypophosphataemia, elevated PTH and alkaline phosphatase levels in the blood. The 25-hydroxyvitamin D level is less than 50 nmol/L. Radiologically, there is cupping and fraying of the metaphyses of the long bones and osteopenia. Treatment with vitamin D 3000 IU daily for 3 months and maintenance of a daily vitamin D intake of 400 IU daily should be continued.

In most developed countries, the most common form of rickets is X-linked familial hypophosphataemia rickets which is caused by loss of function mutation of the phosphate regulating gene with homologies to

Table 21.6: Clinical features of rickets
1. Expanded wrist, knee and ankle joints
2. Rachitic rosary (swelling of costochondral junctions of the anterior chest cage)
3. Bowing deformity of lower limbs in weight bearing children
4. Craniotabes
5. Hypotonia, muscle weakness and delayed motor development
6. Enamel hypoplasia and delayed tooth eruption

endopeptidases on the X-chromosome gene (PHEX). Apart from clinical features of rickets, these patients present with short stature, bone pain, join stiffness, dental abscess but craniotabes and muscle weakness are not present. Biochemical abnormalities include low normal serum calcium, low serum phosphate and elevated alkaline phosphatase levels. The serum PTH and vitamin D levels are normal but the $1,25(OH)_2D_3$ concentration is inappropriately low for the degree of hypophosphataemia. Treatment include phosphate supplement (not more than 70mg/kg/day) and rocaltrol (20-70ng/kg/day) and regular monitoring is required to avoid hypercalcaemia, hypercalciuria (calcium/creatinine ratio >0.7 mmol/ mmol) and nephrocalcinosis.

THE GONADS

The development of the pituitary gland, the control of pubertal development and development of secondary sexual characteristics have already been described. Secretion of GnRH by GnRH neurons are inherently pulsatile. GABAergic receptors mediate inhibitory and NMDA receptors mediate facilitatory input. Oestradiol directly stimulates or inhibits GnRH gene expression under different conditions and the stimulation of GnRH and LH surge in mid-cycle by oestrogen seems to involve induction of progesterone receptors in the hypothalamus. Prolactin suppresses both hypothalamic and gonadotrope GnRH receptor expression. Hypothalamic endorphins suppress GnRH secretion and interleukines inhibit gonadotropin release.

Hypogonadism

Adolescents without signs of puberty by 13 years in girls and 14 years in boys, or failing to progress in the development of secondary sexual characteristics warrant further assessment. Primary amenorrhoea is defined by the absence of menstruation by 14 years of age in a girl with no secondary sexual characteristics or by 16 years in a girl with some development of secondary sexual characteristics. The causes of hypogonadism are shown in Table 21.7.

Clinical Features

With the exception of cryptorchidism and micropenis suggestive of congenital hypopituitarism, the features of hypogonadism in the male only become manifest after the time of normal puberty. Growth continues for an abnormally long period because of delay in fusion of the epiphyses. There is a fall off in the growth velocity in hypogonadal adolescence and this pattern of growth is different from that seen in adolescents with constitutional delay in growth and puberty (CDGP). Children with CDGP grow at a normal rate below the 3rd percentile and the

Table 21.7: Causes of hypogonadism

Hypogonadotropic hypogonadism
1. Congenital defects in hypothalamic – hypophyseal formation associated with midline facial defects.
2. Mutations in genes of pituitary transcription factors, GnRH receptor and gonadotropin.
3. Genetic hypothalamic defects (Kallmann syndrome, Prader Willi and Bardet Biedl syndrome)
4. Acquired
   suprasellar tumours
   infiltrative disease
   damage from radiation, trauma, haemosiderosis, intracranial infection
5. Functional hypothalamic hypogonadism
   drugs and contraceptive pills
   systemic illness and eating disorder
   exercise induced amenorrhoea in girls
   stress and cortisol excess
Hypergonadotropic hypogonadism in girls
1. Gonadal dysgenesis: Turner (45X) and trisomy syndromes, WT1 mutation
2. Autoimmune ovarian failure
3. Damage by radiation, cytotoxic drugs and infection
4. Genetic causes due to mutations of SF1, gonadotropin receptor gene, fragile X premutation, Noonan syndrome
Hypergonadotropic hypogonadism in Males
1. Klinefelter syndrome (47XXY)
2. Damage from orchitis, radiation and chemotherapeutic agents
3. Noonan syndrome, cystic fibrosis and rare genetic causes.

onset of puberty is delayed. The bone age is frequently delayed by more than 2 years when compared to chronological age. Both males and females with hypogonadism have a low upper to lower segment ratio. Clinicians should be aware of the clinical features of syndromes associated with hypogonadism like Prader-Willi, Noonan, Bardet-Biedl, Klinefelter and Turner syndromes. Gynaecomastia is usually seen in hypergonadotropic hypogonadism. Hypogonadotropic hypogonadism associated with anosmia is suggestive of Kallmann syndrome which can be inherited in the X-linked (KAL1 mutation) or autosomal recessive (FGFR1 mutation) fashion. Clinical evaluation should be done to exclude acquired hypogonadism (Table 21.7). Suggested investigations for hypogonadism are shown in Table 21.8.

Table 21.8: Investigations of hypogonadism

1. Serum LH, FSH, prolactin, oestradiol or testosterone levels
2. Morning cortisol, fT4, TSH concentrations
3. X-ray for bone age
4. Karyotype
5. GnRH/GnRH analogue test to distinguish hypogonadotropic hypogonadism from constitutional delay in growth and puberty
6. Combined pituitary stimulation test and MRI scan of the brain, hypothalamus and pituitary gland if indicated.

Treatment

In adolescents with hypogonadism, induction of puberty should be started no later than 14 years in girls and 15 years in boys. The dose of oestrogen (2.5 µg of ethynylo-estradiol daily or premarin 0.3 mg alternate days) can be progressively increased over 2.5 to 3 years. Cyclical oestrogen and progestagen should be initiated when the dose of oestrogen has reached 15-20 mg of oestradiol or 0.625 mg of Premarin daily or when break through bleeding occurs. In boys, puberty can be induced by oral testosterone undecanoate or more commonly by monthly intramuscular injection of testosterone enanthate, starting from 50 mg and slowly increasing to 250 mg every month. Intra-muscular testosterone can be associated with mood swings and cyclical aggression and depression. Testesterone sub-cutaneous implants can provide a more steady testosterone level over months. It is now possible to restore menstruation and induce ovulation in females and induce puberty and spermatogenesis in males with hypogonadotrophic hypogonadism by pulsatile administration of GnRH with a portable pump.

Precocious Puberty

Pubertal development in girls have been reported to occur earlier in recent years in many populations but there has been a less dramatic change in the age of onset of menarche. They age of onset of puberty in boys have not advanced significantly in recent years. Precocious puberty is defined as breast development before the age of 7 years and menstruation before the age of 10 years in girls and testicular or penile enlargement before the age of 9 years in boys. The causes of precocious puberty are shown in Table 21.9.

Clinical Features

In premature thelarche, there is isolated development of the breasts without significant acceleration of growth or skeletal maturation or the development of other secondary sexual characteristics. The condition frequently occurs in the first 18 months of life. There may be fluctuations of the breast size but the condition is not progressive. Occasio-nally non-progressive breast development can occur in girls in the peripubertal age group (5 to 7 years of age) and the condition is sometimes referred to as thelarche variant but should be distinguished from the early stage of central precocious puberty. Premature adrenarche refers to early isolated development of sex hair without other signs of puberty. Premature adrenarche are more prevalent in African Americans and East Asian Indians. Care must be taken to exclude the possibility of late-onset congenital adrenal hyperplasia or androgen secreting tumour from the adrenal glands or gonads.

Table 21.9: Causes of precocious puberty
Gonadotrophin dependent or central precocious puberty
1. Idiopathic
2. Intracranial tumours: hypothalamic hamartoma, pineal region tumour, tumour in posterior hypothalamus, germinoma, craniopharyngioma (rare), optic nerve glioma
3. Cranial irradiation
4. Head trauma
5. Neurological disorders: hydrocephaly, intracranial infection, cerebral palsy, epilepsy
6. Hypothyroidism
7. Neurofibromatosis type 1
Gonadotrophin independent sexual precocity
1. McCune Albright syndrome
2. Familial testotoxicosis
Pseudoprecocious puberty
1. Congenital adrenal hyperplasia
2. Oestrogen or androgen secreting tumours from the gonads or adrenal glands
3. HCG-secreting tumour (boys)
4. Autonomously functioning ovarian cysts in girls
Incomplete precocious puberty
1. Premature thelarche
2. Premature adrenarche

Patients with true precocious puberty have rapid physical growth and advanced skeletal maturation. In addition to the development of secondary sexual character-istics, behavioural change like emotion lability and aggression may occur. The behaviour of children with precocious puberty are more appropriate to their chronological age rather than the degree of sexual development. Other changes include increased sebaceous gland secretion (greasy skin and hair), acne and body odour. Children with precocious puberty who are untreated usually have an increased upper to lower segment ratio. Most cases of precocious puberty in girls are idiopathic but about 10% of girls and 80% of boys with precocious puberty have an occult or known intracranial pathology.

Patients with the McCune Albright syndrome have the characteristic triad of irregular café-au-lait pigmentation, gonadotrophin independent sexual precocity and polyostotic fibrous dysplasia but sometimes, the complete triad is not present. The condition is due to a somatic activating mutation of the GNAS1 gene. The patients typically having breast development due to oestrogen production from an autonomously functioning ovarian cysts. When the cyst ruptures, menstruation occurs as a result of acute oestrogen withdrawal.

Familial testotoxicosis is inherited in an autosomal dominant male limited fashion. There is autosomal dominant presentation of early sexual development in males of the affected families. The condition manifests itself usually by 2 to 3 years of age and is due to activating

Table 21.10: Investigations for precocious puberty
1. Baseline oestradiol or testosterone, LH, FSH levels and the LH and FSH response to GnRH (2.5 µg/kg intravenously)
2. X-ray for bone age
3. Ultrasound examination of the pelvis in girls for ovarian volume and cysts, uterine size, and cervix to uterus ratio
4. Magnetic resonance imaging of the brain
5. Investigations for involvement of other pituitary hormones where indicated: fT4, TSH, prolactin levels, and cortisol and growth hormone reserve.

mutations of the luteinizing hormone receptor gene. Females carrying the mutation will not develop precocious puberty. There is some seminiferous tubule development and spermatogenesis because of the high intra-testicular concentrations of testosterone present in affected patients even though the gonadotropin levels are suppressed.

A germ cell tumour producing HCG can lead to pseudoprecocious puberty in boys only. However germ cell tumours can also cause true precocious puberty due to the location of the tumour in the posterior hypothalamus distorting the hypothalamic "gonadostat". An autonomously functioning ovarian cyst producing oestrogen can cause premature breast development. These cysts should be distinguished from juvenile granulosa tumours of the ovaries by serial ultrasound assessment. Persistence of cystic lesions with a significant solid component and persistent elevation of serum oestradiol concentration for more than 3 months should alert the doctor to the possibility of an ovarian tumour. Congenital adrenal hyperplasia (CAH) can cause isosexual pseudoprecocious puberty in boys and heterosexual pseudoprecocious puberty in girls (refer to subsequent section of this chapter). Differentiation of virilization due to CAH from an adrenal tumour is important in virilized patients.

Investigations

Suggested investigations and interpretation of the hormonal tests are shown in Tables 21.10 and 21.11 respectively.

Treatment

Patients with precocious puberty are at risk of being short as adults because of early skeletal mutation. Treatment with a long-acting GnRH analogue given either monthly or 3-monthly offers the greatest advantage for those children in whom the onset of puberty occurs at a very early age, those who demonstrate rapidly accelerating bone age and those with lower genetic height potential or those with the largest difference between the target and predicted height. Patients with gonadotropin independent precocious puberty require treatment with an aromatase inhibitor in girls or a drug that blocks testosterone biosynthesis like ketoconazole in boys. The underlying condition leading to pseudoprecocious puberty should be managed appropriately.

THE ADRENAL GLAND

Adrenal steroidogensis is controlled by a number of Cytochrome P450 and hydroxysteroid dehydrogenase enzymes (Fig. 21.6). The adrenal cortex produces cortisol, mineralocorticoid (aldosterone) and sex steroids (androgens) whereas the adrenal medulla secretes adrenaline, noradrenaline, catecholamines and dopamine.

Cushing's Syndrome

Cushing's syndrome in children is commonly iatrogenic in nature due to steroids given by the oral, topical or inhalational routes. Rarely steroid excess state can become manifest because of adrenal tumour, ectopic ACTH-secreting malignancy or Cushing disease (ACTH-secreting pituitary adenoma)

Clinical Features

The clinical features of Cushing's syndrome result from the secretion of adrenal hormones and are dominated by the effects of cortisol. Growth retardation, fatigue and emotional liability are common symptoms. Those due to an increased production of glucocorticoids include buffalo hump fat pad over the back of the neck, obesity, moon face, purple striae over abdomen, flanks and thighs, easy

Table 21.11: Sex steroids and gonadotrophins in precocious puberty				
	E$_2$/testosterone	LH (basal)	LH (peak)	FSH (peak)
Premature thelarche (girls)	prepub	<0.5IU/L	prepub	↑↑↑
Early precocious puberty	prepub or ↑	<0.5IU/L	<7IU/L	↑↑
Established precocious puberty	↑-↑↑	>0.6IU/L	>9.6IU/L ♂ >7IU/L @ ♀	↑
Pseudoprecocious puberty	↑-↑↑	↓↓	↓↓	↓↓
Gonadotrophin independent sexual precocity	prepub - ↑	↓↓	↓↓	↓↓
HCG tumour (boys)	↑	slight ↑	no change	↓↓

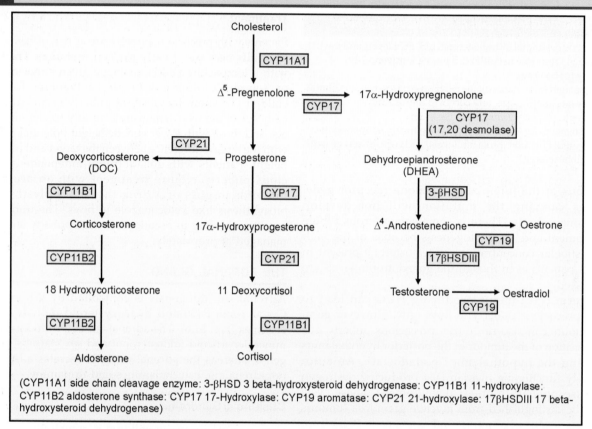

Cholesterol

CYP11A1

Δ^5-Pregnenolone → 17α-Hydroxypregnenolone

CYP17

CYP17
(17,20 desmolase)

CYP21

Deoxycorticosterone ← Progesterone
(DOC)

Dehydroepiandrosterone
(DHEA)

CYP11B1

CYP17

3-βHSD

Corticosterone

17α-Hydroxyprogesterone

Δ^4-Androstenedione → Oestrone

CYP19

CYP11B2

CYP21

17βHSDIII

18 Hydroxycorticosterone

11 Deoxycortisol

Testosterone → Oestradiol

CYP19

CYP11B2

CYP11B1

Aldosterone

Cortisol

(CYP11A1 side chain cleavage enzyme: 3-βHSD 3 beta-hydroxysteroid dehydrogenase: CYP11B1 11-hydroxylase: CYP11B2 aldosterone synthase: CYP17 17-Hydroxylase: CYP19 aromatase: CYP21 21-hydroxylase: 17βHSDIII 17 beta-hydroxysteroid dehydrogenase)

Fig. 21.6: Flow diagram showing pathways of steroid metabolism

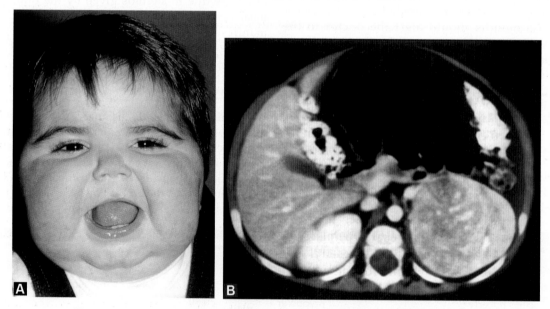

Figs 21.7A and B: (A) A child with Cushing's syndrome; (B) CT scan showing a large well encapsulated tumour with calcification of the left adrenal gland

bruising, muscle wasting and weakness, osteoporosis, latent diabetes mellitus and polycythaemia (Figs 21.7A and B). Increased output of mineralocorticosteroids and aldosterone accounts for the hypertension and hypokalaemic alkalosis. Excessive secretion of androgens may cause hirsutism and clitoral enlargement in females, baldness and acne. These patients are, in addition, highly susceptible to infections.

Diagnosis

In patients with Cushing syndrome due to exogenous steroids given in excess (greater than 6-8 mg/m^2/day of hydrocortisone equivalent), the endogenous secretion of glucocorticoids will be suppressed. Excessive doses of glucocorticoids like prednisolone or dexamethasone (1 mg prednisolone equivalent to 4 mg hydrocortisone) will result in features of Cushing syndrome but the morning plasma cortisol and 24-hour urine free cortisol and 17-oxogenic steroids will be suppressed. Endogenous excessive secretion of glucocorticoids due to an adrenal tumour or ACTH-secreting pituitary tumour will result in loss of diurnal cortisol rhythm with elevated morning and evening plasma cortisol levels. The urinary free cortisol will be elevated more than four times the upper limit of normal corrected for the creatinine level. Frequently the 24-hour urinary oxogenic steroids concentration is also elevated. The change in plasma cortisol and urinary free cortisol levels to low dose (30 µg/kg/day in four divided doses) and high dose (120 µg/kg/day in four divided doses) dexamethasone suppression is a useful test. Failure of adrenocortical suppression by high dose dexamethasone is strongly suggestive of an adrenal tumour. In difficult cases, the corticotrophin releasing hormone test and bilateral inferior petrosal sinus venous sampling may be required to localize a pituitary ACTH-secreting adenoma. Biochemical diagnosis must be complemented by MRI scan with gadolinium enhancement of the pituitary and adrenal glands.

Treatment

Iatrogenic Cushing syndrome should be managed by withdrawal of steroid therapy or to use a minimal effective dose if discontinuation of steroid treatment is not possible. A tumour of the adrenal gland should, of course, be excised when this is possible. In most cases of adrenal hyperplasia a satisfactory result can only be obtained by total bilateral adrenalectomy followed by replacement therapy (as in Addison disease). Unfortunately, it appears that this treatment may be followed by the subsequent appearance of pituitary tumours and severe hyperpigmentation (Nelson syndrome). The prognosis of Cushing syndrome when the cause is tumour will depend upon its nature (e.g., adrenal carcinoma), extent and removability. Pituitary Cushing syndrome is best treated by trans-sphenoidal surgical removal of the pituitary adenoma.

Adrenal Insufficiency

Adrenal insufficiency can be caused by disorders involving the hypothalamus and pituitary gland (Table 21.1) or those

---

Table 21.12: Causes of primary adrenal insufficiency

1. Congenital
   - Adrenal hypoplasia including DAX-1 and SF-1 mutations
   - Congenital adrenal hyperplasia
   - Familial glucocorticoid deficiency
   - Allgrove (Triple A) syndrome
2. Acquired
   - Autoimmune adrenalitis associated with autoimmune polyendocrine syndromes
   - Adrenoleucodystrophy
   - Infections e.g., tuberculosis
   - Adrenal haemorrhage, thrombosis
   - Surgery and drugs (cyproterone, ketoconazole, mitotane)

---

affecting primarily the adrenal gland. The causes of primary adrenal insufficiency are shown in Table 21.12.

Clinical Features

In the most common form of autoimmune polyendocrine syndrome, the children present with cutaneous candidiasis, hypoparathyroidism (tetany and convulsions) and adrenal insufficiency. Allgrove syndrome is characterized by alachrima, achalasia, ACTH-resistance and neurological symptoms. In the older child the manifestations closely resemble those seen in the adult – extreme asthenia, cachexia, hypotension and microcardia. Pigmentation of skin and mucous membranes tends to be less marked in children. Dangerous adrenal crises may occur, often precipitated by infections. Hypoglycaemic convulsions may first bring the child to the physicians.

In the congenital form of the disease, acute adrenal failure may develop with alarming rapidly during the neonatal period. Newborn infants with adrenal insufficiency frequently present with hypoglycaemia and prolonged neonatal jaundice. Increased skin pigmentation is also seen. Vomiting, diarrhoea and extreme dehydration can lead easily to an erroneous diagnosis such as pyloric stenosis, high intestinal obstruction or gastroenteritis. The pointer to adrenal insufficiency is the presence of abundant sodium and chloride in the urine, and hyponatremia, hyperkalaemia in the serum. Tuberculous adrenalitis is now a rare cause of primary adrenal insufficiency in childhood. Exogenous corticosteroid therapy can induce adrenal suppression in patients if used in dosages above the cortisol secretion rate for over three weeks.

Diagnosis

During a crisis, characteristic blood chemical changes include low serum chloride and sodium, elevated serum potassium (with changes in the ECG) and hypoglycaemia. In the absence of a crisis the blood chemistry may not be grossly abnormal and more refined tests are necessary. In primary adrenal insufficiency, the plasma ACTH concentration will be elevated. The early morning plasma cortisol level will be low and fails to rise in response to low dose Synacthen stimulation (1 microgram/1.73 m² intravenously). Failure of the plasma cortisol to increase by 200 nmol/L and reach an absolute level of more than 500 nmol/L in response to Synacthen is suggestive of adrenal insufficiency. If secondary adrenal insufficiency is suspected, appropriate investigations of the hypo-thalamic pituitary axis like the glucagon stimulation test or insulin tolerance test should be performed.

In further assessment of the etiology of primary adrenal insufficiency, recommended investigations include:
(1) plasma very long chain fatty acids
(2) autoantibody levels against adrenal, thyroid, gastric parietal cell, islet cell
(3) serum thyroid hormones, calcium, phosphate, vitamin B$_{12}$ and folate concentrations
(4) recumbant and erect plasma renin activity, aldosterone, electrolytes and urine sodium concentrations to assess mineralocorticoid activity
(5) plasma lactate

Treatment

In the management of acute adrenal crisis, there should be adequate replacement of fluid, sodium and glucose and hydrocortisone by the intravenous route. In situations of stress, it has been suggested that the dose of hydrocortisone (25-30mg/m² every 6 hours) be given by continuous infusion rather than by bolus. The usual oral replacement dose of hydrocortisone is 8-10 mg/m²/day in divided doses and the fludrocortisone dosage is 100-200 μg per day. If a child is unwell during an intercurrent illness, the oral hydrocortisone replacement dosage should be tripled until the child is better. Excessive replacement steroid dosage will stunt physical growth and should be avoided.

Congenital Adrenal Hyperplasia (CAH)

Deficiencies of the enzymes involved in adrenal stero-idogensis will lead to different varieties of congenital adrenal hyperplasia (Fig. 21.6). 21α-hydroxylase deficiency accounts for 95% of the cases of CAH seen in childhood and will be discussed in detail. The incidence varies between 1:15,000 to 1:20,000 births and is inherited in an autosomal recessive manner. 21α-hydroxylase deficiency results from mutations of the CYP21B gene which is situated on chromosome 6 in close proximity to the HLA genes. There is a reasonable genotype-phenotype correlation with drastic mutations causing salt-wasting 21 hydroxylase deficiency (21OHD) and severe mutations leading to virilising form of the disease. Non-classic form of 21α-hydroxylase deficiency occurs if one of two mutations is mild and female patients present with premature adrenarche or hyperandrogenism in ado-lescence.

Clinical Features

Male infants with 21α-hydroxylase deficiency appear normal at birth apart from rather marked pigmentation of the scrotum. After a short time virilization is revealed in the virilising form of 21OHD by enlargement of the penis, growth of pubic hair, excessive muscular development and advanced skeletal maturation due to the action of the excess androgens. The testes, however, remain small and undeveloped. The increased stature ultimately gives way to short adult stature due to premature fusion of the epiphyses. In the salt wasting form of the disease, male patients present in a salt-losing crisis at the end of the first week or in the second week of life with vomiting, diarrhoea, severe dehydration and shock. The correct diagnosis is easy enough in the virilised female infant but in the male an erroneous diagnosis of pyloric stenosis, gastroenteritis or septicaemia is easily made. The serum sodium and chloride levels are reduced, and the serum potassium level is high with corresponding ECG changes. There is also metabolic acidosis, elevated serum urea and increased fractional excretion of sodium. The salt-losing form of 21OHD accounts for 60% to 75% of cases. In all types of adrenal hyperplasia excessive skin pigmentation is common.

In female infants the excessive androgenic effects upon the fetus produce more striking and unwelcome changes. In mild cases there is marked clitoral enlargement. In an extensively virilized newborn female, there is marked clitoral enlargement, fusion of the labia majora and the vagina and urethra may enter a single common urogenital sinus (Fig. 21.8). An extensively virilized infant can readily be mistaken for a cryptorchid male. Similarly, females with drastic CYP21B mutations present in salt-losing crisis in the neonatal period. Without treatment, a girl with virilising 21OHD becomes progressively masculinized with hirsutism, clitoromegaly, muscularity and advanced bone age.

Diagnosis

In countries where there is screening for congenital adrenal hyperplasia in the neonatal period, patients with the salt-losing form but not necessarily the virilzing form of 21 OHD will be identified. Biochemical confirmation of a clinically diagnosed case is shown by elevated plasma ACTH, 17α-hydroxyprogesterone (17 α OHD), high plasma renin activity levels and low plasma cortisol and aldosterone levels in patients with salt-wasting 21OHD. In simple virilising 21OHD, the morning 17α-hydroxy-progesterone levels are high but the plasma renin activity and serum electrolytes may be normal. Advanced skeletal maturation is seen in untreated or undertreated patients with 21OHD. In a virilized female, chromosomal analysis and ultrasound examination of the pelvis for the presence of female internal genital organs are necessary.

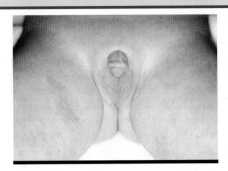

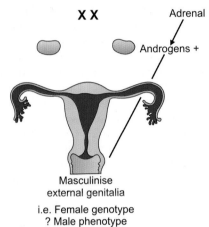

X X   Adrenal

Androgens +

Masculinise
external genitalia

i.e. Female genotype
? Male phenotype

Fig. 21.8: Masculinisation of female genitalia
due to congenital adrenal hyperplasia

Treatment

Hydrocortisone is administrated to children in a dose of
10-20 mg/m^2/day divided into two or three doses. Patients
are monitored by measuring serum electrolytes and 17α
OHP levels every 3 to 4 months. In children and young
adolescents growth velocity and bone age (annually) are
followed over time to ensure that they are receiving the
proper dose. In the salt-wasting form of congenital adrenal
hyperplasia mineralocorticoid replacement is also
necessary. 9α-fludrocortisone in a dose of 0.05-0.2 mg daily
orally is required with careful monitoring of blood
pressure, plasma renin activity, serum and urine
electrolytes. In addition, it is recommended that salt
supplement of 3-5 mmol/kg/day be given to salt-losing
21OHD patients in the first 2-3 years of life. Higher dosages
of hydrocortisone is required in times of stress. In
most virilised females who have been treated with
suppressive glucocorticoids from an early age it is
important to correct the external genitalia, by 2 to 6 months
of age (recession clitoroplasty and feminizing vaginoplasty). Vaginal dilatation is contraindicated in childhood.
Examination of the genitalia should only be done to
assess pubertal development or if under-treatment is
suspected.

DISORDER OF SEX DEVELOPMENT

Sexual development is a complex process which is
dependent on a variety of molecular signals working in
concert to specify sex-specific differentiation and
organogenesis. Genes of several transcription factors
including steroidogenic factor 1 (SF1) and Wilm's tumor 1
(WT1) are required for the formation of the indifferent
genital ridges in humans. The sex determining region of
the Y chromosome gene (SRY) expression must reach a
threshold level at a critical time in the cascade of early
events leading to testis differentiation, before male sex
determination can occur. SOX9 encodes a transcription
factor downstream of SRY and is a crucial component of
the male sex-determining pathway. Loss of function
mutation in SOX9 results in gonadal dysgenesis and
campomelic dysplasia. Other transcription factors and
signalling molecules are important in the differentiation
of peritubular myoid cells, endothelial cells, Leydig cells,
Sertoli cells and germ cells within the developing testes.
Both the Mullerian and Wolffian ducts are present in male
and female embryos. Antimullerian hormone (AMH)
which is secreted by Sertoli cells of the testes, stimulates
the production of matrix metalloproteinase 2 (MMP2)
which induces apoptosis in the Mullerian duct epithelial
cells. The Wolffian ducts develop into the epididymis, vas
deferens and seminal vesicles under the influence of
testosterone produced by Leydig cells of the developing
testes. A number of enzymes are responsible for testosterone biosynthesis (Fig. 21.6) and mutations in these
genes will result in under-masculinization of a genetic
male. Testosterone is converted to dihydrotestosterone
(DHT) by 5α-reductase encoded by the SRD5A2 gene. DHT
signals through the androgen receptor present in the
developing external genitalia to bring about the development of the phallus and scrotum which is completed by
about 8 weeks gestation. Further development of the penis
in males is stimulated by gonadotropin secreted from the
foetal pituitary from mid-gestation onwards. The trans-
abdominal phase of descent of the testes is controlled by
the enlargement of the caudal genito-inguinal ligament
and the gubernaculum mediated by the hormone insulin-
like 3 produced by the Leydig cells. The inguinoscrotal
phase of descent of the testes is controlled by the
neurotransmitter calcitonin gene-related peptide produced
under the control of androgens.

In the absence of SRY, the Wolffian ducts regress and
the Mullerian ductal system develops into the uterus,
fallopian tubes and part of the vagina. Although ovarian
and female genital development has been regarded as a
default pathway, recent evidence suggests that there are
genes important in female sexual development.

A recent suggested classification of disorder of sex
development is shown in Table 21.13.

Table 21.13: Classification of disorder of sex development (DSD) [adapted from Lee PA et al. Pediatrics 2006;118:e488]

Sex Chromosome DSD	Turner syndrome 45X and variants Klinefelter syndrome 47XXY45X / 46XY mixed gonadal dysgenesis 46XX/ 46XY ovotesticular DSD
46XY DSD	Disorders of gonadal development • Complete gonadal dysgenesis • Partial gonadal dysgenesis • Ovotesticular DSD Disorder of androgen synthesis or action • Defect in androgen action • Androgen biosynthetic defects • Luteinising hormone receptor gene mutations • Mutations of AMH or its receptor gene
46XX DSD	Disorder of gonadal development ovotesticular DSD • Ovotesticular DSD • Testicular DSD (SRY+, SOX9 mutation) • Gonadal dysgenesisAndrogen excess e.g. 21OHD

A newborn with disorder of sex development should be referred for assessment and management by a multi-disciplinary team of surgeon, paediatric endocrinologist, geneticist, neonatologist, psychologist and nurse specialist in a tertiary centre. Although not easy, an attempt should be made to decide whether the newborn infant is a virilized female or an undermasculinized male. The degree of masculinization can be assessed according to the Prader staging. Whenever a gonad is palpable, then the newborn is a genetic male. The nature of the opening below the clitorophallus, position of the anus should be noted and the urethral and vaginal opening identified if possible. Increased skin pigmentation in a virilized female newborn is suggestive of 21OHD and the circulatory and hydration status should be assessed. Any dysmorphic feature should be noted.

Diagnosis

Most of the virilized female infants will have 21OHD while a definitive molecular diagnosis can only be reached in less than half of the children with 46XY DSD. Initial investigations should include karyotyping with X- and Y-specific probe detection and measurement of plasma 17α-hydroxyprogesterone, testosterone, DHT, gonado-tropins, antiMullerian hormone, ACTH, cortisol and serum electrolytes concentrations. An ultrasound examination of the pelvis should be performed to assess the presence or absence female internal genital organs. Further assessments of urinary steroid profile or androgen levels after human chorionic gonadotropin stimulation may be required beyond the first one to two months of life.

Management

Gender assignment should be based on the diagnosis, likely functional outcome to the genital organ, testosterone responsiveness, potential for fertility, surgical options and views of the parents. Existing data favour male rearing in all males with isolated micropenis. Testosterone enanthate 25mg intramuscularly monthly for three doses will establish testosterone responsiveness and increase phallus size to facilitate surgical repair of chordee and urethral reconstruction. Virillzed females should have recession clitoroplasty and vaginoplasty by 6 months of age. The timing of genital surgery in a 46XY DSD patient assigned the female sex of rearing remains controversial. Some people are of the view that despite gender assignment early in life, genital surgery should be deferred and only be performed after consent from the patient "herself". However with proper counselling and frank discussion after adequate information has been given to the parents, a decision to have genital surgery in a patient with 46XY DSD in infancy can usually be reached by the multi-disciplinary team and the parents. Sex hormone replace-ment should be initiated at the appropriate age when indicated.

Psychological support should be provided to the family. Assessment of gender identity, gender role and sexual orientation should be performed when the child is sufficiently psychologically developed. Support groups have an important role in the care of patients with disorders of sex development. Transition care is important and the patients must be provided with detailed information on their diagnosis, previous treatment and expected outcome.

DIABETES MELLITUS

Diabetes Mellitus is a common chronic childhood disorder in the Western World but is less common among Asians. A classification of diabetes is shown in Table 21.14 and diabetes mellitus can develop as a result of several pathogenic processes. The diagnostic criteria for diabetes mellitus are shown in Table 21.15.

Type 1 Diabetes Mellitus

The aetiology of type 1 diabetes mellitus has remained elusive but genetic and environmental influences are thought to be important. In Caucasians, there is an association between type 1 diabetes mellitus and the HLA histocompatability complex on chromosome 6 and the insulin gene variable number of tandem repeats (VNTR) polymorphism on chromosome 11. These associations are less strong in Asian diabetic patients. It is likely that type 1 diabetes is a polygenic disorder. Ethnic groups with low incidence of disease take on a higher incidence when they emmigrate to another country where the incidence of diabetes is higher. This suggests that environmental factors

Table 21.14: Classification of diabetes mellitus

I   Type 1 diabetes mellitus (absolute insulin deficiency) auto-immune idiopathic

II   Type 2 diabetes mellitus (insulin resistance with relative insulin deficiency)

III   Other specific types genetic defects of β-cell function genetic defects of insulin action diseases of the endocrine pancreas endocrinopathies drug - or chemical-induced infections uncommon immune-mediated diabetes genetic syndromes

IV   Gestational diabetes

Table 21.15: Diagnosis of diabetes mellitus

I   Classical symptoms of polyuria, polydipsia and presence of glycosuria and ketonuria, a random sugar greater than 11 mmol/L

II   In cases of asymptomatic glycosuria
     (a) Fasting blood sugar greater 7 mmol/L
     (b) 2-hr blood sugar after oral glucose load (1.75 G/kg) greater than 11 mmol/L

III   Pre-diabetes
     (a) Impaired fasting glycaemia (IFG) if fasting blood sugar between 5.6 mmol/L and 6.9 mmol/L
     (b) Impaired glucose tolerance (IGT) if blood sugar two hours after oral glucose load of 7.8 mmol/L to 11 mmol/L

are important. There is a wide geographic difference in the incidence of childhood and adolescent diabetes mellitus. The lowest incidence is found in Asia (0.23 to 1.4 per 100,000 children in China) and highest in Sardinia and Finland (over 40 per 100,000 children). A significant increase in the incidence in recent years has been documented in 65% of the populations worldwide and the relative increase is more evident in populations with a low incidence of type 1 diabetes mellitus.

Clinical Features

Diabetes mellitus is potentially a much more acute disease in the child than in the adult. The onset is marked by polyuria, excessive thirst and rapid loss of weight. Other patients may present with secondary nocturnal enuresis, vomiting, abdominal pain and abdominal distension which can mimic an acute abdomen. In females, pruritis vulvae may be a presenting complaint. The presentation of diabetes mellitus can be preceded by an intercurrent infection. In the untreated state, a child can present with diabetic ketoacidosis and be admitted in a state of profound dehydration with sunken eyes, dry tongue, and scaphoid abdomen. The child can lapse into a coma. Respiration is rapid, sighing and pauseless. The blood pH is reduced. The serum sodium and chloride levels are also reduced.

Diagnosis

In the presence of classical symptoms of polyuria, polydipsia and the documentation of glycosuria and ketonuria, a random blood sugar more than 11 mmol/L is diagnostic of type 1 diabetes mellitus. A glucose tolerance test is not usually necessary for diagnosis. Diabetic ketoacidosis is present if the blood pH is <7.3, bicarbonate <15mmol/L in the presence of hyperglycaemia (blood sugar >11mmmol/L) and heavy glycosuria and ketonuria. At diagnosis, the serum electrolytes, acid base status, haemoglobin $A_{1C,}$ glutamic acid decarboxylase (GAD), anti-islet cell (ICA) and anti-insulin (IAA) antibodies should be measured. These antibodies are present in 85% to 90% of newly diagnosed Caucasian diabetic children and adolescents but the autoimmune form of diabetes is less common in Asians. Tests for thyroid function, thyroid antibodies and antigliadin and anti-endomyseal antibodies for coeliac disease should also be performed. Children may have evidence of infection at presentation and appropriate investigations should also be undertaken.

Management

Diabetic ketoacidosis require prompt recognition and treatment and carries a small risk of death from cerebral oedema, aspiration and cardiac arrhythmia. In a semiconscious or unconscious patient, the gastric contents should be emptied by nasogastric suction. If a patient is severely dehydrated and suspected to be in insipient shock, resuscitation with bolus normal saline (10-20 ml/kg intravenously) should be instituted. Otherwise the fluid deficit should be replenished over 48 hours with normal saline initially and changed to half normal saline in 10% dextrose when the blood sugar has been brought down to 12 to 15 mmol/L by intravenous insulin infusion (0.1 unit/kg/hour). The insulin infusion should be maintained until the ketoacidosis is controlled. There is no evidence that bicarbonate is necessary for the treatment of diabetic ketoacidosis. Potassium replacement (40 mmol per litre of fluid) is only started when a good urine output is established. The treatment can be switched to subcutaneous insulin once the patient is fully conscious, out of ketoacidosis and able to tolerate oral feeding.

The cornerstones of diabetes management include patient education, insulin, diet, exercise and monitoring of metabolic control. The initial education can be done either as an inpatient or on an outpatient basis. At diagnosis, the patient and parents should be taught the survival skills including insulin injection, home blood glucose monitoring, recognition of hypoglycaemia, ketoacidosis and their management, diet, adjustment of insulin dosage especially during illness and for activities. Continued support should be given to the patients and their parents with a continuing educational curriculum and through the diabetes management telephone hotline.

Table 21.16: Actions of commonly used insulin preparations			
Insulin Preparations	Onset	Peak	Duration
Insulin lispro (Lilly)	15 min	30-70 min	2-5 hr
Insulin aspart (NovoNordisk)	15 min	60-180 min	3-5 hr
Actrapid HM (NovoNordisk)	30 min	2-4 hr	5-8 hr
Humulin S (Lilly)	30 min	2-4 hr	5-8 hr
Humulin N (Lilly)	1-2 hr	4-12 hr	12-18 hr
Protaphane HM (NovoNordisk)	1-2 hr	4-12 hr	12-18 hr
Insulin glargine (Aventis)	1-2 hr	No peak	18-24 hr
Insulin determir (NovoNordisk)	1-2 hr	No peak	18 hr
Premixed insulin containing different proportion of soluble neutral insulin and isophane insulin			

Insulin Treatment

The patients and their parents should be knowledgeable about the action of the various types of insulin that are available (Table 21.16)

Insulin can be given subcutaneously into the thighs and lower abdominal wall by fine needle syringes, pen injectors, jet injectors or by insulin infusion pump. Common insulin regimes include a mixture of short-acting and intermediate-acting insulin given before breakfast and the evening meal. In recent years, basal-bolus regime with multiple injections of insulin are preferred with a peakless long acting insulin analogue given once or twice a day together with a short-acting insulin analogue given before the three main meals. Insulin pump treatment is increasingly used in motivated patients who desire tight control and has been used successfully even in young children with brittle diabetes. Prepubertal diabetic children will require 0.7 to 1 unit of insulin/kg/day. Children in puberty will require 30% to 50% more insulin.

Nutritional Management

The diet should provide adequate nutrition and calories for optimal growth. The total energy intake should comprise 55% complex unrefined carbohydrates, 15% protein and 30% fat with less than 10% in both saturated and polyunsaturated fat. Children with diabetes should be educated on healthy eating with a diet high in vegetables, fruits and fibre. In patients on twice daily injections of short-acting and intermediate-acting insulin, the carbohydrate intake should be distributed into three main meals and three snacks in order to avoid hypoglycaemia between the main meals. Snacks may not be needed in patients on basal-bolus regime using peakless long-acting and short-acting insulin analogue before meals.

Monitoring of Metabolic Control and Complications

Self monitoring of blood sugar regularly before and two hours after meals and occasionally at 3 am are necessary for adjustment of insulin dosage. Patients and their parents should be educated and empowered to make day to day dietary and insulin adjustments to optimize metabolic control and in response to illness or physical activity. In young children under 6 years of age, tight metabolic control will result in frequent hypoglycaemia and the aim of management is to achieve reasonable symptomatic control without hypoglycaemia. Children and their parents should be seen regularly every two to three months by the diabetes care team of nurse educator, dietitian and paediatrician. Short and medium term metabolic control can be reflected by measurements of serum fructosamine or plasma haemoglobin A_{1C} concentrations. The paediatrician should also monitor for any psychological issues experienced by the patients or their family members and make appropriate referral for psychological counselling.

Annual screening for complications of diabetes including retinopathy, neuropathy, nephropathy, dyslipidaemia, hypertension, thyroid dysfunction and the development of other associated disorders like coeliac disease should be initiated after 5 years of disease in prepubertal children and after 2 years of disease in pubertal children. Screening for retinopathy is best done by annual fundus photography or by ophthalmoscopic examination after pharmacological dilatation of the pupils by an experienced ophthalmologist. Albumin excretion rate greater than 200 μg/min in two timed overnight urine collections indicates early diabetic nephropathy. Impairment of fine touch, vibration threshold and tendon jerks should be looked for.

Type 2 Diabetes Mellitus

Type 2 diabetes is usually regarded as a disease of people older than 40 years of age. However, with the increase in prevalence of obesity in childhood and adolescence, type 2 diabetes is increasingly reported in adolescents especially of minority or Polynesian origins. In countries where there is annual screening for type 2 diabetes in childhood and adolescence like Japan and Taiwan, the incidence of type 2 diabetes has surpassed that of type 1 diabetes. It has been recommended that obese children and adolescents with a family history of type 2 diabetes and presence of acanthosis nigricans or other cardiovascular risk factors be screened for type 2 diabetes every one to two years.

Clinical Features

Although most of the children and adolescents with type 2 diabetes do not have any symptoms, 5 to 25% can present with ketoacidosis. Up to 85% of the patients have first or second degree relatives with type 2 diabetes. Acanthosis nigricans, polycystic ovary syndrome are common associated disorders. Most patients have absent β-cell autoantibodies and high fasting insulin and C-peptide concentrations. A rarer form of maturity onset diabetes of youth (MODY) is characterised by onset of non-insulin dependent diabetes before 25 years of age with autosomal dominant mode of inheritance involving a minimum of two but preferably three consecutive generations affected by type 2 diabetes in the family. The majority of the individuals with insulin resistance who can compensate by an adequate insulin secretion do not develop type 2 diabetes mellitus but they are still prone to the complications associated with type 2 diabetes.

Management

Patients are encouraged to undertake regular exercise of at least 30 to 40 minutes per day. Obese individuals should seek dietary advice from a dietitian for a caloric and carbohydrate restricted diet to achieve a gradual weight loss of 0.5 to 2.0kg per month. The importance of glycaemic control in the prevention of diabetes complications has been shown in both types 1 and type 2 diabetes. Patients who are not adequately controlled (HbA$_{1C}$ > 7%) on life-style changes and diet should be treated with oral antidiabetic agents (biguanides, sulphonyureas, thiazolidenediones, glucosidase inhibitors). Insulin therapy should be initiated if metabolic control cannot be achieved by diet and oral antidiabetic drugs. Hypertension and dyslipidaemic should be aggressively managed.

HYPOGLYCAEMIA

Blood glucose is the main metabolic fuel of the brain and it is maintained in a relatively narrow normal range of 4.4 mmol/L to 6.7 mmol/L by a number of hormones including insulin, glucagon, cortisol, growth hormone and catecholamines. Hypoglycaemia is defined as a blood sugar below 2.6 mmol/L and would require further investigation but autonomic and neuroglycopenic symptoms will appear when the blood sugar falls below 3.5 mmol/L. The common causes of hypoglycaemia in infants and children are shown in Table 21.17.

Clinical Features

Mild to moderate hypoglycaemia can result in autonomic nervous system activation including hunger, trembling of extremities, pallor, sweating and palpitations and manifestation of neuroglycopenic symptoms. Neuroglycopenia leads to confusion, irritability and abnormal behaviour, jitteriness, headaches, paraesthesia of the extremities and dizziness. Severe hypoglycaemia can result in coma and convulsion. Prolonged and severe hypoglycaemia with coma and convulsion can lead to permanent neurological sequelae.

Investigations

Although hypoglycaemia require prompt treatment once identified (usually by a low glucometer sugar reading at the bedside), it is important to document the true blood sugar and obtaining critical samples (blood for growth hormone, cortisol, insulin, free fatty acids, blood ketones and β-hydroxybutyrate, lactate, ammonia and urine for ketones and toxicology). Non-ketotic hypoglycaemia is due to hyperinsulinism or fatty acids oxidation defects. Hyperinsulinaemic hypoglycaemia is diagnosed when in the presence hypoglycaemia, insulin level is inappropriately elevated (>3 mU/ml), plasma free fatty acids (<1.5 mmol/L) and β-hydroxybutyrate (<2.0 mmol/L) are low, a high glucose infusion rate is required to maintain euglycaemia (>10-12 mg/kg/min) and the presence of an

Table 21.17: Causes of hypoglycaemia in infants and children

1. Intrauterine growth retardation and prematurity
2. Perinatal asphyxia
3. Infant of diabetic mother
4. Intrauterine infection and sepsis
5. Rhesus incompatibility
6. Inborn errors of metabolism
   (a) amino acids and organic
   (b) disorders of carbohydrate metabolism e.g., glaucoma storage disease, fructose intolerance, lactosaemia
   (c) fatty acid oxidation defects
   (d) urea cycle defects
7. Endocrine causes
   (a) hypopituitarism
   (b) growth hormone or adrenal insufficiency
   (c) persistent hyperinsulinaemic hypoglycaemia of infantry
   (d) Beckwith-Wiedemann syndrome
   (e) Insulinoma
8. Ketotic hypoglycaemia
9. Drugs including alcohol, aspirin, β-blockers
10. Sepsis especially due to gram-negative organisms

exaggerated glucose response to glucagon. Hyper-insulinaemic hypoglycaemia with hyperammonaemia is suggestive of a gain of function mutation of the glutamate dehydrogenase gene. Fatty acid oxidation defect can be diagnosed by measurement of plasma acylcarnitine profile and urine organic acids. Ketotic hypoglycaemia commonly occurs in young children following prolonged fasting, decreased intake or repeated vomiting. It is always important to look for sepsis (especially with gram-negative organisms) as a treatable cause of hypoglycaemia. Further assessment for hypopituitarism should be carried out where indicated.

Management

Hypoglycaemia should be treated promptly after obtaining the critical samples by intravenous infusion of 2-4 ml/kg of 10% dextrose followed by an adequate glucose infusion to maintain euglycaemia. Treatment should also the aimed at the underlying cause of the hypoglycaemia. Oral diazoxide (10-15 mg/kg/day) and octreotide given by subcutaneous injection have been successfully used to manage the persistent hyperinsulinaemic hypoglycaemia of infancy and near total pancreatectomy is the only option in drug resistant cases. Patients with ketotic hypoglycaemia should avoid prolonged fasting.

Chapter 22

Paediatric Orthopaedics

Benjamin Joseph

INTRODUCTION

Children may present with a variety of symptoms related to the musculoskeletal system (Box 22.1). It is important to be aware of symptoms that are likely to be innocuous and those that may herald serious underlying disease that requires early treatment. Several conditions need no active treatment; reassurance to allay parental anxiety is all that is required. Another group of conditions may need to be monitored as spontaneous improvement occurs with growth in most cases but in a few instances deterioration may occur, warranting some intervention. The third group of conditions always needs elective, early or urgent immediate treatment. In other words, the children may be managed in one of three ways;

1. Reassurance (no active intervention),
2. Observation (often no treatment is needed but treat later in selected situations),
3. Active intervention (elective intervention, early intervention or urgent intervention).

It is vitally important that this third group is identified and referred to the Paediatric Orthopaedic Surgeon without any delay. In order to try to work out which of these groups the symptom of a particular child would fall into, there are some basic questions that need to be answered. Throughout this chapter the relevant questions to be asked regarding each symptom would be indicated and an attempt will be made to clarify which of these three approaches is appropriate for the particular condition.

> **Box 22.1: Common symptoms with which children may be brought to an orthopaedic surgeon**
>
> - Deformities
> - Gait abnormalities
> - Musculoskeletal pain
> - Paralysis and pseudoparalysis
> - Joint stiffness and limitation of movement
> - Other e.g. Soft tissue swelling/bony swelling/frequent fractures/ limb deficiencies

DEFORMITIES

By far the commonest reason for a child being referred for an orthopaedic opinion is the presence of a deformity. The questions that need to be asked regarding a child with a deformity of the upper or lower limbs are listed in Table 22.1.

Some of the common deformities seen in Paediatric Orthopaedic clinics are shown in Table 22.2. It is clear that a quarter of these conditions need no active treatment. However, it needs to be emphasised that these benign conditions form a much larger proportion of the cases seen in the clinic.

GAIT ABNORMALITIES

The common gait abnormalities seen in children are shown in Box 22.2. The questions that need to be asked while evaluating a child with a gait abnormality are listed in Table 22.3. With the exception of a painful limp, all other gait abnormalities do not require urgent intervention and hence can be evaluated without undue haste.

Table 22.1: Questions to be asked regarding a limb deformity in a child	
Question	*Relevance*
Is the deformity unilateral or bilateral?	Unilateral deformity is more likely to be pathological.
Was the deformity present from birth?	Most deformities that are present from birth either resolve or remain static; only a few progress.
Is the deformity remaining static or is it resolving or progressing?	A deformity that is progressing may indicate that the growth mechanism is affected and would probably need early treatment. A deformity that is resolving just needs to be periodically observed.

Table 22.2: Common deformities seen in the Paediatric Orthopaedic clinic

Region	Aetiology	Condition	Management
Foot	Congenital	Clubfoot	Treat early
		Metatarsus adductus	Observe/Treat electively
		Calcaneovalgus	Observe
		Vertical talus	Treat electively
	Developmental	Mobile flatfoot	Observe
		Rigid flatfoot	Treat electively
	Paralytic	Equinus	Treat electively
		Equinovarus or equinovalgus	Treat electively
		Calcaneus or calcaneovalgus	Treat early
		Cavus	Treat electively
Leg	Congenital	Anterolateral bowing	Treat early
		Posteromedial bowing	Observe
		Internal tibial torsion	Observe
Knee	Congenital	Hyperextension	Treat early
		Flexion	Treat electively
	Developmental	Physiological genu varum or valgum	Observe
		Unilateral genu valgum or varum	Treat electively
Hip	Congenital	Acetabular dysplasia with neonatal hip instability	Treat early
		Femoral anteversion	Observe
	Developmental	Coxa vara	Treat electively
Spine	Congenital	Scoliosis	Treat electively
	Developmental	Infantile scoliosis	Observe
		Adolescent scoliosis	Treat early
	Paralytic	Scoliosis	Treat early

Table 22.3: Questions to be asked while evaluating a child with a gait abnormality

Question	Relevance
Does the child have pain on walking?	If there is pain on walking, urgent investigations are needed to establish the definitive diagnosis as some conditions that cause a painful limp require immediate treatment.
Is the gait abnormality unilateral or bilateral?	Unilateral gait abnormality is more likely to be pathological.
Has the gait abnormality been present from when the child started to walk?	If present from when the child started to walk it is likely to be due to a congenital abnormality.
Does the child run, play and do normal activities with peers?	If the child does play normally it indicates that there is negligible pain and that the underlying problem is probably not serious.
Is there an improvement in the gait pattern with growth?	If the gait improves as the child grows the underlying problem is likely to be "physiological".
Is there a deterioration of the gait pattern with growth?	If gait deteriorates as the child grows there is some underlying pathology.

Box 22.2: Common gait abnormalities seen in children

- Delayed walking
- Toe-walking
- In-toeing gait
- Out-toeing gait
- Short-limbed gait
- Waddling gait
- Painful (antalgic gait)
- Paralytic gait patterns: High stepping gait/hand-to-knee gait/crouch gait/scissor gait etc.

Delayed Walking

Delayed walking is quite alarming for parents and a thorough examination of these children is warranted to determine if there is global developmental delay. The most common cause of delayed walking that is associated with global developmental delay is cerebral palsy. Some children with some forms of severe ligament laxity syndromes tend to walk late without demonstrating any other developmental delay. It had been assumed in the past that developmental dysplasia of the hip with an established dislocation delays walking. However, there is little evidence to support this assumption.

Toe-walking

Children who walk on their toes again need to be evaluated carefully. Among causes for toe-walking are cerebral palsy, some forms of myopathies and muscular dystrophies and a very benign condition known as habitual toe-walking. Habitual toe walking is a diagnosis of exclusion and it is important that the more serious causes of toe-walking are definitely excluded before this diagnosis is made. Initially these children can bring their heels down to the ground while standing but go onto their toes when they start walking. In due course the Achilles tendon may get contracted and then they would also stand on tip toe. At this stage lengthening of the Achilles tendon is indicated.

In-toeing Gait

This is a very common complaint and parents are often very concerned about this gait abnormality. The child typically sits in the "W" position (Fig. 22.1) and examination of the range of passive hip motion would demonstrate excessive internal rotation of the hip with a reduction in the range of external rotation. This is characteristic of excessive femoral anteversion. The anteversion tends to reduce spontaneously as the child grows. There is no functional disability though these children tend to be a bit clumsy and some parents feel that they tend to trip more frequently. The parents need to be reassured that gradual resolution of the torsional deformity

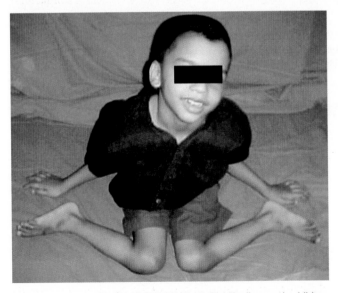

Fig. 22.1: This posture while sitting is characteristically seen in children with excessive femoral anteversion. It is referred to as the "W" pattern because the legs and the thighs of both the limbs together are aligned in the form of a "W"

will occur. Bracing and shoe modifications that have been tried in the past have been quite clearly shown to be totally ineffective and should not be used. Surgical intervention is not justified in these children except in the very rare instance where the deformity persists till the age of ten years and is still severe at this age.

Out-toeing Gait

This is less frequently seen and may be due to retroversion of the femur or external tibial torsion. Again, there is no functional disability in these children and no active treatment is required.

Short-limbed Gait

A short-limbed gait indicates that there is a structural abnormality of one limb. While more commonly the shorter limb is at fault due to reduced growth, occasionally the longer limb may be abnormal. Lengthening of one limb is often seen in association with vascular malformations such as hemangioma, lymphangioma and arterio-venous fistula. The decision to correct the limb-length inequality is governed by the magnitude of the discrepancy that is likely to be present at skeletal maturity. If the difference at skeletal maturity is likely to exceed 2 to 3 centimeters, intervention may be considered.

Waddling Gait

A waddling gait or a Trendelenburg gait is characteristically seen when the hip abductor power is weak. This may be seen in the relatively uncommon situation where there is actual paralysis of the hip abductors. Far more commonly, this gait pattern is seen when the hip abductor mechanism is rendered ineffective either due to dislocation of the hip or due to a reduction of the angle between the neck and shaft of the femur as in coxa vara deformity. This gait pattern signals serious hip pathology and so children with a waddling gait must be evaluated carefully and must have radiographs of the pelvis to exclude these conditions that require surgical intervention.

Antalgic Gait

An antalgic gait or painful gait signifies that bearing weight on the affected limb causes pain. Children who demonstrate this abnormality of gait should undergo a meticulous examination to identify the source of pain and in the vast majority of instances the site of pain can be located by clinical examination alone. Appropriate imaging may then be done to confirm the nature of underlying pathology. Treatment would depend on the nature of the pathological process that is producing pain. Of all conditions that can manifest with a painful limp the one that requires immediate surgical invention is osteo-

	Table 22.4: Causes of musculo-skeletal pain in children		
Region	Condition	Imaging modality to supplement clinical examination	Management approach
Foot	Sever's disease	X-ray	Observe
	Kohler's disease	X-ray	Observe
	Tarsal coalition	X-ray/CT scan	Treat electively
Calf	Growing pains	No imaging	Reassure
Tibia	Osteoid osteoma	X-ray/CT scan	Treat electively
	Acute osteomyelitis	No imaging/Ultrasound scan	Treat urgently
	Osteosarcoma	X-ray/CT/MRI	Treat urgently
	Ewings tumour	X-ray/CT/MRI	Treat urgently
Knee	Osgood-Schlatter	X-ray	Observe
	Septic arthritis	No imaging	Treat urgently
	Tubercular arthritis	X-ray	Treat early
	Referred Pain from the hip		
Hip	Transient synovitis	Ultrasound scan	Treat early
	Perthes' disease	X-ray	Treat early
	Slipped capital femoral epiphysis	X-ray	Treat urgently
	Septic arthritis	No imaging	Treat urgently
	Tubercular arthritis	X-ray	Treat early
Back	Disc prolapse	MRI	Treat early
	Pyogenic discitis	X-ray/CT/MRI	Treat early
Generalised bone pain	Osteogenesis impefecta	X-ray	Treat early
	Adolescent osteoporosis	X-ray/CT/Dexa	Treat early

It will also be evident that several of the conditions listed in Table 22. 4 require urgent or early treatment. This is distinctly different from that seen in the conditions listed in Table 22. 2.

The questions that need to be asked while evaluating a child with musculoskeletal pain are shown in Table 22.5.

Table 22.5: Questions to be asked while evaluating a child with musculoskeletal pain	
Question	Relevance
Can the pain be localised consistently?	Likely to be caused by localised pathology
Is the pain brought on by movement of a joint?	Likely to be due to pathology in the joint
Is the pain present at rest and on bearing weight on the limb?	Likely to be due to disease of bone
Is the child able to run and play normally but has pain at rest after physical activity?	The cause is likely to be innocuous.
Is the child unable to bear weight on the limb?	If the child cannot bear any weight on the limb, it is likely that there is serious underlying pathology.

articular infection. The urgency for establishing a diagnosis and the need for immediate intervention cannot be overemphasised.

Paralytic Gait Patterns

Depending on the pattern of paralysis, typical gait aberrations may occur. Paralysis of the ankle dorsiflexors will produce a high-stepping gait. A hand-on-thigh gait is seen when there is paralysis of the quadriceps muscle. Characteristic abnormal gait patterns such as scissor gait, crouch gait, stiff-knee gait and toe-toe gait are seen in cerebral palsy depending on which muscles are most spastic.

MUSCULOSKELETAL PAIN

When a child complains of pain in the limbs or back, it is imperative that a careful examination is performed and this should be followed by appropriate imaging. It will become clear from the list of painful conditions seen in children (Table 22.4) that most of these conditions can be confirmed by a combination of clinical examination and imaging.

PARALYSIS AND PSEUDOPARALYSIS

When an infant stops moving a limb, a distinction needs to be made between true paralysis and pseudoparalysis.

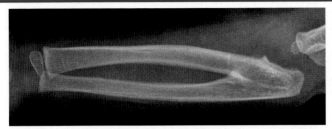

Fig. 22.2: Radiograph of a child's elbow showing congenital synostosis of the radius and ulna

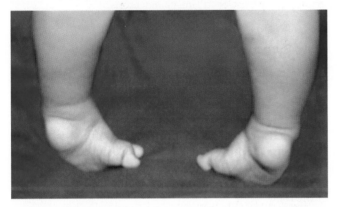

Fig. 22.3: Appearance of congenital clubfoot – equinus and varus deformities of the hindfoot and forefoot adduction are clearly seen

The later phenomenon is on account of pain and this is typically seen when there is osteo-articular infection. Since the infant cannot indicate the site of pain it is important to do a meticulous examination to try to ascertain the site of pain. In the older child with true paralysis, it is necessary to differentiate between flaccid, lower motor-neuron paralysis and spastic, upper motor-neuron paralysis.

JOINT STIFFNESS

Stiffness of a joint or limitation of joint movement can occur on account of abnormalities within the joint itself (intra-articular pathology) or due to contracture or shortening of soft tissue structures outside the joint (extra-articular). Intra-articular stiffness can be caused by adhesions between the articular surfaces or due to actual bony continuity between the bones that form the joint. Bony continuity can be of congenital origin due to failure of segmentation and formation of a joint space resulting in a synostosis. The common sites of synostosis include the proximal radio-ulnar joint, the carpus and the tarsus (Fig. 22.2). If the articular cartilage is dissolved in septic arthritis, the raw bony surfaces may fuse together. This is referred to as bony ankylosis. When either a congenital synostosis or an acquired bony ankylosis is present no movement will be present at all in the affected joint.

CONGENITAL ANOMALIES

Congenital Clubfoot

Treatment Approach: Treat Early

Congenital clubfoot (congenital talipes equinovarus) is probably the most common congenital anomaly of the musculoskeletal system that requires treatment (Fig. 22.3). Clubfoot may occur as an isolated anomaly (idiopathic clubfoot) or may occur in association with spina bifida or with multiple congenital contractures (MCC – formerly called arthrogryposis multiplex congenita). Idiopathic clubfoot is far more common than the neurogenic form that occurs with spina bifida or MCC. Idiopathic clubfoot may either be postural or rigid. The postural variety is due to intrauterine molding; the foot is structurally normal and responds well to non-operative management. On the other hand, the rigid variety is characterised by contractures of muscles and joint capsules and the bones of the foot are structurally abnormal. Despite this, a proportion of these rigid feet do respond to non-operative treatment.

The deformity is a complex one with individual deformities at the ankle, subtalar and the mid-tarsal joints (the calcaneo-cuboid joint and the talo-navicular joints function together in unison and are referred to as the mid-tarsal joint). These individual deformities are caused primarily by contractures of muscles that act on these joints; and secondary contractures of the joint capsules make the deformities more rigid (Table 22.6).

Management of clubfoot should first begin with a careful examination to determine whether the deformity is associated with a swelling in the lumbo-sacral region (spina bifida) or with symmetrical deformities of the knees, elbows and wrists (MCC). Once these conditions have been excluded an attempt is made to gently correct the deformity (Fig. 22.4). If the deformities can be completely corrected by passive stretching, the clubfoot is likely to be a postural clubfoot.

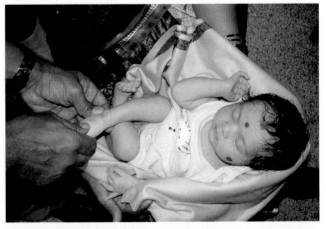

Fig. 22.4: Gentle passive correction of clubfoot in a neonate should be done without causing any pain

Table 22.6: Deformities of clubfoot and the underlying contractures that contribute to these deformities

Region of the foot	Joint	Deformity	Primary muscle contracture	Secondary contracture
Hindfoot	Ankle	Hindfoot equinus	Gastrocsoleus	Posterior capsule of ankle joint
	Subtalar joint	Hindfoot varus (a combination of adduction and inversion)	Tibialis posterior	Medial capsule of the subtalar joint
Mid-foot	Mid-tarsal joint	Forefoot adduction	Abductor hallucis	Medial capsule of the talo-navicular and calcaneo-cuboid joints
		Forefoot inversion	Tibialis posterior	
		Forefoot equinus	Short plantar muscles	Plantar aponeurosis

Serial Manipulation

To begin with, all idiopathic clubfeet should be given a trial of serial manipulation. Treatment should be started as soon as possible after birth. The feet are manipulated without sedation or anaesthesia to ensure that excessive force is not used. At the first sitting, partial correction of the deformity is achieved and with each subsequent sitting more and more correction is achieved. After each manipulation a plaster of Paris cast that extends from the tips of the toes to the groin is applied with the foot in the position of correction that has been achieved. The forefoot deformities and the hindfoot varus are corrected first. Only after these deformities are well corrected should any attempt be made to correct the hindfoot equinus. Full correction of the deformity may be achieved after four or five manipulations. If the hindfoot equinus cannot be corrected by manipulation, percutaneous tenotomy of the Achilles tendon would be needed. A small proportion of feet will not respond to this treatment and these feet would need surgical correction. The success with this method of manipulative correction steadily decreases with increasing age and often this method will not be effective in infants over six to nine months of age.

Soft Tissue Release

Soft tissue release is indicated in children who have not responded well to serial manipulation and in children who are too old for serial manipulation. Soft tissue surgery entails lengthening of the tendons of the contracted muscles and division of the contracted capsules. Since structures on the back and medial aspect of the foot need to be released, the operation is referred to as a postero-medial soft tissue release.

Ideally, soft tissue release should be performed by 9 months of age so that by the time the postoperative plaster immobilisation for three months is over the child will be able to start walking.

Satisfactory correction of the deformity should result in a supple, normal looking foot that functions well throughout life.

Bony Surgery

Children with clubfoot who present after four or five years of age would need additional surgery on the bones of the foot in order to correct the deformity as the tarsal bones would have been deformed by weight-bearing. The common operations include osteotomies of the calcaneum to correct the hindfoot varus and osteotomies of the cuboid and cuneiform bones aimed at shortening the lateral border of the foot or lengthening the medial border of the foot.

Occasionally one may encounter an older child or an adolescent with untreated clubfoot. It is possible to correct the deformity even at this age by either resecting wedges of bone from the dorso-lateral aspect of the foot or by distracting the contracted soft tissues with the help of an external fixator mounted on the limb through wires that pass through the leg and foot. It needs to be emphasised that any form of surgery to correct clubfoot in the older child will result in a stiff foot even if the deformity can be completely corrected.

Clubfoot in Spina Bifida

Clubfoot in spina bifida is more difficult to treat. Manipulation and plaster casts are better avoided on account of the risk of producing pressure sores on the anesthetic feet. There may also be muscle imbalance due to paralysis of some muscles acting on the foot and ankle and this must be addressed or else the deformity will recur.

Clubfoot in MCC

Clubfoot in MCC is far more rigid than idiopathic clubfoot and hence non-operative methods are not likely to succeed. There is also a very high chance of relapse of the deformity following surgical correction. In view of this, surgery should be more radical with excision of segments of the contracted tendons rather than mere lengthening as done in idiopathic clubfoot.

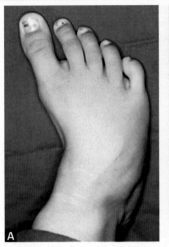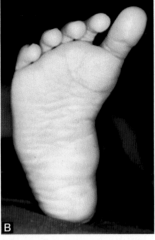

Figs 22.5A and B: Clinical appearance of the foot of a child with metatarsus adductus

Metatarsus Adductus

Treatment Approach: Observe/Treat Electively

Metatarsus adductus is a congenital anomaly where the forefoot is adducted. It resembles the forefoot adduction component of clubfoot; but the deformity is at the tarso-metatarsal joints rather than at the mid-tarsal joint as in clubfoot (Figs 22.5A and B). Metatarsus adductus may be associated with other deformities such as infantile scoliosis, torticollis and plagiocephaly all of which may be part of the molded baby syndrome.

Milder degrees of metatarsus adductus tend to resolve and hence one can wait for a few years to see if resolution of the deformity occurs. The more severe deformity may need release of the abductor hallucis muscle or osteotomies of the bases of the metatarsal bones.

Calcaneovalgus

Treatment Approach: Observe

Congenital calcaneovalgus deformity may occur in isolation or with congenital posteromedial bowing of the tibia. Calcaneovalgus deformity is a postural deformity that develops on account of intra-uterine molding. At birth, the foot is dorsiflexed and everted; the dorsum of the foot may be in contact with the shin (Fig. 22.6). Despite this apparently severe deformity, rapid spontaneous resolution occurs. Spontaneous resolution can be facilitated by gentle stretching of the foot into plantar flexion and eversion by the mother several times a day. Very occasionally, a few casts holding the foot in plantar flexion and inversion may be needed.

If there is an associated postero-medial bowing of the tibia, the parents need to be reassured that the tibial deformity again is likely to resolve spontaneously.

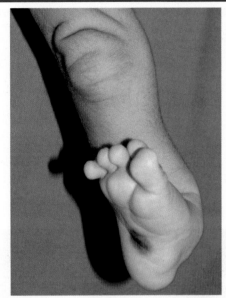

Fig. 22.6: Calcaneovalgus deformity of the foot in a newborn infant

However, these children do need to be followed up as residual tibial deformity and shortening of the limb that may occur in some children may need to be addressed later in childhood.

Congenital Vertical Talus

Treatment Approach: Treat Electively

Congenital vertical talus is a complex, rigid deformity of the foot that is often associated with spina bifida, chromosomal anomalies (Trisomy 13 and18) and MCC. The ankle is plantarflexed and the forefoot is dorsiflexed; consequently there is a total reversal of the normal longitudinal arch of the foot. This is referred to as a rocker-bottom deformity (Fig. 22.7). The talus is severely plantarflexed (hence the name of the condition) and the talonavicular joint is dislocated. There is also a valgus deformity of the foot (Table 22.7). The deformities will not respond to non-operative treatment and surgery is needed to release the contracted structures and to restore normal tarsal relationships. While it may be tempting to get the correction done before the child is one year old, it is easier to perform the operation if the foot is a little larger; for this reason, surgery may be deferred for six to twelve months.

Anterolateral Bowing of the Tibia

Treatment Approach: Treat Early

Bowing of the tibia may be present at birth. The location and the direction of the convexity of the bowing should be identified. When the child is born with anterolateral bow of the tibia, a careful examination must be made to look for

Table 22.7: Deformities of congenital vertical talus and the underlying contractures that contribute to these deformities

Region of the foot	Joint	Deformity	Primary muscle contracture	Secondary contracture
Hindfoot	Ankle	Hindfoot equinus	Gastrocsoleus	Posterior capsule of ankle joint
	Subtalar joint	Hindfoot valgus (a combination of abduction and eversion)	Peroneus longus and brevis	Lateral capsule of the subtalar joint
Mid-foot	Mid-tarsal joint	Forefoot abduction	Peroneus brevis	Lateral capsule of the calcaneo-cuboid joint
		Forefoot dorsiflexion	Tibialis anterior, extensor hallucis, extensor digitorum, peroneus tertius	Dorsal capsule of the talo-navicular joint

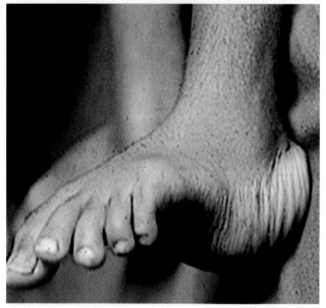

Fig. 22.7: In congenital vertical talus the medial longitudinal arch of the foot is reversed and this is described as a rocker-bottom deformity

pigmented spots (café-au-lait spots) on the trunk or limbs. These spots suggest that the child has neurofibromatosis. If these spots are not present on the baby, examination of the parents may show features of neurofibromatosis in either of them. The radiograph of the limb may show narrowing of the tibia at the junction of the middle and lower third of the leg with obliteration of the medullary cavity. If these changes are noted, the limb needs to be protected in a splint to prevent the tibia from fracturing. If the tibia does fracture, union will not occur by simple immobilisation (fractures in infants and young children normally heal quite quickly by immobilisation in a cast) and will go on to develop a pseudarthrosis that is exceedingly difficult to treat.

In contrast to anterolateral bowing of the tibia, posteromedial bowing is far more benign and spontaneous resolution of the bowing will occur. It is important to clearly identify the direction of the bowing as the natural history and the prognosis are so different in the two types of bowing.

Developmental Dysplasia of the Hip

Treatment Approach: Treat Early

The term "developmental dysplasia of the hip" has replaced the older term "congenital dislocation of the hip" since true dislocation of the hip is not present at birth though the factors that predispose to dislocation are present at birth. Developmental dysplasia of the hip (DDH) covers a spectrum of hip abnormality that includes neonatal hip instability, subluxation and dislocation of the hip and acetabular dysplasia without hip instability. The cause of DDH is multifactorial and among the causes are two clearly defined heritable predisposing factors, namely, ligament laxity and acetabular dysplasia. DDH occurs six times more commonly in girls than in boys; it occurs far more frequently in breech deliveries and in those with a definite family history of DDH.

Unlike most other musculoskeletal congenital anomalies, DDH is not apparent unless one specifically examines the newborn for signs of neonatal hip instability. If the diagnosis of neonatal hip instability is not made, the hip may dislocate in early infancy and this too may remain undetected till the child begins to walk with a limp. Treatment of neonatal instability is relatively simple both for the baby and the treating surgeon, while treatment becomes increasingly difficult as the child grows older. Furthermore, the results of treatment deteriorate as the age at treatment increases; the best chance of obtaining an excellent outcome is if treatment is instituted in the neonatal period itself. Hence, it is imperative that every newborn child is screened for hip instability.

Screening for DDH

The two main methods of screening are clinical and ultrasonographic. For obvious logistic and economic

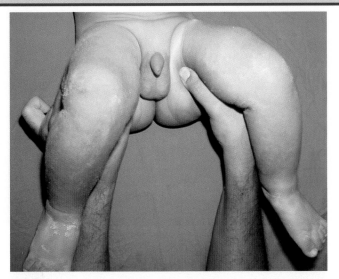

Fig. 22.8: The method of holding the infant's thighs while performing the Barlow and Ortolani tests for detecting neonatal hip instability

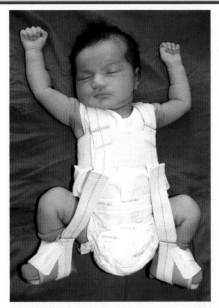

Fig. 22.9: The hips of a neonate with neonatal hip instability are splinted in flexion and abduction in a Pavlik's harness

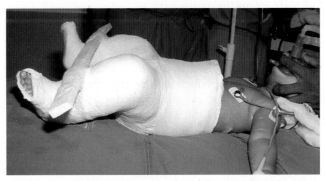

Fig. 22.10: Spica cast applied after closed reduction in an infant with developmental dysplasia of the hip

reasons, it would just not be feasible to screen every newborn in a developing country by ultrasound and hence clinical screening will remain the mainstay of diagnosis of DDH for a long time to come. It is important that every clinician who attends to the newborn is adept at performing the screening tests for neonatal hip instability. This is particularly vital in situations where a paediatric orthopaedic surgeon may not be available.

The two clinical tests for detecting hip instability in the newborn are the Barlow's test and the Ortolani's test. Both these tests should be performed with the baby lying on its back. The thigh is grasped with the thumb of the examiner on the medial side of the thigh and the index and middle fingers over the greater trochanter (Fig. 22.8). The hip is flexed to 90 degrees and the Barlow's test is first performed.

The hip is adducted and at the same time, pressure is applied by the thumb on the medial aspect of the thigh to attempt to push the femoral head posteriorly and laterally. If the hip is unstable the femoral head can be clearly felt moving out of the acetabulum. This provocative test, if positive, signifies that the hip is "dislocatable". Then the Ortolani's test is performed. Pressure is applied on the greater trochanter by the index and middle finger attempting to push the femoral head medially and anteriorly while the hip is abducted. The femoral head can be felt reducing into the acetabulum with palpable click. This is the Ortolani's test which when positive implies that the hip is "reducible".

Treatment of Neonatal Hip Instability

If either of these tests is positive the hips are splinted in flexion and abduction in a Pavlik harness (Fig. 22.9). The

harness is maintained for six weeks, by which time the hip ought to have become stable. If the hip has not stabilised by this time, closed reduction must be performed under anaesthesia as outlined below. In infants over six months of age the Pavlik harness is not likely to be effective.

Treatment of DDH in Infants under 6 Months of Age

If the hip does not become stable in spite of splinting in a Pavlik harness, the child needs to be anaesthetised and then the hip is examined, to see if it will reduce. In the vast majority of instances the hip will reduce. Once it is noted that the hip does reduce, a careful assessment is made to determine the position in which the hip remains reduced. If the hip remains reduced in around 45 degrees of abduction and neutral rotation of the hip, a spica cast extending from well above the costal margin to the tips of the toes is applied with the hips flexed to 90 degrees and abducted to 45 degrees (Fig. 22.10). The spica is changed under anaesthesia at monthly intervals and at each change the stability of the reduction is assessed. Usually, the hip will become quite stable within three to four months, at which time the spica cast can be abandoned. If the hip has to be abducted over 60 degrees or if the hip has to be internally rotated a great deal in order to keep the hip reduced, surgical open reduction if the hip should be undertaken as immobilisation in these positions of excessive abduction and internal rotation can jeopardize the blood supply to the femoral head. Open reduction is also indicated in children under six months of age if the hip cannot be reduced by closed reduction under anaesthesia.

Treatment of DDH between the Age of 6 Months and 18 Months

Once the hip dislocates and remains dislocated, soft tissue contractures will develop and they would prevent the hip from being reduced. This is seen in a proportion of children over six months of age. These children would have to undergo an open reduction of the hip. During the operation, the soft tissue impediments to reduction need to be identified and removed; these include contracture of the inferomedial capsule, iliopsoas tendon, the ligamentum teres and fibrofatty tissue in the floor of the acetabulum. The hip is immobilised in a spica cast for three months following the open reduction. If on the other hand, the hip does reduce when examined under anaesthesia the treatment can be as for children under six months of age.

Treatment of DDH in Children between 18 Months and 3 Years

Adaptive changes will develop in the femur and the acetabulum in a child who has been walking with a dislocated hip, and these would need to be addressed in order to obtain a stable reduction. The femur may be excessively anteverted and the neck may develop some degree of valgus. The acetabulum may become even more dysplastic and sloping. In addition, the muscles that cross the hip would become excessively contracted. Consequently the femur may need to be shortened in order to reduce the hip. Varus de-rotation osteotomy may be needed to ensure that the femoral head is directed towards the centre of the acetabular floor. The normal slope of the acetabulum may need to be restored in order to prevent the hip from subluxating again after the reduction has been achieved (Fig. 22.11). All or some of these bony operations may be needed in addition to an open reduction in these older children.

It is important to follow up all children who have been treated in early childhood for DDH till they are skeletally mature as late subluxation and acetabular dysplasia may occur in a few children. These problems can be promptly

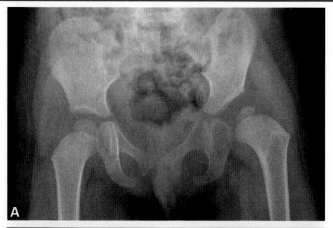

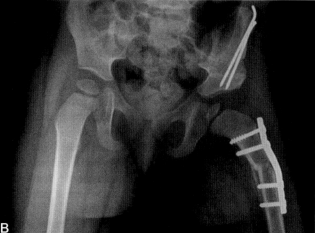

Figs 22.11A and B: Acetabular dysplasia in a child (A) has been corrected by an osteotomy of the pelvic bone (B)

addressed if children are reviewed on a regular basis through their childhood.

Congenital Scoliosis

Treatment Approach: Treat Electively

Congenital scoliosis occurs on account of anomalous development of the vertebral column; this may be failure of development of a part of the vertebra or failure of segmentation. Failure of formation of part of the vertebra results in a hemivertebra, while failure of segmentation can result in block vertebrae or unsegmented unilateral bars. The embryonal mesodermal tissue of the sclerotomes from which the vertebrae develop, is very close to the mesoderm that goes to form the urogenital tract. Consequently, very often, children with congenital scoliosis have associated anomalies of the renal tract. This must be borne in mind and children with congenital scoliosis should be screened for renal and other visceral anomalies.

Due to asymmetric growth of the spine, the deformity may progress relentlessly and neurological deficit may develop in the limbs on account of stretching of the spinal cord. Surgical intervention may be needed in early childhood to prevent rapid progression of the scoliosis. This may involve excision of the hemivertebrae, and spinal fusion.

DEVELOPMENTAL PROBLEMS

FLATFOOT

Flatfoot is a condition where the medial longitudinal arch of the foot is not well formed or has collapsed. At the outset it is imperative that a distinction is made between a mobile, flexible flatfoot and a rigid flatfoot. This distinction can be made very easily by simply asking the child to stand normally and then to stand on tip-toe. While the child is

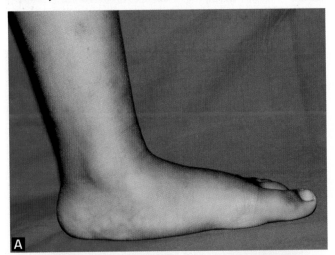

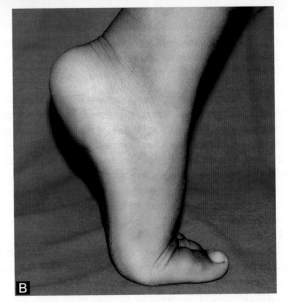

Figs 22.12A and B: The arch of the foot of a child with flexible flatfoot (A) is restored on standing on tip-toe (B)

standing normally it would be seen that the medial longitudinal arch is collapsed and the instep of the foot is resting on the ground. However, as the child stands on tip-toe the arch is completely restored (Figs 22.12A and B). Such a flatfoot is a mobile or flexible flatfoot. In children with rigid flatfeet no restoration of the arch will be noted on standing on the toes.

It is important to be aware that the foot appears flat in the vast majority of infants on account of fat in the instep region. In addition to this the joints of young children are more lax and consequently the ligaments that support the arch, are not taut and the arch flattens when the child bears weight on the foot. By around five or six years of age the ligaments of most children tighten up and the medial longitudinal arch forms. There is evidence to suggest that the arch develops better in children who do not wear footwear. Among children who use footwear from early childhood, those that wear closed-toe shoes appear to have poorer development of the arch than children who wear sandals or slippers.

Flexible Flatfoot

Treatment Approach: Reassurance

Flexible flatfoot is far more common in children who have hypermobile joints and in children who are obese. Less than 1% of children with flexible flatfeet have any symptoms related to the foot. Yet parents are often very concerned about flatfeet in their children. There is also an unsubstantiated notion that flatfeet function badly and limit the activity of the child. It is important that parents are counselled and informed that there is no need to treat asymptomatic flatfeet. The tendency to prescribe shoe modifications for young children with asymptomatic flexible flatfoot should be strongly discouraged for two very compelling reasons. Firstly, there is no evidence at all to show that the use of any form of shoe inserts or shoe modification corrects flatfoot. Secondly, in the light of evidence that shoe-wearing may actually be detrimental to development of the arch the wisdom of prescribing a modified shoe would be questionable. In the very rare situation where there is pain in the foot on standing or walking, an arch support may be worn.

Rigid Flatfoot

Treatment Approach: Treat Electively

The common cause for rigid flatfoot is tarsal coalition or an abnormal bony bar between two tarsal bones. The two most common coalitions are talo-calcaneal coalition and calcaneo-navicular coalition. The coalition may be cartilaginous to begin with and then may ossify. Pain often appears when the child reaches ten to twelve years of age. Examination will reveal that the arch cannot be restored

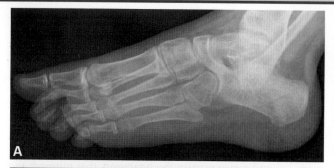

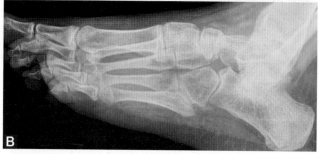

Figs 22.13A and B: Oblique radiograph of the foot of a child with calcaneo-navicular coalition (A). The radiographic appearance of the same foot after excision of the coalition was performed (B)

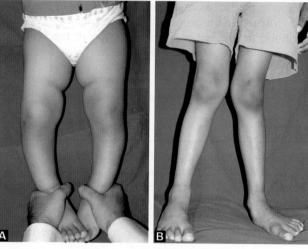

Figs 22.14A and B: Physiological genu varum (A) and genu valgum (B)

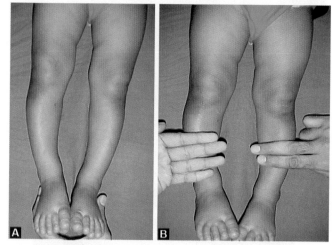

Figs 22.15A and B: The cover-up test showing valgus alignment of the proximal tibia in a child with bow-legs. This indicates that the child does not have Blount's disease

by standing on tip-toe and that there is limitation of movement of the subtalar or mid-tarsal joints. Calcaneo-navicular coalitions can be demonstrated clearly on an oblique-view radiograph of the foot (Figs 22.13A). CT scans may be needed to clearly demonstrate a talo-calcaneal coalition. If pain has developed the coalition can be excised and fat or muscle tissue needs to be interposed into the gap to prevent the coalition from reforming (Fig. 22.13B). This form of surgery usually relieves pain but the movements of the subtalar and mid-tarsal joints are seldom restored to normal. Occasionally, painful arthritis may develop in the adjacent joints; excision of the coalition will be ineffective at this stage and the arthritic joint would need to be arthrodesed.

Physiological Genu Varum and Genu Valgum

Treatment Approach: Reassurance

Several children between the ages of one and three years have genu varum (bowlegs) and children between three and seven years of age often have genu valgum (knock-knees). These deformities spontaneously resolve completely in the vast majority of instances and hence are referred to as physiological genu varum and valgum (Figs 22.14A and B). However, one needs to be certain that the deformities are not due to any underlying pathology. Among the various causes of genu varum and valgum, rickets is a common cause in developing countries and must be excluded before assuming that one is dealing with physiological genu varum or valgum. Plain radiographs

and biochemical investigations can exclude active rickets. Physiological genu varum also needs to be differentiated from infantile Blount's disease which requires early treatment. A clinical sign that appears to be quite reliable in making this distinction is the cover-up test (Fig. 22.15). While the examiner covers the middle and lower third of the bowed leg with the palm the alignment of the proximal third of the leg in relation to the thigh is noted. If the proximal third of the leg is in valgus, Blount's disease is excluded.

Children with physiological genu varum and valgum need to be periodically reviewed to ensure that resolution of the deformity is occurring. The parents can be reassured that the deformity is likely to correct over time. Bracing, night splints and shoe modification have no effect on the natural history of these deformities and are not warranted.

Adolescent Idiopathic Scoliosis

Treatment Approach: Treat Early

Scoliosis or lateral bending of the vertebral column often develops in adolescent girls. The deformity is not merely lateral curvature of the spine but has rotational and sagittal plane components also. The rotation of the spinal column results in an asymmetry of the rib cage; a prominence or rib hump develops on the side of the convexity of the spinal curvature. It is the rib hump that attracts the attention of the parents. The deformity tends to progress during the pubertal growth spurt. If diagnosed early, spinal instrumentation and fusion can correct the deformity satisfactorily. However, if treatment is delayed, surgery may succeed in reducing the deformity but seldom completely corrects it. For this reason the diagnosis needs to be made early. In conservative societies where it is uncommon for the parents or friends to see the adolescent girl's bare back the diagnosis may be delayed till the rib hump is severe enough to attract attention through the girl's loose clothing. For this reason, school-screening for scoliosis is recommended. The screening test is the forward bending test where each student bends forwards and the examiner views the back to identify a rib hump (Fig. 22.16).

PARALYTIC CONDITIONS

Obstetric Brachial Plexus Palsy

Treatment Approach: Treat Early

Injury to the brachial plexus commonly follows shoulder dystocia during labour. Loss of spontaneous movements of the upper limb would be apparent soon after birth. Often

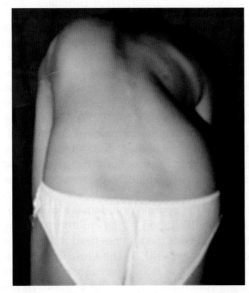

Fig. 22.16: Forward bending test used to detect scoliosis. The rib hump that is evident indicates that there is thoracic scoliosis

what initially appears to be a whole-arm type of paralysis will turn out to be a more localised paralysis; most commonly the upper two roots (C5 and C6) or the upper trunk of the brachial plexus is involved. The severity and the location of the injury determine the extent of recovery. If the injury involves avulsion of the roots of the plexus within the spinal canal (pre-ganglionic injury) no recovery can be anticipated, while if the injury is an extraforaminal (post-ganglionic) neuropraxia complete recovery can be anticipated. Electrodiagnostic tests are unreliable in accurately differentiating between the different grades of severity of injury in the first few weeks and hence are not recommended. A careful clinical recording of the muscle function of each muscle group is made periodically to map the recovery. If shoulder abduction and elbow flexion of more than Grade III power (antigravity function) is restored within two months of birth the prognosis for full recovery is excellent. If antigravity function of the elbow flexors is restored by three to six months some useful recovery of function would occur. However, if no elbow flexor power is restored within three months the prognosis for recovery is poor. In such a child electrodiagnostic tests need to be done at this stage to determine if the injury is pre-ganglionic or post-ganglionic and exploration and repair of the brachial plexus needs to be considered.

Fortunately, in the majority of instances elbow flexor power does return by three months. Several of these children will have some residual weakness and many develop contractures of the shoulder. The commonest contracture that develops is an internal rotation contracture, which can result in posterior dislocation of the shoulder. Since these contractures can develop within a few months, it is imperative that passive stretching exercises to prevent contractures are begun soon after birth and continued regularly for several months. In the past, splints that held the arm abducted and externally rotated were used but currently no form of splintage is recommended. If an internal rotation contracture develops, it needs to be identified early and surgery done in order to correct it and prevent it from going on to produce a dislocation of the shoulder.

Poliomyelitis

Treatment Approach: Treat Electively

Though the incidence of polio has reduced in most parts of the developing world, children with post-polio residual paralysis would be encountered for several years to come. The vast majority of children with post-polio residual paralysis have deformities in addition to paralysis. The two causes of deformity in these children are abnormal posture and muscle imbalance. It follows that deformities in polio can be prevented by ensuring proper posture and by recognizing muscle imbalance early and restoring muscle balance before the deformity develops. The fact that most children do develop deformities clearly indicates that sufficient attention has not been paid to prevention of deformities.

Prevention of Deformities

During the acute paralytic phase of polio, the paediatric orthopaedic surgeon should be involved in planning appropriate bracing to prevent postural deformities. During the stage of recovery again bracing of the paralysed extremity can minimize the onset of deformity. Once the stage of recovery is over, careful muscle charting needs to be done in order to identify if muscle imbalance exists. At this stage, if muscle balance is restored by surgery, deformities can be avoided.

Correction of Established Deformities

Deformities secondary to poor posture result in contracture of fascia, muscles and joint capsules. Muscle imbalance primarily results in joint deformity due to contracture of the stronger muscle group acting on the joint. Secondarily, the joint capsule may get contracted. If the deformity remains uncorrected adaptive bony changes take place. This emphasizes the need to intervene before bony changes develop.

The milder degrees of deformity will get corrected by releasing the contracted fascia and lengthening the tendons of the contracted muscles. In moderately severe deformities the contracted capsule would also have to be released; additional osteotomies of the bone adjacent to the joint would be needed to correct severe deformities.

Dealing with Paralysis

The best option for restoring function of a paralysed muscle is to perform a tendon transfer. However, in order to do so, a muscle that is transferred should have normal (Grade V) muscle power and transferring the muscle should not cause secondary disability. Tendon transfers are most commonly done around the foot and ankle in polio.

Treating Joint Instability

When all the muscles acting on a joint are paralysed, the joint is rendered flail and unstable. Unstable joints need to be stabilised either externally by the use of an orthosis or by fusing the joint. Such an intentional fusion of a joint is referred to as an arthrodesis.

Bracing

If there are no muscles available to consider a tendon transfer, an orthosis may be needed to facilitate ambulation. The extent of bracing would depend on the extent

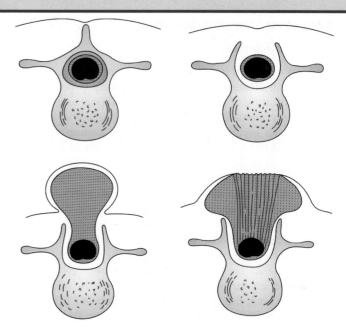

Fig. 22.17: Meningocele in a newborn infant

of paralysis. An orthosis that stabilizes the paralysed foot and ankle (below-knee brace) is referred to as an ankle-foot orthosis or AFO; an orthosis that stabilises the knee, ankle and foot is called a knee-ankle-foot orthosis or KAFO. In the past these braces were made of metal uprights and leather belts. Currently there are made of light-weight thermoplastic materials like polypropylene.

Spina Bifida

Treatment Approach: Treat Early (Incipient Neuropathic Ulcer: Treat Urgently)

Spina bifida is primarily a congenital anomaly of development of the neural tube. Secondarily the neural arches of the vertebrae at the level of the neural tube defect fail to fuse in the midline. Either the meninges alone bulge through the vertebral defect (meningocele) or neural tissue of the spinal cord and the meninges protrude through the defect (myelomeningocele) (Fig. 22.17). Varying degrees of neurological deficit will be present in these children depending on the level of the defect. Motor deficit, sensory loss and autonomic dysfunction, that affects bowel and bladder continence, may all be present in children with myelomeningocele.

The level of the neurological damage, to a large extent, determines the likelihood of the children retaining their ability to walk outside their homes in adult life (community ambulators). In general, if the child has functioning quadriceps muscles of both lower limbs, the potential for remaining a community ambulator is good. If, however, the level of the damage is higher and the quadriceps muscles are paralysed, the child is likely to end up in a wheel chair by adolescence even if the child does walk with braces in early childhood.

Management of Paralysis

The management of paralysis in children with spina bifida is very similar to that in polio. Wherever tendon transfers are feasible, they should be considered and when there are no tendons available for transfer bracing is needed.

Correction of Deformities

In spina bifida, deformities of the spine, hips, knees and feet are all common. Scoliosis and kyphosis occur frequently in these children and their management is particularly difficult. Once the scoliosis becomes severe sitting balance may be lost and the child may only be able to sit with the support of both hands on the cot or chair. The scoliosis must be corrected if this happens or else the child would not be able to use the hands for any other useful activity while seated.

The deformities of the lower limbs in spina bifida again are largely due to muscle imbalance. These deformities can be minimised if muscle balance is restored by appropriate surgery.

In a child who is wheel chair bound, any deformity of the lower limb that precludes sitting should be corrected. In a child who needs to use an orthosis, any deformity that interferes with the fitting of the orthosis must be corrected. Any deformity of the foot that prevents the foot from resting flat on the ground (plantigrade tread) should be corrected in all children with spina bifida who can walk.

Preventing Neuropathic Ulcers

One of the most distressing complications of spina bifida is neuropathic ulceration or pressure sores. These occur in regions of sensory loss over bony prominences. The two

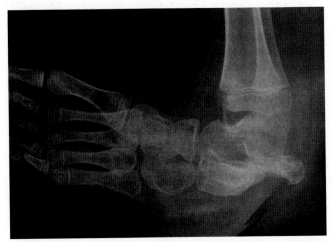

Fig. 22.18: Radiograph of a child with spina bifida who developed osteomyelitis of the calcaneum

common regions where these ulcers develop are the ischial region and the soles of the feet. It is important to understand how these ulcers develop and plan strategies to prevent them because getting an ulcer to heal once it develops is often very difficult. If the ulcer does not heal the underlying bone can get infected (Fig. 22.18).

Neuropathic ulcers develop when insensate tissue overlying a bony prominence is either subjected to excessive pressure or to shearing forces. Since pressure is force per unit area any reduction in the area of contact will result in excessive pressure. This is typically seen when the foot is deformed and not plantigrade; the entire sole will not rest on the ground. Since a smaller area of the sole rests on the ground when the foot is deformed, greater pressure is borne on the sole than when the child stands on a normal plantigrade foot. Hence it is vitally important to correct any deformity that may be present and restore a plantigrade tread. However, it is also important to be aware that operations performed to get the foot plantigrade should not make any joint of the foot stiff. It is important to restore a plantigrade tread while retaining the suppleness of the foot. This is because the frequency of neuropathic ulceration is high if the feet are stiff and rigid even if they are plantigrade.

Similarly, a lumbar scoliosis will cause pelvic obliquity and then more pressure will fall on the ischial tuberosity that is lower when the child is seated and this increases the risk of development of an ischial pressure sore. This underscores the importance of correcting the spinal deformity to overcome the pelvic obliquity.

The second factor that can cause a neuropathic ulcer is shearing forces on tissue overlying a bony prominence. If a child shuffles on its bottom the tissue overlying the ischial tuberosity is subjected to shearing forces and so it is important to educate the parents of the potential risk of ulceration and ensure that the child does not bottom-shuffle. Another example of a situation where shearing forces cause neuropathic ulceration is a calcaneus deformity in an ambulant child. A child with paralysed plantarflexors of the ankle with functioning dorsiflexors will develop a calcaneus deformity. When such a child walks, there is uncontrolled dorsiflexion of the foot during the latter part of the stance phase of gait; quite significant shearing forces develop under the heel when this occurs. Consequently, these children are very prone to develop ulcers on the heel (Fig. 22. 19).

Apart from correcting deformities that predispose to neuropathic ulcers and avoiding activity that can cause abnormal stresses on the insensate tissue in susceptible areas, the parents and the child need to be educated about the care of the anaesthetic regions. Children with anaesthetic feet should use soft-lined foot wear and should not walk without this foot wear. Any orthotic that is used should be lined with soft lining material. Parents (and

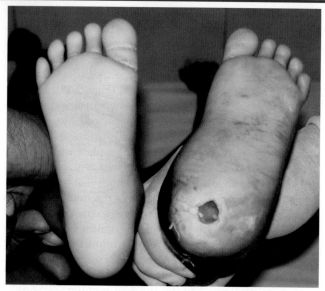

Fig. 22.19: Neuropathic ulcer of the heel in a child with spina bifida and paralysis of the gastroc-soleus.

children who are old enough to co-operate) should be taught to inspect the soles of the feet every day. If redness or early blistering is noted, a day's bed rest should be enforced to enable the incipient ulcer to heal. If the redness does not resolve with rest the orthopaedic surgeon must be consulted immediately.

Cerebral Palsy

Treatment Approach: Treat Early

Though the motor system involvement in cerebral palsy is the most overt, it is extremely important to note that there are several other impairments in children with cerebral palsy including speech defects, visual disturbances, hearing defects, behavioural disorders and epilepsy. Several of these associated impairments often need to be addressed before dealing with the motor deficit (These issues are dealt with in Chapter 18).

Motor system involvement in cerebral palsy compromises upper limb function and the activities of daily living (ADL). Involvement of the lower limb in cerebral palsy results in abnormalities of gait. The manifestations of motor system damage include spasticity, in-coordination, paresis, muscle imbalance, lack of selective motor control and involuntary movements. Uncontrolled spasticity will lead to contracture of the spastic muscle and this in turn will lead to deformities. Among these specific problems, spasticity, muscle imbalance and deformities can be modulated by treatment. It needs to be emphasised that treatment can frequently improve these problems but the function can never be made normal.

The ideal aim of treatment of cerebral palsy is to make the child totally independent. However, in several instances this may not be feasible. It is important to clearly spell out the aims of treatment and communicate these aims to the parents of the child. Every effort must be made to minimize dependence in children who cannot be made totally independent. In children who are severely affected and are likely to remain totally dependent for life, the aim of treatment would be to facilitate care of the child and to make the caregiver's job a bit easier. In addition to these aims of treatment, in all children with cerebral palsy complications such as hip dislocation should be prevented.

Management of Spasticity

There are several ways to reduce spasticity of muscles. These include physiotherapy, myoneural blocks, oral or intrathecal medication, splinting and casting, surgery on the muscles and tendons and neurosurgical procedures such as selective dorsal rhizotomy. Among these different options, physiotherapy, myoneural blocks and surgery on muscles and tendons are the most widely used.

Physiotherapy needs to be done every day throughout the period of growth. The need for regular physiotherapy till skeletal maturity needs to be emphasised at the outset. Often parents abandon physiotherapy when they do not see any dramatic improvement. The compliance can be improved if the patients are reviewed on a regular basis in a special clinic. This would give the opportunity to remind the parents for the need for pursuing with physiotherapy; and interaction with parents of other children can also have very positive effect in this regard.

Myoneural blocks either into the muscle belly or in the vicinity of the nerve supplying the spastic muscle can appreciably reduce spasticity. Currently injection of Botulinum toxin into the muscle at the motor point is widely practiced. This reduces spasticity and the effect lasts up to six months or more. Unfortunately the cost of Botulinum toxin is prohibitive. Alcohol (40%) has a comparable effect and is a great deal cheaper.

The aim of surgery on the muscles or tendons is to weaken the spastic overactive muscles. The force of muscle contraction can be reduced if the resting length of the muscle fibers can be reduced and this can be achieved by either lengthening the tendon or aponeurotic insertion of the muscle or by erasing the muscle from its origin and permitting the muscle to slide distally.

Restoring Muscle Balance

Spastic muscles that are overactive cause reciprocal inhibition of the antagonistic muscles and this results in muscle imbalance. Once the spastic muscle is weakened, the antagonistic muscle can be strengthened by physiotherapy.

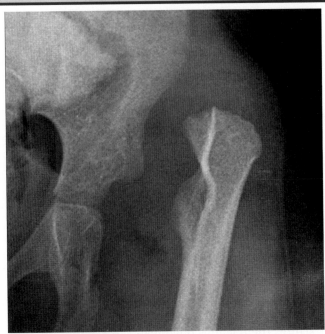

Fig. 22.20: Destruction of the head and neck of the femur following acute septic arthritis in infancy

INFECTIONS OF BONE AND JOINTS

Acute Septic Arthritis

Treatment Approach: Treat Urgently

Acute septic arthritis is a surgical emergency that develops following haematogenous seeding of bacteria in the synovium. The bacteria and the macrophages secrete very potent proteolytic enzymes which can degrade and destroy hyaline cartilage of the articular surfaces, the epiphysis and the growth plate. Enzymatic degradation of cartilage can begin within eight hours of colonisation of bacteria in the synovial tissue. If adequate treatment is delayed beyond three days after the onset of symptoms damage to the joint is almost inevitable (Fig. 22.20).

The most common causative organism is Staphylococcus aureus. Neonates and children under the age of five years are most susceptible to developing septic arthritis, though septic arthritis can occur at any age. The hip and the knee are the most commonly involved joints. In neonates it is not uncommon to have more than one joint simultaneously affected.

In neonates the commonest presentation is pseudo-paralysis; no spontaneous movement of the affected limb will be seen. True paralysis, fracture of a bone in the limb or septic arthritis may all present with lack of spontaneous movement of the limb. A careful examination can help the clinician to differentiate these conditions. Attempting passive movement of the affected joint causes the baby to cry and there may be some swelling around the joint.

X-rays and other imaging modalities are not helpful in confirming the diagnosis of septic arthritis. Similarly, no laboratory test apart from actual demonstration of bacteria in the synovial fluid is diagnostic of septic arthritis. In a sizeable proportion of cases of true septic arthritis bacteria may not be demonstrable on a Gram's stain of the synovial fluid and on culture. On account of the unreliability of laboratory tests and imaging studies in confirming the diagnosis of septic arthritis, treatment needs to be instituted on the basis of the clinical features. Treatment should not be withheld for want of laboratory confirmation.

Intravenous antibiotics that are effective against Staphylococci should be started immediately. If clear improvement in the swelling of the joint and reduction in pain on passive movement are not noted within 8 to12 hours the joint must be explored and drained. Lavage of the joint with copious quantity of saline at the time of surgery will help to reduce the bacterial load. Joints such as the hip that have a propensity to dislocate need to be immobilised in a plaster cast for a few weeks while other infected joints should be immobilised till the inflammation subsides. The intravenous antibiotics may be replaced by oral antibiotics once clinical improvement is noted.

Acute Osteomyelitis

Treatment Approach: Treat Urgently

Acute pyogenic osteomyelitis again most commonly is due to haematogenous spread of bacteria from a source elsewhere in the body. The infection starts in the metaphysis due to peculiarities of the blood vessels in this region. If the infection is not controlled, pus will collect in the metaphysis and then track under the periosteum. Gradually, pus will fill the entire medullary cavity and the endosteal blood vessels will get occluded. At the same time the periosteum will get elevated circumferentially over the entire length of the diaphysis by pus, resulting in loss of the periosteal blood supply to the cortex. The diaphysis which now is devoid of both endosteal and periosteal sources of blood supply will undergo necrosis and become a sequestrum. It is of paramount importance to diagnose osteomyelitis early and prevent this catastrophic complication.

The femur and tibia are most commonly affected. If the metaphysis is situated within a joint, as in the proximal femur, arthritis may ensue very soon and then the clinical features would be those of the arthritis.

The initial mode of presentation in neonates is the same as for acute septic arthritis—as pseudoparalysis. Careful examination of a child with acute osteomyelitis may demonstrate tenderness in the region of the metaphysis with no aggravation of pain on gently moving the adjacent

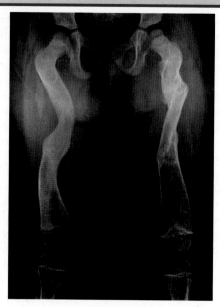

Fig. 22.21: Severe deformities of the femur and tibia seen in osteogenesis imperfecta

joint. As in the case of septic arthritis, imaging modalities and laboratory investigations are not useful in the first few days after the onset of osteomyelitis. Aspiration of the metaphysis with a wide-bore needle may yield pus if frank suppuration has begun. Ultrasonography and MRI scans can delineate the extent of a sub-periosteal abscess if it has formed. However, ideally a diagnosis of acute osteomyelitis should be made on clinical grounds even before the sub-periosteal abscess forms and appropriate treatment should be instituted without any delay. Intravenous antibiotics that are effective against the most likely pathogens should be started immediately. Staphylococci are the most common group of organisms responsible for acute haematogenous osteomyelitis, while in children with sickle cell disease, Salmonella may be the causative organism. If the pain and fever subside and the local warmth and tenderness reduce within 24 to 48 hours, antibiotics and best rest may suffice. If, on the other hand, there is no definite clinical improvement within 48 hours surgery should be undertaken. The involved metaphysis (the diaphysis in Salmonella osteomyelitis) is explored. If a sub-periosteal abscess is present, it is drained. A couple of drill holes are made in the underlying bone and a small quantity of pus may exude through the drill holes. This serves as effective decompression of the bone if the infection is localised. If a large quantity of pus is evacuated, a small cortical window is made in the bone to facilitate irrigation of the medullary cavity. The limb is protected in a plaster-of-Paris cast to prevent a pathological facture. Once clinical improvement is documented intravenous antibiotics may be replaced by oral antibiotics which are then continued for four to six weeks.

INHERITED DISORDERS OF BONE

Osteogenesis Imperfecta

Treatment Approach: Treat Electively

Osteogenesis imperfecta is an inherited disorder of the skeleton characterised by frequent fractures. The frequency of fractures varies with the severity of the disease. There may be associated ligament laxity, blue sclera and abnormal dentition. In the most severe variety, fractures occur in-utero and the baby is often still born. In the less severe varieties fractures may commence soon after birth and in the mild form may not occur till early childhood. The child may be unable to stand or walk as the femur or tibia may fracture. The fractures often malunite and over a period of time quite horrendous deformities may develop (Fig. 22.21). Generalised bone pains and the pain of repeated fractures make the quality of life very poor.

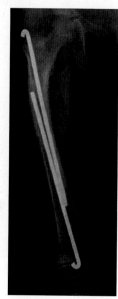

Fig. 22.22: Fractures in osteogenesis imperfecta can be minimised by inserting intra-medullary rods into the long bones

Bisphosphonates appear to reduce the pain and the frequency of fractures. In addition, correction of the deformities and insertion of rods into the medullary cavity of the bones of the limbs markedly reduce the frequency of fractures (Fig. 22.22). Since the bones outgrow the rods as the child grows the rods would have to be removed and longer rods need to be inserted or else, fractures will occur in the unsupported part of the bone. The propensity for fractures tends to reduce as the child approaches skeletal maturity.

Skeletal Dysplasias

Treatment Approach: Treat Electively

Skeletal dysplasias include a large variety of genetically determined abnormalities of the skeleton that manifest as abnormalities in growth of part or the entire skeleton. In some forms, the appendicular skeleton is predominantly involved with little abnormality in the spine, while in other forms both the axial skeleton and the limbs are involved. The pattern of involvement of the skeleton varies with the form of skeletal dysplasia. In some forms the proximal segments (femur and humerus) are most affected, while in other forms the tibia, fibula, radius and ulna are the most severely affected and in a few types, the hands and feet are most affected. The abnormalities of growth may also result in dwarfism or angular deformities due to asymmetric

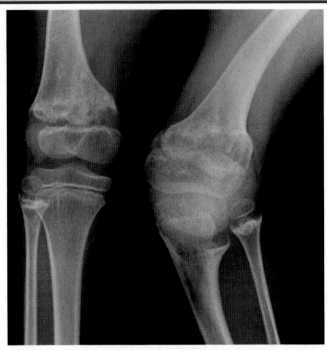

Fig. 22.23: Deformity of the knee seen in a form of skeletal dysplasia

growth at the growth plates of long bones (Fig. 22.23). These deformities result in abnormal stresses on joints and this contributes to very early onset of secondary degenerative arthritis of the weight-bearing joints. In addition to aberrant growth, joint instability or joint stiffness may be present in some dysplasias.

Whenever there is evidence of dwarfism or abnormal body proportions radiographs of the skeleton need to be obtained to exclude skeletal dysplasia. Some skeletal dysplasias can be diagnosed at birth (e.g. achondroplasia) while in some dysplasias the growth abnormality may only become evident in early or even late childhood (e.g. spondylo-epiphyseal dysplasia tarda).

TUMOURS OF BONE

Benign Tumours

Treatment Approach: Treat Electively

One of the common benign tumours of bone is osteochondroma, which as the name implies has a cartilaginous and a bony component. The tumour typically occurs in the metaphyseal region of long bones and may be either solitary or multiple (Fig. 22.24). Multiple osteochondromatosis is an inherited disorder which is associated with a remodeling defect of the long bones and growth abnormalities. The solitary variety, on the other hand is not associated with growth abnormalities or a remodeling defect. The osteochondromata grow till skeletal maturity and then cease to grow unless they have undergone

malignant transformation. Malignant transformation to a chondrosarcoma is very rare in solitary osteochondromas but may occur in about 10% of patients with multiple osteochondromatosis. Unless the osteochondroma causes pressure on an adjacent nerve or impairs movement of a joint it can be left alone. If symptoms warrant it, the osteochondroma may be excised along with the periosteum surrounding the base of the osteochondroma.

Malignant Tumours

Treatment Approach: Treat Urgently

The two important malignant tumours of bone seen in children are osteosarcoma and

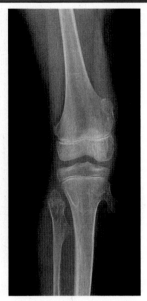

Fig. 22.24: Multiple osteochondromata seen in the distal femur and proximal tibia of both limbs

Ewing's tumour. Ewing's tumour occurs most commonly in the first decade of life while osteosarcoma occurs in the second decade of life. The presenting features may be pain or swelling in the thigh, leg or arm which are the common sites for these tumour to occur. Unexplained pain or swelling of the limb should be investigated carefully. A radiograph of the limb is mandatory and if either of these tumours is present, characteristic changes may be seen. In the case of Ewing's tumour, a lesion would be seen more commonly in the diaphysis with areas of patchy osteolysis, cortical erosion and periosteal reaction that may have a very typical "onion peel" appearance (Fig. 22.25A). Osteosarcoma, on the other and is metaphyseal and the lesion is predominantly sclerotic in appearance; early breach of the cortex with extension of the tumour under the periosteum produces a typical "sun ray" appearance (Fig. 22.25b). Though these radiographic appearances are quite characteristic of these tumours, similar appearances can occur in other less morbid conditions. Radiographic changes in the bone that are similar to those of Ewing's tumour may occur in osteomyelitis, while changes akin to those of osteosarcoma may occur with exuberant callus formation after a fracture in spina bifida or osteogenesis imperfecta. Therefore, it is mandatory to perform a biopsy to confirm the diagnosis. Unless a pathologist who is experienced in interpreting needle biopsies is available, it is preferable to perform an open biopsy.

Ewing's tumour is treated with cyclical chemotherapy and in some instances with additional radiotherapy and surgery. Osteosarcoma is treated with adjuvant chemotherapy followed by surgery. If strict criteria are fulfilled,

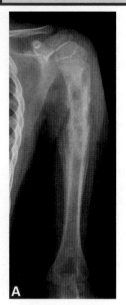
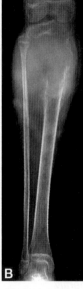

Figs 22.25A and B: Radiographic appearance of
Ewing's tumour (A) and osteosarcoma (B)

Table 22.8: The typical ages at which painful conditions of the hip occur	
Condition	*Common age at presentation*
Septic arthritis	Under 5 years
Transient synovitis	5 to 10 years
Perthes' disease	5 to 12 years
Slipped capital femoral epiphysis	12 to 15 years

limb salvage surgery may be considered or else an amputation is performed. Cyclical chemotherapy is resumed again following surgery. Limb salvage surgery would require some form of reconstruction after resection of the diseased bone segment.

HIP PAIN IN CHILDREN AND ADOLESCENCE

Among all the joints of the body that may be a source of pain in children, the hip joint is most frequently affected. Apart from trauma and bone and joint infection, there are some other causes of hip pain that warrant a brief mention; these include transient synovitis, Perthes' disease and slipped capital femoral epiphysis. The age at which each of these conditions occurs varies (Table 22.8) and the knowledge of the typical ages at presentation can alert the clinician to the possible diagnosis. Though the pathology in these conditions is in the hip, the child may complain of pain in the knee as pain arising from the hip may be referred to the knee. This emphasizes the need to carefully examine the hip in addition to examining the knee when a child complains of knee pain.

Transient Synovitis

Treatment Approach: Treat Early

Transient synovitis affects children between 5 and 10 years of age. The child presents with a limp and pain in the hip or knee. The onset of pain may be preceded by an upper respiratory infection in a proportion of cases. Extremes of hip movement are painful and there may be a mild flexion or abduction deformity. All these signs point to the presence of an effusion in the hip which can be clearly

demonstrated by ultrasonography. The clinical features, including the absence of fever, normal blood counts and ESR help to exclude septic arthritis. A few days of bed rest and traction usually relieves the pain completely and the synovitis settles without any permanent sequelae. However, since Perthes' disease may present in the same manner in the very early stages, these children should be followed up with a radiograph of the hips after six to eight weeks to see if the changes of Perthes' disease are visible.

Perthes' Disease

Treatment Approach: Treat Early

Perthes' disease is a form of osteochondrosis that affects the capital femoral epiphysis (Fig. 22.26). Part or all of the femoral epiphysis becomes avascular, the precise cause of which is unknown; the blood supply gets restored spontaneously over a period of two to four years. The prevalence of Perthes' disease varies profoundly from region to region. In India, the disease is exceedingly common in the south-west coastal plain but is quite uncommon in other parts of the country. In India, the disease affects children mainly between the ages of 5 and 12 years; the peak age at onset of symptoms is around nine years. This is distinctly older than the age of onset reported in the Western literature. The classical presentation is with a limp and pain of insidious onset and moderate limitation of passive abduction and internal rotation of the hip. The X-rays will show characteristic changes of flattening and sclerosis of the capital femoral epiphysis. In the younger child the prognosis is generally good; the blood supply

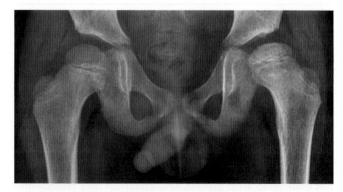

Fig. 22.26: Radiographic appearance of a boy with Perthes' disease. The epiphysis is sclerotic and flattened

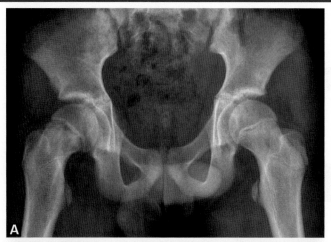

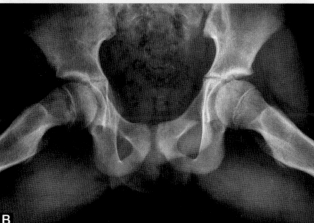

Figs 22.27A and B: The appearance of a slipped capital femoral epiphysis in an adolescent

gets restored and healing of the epiphysis occurs without any deformation of the femoral head. In the older child, however, the femoral head tends to get deformed during the process of healing. Consequently, surgery aimed at preventing femoral head deformation is often needed in the older child. It is important that such surgery is performed early in the course of the disease if it is to be effective. If the femoral head does get deformed, secondary degenerative arthritis may develop by the third or fourth decades of life.

Slipped Capital Femoral Epiphysis

Treatment Approach: Treat Urgently

Slipped capital femoral epiphysis or adolescent coxa vara occurs commonly between 12 and 15 years of age. There may be an underlying endocrine disorder or chronic renal disease in a proportion of these patients and it is important that these are excluded. Majority of the patients are obese though the epiphyseal slip can occur in children with a normal body habitus.

The growth plate of the proximal femur gets disrupted and the epiphysis slips medially and posteriorly off the neck of the femur (Figs 22. 27A and B). The slip is heralded by pain in the hip and in the majority of instances tends to occur gradually. The patient continues to walk albeit with a limp and the slip is referred to as a stable slip. On the other hand if the slip occurs suddenly the pain is severe and the patient will be unable to bear weight on the limb; this is an unstable slip. Complications are far more common in patients with unstable slips and hence the importance of this classification. Complications of slipped femoral epiphysis include progression of the slip, avascular necrosis of the femoral epiphysis and chondrolysis which results in extreme hip stiffness. Secondary degenerative arthritis may occur in early adult life. The aim of treatment is to prevent the slip from progressing and to prevent other complications listed above. Since the risk of complications increase with delay in treatment, it is recommended that the femoral epiphysis is fixed to the femoral neck with a screw as soon as possible. There is a risk that a slip can occur in the opposite hip and because of this some surgeons fix the opposite epiphysis also prophylactically. If prophylactic fixation of the unaffected hip is not done, these patients should be periodically reviewed to ensure that a slip of the epiphysis has not occurred in the second hip.

DENTAL ANATOMY

Introduction

The teeth start to form during the fifth week of embryonic life and the process of tooth formation continues until the roots of the third permanent molars are completed at about the age of 20 years. The stages of tooth formation are the same whether the tooth is of the primary or the permanent dentition.

The tooth is composed of an enamel crown covering an inner layer of dentine, which also forms the root. The external surface of the root is covered in cementum into which the periodontal ligament is attached; the insertion of this ligament is into the alveolar bone. The innermost part of the tooth has vital tissue and is known as the pulp.

The Primary Dentition

The sequence and timing of eruption of the primary dentition has great individual variation (Fig. 23.1). The first tooth to erupt is usually the lower central incisor, which can sometimes be present at birth; the average age

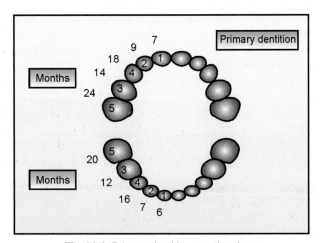

Fig. 23.1: Primary dentition eruption dates

for its eruption is between 4 and 8 months. The upper central incisors erupt at about 10 months followed by the upper lateral incisors at 11 months and the lower lateral incisors at 13 months. At about the age of 16 months the first primary molars erupt, followed by the primary canine teeth at 19 months. The second primary molars erupt around 27-29 months and the lower teeth usually erupt before the uppers. In essence there is an almost continuous process of tooth eruption between the ages of 4 and 29 months. Exfoliation is the process of elimination of primary teeth associated with the eruptive process of the permanent successor at the apex of the primary tooth root. The eruptive process stimulates the development of osteoclasts, which lead to a progressive resorption of the primary tooth root, dentine, and cementum.

The Permanent Dentition

The permanent dentition erupts in two stages (Fig. 23.2). The lower central incisor and the first permanent molars erupt at about the age of 6 years. The upper central incisor and the lower lateral incisor erupt at about the age of 7 and the upper lateral incisor at about the age of 8 years. As with the primary teeth, while some variation in the timing of tooth eruption is only to be expected, this eruption sequence should not vary. In particular, the upper central incisor should erupt before the upper lateral incisor. If the upper lateral incisor erupts before the central then, almost certainly, there is something impeding the eruption of the central incisor, for example: a supernumerary tooth, or dilaceration of the root of the central incisor.

The lower canine usually erupts at around 9 years followed by the premolar teeth at 10 years. The upper canine erupts at age 11 years with the second molar teeth at about the age of 12 years. Third molar teeth start to erupt from about the age of 16 years onwards, but the eruption of third molars is very variable; not uncommonly, these teeth are impacted against their neighbours and fail to erupt at all, in many cases they are congenitally absent.

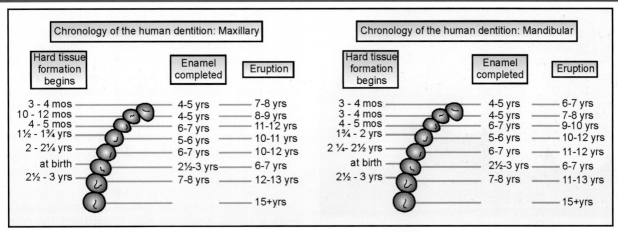

Fig. 23.2: Primary dentition eruption dates

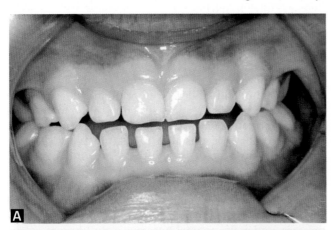

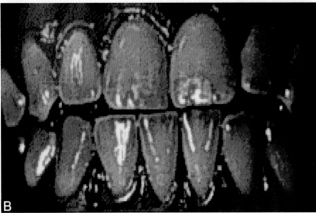

Figs 23.3A and B: Difference in appearance between primary and permanent dentition

Differences between Primary and Permanent Teeth

In comparison to the permanent dentition the crowns of the primary teeth are short and the biting surfaces narrow (Fig. 23.3). They are bulbous in shape and have thin enamel and dentine layers. The primary molars contact each other in broad, flat areas and the internal arrangement of the

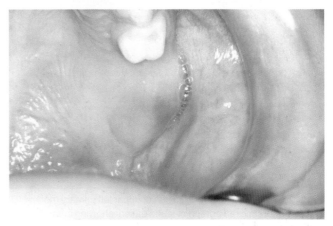

Fig. 23.4: Eruption cyst

enamel differs from permanent teeth. The roots of the primary teeth are long and slender in comparison to the crowns. They have a much larger pulp, which is closer to the outer surface.

Problems Associated with Eruption

An Eruption Cyst presents as a bluish swelling of the gingivae (Fig. 23.4) prior to eruption of a tooth. These rarely require intervention and spontaneously resolve on eruption of the tooth.

Ankylosis is caused by the fusion of the cementum of the root to the bone and accompanying loss of periodontal ligament attachment. Prevalence is between 7-14% in the primary dentition. The most commonly affected teeth are the mandibular primary first molar, mandibular primary second molar, maxillary first molar and maxillary primary second molar in that order (Figs 23.5A and B). This condition can lead to loss of arch length, extrusion of opposing teeth, and abnormal positioning of adjacent teeth.

Ectopic eruption is where the tooth, usually due to a deficiency of space does not take up its normal position within the arch.

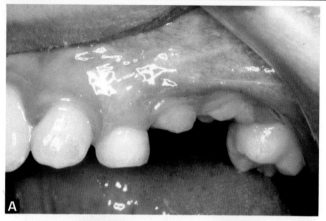

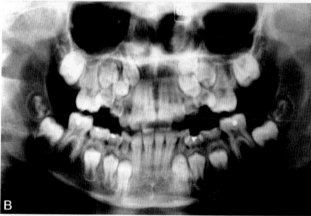

Figs 23.5A and B: (A) Infraocclusion of upper left primary molars; (B) Dental panoramic radiograph of same patient showing infraocclusion of primary molars in each quadrant

CARIES

Aetiology of Caries

Dental caries is one of the most prevalent diseases and yet it is completely preventable.

Dental caries is caused by the fermentation of dietary sugars by microorganisms in plaque on the tooth surface, this produces acid. Rapid acid formation lowers the pH of the mouth and dissolves the enamel. When sugar is no longer available to the plaque microorganisms, the pH within plaque will rise due to the outward diffusion of acids and their metabolism and neutralization in plaque, so that remineralisation of enamel can occur, enamel caries progresses only when demineralisation is greater than remineralisation.

Dental plaque forms on tooth surfaces that are not properly cleaned. Dental plaque is made up of about 70 per cent microorganisms. The types of microorganism present in the plaque changes with its increasing age. When plaque is young, cocci predominate but as plaque ages the proportions of filamentous organisms and veillonellae increase. Diet influences the composition of the plaque flora considerably with mutants streptococci much more numerous when the diet is rich in extrinsic sugar. If the process of dental caries continues, support for the surface layer will become so weak that it will crumble to leave a cavity. Once a cavity is formed, the process of dental caries continues in a more sheltered environment and the protein matrix of dentine is removed by proteolytic enzymes produced by plaque organisms. In the general population it commonly takes 2-4 years for caries to progress through enamel into dentine.

Caries Prevention

The most important of the natural defences against dental caries is saliva. If salivary flow is impaired, dental caries can progress very rapidly. Saliva physically washes away food debris and sugars, it neutralises acids from the diet and those produced by plaque organisms, it also has antibacterial properties.

In terms of preventive treatment the patient should receive: dietary advice to reduce the amount and especially the frequency of sugary intakes; instruction on effective tooth cleaning; and advice on fluoride intake as fluoride incorporation into the enamel structure of the tooth is the most important chemical intervention that can be made. In some cases it is possible to restoratively seal the vulnerable surfaces of the tooth to prevent ingress of bacteria (fissure sealants).

Early caries is difficult to detect, as it is invisible to the eye. The first visible sign may be a faint white mark on the surface of the enamel (Fig. 23.6). As the process progresses the area under the enamel becomes a dull brown colour and as mineral loss under the surface extends the surface layer becomes unsupported and this eventually leads to breakdown and cavitation (Fig. 23.7).

Dental caries can be confused with developmental defects of tooth formation and there are numerous causes of interruption of tooth development with defects varying from very minor whiteness of enamel to gross abnormalities of tooth structure (see tooth anomalies section).

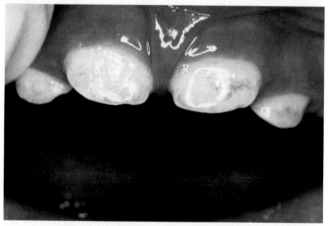

Fig. 23.6: White demarcation of early decay

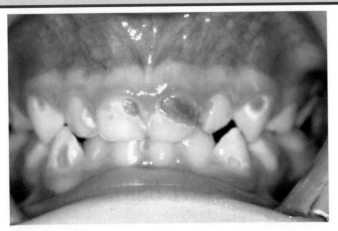

Fig. 23.7: Cavitation of primary dentition

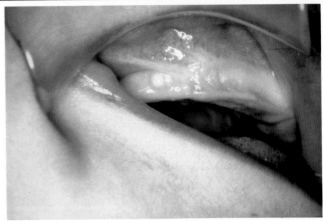

Fig. 23.9: Gingival cyst of the newborn

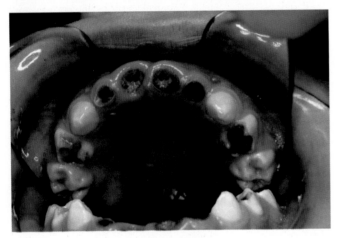

Fig. 23.8: Early childhood caries

Early Childhood Caries/Nursing Caries

This is a particular pattern of caries seen in very young children. It involves early caries of the upper incisor teeth along with the first primary molar in accord with the order of tooth eruption (Fig. 23.8). The disease is caused by inappropriate bottle or breastfeeding. If the child takes a bottle filled with juice or sweetened milk this will result in early caries. This is often compounded by inappropriate timing were the child is given access to this sweetened liquid around the clock, especially at night time where the substance may lie unswallowed in the mouth. At night there is a decrease in the salivary flow rate and hence decreased protection. Prolonged and constant breast-feeding at night may also cause this caries pattern, as human breast milk is cariogenic. The lower anterior teeth tend to be spared in nursing caries as they are covered by the tongue and are washed in whatever saliva is available due to their proximity to the opening of the salivary glands. Advice to give:

- All sweetened drinks should be consumed at mealtimes only.

- Once a baby has been weaned water should be the only night-time feed (after 12 months).
- For good dental health all breastfeeding should be discontinued by 2 years.
- Milk in bottle is safe for daytime feeds but can cause caries if taken during the night.

ORAL PATHOLOGY/ORAL MEDICINE

This section deals with those conditions that occur exclusively, or more commonly in children. It is not an exhaustive guide to paediatric oral pathology/medicine for which readers should refer to oral pathology/medicine textbooks.

Oral Lesions in Neonates and Young Infants

Bohn's Nodules

These gingival cysts arise from remnants of the dental lamina (stage in early tooth formation). They are found in neonates and usually disappear spontaneously in the early months of life (Fig. 23.9).

Epstein's Pearls

These small cystic lesions are located along the palatal mid-line and are thought to arise from trapped epithe-lium in the palatal raphe). They are present in about 80 per cent of neonates and disappear within a few weeks of birth.

Congenital Epulis

This is a rare lesion that occurs in neonates and normally presents in the anterior maxilla or mandible (Fig. 23.10). It consists of granular cells covered by epithelium and is thought to be reactive in nature. It is benign and simple excision is curative.

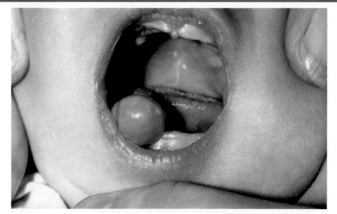

Fig. 23.10: Congenital epulis

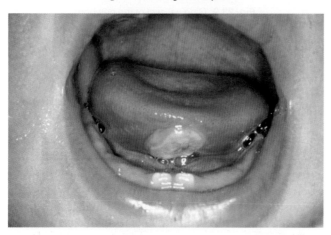

Fig. 23.11: Neonatal teeth causing ulceration of the tongue

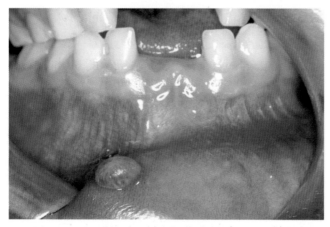

Fig. 23.12: Lower lip mucocele

Melanotic neuroectodermal tumour

This rare tumour occurs in the early months of life usually in the maxilla. The lesion consists of epithelial cells containing melanin with a fibrous stroma. Some localised bone expansion may occur. The condition is benign and simple excision is curative.

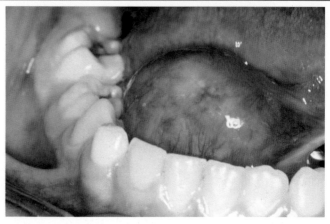

Fig. 23.13: Ranula

Candidiasis

Neonatal acute candidiasis (thrush) contracted during birth is not uncommon.

Natal/Neonatal Teeth

Present at birth (Natal) or erupt within the first month of life (Neonatal). Usually teeth of the normal series that have erupted early, rarely supernummary teeth (Fig. 23.11). Require removal if excessively mobile, causing traumatic ulceration or preventing breastfeeding.

Pathological Findings in Children and Adolescents

Mucocele

The peak incidence of mucoceles is in the second decade of life: however, they are not uncommon in younger children including neonates. Mucoceles are caused by trauma to minor salivary glands or ducts and are most commonly located on the lower lip (Fig. 23.12). They are the commonest non-infective cause of salivary gland swelling in children, as salivary tumours are rare in this age group.

Ranula

This is a bluish swelling of the floor of the mouth (Fig. 23.13). It is essentially a large mucocele and may arise from part of the sublingual salivary gland.

Haemangioma

Haemangiomas are relatively common in children. They are malformations of blood vessels and are divided into cavernous (Fig. 23.14) and capillary (Fig. 23.15) variants although some lesions contain elements of both. Capillary haemangiomas may present as facial birthmarks. The cavernous haemangioma is a hazard during surgery if involved within the surgical site, as it is a large blood filled sinus, which will bleed profusely if damaged. The extent

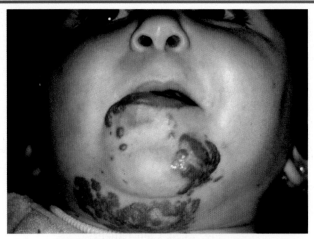

Fig. 23.14: Cavernous haemangioma

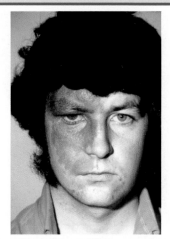

Fig. 23.16: Sturge-Weber syndrome

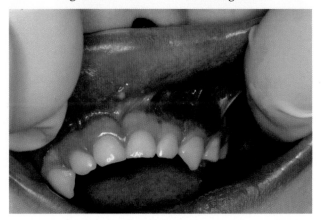

Fig. 23.15: Capillary haemangioma

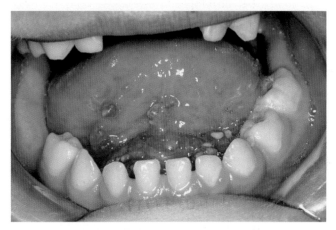

Fig. 23.17: Mixed haemangioma/lymphangioma

of a cavernous haemangioma can be established prior to surgery using either angiography or MRI scanning. Small haemangiomas are readily treated by excision or cryotherapy. Larger lesions are amenable to laser therapy.

Sturge-Weber Syndrome

Sturge-Weber angiomatosis is a syndrome consisting of a haemangioma of the leptomeninges with epithelial facial haemangioma closely related to the distribution of branches of the trigeminal nerve (Fig. 23.16). Mental deficiency, hemiplegia and ocular defects can occur. Intraoral involvement may interfere with the timing of eruption of the teeth (both early and delayed eruption have been reported).

Lymphangioma

Lymphangiomas are benign tumours of the lymphatics. The vast majority are found in children and the head and neck region is a common site.

The cystic hygroma is a variant, which appears as a large neck swelling that may extend intra-orally to involve the floor of mouth and tongue.

Mixed haemangioma/lymphangiomas may also present (Fig. 23.17).

Fibrous Epulis/Fibroepithelial Polyp

These lesions vary in appearance from red, shiny and soft enlargements of the oral mucosa to those that are pale, stippled, firm and pedunculated (Fig. 23.18). They usually arise from marginal or papillary gingivae and are often the result of an initial traumatic incident or continued gingival irritation. Excision is usually indicated and recurrence unlikely.

Drug-induced Gingival Overgrowth

The three drugs most commonly associated with the induction of gingival overgrowth (Fig. 23.19) are the anticonvulsant phenytoin, the immunosuppressant cyclosporin and the calcium channel blocker nifedipine.

Poor oral hygiene exacerbates the overgrowth, which tends to appear interdentally 2-3 months following the introduction of the drug. Excellent oral hygiene is essential to minimise the effects but often-surgical excision will be required in patients whose medical condition does not allow for a change in drug regime.

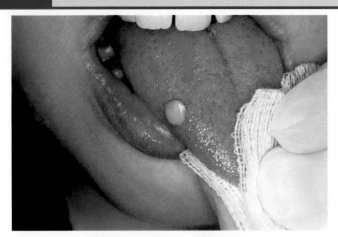

Fig. 23.18: Fibroepithelial polyp

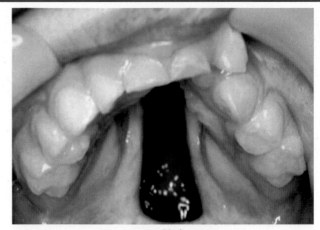

Fig. 23.20: Cleft patient

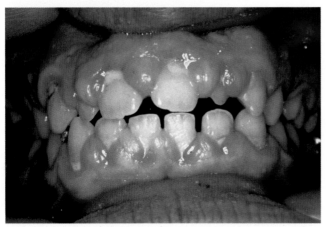

Fig. 23.19: Gingival overgrowth

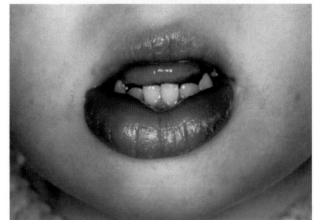

Fig. 23.21: Lip swelling in orofacial granulomatosis

Dental Effects of Cleft Lip and Cleft Palate

Aetiology and early surgical repair is discussed in Chapter 9.

These children should be under the care of a multidisciplinary team. Much of the long-term care for these children is dependent on the maintenance of a healthy dentition. Early advice regarding oral hygiene and non-cariogenic diet is essential if we are to instigate good lifelong habits, this advice is best started ante-natally or during the neonatal period. Children with clefts of the palate often have missing or extra teeth at the cleft site (Fig. 23.20). Teeth at this site may fail to erupt or erupt in an ectopic position due to lack of bone in the area. Many of these patients have very narrow palates as a result of surgical scaring and extensive orthodontic treatment for malocclusion is required.

Orofacial Granulomatosis (Crohn's Disease)

Orofacial granulomatosis (OFG) is not a tumour in the true sense nor a distinct disease entity but describes a clinical appearance. Typically there is diffuse swelling of one or

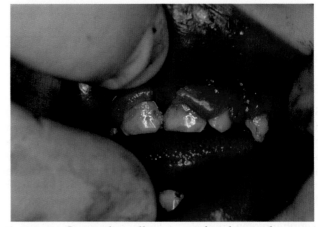

Fig. 23.22: Gingival swelling in orofacial granulomatosis

both lips and cheeks (Fig. 23.21), folding of the buccal reflected mucosa and occasionally gingival swelling and oral ulceration (Fig. 23.22). This may represent a localised disturbance due to an allergic reaction to foodstuffs. Treatment often includes avoidance of dietary allergens and use of anti-inflammatory or steroid mouthwashes.

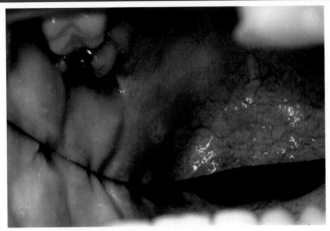

Fig. 23.23: Aphthous ulceration at border of hard and soft palate

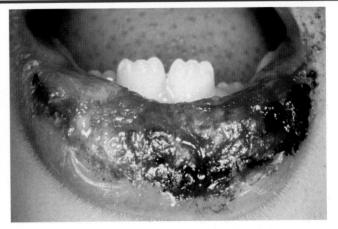

Fig. 23.25: Lip crusting in erythema multiforme

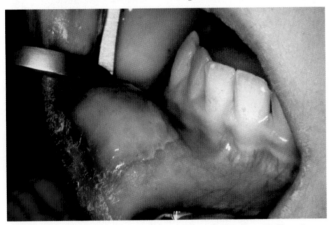

Fig. 23.24: Self induced traumatic ulceration following local anaesthetic administration

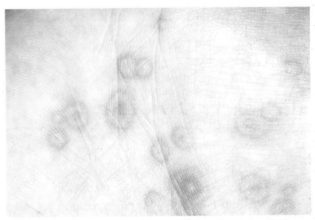

Fig. 23.26: "Target" skin lesions in erythema multiforme

Alternatively the appearance may be due to an underlying systemic condition such as Sarcoidosis or Crohn's disease. These patients may be prescribed various immunosuppresant drugs or offered surgery.

Melkersson-Rossenthal Syndrome

This is a condition that generally begins during childhood and consists of chronic facial swelling (usually the lips), facial nerve paralysis and fissured (scrotal) tongue.

Aphthous Ulceration

Typically these recurrent lesions are multiple, ovoid or round in shape and have a yellow coloured depressed floor with inflamed border, and commonly are not associated with systemic disease (Fig. 23.23). Possible aetiology includes familial, immunological or microbial. One or more small ulcers in the non-attached gingiva may occur at frequent intervals. In a young child, pain associated with this ulceration may be mistaken for toothache. Most aphthous ulcers in children are of the minor variety (less than 5 mm in diameter) and usually

heal within 10 - 14 days. Occasionally a child may present with major aphthae, which can be up to 10 mm in diameter and persist for 2-3 weeks. Treatment other than reassurance is often not necessary however in severe cases the use of topical steroids (adcortyl in orobase or betnesol mouthrinse) may be prescribed. Older children may benefit from the use of antiseptic and anti-inflammatory rinses to prevent secondary infection and increase comfort. In the absence of a history of major aphthous ulceration any ulcer lasting for longer than two weeks should be regarded with suspicion and biopsied.

Traumatic Ulceration

Traumatic ulceration of the tongue lips and cheek may occur in children following the administration of local anaesthetic (Fig. 23.24).

Vesiculo-bullous Disorders

Erythema multiforme (Fig. 23.25) can produce oral ulceration in children and may be associated with viral infection or drug reaction. Oral lesions affect the lips and anterior oral mucosa and distinctive lesions on the skin

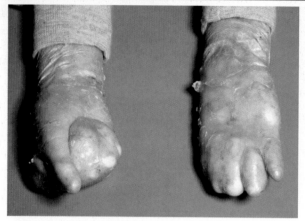

Fig. 23.27: Skin fragility in epidermolysis bullosa

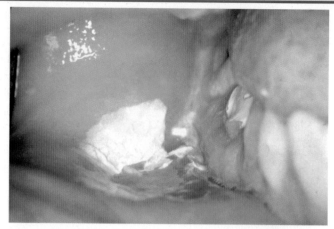

Fig. 23.29: Aspirin burn in buccal mucosa

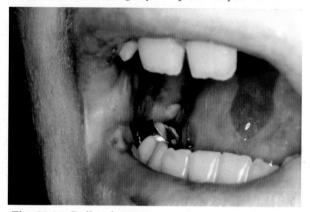

Fig. 23.28: Bullae formation on the tongue of patient
with epidermolysis bullosa

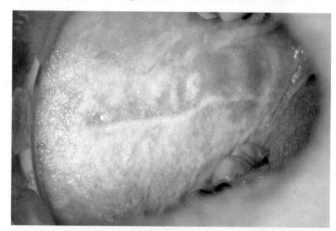

Fig. 23.30: White sponge naevus

may also be present (Fig. 23.26). Initial erythema is followed
by bullae formation and ulceration. Treatment includes
the use of steroids and oral antiseptic and analgesic rinses
to ease the pain.

Epidermolysis Bullosa

Epidermolysis bullosa is a term that covers a number of
syndromes some of which are incompatible with life. The
skin is extremely fragile (Fig. 23.27) and mucosal
involvement may occur. The act of suckling may induce
bullae formation in babies and in older children effective
oral hygiene may be difficult as even mild trauma can
produce painful lesions (Fig. 23.28).

The major vesiculo-bullous conditions such as
pemphigus and pemphigoid are rare in young patients.

White Lesions

- Chemical or physical trauma can lead to intra-oral
  white lesions. Figure 23.29 shows the appearance of
  an aspirin burn.
- A white sponge naevus (Fig. 23.30) is a benign lesion
  often detected in early infancy. It has a rough and folded
  appearance.

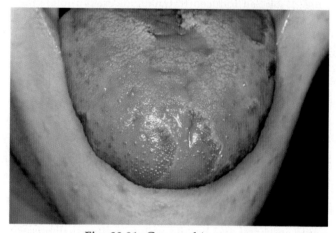

Fig. 23.31: Geographic tongue

- Leucoderma also has a folded appearance. It is a
  normal variant found in children of races who exhibit
  pigmentation of the oral mucosa.
- Geographic tongue (Fig. 23.31) has the characteristic
  appearance of red patches surrounded by a white
  border. The red areas occur where there has been loss
  of the filiform papillae. The patches disappear and then

reappear on other areas of the tongue. Spicy foods may cause discomfort but this is an otherwise symptomless condition of unknown aetiology for which reassurance should be given.

Tumours

- A squamous cell papilloma (Fig. 23.32) is a benign condition characterised by small cauliflower-like growths. These growths vary in colour from pink to white, are usually solitary and may be due to human papillomavirus.
- Verruca Vulgaris (common warts) may present intra-orally. They are probably caused by the human papillomavirus.
- Focal epithelial hyperplasia is a rare condition also known as Heck's disease. It is associated with human papillomavirus and presents as multiple small elevations of the oral mucosa especially in the lower lip.
- Giant cell granuloma (Fig. 23.33) is a dark red swelling of the gingiva. The peripheral form often arises

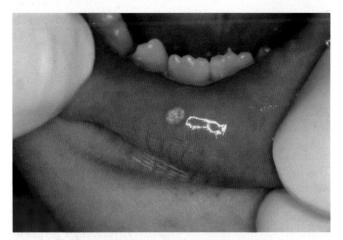

Fig. 23.32: Squamous cell papilloma

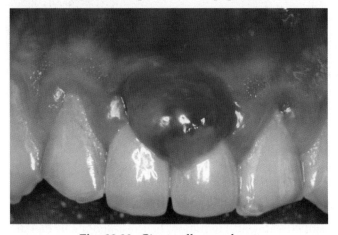

Fig. 23.33: Giant cell granuloma

interdentally and radiographs may reveal some loss of interdental bone. The central giant cell granuloma shows much greater bone destruction. This condition is thought to be a reactive hyperplasia. Unless excision is complete it will recur.
- Neurofibromas may present as solitary or multiple lesions. They are considered hamartomas and present intra-orally as mucosal swellings on the tongue or gingivae. Multiple oral neuromas are a feature of the multiple endocrine neoplasia syndrome, and as the oral signs may precede the development of more serious aspects of the condition (such as carcinoma of the thyroid), children presenting with multiple lesions should be referred to an endocrinologist.

Malignant Tumours of the Oral Soft Tissues

- Epithelial tumours such as squamous cell carcinoma are rare in children. Malignant salivary neoplasms are also rare although muco-epidermoid carcinomas have been reported in young patients.
- Hodgkin's and non-Hodgkin's lymphomas have been reported in children however they are relatively rare in the paediatric age group. An exception is Burkitt's lymphoma, which is endemic in parts of Africa and occurs in those under 14 years of age, indeed in these areas the condition accounts for almost half of all malignancy in children. Burkitt's lymphoma is multifocal, but a jaw tumour (more often in the maxilla) is often the presenting symptom. Burkitt's lymphoma is strongly linked to the Epstein-Barr virus as a causal agent.
- Rhabdomyosarcomas are malignant tumours of skeletal muscle and present in patients around 9 to 12 years of age. The usual site is the tongue. Metastases are common and the prognosis is poor.

Jaw Cysts

- The dentigerous cyst is the most common jaw cyst in children. Its origin is the reduced enamel epithelium (early stage of tooth formation) and attachment to the tooth occurs at the amelo-cemental junction (where the enamel of the crown and the cementum of the root meet). There are often no symptoms but eruption of the affected tooth will be prevented.
- Radicular cysts are related to the apex (root tip) of a non-vital tooth, they rarely occur in the primary dentition. They are often symptomless and are discovered radiographically. Extraction, apicectomy or conventional endodontics will affect a cure.
- Lateral periodontal cysts are very rare in children.
- The odontogenic keratocyst (Fig. 23.34) is the most aggressive of the jaw cysts. It has a high rate of recurrence due to the fact that remnants left after

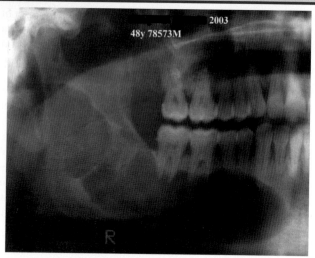

Fig. 23.34: Odontogenic keratocyst

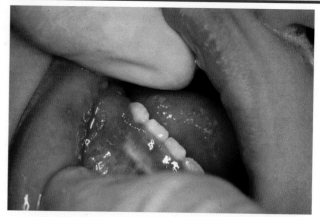

Fig. 23.35: Gingivitis in acute herpetic gingivostomatitis

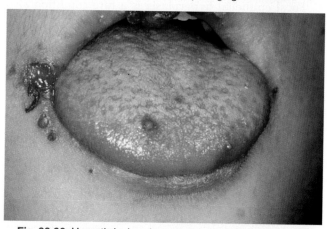

Fig. 23.36: Herpetic lesions in acute herpetic gingivostomatitis

incomplete removal will regenerate. These cysts may be found in children and may be associated with the Gorlin-Goltz syndrome. Keratocysts associated with this syndrome appear in the first decade of life whereas the syndromic basal cell carcinomas are rare before puberty. Other signs and symptoms include: multiple basal cell carcinomas, bifid ribs, calcification of the falx cerebri, hypertelorism, and frontal and temporal bossing.

*   Non-odontogenic cysts include the nasopalatine duct cyst, which may occur clinically as a swelling in the anterior mid-line of the hard palate and radiographically as a radiolucency of greater than 6 mm diameter in the position of the nasopalatine duct. The anterior teeth commonly have vital pulps. Surgical excision is curative.

*   The globulo-maxillary cyst, which occurs between the upper lateral incisor and canine teeth, is now thought to be odontogenic in origin: either a radicular cyst, or an odontogenic keratocyst.

*   The haemorrhagic bone cyst is a condition that may be found in children and adolescents. It occurs most commonly in the mandible in the premolar/molar region and is often a chance radiographic finding and normally asymptomatic. Radiographically it appears as a scalloped radiolucency between the roots of the teeth and regresses either spontaneously or after surgical intervention.

INFECTION

Viral Infections

Herpes Simplex

Initial infection with the herpes simplex virus type 1 (HSV-1) usually occurs in children between the ages of 6 months and 5 years. Younger infants are thought to be protected due to levels of circulating maternal antibodies. This initial infection is commonly known as acute herpetic gingivostomatitis.

Almost 100 per cent of urban adult populations are carriers of the virus, which would suggest that the majority of childhood infections are subclinical. The virus is spread via droplet transmission and has an incubation period of around 7 days.

Early symptoms include: Pyrexia; headache; general malaise; oral pain; mild dysphagia; and cervical lymphadenopathy. Later signs include: Severe oedematous marginal gingivitis (Fig. 23.35); fluid-filled vesicles on the gingivae, tongue, lips (Fig. 23.36), buccal, and palatal mucosa; and yellow ulceration with red inflamed margins (due to rupture of vesicles after a few hours).

Severe but very rare complications of the infection are encephalitis and aseptic meningitis.

The presentation of this infection is so characteristic that diagnosis is rarely a problem. Smears from newly ruptured vesicles can be taken if diagnosis is in doubt.

Herpetic gingivostomatitis does not respond well to active treatment. Hydration, bed rest and a soft diet are recommended during the febrile stage. Pyrexia can be controlled using paracetamol or ibuprofen paediatric suspension. Secondary infection of ulcerated areas may be prevented by the use of chlorhexidine. Chlorhexidine mouthrinse (0.2 per cent, two to three times a day) may be used in older.

Children (>6 years) who are able to expectorate, but in younger children a chlorhexidine spray can be used (twice daily) or the solution applied by the parent using a cotton swab. In severe cases where diagnosis has been made early, systemic acyclovir can be prescribed as a suspension (200 mg) and swallowed, five times daily for 5 days. In children under 2 years the dose is halved. Acyclovir is active against the herpesvirus but is unable to eradicate it completely.

Oral lesions heal without scaring and the clinical signs and symptoms of the infection subside in around 14 days.

Following primary infection, the herpes virus remains dormant in the host's epithelial cells. The latent virus may become reactivated with this recurrent infection presenting as herpes labialis, the common "cold sore" (Fig. 23.37). This vesicular lesion presents on the mucocutaneous border of the lips and vesicles rupture to produce crusting. Intraoral recurrence is also possible presenting as an attenuated form of the primary infection. Cold sores can be treated by applying acyclovir cream (5%, five times daily for about 5 days); again best results are with early treatment.

Herpes Varicella-zoster

- Chickenpox is a presentation of varicella-zoster virus infection mainly affecting children. The virus produces a vesicular rash on the skin and intra-oral lesions that resemble those of primary herpetic infection. The condition is highly contagious but self-limiting.
- Shingles occurs as a reactivation of the latent virus within a skin dermatome (Fig. 23.38), it is far more common in adults. Orofacial presentation of the virus may lead to vesicular lesions within the peripheral distribution of a branch of the trigeminal nerve.

Mumps

Mumps produces a painful enlargement of the parotid glands, it is usually bilateral. The causative agent is a myxovirus. Associated complaints include headache, vomiting and fever. Symptoms last for about a week and the condition is contagious.

Measles (Rubeola)

The intra-oral manifestation of measles (Koplik's spots) occurs on the buccal mucosa as white speckling surrounded by a red margin. The oral signs usually precede the skin lesions and disappear early in the course of the disease. The skin rash of measles normally appears as a red maculopapular lesion. Fever is present and the disease is contagious.

German Measles (Rubella)

German measles does not usually produce signs in the oral mucosa: however, the tonsils may be affected.

Protection against the diseases of mumps, measles and rubella can be achieved by vaccination of children in their early years.

Herpangina

This is a coxsackie A virus infection that can be differentiated from primary herpetic infection by the different location of the vesicles. These are found in the tonsillar or pharyngeal region and in addition herpangina lesions do not coalesce to form large areas of ulceration. The condition is short-lived.

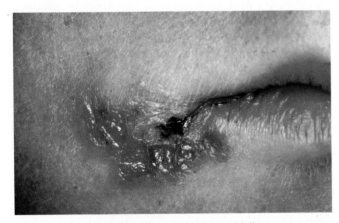

Fig. 23.37: Recurrent herpes labialis

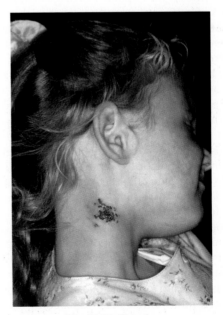

Fig. 23.38: Shingles

Hand, Foot and Mouth Disease

This coxsackie A virus infection produces a maculo-papular rash on the hands and feet. Intra-orally vesicles rupture to produce painful ulceration similar to apthous ulcers. The condition lasts for 10-14 days.

Infectious Mononucleosis

This condition, caused by the Epstein-Barr virus, is not uncommon amongst teenagers and the usual form of transmission is by kissing. Oral ulceration and petechial haemorrhage at the hard/soft palate junction may occur. There is lymph node enlargement and associated fever. There is no specific treatment, however it should be noted that the prescription of ampicillin and amoxycillin could cause a rash in those suffering from infectious mono-nucleosis and so these antibiotics should be avoided during the course of the disease.

Treatment of all the above viral illnesses is symptomatic and relies mainly on analgesia and maintenance of fluid intake. Aspirin should be avoided in children less than 12 years of age in order to avoid Reye's syndrome.

Bacterial Infection

Acute Orofacial Infection

Acute orofacial infection is usually the result of an untreated carious tooth, which has resulted in abscess formation with subsequent dissemination of infectious organisms into the surrounding tissues.

A rapidly spreading extra-oral infection is a surgical emergency, which merits immediate treatment and may require admission for in-patient management (Fig. 23.39). Two areas of extra-oral spread are of special importance. These are the submandibular region and the angle between the eye and nose. Swelling in the submandibular region arising from posterior mandibular teeth can produce raising of the floor of the mouth. This can cause a physical obstruction to breathing and spread from this region to the parapharyngeal spaces may further obstruct the airway. The progression from dysphagia to dyspnoea can be rapid and a submandibular swelling should be decompressed as a matter of urgency in children. A child with raising of the floor of the mouth requires immediate admission to hospital. The fact that trismus is invariably an associated feature makes expert anaesthetic help essential for safe management.

Infection involving the angle between eye and nose has the potential to spread intracranially and produce a cavernous sinus thrombosis. This is a potentially life-threatening complication. The angular veins of the orbit have no valves and connect the cavernous sinus to the external face. If the normal extra-cranial flow is obstructed due to pressure from the extra-oral infection then infected

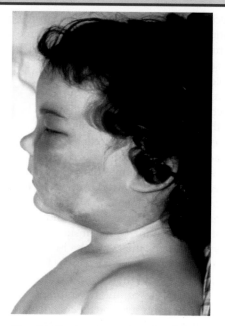

Fig. 23.39: Acute orofacial infection

material can enter the sinus by reverse flow. To prevent this complication infection in this area (which arise from upper anterior teeth, especially the canine) must be treated quickly.

The principles of the treatment of acute infection are:
1. Remove the cause
2. Institute drainage
3. Prevent spread
4. Restore function.

In addition analgesia and adequate hydration must be maintained. Removal of the cause is essential to cure an orofacial infection arising from a dental source. This usually means extraction or endodontic therapy.

Institution of drainage and prevention of spread are supportive treatments—they are not definitive cures. Drainage may be obtained during the removal of the cause, for example a dental extraction, or may precede definitive treatment if this makes management easier, for example incision and drainage of a submandibular abscess.

Prevention of spread may be achieved surgically or by the use of antibiotics. In severe cases intravenous antibiotics will be used. The antibiotic of choice in children is penicillin.

It is important to remember that acute infections are painful and that analgesics, as well as antibiotics, should be prescribed. The use of paracetamol elixir is usually sufficient. Similarly it is important that a child suffering from an acute infection is adequately hydrated. It the infection has restricted the intake of oral fluids due to dysphagia then admission to hospital for intravenous fluid replacement is required.

Staphylococcal Infections

Impetigo may be caused by staphylococci and streptococci and can affect the angles of the mouth and the lips.

It presents as a crusting vesiculo-bullous lesion. The vesicles coalesce to produce ulceration over a wide area. Pigmentation may occur during healing. The condition is self-limiting although antibiotics may be prescribed in some cases.

Staphylococcal organisms can cause osteomyelitis of the jawbone in children. Although the introduction of antibiotics has reduced the incidence of severe forms of the condition it can still be devastating. In addition to aggressive antibiotic therapy surgical intervention is required to remove bony sequestra.

Streptococcal Infection

Streptococcal infections in childhood vary from a muco-purulent nasal discharge to tonsillitis, pharyngitis and gingivitis.

Scarlet fever is a beta-haemolytic streptococcal infection consisting of a skin rash with maculopapular lesions of the oral mucosa associated with tonsillitis and pharyngitis. The tongue shows characteristic changes from a strawberry appearance in the early stages to a raspberry-like form in the later stages.

Congenital Syphilis

Congenital syphilis is caused by transmission from an infected mother. Oral mucosal changes such as rhagades, which is a pattern of scarring at the angle of the mouth, may occur. In addition this disease may cause characteristic dental changes such as Hutchinson's incisors (the teeth taper towards the incisal edge rather than the cervical margin) and mulberry molars (globular masses of enamel over the occlusal surface).

Tuberculosis

Tuberculous lesions of the oral cavity are rare however tuberculous lymphadenitis affecting submandibular and cervical lymph nodes is occasionally seen. These present as tender enlarged nodes that may progress to abscess formation with discharge through skin. Surgical removal of infected glands produces a much neater scar than that caused by spontaneous rupture through skin if the disease is allowed to progress.

Cat-Scratch Disease

This is a self-limiting disease, which presents as an enlargement of regional lymph nodes. It is caused by rickettsiae like agent (Rochalimaea quintana). After successful cultivation, the new species has been named R henselae. The nodes are painful and enlargement occurs up to 3 weeks following a cat-scratch. The nodes become suppurative and may perforate the skin. Treatment often involves incision and drainage.

Fungal Infection

Candidiasis

Neonatal acute candidiasis (thrush) contracted during birth is not uncommon. Likewise young children may develop the condition when resistance is lowered or after antibiotic therapy. The white patches of *Candida* are easily removed to leave an erythematous (Fig. 23.40) or bleeding base. Treatment with nystatin or miconazole is effective (those under two years of age should receive 2.5 ml of a miconazole gel (25 mg/ml) twice daily; 5 ml twice daily is prescribed for those under 6 years of age, and 5 ml four times a day for those over 6 years of age).

Actinomycosis

Actinomycosis can occur in children and may follow intraoral trauma including dental extractions. The organisms spread through the tissues and can cause dysphagia if the submandibular region is involved. Abscesses may rupture onto the skin and long-term antibiotic therapy is required. Penicillin should be prescribed and maintained for at least two weeks following clinical cure.

Protozoal Infections

Infection by Toxoplasma gondii may occasionally occur in children. The principle reservoir of infection being cats. Glandular toxoplasmosis is similar in presentation to infectious mononucleosis and is found mainly in children and young adults. There may be a granulomatous reaction in the oral mucosa and there can be parotid gland enlargement. The disease is self-limiting although in severe infection an anti-protozoal such as pyrimethamine may be used.

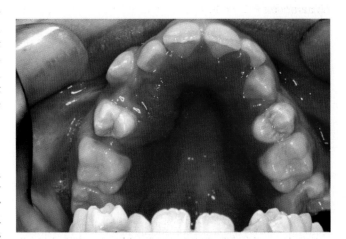

Fig. 23.40: Candidal infection

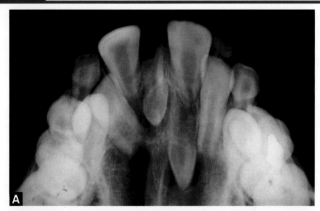

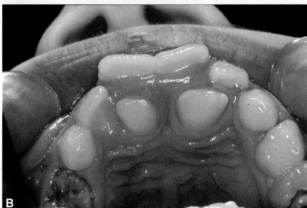

Figs 23.41A and B: (A) Radiograph showing unerupted supernumerary teeth, (B) Clinical picture showing erupted supernumerary teeth

ANOMALIES

Anomalies in Number of Teeth

Alterations in tooth number result from problems during dental development. In addition to hereditary patterns producing extra or missing teeth local aetiological factors can also affect tooth number.

Hyperdontia

Hyperdontia (supernumerary teeth) occurs in both primary and permanent dentition, its incidence in the permanent dentition is around 1-3% and affects male twice as often as females. The most common position for an extra tooth is the maxillary midline (Figs 23.41A and B). Several syndromes are associated with hyperdontia and the following conditions all require referral to a dental surgeon.
• Cleidocranial dysostosis
• Gardner syndrome
• Crouzon's syndrome (Craniofacial dysostosis)

Hypodontia

Hypodontia is the term given to the congenital absence of teeth (Fig. 23.42) it is most commonly hereditary and affects between 3-6% of the population (excluding 3rd molars).

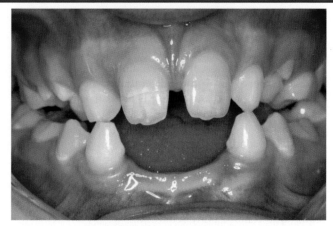

Fig. 23.42: Congenitally absent teeth

The mandibular second premolar is the most commonly missing tooth. Syndromes associated with hypodontia include: Ectodermal dysplasia; Achondroplasia; and Rieger syndrome.

Anomalies in Size of Teeth

Microdontia

Three types of microdontia (small teeth) are recognised:
1. True generalized microdontia—All teeth are normally formed but smaller than normal. Occurs in pituitary dwarfism.
2. Relative generalized microdontia—Normal or slightly smaller teeth present in jaws that are larger than normal.
3. Microdontia—Usually only one tooth is involved. Affects maxillary lateral incisors and third molars. May occur after chemotherapy for neoplastic disease.
   Conditions associated with microdontia include Down syndrome, ectodermal dysplasia and Ellis-van Creveld syndrome.

Macrodontia

Macrodontia (large teeth) can also be classified as three types:
1. True generalized macrodontia—Several teeth are larger than normal. Seen in pituitary gigantism.
2. Relative generalized macrodontia—Teeth are normal or slightly larger than normal in small jaws.
3. Macrodontia of a single tooth is relatively uncommon. An isolated tooth displaying macrodontia can result from twinning abnormalities that originate during the proliferation phase of development. Fusion and gemination are the most common twinning abnormalities, and both demonstrate enlarged crowns.

Double Teeth

Fusion is said to occur when there has been union of two embryonically developing teeth and occurs more commonly in the primary dentition. The majority of these

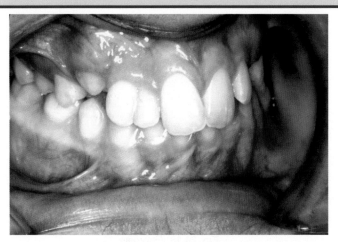

Fig. 23.43: Double lateral incisor

teeth have large bifid crowns with one pulp chamber. Gemination is said to occur when there has been incomplete division of a single tooth bud and again occur more commonly in the primary dentition. Again the appearance is of a large bifid crown with one pulp chamber. As it is difficult to distinguish clinically between these two entities, fusion and germination, the favoured term of "double teeth" (Fig. 23.43) has now more commonly been adopted.

Anomalies in Tooth Shape

Abnormalities of shape originate during the morpho-differentiation stage of teeth development and are manifested as alterations in crown and root form.

Dens Evaginatus

Dens envaginatus (extra cusp) occurs due to an evagi-nation of enamel. It occurs most commonly in the central groove of posterior teeth or on the cingulum of anterior teeth, this is sometimes known as a Talon cusp. The extra cusp contains enamel, dentine and pulp tissue.

Dens in Dente/Dens Invaginatus

Dens in dente/dens invaginatus (Fig. 23.44) occurs due to an invagination of enamel and usually affects the maxillary lateral incisor tooth. Enamel and dentine can be missing in the invaginated area leading to pulpal exposure.

Taurodontism

Taurodontism occurs when there has been an abnormality in root formation. It occurs in 0.5- 5.0% of the population. Teeth appear to have elongated pulp chambers and short blunt roots. This condition may be associated with a number of syndromes: Klinefelter syndrome; Trichodento-osseous syndrome; Oraofacialdigital syndrome II;

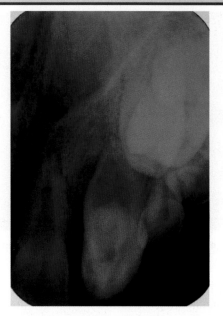

Fig. 23.44: Radiograph showing dens invaginatus

Hypohidrotic Ectodermal dysplasia; Amelogenesis Imperfecta-Type IV; and Down syndrome.

Tooth Dilaceration is seen in 25% of permanent teeth commonly following an intrusion injury to the primary dentition. These teeth have an abnormal bend in the crown or root. Children with Congenital ichthyosis may show this phenomenon.

Anomalies in Enamel and Dentine

Amelogenesis Imperfecta (AI)

This is a group of hereditary defects of enamel, which are unassociated with any other medical condition. Amelo-genesis is an entirely ectodermal disturbance with an incidence of 1 in 14, 000. Both primary and permanent dentitions are affected and the condition can be classified into four major categories.

Type I: Hypoplastic AI

This defect occurs during the histodifferentiation stage. Enamel is not formed to full thickness because ameloblasts fail to lay down sufficient matrix. The resulting disorder may include a localized defect, localized pitting, or generalized lack of enamel formation. Affected teeth appear small with open contacts due to very thin or non-existent enamel causing thermal sensitivity.

Type II: Hypomaturation AI

This defect occurs during matrix apposition. Enamel is softer and chips from the underlying dentin (Fig. 23.45). Enamel has a mottled brown-yellow-white colour. Interproximal contact points between teeth are present as enamel is of normal thickness. Radiographically enamel approaches the radiodensity of dentin.

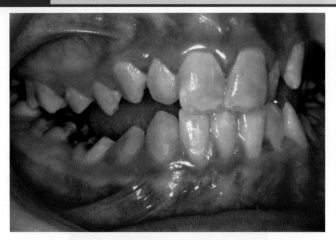

Fig. 23.45: Hypomaturation form of amelogenesis imperfecta

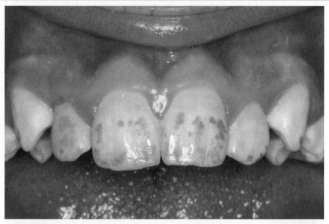

Fig. 23.46: Fluorosis

Type III: Hypocalcified AI

Defect occurs during the calcification stage. Most common type of amelogenesis imperfecta. Enamel is of normal thickness but soft, friable, and easily lost by attrition. Enamel appears dull, lustrous, honey coloured and stains easily.

Type IV: Hypomaturation-hypoplastic with Taurodontism

Defects occur during both the apposition and histo-differentiation stages. Most rare type of enamel defect. Features include patchy areas of reduced enamel thickness leading to loss of interproximal contacts, taurodontism and severe attrition. Radiographically the radiodensity of enamel resembles dentine.

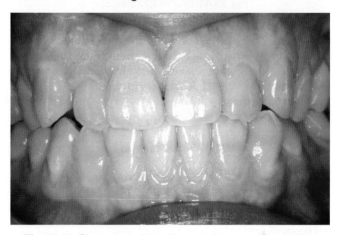

Fig. 23.47: Chronological banding seen in tetracycline staining

Environmental Enamel Hypoplasia or Hypomineralisation

These are defects in the quantitative or qualitative characteristics of the enamel, which can be caused by various systemic factors present during the period of enamel formation such as:
- Nutritional deficiencies in Vitamin A, C, D, calcium and phosphorus
- Severe infections such as Rubella, Syphilis, and high fever
- Neurologic defects such as Cerebral palsy and Sturge-Weber syndrome
- Prematurity and birth injuries
- Radiation.
- Fluorosis (Fig. 23.46)(excessive ingestion of fluoride)
- Tetracycline induced hypoplasia and discolouration (Fig. 23.47).
- Increasing incidence.

All teeth forming during these periods of environmental upset will be affected. The effect can often be seen as chronological banding of the teeth.

Localized Enamel Hypoplasia (Turner's Teeth)

Infection of individual primary teeth may affect the developing permanent tooth leading to localised patched of hypoplasia/hypomineralisation (Fig. 23.48). This effect can also result following trauma to primary tooth, which disturbs the permanent tooth bud.

Dentinogenesis Imperfecta (DI)

These are a group of inherited dentine defects originating during the histodifferentiation stage of dentine formation. The condition affects 1 in 8000 and can be subdivided into three basic types:
- **Shields Type I (Associated with Osteogenesis Imperfecta)**—Inherited defect in collagen formation resulting in osteoporotic brittle bones, these patients commonly have blue sclera (Fig. 23.49). Primary teeth more affected than permanent teeth. Other features include periapical radiolucencies, bulbous crowns, obliteration of pulp chambers, root fractures and amber translucent tooth colour (Fig. 23.50).

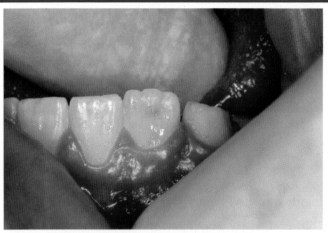

Fig. 23.48: Localised enamel hypoplasia

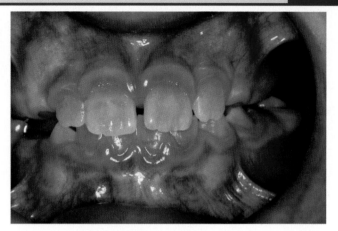

Fig. 23.50: Dentinogenesis imperfecta

Odontodysplasia (Ghost Teeth)

These teeth show a localized arrest in tooth development due to regional vascular developmental anomaly. The teeth have a "Ghost-like" appearance with short roots, shell-like crowns and large diffusely calcified pulp chambers.

Anomalies in Cementum

Developmental defects involving cementum are uncommon.

Hypophosphatasia

This is a rare cause of premature mobility of the teeth. Other features are: low serum alkaline phosphatase levels; osteoporosis with bone fragility; and failure of cememtum formation leading to premature loss of primary incisors.

DENTOALVEOLAR TRAUMA

Prevalence and Aetiology

Dental trauma in childhood and adolescence is common. At 5 years of age 31-40% of boys and 16-30% of girls, and at 12 years of age 12-33% of boys and 4-19% of girls will have suffered some dental trauma. Boys are affected almost twice as often as girls in both the primary and the permanent dentitions.

The majority of dental injuries in the primary and permanent dentitions involve the anterior teeth, especially the maxillary central incisors. The mandibular central incisors and maxillary lateral incisors are less frequently involved.

The most accident-prone times are between 2 and 4 years for the primary dentition and 7 and 10 years for the permanent dentition. In the primary dentition co-ordination and judgement are incompletely developed and the majority of injuries are due to falls in and around the home as the child becomes more adventurous and explores

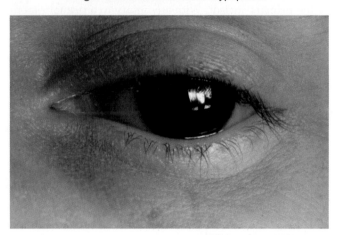

Fig. 23.49: Blue sclera seen in osteogenesis imperfecta

- **Shields Type II (Hereditary Opalescent Dentine)**—Primary and permanent dentition are equally affected. Features are same as Shields Type I except there is no osteogenesis imperfecta.
- **Shields Type III (Brandywine Type)**—Teeth have a shell-like appearance with bell-shaped crowns. Occurs exclusively in an isolated group in Maryland USA called the Brandywine population.

Dentine Dysplasia

These are inherited dentine defects involving circum-pulpal and root morphology. Classified into two types:
- **Shields Type I**—Both primary and permanent teeth exhibit normal crown morphology, multiple periapical radiolucencies, short roots and absent pulp chambers
- **Shields Type II**—Amber coloured primary teeth. Permanent teeth are normal in appearance but radiographically demonstrate thistle-tube shaped pulp chambers.

its surroundings. In the permanent dentition most injuries are caused by falls and collisions while playing and running, although bicycles are a common accessory. The place of injury varies in different countries according to local customs but accidents at school remain common.

Sports injuries usually occur in teenage years and are commonly associated with contact sports such as soccer, rugby, ice hockey, and basketball.

Injuries due to road traffic accidents and assaults are most commonly associated with the late teenage years and adulthood and are often closely related to alcohol abuse.

One form of injury in childhood that must never be forgotten is child physical abuse or non-accident injury. Up to 50 per cent of these children will have orofacial injuries.

Patients with protrusion of upper incisors and insufficient lip closure are at significantly greater risk of traumatic dental injuries.

Dental History

- When did injury occur? The time interval between injury and treatment significantly influences the prognosis of avulsions, luxations, crown fractures with or without pulpal exposures, and dento-alveolar fractures.
- Where did injury occur? May indicate the need for tetanus prophylaxis.
- How did injury occur? The nature of the accident can yield information on the type of injury expected. Discrepancy between history and clinical findings raises suspicion of non-accidental injury.
- Lost teeth/fragments? If a tooth or fractured piece cannot be accounted for when there has been a history of loss of consciousness then a chest radiograph should be obtained to exclude inhalation.
- Previous dental history? Previous trauma can affect future prognosis. An idea of previous dental treatment carried out will help decide on what treatment is possible.

Intra-oral Examination

This must be systematic and include the recording of:
- Laceration, haemorrhage, and swelling of the oral mucosa and gingiva. Any lacerations should be examined for tooth fragments or other foreign material. Lacerations of lips or tongue require suturing but those of the oral mucosa heal very quickly and may not need suturing. Orofacial signs of non-accidental injury (NAI) may present in this manner.
- Abnormalities of occlusion, tooth displacement, fractured crowns or cracks in the enamel.

The following signs and reactions to tests are particularly helpful:

- Mobility. Degree of mobility is estimated in a horizontal and a vertical direction. When several teeth move together a fracture of the alveolar process is suspected. Excessive mobility may also suggest root fracture or tooth displacement.
- Reaction to percussion. In a horizontal and vertical direction and compared against a contralateral uninjured tooth. A duller note may indicate root fracture.
- Colour of tooth. Early colour change is visible on the palatal surface of the gingival third of the crown.

Injuries to the Primary Dentition

During its early development the permanent incisor is located palatally to and in close proximity with the apex of the primary incisor. With any injury to a primary tooth there is risk of damage to the underlying permanent successor (Fig. 23.51).

Due to the patients age few restorative procedures will be possible and in the majority of cases the decision is between extraction and maintenance without performing extensive treatment. A primary incisor should always be removed if its maintenance will jeopardize the developing tooth bud.

Injuries to the Permanent Dentition

Most traumatized teeth can be treated successfully. Prompt and appropriate treatment improves prognosis.

Emergency Treatment

- Retain vitality of fractured or displaced tooth;
- Treat exposed pulp tissue;
- Reduction and immobilization of displaced teeth;
- Antiseptic mouthwash, antibiotics, and tetanus prophylaxis;
- Advise soft diet.

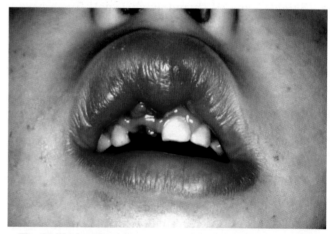

Fig. 23.51: Avulsion injury to upper right primary central incisor

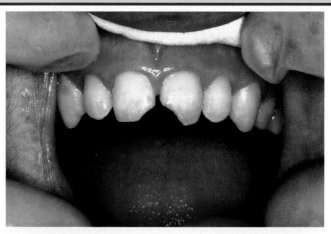

Fig. 23.52: Enamel dentine fractures of permanent incisors

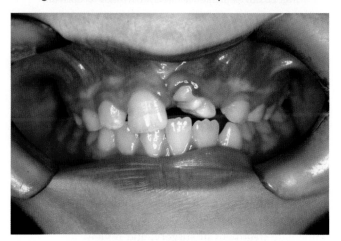

Fig. 23.53: Enamel, dentine and pulp fracture

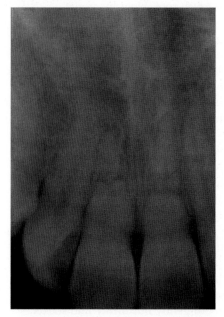

Fig. 23.54: Radiograph showing root fractures

Injuries to the hard dental tissues and the pulp

Enamel-dentine fracture: Immediate treatment is necessary due to the involvement of dentine (Fig. 23.52). The pulp requires protection against thermal irritation and from bacteria via the dentinal tubules. Restoration of crown morphology also stabilizes the position of the tooth in the arch. Emergency protection of the exposed dentine should be carried out as soon as possible, refer to a dental surgeon.

Enamel, dentine, pulp fracture: Immediate treatment is required which will involve treatment of the pulpal tissue; refer to a dental surgeon (Fig. 23.53).

Root fracture: Root fractures occur most frequently in the middle or the apical third of the root (Fig. 23.54). The coronal fragment may be extruded or luxated. Luxation is usually in a lingual or palatal direction.

If displacement has occurred the coronal fragment should be repositioned as soon as possible by gentle digital manipulation and referred as soon as possible to a dental surgeon.

Splinting

Trauma may loosen a tooth either by damaging the periodontal ligament or fracturing the root. Splinting immobilizes the tooth in the correct anatomical position so that further trauma is prevented and healing can occur. Different injuries require different splinting regimens. A functional splint involves one, and a rigid splint two, abutment teeth either side of the injured tooth. There are a number of types and methods of splinting, the most effective of which require materials generally only held in a dental surgery.

Injuries to the periodontal tissues

Subluxation: In addition to the above there is rupture of some periodontal ligament fibres and the tooth is mobile in the socket, although not displaced. All these injuries should be referred to a dental surgeon. The treatment for both these injuries is:
- Occlusal relief;
- Soft diet for 7 days;
- Immobilization with a splint if tenderness to percussion is significant;
- Chlorhexidine 0.2 per cent mouthwash, twice daily.

There is minimal risk of pulpal necrosis following this injury, and in over 97 per cent of cases there is no evidence of resorption.

Extrusive luxation: There is a rupture of periodontal ligament and pulp (Fig. 23.55).

Lateral luxation: There is a rupture of the periodontal ligament, pulp, and the alveolar plate. Refer patient to a dental surgeon as soon as possible. You may wish to

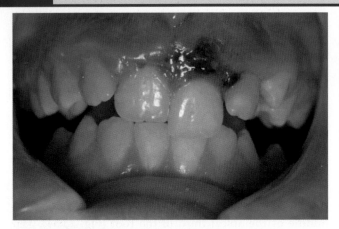

Fig. 23.55: Extrusive and lateral luxation injury

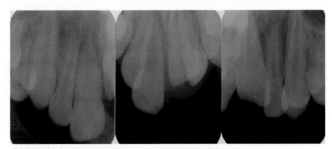

Fig. 23.56: Radiograph showing intrusive luxation injury

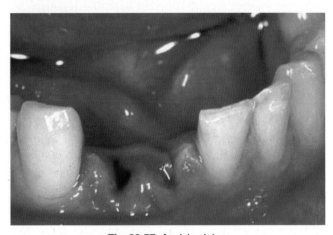

Fig. 23.57: Avulsion injury

prescribe chlorhexidine mouthwash and amoxycillin and advise a soft diet.

Antibiotics may have a beneficial effect in promoting repair of the periodontal ligament. They do not appear to affect pulpal prognosis.

Intrusive luxation: These injuries are the result of an axial, apical impact and there is extensive damage to the periodontal ligament, pulp and alveolar plate (Fig. 23.56).

Avulsion and replantation: Avulsion is when a tooth has been completely removed from its socket (Fig. 23.57)

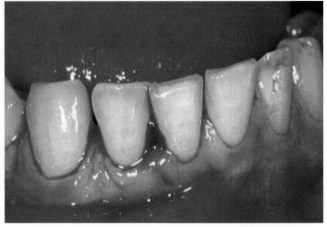

Fig. 23.58: Replanted avulsed teeth ready for splinting

Replantation (Fig. 23.58) should nearly always be attempted even though it may offer only a temporary solution due to the frequent occurrence of external inflammatory resorption. Even when resorption occurs the tooth may be retained for years acting as a natural space maintainer and preserving the height and width of the alveolus to facilitate later implant placement.

Successful healing after replantation can only occur if there is minimal damage to the pulp and the periodontal ligament. The type of extra-alveolar storage medium and the extra-alveolar time, i.e. the time the tooth has been out of the mouth are critical factors. The suggested protocol for replantation can be divided into: advice on phone; immediate treatment in surgery; and review.

Advice on phone (to teacher, parent, etc.)
• Do not touch root. Hold by crown.
• Wash gently under cold tap water for a maximum of 10 seconds.
• Replace into socket or transport in milk to surgery.
• If replaced bite gently on a handkerchief to retain it and come to surgery.

The best transport medium is the tooth's own socket. Understandably non-dentists may be unhappy to replant the tooth, but milk is an effective iso-osmolar medium. Saliva, the patient's buccal sulcus, or normal saline are alternatives.

Immediate surgery treatment
• Do not handle root. If replanted remove tooth from socket.
• Rinse tooth with normal saline. Note state of root development. Store in saline.
• Local analgesia.
• Irrigate socket with saline and remove clot and any foreign material.
• Push tooth gently but firmly into socket.
• Non-rigid functional splint for 7-10 days.

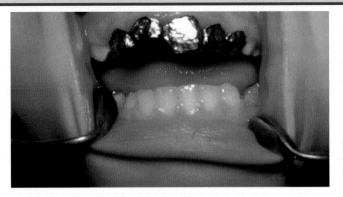

Fig. 23.59: Foil splint

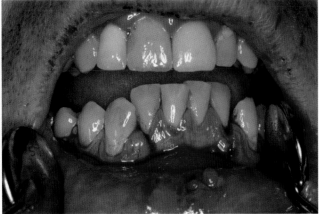

Fig. 23.60: Alveolar bone fracture

- Check occlusion.
- Baseline radiographs: periapical or anterior occlusal. Any other teeth injured?
- Antibiotics, chlorhexidine mouthwash, soft diet as previously.
- Check tetanus immunization status.

For adequate splinting the patient will need urgent referral to a dental surgeon. If dental services are unavailable the tooth can be held in place with some moulded cooking foil (Fig. 23.59) or sutured into position, this will ensure safety from dislodgement or inhalation until dental treatment is obtained.

Injuries to the supporting bone

The extent and position of the alveolar fracture should be verified clinically and radiographically (Fig. 23.60). If there is displacement of the teeth to the extent that their apices have risen up and are now positioned over the labial or lingual/palatal alveolar plates (apical lock) then they will require extruding first to free the apices prior to repositioning.

The segment of alveolus with teeth requires only 3-4 weeks of ridged splinting with two abutment teeth either side of the fracture, together with antibiotics, chlorhexidine, soft diet, and tetanus prophylaxis check.

Pulpal survival is more likely if repositioning occurs within 1 h of the injury. Root resorption is rare.

Child Physical Abuse (Non-accidental Injury)

A child is considered to be abused if he or she is treated in a way that is unacceptable in a given culture at a given time (Fig. 23.61). Child physical abuse is now recognised as an international issue and has been reported in many countries. Each week at least 1-2 children in Britain and 80 children in the United States will die as a result of abuse or neglect. At least one child per 1000 in Britain suffers severe physical abuse; for example fractures, brain haemorrhage, severe internal injuries or mutilation and in the United States more than 95 per cent of serious

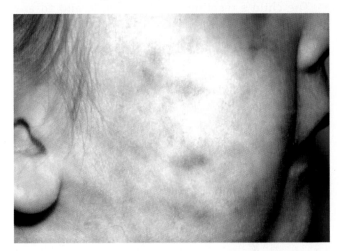

Fig. 23.61: Slap mark on face of physically abused child

intracranial injuries during the first year of life are the result of abuse. Although some reports will prove to be unfounded the common experience is that proved cases of child abuse are four to five times as common as they were a decade ago.

Child abuse is not a full diagnosis; it is merely a symptom of disordered parenting. The aim of intervention is to diagnose and cure the disordered parenting. Simply to aim at preventing death is a lowly ambition. It has been estimated in the United States that 35-50% of severely abused children will receive serious re-injury and 50 per cent will die if they are returned to their home environment without intervention. In some cases the occurrence of physical abuse may provide an opportunity for intervention. If this opportunity is missed, there may be no further opportunity for many years.

Approximately 50 per cent of cases diagnosed as child physical abuse have extra- and intra-oral facial trauma and so the dental practitioner may be the first professional to see or suspect abuse. Injuries may take the form of contusions and ecchymoses, abrasions and lacerations, burns, bites, dental trauma, and fractures.

The following 10 points should be considered whenever doubts and suspicions are aroused.

- Could the injury have been caused accidentally and if so how?
- Does the explanation for the injury fit the age and the clinical findings?
- If the explanation of cause is consistent with the injury, is this itself within normally acceptable limits of behaviour?
- If there has been any delay seeking advice are there good reasons for this?
- Does the story of the accident vary?
- The nature of the relationship between parent and child.
- The child's reaction to other people and to any medical/dental examinations.
- The general demeanour of the child.

- Any comments made by child and/or parent that give concern about the child's upbringing or lifestyle.
- History of previous injury.

ORAL MANIFESTATIONS OF SYSTEMIC DISEASE

In addition to specific pathological oral conditions, diseases that affect other systems of the body can present oral manifestations for example Crohn's disease. Disorders such as chronic renal failure and diabetes can predispose to periodontal disease and there may be poor resistance to spread of odontogenic infection.

The temporomandibular joint can be involved in juvenile idiopathic arthritis and the jaws can be affected in hyperparathyroidism (giant cell tumours).

Not only can the oral soft tissues be affected by systemic conditions but also the physician should always be alert to the fact that the oral mucosa may exhibit signs that help to diagnose a systemic condition.

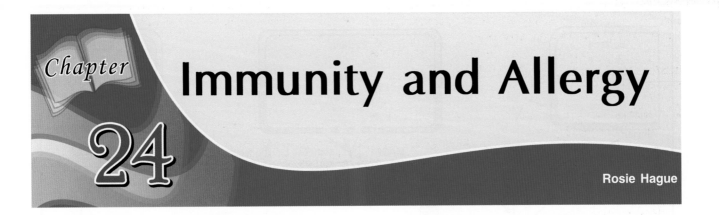

Immunity and Allergy

Rosie Hague

In order to grow and develop normally, we have to develop methods of protecting ourselves from organisms which have the potential for invasion and to cause damage. Pathogenesis of infectious disease is not only dependent upon characteristics of the pathogen, but also upon our immune response to it. As children develop from fetal life through infancy into childhood, so their immune systems are continuing to mature. Hence susceptibility to different infectious agents varies with age.

COMPONENTS OF THE IMMUNE SYSTEM

The first line of defence against infection is the physical barrier formed by the skin and mucous membranes.

The Skin

The epidermis is made up of 4 layers of densely packed cells, through which bacteria cannot penetrate. The outer layers are shed, taking organisms with them. Its dryness, together with the high salt content due to sweat, and low pH due to sebum and lactobacilli inhibits bacterial growth. Sweat also contains lysozyme, which is an antimicrobial enzyme particularly for gram-positive organisms. Sebum from hair follicles contains lipids and salts and proteins which have antimicrobial properties, but it also provides nutrition for commensal organisms such as corynebacteria. Skin cells can also secrete antimicrobial peptides such as cathelicidins and defensins and dermcidins. These peptides do not only have a direct effect, but they also stimulate components of the innate and adaptive immune system. Organisms which are able to colonise the skin surface inhibit pathogens, and many secrete proteins toxic to other species, known as bacteriocins.

Cells of the innate immune systems (Langerhans' cells, mast cells) and adaptive immune system (lymphocytes) are also found in the dermis should the superficial epidermis be penetrated.

Mucous Membranes

These are body surfaces not covered by skin. They are therefore protected by viscous mucus which traps microorganisms, and by washing. For example, tears wash organisms from the conjunctiva, and saliva and chewing of food has the same function in the mouth.

The Respiratory Tract

The nasal turbinates are designed to trap large particles, preventing their travelling down the respiratory tract. Smaller particles get further down, but cough and irritant receptors stimulate cough and bronchoconstriction, enabling them to be cleared. The mucociliary blanket is the chief means of clearing the respiratory tract from the smallest bronchioles to the larynx. In addition, compounds secreted onto the surface of the respiratory epithelium enhance bacterial killing. These include lysozyme, transferrin, alpha 1 antitrypsin, opsonins, interferon, as well as immunoglobulins and complement .

The Gastrointestinal Tract

In contrast to the respiratory tract, where potential pathogens are swept proximally, in the gut, peristalsis keeps bacteria moving distally to be eliminated. Gastric acid creates a stomach pH which is toxic to many bacteria, and those surviving to pass into the small intestine encounter bile and pancreatic secretions. The gut is not a sterile environment, and the normal gut flora is important in keeping pathogenic bacteria at bay. The intestinal wall is protected from invasion by these organisms by intestinal mucins, which bind potential pathogens. Molecules such as lysozyme and immunoglobulins are secreted onto the epithelial surface. The epithelial cells themselves are joined by tight junctions, which limit the passage of antigens across the barrier.

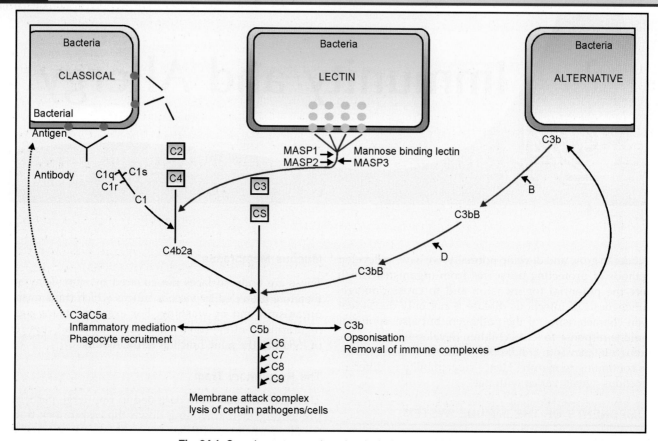

Fig. 24.1: Complement cascade—classical, all ± lectin pathways

Urogenital Tract

The flow of urine washes microorganisms away from the mucosal surface. Vaginal mucus performs the same function. In addition, the vesicoureteric junction acts as a one way valve, preventing urine (and microorganisms) flowing towards the kidneys.

THE NEXT LINE OF DEFENCE: INNATE (NON-SPECIFIC) IMMUNITY

Both humoral (chemical) agents and cells play major roles.

Humoral Agents

These agents are as follows.

Acute Phase Proteins

These are proteins produced by the liver whose plasma levels rise in response to inflammation.

C-reactive protein assists complement in binding to foreign or damaged cells.

Mannose binding lectin binds to carbohydrate moieties on the surface of bacteria and fungi, thus activating the lectin pathway of the complement system.

Alpha 1 antitrypsin and alpha 2 macroglobulin inhibit the activity of harmful proteases produced by bacteria.

Ferritin binds iron which is necessary for bacterial growth.

Others include coagulation factors (fibrinogen, plasminogen, factor VIII, von Willebrand factor), components of complement, amyloid P and amyloid A.

Antibacterial Agents

These include lysozyme, defensins, lactoferrin, and myeloperoxidase.

Complement

This is a series of blood proteins which, when activated, lead to lysis of bacteria, and also stimulate chemotaxis and phagocytosis.

The *classical pathway* is activated by bacterial antigen bound to antibody. The *alternative pathway* is activated directly by bacterial or fungal oligosaccharide, endotoxin, and immunoglobulin aggregates. The *lectin pathway* is activated by Mannan binding lectin bound to its receptor on the bacterial surface (Fig. 24.1).

CELLS OF THE INNATE IMMUNE SYSTEM

Phagocytes

These include monocytes/macrophages and neutrophils. They engulf opsonised bacteria and kill them within the phagosome. The most important mechanism for bacterial killing is the oxidative burst, illustrated in the Figure (Fig. 24.2). The oxygen radicals, hydrogen peroxide and hydroxyl ions all mediate killing.

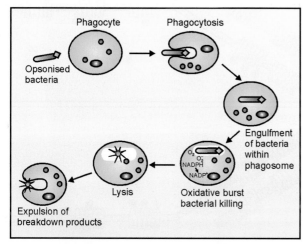

Fig. 24.2: Phagocytosis with oxidative burst

Eosinophils

These comprise 1-3% of circulating white blood cells. They are less efficient at phagocytosis and bacterial killing than neutrophils. They can kill parasites opsonised by antibody or complement. Eosinophil granule protein contains some powerful inflammatory mediators which can kill helminths directly, and induce basophil histamine release. It has long been assumed that they have a major role in defence against parasites, but their true function is unclear. When activated during an allergic response, these mediators cause tissue damage, particularly to the respiratory epithelium, causing chronic inflammatory change.

Basophils

These cells develop from promyelocytes in the bone marrow. They have granules containing many of the same mediators of immediate hypersensitivity as mast cells, but do not release heparin or arachidonic acid metabolites. They are found in the circulation. Again, it is assumed that they have some role in defence against parasitic disease.

Mast Cells

These cells develop from pluripotential stem cells (CD34+ cells) which migrate into tissues, and mature into mast cells which are differentiated from each other, depending on their site. They are activated in allergy, but can also be activated by pathogens or their products, peptide mediators, such as substance P, endothelin, and components of complement. They have high affinity for IgE and release chemicals such as histamine, neutrophil chemotactic factor, inflammatory proteases and heparin, which are pre-formed inflammatory mediators contained in granules. When stimulated they also produce arachidonic acid metabolites and platelet activating factor.

Natural Killer Cells

These are large lymphocytes which recognise and kill cells infected with viruses or intracellular pathogens, such as *Listeria* and *Toxoplasma*. They also recognise tumour cells. They recognise these cells either because of reduced expression of class I HLA molecules on their surface, or by binding to CD16 receptor on an antibody coated target cell (antibody dependent cellular cytotoxicity). They release granules which increase the permeability of the target cell (perforin) and cytokines which promote apoptosis.

THE ADAPTIVE (ACQUIRED) IMMUNE SYSTEM

Humoral Agents: Immunoglobulins

These are proteins which mediate antibody responses, and are found in blood, tissues, secretions, and also as part of the surface membrane of B cells. They combine with antigen to form immune complexes, and can opsonise bacteria, fix complement, and neutralise viruses.

Figures 24.3A to E show the basic structure of immunoglobulin. Each molecule consists of two heavy chains and two light chains, joined by disulphide bridges. The characteristics of the 5 classes are shown.

IgG activates complement via the classical pathway, opsonises organisms, and mediates antibody dependent cytotoxic responses.

IgM is important for clearing bacteria from the blood stream by agglutination and opsonisation. It is the most efficient fixer of complement by the classical pathway.

IgA in its secretory form is important for antiviral and antibacterial activity on mucosal surfaces. It can fix complement via the alternate pathway, and has bactericidal activity when combined with lysozyme and complement.

The majority of **IgD** is bound to B cell membranes, where it acts as an antigen receptor, and is important in the development of B cell responses.

IgE triggers immediate hypersensitivity. This may be important in defence against worm infection, by binding to the worm, and stimulating mast cell degranulation, leading to the worm being flushed from the mucosal surface.

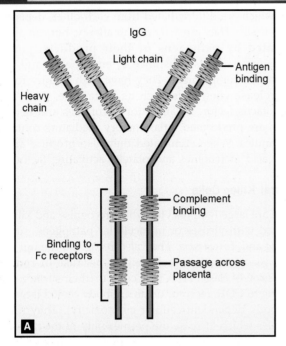

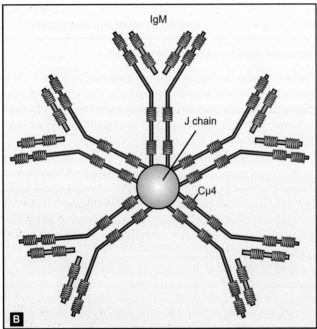

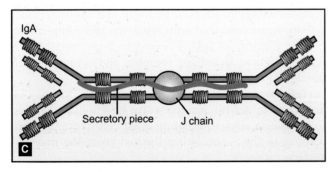

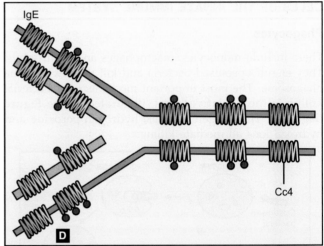

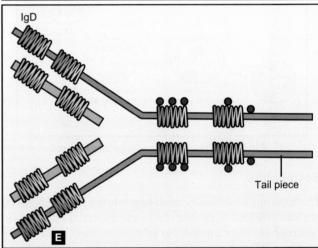

Figs 24.3A to E: Basic structure of immunoglobulin and classes

CELLS OF THE ADAPTIVE IMMUNE SYSTEM

T Cells

These are the coordinators and regulators of specific immunity. They interact with cells of the innate immune system (antigen presenting cells) and with B cells, and produce cytokines which stimulate or suppress the activity of other inflammatory cells.

Antigen Presentation and T Cells

In the process of phagocytosis and elimination of organisms within the phagosome, not all foreign protein is destroyed. A small portion is preserved and then presented on the surface of the cell associated with molecules of the major histocompatibility complex (MHC). The T cell receptor binds to this complex, and is activated, as illustrated in Figure 24.4. Macrophages function both as phagocytes and antigen presenting cells, whereas the

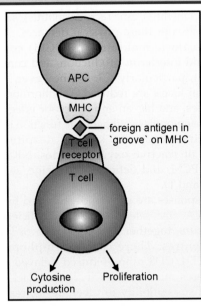

Fig. 24.4: Antigen presentation

major role of dendritic cells is to capture antigen for presentation. Other cells, such as B cells and virus infected cells can also present antigen + MHC.

T cells are classified according to their surface markers and function.

T Helper Cells

These have the CD4 marker. They recognise antigen associated with class II MHC.

Th1 cells differentiate under the influence of interferon gamma and IL12. Activation leads to release of IL2, interferon gamma and tumour necrosis factor (TNF). These stimulate cytotoxic T cells and cell mediated immune responses, including delayed hypersensitivity.

Th2 cells are the main co-ordinators of B cell responses. They possess CD40 ligand which binds to CD40 on the immature B cell surface. This lead to B cell isotype switching and production of B cell memory cells. The main cytokine involved is IL4. Activation of Th2 also leads to stimulation of IgE production, and so mediates immediate hypersensitivity.

Th0 cells initially produce both Th1 and Th2 cytokines. However, either response may predominate, depending on genetic predisposition, type of antigen exposure, and influence of co-stimulatory molecules.

Cytotoxic T Cells

These are characterised by the CD8 marker, which binds to MHC class I. They are responsible for killing virus infected cells.

The Thymus and T Cell Immunity

Early in fetal life, immature lymphocytes enter the thymus. Once within, the genes which encode for the variable region of the T cell receptor are sequentially rearranged. This results in thousands of T cells with different receptors, recognising different MHC/antigen combinations. Those which recognise foreign antigen bound to self MHC are preserved, while those recognising non-self MHC or self antigen are eliminated.

During the maturation process T cells acquire the surface markers CD3, CD4, CD8 and differentiate into helper and cytotoxic/suppressor cells.

B Cells

These bone marrow derived cells are the immunoglobulin factory. The immunoglobulin which is bound to the surface binds antigen, and with T cell help, the B cells proliferate. Once stimulated with antigen, IgM producing plasma cells are formed, while other B cells become memory cells. If exposed to the same antigen again, these produce mature plasma cells, and a larger IgG response. B cells respond to polysaccharide antigen (surrounding encapsulated organisms) without T cell help, but the response is limited, resulting mainly in IgM, and no B cell memory.

Why are Neonates and Infants Prone to Infection?

Cells of the immune system develop early in fetal life. However, the main defences at this stage are the physical barriers of the uterus and the placental barrier. Infants born prematurely lack the same degree of physical protection, with thinner skin and less effective mucous membranes, in addition to immature immune responses.

By the time of birth at term, physical barriers have matured. Acute phase proteins are present, but neonates lack terminal components of complement activation, particularly C9. These are important for lysis of gram-negative bacteria, such as *E. coli*, to which infection they are particularly susceptible.

Neutrophils comprise only 10% circulating white cells in the second trimester, but 50-60% by term. However, neonates often respond to sepsis with neutropoenia. Their neutrophils do not adhere as well to the endothelium, inhibiting migration. Chemotaxis and phagocytosis are less efficient, but bacterial killing and antigen presentation is as good as in adults.

T cell numbers are greater in infancy than in adult life, but the majority of them are naïve, whereas in adults, they are primed to proliferate rapidly following repeated antigen exposure. Cytokine production, cytotoxicity, delayed hypersensitivity, and B cell help are all reduced.

During the last trimester, maternal immunoglobulin (IgG) crosses the placenta, conferring passive immunity to

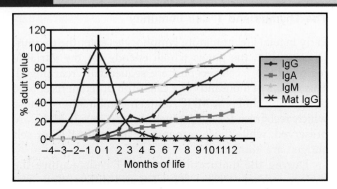

Fig. 24.5: Normal level of immunoglobulin with age

the neonate. B cells are present at birth, and can differentiate into IgM producing plasma cells. The ability to produce T cell dependent responses to protein antigens such as tetanus toxoid, and Hib conjugate is also present at birth. However, development of IgG producing plasma cells, and T independent responses are delayed until around 2 years of age. As the normal response to polysaccharide antigens, such as those in the cell wall of encapsulated organisms requires B cells to work without T cell help, this may account for the increased susceptibility of infants to infections with organisms such as *Pneumococcus*, *Neisseria meningitides*, and *Hamophilus influenzae*. Normal immunoglobulin levels rise with age (Fig. 24.5). IgA is the latest antibody to be produced, and IgA producing plasma cells are not found until around the age of 5.

Nutrition and Immunity

The association of under-nutrition and increased susceptibility to infections, particularly respiratory and gastro-intestinal infection, has long been recognised. The reasons are multi-factorial, in that conditions leading to under-nutrition are also associated with over-crowding, lack of sanitation and access to clean water, increased risk of prematurity, and lack of vaccination. In turn, episodes of infection increase metabolic demand for nutrients and decrease appetite and intake, thus increasing malnutrition in a vicious cycle.

Bacterial infections, such as pneumonia, tuberculosis, gram-negative gastrointestinal infections are particularly common in children sufficiently malnourished to be hospitalised. Mortality from measles due to giant cell pneumonia is high. These children may suffer severe herpes fungal and parasitic infections.

Under-nutrition has adverse effects on all parts of the immune response. Protein-calorie malnutrition leads to atrophy of the skin and mucous membranes. Vitamin deficiencies, particularly A (xerosis), C (scurvy), E and B (dermatitis, cheilitis), and deficiencies of trace elements

such as iron (cheilitis), zinc (acrodermatitis), selenium and copper can disrupt these physical defences.

Protein-calorie malnutrition (PCM) compromises lysozyme and interferon production, and components of complement, particularly C3. C4, however, tends to be raised. Leptin levels are reduced. This hormone promotes Th1 responses, and has an anti-apoptotic effect, important for normal haemopoiesis. Phagocytic function is decreased, with impaired bacterial killing, despite increased production of reactive oxygen species. NK function is reduced in PCM, and deficiencies in zinc, selenium and vitamins A and D.

T cell responses are profoundly affected by PCM, and also vitamin A, zinc, selenium and iron deficiency. Thymic atrophy occurs, together with depletion of lymph node germinal centres. There can be lymphopoenia with decreased CD4/CD8 ratio. Reduced delayed hypersensitivity responses and T cytotoxicity leads to lack of response to BCG and susceptibility to tuberculosis, reactivation of viral infections and other opportunistic infections.

In contrast, levels of immunoglobulin are usually well maintained. There can be particularly high levels of serum IgE, which is not necessarily related to helminth infestation, but probably represents dysregulation. Antibody responses are usually preserved, although some studies suggest decreased response to vaccines in severe PCM.

PROBLEMS WITH THE IMMUNE SYSTEM

How Many Infections is too Many?

The normal range for number of infectious episodes/year in an immunocompetent child is extremely wide, and dependent on factors including the risk of exposure to environmental pathogens (e.g. water-borne organisms, malaria), over-crowding, and exposure to other children, either at home or in nurseries or school. Lack of breast feeding and parental smoking influence rates. Children with medical conditions such as sickle cell syndrome, nephrotic syndrome, cystic fibrosis, are atopic, have injuries breeching physical barriers, such as compound fractures or burns, or who have implanted foreign bodies will have an increased risk. Immune dysfunction may also be secondary to malignant disease, immunosuppressive agents, infections such as HIV, EBV, or result from splenectomy.

When to Suspect Immune Deficiency

An underlying problem with immunity should be suspected in children who have more frequent episodes of infection than expected, given the factors above. Children may suffer recurrent infections with a particular type or organism, or the course of an infectious episode with a particular pathogen is unusual in length, severity, or character. Children may become infected with organisms which would not usually be pathogenic (opportunistic organisms).

Immune deficiency should also be considered in children who have other features of a syndrome known to be associated with immune problems, such as di George, ataxia telangiectasia, Wiskott Aldrich. Early diagnosis (before the onset of severe infections) can sometimes be achieved by taking note of abnormal results of tests performed for other reasons, for example, neutropenia or lymphopenia from a full blood count.

The Diagnosis of Immune Deficiency

The History

From this information, a number of patterns may emerge: Invasive bacterial infections: problems with opsonization (complement, immunoglobulin), phagocyte numbers or function (chemotaxis, phagocytosis, killing). Recurrent infection with encapsulated organisms.

A careful history is the key to diagnosis throughout medicine, and immune deficiency is no exception. A detailed history should include:

- Documentation of episodes of infection, their frequency, their course, character, duration, treatment given, effect of treatment, necessity for hospitalisation, clinical diagnosis given, and whether confirmatory tests performed.

From this information, a number of patterns may emerge: immunoglobulin), phagocyte numbers or function (chemotaxis, phagocytosis, killing).

Recurrent infections with encapsulated organisms: antibody deficiency, complement defects (especially recurrent meningococcal disease).

Recurrent/persistent/severe viral infections: cytotoxic T cells, NK cells.

Fungal infections: neutrophil number/function, T cell function.

Opportunistic pathogens, e.g. pneumocystis: T cell function.

- Periodicity of infections: problems occurring at 3 weekly intervals, particularly associated with mouth ulcers is suggestive of cyclical neutropoenia
- Age of onset:
  o from birth suggestive of cellular defect, e.g. congenital neutropenia, T cell immunodeficiencies.
  o 6-9 months: recurrent sino-pulmonary infection suggestive of antibody deficiency
  o after 2 years of age – consider common variable immune deficiency
- Birth history
  o Gestation
  o Birth weight: intrauterine growth retardation is associated with nutritional immune dysfunction and specific syndromes.

  o Neonatal problems:
    - jitteriness/seizures due to hypocalcaemia or heart failure/cyanosis due to congenital heart disease may indicate di George's
    - petechiae/bleeding from cord in Wiskott Aldrich's
    - severe erythroderma in congenital graft versus host disease
    - neonatal sepsis in reticular dysgenesis and severe neutropoenia and severe T cell defects
  o Time of cord separation: delay associated with lymphocyte adhesion defect.
- Other medical problems:
  o Growth problems
    - Severe failure to thrive in T cell defects
    - Short stature in Bloom syndrome
  o Developmental delay/neurological problems
    - Ataxia telangiectasia
    - Purine nucleoside phosphorylase deficiency
    - HIV
  o Skin problems
    - Eczematoid dermatitis and abscesses in Hyper-IgE
    - Recurrent abscesses in CGD
    - Eczema and petechiae in Wiskott Aldrich's
    - Skin sepsis in antibody deficiency, neutrophil disorders, complement defects
- Immunisations given and reactions
  o Neonatal BCG: reaction/dissemination – T cell deficiency, interferon gamma/IL12 dysfunction
  o Symptomatic disease following live vaccine, e.g. measles – T cell function
  o Abscess/reaction at site; neutrophil function complement
- Allergies
- Current and past medication, including "over the counter" and alternative/herbal remedies.
- Family history
  o Family members with similar features
  o Deaths early in life
  o Consanguinity
- Social history
  o Housing
  o Occupants of house
  o Attendance at nursery/school
  o Risk behaviours for blood-borne virus infection
  o Parental occupations
  o Smoking
  o Pets/animals/birds.

Diagnostic Tests

Selection of appropriate tests should depend upon the differential diagnosis obtained as a result of the history and examination, and also on the resources available.

Full Blood Count

Haemoglobin is reduced in chronic infection and inflammatory conditions.

Neutrophil count will identify chronic neutropenia. Serial tests over a 3 weeks period are needed to diagnose cyclical neutropenia. A neutrophil leucocytosis is seen in disorders of neutrophil function, such as chronic granulomatous disease and lymphocyte adhesion defect.

Lymphocyte count is low in T cell immunodeficiencies such as Severe Combined Immunodeficiency. Note that the lymphocyte count is normally higher in infants, so values persistently below $2.8 \times 10^9/L$ should prompt further investigation.

Platelet count and platelet size is reduced in Wiskott Aldrich syndrome.

Blood film microscopy may identify Howell Jolly bodies in asplenia.

TESTS OF CELL MEDIATED IMMUNITY

Skin Testing

Delayed hypersensitivity is mediated by cell mediated responses, and so it is possible to test for this *in vivo*. The problem in infants and children under 2 years is to find a suitable antigen to which they have previously been exposed and sensitised. Children who had BCG may respond to tuberculin, and those who have had tetanus immunisation may respond to tetanus toxoid. Candidal antigen may also be used. Testing involves an intradermal injection of the antigen, and recording of the resulting erythema and induration at 24-48 hours.

Lymphocyte Subset Quantification

If monocloncal antibodies labelled with fluorochrome are generated against lymphocyte surface markers, they can be used to identify lymphocyte subsets using a flow cytometer or FACS (fluorescence activated cell scanner) machine. The commonest monoclonals used are against CD3 (all mature T cells), CD4, CD8, CD19/20 (B cells) and CD16/56 (NK cells). Normal ranges for numbers and proportions vary with age.

Lymphocyte Function

In vitro, this can be assessed by incubating lymphocytes with mitogens such as phytohaemagglutinin and pokeweed mitogen. The degree of proliferation is measured by assessing the uptake of tritiated thymidine, compared to that of a normal control sample.

Cytokine and Receptor Assays

These are not widely available, but they can diagnose rare immunodeficiencies.

TEST FOR HUMORAL IMMUNITY

Immunoglobulin Assays

Normal plasma concentration of immunoglobulin classes also vary with age. Low levels of all classes are found in T cell immunodeficiencies, such as severe combined immunodeficiency, and in antibody deficiencies such as X-linked agammaglobulinaemia. High levels are found in chronic infection, chronic granulomatous disease and HIV.

B Cell Function

B cell function can be assessed by measuring the titre of antibody to a specific antigen following exposure to the antigen. For example, anti-tetanus antibody, pre- and post vaccination. Antibody to *Pneumococcus* can also be measured, but as this is a polysaccharide antigen, children under 2 years do not normally respond.

Phagocyte Function

There are no reliable tests of chemotaxis. The respiratory burst can be measured using the nitroblue tetrazolium test (NBT) during which normal cells phagocytose the colourless dye and reduces it to a purple compound. Neutrophils from children with CGD phagocytose normally, but there is no colour change.

Complement Function

It is possible to measure levels of individual complement components—the most straightforward being C3 and C4. CH50 is a dynamic assay of total haemolytic complement, and is reduced in defects of the classical pathway.

Genetic Tests

Chromosome analysis can diagnose conditions such as di George syndrome, which is associated with a deletion on q22. The exact genetic defect has been identified for some inherited immune deficiencies, and in these analysis of DNA or assay of the gene product (e.g. B tyrosine kinase in X-linked agammaglobulinaemia). Can be performed.

PRIMARY IMMUNODEFICIENCY DISORDERS

These conditions are individually quite rare, with an estimated prevalence of 1 in 5000 population. The commonest are antibody deficiencies, accounting for approximately 65% total, cellular deficiencies comprise 20%, phagocytic disorders, 10% and complement disorders, 5%. Those with an autosomal recessive mode of inheritance may be more common in societies with a high incidence of marriage within the extended family.

Severe Combined Immune Deficiency (SCID)

This is a group of conditions characterised by low or absent T cells and hypogammaglobulinaemia. B and NK cell numbers may be normal or absent, depending on the type. It may present with congenital graft versus host disease due to engraftment of maternal T cells, or following neonatal transfusion of non-irradiated blood. More commonly, the infant develops recurrent or chronic mucocutaneous candidiasis, chronic diarrhoea and failure to thrive due to persistent viral gastroenteritis, and chronic respiratory viral infection (e.g. RSV, adenovirus) leading to respiratory failure. Acute sepsis can occur, as can opportunistic infection with agents such a pneumocystis and cytomegalovirus. Without treatment (bone marrow transplantation) it is unusual to survive beyond the first year of life. There are X-linked (e.g. common gamma chain deficiency) and autosomal recessive (e.g. ADA deficiency) forms of the condition, and for some the underlying defect is unknown.

Di George Syndrome

The main features of this syndrome are cono-truncal cardiac anomalies (e.g. interrupted aortic arch, truncus arteriosus), hypocalcaemia, and hypoplastic or absent thymus. Children with this syndrome have characteristic facies, with hypertelorism, antimongoloid slant of the eyes, micrognathia, cleft or high-arched palate, and ear malformations. These defects are due to failure of migration of neural crest cells into the 3rd and 4th pharyngeal pouches early in embryological life. This is commonly associated with a microdeletion on chromosome 22 (q2211). Many cases are sporadic, but there is therefore an autosomal dominant inheritance.

Most children present with symptoms of their congenital heart disease or with neonatal hypocalcaemia, and although they may have low T cell numbers compared with normal infants, immune function is well-preserved. However, those with absent or severely hypoplastic thymus can have features of severe T cell immunodeficiency similar to SCID. They can have normal immunoglobulin levels, but reduced specific antibody production. There is also an increased risk of autoimmune disease.

X-linked Agammaglobulinaemia (XLA)

This condition is due to a lack of the enzyme B tyrosine kinase (btk) which is essential for B cell maturation. Circulating B cell numbers are very low or absent, as are levels of circulating immunoglobulin. Children are normal at birth, protected by passive maternal antibody, but develop recurrent bacterial infections, particularly sino-pulmonary infections, usually becoming symptomatic between 6 and 18 months of age. As T cell function is normal, they cope with childhood exanthemata such as varicella normally. Immunoglobulin can be replaced with regular intravenous or subcutaneous infusions, and in those who are treated adequately, prognosis is good. Ongoing problems with chronic sinusitis, purulent rhinitis, and conjunctivitis, can occur despite replacement, and chronic lung disease is particularly likely in those not maintaining adequate trough levels of immunoglobulin.

CD40 Ligand Deficiency

This condition is also X-linked and shares many characteristics with XLA. However, CD40 ligand is a T cell receptor, binding with CD40 on the B cell to enable B cell proliferation and isotype switching. Children with this condition have normal numbers of circulating B cells, and normal or high levels of serum IgM, but absent IgG, IgA and IgE. This T cell ligand has other functions in host defence, in addition to B cell stimulation, so unlike XLA, children can present with pneumocystis carinii pneumonia and fail to clear pathogens such as cryptosporidium. Even with immunoglobulin replacement, the prognosis is much poorer. This is due to the risk of liver failure due to sclerosing cholangitis, which may result from chronic biliary infection with organisms such as *Cryptosporidium*, and of malignancy, particularly abdominal malignancies.

Common Variable Immunodeficiency

This is another form of antibody deficiency, but unlike XLA, symptoms can start at any age, but after 2 years at the earliest. The most common presentation is with recurrent or chronic sino-pulmonary infection, which can lead to chronic lung disease. These children have B cells, but low levels of immunoglobulin, and poor or absent specific antibody responses. In addition to infections, they may develop granulomatous disease or autoimmune features, and have an increased risk of malignancy. Treatment is with immunoglobulin and antibiotic prophylaxis.

Chronic Granulomatous Disease (CGD)

This is a disorder of phagocytes in which there is a defect in NADPH oxidase, the enzyme involved in the respiratory burst. There are both X-linked and autosomal recessive forms of the disease. Children with CGD are at particular risk of infection.

With catalase positive bacteria (such as *Staphylococcus* organisms and coliforms) and fungi such as *Aspergillus*. They can present with recurrent lymphadenitis, invasive bacterial infection, such as pneumonia, liver abscess, osteomyelitis, or life-threatening sepsis. Prophylactic antibiotics and anti-fungals have improved prognosis, but many succumb to invasive fungal infection in the second and third decades of life.

Complement Deficiencies

These are individually very rare, and tend to present with recurrent bacterial infection, due to poor opsonisation, glomerulonephritis, or features suggestive of rheumatological disease. Some, such as properdin deficiency lead to increased susceptibility to infection with encapsulated organisms, particularly *Neisseria meningitidis*, which should be considered if children present with recurrent meningococcal disease. It has X linked inheritance.

Wiskott Aldrich Syndrome

This results from a mutation on the X chromosome of a gene encoding for WAS protein. This protein is important for the normal development of the cytoskeleton, and plays a role in apoptosis. The main features are thrombocytopenia, recurrent infections and eczema. Those affected often present in the neonatal period with petechiae and bleeding. Not only are platelet numbers reduced, but they are smaller than normal, and function less well, so bleeding may be more severe than would be expected from the platelet count alone. Boys suffer recurrent bacterial infections, such as otitis media, pneumonia, and meningitis, particularly with encapsulated organisms. They also suffer from viral infections, such as recurrent herpes simplex and severe varicella. Their eczema has the same characteristics as classic atopic eczema. Other atopic symptoms such as food allergy can develop. Some boys develop autoimmune problems, and the long-term risk is from malignancy, particularly EBV driven B cell lymphoma. Treatments include splenectomy, intravenous immunoglobulin, and antibiotic prophylaxis. However, bone marrow transplant can be curative.

Hyper IgE (Job's) Syndrome

Children with this condition suffer from recurrent severe staphylococcal infection, particularly skin abscesses and pneumonia. They have a dermatitis which may be diagnosed as eczema, but the characteristics and distribution of the lesions are different from atopic eczema. Children can have coarse facies and skeletal abnormalities. As the name suggests, levels of serum IgE are extremely high (often many thousand IU/l). The gene and underlying defect for this condition are unknown, and there is no specific treatment apart from long-term prophylactic anti-staphylococcal antibiotics.

Ataxia Telangiectasia

This is caused by a mutated gene on chromosome 11, which encodes for a protein which is important for repair of double stranded DNA. The cells of those affected are therefore abnormally sensitive to irradiation. Children are normal at birth, and early development is normal. They tend to drool, and speech is slow. They begin walking at the usual age, but become more wobbly. Unlike many other cerebellar disorders, the ataxia of AT results in a narrow based gait, and children have difficulty keeping their head and trunk still when standing. From around the age of 7 there is progressive neurological deterioration. Conjunctival teleangiectasia are often the first to appear, with cutaneous lesions appearing between the ages of 3 and 6.

The immunodeficiency associated with condition is variable, both in clinical manifestation and laboratory findings. Children with AT may suffer from severe or recurrent sino-pulmonary infection, and also chronic or recurrent warts. They commonly have low or absent IgA levels, but can have low specific antibody responses to polysaccharide antigens, or T lymphopenia. They have a very high risk of cancer, chiefly leukaemias and lymphomas, but other solid tumours can occur. Most sufferers die in the second or third decade from chronic lung disease or malignancy.

ALLERGY

Allergy can be defined as an immunologically mediated response whose effects are detrimental to the host.

These responses are much more common in individuals described as **atopic. Atopy** is highly genetic and characterised by an individual or familial tendency to become sensitised to common protein allergens at normal levels of exposure. This response is usually mediated by IgE. Atopic individuals tend to have higher levels of circulating IgE than those who are non-atopic.

Hypersensitivity can be defined as the development of reproducible symptoms and signs following exposure to a particular stimulus at a dose which would normally be tolerated (for example, peanut allergy). However, it can also be used more widely to describe allergic reactions, some of which are universal (for example, reaction to mixmatched blood).

THE IMMUNOLOGY OF ALLERGIC DISEASES

Traditionally, hypersensitivity reactions have been classified into four types. Although we now recognise that many complex interactions occur between different parts of the immune system, it is still a useful way of understanding allergy.

Type I (Immediate/Anaphylactic)

Symptoms occur within minutes/hours of exposure to the allergen, which forms a complex with specific IgE and is bound to the surface of effector cells, such as mast cells

(Fig. 24.6A). This leads to the release of chemical mediators which cause the changes associated with observed symptoms and signs, for example, vasodilatation, capillary leak, bronchoconstriction, increased gut peristalsis. This is the mechanism behind peanut allergy, drug reactions, allergic rhinitis and acute asthma.

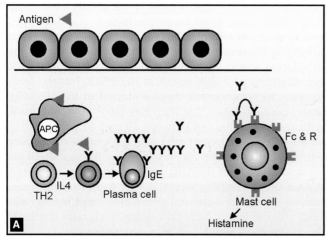

Fig. 24.6A: Type I reaction. Pathogenesis of type 1 hypersensitivity. Exposure to antigen IgE production, mast cell sensitisation

Type II (Cytotoxic)

In this reaction, antibody (IgG or IgM) binds directly to tissue bearing the specific antigen, resulting in complement activation and tissue damage (Fig. 24.6B). Examples are transfusion reactions, to which all are susceptible, but they also occur in diseases such as auto-immune haemolytic anaemia, Goodpasture's syndrome, and some drug induced cytopenias.

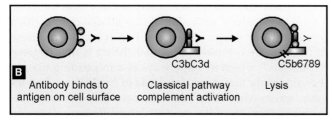

Fig. 24.6B: Type II reaction. Pathogenic mechanism in type II H

Type III (Arthus/Immune Complex)

In these reactions, antibody is bound to antigen to form immune complexes, some of which are cleared by the reticuloenothelial system. However, some are deposited in blood vessels or tissues, inducing complement activation and tissue damage (Fig. 24.6C). This is the pathogenesis of serum sickness and glomerulonephritis.

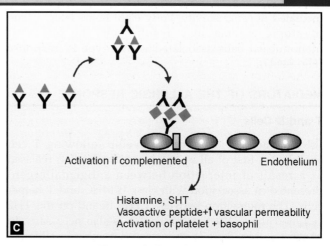

Fig. 24.6C: Type III reaction

Type IV (Delayed/Cell Mediated)

Unlike the first 3 types, delayed hypersensitivity is not mediated by antibody, but by T cells. The maximum inflammatory response may not occur until 48-72 hours after exposure. As a result of interaction between local antigen presenting cells (principally dendritic cells) and T cells, T cells proliferate and produce cytokines which mediate a local inflammatory response. Reactions are universal following exposure to antigen such as poison oak or poison ivy. Induction of this type of reaction is the basis of the tuberculin skin test (Mantoux).

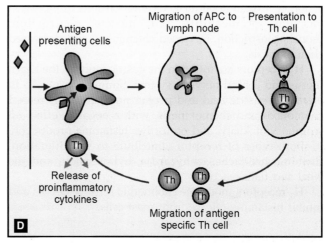

Fig. 24.6D: Type IV reaction

Some allergic conditions involve both immediate and delayed hypersensitivity responses to the same stimulus. For example, exposure to egg in a young child may cause urticaria and angio-oedema within minutes, due to IgE mediated hypersensitivity. Forty eight hours later, a flare of atopic eczema may result from the influx of mononuclear cells associated with a type IV response (Fig. 24.6D).

MEDIATORS OF THE ALLERGIC RESPONSE

T and B Cells

IgE producing plasma cells develop following T cell stimulation, first of all by cytokines (chiefly IL4) released as a result of interaction between antigen(allergen) presented in association with class II MHC and T helper cells. The interaction between CD40 ligand on the TH2 cell, and the CD40 B cell receptor is also necessary. In atopic children, there is an increased number of allergen-specific T cells, which when stimulated, produce IL4, IL5 and IL13. These cytokines induce allergic inflammation by their action on mast cells, basophils and eosinophils.

Mast Cells, Basophils and Eosinophils

These play a large role in the allergic response and resulting inflammation. Their functions have already been outlined.

Histamine

This is the major mediator of type I hypersensitivity. Different tissues have different histamine receptors, determining the response.

H_1 **receptors** are found in blood vessels, and smooth muscle of the respiratory and gastrointestinal tract. The action of histamine on these receptors results in increased vascular permeability, GI muscle contraction, bronchoconstriction, increased chemotaxis, and decreased chemokinesis.

H_2 **receptors** are found in the gastric mucosa, the heart, uterus and central nervous system. Stimulation results in increased gastric acid and pepsin production, increased chemotaxis and chemokinesis, with a negative effect on lymphocytotoxicity, and on further histamine production. Both types of receptor contribute to vasodilatation, flushing, headache, tachycardia, hypotension, and the weal and flare reaction.

H_3 **receptors** modulate cholinergic sensory nerves and inhibit histamine release from mast cells.

Leukotrienes

These are fatty acids whose active inflammatory metabolites cause vasodilatation, swelling of the mucosa, increased mucous production and bronchoconstriction. Metabolism is governed by the 5 lipoxygenase pathway, which can be stimulated by certain antigens. They have an important role in the pathogenesis of asthma and allergic rhinitis.

Other Chemical Mediators

These include kinins, complement, interleukins and cell adhesion molecules.

EPIDEMIOLOGY

The prevalence of atopic disease varies greatly throughout the world, being much more common in the developed world with "Western" lifestyle. There has also been a dramatic increase in prevalence, particularly in the developed world over time. The rise in sensitisation to aeroallergens probably began in the 1920s, but the large increase in symptomatic disease started in the 1960-70s, with some evidence that the rates have now stabilised, with rates of asthma of between 20 and 40%, depending on the criteria used, compared with 2-3% in the developing world. Similarly rates for hay fever, at the age of 16 are around 20-25% in the UK, and 6% for atopic eczema. Within the developing world, a shift from rural to urban habitat results in increased prevalence, and immigrants from areas of low to high prevalence reach rates similar to the indigenous population in a generation.

Why is Atopic Disease Increasing?

We believe that the immune system is "primed" to generate predominantly Th1 or Th2 responses to a given stimulus early on in life. This process may therefore be influenced by the nature of the antigens to which the infant is exposed at this stage. In the West, the burden of infectious disease is much lower than in the developing world now, and in Western society in the past. Moreover, even in developing countries where the overall prevalence is still low, there is an increased risk associated with change from rural to urban environment. Some studies have suggested that large family size, attendance at day nursery, and living on a farm, particularly with animals are all associated with a lower rate of atopic diseases. The reasons for these differences are complex. A popular theory is the "hygiene hypothesis", which in some ways is a misleading title, as it could imply that good standards of hygiene are bad for your health, which is far from the case. It is certainly true, however, that one of the most striking differences between rural life in a developing country, and Westernised society, is in the nature of exposure to microbial and parasitic organisms. The degree of exposure early in life to agents such as bacterial endotoxin, environmental mycobacteria, and to helminths, particularly hookworm, may be important for the manner in which mechanisms which regulate the immune response develop.

Clinical Presentation of Allergic Disease

These include acute anaphylaxis, food allergy and atopic diseases such as asthma, eczema, allergic rhinitis, and conjunctivitis. Allergic asthma and eczema have been described elsewhere in the sections on respiratory medicine and dermatology respectively(see Chapters 6 and 14).

Acute Immediate Hypersensitivity and Anaphylaxis

In some references, the term anaphylactic is used to describe type I hypersensitivity reactions of any severity. Here anaphylaxis is defined as a sudden life threatening systemic reaction which is immune mediated. As such it is an acute medical emergency. It usually results from a type I hypersensitivity reaction, mediated by histamine, and other active chemicals released during IgE associated mast cell degranulation. Type III reactions can sometimes give a similar clinical picture.

If exposure to the allergen has been cutaneous or mucosal, there may initially be local symptoms at the site of contact, such as tingling lips and tongue with local swelling, sneezing, conjunctival irritation, or localised urticaria. Urticaria may progress to become widespread, with intense itch. There may be angio-oedema with facial swelling, and hoarse voice, a feeling of a lump in the throat, with coughing and choking, if this affects the upper airways. Bronchospasm may also lead to audible wheeze. Some children vomit profusely or complain of abdominal cramps, or diarrhoea.

In the most severe cases, the onset is sudden and heralded by a "sense of impending doom", and a sudden feeling of weakness. The child experiences palpitations, becomes cold and clammy, with poor peripheral perfusion. They may develop severe difficulty breathing, either secondary to upper airways obstruction, or to severe bronchospasm. This is followed by circulatory collapse and unconsciousness. Although uncommon, particularly in childhood, deaths do occur.

Anaphylaxis can result from exposure of the sensitised child to food allergens, such as peanut. It can also be triggered by venoms, such as bee and wasp, or plants, such as strawberry and natural rubber latex. A wide variety of drugs can cause it, particularly antibiotics, such as penicillin, sulphonamides, or anaesthetic agents.

Anaphylactoid Reactions

The term anaphylactoid is used to describe a clinical picture which closely resembles anaphylaxis, i.e. urticaria/ erythema, respiratory difficulty, shock, but in which the pathogenesis is not immune mediated. It may result from direct action of chemicals such as drugs on cells, leading to the release of vaso-active peptides. Vaso-active agents may also be released through stimulation of intermediate pathways, such as the complement cascade. It may result from drug interactions, or from infusion of large volumes of plasma products, in which immunoglobulins form aggregates in the circulation. Reactions due to underlying pathology (e.g. tumours), or surgical stimulation causing release of vasoactive peptides is very rare in children. Very occasionally, the cause may be psychosomatic, and the possibility should be considered in teenage patients, when no other explanation can be found.

FOOD ALLERGY

While food is essential to our survival, it can also cause a number of well-recognised adverse events. Moreover, children and their families may attribute all sorts of symptoms which they suffer to "food allergy". Some beliefs regarding the association of certain foods and ill-health are routed deep in the culture of the society to which the family belongs. Many have their base in philosophies other than "conventional" medicine, and are not amenable to application of the scientific method to explore.

There is a number of recognised mechanisms for adverse reactions to food, only one of which is IgE mediated immediate hypersensitivity. Others are immune mediated, but not through IgG. Examples include cow's milk protein intolerance, and gluten enteropathy (coeliac disease). Some foods can lead directly to histamine release, or actually contain histamine, such as strawberries and tomatoes. Localised urticaria after ingestion is commonly described in atopic children, particularly those with eczema, who show no evidence of IgE mediated sensitivity. In some cases symptoms are due to pharmacological effects of ingredients, such as caffeine in soft drinks, leading to vomiting and diarrhoea, or tartrazine (yellow colouring also used in soft drinks) causing bronchospasm, particularly in those with underlying asthma. Reactions can reflect lack of necessary enzymes, such as disaccharidase deficiency in lactose intolerance, or in inborn errors of metabolism, such as galactosaemia. Neurological symptoms following food ingestion can result from build up of a toxin within the food, such as in scombrotoxic fish poisoning, or in botulism, due to contamination of food with *Clostridium*. To some children, certain food smells act as noxious stimuli leading to retching and vomiting and aversion to that food. However, for the purpose of this discussion, we will concetrate on "true" IgE mediated allergic reactions.

Like other atopic disorders, the incidence of food allergy has been increasing. This is reflected in the number of children presenting to clinics with symptoms, but also in admissions to hospital with significant reactions or anaphylaxis. Death from such reactions can occur, but is extremely rare in childhood (0.006/100,000 children aged 0-15/year in the UK). The prevalence in the UK is quoted in the region of 2-6%, with peanut allergy at 0.8%. Many children with food allergies have other atopic diseases. A third of children with atopic eczema in infancy and 1 in 10 children with asthma report food related symptoms.

In many parts of the world, the commonest food allergens in infants and young children are eggs and milk. There is, however, a wide geographical variation, not only in the incidence of food allergy, but also in the foods causing these reactions. In the UK and Australia, peanuts and tree nuts are the next most common. Fish is the commonest allergen in Italy. Sesame allergy is common in the middle east, seafood in Japan and Singapore, and legumes (lentils, peas, beans) in India and Pakistan.

Children who are allergic to one food allergen have an increased likelihood of also being allergic to related foods. For instance, the majority of milk allergic children are also allergic to egg. Allergy to pulses can be associated with peanut allergy. Those with peanut allergy may also be allergic to other nuts and seeds (e.g. sesame seed); although an allergy to one individual nut (e.g. brazil nut) can occur. There can also be cross-reactivity between sensitivity to inhaled allergens, and foods. For example, allergy to birch pollen is associated with reactions to apples, pears and other fruit, and also to hazelnuts. Reactions to melon and banana and ragweed sensitivity are similarly related.

The prognosis for food allergy varies, depending on the allergen. 90% cow's milk allergic infants will become tolerant by the age of 3 years. Egg allergy commonly resolves before school age. However, allergies to pulses and nuts are usually life long, with only around 5% resolving by the age of 7.

The Oral Allergy Syndrome

Children with this condition develop and itchy mouth and tongue, sometimes with localised urticaria and swelling after eating a variety of fresh fruit or vegetables. The same foods may be eaten if they are peeled and/or cooked, as the sensitivity is to proteins which are destroyed by this process. A common association is that of hay fever symptoms in the spring and early summer due to allergy to birch pollen and symptoms on eating whole apple, while the child can still drink apple juice. Although symptoms can be unpleasant, and their precipitants best avoided, these reactions do not carry a risk of anaphylactic shock.

Exercise Induced Anaphylaxis

This is very unusual before teenage years. It occurs when ingestion of a particular food is followed within a few hours by moderate to intense exercise. Both elements are necessary to produce the reaction, and so the causal relationship with the food allergen may not be made, if a history of tolerating the same food on other occasions (when such exercise has not taken place) is elicited. Changes in metabolism associated with the exercise result in the mast cells becoming more activated, and thus more likely to degranulate after a given IgE/allergen stimulus. This effect can also be seen in children who normally suffer only mild reactions after exposure to a food allergen but who may develop anaphylaxis following the same degree of exposure, following exercise.

Latex Allergy

Allergy to natural rubber latex is strongly associated with exposure to settings where a lot of latex material is used. Thus health care workers and those exposed to industrial latex have a high risk of developing sensitivity. In children, high risk groups are those with spina bifida or with genito-urinary abnormalities, which is likely to be due to repeated exposure of mucous membranes to latex urinary catheters. Children with a history of repeated surgery in the first year of life are also at risk, presumably because of repeated exposure to latex gloves and other latex containing equipment. Because of this problem, other materials, such nitrile, are being substituted for latex where this is possible.

Around half of the children with latex allergy also experience symptoms on exposure to various foods. These include banana, avocado, chestnut, potato, kiwi, and other tropical fruits. In children with allergies to these foods, the possibility of latex allergy should therefore be considered.

Latex is used very widely in clothing, for mattresses, bicycle or wheelchair tyres, balls, erasers, computer mouse mats, etc. Total avoidance of all such products is almost impossible, but thankfully seldom necessary. While contact with the skin can lead to urticaria, or contact dermatitis, severe reactions usually occur only after significant mucosal or systemic exposure. The main risks therefore surround episodes of medical or dental care. If latex allergic children need such care, it is very important that every effort is made to ensure the environment is latex free. Where the risk of exposure cannot absolutely be eliminated, for example, during major surgery, pre-medication with hydrocortisone and antihistamines is advised, with careful observation peri-and postoperatively.

Allergic Rhinitis

Allergic rhinitis is very common in industrialised societies, with a prevalence of up to 40% in children. Some suffer symptoms all year round (perennial rhinitis), whereas for others the problem is restricted to times of year when there is exposure to the causal allergen (seasonal rhinitis). The allergens responsible for perennial rhinitis tend to be those encountered in an indoor environment, such as house dust mite, animal dander. Those developing seasonal rhinitis in the spring are allergic to tree pollen, whereas symptoms of grass pollen allergy peak in the mid-summer. Those who have their main problems in the autumn may be allergic to leaf mould or weed pollen.

There are two phases of response. After exposure in a sensitised child, there is a type I reaction, which in the nasal passages leads to nasal vasodilatation, capillary leak, and increased mucus production. This leads to nasal congestion, and a watery runny nose, with itching and sneezing. In around 50% of sufferers, this is followed by a late response, induced by inflammatory cells, causing ongoing nasal congestion, with runny nose and post-nasal drip, which may last for days. Nasal symptoms are often accompanied by itching of the eyes (allergic conjunctivitis), ears, throat and palate.

Although the consequences are rarely life-threatening, these symptoms are a major cause of morbidity in school aged children. Those who are severely affected with chronic nasal obstruction suffer recurrent or chronic headache, tiredness and sleep disturbance, sometimes resulting in sleep apnoea. It can lead to day time somnolence, poor concentration, and poor school performance. The effect on children's emotional and psychological development can therefore be profound.

There is a close association between allergic rhinitis and asthma. Half of children with asthma also have rhinitis, and around a third of children with rhinitis also have asthma. Furthermore, allergic rhinitis is a risk factor for the subsequent development of asthma.

DIAGNOSIS OF ALLERGY

History

Once again, a careful history is the key to diagnosis of allergy. This should include the nature of symptoms experienced, the evolution of symptoms, from the first symptom experienced onwards, time taken to resolution, and whether any treatment was administered. Details of exposure to potential allergens should be obtained, and the length of time between the suspected exposure and onset of symptoms. It is important to take a history of any previous reactions, and their suspected precipitants in a similar way. Also, a history of any previous exposure to the same potential allergen, and whether or not any symptoms developed is important. It should be noted whether or not related allergens are tolerated. If the suspected allergen is a food, whether the food was raw or cooked may be relevant, as may the circumstances in which the reaction took place (e.g. following exercise).

A common acute presentation is urticaria. Although urticaria is one of the signs of immediate hypersensivity, this is not the only mechanism. Many viral and other infectious agents are associated with an immune reaction leading to urticaria which is not IgE mediated. Children developing such rashes are often diagnosed with "allergy". In general, if a child wakes up in the morning in his usual environment with an urticarial rash which lasts for a number of days, and does not resolve with antihistamine, the rash is not due to immediate hypersensitivity, and a "trawl" for possible precipitants is unlikely to be helpful.

In children suspected of allergic rhinitis or asthma, a history of nasal and respiratory symptoms should be taken. These include itching, sneezing, rhinorrhoea, nasal congestion, worsening symptoms first thing in the morning after exposure to allergen the night before, cough, (including nocturnal cough), sleep disturbance, mouth breathing and snoring. Any seasonal variation should be noted.

A past history of any other atopic conditions, e.g. eczema, asthma, rhinitis should be taken. In particular, if the child has asthma, it is important to assess how well controlled the asthma is, in terms of frequency and severity of symptoms, precipitants of symptoms, and what prophylactic and rescue medication the child is using. Any current medication should be noted, together with details of any adverse reactions to medications in the past. A picture should be built up of the child's home environment, or any other place where they regularly spend time, including pets, other animal or bird exposure, dust, mould, vegetation, etc.

Examination

A full general examination may reveal the skin features of eczema. Those with allergic rhinitis may be obvious mouth-breathers with dark rings round the eyes due to sub-orbital oedema. They can also develop an "allergic crease" across the nose just above the tip, formed after constant rubbing, redness around the eyes, again due to rubbing, and excoriation above the upper lip, caused by nasal drip.

Those with asthma may show signs of chronic chest deformity with increased antero-posterior diameter of the chest, and splaying of the lower ribs (Harrison's sulcus). There may be signs of hyper-inflation or wheeze on auscultation.

Investigations

Investigation of Acute Anaphylaxis

For children who present with severe symptoms, it can be difficult to establish clinically whether this is a type I reaction, or whether the reaction is anaphylactoid. True anaphylactic reactions are associated with histamine release, which therefore could be measured. However, the rise and fall in histamine levels following an anaphylactic reaction is very steep and short-lived, and therefore likely to escape detection by the time the child presents.

True anaphylactic reactions are caused by mast cell degranulation. While it is histamine which is the major mediator of the resulting symptoms, other chemicals, such as tryptase are also released. The half-life of mast cell tryptase in the circulation is considerably longer than

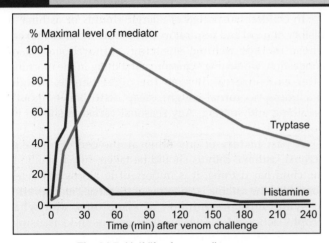

Fig. 24.7: Half-life of mast cell tryptase

histamine (see Fig. 24.7). Serial measurements can therefore be taken over the first 12 hours after the reaction, a rise and subsequent fall to baseline being indicative of true anaphylaxis. If no such change is demonstrated, an alternative mechanism for the symptoms should be sought, and further investigation to identify a particular allergen is likely to be fruitless.

Skin Prick Testing

This is a quick method of diagnosing immediate hypersensitivity. A drop of a standard solution containing the allergen is put on the skin. The most common sites used are the forearm in older children, and the back in younger children, avoiding skin affected by eczema. A calibrated lancet is used to prick the epidermis to a depth of a couple of millimetres only. Excess solution is removed, and after 15-20 minutes, any resulting wheal is measured, and compared with a positive and negative control. A positive test should have a wheal at least 3 mm greater than the negative control or equivalent to the positive control. For some foods, such as fruits, the fruit itself can be pricked, and then the skin pricked in a similar way ("prick prick test"). False-negatives can occur if the child has recently taken an antihistamine. While it is extremely rare for a systemic reaction to occur as a result of this degree of allergen exposure, these test should always be performed where staff are trained in the management of anaphylaxis and appropriate equipment for resuscitation is available.

Serological Testing

Titres of specific IgE directed against a wide variety of allergens can be assayed in the blood using "RAST" or similar techniques. Such tests are more invasive, and often more traumatic for children, but can be performed in settings where no trained staff are available, and the results are not influenced by antihistamine usage. The concentration of specific IgE with a high positive predictive value for clinical hypersensitivity varies between different allergens. For example a titre of 14 kU/l has a 95% positive predictive value for peanut allergy. Care should be taken not to over-interpret results reported as positive, but with lower titres, as highly atopic children may have detectable specific IgE to many potential allergens which they tolerate with no obvious adverse effects.

Provocation Test

This is usually performed to investigate food allergy, but can be used for other potential allergens, such as latex or drugs. It can be used when the diagnosis remains uncertain following the other tests detailed above. It is also useful to determine whether a child with a history of allergy has become tolerant (e.g. in milk allergy), or to investigate possible non-IgE mediated or delayed reactions.

In an open challenge, the child is gradually exposed to increasing amount of the allergen until either a reaction occurs, or until they have tolerated an amount as large as a normal exposure would be expected to be. This should only be performed by staff trained in the early recognition and treatment of reactions and where there are facilities for the management of anaphylaxis. In a food challenge, the food is first applied to the skin, then the lips, before small amounts are ingested.

In a double blind placebo controlled challenge the allergen is "hidden" , so that the child, the parents and the administering staff are unaware which of two foods/ solutions contains the potential allergen. The procedure for each arm is the same as in the open challenge. A sufficient interval between the two arms is necessary to ensure that any delayed symptoms can be attributed to one arm or the other.

Patch Testing

This is often confused with skin prick testing, but this technique is used for the diagnosis of delayed (type IV) reactions, particularly involving the skin, such as contact dermatitis due to perfumes, metals and other chemicals. Adhesive patches containing the allergen are applied to the skin (usually on the back) and left in place for 24 hours. Positive and negative controls are applied to distinguish between true hypersensitivity and irritant reactions. Erythema and induration at the site of contact at 48-72 hours is indicative of sensitivity.

MANAGEMENT OF ALLERGY

Management of Anaphylaxis

If a child presents with symptoms which include severe difficulty breathing or shock, they should be given high flow oxygen via a face mask and epinephrine 1:000 IM. A second dose of epinephrine can be given after 5 minutes if there is no improvement after the first. Antihistamine (e.g. chlorphenamine) should also be given parenterally. Hydrocortisone is useful in helping to prevent recurrence of reaction, particularly if the precipitating cause has not been completely removed. All children with wheeze as part of the reaction, or who have underlying asthma should also have hydrocortisone to prevent an acute asthma exacerbation. Its effects are not seen for four to six hours, however, so it has a limited role in immediate resuscitation. Children with severe shock will benefit from a bolus of intravenous fluid once IV access can be established (the intraosseus route may be used in young children).

It is essential that epinephrine is given by the intramuscular route, the lateral thigh being the most appropriate site. Its mode of action is to stimulate alpha adrenoreceptors, which cause vasoconstriction, thus reducing the excess peripheral blood flow and preventing capillary leak. However, beta receptor stimulation is also required for the bronchodilator effect, and also to stimulate myocardial contractility, and suppress further release of histamine and other mediators. In addition beta 2 receptor stimulation leads to vasodilatation. These receptors are found in muscle, allowing increased blood flow to muscles (for "fight or flight"). This means that epinephrine administered via this route enters the circulation rapidly, enabling its systemic effects. In contrast, subcutaneous tissue only has alpha receptors. The resulting local vasoconstriction inhibits the circulation of epinephrine from the point of injection, limiting its action. It is therefore important to choose a needle of sufficient length to ensure that the muscle is reached.

In profound shock intravenous epinephrine can be given. However, it is potentially very dangerous. A more dilute solution (1:10,000) is used, and it is extremely important that it is given slowly by a doctor experienced in its use.

Allergen Avoidance

The most important measure in all allergic conditions is to avoid the allergen as far as is possible. In food allergic children, they and their parents need detailed information regarding which foods may contain the allergen, and how to avoid them. If children have multiple food allergies, or are allergic to major sources of essential nutrients, such a milk, it is also important to ensure that their restricted diet is nutritionally replete, and they have access to appropriate substitutes. The input of a paediatric dietician is therefore invaluable.

In children allergic to inhaled allergens, such as animal dander, house dust, etc, total avoidance can be impossible. Measures to reduce exposure can, however, be effective in controlling symptoms. For those allergic to house dust mite, these include using impermeable covers for mattresses and pillows, and washing bed linen frequently in hot water (60°C), removing soft toys, replacing carpet with hard flooring and minimising soft furnishings.

Exposure to pollens can be reduced by shutting windows and doors and limiting outdoor activities on days with high pollen counts. If the child is allergic to animal dander, if possible the pet should be removed. If this is not feasible, then dogs and cats should be washed frequently (which may not be popular with the animal!) and it should not be allowed in the child's bedroom. The animal should be kept outside as much as possible. Hands should be washed immediately if the pet is handled.

Antihistamines

For conditions where the allergen cannot be completely avoided, such as seasonal rhinitis and conjunctivitis (hay fever), regular long-acting antihistamines such as cetirizine and loratidine can be used. These are less sedative than first generation anti-histamines, and so have less effect on cognition, which is important particularly for school aged children who need to use these on a long-term basis.

For conditions where the allergen can usually be avoided, but accidental exposure can occur, such as food allergy, it is important to have antihistamine, such as chlorphenamine immediately available, so that it can be given at the first hint of symptoms of immediate hypersensitivity. This means in practice that children or their carers should carry the medication at all times. It should also be available in schools and other settings where the child spends time, where those responsible for the child's care should be trained to recognise and treat the signs of a reaction.

PROPHYLACTIC MEDICATIONS

Cromoglycate

Cromoglycate is a mast cell stabiliser which also has other anti-inflammatory properties. It is no longer as widely used for the prophylaxis of asthma, as it has limited efficacy compared with inhaled corticosteroids. For those who can tolerate the irritation on initial application, it is a useful agent in allergic conjunctivitis when used regularly.

Corticosteroids

Steroids have a broad anti-inflammatory action. As well as reducing inflammation, they decrease vascular permeability, increase the responsiveness of smooth muscle to B agonists, and reduce arachadonic acid metabolite production. Their effects can be seen 4-6 hours after administration, so they are mainly useful in modifiying late phase or delayed responses, and resulting chronic inflammation. Used systemically, they prevent late phase response following anaphylaxis, particularly where wheeze is part of the presentation. They are also used in the treatment of acute exacerbations of asthma, and occasionally in severe allergic rhinitis or dermatitis. The disadvantages of systemic use are the unwanted side effects, such as growth retardation, immunosuppression and adrenal suppression.

Topical steroids are the mainstay of management of chronic allergic conditions such as asthma (inhaled), rhinitis (nasal spray) and eczema (topical creams). Given in sufficiently high doses they can have the same side effects as systemic steroids, but even in lower doses may predispose to local infection, such as candidiasis and herpes simplex, and impair wound healing.

Leukotriene Antagonists

These agents have a more specific anti-inflammatory action than corticosteroids, and also directly inhibit broncho-constriction. They reduce bronchial responsiveness in both immediate and delayed reactions, including drug and exercise induced symptoms. An example is montelukast, which has been used as a single agent for prophylaxis of asthma, but is recommended as second line treatment for asthma in those not well controlled on moderate doses of inhaled steroids. Montelukast is also effective in the treatment of allergic rhinitis, by causing mucosal vasoconstriction, and reducing oedema and mucous production. It has fewer side effects than steroids, but is not as effective in all patients.

Injectable Epinephrine

Epinephrine auto-injectors, such as the Epipen or Anapen are now available. They can be carried by children (or their carers) who are at significant risk of anaphylaxis following accidental exposure to an allergen to which they are sensitised. These may include bee or wasp venom, latex or food allergens such as peanut. They administer a single dose, which delivers 0.15 mg, or 0.3 mg epinephrine, the "pen" used being determined by the weight of the child (15-30 kg, or >30 kg respectively). They are designed for use in the emergency situation, to "buy time" until medical help can be obtained, rather than to be a substitute for it.

Who should Carry Epinephrine?

The answer to this question involves a risk assessment for the individual child. Factors to be taken account include the following:

- Risk of inadvertent exposure to the allergen, despite reasonable precautions being taken to avoid it.
- Severity of reaction after previous exposure. The child with a history of previous anaphylaxis after minimal

exposure would be considered at high risk compared with a child who developed localised symptoms only.

- Concomitant asthma. Those with severe or poorly controlled asthma are at greater risk of developing severe breathing difficulties following allergen exposure.
- Lifestyle where co-factors may increase the risk, e.g. competitive aerobic sport.
- Adolescence—risk taking behaviour and use of alcohol or other drugs which may impair judgement.
- Proximity to back-up medical help. Those in remote areas need to "buy more time".
- Parental anxiety.

Those for whom an auto-injector is prescribed must undertake to carry both anti-histamine and epinephrine at all times, and all carers must be trained in the management of reactions, and in the technique for use of the auto-injector. As it will be used only rarely, if ever, regular updates need to be given to maintain proficiency. The training is required not only for parents, but day care, nursery or school staff, and any adult who undertakes the supervision of the allergic child. This may mean that the child's life is restricted as some people may be unwilling to undertake this responsibility, and therefore the child may be excluded from certain activities. For these reasons it is important that the advantages and disadvantages of such medication should be carefully weighed up before it is prescribed.

Immunotherapy

The aim of specific immunotherapy is to modify the immune response following allergen exposure. The mechanism by which this is achieved is known as immune deviation. Therapy leads to the reduction of activity of the allergen specific Th2 cells, which mediate allergic inflammation, and producing alternative responses, including the up-regulation of Th1 responses, and the production of interferon gamma, and the induction of regulatory T cells, which produce IL10. At one time it was thought that blocking IgG antibodies had a major role in this process, but it is now thought that the cellular mechanisms are more important.

Traditional specific immunotherapy involves the subcutaneous injection of allergen once or twice weekly, starting with a dose below that required to cause a reaction, and gradually building up until a maintenance dose is achieved, which is greater than that likely to be encountered by natural exposure. This can take a considerable amount of time, and even when the maintenance dose is achieved, periodic injections need to be continued for 2-3 years. There is a risk of both local and systemic reaction, and rarely anaphylaxis, and so immunotherapy should only be performed in a setting where staff are trained to deal with anaphylaxis, and resuscitation facilities are readily available. It also entails multiple injections, which limits its tolerability, particularly in young children, and so this restricts its use in this age group.

This form of immunotherapy has been shown to be effective in allergy to bee and wasp venom, and also in allergies to inhaled allergens, such as tree and grass pollen, and animal dander, such as cat. The benefits can last for many years after discontinuation of treatment. There is some evidence that early treatment can prevent further sensitisation to other allergens. Therapy in children with allergic rhinitis can also prevent the subsequent development of asthma. It would appear that it is less effective in children who are allergic to multiple allergens at presentation. It has been tried in food allergies, such as peanut allergy, but the problem is finding a small enough starting dose to which the child does not react. There have been attempts made to modify the peanut protein in order to reduce the undesirable IgE mediated response, while still inducing the immune deviation. So far, there has been limited success with these attempts.

Because of the difficulties inherent in repeated injections, alternative routes have been tried. The most successful of these has been sub-lingual immunotherapy. The allergen is placed under the tongue, and subsequently swallowed. Although some patients do describe itching of the mouth and tongue, and sometimes abdominal pain after swallowing the allergen, systemic effects are rare. Preparations are available for use via this route for inhaled allergens such as pollens. Studies suggest that the beneficial effect may be long-lasting as is the case for subcutaneous therapy, and that there may be a similar effect on the subsequent development of asthma.

FUTURE DEVELOPMENTS

DNA Vaccines

An alternative approach to injecting allergen, is to give the cDNA of allergens directly. This approach has been used to develop vaccines against infectious diseases and cancer. It has been shown that if a plasmid containing sequences encoding for the allergen, a specific immune response involving Th1 and CD8 cells can be induced. Potentially this would mean that that a short course of only one or two doses would be needed to produce the desired clinical outcome.

Anti-IgE

Humanised monoclonal antibodies have been produced, which bind to the high affinity binding site on the IgE molecule. Trials have been performed with such products in asthma, and also in peanut allergy. In asthma, a beneficial effect on symptoms and also on the requirement for corticosteroids was seen. The role of this mode of therapy in asthma management is not yet clear.

In peanut allergy, treated patients could tolerate a much larger amount of peanut protein before reacting than they were previously able to do. While this is certainly not a "cure" as the effect only lasts while the passive antibody remains in the circulation, such treatment may allow the administration of allergen and escalation of therapy in conventional immunotherapy in children who would previously not have been able to tolerate sufficient exposure.

At the present time we have little influence over the underlying disease process, and concentrate mainly on avoidance of the precipitating allergen, and treating symptoms which arise. We would hope that in the future, research in this field may lead to developments which enable us to offer our patients a true cure, or preferably better strategies for prevention of atopic disease.

Chapter 25

Immunisation against Infectious Diseases

Jugesh Chhatwal

IMMUNISATION

Immunisation is one of the most important weapons for protecting individuals and the community from serious diseases.

Immunity to an infectious disease can be acquired through a natural process, e.g. active clinical infection by a microorganism or a subclinical inapparrent infection. Immunisation is a process of inducing immunity against an infectious agent and is generally used in reference to the artificial means of inducing immunity by giving vaccines, i.e. vaccination. Immunisation can also be achieved by a passive process wherein antibodies to the infectious agent produced by another individual or animal who has been exposed to it are extracted and are used to provide protection. These antibodies provide protection for a short duration as their level decreases over a period of time leading to waning of immunity. Also the level of protection provided by such methods is not as good as by the individuals own response.

The examples of passive immunisation are:

(a) Immunoglobulin from human source
1. General non-specific pooled immunoglobulin, e.g. Intravenous Immunoglobulin
2. Specific antibodies against an infectious agent, e.g. Anti-rabies or Anti-tetanus globulins.
3. Transplacental transfer from mother to fetus of various immune globulins.

(b) From animal sources
- Pooled sera, e.g. Anti-diphtheritic serum (ADS – diphtheria antitoxin).

Various types of vaccines used for active immunisation are:

(1) Killed Vaccines

The whole infectious agent is killed artificially and made into a suitable vaccine, e.g. Whole cell pertussis vaccine, cholera vaccine.

(2) Live Attenuated Vaccines

In this type of vaccine the microorganism are subjected to processes which attenuate their disease causing capabilities while retaining the immunity generating components. After administration the microorganisms multiply in the recipient and thus generate an immune response similar to a natural infection, e.g. BCG, measles vaccine

(3) Toxoids

Toxoids are detoxified toxins with the capacity to stimulate formation of antitoxin in the recipient. e.g. tetanus toxoid, diphtheria toxoid.

(4) Sub-unit Vaccines

A part of the microorganism which has the capability to generate the immune response is utilized for making the vaccine, e.g. Acellular pertussis, Vi antigen typhoid vaccine.

(5) Recombinant Vaccines

The recombinant vaccines are synthesized using a nonpathogenic organism carrying immunogenic components of the pathogenic organism, e.g. Hepatitis B vaccine.

Mechanism of Immune Response

Lymphocytes play a vital role in generating the immune response following exposure to an antigen which may be either a microorganism or an exotoxin. For the immune response both types of lymphocytes, i.e. B and T lymphocytes maybe activated and only the B cells may be involved. When the immune response is generated through B lymphocytes only and it is termed as T cell independent and when both B and T cells are involved it is termed T cell dependent. Majority of the antigen however require both B and T cells to generate antibody production and are hence T cell dependent. In children below 2 years of age T independent response is poorly initiated.

After introduction of the antigen into the body, T- helper cells (CD4) are activated, following which a cascade of mediators is triggered. After the first exposure to the antigen, as in a primary vaccination, there is a latent period of 7-10 days followed by detectable antibodies in the serum, usually after about 2 weeks. Initially it is mainly IgM antibodies followed by IgG. IgG antibodies are produced in peak concentration after about 2-6 weeks and are the most critical for protection against infection. Repeat exposure to the same antigen, as in booster vaccination, leads to humoral or cell mediated response rapidly within the first week.

The vaccines given orally are usually live attenuated and hence after ingestion the infecting agent multiply in the intestinal mucosa. This induces an IgA response locally. After multiplication in the mucosa, the microorganisms invade the body further to generate other antibodies.

Factors Affecting Immune Response

Host Factors

Age: Age is one of the critical factors to be considered for immunisation. In young infants presence of placentally transferred maternal antibodies can interfere with the immune response to an antigen, e.g. Measles. Also a relatively immature immune system may not be able to initiate an adequate response to the vaccinated antigen. Another factor is the poor immunogenicity of T cell independent antigens in children less than 2 years of age. Vaccines containing such antigens have to be conjugated with a compound which has the ability to generate T cell response, e.g. HiB conjugate vaccines.

Nutrition: Malnutrition of severe degree can decrease the capability of the host to activate the immune system adequately.

Pre-existing antibodies: Presence of antibodies to the specific vaccinated antigen may interfere with the immune response, e.g. maternal antibodies.

Immunocompromised status: Any condition leading to an immunocompromised state either due to a disease, e.g. malignancy or due to treatment, e.g. prolonged steroid use can impair the immune response to a vaccine.

Key Learning Points
Live vaccines should not be given to children with impaired immune response, whether caused by disease or treatment with high doses of corticosteroids or other immunosuppressive drugs. In fact live vaccines should be postponed until at least 3 months after stopping corticosteroids or other immunosuppressive drugs and 6 months after stopping chemotherapy or generalized radiotherapy.

Vaccine Related Factors

a. Type of vaccine

Live vaccines are much more likely to induce an immune response similar to a natural infection and confer longer period of immunity.

b. Route of administration

The optimal route of administration as specified for a particular vaccine should be used. Alternative routes may not be equally effective. Orally administered vaccines lead to a secretary IgA response in gut mucosa which cannot be induced by parenteral vaccine, e.g. Oral polio vaccine.

c. Storage conditions

Appropriate temperature and other storage conditions are an absolute essential requirement to maintain potency of the vaccine. Cold chain, i.e. maintaining the required temperature from the manufacturer to the recipient is an essential pre-requisite for effective vaccination.

Key Learning Points
The intramuscular route should not be used in children with bleeding disorders such as haemophilia or thrombocytopenia. Instead they may be given vaccines by subcutaneous injection.

ADVERSE EVENTS

The present day vaccines which have been approved for use in children are expected to be safe. Sometimes they can cause certain mild adverse reactions and rarely serious events. Various components of the vaccine can lead to an allergic reaction, e.g. the microorganism, antibiotics or other stabilizing agents used in the vaccine. The usual adverse events and the causative vaccines are shown in Table 25.1.

Table 25.1: Common adverse events of vaccines	
Fever of short duration	**Shock like state**
• DPT	• DPT
• Measles	• Measles (contaminated)
• Typhoid	**Rare events**
• T. toxoid	• Seizure DPT
Local reaction	• Paralysis OPV
• DPT	• Anaphylaxis Measles
• Typhoid	• Guillian Barre T. toxoid
• T. toxoid	• Inconsolable crying DPT
Transient rash	
• Measles	
• Varicella	

Contraindications

Every child has a right for immunisation and withholding it for some common minor illness or for any other reason is not justifiable. There are few contraindications to vaccination and one must apply them judiciously so as not to have a missed opportunity for immunisation in a child.

- Severe acute illness—Infectious or noninfectious
- Immunocompromised states especially for live vaccines.
- History of allergic reaction to vaccine
- Egg allergy in case of egg/chicken protein containing vaccines
- History of previous severe reaction to DPT

Box 25.1: Post Immunisation Pyrexia in Infants

The parent(s) should be advised that if pyrexia develops after childhood immunisation, the infant can be given a dose of paracetamol and if necessary, a second dose given 6 hours later; ibuprofen may be used if paracetamol is unsuitable. For post-immunisation pyrexia in an infant aged 2-3 months, the dose of paracetamol is 60 mg; the dose of ibuprofen is 50 mg.

Less Frequently Used Vaccines

Pneumococcal Vaccine

Pneumococci cause significant morbidity of upper as well as lower respiratory tract as well as invasive disease especially in children below 2 years of age. A polyvalent polysaccharide pneumococcal vaccine is available which has poor immunogenicity in children <2 years old as it is T-cell independent. Another heptavalent conjugate vaccine is also available which is effective in the target population of <2 years age. The pneumococcal vaccines are specially indicated in splenectomized or likely to undergo splenectomy or those with chronic diseases or immunocompromised.

The vaccine is given in dose of 0.5 ml intramuscularly with revaccination after 3-5 years for polyvalent vaccine.

Meningococcal Vaccine

Meningococci are capable of causing epidemics of meningitis or severe meningococcemia. In view of these, the vaccine is indicated for contacts of the patient or in outbreak situations. There are mainly 5 disease causing sero groups namely A, B, C, Y, W135. As immunity is specific for sero groups, the vaccine use is dictated by the isolation of a particular serotype during outbreaks/epidemics. Meningococcal vaccine is also indicated for immunocompromised children. Unconjugated bivalent (A + C) vaccine is more freely available as compared to conjugated quadrivalent (A, C, Y, and W135) which is more expensive also.

Influenza Vaccine

Influenza viral disease is a frequent respiratory morbidity which can become serious in certain patients. Influenza virus is characterized by frequent mutations, antigenic drifts and shifts. The immunity for the various strains is specific and hence to be effective the vaccine has to incorporate the prevalent antigenic strain. For this vaccine, WHO reviews and recommends the inclusion of prevalent strains annually. The vaccine is given intramuscularly/subcutaneously to children at high risk for Flu related morbidity, e.g. those with chronic lung/heart disease or immunocompromised.

Box 25.2: Vaccines and Asplenia

The following vaccines are recommended for asplenic children or those with splenic dysfunction.
Haemophilus inflenzae type b (Hib) vaccine, meningococcal group conjugate vaccine, pneumococcal polysaccharide vaccine, influenza vaccine.

Rabies Vaccine

Rabies caused by a bite/lick/scratch of a rabid animal is a fatal disease. The vaccine is usually used as a post exposure prophylaxis but can be given for routine immunisation for those at higher risk, e.g. handling susceptible animals (veterinarians, wild life workers, etc.). The older nerve tissue vaccine is no longer recommended or used. The tissue culture vaccines can be: **a.** Chick embryo cell, **b.** Human diploid cell, **c.** Duck embryo cell, **d.** Vero cell vaccine. All have almost equal efficacy. For post-exposure prophylaxis, as per WHO guidelines, the vaccine is given on day 0, 3, 7, 10, 14 and 28.

Inactivated Polio Vaccine (IPV)

This contains killed virus of all three serotypes. It is an effective vaccine with good safety profile and can be combined with other vaccine like DPT and HIB.

Newer Vaccines

Japanese Encephalitis

Viral encephalitis caused by Japanese B virus is endemic in some parts of India (Uttar Pradesh, Andhra Pradesh). As there is no specific treatment and it is associated with high mortality and morbidity, there is a definite indication for this vaccine. Presently there are three types of vaccines for Japanese encephalitis – 2 inactivated and 1 live attenuated, and better ones are in investigational stage.

Acellular Pertussis (DPaT)

Acellular pertussis vaccine has been synthesized to decrease the reactogenicity of the whole cell vaccine. In these, components of the pertussis bacillus with good immunogenic properties have been incorporated instead of the whole killed bacillus. It is equally effective but more expensive.

Some Important Vaccines under Investigation

Shigella vaccine	Rota Virus
Cholera vaccine	RSV
Streptococcal vaccine (Rheumatic fever)	HIV
Malarial vaccine	Hepatitis C

Some Important Issues

Simultaneous multiple vaccines are sometimes required for a child with incomplete schedule and poor compliance. Most of the vaccines can be given without the risk of losing efficacy or compromising safety. Combination vaccine should be used as per the manufacturer's guidelines.

Delayed doses of a particular vaccine do not necessarily indicate restarting the series but number of scheduled doses must be completed.

Interval between vaccines is an important issue for most live vaccines as they invade the host and multiply in the body to generate the immune response. Either the live vaccines should be administered together or 4 weeks apart.

International Immunisation Endeavours

Immunisation has been one of the most cost effective public health strategies the world over. Immunisation alone has saved many more lives than any other preventive strategy. Small pox has been eradicated from the world, poliomyelitis is in the process of being eradicated and many other diseases like measles, tetanus, and diphtheria have been hit.

At the international level, immunisation has been a key strategy for all health organizations. The first organized programme launched by World Health Organization (WHO) was the Expanded Programme of Immunisation (EPI) in 1974. EPI covered children less than 5 years of age for the vaccines viz: BCG, DPT, OPV, Measles and TT. In India, typhoid was included. As this did not meet the desired goals, it was changed to Universal Immunisation Programme (UIP) which targeted children less than 1 year of age along with infrastructural issues like vaccine production, cold chain system and monitoring.

Globally, many international agencies (WHO, UNICEF, World Bank, Rockefeller foundation) launched the childhood vaccine initiative (CVI) in 1991. This was further consolidated into a Global Alliance for Vaccine and Immunisation (GAVI).

The immunisation schedule is shown in Table 25.2.

Box 25.3: Prematurity

Children born prematurely should receive all routine immunisations based on the actual date of birth. There is no evidence of adverse reactions from vaccines.

TRAVEL IMMUNISATION

In these days of international travel it is essential that a child should be particularly immunized against those diseases which he may be exposed to in the country of his visit. This will be in addition to the routine childhood immunisations being up to date. There are countries in the world where no special immunisation is required for travellers such as the United States, Europe, Australia or New Zealand although all travellers should have immunity to tetanus and poliomyelitis. But certain precautions are required in Non-European areas surrounding the Mediterranean, in Africa, the Middle East, Asia, and South America. Many countries require an international certificate of vaccination from individuals arriving from or who have been travelling through endemic areas, whilst other countries require a certificate from all entering travelers.

Long-term travellers to areas that have a high incidence of poliomyelitis or tuberculosis should be immunized with the appropriate vaccine. Protection against hepatitis A is recommended for travellers to high-risk areas outside Northern and Western Europe, North America, Japan, Australia and New Zealand. Hepatitis A vaccine is preferred and it is likely to be effective even if given shortly before departure; normal immunoglobulin is no longer given routinely but may be indicated in the immuno-compromised.

Hepatitis B vaccine is recommended for those travelling to areas of high prevalence and plan to stay there for long periods. Short-term tourists are not generally at increased risk of infection. Prophylactic immunisation against rabies is recommended for travellers to enzootic areas on long journeys or to areas out of reach of immediate medical attention.

Typhoid vaccine is indicated for travelers to those countries where typhoid is endemic. There is no requirement for cholera vaccination as a condition for entry into any country, but oral cholera vaccine may be considered for those travelling to situations where the risk is greatest. Yellow fever immununisation is recommended for travel to the endemic zones of Africa and South America.

Immunisation against meningococcal meningitis is recommended for children travelling to countries of risk. They should be immunized with a meningococcal polysaccharide vaccine that covers serotypes A,C,W135 and Y. Vaccination is especially important for those living

Table 25.2: Immunisation schedule

Vaccine name	Type	Contents	Route	Dose	Efficacy	Storage temperature	Age of admin
BCG (Bacillus Chalmette Guerin)	Live attenuated, freeze dried, bovine strain	0.1-0.4 million bacilli/dose	ID	0.1ml	0-80%	2-8°C	Birth
Polio Vaccine Oral (Sabin)	Live attenuated	Trivalent I 106 TCID 50 II 105 TCID 50 III 105.8 TCID 50	O	2 drops	80-90%	=<-20°C	5 doses in 1st year starting at 0 mth & then at 4-8 wk interval; Boosters with DPT
Injectable (Salk)	Killed	I 40D II 8D III 32D	IM	0.5 ml	>95%		
DPT as		20-30 lf			95%	2-8°C	
Diphtheria Toxoid	Toxoid		IM	05 ml			3 doses in 1st year starting at 6-8 wk & then 4-8 weeks apart; Boosters at 18 months & 5yr
Pertussis	Killed	20 million bacilli 5-10 lf	"	"	85%		
Tetanus	Toxoid			"	100%		
Hepatitis B	Recombinant subunit	10 mcg (up to 19 yrs.) 20 mg (>19 yrs)	IM	0.5 ml	94%	2-8°C	0,1,6 months
HiB *H.influenza B*	Conjugate capsular polysaccharide vaccine	10 mcg	IM	0.5 ml	97%	2-8°C	Same as DPT; only 1 booster at 18 mths
Measles	Live attenuated	1000TCID50	SC	0.5 ml	95%	2-8°C	6-9 months
MMR(Measles Mumps Rubella	Live attenuated	1000TCID50 5000TCID50 1000TCID50	SC	0.5 ml	95%	2-8°C	At 15 months age
Typhoid Vi antigen	Capsular polysaccharide Subunit	25-30 mcg	SC, IM	0.5 ml	70%	2-8°C	After 2 yrs. Age; booster every 2-3 years Above 6 yrs. age; booster every 3 years
Oral typhoid vaccine Ty21a	Live attenuated		O	3 Capsules	70%	2-8°C	
Chickenpox	Live attenuated	103.3PFU	SC	0.5 ml	95-100%	2-8°C	1-13 yrs age single dose, >13 yrs age 2 doses 1 month apart
Hepatitis A	Live attenuated	720 ELU(up to 19yr)	IM	0.5 ml	90-100%	2-8°C	2 doses six months apart

with local people or visiting an area of risk during outbreaks.

Malaria chemoprophylaxis should generally be started one week before travel into an endemic area and should be continued for 4 weeks after leaving. It is important to be aware that any illness that occurs within 1 year and especially within 3 months of return might be malaria even if all recommended precautions against malaria were taken.

Key Learning Point

Those children who cannot receive live vaccines, the use of normal immunoglobulin should be considered after exposure to measles and varicella-zoster immunoglobulin after exposure to chickenpox or herpes zoster.

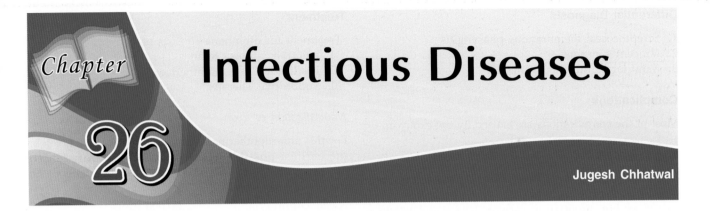

Infectious Diseases

Chapter 26

Jugesh Chhatwal

DIPHTHERIA

Aetiology

Diphtheria is caused by Corynebacterium diphtheriae also known as Klebs-Löeffler bacillus. C diphtheriae is an aerobic, polymorphic, gram-positive bacillus. The disease causing potential is in the exotoxin produced by the bacillus. Three biotypes of the bacillus namely mitis, intermedius and gravis have been differentiated with varying disease causing capabilities.

Epidemiology

C diphtheriae resides mainly on human mucous membranes and skin although it can be viable in dust or on fomites for about six months. The disease is transmitted from man to man, either through carriers or patients. It spreads primarily by airborne droplets or direct contact with respiratory secretions. The most susceptible age group is unimmunised children below 15 years but can occur in unprotected adults also. Asymptomatic carriers are an important source of infection.

Pathogenesis

After infection, C diphtheriae remains in the respiratory mucosa. They induce a local inflammatory reaction and elaborate an exotoxin, which is responsible for the virulence of the disease. Locally, there is necrosis of the mucous membrane along with collection of fibrin, leucocytes and RBCs. Together they form the characteristic dirty grey coloured membrane seen in the upper airways of a patient with diphtheria. Attempts to remove this thick adherent membrane lead to bleeding, as superficial epithelium is part of the membrane. The membrane can cause life threatening obstructive respiratory symptoms by blocking the air passages from pharynx to larynx and even trachea. The toxin affecting the nervous tissues, cardiac muscles, renal tubules and platelets causes the other serious manifestations.

Clinical Features

The usual incubation period of diphtheria is 2-5 days. The major symptoms and signs are related to the respiratory tract but other parts of the body can also be affected viz. skin (Cutaneous diphtheria) ears, eyes or genital tract. The presentation due to the local involvement varies according to the site whereas the features due to exotoxin occur irrespective of the site. The commonest site of involvement is tonsillopharyngeal area followed by nose and larynx.

Nasal

Frequently resembles common cold. It is seen more often in infants. There is serosanguineous nasal discharge which maybe unilateral with mild constitutional symptoms. Often there is a membrane seen on the nasal septum.

Tonsillopharyngeal

The typical membrane is the hallmark of the disease. This can have a variable extent from unilateral to bilateral involving all the pharyngeal structures and can lead to respiratory obstruction. Accompanying symptoms maybe mild initially but toxaemia can set in early. The surrounding soft tissue and the draining lymph nodes can enlarge and give the appearance of 'Bull-Neck'.

Laryngeal

The membrane can extend from pharynx to larynx causing severe respiratory obstruction or difficult, noisy breathing with hoarse voice and stridor. From larynx the membrane can further extend to trachea and the respiratory symptoms can become more severe.

Differential Diagnosis

1. Streptococcal membranous pharyngitis
2. Vincent's angina
3. Viral laryngotracheobronchitis

Complications

Most of the complications are caused by the exotoxin.

Toxic Myocarditis

It occurs in 10-25% of patients and is responsible for almost half the deaths due to diphtheria. Typically it is seen during 2nd-3rd wk but can occur as early as 1st wk and as late as 6th wk. Tachycardia with soft heart sounds, heart failure or sudden respiratory distress may indicate the onset. Cardiac dysrhythmias may also occur.

Toxic Neuropathy

Diphtheria toxin can lead to a variety of neurological involvements in a multiphasic manner. The different manifestations are shown in Table 26.1. The recovery from most of these is likely although residual weakness may sometimes persist.

Table 26.1. Neurological complications of diphtheria		
Site of involvement	Time of onset	Clinical presentation
a. Palatal paralysis	2-3 wks	Weakness of pharyngeal muscles, hoarse voice, nasal twang, swallowing difficulty, aspiration.
b. Ocular paralysis (Oculomotor ciliary paralysis)	3-5 wks	Strabismus, blurred vision, accommodation paralysis
c. Polyneuropathy (Symmetric)	2 wks to 3 months	Proximal muscle weakness, motor deficits with decreased deep tendon reflexes
d. Phrenic nerve paralysis	2 wks to 3 months	Diaphragmatic paralysis
e. Vasomotor Centre	2-3 wks	Hypotension, cardiac failure.

DIAGNOSIS

The diagnostic investigation for diphtheria is the demonstration of *C diphtheriae* either by smear examination or by culture. For this purpose a swab should be taken from under the edges of the membrane or the membrane itself. The smear is preferably stained by Albert stain. A negative smear is not reliable and culturing the organism is necessary. For culture, selective media, potassium tellurite, should be used.

Treatment

Treatment for diphtheria consists of
 I. Neutralization of toxin
 II. Eradication of C diphtheriae
 III. Supportive Therapy

Neutralization of toxin

For this anti-diphtheritic serum (ADS) should be given at the earliest possible. ADS is given after intradermal sensitivity testing by IM or IV route. The dose depends on the site of involvement.

Nasal Diphtheria	20,000 units
Tonsillar/Pharyngeal	40,000-80, 000 units
Laryngeal	80, 000-1, 20, 000 units

Diphtheria immune globulin (human) if available can also be used in the dose of 0.6 ml/kg.

Eradication of C diphtheriae

It is equally important to stop further production of toxin by eliminating the organism. The antibiotic of choice is Penicillin or Erythromycin. IV crystalline penicillin 1 lac units (=100,000 units)/kg/day in 6 hourly doses is given for 10-14 days. The dose of erythromycin is 40-50 mg/kg/day in 4 divided doses orally for the same duration. Elimination of *C diphtheriae* is documented by 2 successive cultures from the site after stopping antibiotics.

Supportive treatment

Isolation of the patient is required to prevent cross infection. Bed rest is mandatory for first 2 weeks and even later in case of cardiac complications followed by graded return of activity. Respiratory obstruction is a frequent occurrence hence careful watch needs to be maintained till the oropharyngeal inflammation and membrane disappear. A tracheotomy set and provision for assisted ventilation should be readily available.

The case fatality rate of 10% is reported from even good centres. The usual cause of death is either respiratory obstruction or myocarditis. After recovery from diphtheria, the child needs to be vaccinated, as the disease does not confer good immunity.

Contacts and carriers

All household contacts should be screened with swab cultures and given prophylaxis with either erythromycin for 7 days or a single injection of long acting benzathine penicillin. This should be followed by appropriate vaccination. If cultures come positive, subsequent cultures after prophylactic antibiotic need to be done to document negative culture.

CASE STUDY

A 4-year-old boy from poor socio-economic strata was brought to the emergency paediatric service with a history of cough and a low-grade fever for 4 days. He had developed difficulty in breathing over 4 hours prior to hospitalisation. His father did not know the child's immunisation status. On arrival he was dysphonic, pale, malnourished and temperature was 38°C. There was a diffuse swelling of his neck. Throat examination revealed a dirty grey membrane over his tonsils, tonsillar pillars and extending to the soft palate. The membrane could not be removed easily and bled from underneath. Pulse 120/min. He had marked suprasternal and subcostal retractions. Otherwise systemic examination was unremarkable. Throat swab for *C diphtheriae* was positive. He was given diphtheria antitoxin intravenously 60,000 units after sensitivity testing and benzyl penicillin. He developed sudden onset acute respiratory distress. He underwent tracheotomy to relieve the obstruction caused by the membrane in the upper airways. Thereafter he made an uneventful recovery.

Diagnosis: Tonsillar diphtheria.

Key Learning Points

The two usual causes of mortality in diphtheria are upper airways obstruction and myocarditis.
After recovery from diphtheria the patient needs active immunisation with appropriate diphtheria vaccine.

PERTUSSIS (WHOOPING COUGH)

Pertussis means intense cough in Latin. Pertussis is an acute infectious disease of the respiratory tract occurring in susceptible hosts of all ages.

Aetiology

The main causative organism for pertussis is Bordetella pertussis. Few cases are attributable to other Bordetella species like B. parapertussis or B. bronchiseptica. These organisms are tiny, gram-negative and cocco-bacillary in shape.

Epidemiology

Pertussis has been prevalent worldwide for many centuries and has been a leading cause of death in children especially in the pre-vaccination era. Whooping cough may occur at any age, even in the first few weeks of life. Placental transfer of antibody does not protect young infants passively. With effective coverage of pertussis vaccine the incidence of the disease as well as attributable mortality have markedly decreased. The immunity conferred by vaccine as well as the disease wanes over a period of time. Hence older children and adults with poor vaccine updates become susceptible to active disease and/or act as reservoir of infection.

Pathogenesis

Bordetella pertussis produces a pertussis toxin as well as few other biologically active substances. All together are responsible for various inflammatory changes with pertussis toxin playing a central role. The mucosal lining of the respiratory tract is inflamed with necrosis and desquamation of epithelial cells leading to obstruction, atelectasis and accumulation of secretions. The resultant hypoxia can affect liver and brain also.

Clinical Features

The incubation period of 3-12 days is followed by three characteristic stages of pertussis. The first stage, Catarrhal stage begins with low-grade fever, nasal symptoms and conjunctival redness with watering of eyes, just like any other upper respiratory infection. Coughing indicates the beginning of Paroxysmal stage, which can last 2-6 weeks. Initially the cough is dry, irritating and hacking and gradually becomes paroxysmal. The paroxysms of cough can soon be accompanied by the characteristic whoop. The whoop is a forceful inspiration through partially closed airways, which follows a bout of coughing. During the paroxysms of cough the child has incessant coughing which increases in crescendo with flushing of face, bulging of eyes and gasps of respiration. During severe bouts of coughing there may be cyanosis also. Very often vomiting follows the bouts of coughing. The infant or young child usually appears quite well in between these paroxysms of coughing although the frequency of such bouts can keep on increasing progressively. Gradually the patient passes into the Convalescent stage where the coughing episodes become less severe and less frequent. The cough can persist for sometime and hence the disease has also been called 'Cough of 100 days'. The young infant or a sick child may not have the characteristic whoop, as they cannot generate enough pressures in their respiratory passage.

Complications

Respiratory system is the site for most complications especially secondary bacterial infections. Otitis media, emphysema, air leaks in the form of pneumothorax or pneumomediastinum and even subcutaneous emphysema can occur. During the paroxysmal stage, serious CNS complications like seizures and encephalopathy can occur. A number of complications associated with the severe cough or whoop can occur. The raised pressure in various blood vessels can lead to subconjuctival haemorrhage, retinal haemorrhage, epistaxis and even intracranial haemorrhage (Fig. 26.1). Increase in intra-abdominal pressure can cause inguinal hernia, rectal prolapse and rarely diaphragmatic rupture. Due to protracted course,

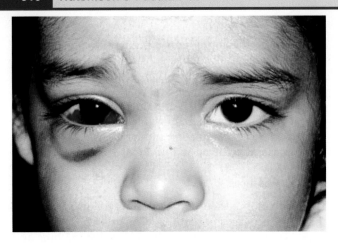

Fig. 26.1: Subconjunctival haemorrhage and black eye in a child with pertussis

vomiting and poor feeding, malnutrition is a frequent occurrence. Flaring of underlying tuberculosis can also occur.

Differential Diagnosis

1. Viral Infections, e.g. Adenovirus, Influenza, RSV
2. Mycoplasma infection
3. Foreign body aspiration
4. Endobronchial tuberculosis

Diagnosis

Diagnosis is mainly based on the history and clinical examination. None of the investigations are very efficient in diagnosing pertussis. Following investigations maybe helpful:

    I. Leucocytosis especially increased lymphocytes.
    II. Low ESR
    III. Isolation of B. pertussis
      - Deep nasopharyngeal swab/cough plate cultures
      - Direct fluorescent antibody testing
      - PCR on nasopharyngeal swab.
    IV. Serological tests during convalescent stage to detect specific antibodies.

Treatment

The aims of treatment are:

    I. Decrease the severity and frequency of cough paroxysms as much as possible.
    II. Maintain nutrition
    III. Identifying the need for assisted / hospitalisation care
    I. Initially the episodes of cough paroxysms should be observed and an assessment of their severity made. The child should be asked to rest in a quiet,

undisturbed environment with minimal essential lighting. A nebulised mist and /or salbutamol can be helpful in some patients. In addition, administration of appropriate antibiotics early in the course of disease can also decrease the severity. The antibiotic of choice is Erythromycin 40-50 mg/kg/day in 4 divided doses orally for 2 weeks.

    II. Small, frequent, easily swalloable and calorie dense foodstuffs should be given. Forced feeding should be avoided. Feeds are better given soon after a bout of coughing.
    III. A child with pertussis should be managed at home if having infrequent paroxysms and able to feed well. Only in young or sick infants hospitalisation may be required.

All patients need to be isolated till they have received at least 5 days of antibiotics.

Contacts

All contacts irrespective of symptoms, age, and immunization status should be given antibiotic for 2 weeks. For unimmunised or incompletely immunised contacts, the schedule should be completed. Those who have received a vaccine dose >6 months back should receive a booster.

Key Learning Point
Diagnosis of pertussis is mainly clinical.

TETANUS

Tetanus, also known as Lock-jaw is an illness caused by Clostridium tetani. Despite the availability of safe and effective immunisation, tetanus is still a serious health problem worldwide especially in many developing countries.

Aetiology

Clostridium tetani is a gram positive, anaerobic organism. It forms spores, which are resistant to boiling but are destroyed by autoclaving. *C tetani* is not an invasive organism. On entering the human body, it elaborates two exotoxins namely tetanospasmin and tetanolysin. Tetanospasmin is responsible for all the manifestations of tetanus. After botulinum toxin, it is the next most poisonous substance known in the world.

Epidemiology

Tetanus occurs all over the world. The resistant spores of *C tetani* are ubiquitous in nature and can be present in several dirty objects. They also inhabit the human intestines or animal oral cavity and intestines.

Tetanus occurs in unimmunised adults and children exposed through dirty or contaminated injuries and wounds. The other susceptible group is pregnant women undergoing unsterile methods of delivery. Along with them, the newborns are another major susceptible population. Neonatal tetanus is reported from many developing countries where unimmunised women give birth in unclean conditions. The umbilical cord is the portal of entry for the neonate born through such a process. Occasionally tetanus occurs with no history of trauma. In such cases chronic supportive otitis media or intestinal colonization with *C tetani* leads to an invasive infection.

Pathogenesis

After entering through a portal, the tetanus spores germinate and the vegetative bacterial cell dies releasing the exotoxin. Tetanospasmin binds the neuromuscular junction and then enters the major nerves and travels to the spinal cord. There it blocks the inhibitor pathways of muscular contraction leading to sustained spasm of muscles. The autonomic nervous system is also affected. *C tetani* by itself causes little local inflammatory reaction.

Clinical Features

The incubation period of tetanus varies from 3-30 days. The presentation is most often generalized but sometimes can be localized also. The usual early symptoms maybe irritability or headache, which is soon accompanied by the classical presentation of Trismus or lockjaw in 50% of cases. These are followed by stiffness of whole body, difficulty in chewing and swallowing and then muscle spasms. The typical Risus sardonicus occurs because of spasm of masseter muscles of face. The stiffness and spasms lead to neck retraction and an extreme opisthotonus position i.e. arching of the back. There can be involvement of laryngeal and respiratory muscles also. With all this, the patient is generally conscious and hence has extreme pain. The spasms can be caused by minor stimuli such as noise, light, touch and even occur spontaneously. The autonomic involvement can cause tachyarrhythmias, hypertension, urinary and bowel involvement. There is accompanying fever of variable level.

Neonatal Tetanus (Tetanus neonatorum)

Tetanus in neonates is an important cause of neonatal mortality. As stated earlier, unimmunised mothers undergoing unclean delivery is the cause, the portal of entry being the umbilicus. The first symptom is sudden inability to suck. The infant rapidly develops stiffness of the body, followed by generalised spasms. Persistent Risus sardonicus is common. Spasms of the larynx occur early in the course of neonatal disease and the infant is unable to swallow. Aspiration pneumonia and gastroenteritis are

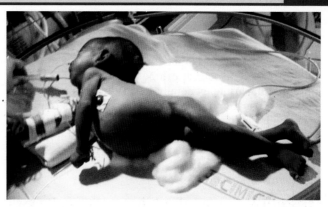

Fig. 26.2: Marked opisthotonus seen in Tetanus neonatorum

common complications. The differential diagnosis includes intracranial injury secondary to birth trauma, meningitis, hypocalcaemic tetany, sepsis and seizures of any other aetiology (Fig. 26.2).

Complications

Respiratory complications occur due to heavy sedation and laryngeal spasms. Cardiac arrhythmias, hypotension are seen in some patients.
Severe spasms can cause rhabdomyolysis, myoglobinuria and fractures.

Differential Diagnosis

1. Abscess in pharyngeal areas can sometimes produce trismus.
2. Acute encephalitis
3. Rabies
4. Strychnine poisoning

Diagnosis

The diagnosis is based on classical clinical picture. Attempts to isolate C tetani are not successful and not required. The routine laboratory investigations are more helpful for assessing secondary bacterial infections.

Treatment

Following are the objectives of treatment of tetanus
A. Neutralization of toxin
B. Control of spasms
C. Eradication of *C tetani*
D. Intensive supportive care
E. Prevention of recurrence

A. Neutralization of toxin

The toxin bound to neural tissue cannot be neutralized. Hence the first priority is to administer antitoxin to render the free available toxin ineffective. For this purpose, animal derived antitoxin Anti-tetanus serum (ATS) as well as human derived tetanus immune globulin (TIG), both, are available. ATS is given in the dose of 50, 000-1,00,000 units after sensitivity testing. It can be given by intravenous or intramuscular route, generally half IV and half IM. It has to be given as a one time dose as repeat doses can cause severe immunological reactions. There is a significant risk of serum sickness with ATS. The dose for TIG ranges from 3000-6000 units, intramuscular.

B. Control of spasms

Spasms and the generalized hypertonia need muscle relaxants and sedatives. Diazepam is used in the dose of 0.1-0.2 mg/kg IV either as intermittent doses 2-4 hourly or as a continuous infusion in severe cases. Prolonged administration is required for up to 6 weeks for muscle relaxation. Other agents used may include chlorpromazine, benzodiazepines, Baclofen and magnesium sulphate. Sometimes IV phenobarbitone may also be helpful. In intensive care settings use of neuromuscular blocking agents like vecuronium and pancuronium along with mechanical ventilation can give better survival rates.

C. Eradication of C tetani

To eradicate *C tetani*, inj. Crystalline penicillin 1 lac units (=100,000 units)/kg/day IV in 4 divided doses for 10-14 days is the antibiotic of choice. Alternative for penicillin hypersensitive patient are Erythromycin, Tetracycline or Metronidazole.

D. Intensive supportive care

Supportive care is an essential part of looking after tetanus patients. A quiet, dimly lit room with minimal handling is important. All care taking activities and medications should be timed to cause as little stimulation as possible. Equipment for emergency ventilatory support must be readily available.

E. Prevention of recurrence

Tetanus does not confer any immunity after recovery and all patients must be fully immunized after recovery irrespective of the age group.

Key Learning Points
Exotoxin produced by tetanus bacilli, tetanospasmin is responsible for the clinical features. A tetanus patient usually remains conscious even with severe spasms and opisthotonus.

Other Clostridial Infections

Clostridium botulinum

C botulinum causes Botulism of which three presentations are known (i) Infantile botulism due to intake of contaminated honey or similar items. (ii) Food borne botulism seen in older age groups or adults due to ingestion of food contaminated with *C botulinum*. This contamination can occur in canned as well as non-canned foods. (iii) Botulism due to wound infection is less common. Botulinum toxin is the most poisonous substance known. It causes neuromuscular blockade leading to motor paralysis of all muscles of body. The diagnosis is mainly clinical. Treatment consists of intensive supportive care and administration of human derived botulinum antitoxin especially in infants. No antibiotics are required for *C botulinum* as the organism undergoes lysis and releases the toxin.

Clostridium Difficile

C difficile has been associated with pseudomembranous colitis or antibiotic associated diarrhoea. It produces two types of toxins, which are responsible for death of intestinal cells, inflammatory response and the formation of a pseudomembrane. The clinical presentation can range from mild diarrhoea to an explosive onset of watery diarrhoea with blood, fever and abdominal pain. Treatment includes stopping the offending antibiotics, if possible and to restore normal gut flora. The accompanying fluids and electrolytes disturbances need correction. The specific treatment is given for severe cases with oral Metronidazole or IV Vancomycin.

ENTERIC FEVER (TYPHOID FEVER)

Enteric fever or typhoid fever is caused by Salmonella group of organisms. Salmonella are gram-negative bacilli with flagellar motility. There are 2463 serovars of salmonella, which are broadly classified, as Typhoidal or Non-typhoidal.

Aetiology

The 'Typhoidal' salmonellae are comprised of *S. typhi, S. paratyphi* A, B and C. The classical Typhoid fever is caused by *S. typhi* while the paratyphi causes a less severe febrile illness.

Epidemiology

Typhoid fever occurs worldwide but incidence differs according to the sanitation and hygiene levels. In developing countries where insanitary conditions are prevalent, it continues to be a significant infectious disease and a public health problem. Man is the only reservoir. Infection occurs through oro-fecal route due to ingestion of contaminated water and food. As asymptomatic persons can continue to excrete the bacilli for months to years, food handlers can be an important source of infection. Contaminated water cultivation of oysters and shellfish can also cause infections. Salmonella can cross the placental barrier in a pregnant mother to infect the fetus.

Pathogenesis

During a variable incubation period ranging from 3-30 days, the organisms invade the intestines through Peyer's patches and then travel via lymphatics to mesenteric nodes to reach blood stream through thoracic duct. This leads to primary bacteraemia followed by proliferation of the bacilli in the reticulo-endothelial organs. From there the organisms re-enter the blood stream causing secondary bacteraemia and the clinical illness. The proliferation in Peyer's patches causes sloughing, necrosis and ulceration of the intestinal mucosa. These typhoid ulcers can become deep and lead to haemorrhage or perforation. During the second phase of bacteraemia, gallbladder is seeded and can become a reservoir of bacilli in carriers from where the organism is excreted through bile into the intestines and faeces. The organism has a somatic antigen (O), flagellar antigen (H) and a capsular antigen (Vi). The Vi antigen interferes with phagocytosis. It also produces an antitoxin, which causes the toxic symptoms of typhoid.

Clinical Features

Typhoid fever occurs at all ages including neonates. The clinical presentation may vary a little with age but fever is a universal symptom. Initially it may be low grade but increases in few days to become high grade and persistent. The fever is soon accompanied by abdominal symptoms like diarrhoea, abdominal pain, vomiting and loss of appetite. There may also be cough and myalgia. The child by the second week appears sick and toxic with a coated tongue, hepatomegaly and a tender abdomen. Soft splenomegaly may also be present. The rashes of typhoid, rose spots, are frequently transient and faint and hence not easily visualized. Some respiratory signs like rales may also appear. A tender mass palpable in right hypochondrium suggests a calculus cholecystitis. Sometimes liver involvement can lead to a clinically manifest hepatitis with jaundice and tender hepatomegaly. In severe cases an encephalopathy like picture- Coma vigil can occur. The patient lies in bed with open eyes but oblivious of surroundings.

Complications

Complications are less frequent in children than adults. Two dreaded intestinal complications, which usually occur in 2nd or 3rd week of illness, are haemorrhage and perforation. In both situations patients can suddenly collapse with shock, tachycardia and drop in temperature. Perforation may be indicated by increase in abdominal pain, distension and features of peritonitis. A surgical

intervention may be required. For both conditions intensive supportive care is required. Repeated blood transfusions may be required for a bleeding typhoid ulcer.

S. typhi can invade any organ of the body to cause inflammation ranging from meningitis, endocarditis, myocarditis to osteomyelitis and arthritis. Certain late neurological complications like acute cerebellar ataxia, chorea, and peripheral neuritis have also been reported.

Diagnosis

Blood culture for *S. typhi* is the confirmatory test. It becomes positive in the 1st week itself. Bone marrow aspirate culture has a higher sensitivity of 85-90%. Polymerase chain reaction has also been used to detect typhoid and has a good specificity and sensitivity. Cultures of urine and stool can be positive for salmonella but are not considered useful in diagnosis.

Widal test, a serological test, used to measure antibodies against O and H antigens is commonly used for aiding in diagnosis. It has a fairly high rate of false positive and negative. In addition, the baseline antibody levels of different communities may differ according to the endemicity of the disease in the region. The immunization may also affect the antibody levels. A careful interpretation of Widal results is required keeping in mind the clinical picture of the patient and the above factors.

Haematological investigations can show anaemia due to infection/ blood loss as well as poor intake. Leucopenia is the usual finding in typhoid but in younger children leucocytosis is more common.

Treatment

Treatment of Typhoid fever has been evolving. Chloramphenicol was and still is the drug of choice in most places. It is given as 50 mg/kg/day in 4 divided doses for 2 weeks. In many developing countries, *S typhi* has become resistant to chloramphenicol and other drugs used like ampicillin, sulphamethoxazole-trimethoprim. Third generation cephalosporins like ceftriaxone are recommended in such situations with or without combination of aminoglycoside. Quinolones like ciprofloxacin, ofloxacin have also been found to be effective but need to be used with caution in young children.

Supportive therapy includes providing adequate fluids and nutrition either orally or parenterally. If child can take orally, a soft low residue diet is advised initially. During hospitalisation hygiene measures must be instituted to prevent cross infection.

Typhoid immunisation is advised for children travelling to areas where sanitation standards may be poor, although it is not a substitute for scrupulous personal hygiene.

Non-typhoidal Salmonellosis

Non-typhoidal salmonellosis is caused by a number of organisms similar to *S typhi* but have different serotypes (e.g. *S dublin, S typhimurium, S cholera-suis, S marina*). Unlike *S typhi*, animals are important source of human infection for non-typhoidal salmonellae. Poultry and related products are responsible for a number of outbreaks. The infection has a short incubation period of 6-72 hours. The common clinical presentation is of acute enterocolitis. In neonates, young infants, malnutrition and other immuno-compromised states they can cause a more invasive disease leading to septicaemia like picture and meningitis. Seeding of bones can lead to osteomyelitis especially in children with sickle cell anaemia. The diagnosis is by culturing the organism from stool or other areas of involvement. Treatment is same as for typhoid fever.

CHOLERA

Cholera, caused by *Vibrio cholerae*, is an acute gastrointestinal infection. It is a major public health problem especially in developing countries.

Aetiology

V cholerae is a gram-negative, motile, comma shaped organism with a flagellum. Two pathogenic strains *V cholerae* 01 and 0139 are known. The 01 strain has two bio groups i.e. Classic and El Tor and there are further serogroups of O antigens viz Ogawa, Inaba and Hikojima.

Epidemiology

Cholera has been known to occur for centuries in various parts of the world. It has not only an endemic or sporadic presence but has caused epidemics as well as pandemics. The route of infection is feco-oral. Contaminated water serves as a reservoir and frequently the source of the infection. Other sources of infection include contaminated foodstuffs, utensils and houseflies. There are no animal reservoirs of infection.

Pathogenesis

Cholera has one of the shortest incubation periods of 6 hours to 5 days. After ingestion, the organisms have to pass through the acid barrier of stomach. Once they survive that, they colonize the upper small intestines. For colonization, a relatively large inoculum of *V cholerae* is required. The organisms produce an enterotoxin, cholera toxin, which causes the symptoms. The toxin enters the intestinal epithelial cells, binds and activates the enzyme adenyl cyclase. As a result, cyclic AMP levels increase. This leads to decreased absorption of sodium and chloride from villous cells and also an active secretion of chloride. As sodium absorption is impaired, water is poured out from intestinal epithelium. The outpouring of fluid and electrolytes produces the watery diarrhoea and the related changes.

Clinical Features

Cholera infection can be a mild self-limiting disorder or even asymptomatic. Severe infection leads to profuse watery diarrhoea accompanied by vomiting. In young children there can be significant fever. The stools are watery with a fishy odour and the mucus flakes give it the typical rice water appearance. The fluid and electrolyte loss can be massive leading to symptoms and signs of severe dehydration and even circulatory collapse and acute renal failure. The outpouring of watery diarrhoea can continue for 5-7 days.

Diagnosis

Examination of fresh stool sample as a hanging drop preparation under the microscope can show the darting motile *V cholerae*. There are generally no fecal leucocytes. Stool culture confirms the diagnosis as well as helps in identifying the type. *V cholerae* is best cultured on thiosulphate citrate bile sucrose media (TCBS).

The estimation of serum electrolytes and blood sugar levels is useful for appropriate management of sick children.

Treatment

The mainstay of treatment is replacement of fluid and electrolytes losses. If the child can take orally then oral rehydration solution (ORS) should be given ad libitum. In case oral intake is not possible or inadequate, intravenous rehydration is essential. Hyponatraemia, hypokalaemia and acidosis need appropriate attention.

Antibiotics can help in shortening the duration of illness and possibly the carrier rate. The drug of choice is oral tetracycline for 3 days. In younger children, trimethoprim- sulphamethoxazole combination can be used. Furazolidone has also been used.

Complications

All the complications and even the mortality are related to the fluid and electrolyte losses. Hence prompt and appropriate treatment can prevent the complications.

Prevention

Besides good hygiene and public health measures no other practical methods are there for prevention of cholera. Three types of vaccines are available in the world. The commonly used one is a parenterally administrated, phenol-killed vaccine with an efficacy of 50% and immunity lasting up to 6 months. There are two oral vaccines; one killed subunit and another live attenuated. Their efficacy is reported to be better but again protection lasts 6 months. None of them protect against 0139 strain.

CASE STUDY

An 8-year-old boy was brought to the emergency service with a history of frequent, profuse watery stools, fever and vomiting for one day. The stools were whitish, watery with a peculiar fishy odour. The child was severely dehydrated and was in shock. He was resuscitated with intravenous fluid therapy. His serum sodium was 265meq/l, potassium 3.5meq/l, chloride 85meq/l. Stool hanging drop preparation showed organisms with Vibrio like morphology and motility. He was given oral doxycycline and continued on IV fluids. He made a complete recovery in 4 days.
Diagnosis: Cholera

Key Learning Points

Cholera has a short incubation period of 6 hours to 5 days.
Typical cholera stools are watery, rice water in appearance with fishy odour.
Appropriate fluid and electrolyte replacement is life saving in cholera.

SHIGELLOSIS

Shigellosis is caused by shigella group of organisms. There are four etiological species namely *Shigella dysenteriae*, *S flexueri*, *S sonnei* and *S boydii*.

Epidemiology

S dysenteriae is endemic in Asia and Africa and can cause epidemics. The infection is more common during warm season and source is contaminated water and food. Shigella can survive in milk for upto 30 days. Flies also excrete shigella. Unlike Cholera, a small inoculum of 10 to 100 bacteria is adequate to cause disease. Asymptomatic individuals can carry shigella organisms and be a source of infection. Person to person transmission due to poor hand washing also occurs.

Pathogenesis

Shigellas are invasive organisms and affect the colon. There is colitis with mucosal edema, ulceration and bleeding. The deeper layer of colonic wall i.e. muscularis mucosa and submucosa can also be affected by the inflammatory process. *S dysenteriae* also produces an exotoxin, shiga toxin, which can cause watery diarrhoea.

Clinical Features

All four types cause similar clinical picture although severity may vary. After an incubation period of 12 hours to several days, the clinical presentation may start with loose stools, abdominal pain, fever and vomiting. Soon the fever becomes higher; there are severe abdominal cramps, tenesmus with blood in stools. Abdominal examination may reveal distension and tenderness. There can be accompanying features of fluid and electrolyte loss. In some children, neurological manifestations like convulsions, headache and lethargy may occur.

Complications

I. Dehydration and dyselectrolytaemia
II. Sepsis and bacteraemia can occur with *S dysenteriae* and organisms may be isolated from blood culture.
III. Haemolytic Uremic syndrome is mediated by shiga toxin.
IV. Persistent diarrhoea and malnutrition
V. Rectal Prolapse- In malnourished children there can be rectal prolapse due to tenesmus.

Diagnosis

Stool examination can show numerous leucocytes. Culture of stool for Shigella proves the diagnosis. There is leucocytosis and in some children leukemoid reaction can also occur. In sick and toxic looking children, blood culture should also be obtained.

Treatment

The priority is on correcting the fluid and electrolyte balance with either oral or intravenous rehydration. Antibiotic therapy is recommended as it shortens the episode and improves the outcome and also decreases carrier state. The choice may depend on culture sensitivity if available. Oral ampicillin, trimethoprim-sulphamethoxazole or Nalidixic acid all are effective. In older children quinolones may also be used.

STREPTOCOCCAL INFECTIONS

Streptococcus pyogenes or group A Streptococcus is known to cause acute infection of the respiratory system and skin. It is also responsible for certain clinical syndromic conditions like scarlet fever, necrotizing fascitis and toxic shock syndrome and post infectious entities like acute rheumatic fever and acute glomerulonephritis.

Aetiology

Streptococci are gram-positive cocci seen in chains. They are categorized into 3 categories depending on their ability to cause haemolysis viz. beta (β)-haemolytic causing complete haemolysis, alpha (α) cause partial haemolysis while gamma (γ) cause no haemolysis. The Beta-haemolytic streptococci are further divided based upon polysaccharide components in their cell wall. These groups known as Lancefield grouping range from A to T.

Epidemiology

Group A streptococci cause highly contagious disease and all persons not having immunity to it are susceptible. Humans are the source of infection and transmission occurs by droplet infection from respiratory passages. Overcrowding, close contact favour the spread of infection. Skin infections occur only after a break in the normal barrier, as streptococci do not penetrate intact skin.

Pathogenesis

The pathogenesis and virulence of group A Streptococcus is related to presence of M proteins. M protein rich streptococci resist phagocytosis and also generate a protective antibody response. The streptococci produce a variety of toxins and enzymes. Streptococcal erythrogenic or a pyrogenic toxin is one of these and responsible for causing invasive diseases. Certain other substances also cause antibody production but not immunity. One of these is streptolysin O (antigen) and the antibody is antistreptolysin O (ASO). The ASO levels are measured as an evidence of a recent streptococcal infection. Another similar antibody is anti-deoxy ribonuclease (anti-DNASe).

Clinical Features

In addition to the common respiratory and skin infections, streptococci A are also associated with a number of other acute infective as well as non-infective conditions (Table 26.2).

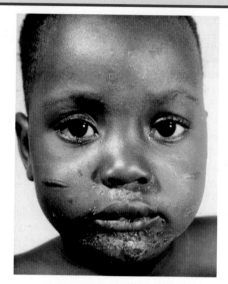

Fig. 26.3: Impetigo lesions

Table 26.2: Diseases caused by Group A Streptococcus	
Infective Conditions	*Non-infective Conditions*
• Acute pharyngitis/pneumonia	• Acute rheumatic fever
• Scarlet fever	• Post streptococcal GN
• Impetigo – Bullous Non bullous (Fig. 26.3)	• Post streptococcal reactive arthritis
• Erysipelas	• Paediatric autoimmune
• Perianal dermatitis	neuropsychiatric disorders
• Vaginitis	associated with Strep
• Toxic shock syndrome	pyogenes (PANDAS)
• Necrotizing fascitis	

Scarlet fever

The illness starts as an upper respiratory infection. Soon, within 24-48 hours, a rash appears, first around the neck and then spreads to trunk and extremities. The rash is brightly erythematous, diffuse, and finely papular giving a sand paper feel of the skin. The face is usually not involved with rash but there is characteristic perioral pallor. The rash fades in 3-4 days leading to desquamation. During the acute stage, the pharynx is also inflamed and tongue is coated and inflamed. Later the papillae appear swollen and red giving rise to the 'strawberry tongue'.

Erysipelas

Streptococcal infection of the subcutaneous deeper layers and connective tissue is known as Erysipelas. The child has fever and other constitutional symptoms. The involved area has the signs of inflammation and is very tender. There may be few overlying blebs. There is a sharp demarcation of the involved area.

Invasive Streptococcal disease

Isolation of streptococci from sterile body sites with serious systemic manifestation is taken as invasive disease. This can be in the form of Toxic shock syndrome, Necrotizing fascitis or other system involvement e.g. meningitis, septicemia, osteomyelitis etc.

Diagnosis

Isolation of Streptococcus A from the site of infection is confirmatory. The only exception to this can be asymptomatic chronic carriers with organism in the pharynx. Rapid antigen detection test with high specificity but medium sensitivity are available and are useful for a quick diagnosis although they are expensive. Evidence of a recent streptococcal A infection can be seen from ASO titres especially increasing titres. ASO titres of 320 Todd unit are significant in children while for anti-DNASe the value is 240 Todd unit or greater. The values in adults are 240 and 120 Todd units respectively.

Treatment

The antibiotic of choice for Streptococcus A is penicillin. Resistance to penicillin is infrequent. It can be given orally or parenterally but must be continued for complete 10 days to eradicate streptococci. In hypersensitive patients, erythromycin can be given for 10 days.

For skin infections, topical antibiotics can be used. Mupirocin is effective but if a child has wide spread infection or systemic features, oral treatment maybe indicated.

PNEUMOCOCCAL INFECTIONS

Pneumococcus or Streptococcus pneumoniae is a frequent inhabitant of upper respiratory tract. It is a common cause of meningitis and acute respiratory infection. It is gram-positive capsulated diplococci and based on capsular polysaccharide, ninety serotypes have been identified.

Epidemiology

More than 90% of children below 5 years of age have pneumococci in their respiratory tract sometime or other. The route of infection is by droplet infection. Children with asplenia, sickle cell disease and immunocompromised states are more susceptible to pneumococcal infections.

Pathogenesis

Normal defence mechanisms of the respiratory passages e.g. ciliary movements, epiglottic reflex etc inhibit infection of lower passages with organisms like pneumococci, which colonize the upper passages. Any conditions altering these mechanisms like a preceding viral infection or allergy can predispose to pneumococcal disease. The commonly involved sites are lungs, ears, CNS. The spread of infection is facilitated by the anti-phagocytic properties of the capsular polysaccharide of bacteria.

Clinical Features

Clinical presentation depends on the site of involvement. Upper respiratory tract infection may present predominantly as an otitis media, tonsillopharyngitis or sinusitis. Lower respiratory tract involvement may be seen as pneumonia. An invasive infection can cause bacteraemia and septicaemia. Pneumococcal peritonitis occurs rarely as a spontaneous infection. Serious systemic involvement can also occur as meningitis, osteomyelitis, arthritis or endocarditis.

Diagnosis

Culturing pneumococci from the site of infection viz. throat, blood or CSF establishes the diagnosis.

Treatment

Penicillin is the drug of choice either parenterally or orally depending upon the severity of the disease. Penicillin resistant pneumococci are becoming common and culture sensitivity is helpful in making a choice of antibiotic easier. Macrolides, trimethoprim-sulphamethoxazole, clinda-mycin, and amoxicillin-clavulanic acid are other alternatives, which can be used for oral therapy.

MENINGOCOCCAL DISEASE

Meningococcal meningitis was described over two centuries back but it still remains a feared public health problem.

Aetiology

The causative organism *Neisseria meningitidis* is gram-negative kidney shaped diplococci. Humans are the only source of infection. Many individuals carry the organism in their nasopharynx. The polysaccharide capsule of the organism has antigen variation and based on that 13 serotypes have been identified. The well-known serotypes are A, B, C, W 135 and Y.

Epidemiology

Meningococcal infections are endemic in many parts of the world and are marked by periodic outbreaks in geographical areas. Overcrowding, low socio-economic status, and viral infections are risk factors for the infection. The route of infection is through respiratory droplet infection. Serotypes A, B and C are variably responsible for endemic disease as well as outbreaks.

Pathogenesis

The meningococci first attach themselves to non-ciliated epithelial cells and gain entry to the blood stream. They are protected by their polysaccharide capsule, which resists phagocytosis. After invasion, there is an acute inflammatory response, diffuse vasculitis, disseminated intravascular coagulation (DIC) leading to focal necrosis and haemorrhage. Any of the organs can be affected. In meningococcemia, myocarditis occurs in more than half the fatal cases. Waterhouse-Friderichsen syndrome due to adrenal haemorrhage can be another fatal complication.

Clinical Features

Meningococci can cause clinical disease in the form of meningitis, septicaemia or meningococcemia.

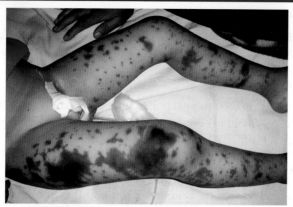

Fig. 26.4: Extensive purpuric lesions in a child with overwhelming meningococcaemia

Acute meningococcaemia is a fulminant disease. The initial presentation is similar to a viral illness with fever, headache, myalgia and pharyngitis. An erythematous generalized maculopapular rash may also be seen. The disease can rapidly progress to hypotension, DIC, septic shock, adrenal haemorrhage, myocarditis or renal failure. Multiple petechiae, purpuric spots and purpura fulminans may be seen. Meningitis is not a necessary feature (Fig. 26.4).

Meningococcal meningitis can occur with or without meningococcemia. All the features of meningitis are seen. Occasionally only cerebral involvement is present. Rarely meningococci can cause pneumonia, osteomyeltis, cellulitis, otitis media and empyema.

Diagnosis

Culturing meningococci from CSF or blood is diagnostic. Rapid diagnostic tests like latex agglutination are helpful especially in seriously ill patients.

Treatment

Parenteral penicillin is the drug of choice. Third generation cephalosporins can also be used. Chloramphenicol is also effective. In sick patients intensive supportive care with vasopressors etc is required. Hydrocortisone supplementation may be helpful in patients with shock. The patient should be kept isolated for at least 24 hours after starting of treatment.

Household and other close contacts of the patient need prophylactic therapy. Rifampicin 10 mg/kg 12 hrly for 4 doses is recommended. Other antibiotic used for chemoprophylaxis is Ciprofloxacin.

HAEMOPHILUS INFLUENZAE

Aetiology

Haemophilus influenzae is a gram-negative, pleomorphic coccobacillus. serotype b is the most common and most virulent strain.

Epidemiology

H influenzae is seen in the respiratory flora of normal healthy persons. Humans are the only reservoirs. The mode of transmission is from droplet infection.

Clinical Features

H influenzae can cause a wide range of illness primarily affecting the respiratory system and meningitis (see Table 26.3).

Meningitis: The clinical presentation is like any other meningitis. It is often associated with post-meningitic sequelae in the form of sensorineural hearing loss, developmental retardation, seizures, ataxia and hydrocephalus.

Table 26.3: Clinical disease caused by *H Influenzae* Type B	
Respiratory	**Miscellaneous**
Epiglottitis	Cellulitis
Sinusitis	Arthritis
Otitis media	Pericarditis
Pneumonia	Septicaemia
Eye	**Neonatal infection**
Conjunctivitis	
Orbital cellulitis	

Diagnosis

H influenzae is a fastidious organism to culture and requires care. The specimens must be promptly transported without drying or at extreme temperatures. Positive culture or smear from the affected site confirms the diagnosis.

Treatment

In a suspected H influenzae b infection, ampicillin or chloramphenicol are recommended. Third generation cephalosporins like cefotaxime or ceftriaxone are also useful. The treatment should be initially given parenterally and after adequate response oral therapy can be considered. In meningitis, parenteral therapy for 10-14 days must be given. Addition of dexamethasone in initial stages of meningitis especially just before antibiotic therapy decreases the incidence of hearing loss.

Prevention

Unvaccinated children below 5 years of age in contact with a case need chemoprophylaxis with Rifampicin in a dose of 20 mg/kg for 4 days.

STAPHYLOCOCCAL INFECTIONS

Staphylococci are gram-positive cocci and are present as normal flora in a ubiquitous manner in humans, animals and on fomites. They are resistant and hardy bacteria. They are broadly classified as *Staphylococcus aureus*, coagulase positive or coagulase negative Staphylococci (CONS).

Staphylococcus aureus

S aureus is a common infective organism. It causes a variety of infections of many organs or a generalized sepsis. The organisms produce various toxins and enzymes, which are largely responsible for the pathogenesis. Different strains produce one or more of these virulence factors, which may have a combination of the following mechanisms of action.

i. Protection of the organism from host defence mechanisms e.g. Leukocidin, Protein A.
ii. Local tissue destruction e.g. Hemolysins, Exfoliations.
iii. Toxins affecting non-infected sites. e.g. Enterotoxins.
iv. Localized infection e.g. coagulase.

Epidemiology

Within a week after birth, the newborn infant is colonized with *S aureus*. Nearly one third of normal individuals carry a strain of *S aureus* in their anterior nares from where it can be transmitted to skin. Autoinfection can commonly cause minor infections. Persons harbouring *S aureus* in nose can be a frequent source of infection to others especially nosocomial infections. Defects in muco-cutaneous barrier like trauma and surgery increase the risk. Defects in immune system like defective chemotaxis or phagocytosis or humoral immunity predispose to infection.

Clinical Features

The clinical presentation depends on the site of infection and virulence of the organism. Skin infections are the commonest. Involvement of the respiratory system is a frequent occurrence. Other systemic involvements also occur (Table 26.4).

Table 26.4: Systemic involvement with *S aureus*		
Skin	**Respiratory system**	**Musculoskeletal system**
Impetigo	Lobar pneumonia	Pyomyositis
Ecthyma	Bronchopneumonia	Osteomyelitis
Folliculitis	Empyema	Arthritis
Furuncle	Pyopneumothorax	
Carbuncle	Necrotizing pneumonia	
Scalded skin syndrome	Bronchopleural fistula	
CNS	**Heart**	**Kidney**
Meningitis	Infective endocarditis	Renal abscess
Brain abscess	Purulent pericarditis	Perinepheric abscess
Gastrointestinal	Septicaemia	Toxic shock syndrome
Enterocolitis		
Food poisoning		

Diagnosis

Isolation of *S aureus* from the affected site is diagnostic. Antibiotic sensitivity testing must be done to plan appropriate therapy.

Treatment

Parenteral antibiotics are used to treat all serious infections. Only for minor skin infections, oral therapy can be given. Treatment should be with a penicilinase resistant antibiotic and in combination with at least one more antibiotic. Serious staphylococcal infections may require more than 2 antibiotics. Prolonged therapy is usually required especially for osteomyelitis and endocarditis, which can be given orally after the features of infection have disappeared. In addition to antibiotics, any localized collection of pus, if present, must be drained.

MRSA (methicillin resistant *Staphylococcus aureus*)

Staphylococcus aureus strains resistant to methicillin and to flucloxacillin have emerged; some of these organisms may be sensitive to vancomycin or teicoplanin. Treatment is guided by the sensitivity of the infecting strain. It is essential that hospitals have infection control guidelines to minimise MRSA transmission, including policies on isolation and treatment of MRSA carriers, and on hand hygiene.

Coagulase Negative *Staphylococcus aureus* (CONS)

S epidermidis is the most well known from this group. These cause sepsis in patients with indwelling devices, surgical trauma and immunocompromised hosts especially small neonates. They can cause septicaemia, endocarditis, urinary tract infection, device infection e.g. shunt infection. As *S epidermidis* is a normal inhabitant, isolation from blood culture may indicate contamination. True bacteraemia is considered if more than one blood culture is positive. For treatment, antibiotic susceptibility reports are helpful. The indwelling device responsible for sepsis must be removed.

TUBERCULOSIS

Tuberculosis, an ancient disease, occurs in all parts of the world with variable frequency. It has been given many names and has a very diverse spectrum of clinical presentation.

Aetiology

The causative organism, *Mycobacterium tuberculosis* belongs to family mycobacteriaceae. The tubercle bacilli are pleomorphic, weakly gram-positive, non-motile, non-sporing organisms. The characteristic feature of all mycobacteria is their resistance to acid decolouration after staining, a property attributed to the mycolic acid in their cell wall. Most mycobacteria are slow growing organisms. Their generation time is 12-24 hours and cultures require at least 3-6 weeks.

Epidemiology

WHO estimates that one third of the world's population is infected with *M tuberculosis*. Out of these, more than 95% of the tuberculosis (TB) cases occur in developing countries. The ongoing HIV epidemic, poverty, crowded populations and inadequate TB control programs have all contributed to this.

The most common route of infection is through respiratory secretions containing TB bacilli. Patients with sputum positive for acid-fast bacilli (AFB) are the source of infection. Persons with copious sputum or a severe, forceful cough and a closed ill ventilated environment increase the likelihood of transmission. There is no transmission from fomites or from direct contact with secretions. Young children are usually not infective. Other possible route of infection is through gastrointestinal system if the bovine strain *M bovis* is ingested. Congenital TB occurs if mother has TB during pregnancy, which is transmitted through placenta to the fetus.

HIV and TB share a symbiotic relationship. TB is more common, widespread and severe in persons with HIV infection. Recently the World Health Organisation has reported that the very rare strain Extremely Drug Resistant TB (XDR-TB) accounts for possibly only 2 per cent of the million cases of tuberculosis in the world, but that it poses a grave public health threat, especially in populations with high rates of HIV and where there are few health care resources. XDR-TB poses a far greater challenge to doctors than MDR-TB (Multidrug Resistant TB), which is resistant to at least the two main first-line tuberculosis drugs, isoniazid and rifampicin. XDR-TB is a form of MDR-TB that is also resistant to three or more of the six classes of second-line drugs. Recent findings from a survey of data from 2004-04 found that XDR-TB had been identified in all regions of the world but was most frequent in the former Soviet Union and Asia.

Pathogenesis

After infection through the respiratory route, the TB bacilli start multiplying in the lung alveoli. Most are killed but some bacilli survive which are intracellular in the macrophages. The macrophages carry them along the lymphatics to the lymph nodes, usually the hilar nodes or in case of upper lobe the paratracheal nodes. The organisms multiply and lymphatic reaction increases over the next 12 weeks. There is also development of tissue hypersensitivity. The whole complex of parenchymal lesion along with the involved lymphatics and the draining lymph nodes are known as the primary complex. The infection at this stage can become dormant with healing of the primary complex by fibrosis or calcification. The tuberculin skin test is positive at this stage. Or there can be progression of the disease, the risk being greatest in children within 2 years of infection. The risk gradually decreases till adulthood.

Immunity

Immunity in TB is an important determinant of the spread of the disease as well as the presentations. The primary immune response is cell-mediated immunity (CMI), which develops 2-12 weeks after infection. Progression from TB infection to TB disease is affected by cell-mediated immunity. In individuals with decreased CMI due to any reason the disease disseminates whereas in those with good CMI and tissue hypersensitivity there is a granuloma formation restricting the infection to a localized area.

Progress of Primary Infection

The primary infection in the form of primary complex can have variable outcome.
A. Progressive primary complex
   The primary complex enlarges with pneumonitis and pleuritis. There can be associated caseation and liquefaction. The radiological appearance shows a segmental lesion with lymph node enlargement.
B. Partial obstruction of a bronchus due to enlarged lymph nodes can cause emphysematous appearances (Fig. 26.5).
C. The caseous nodes can erode through a bronchus and empty into the distal lung giving rise to a bronchopneumonia.
D. The bronchi adjacent to the tuberculous nodes can get thickened and develop endobronchial tuberculosis.

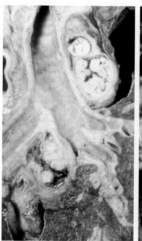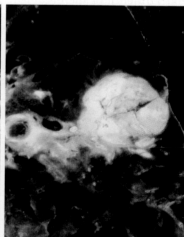

Fig. 26.5: Tuberculous lymph nodes compressing the trachea

E. The haematogenous spread from a primary infection can cause miliary tuberculosis.

During the primary infection, the TB bacilli seed various organs through blood borne or lymphatic spread. If the number of bacilli are more and the host immunity inadequate, disseminated TB occurs. In children with good immunity and less bacilli, the seeding of the organs becomes dormant. This can get reactivated at any time when the balance of immunity changes. The presentation of the involvement of these organs can be variable (Table 26.5).

Table 26.5: Time interval from primary infection	
Disseminated TB	2-6 months
TB meningitis	2-6 months
Osteomyelitis/Arthritis	Several years
Renal TB	Decades

Clinical Features

The clinical presentation of TB can be either of pulmonary symptoms and signs only or of any other organ system involvement or a mixed picture. In children, approximately 25-30% cases are of extrapulmonary TB.

Pulmonary TB: The symptomatology of pulmonary TB is almost uniform across various types of involvement in the lungs. Children tend to have more non-specific symptoms. Cough, low-grade fever, loss of appetite, lethargy and weight loss are usual symptoms. Failure to thrive is one of the commonest presentations. The additional clinical signs of the disease depend upon the type and extent of the involvement. There may be no clinical signs or range from findings of pleural effusion, consolidation and bronchopneumonia. In military type of pulmonary TB, there may be high-grade fever, toxic look and splenomegaly.

Extrapulmonary TB: Any organ can be involved by tuberculous infection. In children, CNS TB is a frequent occurrence. Depending upon the extent of involvement, CNS tuberculosis can have variable clinical picture (see chapter 18).

TB lymphadenitis: Lympadenitis due to *M tuberculosis* is one of the common forms of extrapulmonary TB seen at all ages. The nodes draining the lungs fields are usually involved. The common groups of nodes involved are cervical and axillary but other groups can also be involved especially secondary to drainage from an infected organ. The node involvement usually occurs 6-9 months after primary infection. The affected nodes are firm, non-tender, fixed and often matted due to periadenitis. There may be accompanying low-grade fever. In case a node breaks down, it leads to sinus formation.

Disseminated TB: Two forms of disseminated spread are seen. In disseminated TB, the organs seeded during the haematogenous spread begin to get active involvement. Usually, there is fever, hepatosplenomegaly and lymphadenopathy. Other organs may also be involved.

In the other more serious disseminated form of TB, there is a large haematogenous spread and in a patient with inadequate immune response there is miliary TB. It can occur at any age but is more common in young children. It usually occurs 2-6 months after primary infection. Miliary TB may start with an insidious fever, malaise and loss of appetite. Soon fever rises and there is lymphadenopathy with hepatosplenomegaly. There can be an acute presentation of miliary TB also. The child looks toxic with high fever, has dyspnoea along with crepitations in the chest and hepatosplenomegaly. There can be extra-pulmonary involvement with meningitis in which there may be characteristically choroid tubercles on fundoscopy. Choroid tubercles indicate end artery embolisation with formation of tubercles.

TB of bones/joints: Skeletal tuberculosis is a late complication. The commonest site of involvement is vertebra leading to the classical Pott's spine with a formation of gibbus and kyphosis. Tuberculosis of any bone can occur. Dactylitis of metacarpals is seen in children. Tuberculous arthritis of any of the joints can occur.

Abdominal TB: In the abdomen there are two major clinical presentations viz, tuberculous peritonitis and tuberculous enteritis.

Tuberculous peritonitis is uncommon in children but can occur due to either haematogenous spread or local extensions from abdominal lymph nodes or intestines. Low-grade fever and pain, ascites, weight loss are the typical features. **Tuberculous infection of the intestines** occur either secondary to haematogenous spread or from ingestion of TB bacilli from sputum. Small intestines and appendix are the usual sites of the involvement. Tuberculous ulcers or later strictures can cause the clinical features. Low-grade fever, weight loss, diarrhoea or constipation or features of sub-acute intestinal obstruction can be the presenting features.

Genitourinary TB: Renal TB has a long incubation period and hence is generally seen in older children or adolescents. Kidneys as well as other parts of the urinary system can be involved. Renal involvement is unilateral and initially present as sterile pyuria and microscopic haematuria. Later abdominal pain and mass, dysuria and frank haematuria with progression to hydronephrosis or urethral strictures may be seen.

Congenital TB: Perinatal transmission of TB can occur as a haematogenous spread through the placenta in mother with active disease. Inhalation/ingestion of infected amniotic fluid or exposure after birth to a positive contact can also cause infection in a neonate. The transplacental infection presents with a primary complex like manifestation in the abdomen. The liver has the focus with the nodes in porta hepatis also involved. If the infection is through inhalation or the haematogenous spread occurs further to lungs then respiratory signs are predominantly present. The neonate can have acute onset respiratory distress, fever, poor weight gain, lymphadenopathy and hepatosplenomegaly. Occasionally meningitis can also occur. The clinical signs and symptoms can be similar to other infections. A maternal history or contact with an AFB positive person should raise the suspicion.

Diagnosis

Diagnosis of TB in children is not simple. A high index of suspicion in the endemic area is important. The modalities most frequently used for diagnosis are:
Mantoux Test (Fig. 26.6)
Radiological examination
Gastric aspirate/sputum AFB smear and culture
Polymerase chain reaction (PCR)
See Table 26.6 for further information.

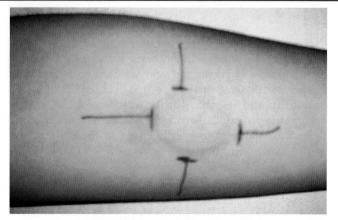

Fig. 26.6: A positive Mantoux test

Treatment

Effective anti-tuberculous therapy requires a combination of anti-tuberculous drugs. The bacillary load is an important determinant of treatment. Children tend to have moderate load of TB bacilli as compared to large bacillary populations among adults with cavitatory disease. The anti TB drugs are listed in Table 26.7. Combination of isoniazid and rifampicin with either pyrizinamide or ethambutol or both is used. The duration of treatment depends on the site of involvement and the response and can range from 6-18 months. In CNS TB and in involvement of serosal tissues like pleura/pericardium addition of corticosteroids may be required. Surgical intervention may be indicated in TB of the spine, bones or abdomen.

WHO has recently recommended directly observed therapy (DOTS) for treating all types of tuberculosis.

Table 26.6: Diagnostic tests in tuberculosis			
Type of disease	*Mantoux test*	*AFB isolation*	*Radiology*
1. Pulmonary TB	+ve except in Miliary TB	Gastric aspirate or Sputum	X-ray Chest Segmental lesions Primary complex Effusion Non specific picture
2. CNS TB	+ve can be neg in TBM	CSF AFB v.rarely PCR+	CT scan or MRI scan
3. Bones and Joints	+ve	Curettage may show AFB	X ray of the affected area MRI
4. Abdominal TB	+ve	Not seen	Ultrasono-graphy or CT scan may show lymph nodes
5. Genito-urinary TB	+ve	Urine AFB	IVP and ultrasono-graphy
6. Congenital TB	May be +ve	Not seen	May not be helpful Biopsy of nodes

Table 26.7: Commonly used Anti TB drugs in children			
Drug	*Dose mg/kg/d*	*Max*	*Side effect /Toxicity*
Bactericidal			
Isoniazid (INH, H)	10-15	300 mg	Pyridoxine deficiency, Peripheral neuritis, hepatotoxicity
Rifampicin (RIF, R)	10-20	600 mg	GI upsets, hepato-toxicity
Streptomycin (STM,S)	20-40	1 gm	Vestibular and auditory toxicity
Bacteriostatic			
Pyrizinamide (PZA, Z)	20-40	2 gm	
Ethambutol (EMB, E)	15-25	2.5 gm	Optic neuritis, colour blindness

DIRECTLY OBSERVED TREATMENT SHORT COURSE (DOTS)

This is a strategy to ensure cure by providing the most effective medicines and confirming its intake regularly. Worldwide it has been documented as an effective strategy to cure TB.

In DOTS, the treatment is given in two phases. During the intensive phase of treatment, a health worker or other trained person watches as the patient swallows the drugs in his presence. During the continuation phase the patient is issued medicines for one week in a multiblister combipack of which the first dose is swallowed by the patient in the presence of the health worker or other trained person. The consumption of medicines in the continuation phase is also checked by return of the empty multiblister combipack when the patient comes to collect medicine for the next week. Sputum microscopy is done at defined intervals during treatment to monitor the patient's progress toward cure. The key to the success of the DOTS strategy is that it places the responsibility for curing TB patients on the health workers – not the patients. This strategy has proven successful throughout the world. The components of the DOTS strategy are:

1. Diagnosis of patients by sputum microscopy.
2. Regular and uninterrupted supply of drugs.
3. Short-course chemotherapy given under direct observation.
4. Systematic evaluation and monitoring.

Category I: New cases that are sputum positive, or seriously ill patients with smear negative or extrapulmonary disease. The intensive phase consists of isoniazid, rifampicin, pyrazinamide and ethambutol given under direct observation thrice weekly on alternate days and lasts for 2 months (24 doses). This is immediately followed by the continuation phase, which consists of 4 months (18 weeks, 54 doses) of isoniazid, rifampicin given thrice weekly on alternate days. The first weekly dose is directly observed.

Category II: Retreatment cases including patients with relapse, failure and those who return to treatment after default. Such patients are generally sputum negative. Phase one consists of two months (24 doses) of isoniazid, rifampicin, pyrazinamide, and ethambutol, all given under direct observation weekly on alternate days. This is immediately followed by the continuation phase, which consist of 5 months (22 weeks, 66 doses) of isoniazid, rifampicin, and ethambutol given thrice weekly on alternate days, the first dose of the week being directly observed.

Category III: Patients who are sputum-negative, or who have extra-pulmonary TB and are not seriously ill. Phase I consist of isoniazid, rifampicin, and pyrazinamide given under direct observation thrice weekly on alternate days and lasts for 2 months (24 doses). This is immediately followed by the continuation phase, which consist of 4 months (18 weeks, 54 doses) of isoniazid and rifampicin given thrice weekly on alternate days, the first dose of the week being directly observed.

A symptomatic child contact with a positive Mantoux test (10mm or more) is to be treated as a case regardless of BCG status. for infants, if the mother or any other household member is smear positive then chemo-prophylaxis should be given for 3 months. At the end of 3 months, a Mantoux test is done. If the Mantoux test is negative, chemoprophylaxis is stopped and BCG vaccine is given. If the Mantoux test is positive, chemoprophylaxis is given for a total duration of 6 months.

LEPROSY

Leprosy also known as Hansen's disease is an ancient disease. It is a chronic infection of skin, peripheral nerves and respiratory system.

Aetiology

The causative organism is *Mycobacterium leprae*, an intracellular acid-fast bacillus from mycobacteriaceae family, closely related to Mycobacterium tuberculosis. Illness usually results from prolonged exposure to infected persons. The bacterium only affects humans under natural conditions. Transmission of the disease to experimental animals is difficult. This fact hampers research into many aspects of the disease.

Epidemiology

World over there has been a steady decline in the prevalence of leprosy. Presently, more than 90% of cases of leprosy are in 10 countries of the world, located in Africa, SE Asia, Central and South America, with 70% in India alone. Transmission occurs from person to person among those in close contact especially the family members. The infection is transmitted through breast milk but nasal and respiratory secretions are the ones with highest bacterial load and are the usual source. Infection rarely occurs in infants but is common in the 5-14 years age group. In utero transmission has been considered a possibility. The incubation period is between two and five years, but may be much longer. Infection is spread only by the lepromatous type of the disease.

Pathogenesis

Most of the persons coming in close contact with *M leprae* develop immunity without an evident disease. *M leprae* and host immunity are two major determinants of the extent and severity of the disease in an individual. After entering through the respiratory mucosa especially nose, the bacilli spread hematogenously to skin and peripheral nerves. The organisms colonize the perineural and endoneural spaces and the Schwann cells. In hosts with good cell mediated immune response the presentation is in form of tuberculoid leprosy (TL). The tissues show granuloma formation with epithelioid cells, lymphocytes and scanty bacilli. There is no caseation or intracellular bacilli in macrophages. The cutaneous nerve fibres are destroyed with extensive cellular infiltration of the dermis.

On the other extreme in the presentation of Lepromatous leprosy (LL) where there is almost no immune response to *M leprae*. A large number of bacilli invade the skin, peripheral nerves, nasal mucosa as well as other organs with the exception of CNS, which is not involved. There are poorly formed granulomas with foamy histiocytes and macrophages with numerous intracellular bacilli. In between the two extremes of the spectrum of presentation of Leprosy lie three other forms of borderline (BB), borderline tuberculoid (BT) and borderline lepromatous (BL) pictures with in between features.

Clinical Features

Tuberculoid Leprosy (TL): The usual presentation is with a large skin lesion (>10 cm). The lesion has a well-demarcated erythematous rim with atrophic, hypopigmented, anaesthetic area. There can be more than one lesion sometimes. The peripheral nerve closest to the area involved is usually thickened. The lesion can continue to enlarge and there is irreversible loss of skin appendages i.e. hair follicle, sweat glands as well as cutaneous receptors (Fig. 26.7).

Indeterminate Leprosy: This is the earliest clinically detectable stage from which most patients will pass. There is a skin lesion, which is a single hypopigmented macule of 2-4 cms size with minimal anaesthesia. A high index of suspicion in close contacts of leprosy patients is required to diagnose this stage. In majority, this lesion may heal without any treatment while in some it progresses to other forms of the disease.

Borderline Leprosy (BL): Features, which do not clearly belong to either TL or LL and are ill defined, are taken as borderline leprosy. There can be 3 further subdivisions borderline tuberculoid (BT), borderline (BB), or borderline lepromatous (BL). There can be shift from one category to the other depending upon host and bacterial factors, which change the clinical picture.

Lepromatous Leprosy: The initial skin lesions are a macule or diffuse skin infiltration. Later they progress, become papular and nodular, and innumerable and confluent. The characteristic facial features – Leonine facies, loss of eyebrows and distorted earlobes develop. There may be

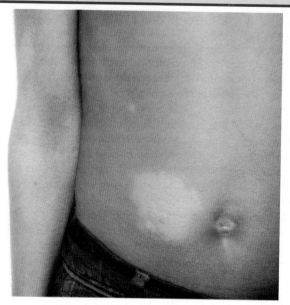

Fig. 26.7: Hypopigmented patch in tuberculoid leprosy

accompanying anaesthesia and later peripheral sensory neuropathy which may go on to deformities such as claw hand, dropped foot, inversion of the feet and claw toes. Trophic ulcerations follow with loss of peripheral tissues, such as the nose or digits.

Reactional states: Changes in the immunological balance between host and bacteria especially on treatment can cause following acute clinical reactions.

A. **Type I (reversal) reactions:** Acute pain and swelling of existing skin and neural lesions occurs. The acute neuritis can cause irreversible nerve injuries e.g. facial paralysis, foot drop, and claw hand. The skin lesions ulcerate and can leave severe scars. This results from a sudden increase in cell-mediated immunity and is seen predominantly in BL. Type I reactions are a medical emergency requiring immediate treatment.

B. **Type II reactions (Erythema Nodosum Leprosum (ENL)):** This reaction is seen in lepromatous leprosy or BL. The skin nodules become red and tender resembling erythema nodosum. There is accompanying fever, polyarthralgia, tender lymphadenopathy and splenomegaly. This is caused by a systemic inflammatory response to the immune complexes.

Diagnosis

Anaesthetic skin lesions are pathognomonic of leprosy. A skin biopsy from an active lesion provides confirmation. To classify patients for treatment categories, slit and smear preparations are made. The disease is classified as Paucibacillary if there are < 5 skin lesions and no bacilli on smear; Multibacillary if > 6 skin lesions with bacilli on smear.

No other investigations are required

Treatment

There are three compounds, which have shown efficacy in treatment of Leprosy. The earliest one, Dapsone (since 1940) is the most important and frequently used. Rifampicin is a rapid bactericidal drug and the third is clofazimine. Multi drug therapy is recommended to prevent resistance and a high cure rate. As per WHO. recommendations, intermittent (weekly/monthly) directly observed treatment is given and the doses for this are higher than daily therapy. The duration of treatment for paucibacillary ranges from 6 months to 1 year and for multibacillary 1-2 years (Table 26.8).

With adequate treatment the prognosis is good but the irreversible changes in skin and nerves remain. For prevention, BCG, the tuberculosis vaccine, has been found to give 50% protection with a single dose and more with second dose.

Table 26.8: Daily Paediatric doses for Leprosy	
Dapsone	1 mg/ kg
Rifampicin	10 mg/ kg
Clofazimine	1 mg/ kg

SYPHILIS

Aetiology

The causative organism for syphilis is Treponema pallidum from spirochaeteae family.

Epidemiology

Syphilis is either an acquired infection or transmitted transplacentally. The acquired infection occurs most commonly through sexual contact with an infected person and very infrequently through blood or blood products.

A pregnant woman who is in either primary or secondary stage of syphilis or less often while in latent stage transmits congenital syphilis.

Clinical Features

Congenital Syphilis: The transplacental transmission rate of syphilis is almost 100% with fetal loss in little less than half of the pregnancies. If the baby is born alive then he goes through early and late signs of congenital syphilis. The infant may be asymptomatic at birth or develop early manifestations. One of the characteristic presentations is a maculopapular rash along with hepatosplenomegaly, lymphadenopathy and bone involvement in the form of

osteochondritis and periosteitis leading to pseudoparalysis. There can be involvement of any of the systems like CNS, renal and gastrointestinal. Late signs of syphilis appear after the first 2 years of life and are primarily related to involvement of the bones and CNS involvement (Table 26.9).

Table 26.9: Late signs of congenital Syphilis	
Olympian brow	Periosteitis of frontal bone and bony prominence of forehead
Higoumenakis sign	Unilateral or bilateral thickening of the sternal head of clavicle
Saber shins	Anterior bowing of tibia
Hutchison's teeth	Peg shaped upper central incisors
Mulberry molars	Excessive cusps in lower molar
Saddle nose	Depressed nasal root
Rhagades	Linear scars around mouth
Juvenile tabes	Spinal cord involvement
Clutton Joints	Unilateral / Bilateral synovitis of lower limb joints esp. knee
Interstitial Keratitis	

Diagnosis

I. Direct examination for *T pallidum* under dark field microscopy from any lesion is diagnostic.
II. Serological tests
    A. Non treponemal serological tests
        i.   VDRL (Venereal disease research laboratory test)
        ii. RPR (Rapid plasma regain test)
    B. Treponemal serological tests
        i.   TPI: Treponema immobilization test
        ii. FTA-ABS Fluorescent Treponemal antibody absorption test
        iii. MHA-TP: Micro haemagglutination assay for antibodies *T pallidum*

The treponemal antibody tests in congenital syphilis have to be interpreted in context of the maternal antibody titers. (If the infant's titer decreases by 3-6 months, it confirms transplacentally transferred maternal antibodies). If initial titers of non-treponemal serology are 4 times more than the maternal levels, it indicates an infected infant. An infected placenta indicated by a large size and histological changes showing endovascular and perivascular arteritis, proliferative villitis is additional evidence of fetal infection.

Treatment

An infant showing early signs of congenital syphilis has to be treated completely. In an asymptomatic infant with maternal history of syphilis or positive VDRL, treatment is indicated if:

i.   Untreated or inadequately treated mother
ii. A non-treponemal serology titer of 4 fold or greater than maternal levels in the infant

The drug of choice is inj. Crystalline penicillin 1 lac (=100,000 units)/kg/ day IV in 12 hourly doses for 7 days and then 8 hourly doses for 7 days.

LEPTOSPIROSIS

Leptospira are aerobic spirochaetes occurring worldwide. It is the most widespread zoonotic disease. There are more than 200 pathogenic sero varieties of Leptospira with clinically overlapping presentations.

Epidemiology

Most of the cases occur in tropical and subtropical areas. Leptospira infects many species of animals but rat has been the principle source of infection for man. Pets especially dogs can also infect if good hygiene is not maintained. Leptospira cause disease in animals as well. The animals excrete the bacteria in urine and contaminate surface water and soil from which infection travels to humans.

Pathogenesis

The portal of entry for leptospira is usually a break in skin like abrasions or mucous membranes. The leptospira after entry into the blood stream, spread to various organs and get lodged in liver, kidneys or CNS for a long time. The primary pathology seen is damage to the endothelial lining of small blood vessels.

Clinical Features

Leptospiral infection can be asymptomatic or a mild illness or a typical biphasic illness with severe organ dysfunction and death. The incubation period is 7-12 days. The initial phase of blood stream invasion is called septicemic phase and lasts 2-7 days. During this time the child has fever with chills, headache, vomiting and myalgia. Lympha-denopathy and hepatosplenomegaly may also occur. The septicemic phase may be followed by a brief asymptomatic period and followed the immune phase. The immune phase is characterized by appearance of antibodies to leptospira while the organism itself disappears from circulation and is present in the organ systems. This phase can last for several weeks. There is a recrudescence of fever and depending on the extent of the organ involvement; the clinical presentation can be variable. Neurological involvement is seen as meningo-encephalitis and neuropathies. Liver involvement is generally a severe disease with jaundice and elevation of enzymes (Weil's disease). Renal dysfunction can range from abnormal urinalysis, azotaemia to acute renal failure. Hemorrhagic manifestations and circulatory collapse are uncommon manifestations.

Diagnosis

During first week, leptospira can be cultured but requires prolonged period. for same. Dark field microscopy of blood (1st week) and fresh urine (2nd week) may show leptospira. Serological tests (a) Microscopic agglutination test is the specific test but difficult to do as involves live cultures of leptospira. (b) ELISA test – tests IgM antibodies and is positive early in disease. (c) Slide agglutination test.

Treatment

Penicillin is the drug of choice especially if given early. Inj. crystalline penicillin IV 6-8 million units/m^2/day is given in 4 divided doses for 1 week. For hypersensitive patients the alternative is tetracycline.

MEASLES

Measles, also known as Rubeola, occurs worldwide and is an important cause of childhood morbidity and mortality.

Aetiology

Measles is caused by an RNA virus belonging to Paramyxoviridae family, genus morbillivirus. There is only one serotype known.

Epidemiology

Measles has been identified to occur in history for a long time. Epidemics have occurred in various parts of the world. With the widespread use of measles vaccine, the epidemiology has changed. The unimmunised children of all ages are susceptible. Infants younger than 6-9 months have protective antibodies transferred from their mothers transplacentally and hence are protected. As the measles vaccination coverage is increasing, it has been suggested that the transplacental antibodies of vaccine-immunized mothers may protect the infant for a lesser time.
Measles is a highly contagious disease with secondary attack rate as high as 90% among susceptible close contacts. The infection occurs through droplets and there are no other hosts or vectors. The period of infectivity is 5 days before and 4 days after the appearance of rash.

Pathogenesis

The measles virus enters the body via respiratory epithelium causing a viraemia and then lodges in the reticulo-endothelial system. A second phase of viraemia occurs infecting various organs. There is an inflammatory reaction in the mucosa of respiratory tract with exudation and proliferation of mononuclear cells. An interstitial pneumonitis can result – Hecht giant cell pneumonia. The intestinal tract is also involved and there can be hyperplasia of lymphoid tissue especially in appendix where multinucleated giant cells (Warthin-Finkeldey cells) are seen. The skin rash (exanthema) of measles is accompanied by a similar reaction (enanthem) in the mucosa characteristically seen as Koplik spots in buccal mucosa. Enanthems occur in the mucosal lining of respiratory and gastrointestinal systems also.

Clinical Features

Three clinical stages have been described in measles including the incubation period, which is of 10-12 days duration. This is followed by the 2nd stage or the prodromal period. During this the child has cough, coryza, conjunctivitis and the pathognomonic Koplik spots. Koplik spots are seen on buccal mucosa opposite lower molar and appear as pale white or greyish tiny dots over reddish mucosa. They are seen for 1-2 days only. The conjunctival inflammation initially has a characteristic erythematous line at the lid margin but later becomes more diffuse. The 3rd stage, the stage of rash is heralded by a sudden rise of fever to 40°C or even higher and the appearance of rash. The erythematous, maculopapular rash first appears behind ears, along hairline and neck, spreads to face, arms and chest within 24 hours (Fig. 26.8A). Rash spreads further to abdomen, back and lower limbs. As it starts appearing on feet, it begins to fade from the face and downwards in the order of appearance. The whole stage takes 3-4 days. The fever drops to normal as the rash reaches the lower limbs. Persistence of fever indicates a secondary bacterial infection. The measles rash on fading leaves a branny desquamation and a brownish pigmentation, which persists for 2 weeks or more (Fig. 26.8B). The clinical appearance of rash can vary from mild to confluent and completely covering the body.

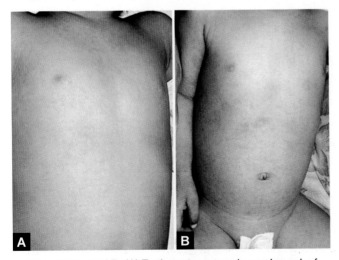

Figs 26.8Aa and B: (A) Erythematous maculopapular rash of measles (B) Post-measles brownish pigmentation

Occasionally there can be a hemorrhagic rash (Black Measles) and this may be accompanied by bleeding from other sites as well.

Involvement of reticulo-endothelial system is apparent clinically as enlargement of Lymphnodes in the neck, splenomegaly and abdominal pain due to mesenteric lymphadenopathy.

Diagnosis

No investigations are required to diagnose measles in a typical case. In doubtful cases, measles IgM antibody can be estimated. Paired sera (acute and convalescent phases) estimation will be more reliable.

Differential Diagnosis

See Table 26.10.

Treatment

The mainstay of treatment is supportive therapy. Maintaining adequate hydration and nutrition are important. Antipyretics and tepid sponging for high fever and humidification for relief of cough should be given. There are no specific antiviral drugs for measles.

Complications

I. **Respiratory complications:** Secondary bacterial infection can cause otitis media and other upper respiratory system involvements. Interstitial pneumonitis can occur due to measles virus itself. Secondary bacterial pneumonia or viral infections are also common.

II. **Myocarditis** is an infrequent occurrence.

III. **Gastrointestinal complications** - Acute diarrhoeal disease is a common complication especially in developing countries. Due to decreased immunity, dysentery can also occur.

IV. **Neurological complications:**
Measles infection has been associated with various types of encephalomyelitis.
(a) Early encephalitis like picture thought to be due to direct viral invasion of the CNS.
(b) A later post-measles encephalitis due to demyelination, may be an immunological reaction.
(c) Chronic encephalitis-subacute sclerosing panencephalitis.
(d) In addition, other neurological complications like Guillain-Barré syndrome, retro-bulbar neuritis can also occur.

V. Ocular involvement can cause keratitis and corneal ulceration

TABLE 26.10. Differential diagnosis of exanthematous fever

Features	Measles	German measles	Roseola infantum	Scarlet fever	Meningo coccemia	Kawasaki disease	Drug rash	Dengue fever
Prodromal illness	Catarrh, conjunctivitis cough, Koplik spots, fever	Mild Catarrh	Mild respiratory symptoms	None	Respiratory symptoms	None	None	None
Onset of rash	Preceding fever x 3-4 days, onset with high fever, rash along hairline, cheeks	Preceded by lymphadeno-pathy, rash begins on face, minimal fever	After 3-5 days of high fever and as fever resolves, rash appears on trunk	Within 1-2 days of fever, around neck	No definite pattern with fever	After about 1 week of fever	Related to the drug	After 1-2 days of defervescence
Spread of rash	Face, neck, trunk and limbs in 2-3 days	Spreads quickly	Spreads to neck, face and limbs	Spreads to trunk and limbs, face is spared	No typical order of spread	No pattern	No specific pattern	Spreads to whole body may spare palms and soles
Type of rash	Erythematous maculopapular	Erythematous maculopapular with flushing	Discrete, raised, pink lesions 2-5 mm	Finely, papular, erythematous sand paper feel	Erythematous maculopapular	Any type	Any type	Erythematous morbilliform or maculopapular
Fading of rash	fever subsides, rash fades in order of appearance leaving branny brownish discoloration	Fades in 3 days, minimal desquamation	Fades in 1-3 days	Fade after 3-4 days with extensive desquamation	No pattern	No pattern	Depend on with-drawal of drug	Fades 1-2 days
Associated features	Respiratory symptoms	Tender lymph adenopathy	Febrile seizures are common	Respiratory symptoms, strawberry tongue	Sepsis, DIC, shock petechiae, purpura	Bulbar conjunctival injection, lymph-adeno-pathy swelling of hands, feet desquamation	Itching	Body aches, leucopenia thrombocytopenia
Diagnostic investigation	None	None	None	Throat swab culture group A streptococci	Culture positive for meningococci		With drawal of drug relieves the rash	Dengue serotology

VI. Skin infection can cause gangrene of cheeks known as Noma.

VII. Malnutrition

VII. Flaring of underlying pulmonary tuberculosis

Subacute sclerosing panencephalitis (SSPE): also known as Dawson encephalitis occurs due to persistent measles virus in CNS. It is a rare disorder occurring worldwide. The onset generally occurs at 5-15 years of age. A higher risk has been seen for measles infection occurring at a younger age, for boys and children from rural or poor socio-economic background.

The pathological picture shows necrosis and inclusion body panencephalitis picture. It has an insidious onset with behaviour changes or declining school performance. This is followed by myoclonic jerks and there may be frank seizures also. Cerebellar ataxia and other abnormal movements may also be seen. There is progressive dementia, stupor and coma. The course is variable ranging from few months to few years (1-3 years).

Diagnosis is by demonstrating IgG and IgM measles antibodies in CSF. The gamma globulins are markedly elevated in CSF. There are no diagnostic EEG or MRI pictures of SSPE. Treatment is symptomatic and supportive. Prognosis is poor as there is slow progression of the degenerative process

MUMPS

Mumps is an acute viral infection of the salivary glands.

Aetiology

Mumps virus, with only one serotype, is an RNA virus from paramyxoviridae family.

Epidemiology

Mumps is known to occur worldwide. Unimmunised children are at risk. The mode of transmission is airborne droplets or contaminated fomites. There is no other reservoir of infection. The infective period extends from 24 hours before the appearance of swelling to 3 days after it has subsided.

Clinical Features

A little less than half of the infections by mumps virus are subclinical. The incubation period is 2-4 weeks. The prodromal features are minimal. The primary manifestations of mumps are related to salivary glands. Parotid salivary gland is the most commonly involved structure. The glands swell and increase in size to obliterate the angle of jaw (mandible) and reach the ear, which gets displaced upwards and outwards. The gland is tender

with pain in the ear and also on salivation. The opening of Stensen's duct near the upper molars may show redness and oedema. The involvement of parotid glands may be unilateral or bilateral. The submandibular salivary glands are affected less frequently. There is swelling and tenderness in the submandibular area and the Wharton's duct opening is inflamed. Sublingual salivary glands are still less commonly involved. There can be accompanying low-grade fever. The swelling of the salivary glands subsides in a week's time.

Differential Diagnosis

1. Other Viruses causing parotitis e.g. Influenza and Parainfluenza, Coxsackie, CMV, HIV
2. Bacterial parotitis
3. Salivary Calculus
4. Cervical lymphadenitis

Diagnosis

Viral confirmation of a diagnosis of mumps depends on isolation of the virus or the demonstration of a significant rise in antibody titre during the illness.

Treatment

No specific treatment is indicated and only supportive treatment is required. Analgesics/antipyretics for pain and fever can be given.

Complications

A. CNS complications are the most frequent in children.
   I. Aseptic meningitis
   II. Mumps encephalitis
   III. Post infectious demyelination encephalitis
   IV. Aqueduct stenosis and hydrocephalus
B. Orchitis and Epididymitis:
   Commonly seen in adolescents or adults. This may follow salivary gland involvement by a week or so. There can be bilateral orchitis. The symptoms of fever, vomiting and lower abdominal pain with testicular swelling and pain last for about 4 days. In 1/3 cases affected testis may undergo atrophy. Infertility is rare.
C. Oophoritis in post pubertal females is seen.
D. Pancreatitis
E. Myocarditis
F. Arthritis
G. Sensorineural deafness

Key Learning Points
CNS involvement in mumps can precede parotitis. Mumps rarely causes sterility in males.

CASE STUDY

A 4-year-old partially immunised child was hospitalised with fever for 3 days, seizures and altered sensorium for one day. Systemic examination was normal except for positive meningeal signs and altered sensorium. A diagnosis of acute meningoencephalitis was made. CSF examination showed pleocytosis of 400 WBCs/cumm with 50% lymphocytes and 50% polymorphs and normal sugar and protein levels. Over the next few days in hospital, the child developed a tender swelling over the left parotid region indicative of parotitis.

Diagnosis: Mumps with meningoencephalitis

RUBELLA

Rubella or German measles is a milder viral infection as compared to measles. The major clinical significance of rubella is in the transplacental transmission to the embryo and fetus from an infected mother leading to Congenital Rubella syndrome.

Aetiology

Rubella virus, the causative agent, is an RNA virus from the family Togaviridae.

Epidemiology

As with measles, human is the only host for rubella virus. It has a worldwide presence. The route of usual infection is through droplet except for congenital rubella. It is also highly contagious with outbreaks occurring in hostels or institutions with closed environment. The period of infectivity is from 7 days before the rash to 7 days after the disappearance. Even subclinical cases can be a source of infection.

Clinical Features

The incubation period of 14-21 days is followed by a prodrome of mild catarrhal symptoms, which are of short duration. Before the appearance of rash, the typical tender lymphadenopathy of rubella is seen. The posterior auricular, post cervical and post occipital groups of lymph nodes are involved. The lymphadenopathy can last up to one week. The rash begins on face and spreads fast to the rest of the body, generally within 24 hours and then fades in the next 1-2 days leaving minimal desquamation. The fever may be absent or low grade.

Diagnosis

Confirmation of the diagnosis, if required, is by serology and sometimes by cultures. Haemagglutination inhibition (HI) antibody test, EIA, fluorescent immunoassay have been found to be sensitive tests.

Treatment

Only supportive treatment is required.

Complications

Unlike measles, few complications occur. A rare progressive rubella panencephalitis similar to SSPE has been described.

Congenital Rubella Syndrome

Active infection during pregnancy can lead to transplacental infection of the embryo or fetus depending upon the gestation. The risk is greatest (90%) during first trimester and decreases to 70% in 2nd and lesser in 3rd trimester. The fetus develops intrauterine growth retardation. The virus infects all the organs (Table 26.11). The diagnosis is confirmed by Rubella IgM antibodies in the neonate or by isolating the virus, as it is present in the tissues and nasopharynx. It is excreted in urine for one year or more. The outcome of congenital rubella is highly unfavourable as disease can progress even after birth.

Table 26.11: Features of congenital rubella	
General	**CNS**
IUGR	Meningoencephalitis
Skin rashes–blueberry muffin	Mental retardation
	Microcephaly
Eyes	**CVS**
Cataracts	Myocarditis
Micro-ophthalmia	Patent
Ears	**Haematological**
Sensorineural hearing loss	Anaemia
Others	Thrombocytopenia
Pneumonia	
Hepatitis	

VARICELLA VIRUS (CHICKENPOX)

Varicella zoster virus is responsible for two clinical entities chickenpox and herpes zoster (shingles).

Aetiology

Varicella virus belongs to human herpes virus group.

Epidemiology

Varicella has a worldwide distribution and is almost a universal infection. Prior to vaccination, by 15 years of age, most of the children were infected with less than 5% remaining susceptible especially in temperate climates. In warmer climates, there may be a shift to older age infection.

It is a highly contagious disease with high secondary attack rates. The source of infection is either droplet or contact with the lesion fluid. The period of infectivity is 1-2 days before the rash and to till all the lesions have crusted. There is usually no asymptomatic infection although the disease maybe very mild in young children. Herpes zoster is caused be reactivation of the virus, which has become latent after the primary infection. It is uncommon in children and is a milder disease in childhood.

Pathogenesis

The varicella virus enters the respiratory epithelium where it multiplies and causes viremia. A second viraemic phase occurs during which the cutaneous lesions appear in crops. The virus enters the sensory ganglia and becomes latent there. The subsequent reactivation of this leads to herpes zoster rash and the neurological features.

Clinical Features

Chickenpox is a febrile exanthematous illness. The incubation period is 10-21 days following which prodromal symptoms of fever, malaise, and headache may occur for 1-2 days. The fever can rise to 104-106°F. The rash starts from face or trunk as erythematous papules. It evolves through the stages of clear fluid filled vesicles, which then become pustules and finally there is crusting of the lesions. The evolution can take 1-2 days. Fresh crops of rashes keep erupting and at a time in the illness one can find all stages of the rash (Fig. 26.9). The rash has a centripetal appearance with more lesions in the trunk. The palms and soles are also involved, as are oropharynx and vagina. There is intense itching of the lesions. By the end of 1 week, usually most lesions are scabbed. The scabs fall off leaving faint scars, which usually disappear.

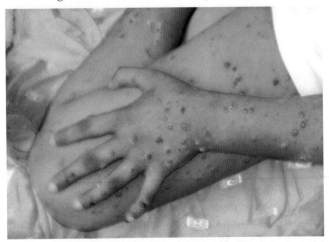

Fig. 26.9: Polymorphic lesions of chickenpox

Diagnosis

The classical skin lesions help in making the diagnosis on clinical basis. There may be leucopenia for few days. Liver enzymes also show transient elevation.

Treatment

In healthy children with mild disease only supportive treatment is recommended. There is a specific and safe anti viral drug, Acyclovir, available. It can be given safely to children in the dose of 20 mg/kg/dose as 4 doses per day for 5 days. The earlier it is started the better is the efficacy in limiting the spread of the disease and eliminating the virus. If Acyclovir is given 3 days or later after the onset of rash, it may not be effective in preventing further spread of the disease. Varicella- zoster immunoglobulin (VZIG) is recommended for those who are at increased risk of severe varicella e.g. neonates and immunosuppressed patients.

Complications

1. Thrombocytopenia
2. Cerebellar ataxia
3. Varicella encephalitis
4. Pneumonia
5. Nephritis/Nephrotic syndrome
6. Haemolytic uraemic syndrome
7. Secondary bacterial infections

Herpes Zoster: In Herpes zoster, the skin rash is similar to chickenpox but has the characteristic dermatomal distribution and the vesicles can coalesce to become large bullae. The rash is accompanied by pruritus, pain and hyperaesthesia. Unlike adults, post-herpetic neuralgia is not common in children. Immunocompromised children e.g. with HIV infection, tend to have severe zoster disease and may even have recurrent episodes. Oral acyclovir is effective in Herpes zoster.

Neonatal Chickenpox: Neonatal chickenpox can be a severe disease with high mortality. It occurs if the baby is born within a week of onset of maternal varicella rash, as the virus will pass to the baby. If maternal illness occurs more than 1 week before delivery the maternal antibodies may form and protect the neonate. Neonatal varicella requires vigorous treatment with IV acyclovir and zoster immune globulin.

Varicella fetopathy: Varicella fetopathy has been described if maternal infection occurs before 20 weeks of gestation. A number of malformations can occur. There are cicatricial skin lesions with limb defects and damage to eyes and CNS.

POLIOMYELITIS

Poliomyelitis is an acute viral illness caused by poliovirus and has a wide spectrum of presentation ranging from a mild disease to acute flaccid paralysis. It is covered in the chapter on Diseases of Nervous System –see Chapter 18.

RABIES

Rabies, a viral infection of warm-blooded animals, has been known to occur for a very long time and finds mention in ancient texts.

Aetiology

The rabies virus belongs to the Rhabdoviridae family and is an RNA virus.

Epidemiology

Rabies virus is present in the susceptible animals through out the world. Although dogs are the most well known vectors, there are many other animals, which transmit rabies including bats, skunks, raccoons, foxes and cats. With the vaccination of pets becoming widespread, other animals are becoming an important source of infection. In areas with substantial population of stray animals, the virus remains in circulation. The main source is the virus shedding in the saliva by the infected animal. The incubation period in the dog ranges from 2 weeks to 6 months. The shedding of virus occurs only 3-6 days before visible symptoms. The viral shedding may be variable and only less than half of bites from proven rabid animals result in rabies. Claw scratches by animals are also considered dangerous as they lick their paws and leave the virus there. Human to human transmission has not been reported except for transplants from infected individuals.

Pathogenesis

After the bite, the virus enters the skeletal muscles, multiplies and enters the nerves, ascends along the axons to the spinal cord and eventually brain causing neuronal destruction. The areas involved include medulla, pons, brainstem, floor of the fourth ventricle, hippocampus, thalamus and basal ganglia. Characteristically the cerebral cortex is spared. The typical Negri bodies are cytoplasmic inclusions of the virus in the neurons. These can be absent in proven cases. The combination of brainstem encephalitis with an intact cerebral cortex is seen in rabies only.

Clinical Features

The incubation period of human rabies is extremely variable. The usual is 20-180 days but the extremes have been 9 days and 7 years. There may be a prodrome of non-specific symptoms for the first week before entering the acute neurological phase. The neurological illness can be of 2 types, the furious variety seen in 80% of cases or the paralytic variety in 20%.

Furious Rabies: The pathognomonic sign of this is Hydrophobia. It is presumed to be occurring due to an inspiratory muscle spasm secondary to destruction of brainstem neurons inhibiting the nucleus ambiguus controlling inspiration. Whenever the patient attempts to swallow liquids, there is possible aspiration into the respiratory passages leading to a respiratory muscle spasm. With this reflex spasm even the sight of water causes distress to the patient. A similar response is seen to the air currents fanning the patient – Aerophobia that is another pathognomonic sign. Along with these two characteristic signs, there are behavioural changes in the form of disorientation, violent behaviour and there may be seizures. The patient may have brief lucid intervals.

Paralytic Rabies: There is an ascending, symmetrical flaccid paralysis.

Differential Diagnosis

The classical signs of rabies help in differentiating from encephalitis due to any other cause. The paralytic rabies may be mistaken for other causes of acute flaccid paralysis like Guillain Barrè syndrome or Poliomyelitis.

Diagnosis

Rabies virus can be isolated from saliva, conjunctival epithelial cells or skin cells at the hairline. The method used can be fluorescent antibody stain or reverse transcriptase PCR. These tests can be done on the brain tissue also after the death of a patient.

Treatment

There is no specific treatment for Rabies. After the onset of neurological symptoms Rabies immunoglobulin also do not help. WHO has given guidelines on post exposure prophylaxis (Table 26.12).

Table 26.12: Guidelines for post-exposure treatment of rabies	
Category Type of contact with suspect/confirmed domestic/ wild animal/animal unavailable for observation	**Recommendations**
1. Touching or feeding of animals, Licks on intact skin	None if reliable history is available
2. Nibbling of uncovered skin	Administer vaccine immediately. Stop treatment if animal remains healthy throughout an observation period of 10 days or if animal is killed humanely and found to be negative for rabies by appropriate laboratory techniques.
3. Single or multiple bites or scratches. Contamination of mucous membrane with Saliva (i.e. licks)	Administer rabies immunoglobulin and stop treatment if animal remains healthy throughout an observation period of 10 days, or if animal is killed humanely and found to be negative for rabies, by appropriate laboratory techniques.

Exposure to rodents, rabbits and hares seldom, if ever, requires specific anti-rabies treatment.

If an apparently healthy dog or cat, in or from a low risk area is placed under observation, the situation may warrant delaying initiation of treatment.

This observation period applies only to dogs and cats. Except in the case of threatened or endangered species, other domestic and wild animals suspected as rabid should kill humanely and their tissues examined using appropriate laboratory techniques.

JAPANESE ENCEPHALITIS

Aetiology

Japanese encephalitis (JE) is caused by an RNA virus from Flaviviridae family and is an Arbo viral disease.

Epidemiology

JE as the name suggests was reported from Japan in late 19th century and the virus identified in early 20th century. It has also been called Japanese B encephalitis to differentiate from another type of viral encephalitis called type A. The distribution of JE is mainly in the eastern part of the world i.e. Japan, Korea, China, Philippines, Indonesia and the Indian subcontinent. The vector for this arbo virus is a mosquito, Culex tritaeniorhynchus that usually bites large animals and birds or humans at nighttime. Culex vishnui is another related species of mosquito, which spreads the disease in India. As mosquito population is closely related to seasonal changes so JE outbreaks also follow the seasonal pattern.

Clinical Features

The incubation period of 4-14 days is followed by four stages of JE.

Prodromal Stage	2-3 days
Acute Stage	3-4 days
Subacute	7-10 days
Convalescence	4-7 weeks

The illness starts with a sudden onset of fever accompanied by respiratory symptoms and headache. This is soon followed by some behavioural changes like disorientation, delirium or excessive sleepiness. Seizures of generalized variety may occur in one fourth of patients. The neurological signs fluctuate from hyperreflexia to hyporeflexia, intention tremors and cogwheel rigidity. Patient may progress to coma. A rapid progression of disease is often seen in young children with high fatality.

Diagnosis

The CSF shows pleocytosis (100-1000/cumm) with initial polymorph predominance followed by lymphocytosis. Confirmation of the diagnosis can be by checking for specific IgM antibodies in the serum or CSF early in the illness or an increase of IgG antibodies in paired sera. EEG shows diffuse slowing. Cranial MRI/CT may show white matter oedema and hypodense lesions in thalamus, basal ganglia and pons.

Treatment

There is only supportive treatment.

Prognosis

Mortality is high especially in children. Neurodevelopmental sequelae are frequently seen in survivors.

DENGUE FEVERS

Dengue fevers comprise a group of febrile illnesses caused by arthropod borne viruses (Arbo viruses) including Dengue hemorrhagic fever and Dengue shock syndrome.

Aetiology

The dengue viruses belonging to family flaviviridae have four distinct antigenic types. In addition, there are a few other arbo viruses, which cause a similar clinical picture.

Epidemiology

The principal vector for all dengue viruses is a mosquito, Aedes aegypti. Other Aedes species have also been reported to carry these viruses. At present the disease is endemic to areas, which have suitable breeding environment for the specific mosquito. Hence it is the tropical areas like Asia, Africa, Caribbeans and South America, which have majority of cases. Explosive outbreaks of dengue occur in urban areas where A. aegypti is breeding. This mosquito lives in areas where stored or pooled water is collected and is a day biting mosquito. The biting rates increase with increase in temperature and humidity. The mosquito does not have a wide flight range so the outbreaks and epidemic are usually due to viraemic humans travelling to different areas.

Pathogenesis

The exact pathogenetic mechanism for the diverse clinical presentations of dengue fevers is not yet known. No single characteristic pathological change has been noticed in the autopsy of patients dying with dengue. It has been observed that a second exposure or infection by the dengue viruses is more likely to lead to a significant disease. There are infection-enhancing antibodies formed as a result of first infection, which on second exposure cause higher degree of viraemia and consequently a more severe disease. The second infections activate the complement system and there are many factors, which together interact to produce increased vascular permeability. This allows fluids to move from intra to extravascular spaces leading to haemoconcentration and hypovolaemia.

The mechanism of bleeding in dengue hemorrhagic fever is not exactly clear. It may be a combination of factors like thrombocytopenia, DIC and liver damage. The cause of thrombocytopenia is also not well established. There is a maturational arrest of megakaryocytes in bone marrow. Other mechanisms like antibodies on platelet surface or cross-reacting antibodies have also been considered.

Clinical Features

The incubation period of dengue fever is 1-7 days. The clinical presentation can be variable.

Dengue Fever

There may be an initial flu-like illness for few days or a sudden rise of temperature even up to 106°F. There is accompanying frontal headache and retro-bulbar pain with severe myalgia and arthralgia. There may also be severe backache before the fever. A transient erythematous rash may also appear early in the febrile phase. Towards the end of first week of illness, there is a typical cutaneous hyperaesthesia and hyperalgesia with marked loss of appetite and taste. As the fever comes down, there is a second phase of rash, which is generalized, erythematous with morbilliform or a lacy appearance. There can be accompanying diffuse oedema especially of palms and soles. The rash lasts 1-5 days followed sometimes by desquamation and intense itching. There may be a slight fever also at this stage. In some patients there is

thrombocytopenia and neutropenia with variable bleeding manifestations ranging from epistaxis to menorrhagia. The platelet count can drop to 10,000 /cu.mm and WBC count to even 1000/cu.mm. Usually the patient makes a quick recovery in 2-4 days.

Dengue haemorrhagic fever (DHF): The initial mild onset of dengue fever may rapidly change its course towards rapid deterioration after 2-5 days. The patient appears ill with flushed and cold extremities, restlessness and has bleeding from venipunctures or spontaneous petechiae and ecchymoses. There is significant hepatomegaly. Few patients may have gastrointestinal bleeding also.

Dengue shock syndrome (DSS): In few patients, the DHF may be complicated by a shock like state due to the accompanying hypovolaemia (Leaky capillaries) and also bleeding.

Some patients have significant extravasations into pleural spaces (pleural effusion, unilateral or bilateral) as well as ascites. The liver involvement occasionally can be clinically manifested as mild icterus also. After 1-2 days of critical illness, the patient can make a quick recovery with return to normal temperature, blood pressure and pulse. There is reabsorption of the intravascular fluid. During this phase, careful attention to fluid intake and balance is required as patient may develop congestive heart failure. There have been few reports of dengue encephalitis also in children similar to other viral encephalitis.

Differential Diagnosis

A clinical suspicion in the setting of dengue fever endemicity is usually used to make a diagnosis. As there are other viruses causing similar diseases, the term Dengue like disease should be used in the absence of specific diagnosis. WHO has given guidelines for diagnosing DHF/DSS.

WHO Criteria for DHF/DSS

DHF

1. Fever
2. Minor /major haemorrhagic manifestations
3. Thrombocytopenia <100,000/cu.mm
4. Increased capillary permeability (increase in hematocrit of >20%)
5. Pleural effusion (X-ray chest)
6. Hypoalbuminaemia

DSS

DHF criteria Plus
Hypotension
Pulse pressure < 20 mmHg

Diagnosis

Complete blood counts including hematocrit and platelets will show the already mentioned changes. Liver function test may show elevation of enzymes, hypoproteinaemia and prolonged prothrombin time. Chest radiographs show pleural effusion in many patients.

Specific virological investigations are based on serological tests or virus isolation. In dengue infection first episode IgM levels rise for 6-12 weeks but in second infection IgG rise is much more. Fourfold rise in paired sera help in diagnosis. A single serum sample for antibodies collected at least 5 days after the onset and up to 6 weeks can also be used.

Treatment

Supportive treatment especially during the critical period of illness is most essential. Bed rest and antipyretics during the febrile period are used. Adequate fluid intake must be insured. Close monitoring is required for further progression into DHF/DSS. For patients with significant bleeding manifestations and thrombocytopenia, platelet transfusions as well as blood transfusions are required. For patients in shock rapid intravenous fluid, normal saline bolus is given. If there is persistent shock or haemoconcentration, colloids in the form of plasma are indicated.

CASE STUDY

A 13-year-old boy was hospitalised with a history of fever with body ache for one week, generalised rash, and epistaxis on the day of admission. On examination he had a low-grade fever, a generalised morbilliform erythematous rash and a few petechiae on limbs. He had tachycardia otherwise examination of respiratory and cardiovascular system was normal. There was hepatomegaly on abdominal examination. Investigations: Hb 14gm/dl, Total white cell count 3,000/cumm, P45%, L42% M5%, E3%, Platelets 20,000/cumm.
Diagnosis Dengue fever.

HUMAN IMMUNODEFICIENCY VIRUS INFECTION (AIDS)

Infection with human immunodeficiency virus (HIV) is one of the recently identified diseases. The first case of HIV infection in paediatric age group was reported in 1983. HIV infection eventually leads to acquired immuno-deficiency syndrome (AIDS), a disease with a very high mortality.

Aetiology

HIV virus is of two types viz HIV-1 and HIV-2. They are both RNA viruses of family Reteroviridae. HIV-2 is a rare cause of infection in children.

Epidemiology

According to WHO year 2005 estimates, 38,600,000 persons are living with HIV or AIDS. Out of these children comprise about 6%. The sub-Saharan Africa, South East Asian countries like India, Thailand, Vietnam and China dominate the picture. In children, >90% of infection is through vertical transmission i.e. from mother to child. A small percentage is through blood or blood products and transmission through sexual contact or IV drug use seen in the adolescent age group.

Perinatal transmission: In HIV positive women, the perinatal transmission rates can very from 16-40% if no protective measures are undertaken. The risk factors for higher rates of transmission are advanced maternal HIV disease, delivery < 37 wks, prolonged rupture of membranes, vaginal delivery, chorioamnionitis, invasive procedures (e.g. amniocentesis) and haemorrhage in labour. The transmission of infection can occur any time during pregnancy or intrapartum period. In utero transmission can occur as a transplacental infection or through inflammation of the membranes or by materno-fetal transfusion. With early infection fetal loss is more likely. The most frequent timing of transmission of infection is intrapartum (60-75%) and occurs through materno-fetal transfusion. Post-partum transmission can occur through breast-feeding. The risk of HIV transmission to baby from breast milk ranges from 12-14%. The risk is higher in babies on mixed milk feeding as compared to exclusive breast-feeding.

Pathogenesis

The first cells to be infected through mucosal entry of HIV are the dendritic cells. These cells transport the virus to the lymphatic tissues where it selectively invades the CD4 lymphocytes, monocytes and macrophages.

After infecting CD4 cells there is progressive viral replication followed by a viraemic phase 3-6 weeks after infection. This is associated with flu like symptoms sometimes. Subsequently there is a decline in the viraemia due to the normal immune response of the body. CD8 cells are of help in containing the initial infection. A variable period of clinical latency follows but during this phase viral multiplication continues. The cytokines play an important role in sustaining viral load during this phase.

Following perinatal transmission of infection, there is little evidence clinically or virologically of HIV infection at birth. The viral load increases after first month and viral isolation by laboratory tests is more likely to be positive between 1-4 months of age. The immunological abnormalities in HIV infected children are similar to changes in adults except that as there is physiological lymphocytosis hence the values for labelling CD4 depletion are different in children. There is also B cell activation leading to an increased antibody production and resultant hypergammaglobulinemia.

Clinical Features

After perinatal transmission, there are three types of clinical presentation described. The first presentation is of rapid progression where the infant presents with features of AIDS in first few months of life. There is a rapid deterioration with poor survival beyond first year of life. Majority of the children have the second type of presentation. The child is asymptomatic during initial 1-2 years and later presents with lymphadenopathy, failure to thrive and other features of AIDS. The median survival in this pattern is about 6 years. The third pattern is of a delayed presentation, which is seen infrequently. The child has no significant features till 8-10 years of age followed by full AIDS presentation.

The usual presenting features in developing countries are chronic or recurrent diarrhoea, failure to thrive and wasting. There may be accompanying chronic or recurrent mucocutaneous candidiasis, lymphadenopathy and hepatosplenomegaly. In infants the initial presentation may be a severe respiratory distress due to Pneumocystis. carinii infection. CNS involvement is also more common in children. The symptoms have been categorized by CDC as shown below.

Staging of Paediatric AIDS (Centres for disease control (1994) criteria)

Category N

Asymptomatic, no signs or symptoms or only one of the conditions listed in Category A

CATEGORY A - Mildly symptomatic or two or more of the following conditions.
- Lymphadenopathy
- Hepatomegaly
- Splenomegaly
- Parotitis
- Dermatitis
- Recurrent or persistent upper respiratory infection

CATEGORY B – Moderately symptomatic conditions attributed to HIV infection
- Severe bacterial infections
- Lymphoid interstitial pneumonia
- Anaemia
- Neutropenia
- Thrombocytopenia
- Cardiomyopathy
- Nephropathy
- Hepatitis

- Diarrhoea
- Candidiasis

CATEGORY C – Severely symptomatic, two serious bacterial infections.
- Encephalopathy (acquired microcephaly, cognitive delay, abnormal neurology)
- Opportunistic infections (*Pneumocystis carinii* pneumonia, cytomegalovirus, toxoplasmosis, disseminated fungal infections)
- Disseminated mycobacterial diseases
- Cancer (Kaposi's sarcoma, lymphomas).

ASSOCIATED INFECTIONS

As HIV causes serious disturbances in immune system, associated infections are almost universal and very often the presenting feature. Any organism bacteria, viruses, protozoa or fungi can cause serious systemic sepsis in HIV infected children. Opportunistic organisms are also frequent causes of serious disease in such children. Various opportunistic infections are listed below.

Opportunistic Infections

Pneumocystis carinii pneumonia
Candidiasis – oesophageal or pulmonary
Tuberculosis
Mycobacterium avium
Cytomegalovirus
Cryptosporidiosis
Non-tuberculous mycobacteria
Herpes zoster
Toxoplasmosis

Mycobacteria and HIV share a symbiotic relationship in HIV infected patients. Both tuberculosis as well as non-tuberculosis mycobacteria, can cause difficult to treat, disseminated and resistant disease.

Candidial infections also occur in a more widespread fashion often involving oesophagus along with oral cavity. Out of viruses, Herpes group, both zoster and simplex are frequent offenders.

Diagnosis

If any one of the parents is known to be having HIV infection, the infant/child must be screened for it. In others, the indications for HIV testing are given below.

In asymptomatic children:
a. Parent at high risk for HIV infection e.g. truck drivers, IVdrug users.
b. Children receiving transfusion or blood products etc.

In symptomatic infants and children:
a. Recurrent, severe bacterial infections
b. Opportunistic infections

c. Poor response to antitubercular treatment

d. Evidence of congenital TORCH infection

e. Unexplained wasting, neuroencephalopathy, myopathy, hepatitis, cardiomyopathy, nephropathy

f. Hyperimmunoglobulinemia

Viral cultures are the gold standard for diagnosis of HIV and have 100% specificity. The culture requires 2-3 weeks, is labour intensive and expensive. The alternative, PCR for viral DNA or RNA, is also specific and sensitive. The assay for p24 antigen of HIV has also been frequently used with good specificity but less sensitivity.

PERINATAL TRANSMISSION

At birth all infants born to HIV positive mothers have placentally transferred antibodies. These decline slowly in 6-12 months time. Only at age 18 months or more, if the antibody test is positive that can be used as an indicator of infection in the child. In a neonate born to an HIV positive mother virological assay (PCR/Culture/p24 antigen) provide reliable results. If antiretroviral therapy is to be started, it is recommended that testing should be done within 48 hrs of birth, at 4-6 weeks of age and or 4-6 months of age. Two positive tests from different samples confirm the transmission of HIV infection to the infant. On the other hand if two different tests of which one should be at 4-6 months of age are negative then HIV infection can be excluded. At 18 months age, in an asymptomatic infant, two negative antibody tests exclude HIV infection.

Older Infants and Children

In older infants and children, two or more HIV antibody tests done by different techniques on different samples are recommended to make a diagnosis. Once HIV infection is diagnosed in a child further evaluation is done by complete blood count along with CD4 and CD8 lymphocyte counts. Additional tests depend on the extent and type of systemic involvement.

Treatment

At present the available anti-viral drugs suppress the virus and help in making the disease less aggressive. There are two broad categories of anti viral drugs viz.

i. Protease inhibitors (PI) e.g.

ii. Reverse transcriptase inhibitors which are further classified as nucleoside (NRTI) or non-nucleoside (NNRTI) e.g.

The basic principle of anti-retroviral treatment is combination therapy with 2 NRTI+ PI or 2 NRTI + 1 NNRTI. Monotherapy is only used in prevention of perinatal transmission. Intiation of therapy in HIV infected asymptomatic children needs appropriate consideration. In symptomatic children or in those with evidence of immunosuppresion treatment is definitely indicated.

Supportive Treatment

Attention must be paid to the nutrition of child; frequent evaluation of growth and development is necessary. All vaccinations except live attenuated ones can be given safely. In asymptomatic infants live vaccine may also be given. In all infants and in immunosuppresed children, *Pneumocystis carinii* prophylaxis with cotrimoxazole must be given. Frequent screening for tuberculosis must be done.

Prevention

Prevention of perinatal transmission of HIV is a unique opportunity for protecting the infant. One of the standard regimens is to give zidovudine to the pregnant woman and continue through intrapartum period followed by 6 weeks therapy in the infant. Recently oral Nevirapine, an NNRTI, has been used effectively for reducing the perinatal transmission. It is given as a single oral dose to the mother during labour followed by a single oral dose to the neonate within first 48 hours. This strategy has been effective in the developing countries as Nevirapine is inexpensive and only two oral doses are required. It has been adopted as a National program in India. In addition to anti-retroviral therapy in mother, caesarean section and preventing prolonged rupture of membrane are also helpful in reducing transmission.

Breast feeding can be responsible for up to 14% risk of HIV transmission but the decision to breast feed or not must be taken after discussion with the mother regarding implications of giving animal milk. Mixed feeding i.e. breast + animal milk should be avoided. If breast-feeding, then at 3 months of age an early and abrupt weaning is recommended.

For prevention in adolescents, sex education and awareness especially regarding condom use must be propagated.

MALARIA

Aetiology

Intracellular protozoa, Plasmodium, cause malaria. There are four species of plasmodium that infect humans viz *P vivax, P falciparum, P malariae* and *P ovale*. Female anopheles mosquitoes transmit it during a blood meal on humans. It can also be a transfusion transmitted infection or a transplacental infection from mother to the fetus.

Epidemiology

Malaria occurs worldwide but the endemicitiy depends on the mosquito population. In areas with suitable environment for mosquito breeding, the incidence of malaria is high e.g. Africa, Asia and South America. *P falciparum* and *P vivax* are more commonly seen in sub-Saharan Africa and Indian subcontinent. *P ovale* is rare and seen mainly in Africa. *P malariae* is the rarest.

Pathogenesis

Plasmodia have two parts of their life cycle, sexual and asexual phase, in vector mosquito and human host respectively. In the humans there are two stages. First stage in the liver, the exoerythrocytic phase and the second one in RBCs, the erythrocytic phase. Mosquito bites the human host and releases sporozoites in the blood stream, which quickly enter the hepatocytes. In the hepatocytes the sporozoites multiply, become schizonts and rupture the cell. On rupture of hepatocytes, thousand of merozoites are released into the circulation. P.vivax has two types of schizonts, a primary type, which follows the above cycle, and a secondary type, which becomes dormant in the hepatocytes for weeks and months causing frequent relapses. The merozoites released into the circulation enter the RBCs and become the ring form, which later grows to become trophozoite. The trophozoite multiplies again and gives rise to merozoites in RBCs, which rupture releasing them in circulation. The release of merozoites is associated with a sharp rise in fever. Some of the merozoites develop into male and female gametocytes, which are ingested by the female anopheles mosquito during a blood meal. The gametocytes undergo the sexual phase of development in the stomach of the mosquito where a zygote is formed and develops into sporozoites, which enter the mosquito salivary glands ready to inject the new host.

In the pathogenesis of malaria, fever results from RBC rupture and release of merozoites. The other common feature, anaemia, is a result of breakdown of RBCs i.e. haemolysis. There are two more mechanisms responsible for other clinical features. An immunopathological process leading to release of cytokines, which cause many features. In P.falciparum, another pathological change is the adherence of infected RBCs to the endothelial lining of blood vessels. This results in damage to various organs like brain, kidneys, intestines etc.

Clinical Features

Incubation period for each species is different (see Box below 26.1)

BOX 26.1: Incubation period of Malaria Species	
P vivax	12-17 days
P falciparum	8-14 days
P malariae	18-40 days
P ovale	16-18 days

The onset of the disease is marked by a sudden rise of fever, which may be periodic. Rigors and sweating, headache, body ache, nausea and vomiting accompany the fever. There may be diarrhoea and cough also

sometime. The gastrointestinal and respiratory symptoms are seen more often in young children and infants. After a few days of fever, the patient begins to appear pale and may even have jaundice. In adults there is a definite periodicity of fever, which is generally not seen in children. The clinical presentation in some children may be different with low-grade fever, hepatosplenomegaly, anaemia and thrombocytopenia.

Congenital malaria is considered in a neonate whose mother was symptomatic during late pregnancy. The neonate may manifest with symptoms between 10-30 days of age. The neonate may or may not have any fever along with poor feeding, lethargy and vomiting. Unexplained anaemia and severe jaundice (indirect hyper-bilirubinaemia) are additional features.

Black water fever is a severe form of falciparum malaria with haemolysis, hemoglobinuria and severe anaemia. The mortality can be high with this presentation of malaria.

Algid malaria is a severe infection with P. falciparum. There is hypotension, shock, shallow respiration, and pallor with a rapid fatality. Gram-negative sepsis is often associated.

Diagnosis

Peripheral blood smear, thin and thick smear, should be examined. From the thick smear the diagnosis can be made more quickly while thin smear helps in identifying the species and the parasitic load. Several smears over different days maybe required to confirm the diagnosis (Fig. 26.10).

The newer diagnostic tests include an antibody test as well as a PCR. A test based on malarial antigen has also been available for sometime although sensitivity and specificity are still a problem.

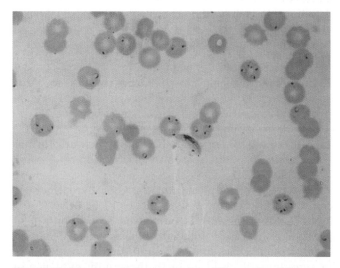

Fig. 26.10: Ring forms and gametocytes of Plasmodium falciparum

Complications

a. Cerebral Malaria

P. falciparum causes this serious life threatening complication especially with a heavy parasitaemia. The child presents with high fever even up to 108°F (hyperpyrexia) accompanied by alteration of sensorium, coma, twitching and seizures. There may be retinal haemorrhages and neurological deficits also. The CSF does not show any significant abnormality except for raised pressure. Cerebral malaria is associated with high mortality and requires intensive treatment at the earliest possible.

b. **Renal Failure** may occur due to haemoglobinuria and tubular damage.

c. **Hypoglycaemia**

d. **Thrombocytopenia**

e. **Splenic** rupture may occur if spleen is greatly enlarged or there is trauma.

Treatment

All Plasmodium Species are treated with oral Chloroquine phosphate10 mg base/kg (maximum: 600 mg base) then 5 mg base/kg (maximum: 300 mg base), 6 hr later, and 5 mg base/kg/24 hr (maximum: 300 mg base) at 24 and 48 hr. Parenteral drug of choice if required is Quinine dihydrochloride 20 mg/kg loading dose over 4 hrs, then 10 mg/kg over 2-4 hrs q8 hrly (max. 1200 mg/24 hrs) until oral therapy can be started. In areas of known Chloroquine resistance Quinine sulfate Plus Tetracycline or plus Pyrimethamine-sulfadoxine combination is given. Another alternative is Mefloquine hydrochloride *Prevention of Relapses*: (**For P vivax** and ovale only)

Primaquine phosphate in the dose of 0.3 mg base/kg/24 hr for 14 days (maximum: 15 mg base) should be given. Primaquine phosphate can cause haemolytic anaemia in patients with glucose-6-phosphate dehydrogenase (G6PD) deficiency. A G6PD screening test should be performed before initiating treatment.

Along with specific treatment, the child may need additional fluids during acute stage. In a severe case, anaemia needs attention. Haematinics to bring up the haemoglobin should be given on recovery. Preventive measures for mosquito breeding as well as from bites must be reinforced.

CASE STUDY

An 8-year-old girl was brought to the paediatric service with a history of fever for 4 days, which went up to 104° F accompanied, by a feeling of chills. She also had mild cough and vomiting. Examination showed pallor and no jaundice. Examination of abdomen revealed a mild hepatomegaly of 3 cms while spleen was enlarged to 4 cm and was firm in consistency. Rest of the systemic examination was normal, Investigations: Hb 9 gm/dl, Total leucocyte count 5,400/cumm, P 60%, L 40%. Peripheral smears showed Plasmodium vivax schizonts.
Diagnosis: Malaria caused by *P vivax*.

Key Learning Points

Malaria can cause respiratory and gastrointestinal symptoms in young children.
P vivax and *P ovale* require a radical cure to eradicate the exoerythrocytic phase.

TOXOPLASMOSIS

Toxoplasmosis is a disease with many varied presentations. It occurs in neonates as a transplacental infection and in immunocompromised older individuals. Healthy immunocompetent persons rarely manifest clinical disease.

Aetiology

The causative organism is an intracellular protozoa, Toxoplasma gondii. The infection occurs after ingesting oocysts, which may be present in the contaminated foodstuff especially infected meat. The oocysts are released in the environment by cats in their faeces. Cats acquire the infection after ingesting mice infected with encysted bradyzoites of T.gondii.

Epidemiology

T gondii occurs as a latent infection among humans throughout the world with a higher prevalence in warmer, humid area. The route of infection is by ingestion of contaminated meat containing oocysts or transplacental or transfusion transmitted. There is no direct person-to-person transmission. The oocysts ingested by cats undergo schizogony and gametogenesis in the intestines and form sporocysts, which are excreted in the faeces and remain viable in a suitable environment for 1 year. They can be destroyed by drying, boiling or by some strong chemicals. Other animals e.g. sheep, pigs and cows become infected by ingesting the cysts and develop viable tissue cysts in muscles and brain. Humans eating partially cooked or uncooked meat of these animals ingest these cysts.

Congenital toxoplasmosis occurs in case mother acquires the infection during pregnancy. In the first trimester, the likelihood of transmission is low but the resultant fetal infection is severe. In 3rd trimester, almost 65% of fetuses are infected but the disease is either mild or inapparent.

Pathogenesis

T gondii can multiply in any mammalian tissue. They cause necrosis and an immunological reaction. In healthy persons, the tachyzoites soon disappear from tissues to become latent. They cause characteristic changes in lymph nodes. In congenital toxoplasmosis, CNS, eyes, heart, lungs, liver, spleen and muscles can be involved with the necrotic lesions.

Clinical Features

Majority of healthy individuals do not have any clinical features. Occasionally, there can be features ranging from fever, myalgia, CNS involvement, rashes, lymphadenopathy which may be present for a variable period of time. Lymphadenopathy can wax and wane for 1-2 years. One of the frequently caused presentations is of chorioretinitis.

Congenital infection can present as intrauterine growth retardation, prematurity, prolonged jaundice. The classical triad is of chorioretinitis, hydrocephalus and cerebral calcification. Severe manifestations include hydrops fetalis and perinatal death. The infants with inapparent infection often present with ocular involvement later in life.

Diagnosis

T gondii can be isolated from body fluids or from tissues. Cultures are done by inoculating into mice or tissue cultures. The tachyzoites of *T gondii* can be demonstrated in bone marrow aspirates, CSF, amniotic fluid or in biopsy specimens.

Serological testing: A number of serological tests are available for toxoplasmosis. It is important that these tests have appropriate quality control measures. Some of the tests used are:

a. Sabin-feldman dye test
b. IgG or IgM indirect fluorescent antibody test
c. Double sandwich ELISA
d. Polymerase chain reaction (PCR)

Treatment

All congenitally infected infants need treatment. The treatment of choice is Pyrimethamine given for 1 year along with sulphadiazine or triple sulphonamides. Acutely infected pregnant women should be treated with spiramycin to prevent transplacental fetal infection.

AMOEBIASIS

Aetiology

Amoebiasis is caused by *Entamoeba histolytica*. There are few non-pathogenic Entamoeba also which are present in the gastro-intestinal tract of human beings e.g. *Entamoeba coli*.

Epidemiology

Amoebiasis is more commonly seen in tropics and in areas of low socio-economic status with poor sanitation. It is estimated that Amoebiasis is the third leading parasitic cause of death worldwide. The transmission is through feco-oral route. The cysts of *E histolytica* are the infectious form while the trophozoites do not transmit infection. The amoebic cysts are nucleated. They are resistant to low temperature and chlorination of water. On ingestion, they are resistant to gastric acidity and the digestive enzymes. Trophozoites succumb to the environmental factors.

Pathogenesis

After ingestion, the amoebic cysts reach the small intestine and give rise to eight trophozoites, which are actively motile and reach the large intestines. In the colon, they attach to the mucosa and cause tissue destruction by various cellular products. This leads to ulceration of the mucosa but surprisingly there is little local inflammatory response. The organisms spread laterally from the ulcerated areas causing further destruction and leading to the typical 'flask-shaped' ulcers. The trophozoites invade liver also producing similar lesions but again with no inflammatory reaction.

Clinical Features

The spectrum of amoebic disease varies from asymptomatic carriers to severe intestinal or extra intestinal disease. More severe disease is likely in young or malnourished children and those on corticosteroid therapy.

Symptomatic intestinal amoebiasis: The symptoms of intestinal amoebiasis can occur anytime after infection and even an asymptomatic carrier can develop invasive disease later on. The presentation starts with abdominal colic, loose stools with or without blood, tenesmus and occasionally there may be fever. In young children, the onset can be of more acute colitis with dehydration and dyselectrolytaemia. Chronic amoebiasis is more commonly seen in adults.

Systemic or extra intestinal amoebiasis: Liver can be affected in amoebiasis as a diffuse hepatitis like picture with hepatomegaly. The more severe and less common is formation of an amoebic liver abscess, which is seen in <1% of infected persons. The abscess is usually in the right lobe and single. There may be a history of associated intestinal symptoms. The presentation is with high fever, abdominal pain and tender hepatomegaly. There may be reactionary changes in the adjacent right lung or pleura. The abscess can rupture into the abdominal or thoracic cavity. The contents of the abscess are characteristically described as 'anchovy sauce' and contain lysed RBCs.

Diagnosis

Detection of the amoebic trophozoites in stool sample is diagnostic. A fresh stool sample i.e. within 30 minutes of passage can show motile trophozoites with ingested RBCs. Repeated stool examination, at least 3, increase the yield.

Serological tests are helpful in diagnosis but may be positive in asymptomatic carriers also. Indirect haemagglutination is the most sensitive serological test.

Treatment

The treatment of intestinal disease is with luminal amoebicides viz Iodoquinol, Paromomycin and Diloxanide furoate. All persons including asymptomatic carriers should receive treatment. In extraintestinal disease or invasive colitis, tissue amoebicides are used. These include Metronidazole and other related compounds, Dihydroemetine and Chloroquine. Metronidazole is given in the dose of 30-50 mg/kg/d in 3 divided doses for 10 days. For giving dehydroemetine, the patient has to be hospitalised. Chloroquine is concentrated in the liver and considered useful for liver abscess. Surgical management of liver abscess is recommended if there is a poor response after a week of treatment with amoebicidal drugs.

CASE STUDY

A 10-year-old boy was hospitalised with a history of high-grade intermittent fever for one week, pain in abdomen for 4 days. He had diarrhoea for about 2-3 weeks previously. On examination, he was mildly icteric, pale, febrile and sick looking. His vital signs were stable. On chest examination, the movements and breath sounds were diminished in the right lower zone but there were no adventitious sounds. Abdomen had an enlarged, tender hepatomegaly of 8 cms in midclavicular line. There was no splenomegaly. Hepatic punch was positive. Investigations: Hb 9 gm/dl, TLC 20,000/cumm, P80%, L20%, blood film showed normocytic, normochronic anaemia. Serum liver function tests were abnormal. Ultrasonography of abdomen showed a large 6 x 8 cms abscess in right lobe of liver near the dome of diaphragm with restricted mobility of diaphragm.

Needle aspiration of the abscess revealed chocolate brown thick fluid.
Diagnosis: Amoebic liver abscess.

GIARDIASIS

Aetiology

Giardia lamblia is a flagellate protozoon, which causes primarily an intestinal infection. Giardia cysts are infective in even small numbers.

Epidemiology

Giardiasis is the commonest intestinal parasitic infection the world over. It is more common in areas of poor sanitation and hygiene and in institutionalised children. Drinking contaminated water is a frequent source of infection but other foodstuffs can also transmit infection. The cysts are resistant to chlorination and ultraviolet radiation but boiling inactivates them.

Pathogenesis

After ingestion, the cysts produce trophozoites, which colonize the duodenum and jejunum. They attach to the brush border of the intestinal epithelium and multiply there. The trophozoites pass to intestines and are encysted to form the cysts, which are then excreted in the stools.

Clinical Features

The incubation period is usually 1-2 weeks but can be longer. Most infections may remain asymptomatic. In children with no prior exposure to giardia the presentation can start as acute diarrhoea. In another manifestation, the child may have intermittent diarrhoea, which is accompanied by abdominal cramps, distension, flatulence and loss of appetite. There may be features of increased gastro-colic reflex. The stools become greasy and foul smelling. There are no blood, mucus or pus cells in stools. Chronic giardiasis can present as malabsorption with significant weight loss.

Diagnosis

Demonstration of giardia cysts or trophozoites in stool sample is diagnostic. A fresh stool sample (within 1 hour of passage) is more likely to be positive and repeated examinations are helpful. In some cases, if necessary, duodenal aspirates or a biopsy can show the trophozoites.

Treatment

A number of drugs are effective for treating giardiasis. Albendazole in a dose of 10-mg/kg/day for 5 days is safe and effective. It is also helpful in treating mixed infection, as it is an antihelminth also. Tinidazole is effective in a single dose of 50 mg/kg. Metronidazole, Furazolidone, Quinacrine are other drugs that are used.

CASE STUDY

A 7-year-old child had history of recurrent diarrhoea for 6 months. The stools were pale yellow foul smelling, greasy and did not contain blood or mucus. He had abdominal pain off and on and an urge to pass stool after every meal. He had lost weight and looked pale. There were no other findings on examination. A fresh stool examination showed trophozoits of Giardia lamblia.
Diagnosis: Giardiasis.

Key Learning Point

Giardiasis can cause a clinical presentation similar to malabsorption syndrome. Examination of fresh stool or duodenal aspirate confirms the diagnosis.

KALA AZAR (VISCERAL LEISHMANIASIS)

Leishmania are a group of organisms causing diverse diseases transmitted by sandflies. There are a number of species, which cause cutaneous or mucosal disease and also visceral disease.

Aetiology

Leishmania are protozoa belonging to trypanosomatidae family. They have two morphological forms, a flagellate organism in the insect known as promastigote and the aflagellate form in the humans, amastigote.

Epidemiology

Leishmaniasis occurs in most parts of the world except Australia and Antarctica. The various types of leishmaniasis are specific to the regions of the world. Leishmania causing cutaneous disease do not cause visceral involvement. Leishmania enters the vector sandfly and change from promastigote to an infective stage and migrate from the gut to mouth of the sand fly. From the mouth they are inoculated into the host during a blood meal. In endemic areas, leishmanial cycle is continued as a zoonosis with humans being incidental hosts. The reservoir for visceral forms is dog.

Pathogenesis

Leishmania after inoculation into the host, enter the macrophages. Inside the macrophages, the promastigote form change to amastigote form and start multiplying. They rupture the cell to infect more macrophages.

Clinical Features

The children may have an asymptomatic infection. Some children develop a symptomatic illness with fever, malaise, fatigue accompanied by a mild hepatomegaly. In all but few this resolves spontaneously. In few it progresses slowly over weeks and months to Kala-azar. There is intermittent fever, weakness and splenomegaly. As the disease progresses fever becomes higher, there is weight loss and hepatosplenomegaly. The patient has severe anaemia and may develop heart failure due to this. Oedema and jaundice are also present. As spleen becomes massive, features of hypersplenism in the form of thrombocytopenia and pancytopenia develop.

Differential Diagnosis

The conditions causing pyrexia with hepatosplenomegaly, anaemia are to be considered in differential diagnosis of visceral leishmaniasis.

Diagnosis

Amastigote forms, also known as Leishmania Donovan (LD) bodies are found intracellularly in tissues like liver, spleen and bone marrow. A positive bone marrow or spleen aspiration for LD bodies provides confirmation of diagnosis (Fig. 26.11). An ELISA test using a recombinant antigen also has high sensitivity and specificity.

Treatment

The specific treatment for visceral leishmaniasis has remained unchanged for more than four decades. Pentavalent antimony compounds, sodium stibogluconate is given as 20 mg/kg/day IV/IM for 3-4 weeks. Complete recovery can take a few months and sometimes even repeated courses. Recently, Amphotericin B especially liposomal variety, has been shown to be highly effective even among those refractory or resistant to antimony compounds. Pentamidine has also been used but higher doses and prolonged treatment is required.

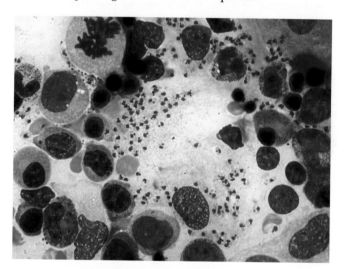

Fig. 26.11: Leishman Donovan (LD) bodies seen in bone marrow

In addition, supportive treatment to improve nutritional status is important. In cases with severe pancytopenia, blood component therapy may prove life saving.

CASE STUDY

A 9-month-old girl was admitted to a children's hospital, with a 10-day history of lethargy, pallor, fever, and poor feeding. On examination she was found to have a mass in the left hypochondrium. She was febrile and miserable. Her Hb was 65 g/l, white cell count 6.3×10^9/l, and platelets 41×10^9/l. Initially she was thought to be suffering from a malignant condition and was investigated accordingly. Bone marrow examination, blood culture, chest radiography, skeletal survey, and urine catecholamines were all normal. Abdominal ultrasound examination showed the mass to be a massively enlarged spleen.

Contd....

Contd....

She was given a blood transfusion and antibiotics after which her general condition improved, although she continued to spike a fever two to three times a day. By the third day after admission, the results of the above investigations were all negative and the possibility of visceral leishmaniasis was raised. The child had been on holiday to an endemic area where leishmaniasis is known to occur. The bone marrow examination showed the presence of Leishman Donovan bodies. Also Leishmania serology became positive five weeks after presentation.

She was treated with sodium stibogluconate 20 mg/kg/day for 10 days followed by 10 mg/kg/day for another 10 days. Her temperature settled within two days of starting treatment. Her platelet count returned to normal within seven days and by the 10th day of treatment her white cell count reached normal values. She made an uneventful recovery.

Diagnosis: Visceral leishmaniasis.

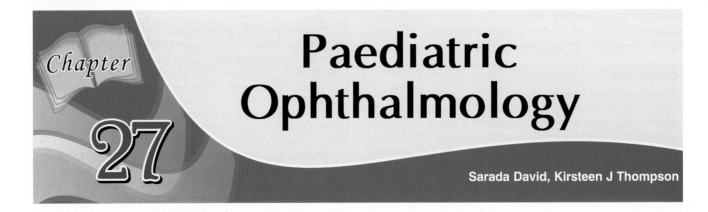

Paediatric Ophthalmology

Chapter 27

Sarada David, Kirsteen J Thompson

VISUAL ASSESSMENT IN CHILDREN

A child's eye is different from that of an adult. It is a growing eye, with the most rapid growth-taking place within the first two years of life. Astigmatism is often present during the first few months of life, and most infants are hypermetropic, becoming normal sighted (emmetropic) during the first few years of life.

The developing immune system results in children responding to inflammation and to other disease conditions differently from adults.

Myelination of the optic nerve and maturation of the fovea continue after birth, as does pigment deposition in the anterior iris stroma.

Visual Acuity

Visual acuity is a measure of the clarity of central vision. It is defined as the measurement of the resolution of the visual system in terms of the angle subtended at the fovea by an object at a distance of 6 metres from the eye, tested at maximum contrast (black on white).

In clinical practice, quantification of visual acuity is required to diagnose abnormality, to chart progress of disease and to determine the results of treatment.

Standard visual acuity measurement in ophthalmology has traditionally been performed using the Snellen's chart. 6/6 is a normal visual acuity. The numerator of this fraction is the distance in metres at which the letters are shown to the patient, and the denominator is the distance at which that letter being read subtends 5 minutes of arc at the eye. The 6/60 letters at the top of the chart therefore subtends 5 minutes of arc at a distance of 60 metres. In the USA the numbers used refer to feet, so that 6/6 acuity is the same as 20/20 acuity.

An alternative, and arguably more logical way to record visual acuity is the Log MAR notation in which 6/6 is an acuity of 0.1 and 6/60 becomes 1.0 with eight intervening steps.

In infants and young children, such methods are not feasible, but quantification of visual acuity is obtained using different methods (below), and equivalent scales of measurement.

Amblyopia

Visual development takes place from birth until the age of 6-7 years, and requires clear visual images to be formed on the retina of each eye.

Amblyopia occurs when there is deficient development of the visual brain due to impaired stimulation of the fovea during the first few years of life. This may occur due to the presence of uncorrected refractive error, squint (deviation of the eye such that the image formed on the retina is extra-foveal, i.e. falls on an area of retina other than the fovea), or any type of occlusion in front of the retina including media opacities (cataract, vitreous opacity, blood or inflammatory cells in the anterior chamber), corneal opacity or abnormal eyelid position (ptosis).

Box 27.1: Types of Amblyopia

1. Refractive
2. Strabismic
3. Stimulus deprivation

Iatrogenic causes of amblyopia may include prolonged use of eye ointment, or of eye padding following injury or surgery to an eye. Prolonged pupil dilatation may also be amblyogenic. The retina appears normal, but visual acuity is reduced. If detected before the age of 7-8 years, amblyopia may be partially or wholly reversible by treating the underlying cause. Amblyopia is usually unilateral or asymmetrical, and occlusion of the better eye (taking care not to induce amblyopia in that eye!) is used to bring about adequate retinal stimulation of the eye with poorer vision (once the refractive error or media opacities etc. have been dealt with) in order to overcome amblyopia. It is, therefore, important to be aware of, and to use, accurate methods for determining vision in young children of different age groups. Appropriate measures for treatment of amblyopia can then be instituted promptly.

Assessing Vision

There are several key factors to be considered when assessing vision in young children.

1. Young children are neither in a position to understand "normality" of visual ability, nor can they articulate what they can or cannot see.
2. A "difficult" examination of a child is usually due to a "difficult" examiner rather than a "difficult" child. Entering a child's mindset, setting them at their ease, and maintaining patience and respect throughout the examination may be a daunting thought for some of us, particularly in the presence of anxious parents. However, it is a skill we ignore at our peril. Once the skill is mastered, or even haltingly attempted, clinic appointments can become something child and examiner alike, look forward to, though fewer are likely to be required, and the final outcome has a much greater likelihood of being successful and satisfying for all parties involved.
3. A child's general demeanour and ability to move around and to communicate is not necessarily a guide to the level of their visual function, as different aspects of general development as well as of visual development, may be impaired in different disease states. A child can have very poor clarity of visual acuity and yet have practically normal mobility.
4. Accommodation of the lens is easily stimulated in children and resting accommodative tone is high. Thus, accurate assessment of refractive error must always be performed after full cycloplegia using cyclopentolate or atropine drops.

Visual Acuity Measurement

Formal visual acuity assessment in children is carried out in the following ways:

1. Infants (0-6 months): Preferential looking, VEPs (visual evoked potentials). (Watching the child's visual behaviour, whether she returns a smile, and at what distance; and spinning the child to find out what speed is required to make the eyes move to and fro, by eliciting the vestibulo-ocular reflex (VOR), gives an index of central visual function. Good vision suppresses the VOR.)
2. Toddlers (7 months -3 years): Cardiff acuity cards,
3. Pre-School children (3-5 years): Kay's pictures
4. Primary School children (5-7 years): Sheridan-Gardiner Acuity cards or Glasgow Acuity cards, with a card of letters to point to.
   Over 7 years: Log MAR chart or Snellen's chart (Figs 27.1 and 27.2).

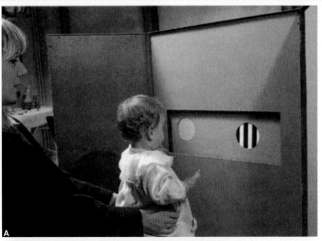

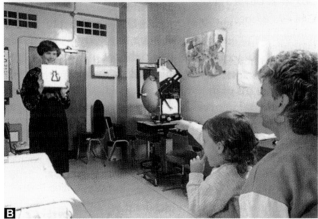

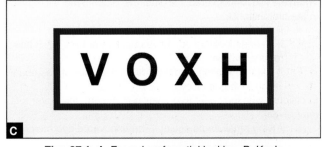

Figs 27.1: A. Forced preferential looking, B. Kay's pictures and C. LogMAR crowded test

Assessment of Eye Movements

Orthoptic assessment of ocular muscle balance and the presence or absence of latent or manifest squint is assessed using the cover/uncover test (Boxes 27.2 and 27.3) and the alternate cover test (Boxes 27.2 and 27.3). A target of interest or a light moved into the 9 directions of gaze, brought about by the action of the 6 extraocular muscles, is then used to examine the adequacy of the muscle actions. Further tests using prism bars are used to record the magnitude and precise type of squint present, and the ability to fuse disparate images.

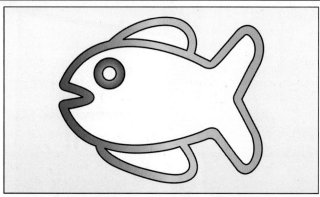

Fig. 27.2: Example of a Cardiff card

Box 27.2: Cover Test

One eye is covered and the other eye is observed to see if it moves to look at a target. (In the absence of squint, no movement takes place.

In children who look as if they have a squint, the cover test shows:

1. A fixation movement if a true squint is present and the eye can see.
2. No fixation movement if
   - There is a true squint and the eye is blind, for example due to a cataract or retinoblastoma
   - The squinting eye is an artificial eye
   - The macula is displaced. This causes the eye to appear to have a squint despite "fixing" with the macula.
   - The image is being viewed with eccentric retina (extra-foveal fixation).
   - The eye is tethered and cannot move.

When the eye is uncovered, the other eye is observed, if it moved in the first instance.

   - If it moves back immediately, it has poor vision.
   - If it keeps looking, but moves back after blinking, it has reduced vision.
   - If it keeps looking, and does not move back, it has equal vision to the other eye.

In children who look as if their eyes are straight, the cover test may reveal:

1. A very small angle squint. (The uncovered eye moves slightly to take up fixation).
2. Latent nystagmus (a to and fro movement of the eyes which only occurs when one eye is covered).

Box 27.3: The Uncover/Alternate Cover Test

This test is done when the eyes have been shown to be straight by the cover test.

One eye is covered, and then observed when it is uncovered. The test is repeated for the other eye. If either eye moves when uncovered, a latent squint (a phoria) is present.

If both eyes see well, the brain can join the images by fusing them (fusion), and this keeps the eyes straight. When an eye is covered, fusion is lost. If that eye has a position of rest which is turned out (exophoria), turned in (esophoria), turned up (hyperphoria) or turned down (hypophoria), then it will do so when covered, but will be seen to straighten up when uncovered.

Other Visual Functions

Colour vision is tested using Ishihara plates for red-green defects, Llantony plates for blue-yellow defects, or the City University test. The child is asked to trace along, or to point to a particular colour.

Central and peripheral visual fields are assessed manually using a target, a light, or a variable number of fingers held up, in the 4 quadrants of each visual field, while watching the child's attentiveness to the target. The target may be moved in order to map the point at which it comes into view. Older children are able to co-operate with Goldmann perimetry or with automated perimetry. Lesions of the occipital cortex or posterior visual pathways cause homonymous visual field defects in both eyes. Lesions affecting the optic chiasm typically cause a bitemporal hemianopia, while lesions of the anterior visual pathways or the retina, cause non-homonymous, or unilateral field defects.

Binocular depth perception or stereopsis, measured in seconds of arc, is tested using the Titmus fly and randot test, where superimposed images, displaced by varying degrees are viewed through polarised lenses, and, with adequate levels of stereopsis, are identified as 3-dimensional. In children younger than 5 years old, the Lang or Frisby tests, where the child identifies an elevated image in a group of otherwise identical images, are used. As in the Titmus test, image disparity is graded in order to quantify the level of stereopsis achieved.

Refractive error is measured using retinoscopy and trial lenses (spherical and cylindrical), while singing (at least, the budding performers among us!), or holding up an interesting target, to hold the child's attention.

Contrast sensitivity is not routinely tested in children, but can be useful for monitoring amblyopia and to quantify visual dysfunction.

A child may perform well in all the above tests and yet have significant visual problems in daily life such as difficulty identifying an object in a crowded scene, difficulty recognising faces or route finding, due to impaired visual integration processes at a cerebral level. Such problems occur more commonly than hitherto acknowledged. They are commonly associated with peri-ventricular leukomalacia, which may occur as a consequence of premature birth, antenatal or postnatal cerebral hypoxic episodes, meningitis or head injury. Typical features can usually be elicited by detailed history taking (see check list in Box 27.4), and by an awareness of the typical patterns of disorder, often suggested by symptoms described by a child or their carers.

Strabismus

Strabismus, or squint, refers to a deviation of an eye due to an imbalance of function of the extra-ocular muscles such that both eyes do not function together. There may be

Box 27.4: Check list of Visual Problems

Features

Dorsal stream dysfunction

Impaired ability to handle complex visual scenes* can cause difficulties with:

Finding a toy in a toy box.

Finding an object on a patterned background (Figure 27.3).

Finding an item of clothing in a pile of clothes.

Seeing a distant object (despite adequate acuity).

Identifying someone in a group.

Tendency to get lost in crowded locations.

Distress in busy shops and crowded places.

Reading.

Impaired visually guided movement (optic ataxia)

Upper limbs: Inaccurate visually guided reach, which may be compensated for by reaching beyond an object then gathering it up.

Lower limbs: Feeling with the foot for the height of the ground ahead at floor boundaries. Difficulty walking over uneven surfaces (Despite full visual field, and looking down.)

Impaired attention

Difficulty 'seeing' when talking at the same time, which may cause a child to trip or bump into obstacles.

Marked frustration at being distracted.

Ventral stream dysfunction

Impaired recognition

Difficulty recognising people and photographs.

Difficulty recognising shapes and objects.

Impaired orientation

Tendency to easily get lost in known locations.

Recommendations

Store toys separately (Figures 27.4 and 27.6).

Use plain carpets, bedspreads and decoration (Figure 27.5).

Store clothes separately in clear compartments.Get close.

Share a zoom video/digital camera view.

Identify through waving and speaking.

Training in seeking and identifying landmarks.

Visit shops when they are quiet.

Determine whether masking surrounding text improves reading ability.

Occupational therapy training.

Provision of tactile guides to the height of the ground ahead. For example pushing a toy pram or holding on to the belt pocket or elbow of an accompanying person.

Limit conversation when walking.

Limit distraction by reducing background clutter and background activity. (Performance may be enhanced at the 'quiet table' at school.)

Family and friends introduce themselves and wear consistent identifiers.

Training to identify and recognise identifiers.

Training in tactile, as well as visual, recognition.Training in orientation.

Reproduced from: Dutton GN, McKillop EC, Saidkasimova S. Visual problems as a result of brain damage in children. *Br J Ophthalmol.* 2006;90:932-3.

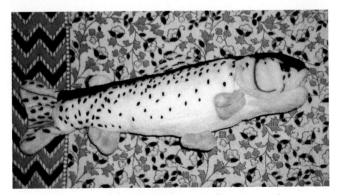

Fig. 27.3: Single toy on patterned background: visual information too complex

eso- or exo-, hyper- or hypo- deviation, representing convergence, divergence, depression and elevation of the eye respectively. Occasionally, a torsional abnormality is present. Most strabismus in children is concomitant, i.e. similar in magnitude in all positions of gaze. Incomitant strabismus varies in magnitude with gaze in different directions, and is associated with paresis or palsy of the third, fourth, or sixth cranial nerves. The commonest type of strabismus encountered in paediatric practice is a concomitant congenital esotropia, which may not present until 2-3 years of age.

Strabismus may be latent (termed a "phoria") and brought out only by dissociating the two eyes by alternate cover testing, or manifest (a "tropia") even before testing. It may be intermittent or constant, and there may be alternate fixation of each eye or, in large angle esotropia, or cross-fixation (in which the child uses the right eye to look to the left and the left eye to look to the right).

Amblyopia is both a cause and a consequence of strabismus, and should therefore be identified and treated as early as possible.

Uncorrected refractive error, particularly hypermetropia in young children, may cause strabismus.

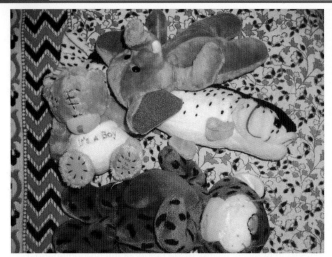

Fig. 27.4: Group of toys on patterned background: visual information too complex

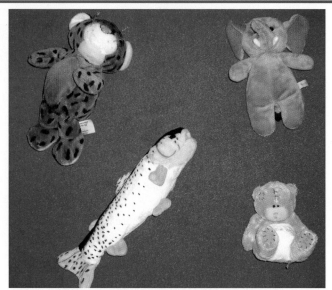

Fig. 27.6: Toys spaced out on plain background to simplify visual information

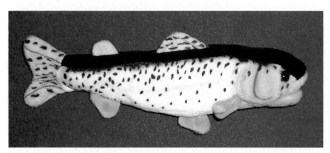

Fig. 27.5: Single toy on plain background: good contrast

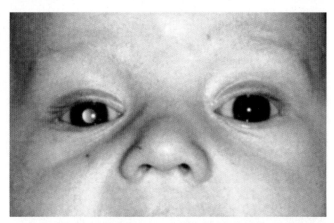

Fig. 27.7: Leukocoria: a white papillary reflex. Retinoblastoma must be excluded

A red reflex should be sought in every child with a squint because conditions such as cataract or retinoblastoma with reduced acuity (with or without amblyopia) can present with squint and may cause a white pupil (leukocoria) (Figure 27.7).

There is a higher incidence of strabismus following premature birth, in individuals with a positive family history of strabismus and in children with other developmental abnormalities.

Management

On diagnosing strabismus, findings on base-line examination are documented, including the magnitude of the deviation in prism dioptres, enabling comparison with future tests. The degree of stereopsis present is also noted as this affects the final prognosis of treatment.

Treatment of strabismus includes the following measures as indicated:

1. Accurate refractive correction, and ensuring that spectacles fit well, and are worn.

2. Treatment of underlying causes of amblyopia such as refractive error (as above) or cataract.

3. Treatment of amblyopia itself (in children under 7-8 years), by occlusion of the other eye, and detailed visual tasks given, such as drawing or reading.

4. Exercises to strengthen accommodative convergence and fusional range.

5. Surgery to re-align the visual axes by weakening and/ or strengthening the appropriate extraocular muscles by recession or resection of the muscle insertions. Due to the dynamic nature of extraocular muscle imbalance, a single surgical procedure may not suffice. Patients and their carers should always be prepared for the possibility of further surgery.

NYSTAGMUS

Nystagmus in children can be congenital or acquired

Congenital nystagmus has the following features:
- Onset during the first month of life.
- The meridian of the nystagmus is the same in each position of gaze (it is uniplanar).
- The nystagmus tends to be greater on distance fixation and least on near fixation.
- There is a position in which the nystagmus is least (the null position).
- There may be a head posture to place the eyes in the null position to optimise vision.
- Compensatory head nodding to stabilise the eyes can occur.

The causes of congenital nystagmus include:
- Idiopathic motor nystagmus, which may be idiopathic or inherited with dominant or recessive inheritance.
- Albinism (look for fair hair, pale complexion, iris transillumination, and macular hypoplasia)
- X-linked ocular albinism (most commonly in boys) (In this condition there is patchy iris transillumination, but the hair may be dark coloured and the skin pigmented).
- Congenital stationary night blindness in which there is poor rod photoreceptor function (ask whether the child can see in dark conditions)
- Achromatopsia in which there is rapid fine horizontal nystagmus (ask whether the child is photophobic and sees better in dark conditions than in daylight)
- Optic nerve hypoplasia (look for small optic nerve heads)
- Achiasmia (look for bitemporal visual field impairment)
- Damage in the occipital area of the brain, in particular damage to the white matter (posterior peri-ventricular leukomalacia).

Acquired nystagmus has the following features:
- The key feature is that the pattern of nystagmus is not uniplanar and is different in different positions of gaze.
- The causes of acquired nystagmus include loss of vision, tumours in the region of the chiasm and posterior fossa tumours.

Clinical Assessment of Patients With Nystagmus

History taking seeks a family history and determines whether vision is worse in dark or daylight conditions. A history of premature birth may suggest periventricular leukomalacia.

As in all patients with an eye problem vision is assessed.

The pattern of nystagmus is assessed in each position of gaze. If the nystagmus is uniplanar then it is very likely to be congenital in origin. If it is not, and the pattern of nystagmus is different in different positions of gaze, imaging of the brain must be carried out to seek evidence of organic pathology such as tumours in the region of the chiasm or brainstem.

Eye examination seeks evidence of blinding pathology such as cataract, iris transillumination, macular hypoplasia, optic nerve hypoplasia and optic atrophy.

Investigation by electroretinography detects rod and cone photoreceptor dysfunction. Visual evoked potentials may be delayed and reduced in amplitude if there is pathology affecting the visual pathways or the brain. Brain imaging is carried out if pathology is suspected.

Management

Vision is optimised by spectacle correction if required for refractive error. Treatable blinding pathology is identified and treated (e.g. cataract). Nystagmus reduces visual function, which may require appropriate action to be taken to ensure that school material is enlarged or magnified.

INTRAUTERINE INFECTIOUS DISEASES

Maternally transmitted infections can be remembered by the acronym TORCHES. Toxoplasmosis, rubella, cytomegalovirus, herpesviruses including the Epstein-Barr virus, and syphilis. These infections have a broad range of presentations, from subclinical forms to severe organ damage. Continuous tissue damage can occur throughout life; therefore long-term follow-up is necessary.

Toxoplasmosis

Toxoplasma gondii is an obligate intracellar protozoan parasite. Feline animals are the definitive hosts. Infected rodents, farm animals, birds, and humans serve as the intermediate hosts. Cats shed millions of oocysts in their faeces, and when these oocysts are then ingested by the intermediate host, the cyst wall dissolves releasing actively dividing tachyzoites. These are transported via intestinal lymphatics to various organs. Dissemination occurs to liver, lung, heart muscles and eyes. Once host immunity is established, the organisms transform to bradyzoites contained within tissue cysts. Bradyzoites lie dormant within the tissues of the intermediate host and when conditions are favourable, cause reactivated infection. The stimulus for local reactivation of an infected cyst is unknown. Humans are infected when they ingest oocysts or contaminated meat containing tissue cysts. Other modes of infection are transplacental transmission, organ transplantation and blood product transfusion.

Clinical features: Systemic infection is mild and usually goes undiagnosed. Clinical features include fever, headache, sore throat and diffuse lymphadenopathy. If the mother is acutely infected during pregnancy, transplacental transmission can occur. Congenital toxoplasmosis is described as a triad of convulsions, cerebral calcification and retinochoroiditis. If the foetus is infected in the first trimester, the resultant illness may be severe, with microcephaly, seizures and hepatosplenomegaly. Ocular manifestations include retinochoroiditis, often involving the macula, iritis, anterior and posterior uveitis, optic atrophy, strabismus and nystagmus. Infections acquired later in gestation are less severe and may be asymptomatic. Strabismus and poor vision are due to macular scarring, which can be bilateral. Many cases of "acquired" toxoplasma retinochoroiditis are due to reactivation of a congenitally acquired infection. The active area of retinochoroiditis is often at the edge of an old flat atrophic scar, a so-called satellite lesion.

Diagnosis: It is primarily clinical-based on characteristic retinal lesions. The presence of IgG or IgM antibodies in serum can be detected by ELISA (Enzyme-linked immunosorbent assay). Any positive testing, even undiluted, is significant. The presence of IgM in the infant serum is evidence of congenital infection because maternal IgM does not cross the placenta. Indications for treatment include a lesion threatening the macula or optic nerve head and severe vitritis. All immuno-compromised patients should be treated.

Treatment: Triple drug therapy is commonly used and consists of pyrimethamine (50 mg loading dose, then 25 mg orally twice daily), sulfadiazine (1g orally four times a day) and prednisolone (20 to 40 mg or more, started 1-2 days after the other drugs). Pyrimethamine can cause thrombo-cytopenia, leucopenia and folate deficiency. The drug is used only in combination with oral folinic acid (3-5 mg orally three times per week) to counteract the side effects. Weekly blood counts are required during therapy. Alternative drugs that can be used are co-trimoxazole (septrin), azithromycin and clindamycin. Atovaquone has been used mainly for immunocompromised patients (Figs 27.8 and 27.9).

Rubella (German measles)

Rubella is a relatively mild illness in the postnatal period, but results in a variety of abnormalities when acquired congenitally. Maternal infection acquired in the first trimester carries the greatest risk of complications. Systemic manifestations include congenital heart diseases, deafness, dental deformities, mental retardation, hydrocephalus, spina bifida, seizures and spasticity. Ocular abnormalities from rubella are microphthalmos, nuclear cataract, glaucoma, optic nerve abnormalities and retinopathy, which vary from salt and pepper retinal pigment epithelial disturbance to an appearance of pseudoretinitis pigmentosa. The incidence of the disease has come down worldwide with the institution of routine vaccination (Figs. 27.10).

Diagnosis: It is based on a characteristic clinical picture, which may include any of the above features, and is supported by positive serum titres of antibody against the rubella virus. However, a negative antibody titre does not rule out rubella as antibodies may disappear with time.

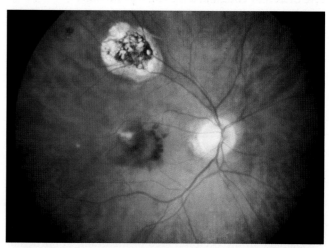

Fig. 27.9: Toxoplasma retinochoroiditis showing active and inactive lesions

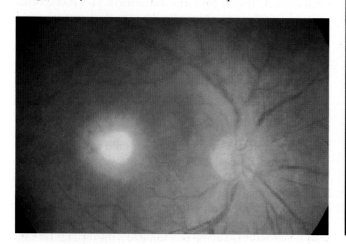

Fig. 27.8: Active toxoplasma retinochoroiditis

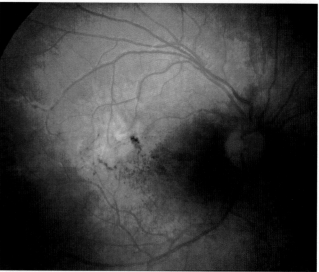

Fig. 27.10: Rubella "salt and pepper" retinopathy – may also be evident in the mid-peripheral retina

Treatment: Rubella cataract is managed by lensectomy. Intense postoperative inflammation may follow and requires adequate control with topical steroids.

Cytomegalovirus

Cytomegalovirus belongs to the herpes family. Infections may occur transplacentally, during birth, through breastfeeding or from other infected children who continue asymptomatic secretion of the virus. Immunocompromised children may acquire the infection through blood transfusion, chemotherapy or organ transplantation.

Congenital CMV presents with jaundice, hepatosplenomegaly, thrombocytopenia and anaemia. Typically there is microcephaly or hydrocephalus. Ocular manifestations include keratitis, uveitis, cataract, retinochoroiditis, optic nerve abnormalities and microphthalmos. The keratitis may manifest as punctate epithelial lesions, or as a dendritic, or geographical ulcer. Stromal keratitis presents as a zone of epithelial oedema with stromal thickening and keratic precipitates. Retinal involvement consists of bilateral progressive white areas of retinitis, exudates associated with haemorrhage, vasculitis, vitritis and necrosis (Fig. 27.11).

Diagnosis: It is based on clinical presentation, confirmed with viral cultures and PCR (Polymerase chain reaction) based assays.

Treatment: Of epithelial keratitis is with topical acyclovir ointment 3%. Ganiciclovir gel 0.15% and trifluorothymidine 1% drops are other effective agents. Stromal keratitis requires combined therapy with topical steroids, anti-viral agents. Disseminated disease and posterior segment involvement require intravenous antivirals such as acyclovir.

Syphilis

Syphilis is a sexually transmitted infection caused by a *Spirochaeta*, *Treponema pallidum*. Transplacental infection occurs following maternal spirochaetaemia.

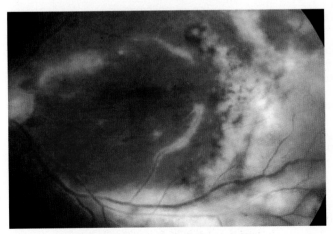

Fig. 27.11: Cytomegalovirus retinitis

Ocular manifestations are anterior uveitis, interstitial keratitis and pigmentary retinopathy. Malformed peg-shaped incisors, with nerve deafness and interstitial keratitis constitute Hutchinson's triad. Other signs include frontal bossing, a short maxilla, prognathism, a high arched palate, a saddle-shaped nose and linear scars around body orifices.

Diagnosis: Is by the Venereal Disease Research Laboratory test (VDRL), the Fluorescent Treponemal Antibody Absorption (FTA-ABS) test, or a Micro-haemagglutination assay with *Treponema pallidum* antigen (MHA-TP).

Treatment: Of congenital syphilis in neonates younger than 1 month consists of aqueous crystalline penicillin G, 50,000 units/kg given intravenously every 12 hours for one week and then every 8 hours for a total of 10-14 days. Infants older than one month require aqueous crystalline penicillin G every 6 hrs for 10-14 days. Serological tests should be repeated and persistent positive titres at 6 months require re-treatment.

Ophthalmia Neonatorum (Neonatal conjunctivitis)

Ophthalmia neonatorum is a conjunctivitis that occurs within the first month of life. Chemical conjunctivitis due to treatment with silver nitrate used to be the commonest cause. However, prophylaxis with silver nitrate is now almost obsolete.

Neonatal conjunctivitis is caused by exposure to organisms in the birth canal. The common pathogens causing this condition are gonococcus, chlamydia and herpes simplex. Other infectious agents include *Streptococcus*, *Staphylococcus, Haemophilus*, etc. Any discharge from a newborn infant's eye is pathological and should be taken seriously. Tear production is present from birth but does not become obvious until the infant is a few weeks of age.

Gonococcal Conjunctivitis

Because of effective antenatal screening and prophylaxis, the incidence of gonococcal conjunctivitis has decreased markedly in affluent countries. In developing countries, however, gonococcal conjunctivitis continues to be a significant problem. Most serious gonococcal conjunctivitis is caused by *Neisseria gonorrhoeae* and presents within forty-eight hours of birth. There is marked lid oedema, mucopurulent discharge, severe chemosis and intense conjunctival congestion. Gonococcus has the power to invade intact corneal epithelium and cause corneal ulceration. Unless effectively treated, ulceration can progress rapidly leading to perforation of the cornea, iris prolapse and lens extrusion. If the corneal ulceration heals with or without perforation, corneal scarring and opacification occur, causing reduced vision or loss of vision.

Diagnosis: Gram staining of conjunctival scrapings reveals gram-negative intracellular diplococci.

Treatment: Topical erythromycin ointment 2-4 hourly and intravenous or intramuscular Ceftriaxone 30-50 mg/kg/day in divided doses, are the treatment of choice. Gentamicin drops hourly and penicillin G injections 50,000 units/kg/day every 12 hours for 7 days are an effective alternative treatment. However, penicillin-resistant gonococci may be involved.

Chlamydia Conjunctivitis

Chlamydiae are a relatively common cause of ophthalmia neonatorum. Onset is usually at age 4-10 days. Causative agents are *Chlamydia trachomatis* and *Chlamydia oculogenitalis* (called trachoma-inclusion conjunctivitis or TRIC). Lid oedema, chemosis and conjunctival congestion are less severe than in gonococcal conjunctivitis. Since infants do not have a subconjunctival adenoid layer, follicles do not appear. Pseudomembranes and superficial keratitis occur.

Diagnosis: Conjunctival scrapings, stained with Giemsa's stain, show intracytoplasmic inclusion bodies. Enzyme-linked immunoassays and direct immunofluorescent antibody tests are available.

Treatment: The treatment of chlamydial conjunctivitis includes topical erythromycin ointment 3-4 times/ day or ciprofloxacin drops 2-3 hourly along with oral erythromycin 30-50/kg/day in divided doses.

Herpes Simplex

Most cases of neonatal herpetic conjunctivitis are due to Herpes simplex type II, but approximately one third are caused by Herpes simplex type I. The onset is usually between 1 and 2 weeks after birth. Presenting signs are a watery discharge and conjunctival injection. Fluorescein staining of the cornea shows punctuate keratitis or dendritic ulceration.

Diagnosis: Diagnosis is clinical, with conjunctival scrapings taken for viral culture and PCR in the absence of dendritic corneal ulceration.

Treatment: Acyclovir 3% eye ointment is instilled 5 times a day. Systemic acyclovir is advised for recurrent viral keratitis and when there is systemic involvement.

Prophylaxis for ophthalmia neonatorum: Agents effective against both gonococci and TRIC, for example, erythromycin ointment, can be used prophylactically in the newborn (Box 27.5).

ORBITAL CELLULITIS

The orbit is a pear-shaped cavity surrounded by bony walls, tapering posteriorly into the orbital apex and the optic canal, which contains the optic nerve. The cavity contains the globe, extraocular muscles, nerves, blood vessels, fibrous tissue and fat. The orbit is surrounded by the paranasal sinuses. The ethmoid air cells begin to develop in the second trimester and maxillary sinuses by 2 years of life. The frontal sinus develops between the fifteenth and seventeenth year. Infection from the sinuses spreads easily to the orbit through incomplete bony walls and the valveless veins of the orbit and sinuses.

Box 27.5: Prophylaxis for Ophthalmia Neonatorum			
Onset	Organism	Diagnosis	Treatment
2-4 days	*N.gonorrhoeae*	Gram negative diplococci	Ceftriaxone IM or IV Penicillin G IV Topical erythromycin Topical gentamicin
4-10 days	*Chlamydia*	Giemsa stains for basophilic inclusion bodies. Positive direct immunofluorescent assay.	Oral erythromycin Erythromycin eye ointment. Ciprofloxacin eye ointment.
4-7 days	Other bacteria (streptococci or staphylococci)	Gram positive cocci in pairs or chains	Neomycin – bacitracin ointment or Gentamicin eye drops
5-7 days	Herpes simplex	Viral culture, PCR Virus (HSV II)	Acyclovir 3% eye ointment Systemic acyclovir

Other sources of infection are facial skin, ear, and teeth direct inoculations after trauma and bacteraemic spread from a distant focus. Since the orbit is surrounded by bony walls. Infection and inflammation cause increase in intra-orbital pressure leading to compromise of ocular and optic nerve is functioning with small complications are cavernous sinus thromboses, intracranial abscess. Therefore, orbital cellulites must be promptly recognised and aggressively treated.

Classification: Orbital cellulitis can be classified into five stages as described by Chandler

1. Preseptal cellulitis: Inflammation confined to the eyelids with mild anterior orbital involvement. Ocular motility and viral function are normal.
2. Orbital cellulitis: The four cardinal signs of orbital involvement are eyelid oedema, chemosis proptosis and loss of motility. Visual impairment may occur.
3. Sub-periosteal abscess: Collection of pus within the sub-periosteal space causes local tenderness,fluctuation and non-axial proptosis.
4. Orbital abscess: Progression of cellulitis leads to intra-conal and extra-conal loculation of pus. Proptosis, inflammatory signs, ophthalmoplegia, visual deficit and systemic toxicity are increased at this stage.
5. Cavernous sinus thrombosis: Proptosis progresses rapidly and frequently becomes bilateral, and changes in mental state occur. Meningitis or intracranial abscess may follow. Inflammatory cells are present on lumbar puncture.

Diagnosis: The commonest organism causing orbital cellulitis is *Staphylococcus aureus*, followed by *H. influenzae* and *M. catarrhalis*.

Management: All children with orbital cellulitis (any stage) must be admitted to hospital and investigations performed to identify the source of infection. Material for culture and gram's stained smear should be taken from the abscesses or nasopharynx. Signs of central nervous system involvement warrant lumbar puncture. Blood cultures are taken if leucocytosis and fever are present.

Treatment: The antibiotic of choice for children with orbital cellulitis is parenteral cefuroxime, 100 mg/kg/day divided into three or four doses. The drug penetrates well into the soft tissues, bones and cerebrospinal fluid. Alternative regimens include Inj. Cloxacillin 100-150 mg/kg/day and gentamicin 3-5 mg/kg/day. If there is no response within 24 hours, the plan of management should quickly proceed to CT scan of the orbit and sinuses. If there is no direct site of inoculation seen, adequate drainage of a sinusitis abscess should be performed to prevent complications. The condition should be managed jointly by the ophthalmologist, paediatrician and neurologist, if necessary (Fig. 27.12).

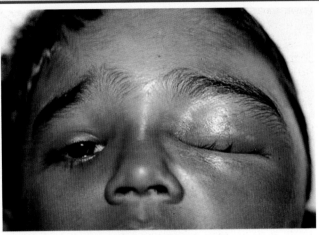

Fig. 27.12: Left orbital cellulites

ALLERGIC CONJUNCTIVITIS

Allergic conjunctivitis is a type I hypersensitivity reaction caused by interaction between allergens and IgE antibodies on the surface of mast cells in the conjunctiva. This interaction causes degranulation of mast cells and release of mast cell mediators. The mediators that are implicated in allergic ocular disease include histamine, leukotrienes, eosinophilic chemotactic factors (ECF), eosinophilic granule major basic protein (EMBP), platelet-activating factor (PAF), prostaglandin D2 (PGD2) and several other less well-defined factors. The hallmark of allergic ocular disease is itching and hyperaemia. The chronic, recurrent and seasonal nature of the disease is characteristic. Affected children often have a history of asthma, allergic rhinitis and atopic dermatitis.

Seasonal allergic conjunctivitis (Hay fever conjunctivitis): Airborne allergens such as pollen, moulds, dander, grasses and weeds trigger a hypersensitivity reaction. As the name suggests the conjunctivitis is seasonal. Patients present with watering, conjunctival hyperaemia and chemosis.

Vernal keratoconjunctivitis: Is a severe form of IgE-mediated mast cell dependent, type I hypersensitivity reaction. The onset of the disease is usually between 3 and 4 years of age. It can last 4- 10 years with exacerbations and remissions. Symptoms include photophobia, severe itching, foreign body sensation and watering of the eyes. Vernal conjunctivitis is divided into two types, palpebral and bulbar. Both types can coexist. The palpebral form has hypertrophied papillae, most prominently over the upper palpebral conjunctiva, the so-called cobblestone appearance. The conjunctiva has a milky hue and thick, ropy, white discharge. The bulbar form has nodules or gelatinous thickening of the conjunctiva along the limbus. Corneal involvement in vernal conjunctivitis includes punctate

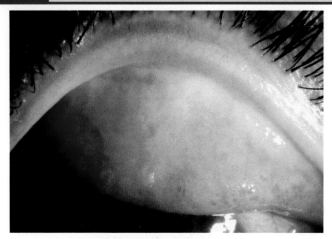

Fig. 27.13: Allergic conjunctivitis

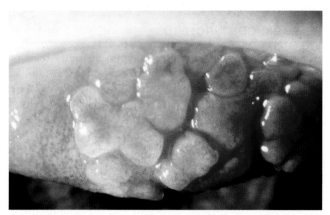

Fig. 27.14: Giant papillae in vernal conjunctivitis

epithelial erosions, which can progress to form a sterile ulcer, called a shield ulcer, on the upper part of the cornea (Figs 27.13 and 27.14).

Atopic keratoconjunctivitis: Atopic keratoconjunctivitis is relatively rare in children, usually affecting young men with atopic dermatitis. Ocular symptoms and signs are similar to vernal keratocojunctivitis. Unlike vernal kerato-conjunctivitis, the inferior palpebral conjunctiva can be involved.

Treatment: Treatment of all ocular allergic diseases is basically similar. It is often impossible to identify and remove the allergens. Therefore, therapy is directed towards relief of symptoms. Topical eye drops are the mainstay of therapy. The therapeutic agents employed are

1. Mast cell stabilizers: e.g.: Sodium cromoglicate, Lodoxamide and Nedocromil sodium.
2. H_1-reception antagonists: e.g.: Emedastine difumarate.
3. Agents with both mast cell stabilizer activity and H_1-receptor blocking activity: e.g.: Olopatadine hydrochloride and Ketotifen fumarate.

Other useful agents include nonsteroidal anti-inflammatory agents (NSAIDS) and topical steroids, although the risk of steroid-induced glaucoma and cataract limits the use of steroids to short intervals. Cyclosporin 2% may be useful in steroid-resistant cases, but is not widely available.

LACRIMAL SYSTEM

Anatomy: The lacrimal system consists of epithelium-lined passages that drain tears from each eye to the nasal cavity. Tears enter a punctum at the medial end of each eyelid, proceed through the upper- and lower-canaliculi, which then form a common canaliculus on each side, and enter the lacrimal sac. This leads to the nasolacrimal duct, which opens into the inferior meatus of the nose beneath the inferior turbinate bone. The opening of the upper and lower canaliculi into the common canaliculus is guarded by one-way valve, the valve of Rosenmüller. The membranous opening into the nose is called the valve of Hasner.

Congenital Abnormalities of the Lacrimal Drainage System

Puncta: The puncta may be absent (atresia), rudimentary, or covered by epithelium.

Canaliculi: The canaliculi may be rudimentary or anomalous in position and number.

Amniocoele (Dacryocystocoele): If there is obstruction at the valve of Rosenmüller and also inferiorly at the nasolacrimal duct, the lacrimal sac becomes distended. This condition may be present at birth or in early infancy and is termed an amniocoele or dacryocystocoele. The distended sac may become secondarily infected, causing dacryocystitis (Fig. 27.15).

Management: Hydrostatic massage and topical antibiotics may resolve the condition. If the condition persists lacrimal probing should be done no later than one month.

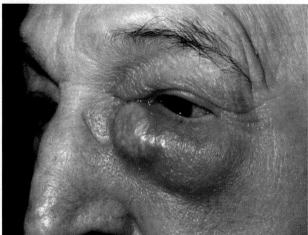

Fig. 27.15: Acute dacryocystitis

Congenital Nasolacrimal Duct Obstruction

Nasolacrimal duct (NLD) obstruction due to delayed canalization may occur, most often at the valve of Hasner. The clinician can elicit regurgitation of mucopurulent discharge with pressure over lacrimal sac area. The differential diagnosis of congenital NLD obstruction includes conditions which present with epiphora: punctal atresia, conjunctivitis, blepharitis, keratitis and congenital glaucoma.

Management: Conservative management includes lacrimal sac massage and administration of topical antibiotics. NLD obstruction resolves spontaneously in the majority of the cases. Beyond one year of age, the rate of spontaneous resolution is significantly reduced.

Surgical treatment: Early probing reduces the burden of conservative management and the potential for infection. However, delaying probing until one year age may avoid surgery altogether in many cases. The success rate of properly performed probing exceeds 90%. There is no convincing evidence that delaying probing until one to two years of age is harmful. However, after two years of age, simple probing may fail in as many as 30% of the cases.

Balloon catheter dilation: A lacrimal drainage system that appears to be blocked by scarring or constriction can be dilated by an inflatable balloon carried on a probe.

Intubation: Silicone tube intubation of the lacrimal system is usually recommended when one or more probings fail. The silicone tube should be left *in situ* for 3-6 months.

Dacryo-cysto-rhinostomy (DCR): DCR is indicated when repeated probings fail, when intubation cannot be accomplished and when significant symptoms recur after tube removal.

In this procedure, the sac wall is anastomosed to the nasal mucosa after creating a bony osteum, or defect, in the lacrimal fossa. The new passage thus opens from the lacrimal sac into the middle meatus of the nose (Fig. 27.16).

CORNEA

Embryology

The primitive cornea develops from surface ectoderm of the optic vesicle, and from neural crest cells, which migrate in waves over the surface of the primitive lens. The lens vesicle separates from surface ectoderm by six weeks gestation, and by four months gestation, the corneal endothelial layer is complete. However, the iris insertion at this stage is anterior to the primitive trabecular meshwork (neural crest cells), and gradual posterior migration continues until the end of the first year of life.

Abnormalities of neural crest cell migration, proliferation or differentiation may occur, and present as a spectrum of anterior dysgenesis syndromes.

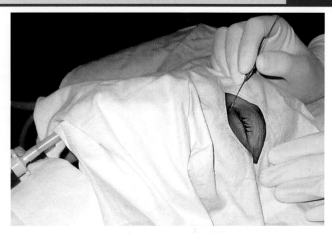

Fig. 27.16: Naso-lacrimal probing

Corneal Size and Shape in Childhood

In the neonate, the normal horizontal corneal diameter is 9.5–10.5 mm, which grows to reach 12 mm, the average adult corneal diameter, by the age of two years. Abnormalities of corneal size or shape may be evident at birth, and may show a characteristic inheritance pattern, or may occur sporadically. They may be associated with other abnormalities of the eye, and may be part of a syndrome affecting other systems of the body also (Box 27.6).

Causes of Corneal Opacity in Childhood

Corneal disease remains the commonest cause of childhood blindness in the world today.

In the developing world, poor nutrition and the inadequacy of public health measures such as the provision of sanitation and immunisation remain key factors. In more affluent countries, congenital anomalies of the cornea form a small but significant proportion of the blinding conditions in childhood.

The normal cornea is avascular and transparent, and the cause of any opacity, which may interfere with vision, must be diagnosed, and if possible, treated, at the earliest possible opportunity, to avoid irreversible damage and visual loss, or the development of amblyopia.

Xerophthalmia and Nutritional Corneal Ulceration or Keratomalacia

Xerophthalmia describes a dry ocular surface due to vitamin A deficiency, which may progress to keratomalacia, an acute keratitis due to untreated vitamin A deficiency, which in turn, if not treated urgently and adequately, progresses rapidly to corneal melting and perforation.

The earliest symptom of vitamin A deficiency is night blindness. This should be specifically asked about in consultations or in paediatric eye screening programmes, in developing countries. If vitamin A remains deficient, the

Box 27.6: Corneal size and shape in childhood

	Megalocornea	Keratoglobus	Keratoconus	Microcornea
Typical Features	Horizontal corneal diameter > 12 mm in neonate, or 13 mm in an older child. Usually bilateral.	Thinned, globular shaped cornea, with deep anterior chamber. Episodes of corneal oedema. Risk of corneal rupture with minor trauma.	Coning of the central or paracentral cornea due to progressive thinning. Often presents in adolescence, with gradual or rapid progression. Undetermined	Horizontal corneal diameter < 9 mm in the neonate, or 10 mm in an older child. In nanophthalmos, other ocular structures as the cornea, are smaller than normal. Sporadic, or autosomal dominant
Inheritance Pattern	X-linked recessive	Autosomal recessive		
Associations	Glaucoma, lens subluxation, iris hypoplasia and ectopic pupil	Ehlers-Danlos type IV syndrome	Down syndrome, other types of mental retardation. Atopy.	Cataract, coloboma, high myopia, persistent hyperplastic primary vitreous, oculo-dento-digital dysplasia syndrome.

conjunctiva becomes dry, with a wrinkled, reddened or pigmented appearance. Bitot's spots may form on the exposed conjunctiva, lateral, and sometimes medial, to the cornea. They appear like a triangular or irregular area of froth or tiny bubbles on the conjunctiva, sometimes with underlying pigmentation. Adequate treatment with vitamin A at this stage, and ensuring that inadequate dietary intake as well as conditions causing diarrhoea and vomiting are properly managed, can prevent the occurrence of keratomalacia and blindness. Conversely, neglect of early signs of vitamin A deficiency results in a high risk of adherent leukoma formation. A dense corneal scar develops, due to corneal perforation with adherence to the iris and lens, causing cataract. Secondary infection may result in endophthalmitis. The latter may be life-threatening, as is continuing, untreated vitamin A deficiency (Figs 27.17 and 27.18).

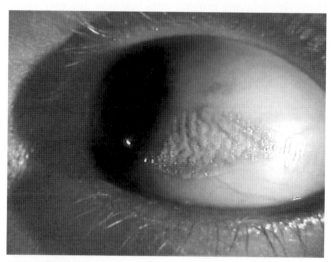

Fig. 27.17: Bitot's spots in vitamin A deficiency

World Health Organisation (WHO) Classification of Xerophthalmia

XN   Night blindness
X1A   Conjunctival xerosis
X1B   Bitot's spots
X2   Corneal xerosis
X3A   Corneal ulcer < one third of corneal surface
X3B   Corneal ulcer > one third of corneal surface
XS   Corneal scar
XF   Xerophthalmic fundus

If the deficiency is progressive, children may go through this spectrum of clinical signs. When there is a sudden increase in metabolic demand, as in the case of infections such as measles or diarrhoea, vitamin A deficiency may rapidly progress to keratomalacia without passing through the whole spectrum of clinical signs. Severe keratomalacia is usually seen in children below 5 years of age. Children between 6 months and 3 years are particularly at risk.

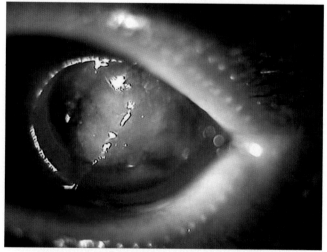

Fig. 27.18: Keratomalacia with corneal melt, due to vitamin A deficiency

Prevention: 2,00,000 IU of vitamin A should be administered orally every 6 months to children from 1 to 6 years of age. The first dose can be given at the time of MMR vaccination. Measles vaccination has played important role in the prevention of vitamin A related blindness. Vitamin A is teratogenic; therefore, administration is not advised in early pregnancy. It can be administered to women at delivery or within one month of delivery, and breast-feeding should be encouraged. Health education and improved nutrition, particularly with foods rich in vitamin A, contribute significantly to prevention of deficiency.

Keratomalacia: Keratomalacia is a medical emergency. The affected child requires hospitalization for adequate treatment.

Treatment schedule for vitamin A deficiency in keratomalacia:

Timing	< 1 year of age	> 1 year of age
On diagnosis	100, 000 IU	200,000 IU
Following day	100,000 IU	200,000 IU
2-4 weeks later	100,000 IU	200,000 IU

In addition secondary bacterial infection should be treated with combination antibiotic therapy (for example, gentamicin drops + cefazolin drops), and protein-calorie malnutrition and diarrhoea should be treated. Small punched out corneal ulcers which occur, usually heal well, but residual scarring may persist.

Infection of the cornea in childhood may be bacterial, viral or fungal.

- Ophthalmia neonatorum refers to neonatal conjunctivitis. If untreated, corneal infection and scarring may be a complication.
- In older children, minor corneal trauma or untreated conjunctivitis, particularly in the presence of malnutrition or other systemic illness, may cause corneal infection and ulceration, with subsequent corneal opacity.
- Measles keratitis remains a significant cause of corneal scarring and blindness in some regions, although measles immunisation and improved childhood nutrition have markedly reduced the incidence of measles and its complications.
- Trachoma, primarily an infection of the conjunctiva, can result in scarring of the tarsal conjunctiva, with consequent mis-directed eyelashes or trichiasis, which constantly rub against the cornea. This causes chronic irritation, sometimes with corneal ulceration and scarring.
- Herpes simplex keratitis is more commonly seen in young adults, but can occur in childhood, particularly in atopic individuals.

Injury due to birth trauma, which usually involves Descemet's membrane (the protective layer of the cornea, adjacent to the endothelium), may resolve spontaneously, or with simple measures to avoid infection if the epithelium is damaged, but may require subsequent correction of astigmatism and patching of the other eye, to overcome amblyopia.

Injury due to accidental trauma may also cause corneal scarring in childhood. Delayed treatment is likely to be associated with secondary infection and a worsening of prognosis. Agricultural injuries with secondary fungal infection and injuries (often gram negative or anaerobic infections) from pet animals may be particularly severe. In penetrating injuries, adequate tetanus immunisation should always be ensured.

Chemical injuries constitute an emergency where time is of essence. Immediate, copious irrigation of the injured eye, including the upper conjunctival fornix (the area under the upper eyelid) with buffered saline or Ringer's lactate where possible, but with clean water if that is all that is available, can save an eye and its sight, which may otherwise be lost. Acids cause coagulation of surface proteins on the cornea with rapid scarring, whereas alkalis penetrate rapidly into the eye causing widespread destruction of intraocular tissues as well as of the ocular surface. Prompt and prolonged irrigation of the eye dilutes and removes such chemicals from the ocular surface, thereby preventing or minimising these types of destruction.

Congenital glaucoma can present with cloudy or opaque corneas, which are usually also enlarged. The raised intraocular pressure initially causes enlargement of the globe, which, in infants, is relatively elastic. Without treatment, however, the disease progresses causing atrophy of the optic nerve, and irreversible visual loss. This condition must always be considered, therefore, in the presence of hazy or opaque corneas, in order that early treatment can be instituted, and blindness prevented (Fig. 27.19).

Dermoids on the cornea, usually extending from across the rim, or limbus of the cornea (most commonly

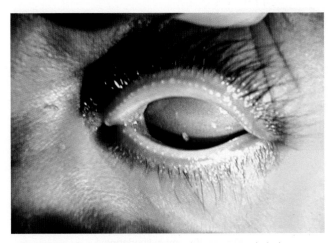

Fig. 27.19: Enlarged, hazy cornea due to congenital glaucoma

infero-temporally), consist of hamartomatous fibrofatty tissue and keratinised epithelium. They sometimes contain skin appendages such as hair follicles, sebaceous glands and sweat glands, and may be up to a centimetre in diameter. They may involve the corneal stroma, but not usually the whole thickness of the cornea. Large dermoids may cover the visual axis, thereby occluding vision. Smaller ones may result in astigmatism (as may surgical excision), which, uncorrected can cause amblyopia (Fig. 27.20).

Anterior segment dysgenesis includes a spectrum of developmental genetic anomalies of peripheral and central anterior segment structures, the more severe of which include corneal scarring. The peripheral developmental anomalies include posterior embryotoxon, and Axenfeld-Rieger syndrome. The central developmental anomalies include posterior corneal depression and Peter's anomaly. In Peter's anomaly, there is a posterior corneal defect with a central stromal opacity, with iris strands often adherent to its posterior surface. The opacity may lessen with time.

Sclerocornea is a congenital condition in which, as its name suggests, the cornea is opaque and appears undifferentiated from the sclera. Flattening of the cornea may also occur. The condition is often associated with other ocular or systemic abnormalities.

Mucopolysaccharidoses and mucolipidoses constitute a varied group of conditions with lysosomal disorders, resulting in a range of mucopolysaccharides or mucolipids not being broken down and therefore accumulating in the tissues. Some of these conditions manifest ocular abnormalities. In Hurler's syndrome (mucopolysaccharidosis IH) and in Scheie's syndrome (mucopolysaccharidosis IS), corneal clouding occurs within the first 6 months to 2 years of life. In mucolipidosis IV, corneal clouding may occur in the first few weeks of life. In these conditions, electron microscopy on conjunctival biopsies reveals abnormal cytoplasmic inclusions.

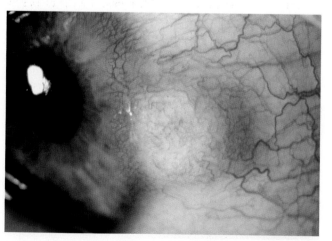

Fig. 27.20: Limbal lipodermoid

Congenital Hereditary Endothelial Dystrophy (CHED) manifests in the early days of life. It is a defect of the endothelial layer of the cornea and of the adjacent Descemet's layer, resulting in diffuse oedema of the epithelial and stromal layers of the cornea. The cornea is, therefore, thickened and hazy, and must be differentiated from congenital glaucoma, where the corneal diameter is usually increased and the intraocular pressure is elevated. CHED is a rare inherited condition, which may be autosomal dominant or autosomal recessive.

Treatment of Corneal Opacities in Childhood

Treatment of corneal injuries, infections and damage due to vitamin A deficiency must be prompt and adequate in order to preserve, or restore sight. In many situations, there may be astigmatism or corneal scarring despite repair, resolution of infection, or restoration of adequate levels of vitamin A in the body. Refractive correction of astigmatism can then be undertaken, or corneal grafting if appropriate.

Corneal grafting requires special care and expertise in children, and the final visual outcome maybe poorer than one would hope. Furthermore, since deprivation amblyopia has been found to be best reversed by treatment of the underlying cause within the first 3 months of life, the surgery, and the anaesthesia required, may be more complex than if performed later. Some studies have shown less corneal rejection, and a better final visual outcome if surgery is delayed until approximately one year after birth.

Where treatment of corneal opacities is not possible, support of the child and the family is essential, with appropriate advice and information given, and all possible rehabilitation measures put in place to enable the child to live as full a life as possible, and to avoid the additional risks and possible harm associated with poor sight.

SYSTEMIC DISEASES WITH CORNEAL MANIFESTATIONS IN CHILDHOOD

Congenital Syphilis

Interstitial keratitis secondary to congenital syphilis may present during the first 10 years of life, with corneal oedema and aggressive vascularisation of the deep stromal layer of the cornea, giving it a pink appearance ("salmon patch"). Blood flow through these vessels gradually stop over a period of weeks to months, leaving greyish white "ghost" vessels visible deep in the stroma, which are evident throughout life.

Leprosy

Although the prevalence of leprosy has diminished dramatically over the past 15 years, new cases continue to be diagnosed in children, and may result in impairments such as lagophthalmos and impaired corneal sensation.

Neurotrophic keratitis, and exposure keratitis may both result in corneal opacity, and secondary infective keratitis can cause more severe corneal damage or corneal perforation and endophthalmitis. Corneal lepromas (granulomatous lesions which develop as a response to the presence of *Mycobacterium leprae*) are now rare, but chronic iritis my result in band keratopathy – a condition that occurs in eyes with chronic inflammation, in which calcific material is deposited in a band-shaped area across the cornea.

The Mucopolysaccharidoses

All of the mucopolysaccharidoses cause varying degrees of corneal haziness due to deposits in the cornea, except for Hunter's syndrome (mucopolysaccharidosis II) (see previous section).

Hepatolenticular Degeneration (Wilson's disease)

Wilson's disease is an inborn error of metabolism in which excess copper deposition occurs in the liver, kidney, and basal ganglia of the brain. Inheritance is autosomal recessive, and clinical features include cirrhosis of the liver, renal tubular damage, and a type of parkinsonism. A copper coloured ring (the Kayser-Fleischer ring) in Descemet's layer of the cornea is a diagnostic feature of established disease, but may not be present in the early stages. Copper deposits are first seen in the 12 and 6 o'clock positions, and then form a complete ring.

Cystinosis

Cystinosis is a rare, metabolic disease in which intracellular cystine levels are elevated, resulting in the deposition of cystine crystals in various parts of the body. In infants, failure to thrive, rickets and progressive renal failure occur, and are known as the Fanconi's syndrome. Ocular features develop in the first year of life, and include the deposition of crystals in the peripheral cornea and throughout Descemet's layer, as well as on the anterior iris surface and in the conjunctiva. Photophobia occurs. Oral cysteamine reduces systemic crystal deposition and is more effective than topical cysteamine, which is also difficult to obtain (Fig. 27.21).

Familial Dysautonomia (Riley-Day syndrome)

This is an autosomal recessive condition seen largely in Ashkenazi Jews. There is autonomic dysfunction with relative insensitivity to pain and temperature instability.

Abnormal lacrimation and decreased corneal sensation result in exposure keratitis and frequent corneal ulceration with secondary opacity. Topical artificial tear preparations and tarsorrhaphies may protect the corneas to some extent.

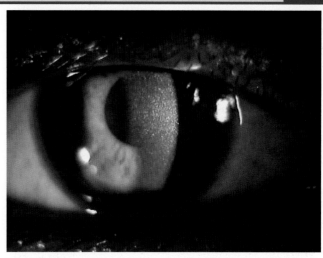

Fig. 27.21: Deposition of cystine crystals in the cornea in cystinosis

CHILDHOOD LENS DISORDERS

Childhood lens abnormalities include cataract, subluxation, and abnormal lens shape and development. These abnormalities continue to be an important cause of visual impairment. Lens disorders can be the presenting sign of systemic abnormalities involving the central nervous system, the urinary tract and the skin.

Paediatric Cataracts

The cause of most cataracts is unknown. They are most commonly inherited in an autosomal dominant pattern, but x-linked and autosomal recessive types have been reported. Trisomy 13, 18 and 21 are associated with cataracts. The onset, location and morphology of cataracts provide important information regarding their cause and likely visual outcome following surgery. Cataracts that present at birth are most serious, because the visual system is still immature. Amblyopia is inevitable unless the visual axis is rendered clear by 6-8 weeks of age. Unilateral cataracts tend to cause denser amblyopia because of the rivalry between the two eyes.

Morphological Classification of Cataracts

Cataracts can be classified as:
- **Anterior** (Anterior polar cataract, anterior subcapsular and anterior lenticonus).
- **Lamellar**
- **Nuclear**
- **Posterior** (Posterior lenticonus, Persistent hyperplastic primary vitreous, posterior subcapsular cataract).

Anterior Cataract

Anterior polar cataract is a small white discrete opacity at the centre of the anterior capsule. These opacities are usually non-progressive and visually insignificant. One third of them are bilateral. Most of them can be managed conservatively. However, because they can be associated with strabismus, anisometropia and amblyopia, follow up is necessary.

Anterior pyramidal cataract is a white conical opacity at the anterior pole. These cataracts are usually bilateral and are not associated with any systemic disease.

Anterior subcapsular cataract lies immediately under the anterior capsule of the lens in the anterior cortex. Such cataracts are usually idiopathic. However, the possibility of trauma or Alport's syndrome should be considered. Lens changes in Alport's syndrome consist of bilateral anterior subcapsular cataract and bilateral anterior lenticonus.

Lamellar Cataract

Lamellar cataracts occupy specific zones in the lens and have spoke-like radial opacities. Most lamellar cataracts progress and require surgery. These may be unilateral or bilateral. Bilateral lamellar cataracts are frequently inherited in an autosomal dominant manner. Metabolic diseases such as neonatal hypoglycemia and galactosaemia can cause bilateral lamellar cataracts (Fig. 27.22).

Nuclear Cataract

Nuclear cataract is an opacity located within the embryonic or foetal nucleus. These cataracts can be unilateral or bilateral. Bilateral nuclear cataracts are often inherited according to an autosomal dominant pattern. Intrauterine rubella infection causes a distinctive nuclear cataract with a "shaggy" appearance. Visual prognosis in these cataracts is only fair, even after early surgery.

Posterior Cataract

Posterior lenticonus is almost always unilateral and can cause myopia and astigmatism. Therefore, it is important to monitor vision and prescribe appropriate optical correction to prevent amblyopia.

Persistent hyperplastic primary vitreous (PHPV) is caused by failure of regression of the primitive hyaloid vascular system. PHPV occurs sporadically, is almost always unilateral and is associated with microphthalmia. Clinically there is a retrolenticular fibrovascular membrane, which extends to the optic disc as a stalk. The membrane may contract, push the lens-iris diaphragm anteriorly and cause glaucoma. **Posterior subcapsular cataracts** in children are often stellate, or rosette-shaped, and secondary to trauma or steroid-induced. They affect vision significantly and require surgery, for which the visual prognosis is excellent (Figs 27.23 and 27.24).

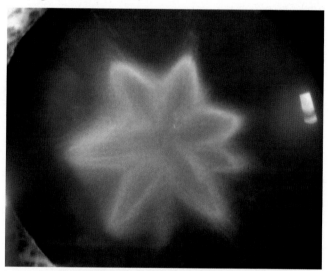

Fig. 27.23: Stellate cataract

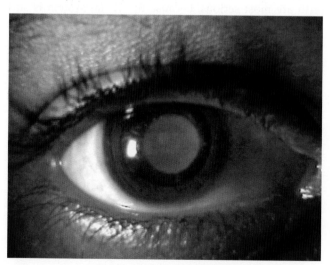

Fig. 27.22: Lamellar cataract

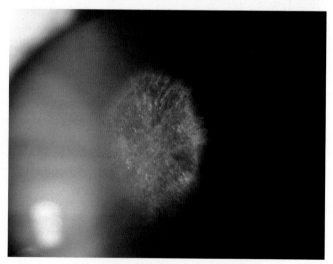

Fig. 27.24: Steroid-induced cataract

Evaluation of Cataract

Examination in a darkened room is performed by shining the light of a direct ophthalmoscope into both eyes simultaneously, in order to detect normal, symmetrical red reflexes. This test is called Bruckner's test. Any central opacity or surrounding cortical distortion more than 3 mm is considered to have a significant effect on vision. Taking a family history is important in order to elicit whether there is an autosomal dominant or X-linked pattern of inherited cataract. General physical examination in addition to examination of the anterior and posterior segments of the eye is required. Unilateral cataracts are generally not metabolic or genetic in origin, and therefore laboratory tests are not helpful, except a TORCHES titre (see intrauterine infectious disease). Laboratory tests, however, can provide valuable information in bilateral cataracts, particularly is Lowe's syndrome and galactosaemia. Recommended tests include: urine test for reducing substances after milk feeding, TORCH titre and VDRL test. Other optional tests include urine test for amino acids, and blood tests for calcium, phosphorus and red-cell galactokinase level.

Surgery

The most important surgical options are lensectomy or the removal of lens matter through a capsulorhexis. Intraocular lens implantation (IOL) at the same time in infants remains controversial. Intraocular lens implantation is recommended in children above age 2 years. Because rapid posterior capsule opacification occurs, a controlled moderate posterior capsulotomy and anterior vitrectomy should be performed at the time of surgery. This allows establishment of a clear visual axis, facilitating accurate retinoscopy and subsequent fitting of an appropriate optical correction. Optical rehabilitation is important to avoid amblyopia. If an IOL is not inserted at surgery, aphakic spectacles or contact lenses are required. Aphakic spectacles are the safest and can be easily changed according to the refractive requirement. Contact lenses provide more constant refractive correction but are less easily changed, may be displaced by eye rubbing, and can pose a risk of infection and corneal ulcer. If an intraocular lens is inserted, it is important to ensure that it is placed within the lens capsule ("in the bag"). Children often require spectacle correction, especially for reading in spite of the intraocular lens. All children need long-term follow-up for changes in refractive status, amblyopia management, intraocular pressure monitoring and posterior segment evaluation.

A good visual outcome depends on the timing of surgery, appropriate optical correction and adequate treatment of amblyopia. In general, children with bilateral cataracts achieve a better final visual outcome than those with a unilateral cataract.

Dislocation of the Lens

When the lens is not in the normal position, it is said to be subluxated or dislocated. The signs of lens subluxation are iridodonesis (a shimmering movement of the iris due to lens movement posterior to it), phakodonesis (a shimmering movement of the lens) and visibility of the lens edge within the pupil. Important systemic conditions associated with subluxated lenses are:

1. Marfan's syndrome
2. Homocytinuria
3. Weill-Marchesani syndrome
4. Hyperlisenemia
5. Sulphite oxidase deficiency
6. Ehlers-Danlos syndrome

Subluxated lenses may remain stable, and satisfactory vision can be achieved with an appropriate astigmatic, or hypermetropic (aphakic) spectacle correction. In other situations, where the subluxation is unstable, or progressive, lens extraction may be indicated to avoid complications such as dislocation into the anterior chamber and secondary glaucoma (Figs 27.25 to 27.27).

PAEDIATRIC GLAUCOMA

Childhood glaucomas may be classified into two groups
1. Primary congenital glaucoma
2. Secondary congenital glaucoma

Primary Congenital Glaucoma

This condition is bilateral in almost two thirds of patients, occurs more frequently in males and has no racial predilection. Inheritance is mostly sporadic or autosomal recessive with variable penetrance.

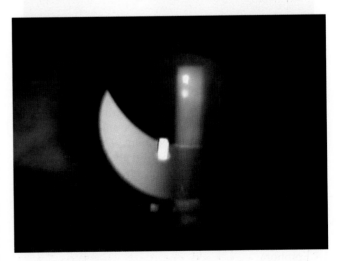

Fig. 27.25: Marfan's syndrome: lens subluxed upwards

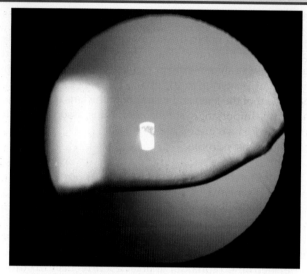

Fig. 27.26: Marfan's syndrome: upward subluxation of lens seen against red reflex

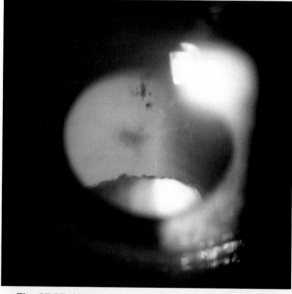

Fig. 27.27: Homocystinuria: lens subluxed downwards

The cause of this type of glaucoma is abnormal development of the anterior chamber angle which causes obstruction to outflow of the aqueous. This in turn causes increased intraocular pressure and the relatively elastic sclera of the infant eye respond with stretching and enlargement of the globe.

Clinical Features

The classic triad of symptoms comprises:
1. Epiphora
2. Photophobhia
3. Blepharospasm

Signs

1. A hazy cornea. Corneal oedema is the presenting sign in most infants, often accompanied by breaks in Descemet's membrane called Haabs striae.
2. Increased corneal diameter. The normal horizontal corneal diameter is 9.5-10.5 mm at birth and 10.5-11.5 mm at one year. A diameter of more than 12.5 mm is suggestive of glaucoma.
3. Deep anterior chamber
4. Increased intraocular pressure
5. Optic disc changes (pallor, atrophy).

Diagnosis

A detailed ocular examination under anaesthesia should be done. The following tests are required.
1. Measurement of corneal diameter.
2. Intraocular pressure recording
3. Gonioscopy
4. Ophthalmoscopy

Differential Diagnosis

1. Megalo-cornea
2. Nasolacrimal duct obstruction
3. Keratitis
4. Trauma
5. Metabolic disorders

Secondary Congenital Glaucoma

Ophthalmologist and paediatrician must be aware of associated systemic and ocular anomalies is an infant with glaucoma. Example of associated systemic abnormalities includes:
1. Sturge-Weber syndrome
2. Neurofibromatosis
3. Oculocerebrorenal syndrome (Lowe's syndrome)
4. Congenital rubella.

Treatment

Medical therapeutic agents
1. Carbonic anhydrase inhibitors.
2. Topical beta-blockers
3. Prostaglandin derivatives

Surgical therapy
1. Goniotomy
2. Trabeculotomy
3. Trabeculectomy
4. Glaucoma implants
5. Cycloablation

All cases of childhood glaucoma require careful, long-term follow-up. Visual loss is not only due to corneal scarring and optic nerve damage, but may also be due to significant astigmatism and amblyopia. Glaucoma that present at birth has a poor visual prognosis. Presentation at 3-12 months age is associated with a better visual prognosis.

UVEITIS IN CHILDREN

Introduction

Uveitis is an inflammatory response to a physical or biological insult, involving part of, or the whole uveal tract. Polymorphonuclear leucocytes and monocytes accumulate in the uvea and stimulate the release of chemical mediators. These may remove the offending stimulant as well as creating further inflammation. Approximately 50% of children presenting with anterior uveitis manifest no obvious cause of the condition. The commonest identifiable cause, however, of anterior uveitis in the paediatric age group, is juvenile rheumatoid arthritis, particularly the pauci articular type.

Uveitis in children accounts for 2-8% of uveitis occurring at all ages. It presents particular challenges to the clinician:
1. Late presentation is common, because children may not be able to express their symptoms.
2. Potential side effects and poor compliance may limit the effectiveness of treatment.
3. Steroid-induced glaucoma, secondary cataract and band keratopathy have a higher incidence rate in children than in adults.

Causes of Uveitis in Children

The majority of uveitis cases in children are bilateral, non-granulomatous and anterior. Intermediate and panuveitis are seen less commonly, and posterior uveitis, least of all.

Causes of each type of uveitis are listed in Box 27.7.

Clinical Features

The symptoms of acute anterior uveitis include pain, redness of the eye and photophobia. There may be watering of the eye. In chronic uveitis, which may be anterior, intermediate or posterior, there is often little in the way of pain or redness, but vision may be blurred, or there may be an awareness of "floaters" in the eye. On examination, in acute anterior uveitis the redness is found to be maximal around the limbus of the cornea. Keratic precipitates (KP), which may be large and clumped together ("mutton fat" KP), or fine and diffuse, are usually present on the corneal endothelium, and cells (inflammatory cells), and flare (protein exudate) are seen on slit lamp examination of the aqueous fluid, and/or the vitreous, when the posterior segment of the eye is involved. In acute anterior uveitis, the pupil may be miosed (constricted), or irregular, due to adhesions of the iris to the anterior lens surface, known as posterior synechiae. (Anterior synechiae refer to adhesions of the peripheral iris to the corneal endothelial surface, which may occur in conditions with severe inflammation or in prolonged shallowing of the anterior chamber).

In intermediate uveitis, creamy, inflammatory exudates are evident in the pars plana of the ciliary body, at the anterior periphery of the retina, and in posterior uveitis, similar lesions may be present elsewhere on the retina, or in the vitreous (Figs 27.28 and 27.29).

Management

Anterior Uveitis

Investigation for an underlying cause of anterior uveitis in children is usually undertaken when the uveitis is bilateral, or recurrent, or does not respond to initial therapy.

Topical steroid and mydriatic drops are usually effective, and the minimum effective doses are used to prevent posterior synechiae and reduce the number of cells in the anterior chamber, while minimising side effects: such as visual blurring in the case of mydriatics, and secondary cataract or glaucoma in the case of steroids.

Periocular depot injections of steroid, oral steroids and systemic immunosuppressives are all reserved for patients in whom topical therapy yields an inadequate response, and they should be used with care due to the occurrence of significant side effects in children.

Box 27.7: Causes of Uveitis			
Anterior uveitis	*Intermediate uveitis*	*Posterior uveitis*	*Panuveitis*
Juvenile rheumatoid Arthritis	Pars planitis	Toxoplasmosis	Sarcoidosis
Trauma	Sarcoidosis	Ocular histoplasmosis	Vogt-Koyanagi-Harada syndrome
Sarcoidosis	Tuberculosis	Herpetic disease	Behcet's syndrome
HLA B27–related	Toxocariasis	Syphilis	Idiopathic
Herpetic disease	Lyme disease	Sympathetic ophthalmia	
Sympathetic ophthalmia	Idiopathic	Lyme disease	
Syphilis		Idiopathic	
Lyme disease			
Fuch's heterochromic cyclitis			
Viral syndromes			
Idiopathic			

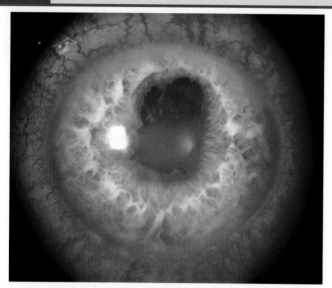

Fig. 27.28: Acute anterior uveitis with posterior synechiae

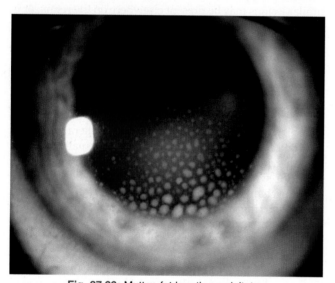

Fig. 27.29: Mutton fat keratic precipitates

Surgery for secondary cataracts may be necessary, and corneal epithelial debridement combined with chelation therapy, for band keratopathy.

Children who present with juvenile rheumatoid arthritis should have regular eye screening, as the associated uveitis is often symptom free in its early stages.

Blunt **trauma** to the eye may present as a mild self-limiting anterior uveitis. More severe blunt trauma, or trauma involving damage to the eye by a sharp object, presents with more severe disruption to the globe, including lens dislocation, retinal detachment or perforation of the globe. In these situations, surgical intervention is required. In penetrating injuries, both infectious and sympathetic endophthalmitis are major risks, particularly if treatment is delayed. Tetanus prophylaxis must also be ensured in all such cases.

Intermediate Uveitis (Pars Planitis)

Due to its chronic nature, treatment is initiated in situations of moderate reduction in visual acuity. Topical or periocular steroids should be tried first, and systemic steroids used only if these do not prove effective. Systemic immunosuppressive therapy is considered if therapy is prolonged to avert steroid-induced cataract and systemic side effects. Other measures including vitrectomy may be indicated in severe, refractory intermediate uveitis.

Posterior Uveitis

Inflammation of the posterior segment occurs in over 50% of childhood uveitis cases. Approximately one third of these are idiopathic, and on exclusion of conditions requiring more specific measures, treatment is administered as for intermediate uveitis. Almost half the cases of posterior uveitis seen in children are caused by toxoplasmosis. The standard treatment for this has hitherto been a combination of sulphadiazine and pyrimethamine, although more recently, azithromycin has also proved to be effective. Additional systemic steroids are sometimes required.

Systemic Infections and Uveitis

Systemic infections, which may include, or may initially present with uveitis include candidiasis, tuberculosis, syphilis and leprosy.

Systemic candidiasis occurs in drug addicts and in individuals with immunosuppression due to diseases such as cancer or other diseases associated with immuno-suppression, or to immunosuppressive therapy. When the eye is involved, typical findings include cells, fibrinous strands and "puff balls" in the vitreous; discrete, and sometimes, haemorrhages and creamy exudative lesions on the retina. Diagnosis is confirmed by vitreous biopsy, and intravitreal and intravenous antifungal agents are required.

Tuberculosis may affect any part of the uvea, and may manifest as a localised mass with surrounding inflammatory reaction, and mutton fat keratic precipitates on the corneal endothelium. In miliary tuberculosis, discrete miliary choroidal tubercles or peripheral exudative "candle wax drippings" may be visible on fundoscopy. Focal retinopathy resembling toxoplasmic retinochoroidopathy may also be seen. Anti-tuberculous treatment is mandatory, and topical steroids should be used with care, only if systemic antituberculous treatment is also given.

Syphilis may cause localised or diffuse uveitis or choroiditis, which resolve leaving areas of iris or choroidal atrophy.

Multibacillary leprosy often causes an acute anterior iritis, particularly as part of a Type II, or erythema nodosum leprosum (ENL) reaction. Chronic, low-grade uveitis is also seen in multibacillary leprosy, and as in juvenile rheumatoid arthritis, may present with secondary features such as cataract, iris atrophy, ocular hypotony or band keratopathy. Thus, regular ocular screening of such patients is recommended. Along with anti leprosy multi-drug therapy, topical steroids and cycloplegics are indicated. Where the corneal epithelial surface is compromised due to impaired corneal sensation or weakness of orbicularis oculi, topical steroids must be used with care, and topical non-steroidal anti-inflammatory agents may be preferable.

Systemic viral illnesses including chickenpox and cytomegalovirus infection are occasionally associated with a posterior uveitis and retinochoroiditis. Inflammatory cells in the vitreous are seen, with foci of exudate and haemorrhage on the retina and sheathing of peripheral retinal vessels.

Onchocerciasis is a parasitic disease caused by Onchocerca volvulus, a filarial worm. The geographical distribution of this disease includes West Africa, central Africa and Yemen, as well as parts of Central America.

The life cycle of the worm includes humans in whom the microfilaria matures into adult worms, and a second vector, the Simulium fly; in which young microfilaria develop into mature ones. The larval microfilaria is found all over the body, and accumulates in the eye in large numbers. Microfilaria may be seen under the conjunctiva, or in the anterior chamber on slit lamp examination. Symptoms occur largely as a result of an inflammatory response to dead or dying microfilaria. A sclerosing keratitis, typically starts peripherally, and spreads to include the whole cornea. Uveitis occurs, with pigmented keratic precipitates and posterior synechiae. Optic atrophy and chorioretinal atrophy are often observed, and glaucoma may occur in the absence of obvious infection, possibly due to obstruction to aqueous outflow by the microfilaria.

Since the ocular changes due to onchocerciasis are by and large irreversible, early treatment of the disease is required to prevent these changes and the resulting sight impairment or blindness. Ivermectin is now the treatment of choice for Onchocerciasis.

Loaiasis, which is caused by the Loa loa filarial worm, occurs in West and Central Africa.

The worm has a similar life cycle to *Onchocerca volvulus*, and often causes inflammation involving the eye, although not usually uveitis. Loa loa worms are often seen under the conjunctiva, and may be removed with forceps after instilling local anaesthetic and incising the conjunctiva at the appropriate site. An acute localised inflammatory response to the worms is recognised, and has been called "Calabar swelling". This commonly occurs in the orbit or eyelids, with a dramatic presentation, but with resolution to normal in a few days. Treatment is with diethyl-carbamazine.

RETINOBLASTOMA

Retinoblastoma is the most common primary, malignant intraocular tumour of childhood. If left untreated it is lethal. The long-term survival rate for retinoblastoma is over 90% in the developed world. The prognosis in developing countries continues to be poor because of late diagnosis and intervention (Fig. 27.30).

Epidemiology

Retinoblastoma occurs equally in males and females. There is no racial predilection.

60–70% of tumours are unilateral and the mean age at diagnosis is 24 months. 30–40% are bilateral, with a mean age at diagnosis of 14 months. Only 6% of patients have a family history of retinoblastoma. Inheritance is autosomal dominant. The predisposing gene (RPE1) is at 13q14. Sporadic cases constitute about 94% of all patients with retinoblastoma.

Clinical Presentation

The possibility of retinoblastoma should be considered with any lesion in the posterior segment of a child less than 5 years of age. Presenting features include:

1. Leukocoria (a white pupil reflex)—most common (Box 27.8; Fig. 27.31).
2. Strabismus- due to a macular lesion causing reduced vision.
3. Uveitis- with a tumour hypopyon (tumour cells or white blood cells in the anterior chamber).
4. Glaucoma – where an eye filled by tumour has raised intraocular pressure.
5. Hyphaema (red blood cells in the anterior chamber)
6. Orbital cellulitis-due to tumour necrosis and inflammation.

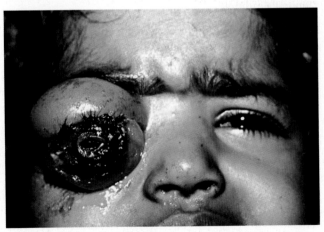
Fig. 27.30: Retinoblastoma with orbital extension

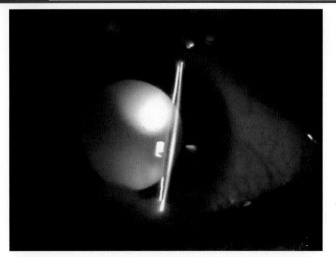

Fig. 27.31: Leukocoria and hypopyon due to retinoblastoma

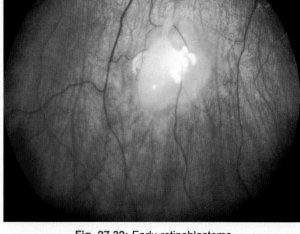

Fig. 27.32: Early retinoblastoma

> **Box 27.8: Differential diagnosis of a white pupil**
>
> • Retinoblastoma
> • Cataract
> • Retinal detachment
> • Severe posterior uveitis
> • Retinopathy of prematurity
> • Persistent hyperplastic primary vitreous
> • Retinal dysplasia (Norrie's disease)
> • Coats' disease

7. Nystagmus
8. Proptosis
9. On routine examination - least common.

Diagnosis

Indirect ophthalmoscopy with scleral indentation must be done on **both eyes** after full mydriasis. Appearances depend on the size of the tumour and on its pattern of growth. Multiple tumours may be present in the same eye.

Clinical Findings

• An *intraretinal* tumour is a flat or round gray to white lesion, fed and drained by dilated tortuous retinal vessels.
• An *Endophytic* tumour projects from the retinal surface as a white, friable mass and may have vitreous seeding.
• An *Exophytic* tumour grows into a cauliflower-like white mass, often associated with a retinal detachment and vitreous haemorrhage.
• As the tumour expands, it undergoes necrosis with areas of calcification (Figs 27.32 and 27.33).

Special Investigations

Ultrasonography – detects calcification and enables measurement of the tumour dimensions.

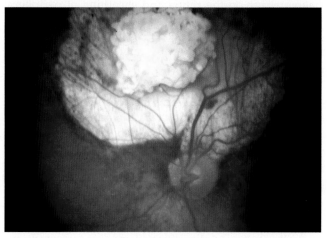

Fig. 27.33: Exophytic retinoblastoma with surrounding chorioretinal atrophy

CT scan – detects calcification, gross involvement of the optic nerve, extension to the orbit or central nervous system and the presence or absence of pinealoblastoma.

MRI – provides the optimum means of evaluation of the optic nerve and of the detection of pinealoblastoma.

Differential diagnosis includes persistent hyperplastic primary vitreous, toxocara granuloma, Coats' disease, retinopathy of prematurity, retinal dysplasia.

Natural history – As the tumour grows, the globe is gradually filled with tumour, which then expands further and involves the periocular tissues. It then extends intracranially. Blood-borne metastases to distant sites can occur.

Histologic Features

Retinoblastoma consists of cells with round, oval or spindle-shaped nuclei, which are hyperchromatic and surrounded by scanty cytoplasm.

Flexner-Wintersteiner rosettes: These are a characteristic feature of retinoblastoma. A single layer of columnar cells surrounds a central lumen lined by a retractile structure, corresponding to the external limiting membrane of the retina.

Homer-Wright rosettes: These do not show features of retinal differentiation and are found in other neuroblastic tumours also.

Fleurettes: Are curvilinear clusters of cells composed of rod and cone inner segments that are frequently attached to abortive outer segments.

Trilateral retinoblastoma: This term refers to bilateral retinoblastoma with ectopic intracranial retinoblastoma, usually located in the pineal gland or the parasellar region.

Treatment: Management of retinoblastoma is highly individualized and is based on age at presentation, laterality, tumour location, tumour staging, visual prognosis, systemic involvement and cost-effectiveness. Decisions regarding treatment should be made after detailed discussion with the child's family, who should be involved at all stages of management.

1 Focal therapy- laser photocoagulation, transpupillary thermotherapy (TTT), cryotherapy, plaque brachytherapy.
2 Local therapy-external beam radiotherapy [EBRT], enucleation.
3 Chemotherapy reduces tumour size and makes it more amenable to laser, cryotherapy, TTT or radiotherapy. Chemotherapy followed by focal treatment is the primary treatment of choice for intraocular retinoblastoma.
4 Primary enucleation is still indicated for advanced intraocular retinoblastoma, especially in unilateral cases.
   On histopathological examination, infiltration of the uvea, sclera and optic nerve beyond the lamina cribrosa imply a high risk of metastasis. Such patients need chemotherapy or radiotherapy. Various combinations of chemotherapeutic drugs are used, the most frequently used agents being vincristine, etoposide and carboplatin.

Genetic counselling is an important part of the management of retinoblastoma.

Follow-up: Children with unilateral disease should be followed up at least until 5 years of age. Those with familial or genetically transmitted disease should undergo life-long follow up.

RETINOPATHY OF PREMATURITY

Retinopathy of prematurity is a proliferative retinopathy affecting premature infants of low-birth weight and young gestational age. Despite improvements in detection and treatment, ROP remains a leading cause of lifelong visual impairment among premature children.

The **International Classification of Retinopathy of Prematurity (ICROP)** provides standards for the clinical assessment of ROP on the basis of severity (stage) and anatomical location (zone) of disease.

Location
   Zone I – posterior retina within a 60° circle centered on the optic nerve
   Zone II – from the posterior circle (Zone I) to the nasal ora serrata anteriorly
   Zone III –the remaining temporal peripheral retina
   Extent – number of clock hours involved

Severity
   Stage 1 – a demarcation line between vascularized and non-vascularized retina
   Stage 2 – the presence of a demarcation line that has height, width, and volume (ridge)
   Stage 3 – a ridge with extraretinal fibrovascular proliferation
   Stage 4 – subtotal retinal detachment
      A. extrafoveal B. retinal detachment including the fovea
   Stage 5 – total retinal detachment

Ophthalmic evaluation of the premature infant may be performed in the nursery or in the office. Examination of the anterior segment is performed with a hand light, with specific attention to the iris vessels, lens and tunica vasculosa lentis. Ophthalmoscopy is performed with an indirect ophthalmoscope and a 28D or 30D condensing lens with scleral indentation when indicated.

Screening for ROP should be performed in all infants with a birth weight with less than 1500 g or a gestational age of 28 weeks or less, as well as infants weighing between 1500 g and 2000 g with an unstable clinical course and who are believed to be at high risk (Figs 27.34 and 27.35).

Differential diagnosis: Retinoblastoma, familial exudative vitreoretinopathy, Norrie's disease, X-linked retinoschisis, incontinentia pigmenti

Treatment: The ultimate goals of treatment of threshold ROP are prevention of retinal detachment or of scarring and optimization of visual outcome.

Treatment Options

- Cryotherapy
- Laser photocoagulation
- Surgery

Threshold or pre-threshold ROP can be treated with laser therapy or retinal cryoablation. Laser therapy is preferred over retinal cryoablation. The treatment is applied in full scatter fashion to the avascular anterior retina with the indirect ophthalmoscope. Laser therapy is believed to be less

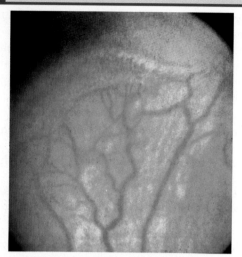

Fig. 27.34: Retinopathy of prematurity: peripheral retinal vessel proliferation and ridge

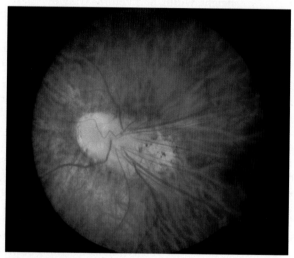

Fig. 27.35: Retinopathy of prematurity: long-term outcome

traumatic systemically than cryoablation; it also appears to yield a better visual outcome.

Surgery may be undertaken for patients with Stage 4 and Stage 5 ROP. The modalities commonly used are scleral buckling and vitrectomy, which relieve the tractional components of the retinal detachment.

Certain problems are more likely to occur in eyes with regressed ROP, including myopia with astigmatism, anisometropia, strabismus, amblyopia, cataract, glaucoma and retinal detachment.

It is important to remember that the sequelae of advanced ROP can cause problems throughout the patient's life, and long-term follow up is warranted.

TRAUMATIC RETINOPATHY

Retinal haemorrhages concentrated at the macula, or spread extensively over the whole retina, sometimes with the presence of Roth's spots (circular haemorrhages with white centres) can be caused in the first two years of life by head injury, for example following road traffic accident. However, such retinal haemorrhages are characteristically seen, sometimes accompanied by subdural haematoma and bruising or injuries elsewhere, in what has been termed the *shaken baby syndrome*. This terminology is best reserved for instances where the aetiology of the injuries has been proved beyond doubt, and the term "traumatic retinopathy" used at all other times, as a descriptor, as other causes such as a coagulation defect must be considered and ruled out. Retinal haemorrhages due to birth injury seldom persist for longer than one month (Figs 27.36 and 27.37).

PREVENTIVE OPHTHALMOLOGY

Childhood Blindness

The WHO definition of blindness is a best-corrected visual acuity of less than 3/60 in the better eye or a field of vision less than 10 degrees. Visual impairment is graded according to intermediate levels of visual acuity less than 6/18. It is estimated that there are about 5 million visually impaired children in the world. Of these, approximately 1.5 million are blind or severely visually impaired, and approximately 1 million of them live in Asia.

Causes of Childhood Blindness

The important causes of preventable childhood blindness in the developing world are vitamin A deficiency, measles, ophthalmia neonatorum, glaucoma, cataract, refractive error, squint, retinopathy of prematurity, trachoma and rubella. Onchocerciasis continues to be a problem in Africa and in parts of the Middle East.

Timely and appropriate intervention in vitamin A deficiency is crucially important in the prevention of blindness in individual patients and, since the condition remains a major public health problem in children (with potentially many years of life ahead) in the developing world, widespread measures of prevention could

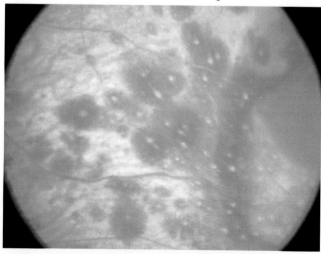

Fig. 27.36: Retinal haemorrhages in traumatic retinopathy

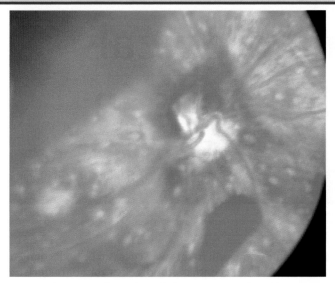

Fig. 27.37: Posterior pole in traumatic retinopathy

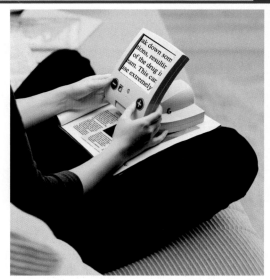

Fig. 27.38: Magnifying aids for reading with visual impairment (Traveller + portable video magnifier, available from Optelec-www.optelec.com)

significantly reduce the burden of blindness, in terms of blind person-years, in these societies.

THE CHILD WITH VISUAL IMPAIRMENT

Vision is required to:

1. Access 'information' in the distance. (It is largely through vision that we learn about the environment).
2. Access to near information. (For example, playing with toys and looking at and reading books).
3. Interacting socially. (Recognising people and their facial expressions and gestures).
4. Guiding movement of the upper limbs. (Picking anything up is usually by means of vision in the sighted person).
5. Guiding movement of the body. (Walking over steps or in a crowd is mediated through vision to give visual guidance).

In children, vision is required to learn these attributes.

Visual impairment can restrict such learning because it imposes limitations on performance.

It is, therefore, essential to measure all aspects of vision and to understand how each child's visual impairment is impacting upon their development. This knowledge is then employed to implement appropriate strategies to minimise the adverse impact of poor vision.

Poor acuity may not impede mobility but can profoundly affect learning if educational material is not enlarged, and can limit social interaction, if friends and relatives are not aware of this.

Visual field impairment may not significantly impair access to information and social interaction but can significantly impair mobility.

Explaining Poor Vision to Parents and Carers

The diagnosis of visual impairment in a child is distressing. The information is conveyed with care and sensitivity, making and giving the requisite time.

Not only do parents and carers need to understand the child's diagnosis and treatment, but if vision is impaired a detailed analysis of how this can adversely impact on day to day life is required, followed by a structured programme for each child, aimed at ensuring that development is not impaired and education is optimised. This may require magnifying aids and the provision of educational material, which is designed either for visual impairment or blindness as appropriate for each child (Fig. 27.38).

BIBLIOGRAPHY

1. Am 18, 2005.
2. Basic and Clinical Science Course, American Academy of Ophthalmology, 2004-2005.
3. David Taylor, Paediatric Ophthalmology – 2nd Edition, 1997. Blackwell Science Ltd.
4. Honover SG, Singh AD. Management of Advanced Retinoblastoma, Ophthalmol Clin N.
5. John Sandford-Smith. Eye Diseases in Hot Climates, J W Arrowsmith Ltd, Bristol, 1986.
6. Kenneth W Wright. Paediatric Ophthalmology and Strabismus, Mosby-Year Book, Inc.1995.
7. Myron Yanoff, Jay S. Duker. Ophthalmology – 2nd Edition 1997, Vol. 2, Mosby, Inc.
8. Principles and Practice of Ophthalmology, 2nd Ed, 2000, Jakobeic: Philadelphia, WB Saunders, 2000.

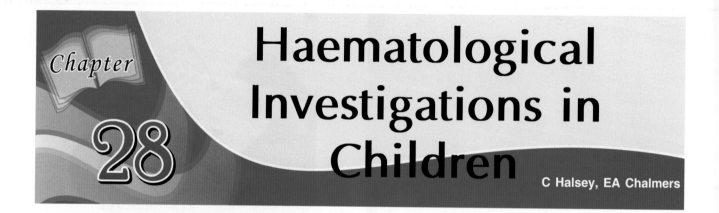

Haematological Investigations in Children

C Halsey, EA Chalmers

The haematology laboratory is able to perform a number of tests to help establish the cause of illness in children. The full blood count (FBC, also known as a complete blood count, CBC) is one of the most basic blood tests performed on children attending hospital or a primary care clinic. All doctors should therefore have an understanding of how the test is performed, possible pitfalls, be able to interpret results and know when more specialised testing or advice is required. Other haematological investigations in routine use include coagulation screens, blood film examination, reticulocyte counts and methods for estimation of iron stores and detection of abnormal haemoglobins. This section will focus on these basic tests and simple algorithms for the subsequent investigation and differential diagnosis of the commonest haematological abnormalities encountered in general paediatric practice. The reader is referred to Chapter 15 for an account of the clinical presentation and management of primary haematological disorders in children.

Full Blood Count

The FBC is a numerical estimate of the number of red cells, platelets and white cells in a given sample of blood along with measurement of the haemoglobin concentration and various red cell indices some of which are directly measured and others derived. Blood is collected into an anticoagulant solution (usually EDTA) and transported to the laboratory. Although counting of each component can be done manually it is now routine to use automated counters in almost all haematology laboratories. These counters recognise cells on the basis of size and physical characteristics. There are two main methods (often used in conjunction). Electrical impedance measurement is based on the fact that blood cells are very poor conductors of electricity. Therefore when cells in a conducting medium are made to flow in single file through an aperture across which an electric current flows, there is a measurable increase in electrical impedance which is proportional to

the volume of the cell. In this way cells can be both counted and sized. The second method relies on characteristic patterns of light scatter and absorbance as cells pass through a laser beam, this is particularly useful for the recognition and counting of the different types of white blood cell (to produce a white cell differential count). In addition counters estimate haemoglobin by lysing the red blood cells and measuring the optical density of the resulting solution at an appropriate wavelength. A typical readout from an automated counter is shown in Fig. 28.1.

Key Learning Points

- Automated blood counters identify cells on the basis of size and laser light scatter patterns. Haemoglobin concentration is measured by lysis of red blood cells and measuring the optical density of the resulting coloured solution
- Because automated machines rely on size as one way to classify cells it is possible to get artefactual results in some situations. For example nucleated red blood cells are often counted as white cells and fragmented red cells are counted as platelets. Any unusual count should be checked manually with a blood film.

Red Cell Indices

In addition to the red cell count and haemoglobin concentration it is clinically useful to know the size of red cells (mean cell volume, MCV) the amount of haemoglobin per cell (mean cell haemoglobin, MCH) and a measure of the variation in size of individual red cells (red cell distribution width, RDW). Collectively these values are known as red cell indices. They are particularly useful in the assessment of likely causes of anaemia (see below).

Blood Film

Examination of a stained blood film is an essential part of the assessment of most haematological disorders. Many haematological diseases have characteristic changes. In

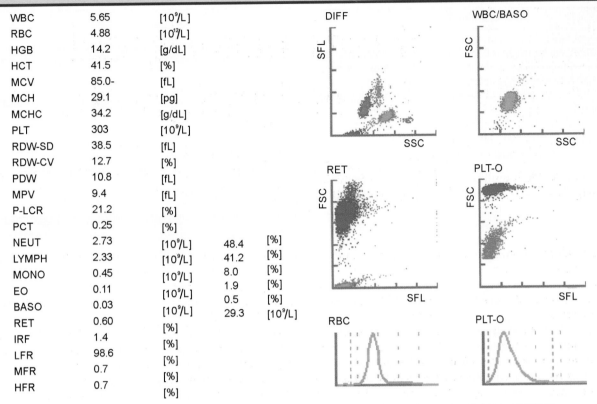

WBC	5.65	[10⁹/L]		
RBC	4.88	[10¹²/L]		
HGB	14.2	[g/dL]		
HCT	41.5	[%]		
MCV	85.0-	[fL]		
MCH	29.1	[pg]		
MCHC	34.2	[g/dL]		
PLT	303	[10⁹/L]		
RDW-SD	38.5	[fL]		
RDW-CV	12.7	[%]		
PDW	10.8	[fL]		
MPV	9.4	[fL]		
P-LCR	21.2	[%]		
PCT	0.25	[%]		
NEUT	2.73	[10⁹/L]	48.4	[%]
LYMPH	2.33	[10⁹/L]	41.2	[%]
MONO	0.45	[10⁹/L]	8.0	[%]
EO	0.11	[10⁹/L]	1.9	[%]
BASO	0.03	[10⁹/L]	0.5	[%]
RET	0.60	[%]	29.3	[10⁹/L]
IRF	1.4	[%]		
LFR	98.6	[%]		
MFR	0.7	[%]		
HFR	0.7	[%]		

Fig. 28.1: A typical computer generated readout from an automated blood cell analyser (Sysmex XT2000i)

some cases it is possible to diagnose a disorder purely from the blood film (e.g. hereditary elliptocytosis) in most cases other confirmatory tests are needed. The blood film may be very useful in identifying artefactual results such as thrombocytopenia caused by platelet clumping. Systemic disease may also produce blood film changes for example sepsis may be accompanied by an increase in immature neutrophils (left shift or band forms), toxic granulation and formation of Döhle bodies (pale blue cytoplasmic inclusions) within neutrophils. These latter changes are particularly useful in assessment of neonates. Figure 28.2 shows some of the characteristic red cell changes seen on the blood film along with common causes for these appearances.

Reticulocyte Count

Reticulocytes are young red cells that have lost their nucleus but still contain substantial amounts of ribosomal RNA, leading to their characteristic bluish purple colour on standard haematoxylin and eosin (H&E) staining of blood films. They can be more easily identified using special stains such as new methylene blue and can be counted manually or on some automated counters. They can be expressed as a percentage of the total red cells or an

absolute count. Reticulocyte numbers are very useful in the evaluation of anaemia as they allow a distinction to be made between inadequate marrow production of red cells (associated with a low reticulocyte count) and excessive destruction or loss of red cells in the periphery (usually associated with increased reticulocyte release from the marrow).

Normal Ranges

The synthesis of blood cells and coagulation proteins go through various changes during development (discussed further in Chapter 15). This is particularly marked in the neonatal period and early infancy because of adaptive changes needed for the transition between the uterine microenvironment and the outside world. Therefore when interpreting any haematological value it is important to be aware of age appropriate normal ranges. Table 28.1 gives approximate values for the FBC from birth to adulthood. Normal ranges should ideally be determined using the local population and the actual instruments in everyday use in the laboratory. In paediatrics it is difficult to obtain sufficient numbers of samples from healthy controls and therefore estimates are usually made using published normal ranges.

Investigation of a Low Haemoglobin in Infancy and Childhood

Although there are a multitude of causes for anaemia in this age range the majority of causes can be ascertained by logical use of relatively few tests. An initial history should focus on the length and speed of onset of symptoms, a dietary history, ethnic origin, any other medical conditions and any family history of blood disorders. When considering the differential diagnosis for any haematological disorder it is useful to divide the causes into those due to underproduction of cells from the bone marrow, those due to peripheral destruction of cells and those due to loss of cells from the circulation (haemorrhage or sequestration). A simple way to narrow down the list of differential diagnoses for anaemia is to look at the red cell indices. There are a limited number of causes of a hypochromic microcytic anaemia or a macrocytic anaemia – the common causes are listed in Table 28.2. When assessing a normocytic anaemia a reticulocyte count is useful to distinguish between marrow production problems and peripheral destruction or haemorrhage. The blood film may also be useful with characteristic changes seen in some red cell haemoglobin or enzyme disorders (see Fig 28.2).

Table 28.2: Causes of anaemia classified on red cell indices

Hypochromic	Normocytic	Microcytic
Iron deficiency	Haemorrhage (acute)	Vitamin B_{12}/Folate deficiency
Thalassaemia	Haemolysis-AIHA	Reticulocytosis
Sideroblastic anaemia	Haemoglobinopathy-sickle cell disease	Myelodysplasia
Chronic disease	Red cell membrane defect- Hereditary spherocytosis	Hypothyroidism
Lead poisoning	Red cell enzyme defect –G6PD, Pyruvate kinase	Drugs
	Marrow infiltration-malignancy	Liver disease
	Aplastic anaemia Transient Erythroblast-openia of childhood Bone marrow failure syndromes Anaemia of chronic disease	Scurvy

Table 28.1: Normal ranges for the FBC in infancy and childhood

Haemo-globin (g/dl)	Hct	MCV (fl)	WBC (x10⁹/l)	Neutro-phils (x10⁹/l)	Lympho-cytes (x10⁹/l)	Mono-cytes (x10⁹/l)	Eosino-phils (x10⁹/l)	Baso-phils (x10⁹/l)	Platelets (x10⁹/l)
14.9-23.7	0.47-075	100-128	10-26	2.7-14.4	2.0-7.3	0-1.9	0-0.85	0-0.1	150-450
13.4-19.8	0.41-0.65	88-110	6-21	1.5-5.4	2.8-9.1	0.1-1.7	0-0.85	0-0.1	170-500
9.4-13.0	0.28-0.42	84-98	5-15	0.7-4.8	3.3-10.3	0.4-1.2	0.05-0.9	0.02-0.13	210-650
10.0-13.0	0.3-0.38	73-84	6-17	1-6	3.3-11.5	0.2-1.3	0.1-1.1	0.02-0.2	210-560
10.1-13.0	0.3-0.38	70-82	6-16	1-8	3.4-10.5	0.2-0.9	0.05-0.9	0.02-0.13	200-550
11.0-13.8	0.32-0.4	72-87	6-17	1.5-8.5	1.8-8.4	0.15-1.3	0.05-1.1	0.02-0.12	210-490
11.1-14.7	0.32-0.43	76-90	4.5-14.5	1.5-8.0	1.5-5.0	0.15-1.3	0.05-1.0	0.02-0.12	170-450
12.1-15.1	0.35-0.44	77-94	4.5-13	1.5-6	1.5-4.5	0.15-1.3	0.05-0.8	0.02-0.12	180-430
12.1-16.6	0.35-0.49	77-92							

Reproduced from Pediatric haematology. 3rd edition. Eds Arceci, Hann & Smith. Blackwell publishing August 2006

Finding		**Causes**
a. Spherocytes		Autoimmune haemolytic anaemia, Hereditary spherocytosis, Haemolytic disease of the newborn
b. Sickle cells		Sickle cell anaemia- HbSS/HbSC
c. Bite cells		G6PD/oxidative damage
d. Pencil cells		Iron deficiency

e. Basophilic stippling

B Thalassaemia trait, lead poisoning

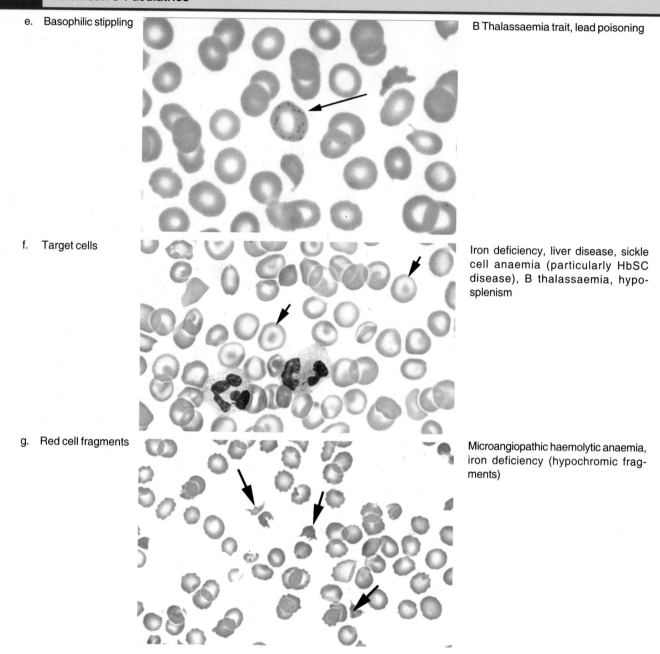

f. Target cells

Iron deficiency, liver disease, sickle cell anaemia (particularly HbSC disease), B thalassaemia, hyposplenism

g. Red cell fragments

Microangiopathic haemolytic anaemia, iron deficiency (hypochromic fragments)

Fig. 28.2: Red cell changes seen on blood films and their common causes (a) Spherocytes (b) Sickle cells (c) Bite cells (d) A pencil cell (e) Basophilic stippling (f) Target cells (g) Red cell fragments. Arrows point to the abnormal cell type

Hypochromic Microcytic Anaemia

The main differential diagnosis is between iron deficiency anaemia and thalassaemia. Thalassaemia major presents in early infancy with a transfusion dependent anaemia and a characteristic blood film and electrophoretic findings (absent haemoglobin A) and usually presents little diagnostic difficulty. Thalassaemia trait does not produce significant anaemia alone but does give hypochromic microcytic indices often in association with a raised red cell count but relatively normal RDW. In contrast iron deficiency usually gives a low red cell count but a raised RDW (this being a measure of variation in red cell width and therefore raised in the presence of anisocytosis). The blood film is often helpful. Beta thalassaemia trait is characterised by basophilic stippling (see Fig 28.2). Alpha thalassaemia trait has few characteristic features. Iron deficiency gives marked anisopoikilocytosis with hypochromic red cell fragments, pencil and teardrop cells and frequent accompanying thrombocytosis.

Tests to Diagnose Iron Deficiency

Iron deficiency can be sub-divided into initial depletion of iron stores followed by iron deficient erythropoiesis and finally the development of anaemia (see Fig 28.3). Serum ferritin is the first marker of depleted iron stores in the body. It is diagnostic if low, but false negative results can be seen because ferritin is an acute phase reactant and therefore can be elevated with acute inflammation or infection even in the presence of iron deficiency. As iron deficiency progresses the transferrin (measured as total iron binding capacity—TIBC) becomes elevated with reduced serum iron. The ratio of these two results can be expressed as the transferrin saturation. Immediate precursors of haem accumulate (zinc (free erythrocyte) protoporphyrin). Finally a hypochromic microcytic anaemia develops. Other tests include measurement of soluble transferrin receptors (increased in iron deficiency). The gold standard test remains Perls' staining of a particulate bone marrow biopsy specimen for iron but this is rarely necessary.

Tests to Diagnose Thalassaemia

In order to understand tests for thalassaemia properly it is necessary to be aware of the composition of haemoglobin and the developmental changes that occur in the use of various globin chains, these are discussed on page xx chapter 15. Diagnosis of thalassaemia is usually made by tests that separate the haemoglobin molecules on the basis of electrical charge; this allows quantitation of the normal haemoglobins HbA ($\alpha_2\beta_2$), HbA$_2$ ($\alpha_2\delta_2$) and HbF ($\alpha_2\gamma_2$) and also detection of abnormal haemoglobins that contain amino acid changes that alter charge (such as sickle cell HbS). The two main methods in use are haemoglobin electrophoresis and high performance liquid chromatography (HPLC). Beta thalassaemia major can be diagnosed by the complete absence of Haemoglobin A on haemoglobin electrophoresis, provided the test is performed before transfusion of the patient. Beta thalassaemia trait usually shows an elevated HbA$_2$ level above 3.5% (normal ranges will vary from lab to lab), care should be taken in the presence of iron deficiency as this may reduce the HbA$_2$ level back into the normal range-results should be repeated after iron replacement in any iron deficient individual. Alpha thalassaemia major is usually diagnosed antenatally or at the time of birth of a severely hydropic infant since all the normal haemoglobins present at birth contain α-chains. Three α gene deletions, so called HbH disease can be diagnosed by electrophoretic detection of Haemoglobin H (β_4 tetramers) or by staining a blood film with brilliant cresyl blue- the β_4 tetramers in the red cells are stained dark blue and produce a golf-ball like appearance. The diagnosis of alpha thalassaemia trait (one or two gene deletions) is suspected by the presence of hypochromia and microcytosis in the absence of iron deficiency and with a normal HbA$_2$ measurement. As it does not produce clinically significant disease, definitive diagnostic investigations (genetic testing for individual mutations) are usually reserved for antenatal patients at significant risk of alpha thalassaemia major in their offspring. Diagnostic investigations for thalassaemia are summarised in Table 28.3.

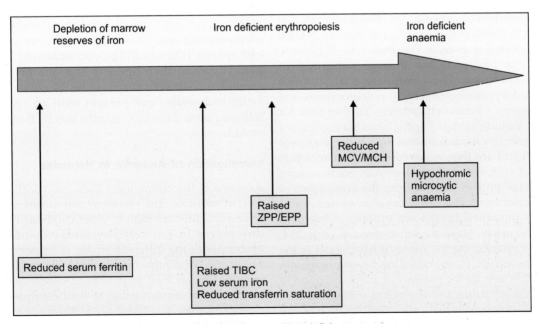

Fig. 28.3: Stages of iron deficiency

Table 28.3: Investigation results in thalassaemia

Diagnosis	Genetic defect	Blood film	Haemoglobin electrophoresis
Beta thalassaemia major	2 β gene mutations	Severe hypochromic microcytic anaemia, nucleated red cells, target cells	Absent HbA (pretransfusion), high HbF
Beta thalassaemia trait	1 β gene mutation	Basophilic stippling, hypochromia and microcytosis but normal or borderline low haemoglobin	Raised HbA_2 >3.5%
Alpha thalassaemia major (incompatible with survival beyond embryonic period)	4 α gene deletions	Very severe anaemia, nucleated red cells	Absent HbA, A2 and HbF Presence of embryonic haemoglobin HbPortland and HbBart's and HbH
Haemoglobin H disease	3 α gene deletions	Anaemia, target cells, teardrop cells and fragments HbH bodies on special staining of film	HbH
Alpha thalassaemia trait	1 or 2 α gene deletions	Hypochromia, microcytosis	2-8% Hb Bart's at birth (may be detected on neonatal screening programmes)

Macrocytic Anaemia

The cause of a macrocytic anaemia in children is often obvious from the history. History of concurrent or past illnesses, symptoms and signs of malabsorption, and a detailed drug history are important. B_{12} and folate, liver function tests, a reticulocyte count and thyroid function should be measured in unexplained cases. Causes are listed in Table 28.2.

Normocytic Anaemia

As mentioned above a reticulocyte count is particularly useful in distinguishing reduced marrow production from increased destruction of red cells. The blood film can also give clues as to the most likely cause and best initial tests. A simple algorithm is given in Fig. 28.4.

Haemolytic anaemias are a large subgroup of normocytic anaemias. The combination of jaundice (unconjugated hyperbilirubinaemia), reticulocytosis and anaemia suggests a haemolytic process. Further tests for haemolysis include serum haptoglobin measurement (proteins present in normal plasma which can bind free haemoglobin and are then removed from the circulation by the reticuloendothelial system), urinary haemosiderin (an iron storage protein derived from the breakdown of free haemoglobin in the renal tubular system) and urobilinogen (a natural breakdown product of bilirubin excreted in the urine). These are summarised in Table 28.4. A key test in establishing the cause of haemolysis is the direct Coombs test (DCT), also called the direct antiglobulin test (DAT). This tests for the presence of antibody bound to the red cell surface by the use of reagents containing anti-IgG and anti-complement that cause agglutination of the cells as shown in Fig. 28.6. A positive DCT indicates a likely immune cause for the anaemia. If the DCT is negative then tests for red cell enzyme defects (G6PD and pyruvate kinase assays), haemoglobinopathies (haemoglobin electrophoresis and sickle solubility test) and membrane disorders (demonstration of increased osmotic fragility of cells, protein analysis by SDS-Polyacrylamide gel electrophoresis or more recent dye binding tests) may need to be performed.

If the reticulocyte count is normal or low it is likely that the anaemia is due to a problem with red cell production in the marrow. A bone marrow aspirate and trephine (see section on white cell disorders below) may be needed to help establish the cause. Lack of red cell precursors in the marrow can be seen as an isolated phenomenon in transient erythroblastopenia of childhood (TEC) or inherited red cell aplasia (Diamond-Blackfan anaemia). If part of a pancytopenia, then aplastic anaemia or hypoplastic myelodysplastic syndrome may be the cause. Occasionally acute leukaemias can present with an aplastic phase followed several weeks to months later by the development of ALL.

Investigation of Anaemia in Neonates

Anaemia is the commonest haematological abnormality seen in neonates. The spectrum and causes of disease are somewhat different than in older children. There are key differences in red cell physiology in neonates that contribute to the different modes of presentation in this age group. Although the haemoglobin tends to be high initially (due at least in part to haemoconcentration and placental transfusion prior to cord clamping), erythropoiesis is then switched off at the time of birth and haemoglobin falls to a nadir of around 10 g/dl by the age

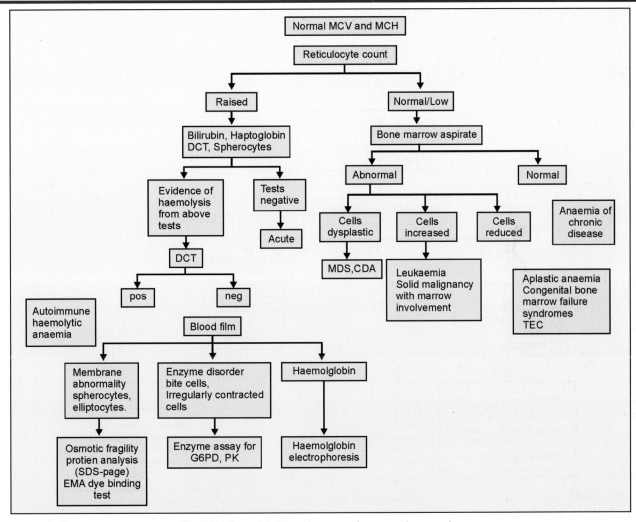

Fig. 28.4: Investigation and causes of normocytic anaemias

Table 28.4: Indicators of haemolysis	
Due to increased red cell destruction	Raised serum unconjugated bilirubin Raised urinary urobilinogen Reduced plasma haptoglobins
Due to increased red cell production	Raised reticulocyte count
Due to presence of damaged red cells	Abnormal morphology – spherocytes, bite cells, fragments Increased osmotic fragility

of 8 weeks. This fall is exaggerated in premature infants – so called anaemia of prematurity. In addition premature babies are particularly vulnerable to iatrogenic anaemia secondary to blood loss associated with frequent blood testing. The MCV is high in neonates and differences in red cell membrane composition can make some haemolytic red cell disorders such as hereditary pyropoikilocytosis and hereditary spherocytosis worse in the neonatal period. In contrast, the enzymopathy glucose-6-phosphate dehydrogenase deficiency (G6PD) is not usually associated with significant haemolysis in the newborn period (unless the baby is exposed to oxidant stress) but may present with severe jaundice which is thought to be haepatic in origin. Haemolysis may also be antibody mediated due to Rhesus or ABO incompatibility between mother and infant. Increased red cell destruction puts the baby at risk of kernicterus caused by high bilirubin levels. Hence it is important to be aware of the possibility of haemolysis in all newborn babies.

Anaemia presenting soon after birth may also be due to haemorrhage pre, during or post delivery. Feto-maternal haemorrhage can be diagnosed by performing a Kliehauer test on the mother – this test looks for the presence of fetal haemoglobin containing cells in the maternal circulation by virtue of their ability to resist acid elution of haemoglobin. In multiple pregnancies that share a placental circulation twin-to-twin transfusion may also occur, producing one polycythaemic twin and one anaemic one. An algorithm for the diagnosis of neonatal anaemia is given in Fig. 28.5.

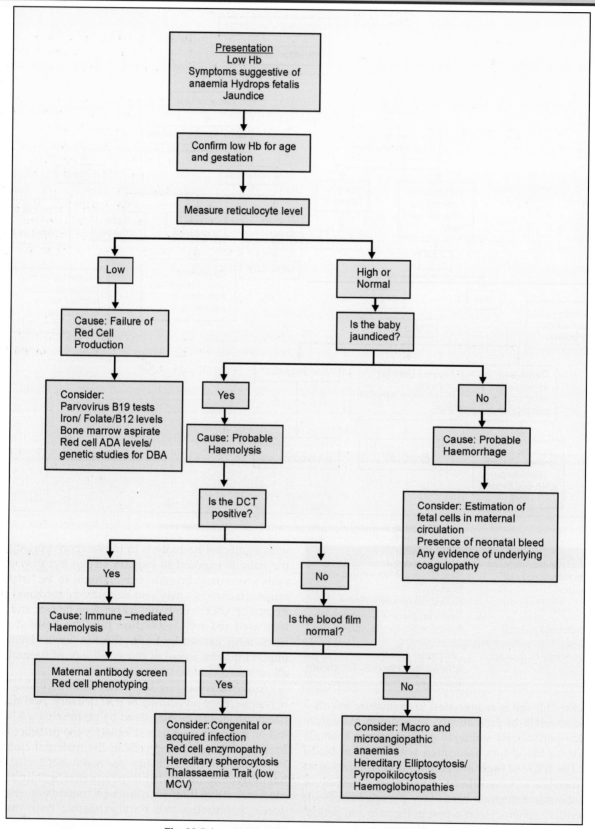

Fig. 28.5: Investigation and causes of neonatal anaemia

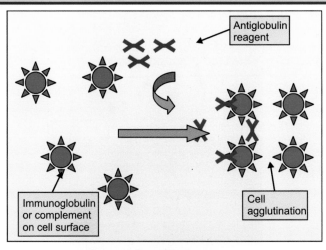

Fig. 28.6: The direct Coombs test

Polycythaemia

High haemoglobins and haematocrits can be due to increased numbers of red cells (true polycythaemia) or dehydration leading to a decreased plasma volume (relative polycythaemia). In children true polycythaemia is usually due to a secondary cause such as hypoxia from cyanotic congenital heart disease leading to increased erythropoietin production. Occasionally kidney tumours can secrete erythropoietin. Primary erythrocytosis (a myeloproliferative disease relatively common in adults) is extremely rare in children. Neonates have higher incidences of polycythaemia usually secondary to placental insufficiency or delayed clamping of the cord. The blood viscosity increases exponentially with haematocrits above 0.65 therefore these infants are often treated with exchange transfusion – the evidence for benefit from this is lacking.

White Cell Disorders

The white cells in the blood can be subdivided into different subpopulations with distinct functions. These are listed in Table 28.5 along with the main causes of high or low counts for these cells.

Table 28.5: White cell types and their disorders			
Cell type	Function	Causes of increased count	Causes of decreased count
Neutrophil	Innate immunity, control of bacterial and fungal infection, Role in phagocytosis of dead and damaged cells as part of inflammation	Bacterial infection Inflammatory disorders and tissue necrosis Severe marrow stress- haemorrhage or haemolysis Steroid therapy Myeloproliferative disorder (rare in children)	Infection – viral or fulminant bacterial Autoimmune Marrow failure Drugs African race
Lymphocyte	Adaptive immunity Control of viral infection	Acute infection especially viral e.g. Epstein Barr virus (glandular fever) Chronic infection- TB, toxoplasmosis Acute leukaemia	Acute stress including acute infection, burns, surgery, trauma Steroids, Cushing's syndrome Immunodeficiency- congenital and acquired including use of immunosuppressive drugs
Monocyte	Part of reticuloendothelail system- macrophage precursors in transit	Chronic bacterial infections (TB) Lymphoma Juvenile myelomonocytic leukaemia Associated with neutropenia	Marrow failure Drugs
Eosinophil	Inflammatory responses Response to parasitic infection	Parasitic infection Allergy, atopy Skin diseases Hodgkin's disease	Marrow failure Cushing's syndrome Acute stress e.g. burns Drugs
Basophil	Largely unknown, blood counterpart to tissue mast cell	Chicken pox Myeloproliferative diseases Hypothyroidism Ulcerative colitis	As above

Low White Cell Counts (Leucopenia)

The commonest and most important white cell deficiency is that involving neutrophils (neutropenia) since this can be associated with an increased risk of serious infection. It can be caused by a defect in bone marrow production either affecting this cell type alone (isolated neutropenia), or as part of a general failure of the bone marrow to produce mature blood cells (pancytopenia). Alternatively neutropenia can result from peripheral destruction of neutrophils by antibodies or their redistribution to the tissues or sites of injury. Normal ranges for neutrophils vary between ethnic groups and are particularly low in black Africans. This is thought to represent a different distribution of neutrophils between the tissues and the circulation, rather than an overall lower total body count. Neutrophil numbers circulating in the bloodstream rise after exercise and as a stress response.

Lymphopenia can follow acute infections or periods of immunosuppression. Lymphocyte counts are generally higher in neonates. In neonates with lymphopenia and serious infections the possibility of an inherited immunodeficiency should be borne in mind.

High White Cell Counts (Leucocytosis)

A high neutrophil count often accompanies infection (neutrophilia) and can be a useful marker of sepsis. Very high neutrophil counts with evidence of immature precursors in the bloodstream are sometimes called a leukaemoid reaction. This can be seen with overwhelming sepsis, marrow infiltration by a solid malignancy, a severe stress response such as status epilepticus or burns. Leukaemia itself can present with high or low white cell numbers and is usually suspected by the combination of an abnormal blood count (white cells high or low, usually with accompanying anaemia and thrombocytopenia) with a blood film that shows a population of immature precursors (blast cells). Blast cells vary in appearance with the different subtypes of leukaemia but are generally larger than normal cells with a large nuclei and open chromatin (see chapter 15, Figs 15.15 and 15.16). Myeloid blast cells may have rod-like inclusions in their cytoplasm called Auer rods.

The definitive diagnosis of leukaemia usually requires bone marrow examination, this allows detailed study of the appearance of the red cells (morphology) as well as analysis of various specific proteins expressed by the cells (immunophenotyping) and genetic abnormalities (molecular genetics and cytogenetics) which help classify the leukaemia further and guide treatment.

Bone Marrow Examination

Bone marrow examination is performed for further assessment of haematological disorders where production

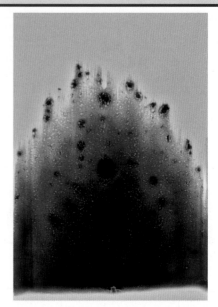

Fig. 28.7: Example of bone marrow aspirate specimen spread on a slide and stained with H&E, note the granular appearance at the top of the smear

of cells from the bone marrow is thought to be abnormal. In children it is often performed under general anaesthesia although local anaesthetic can be used if appropriate. The usual site for aspiration is the posterior iliac crest. A large bore needle is used to penetrate the bony cortex and enter the marrow cavity. Bone marrow is then aspirated and spread on glass slides, preferably immediately. If a good specimen is obtained then a granular appearance should be seen (see Fig 28.7). Further samples can be taken in appropriate anticoagulant or medium for cytogenetics, immunophenotyping and molecular genetic tests. In many cases a bone marrow trephine can also be taken – this involves introducing a longer needle below the cortex and taking a core of tissue that can then be fixed in formalin and sectioned for pathological examination.

Platelet Disorders

Platelets are small cytoplasmic fragments produced from megakaryocytes in the bone marrow and are important for the initiation of haemostasis and may have as yet poorly understood roles in inflammation. As with white and red cells, platelet disorders can be subdivided on the basis of high and low numbers.

High Platelet Counts (Thrombocytosis)

High platelet counts are usually reactive i.e. not primary bone marrow disorders but secondary to iron deficiency, ongoing inflammatory processes or infection. Very high platelet counts ($>1500 \times 10^9$/l) can be associated with an increased risk of thrombosis. Primary thrombocytosis (essential thrombocythaemia) is rare in children.

Low Platelet Counts (thrombocytopenia)

Again these can be classified according to the underlying problem ie inadequate bone marrow production or peripheral destruction/consumption (see Table 15.3 chapter 15). Unexpectedly low platelet counts should always be confirmed by examination of a blood film as artefactually low platelet counts are not uncommon either due to partial clotting of the sample or platelet clumping, the latter is often an *in vitro* phenomenon due to EDTA dependent antibodies. The commonest cause of true thrombocytopenia in children is immune mediated peripheral destruction – idiopathic thrombocytopenic purpura (ITP). Unfortunately there is no diagnostic test for this condition so it remains a diagnosis of exclusion. It is characterised by the sudden onset of bruising and/or bleeding in an otherwise well child, often with a history of an antecedent viral infection or more rarely post immunisation. There should be no other abnormalities in the blood count and no lymphadenopathy or organo-megaly on examination. In these cases careful examination of a peripheral blood film is sufficient but in the presence of any abnormal or suspicious features a bone marrow examination should be performed to exclude leukaemia. The bone marrow in ITP shows increased numbers of normal megakaryocytes (as shown in chapter 15 Fig. 15.11). Although the disease is immune mediated platelet associated antibodies show high false positive and negative results and are therefore not useful in making or excluding the diagnosis.

Platelets may also be consumed in the periphery and a low platelet count almost always accompanies established disseminated intravascular coagulation (see Table 28.6). Giant haemangiomas (Kasabach–Merritt syndrome) or splenomegaly may also sequester and destroy platelets.

Lack of marrow production of platelets often accompanies marrow infiltration by diseases such as leukaemia. Other bone marrow failure syndromes such as Fanconi's anaemia can also present initially with low platelets.

It is also possible to have a platelet function disorder. The commonest of these are Glanzmann's thrombae-sthenia, usually associated with a normal platelet count, and Bernard-Soulier syndrome, associated with a moderate to severe thrombocytopenia. Both are due to

Table 28.6: Haematological finding in disseminated intravascular coagulation
1. Prolonged APTT
2. Prolonged PT
3. Prolonged thrombin time
4. Low fibrinogen
5. Low platelet count
6. Raised fibrin degradation products or D-Dimers
7. Red cell fragmentation on the blood film

different platelet glycoprotein defects and can be diagnosed by platelet function testing and flow cytometry.

In neonates causes of thrombocytopenia vary depending on the gestation and clinical condition of the baby. In well term neonates alloimmune thrombocytopenia due to the transplacental passage of maternal anti-platelet antibodies directed against foreign paternal antigens on the babies platelets (akin to the red cell disorder Rhesus haemolytic disease of the newborn) needs to be excluded. In preterm neonates benign gestational thrombocytopenia may be seen soon after birth but later appearance of thrombocytopenia often heralds sepsis.

Coagulation Testing in Infants and Children

Interpreting the results of coagulation screening requires some basic knowledge of the coagulation cascade. Coagulation tests are performed in the laboratory (*in vitro*) and do not faithfully replicate the circumstances seen in the body (*in vivo*). The interpretation of laboratory tests often places a lot of emphasis on extrinsic and intrinsic pathways but these sequences of activation probably do not play a major role in the initiation of clotting *in vivo*. Despite this the concept of extrinsic and intrinsic pathways is useful to be aware of when faced with an abnormal coagulation screen and is shown in Fig. 15.12.

It is now thought that the key initiating event *in vivo* is exposure of tissue factor in response to endothelial damage. Tissue factor activates factor VII to form a complex, TF-VIIa, which cleaves factor X to its active form Xa. Xa can convert prothrombin to thrombin with low efficiency but this generation of small amounts of thrombin then activates feedback loops to increase coagulation factor activation. Factor VIII (activated by thrombin) and factor IX (activated by TF-VIIa and factor XI) form a complex VIIIa-IXa known as tenase. Tenase generates activated factor X with great efficiency. Thrombin also activates factor V and a Xa-Va complex is formed which cleaves prothrombin to form thrombin. Thrombin generation leads to conversion of fibrinogen to fibrin with subsequent crosslinking by factor XIII. This pathway is summarized in Table 28.6.

When to perform a coagulation screen

Coagulation screens should not be a routine blood test. They should be performed in any child with unusually severe or unexplained bleeding or in very unwell children with suspected disseminated intravascular coagulation. They can also be performed prior to high-risk invasive interventions. A good bleeding history needs to be taken to determine the need for investigation and to help guide appropriate tests. This includes a history of abnormal bleeding in the patient or relatives in response to haemostatic challenges such as tooth extraction, cuts and minor operations as well as a history of maenorrhagia in older females. Some clinically significant bleeding disorders can have a normal coagulation screen (in

Table 28.7: Bleeding disorders that may present with a normal coagulation screen and platelet count

- Factor XIII deficiency
- Glanzmann's Thrombaesthenia / other platelet function disorders
- von Willebrand's disease
- Vascular disorders

particular some von Willebrand's disease and Factor XIII deficiency see Table 28.7) and some abnormal coagulation screens do not lead to a clinical risk of bleeding (e.g. Factor XII deficiency or lupus anticoagulant). Therefore the results of testing always need to be interpreted in the light of a clinical history.

Key Learning Point
Do not rely on coagulation screening as the sole indicator of bleeding risk. History of bleeding in response to a haemostatic challenge is just as important

Coagulation Tests

When performing a clotting screen care should be taken during venepuncture to avoid activation of clotting as this can produce artefactually low results. Samples should be from a free flowing vein, in particular heel prick samples are unsuitable in neonates. Care should be taken to avoid contamination with heparin – a particular problem when sampling is from an indwelling venous catheter. Like the FBC it is very important to be aware of normal ranges for the clotting screen especially in neonates who tend to have significantly prolonged values compared to older children. In addition values vary considerably between different automated analysers and may therefore vary between hospitals, local normal ranges should always be used.

Initial screening tests should comprise:

1. *Prothrombin time* (PT) –this is a test of the overall activity of the extrinsic pathway. It measures the activity of factors II, V, VII and X and is also dependent on adequate fibrinogen levels.
2. *Activated partial thromboplastin time* (APTT) – this is a test for the overall activity of the intrinsic pathway and measures factors II, V, VIII, IX, X, XI and XII, it also requires adequate fibrinogen levels.
3. *Thrombin time* (TT) – prolonged by quantitative and qualitative disorders of fibrinogen, the presence of inhibitory factors such as fibrin/FDPs and the presence of heparin.
4. Fibrinogen level.
5. Platelet count.

Results of these tests along with clinical history can guide subsequent investigation. Bleeding times are generally unhelpful. A diagnostic algorithm is shown in Table 28.8.

The typical findings in disseminated intravascular coagulation are shown in Fig. 28.6, although coagulation screening is useful in this disorder the primary therapy for DIC is treatment of the underlying cause. Replacement of coagulation factors with fresh frozen plasma or cryoprecipitate should be guided by the patient's clinical condition and presence of other risk factors for bleeding rather than treating the abnormal clotting screen *per se*.

Factor Assays

Clinical aspects of inherited coagulation disorders are discussed in chapter 15. Inherited factor deficiencies may initially be suspected on the coagulation screen and confirmed by direct assay of the clotting factor. In the case

Table 28.8: Causes of abnormal coagulation tests					
APTT	*PT*	*TT*	*Fibrinogen*	*Platelets*	*Possible Diagnosis*
Prolonged	Normal	Normal	Normal	Normal	Factor VIII, IX. XI deficiency (Haemophilia A, B or C) von Willebrand's disease Lupus Anticoagulant Factor XII/ Contact factor deficiency
Prolonged	Prolonged	Prolonged	Normal or low	Normal or low	Heparin Liver disease Fibrinogen deficiency Vitamin K deficiency DIC
Prolonged	Prolonged	Normal	Normal	Normal	Vitamin K deficiency Warfarin Factor II, V, VII, X deficiency
Normal	Prolonged	Normal	Normal	Normal	Warfarin therapy Factor VII deficiency

of suspected von Willebrand's disease, von Willebrand Factor (vWF) should be measured both quantitatively (vWF antigen) and qualitatively (a functional test such as a ristocetin cofactor assay). This is because low levels of vWF or normal levels of dysfunctional vWF can cause the disease. vWF can also rise with stress and therefore repeated testing may be needed to exclude disease especially in young children who are difficult to venepuncture.

Platelet Function Testing

Besides a platelet count and assessment of platelet morphology by light microscopy it is possible to assess platelet function in a number of ways. Historically a bleeding time has been used as a global test of platelet function but it is difficult to standardize and not very predictive of bleeding risk. Currently the three commonest techniques in use are platelet aggregation studies (looking at aggregation in response to various stimulants such as epinephrine), flow cytometry (to assess expression of glycoproteins on the platelet surface) and use of a platelet function analyzer (PFA-100, an automated machine that measures the ability of platelets to form a plug under shear stress).

Heparin

The presence of contaminating heparin in a sample is often initially suspected by the combination of a prolonged APTT with a significantly prolonged thrombin time (this test is exquisitely sensitive to heparin). A number of methods exist to try and confirm whether the abnormal result is due to heparin or not. These include a reptilase time (which measures the same pathway as the TT but is unaffected by heparin) or methods to neutralize the heparin using protamine sulphate.

Monitoring of Anticoagulant Therapy

Therapeutic anticoagulation in children is used to prevent or treat thrombosis. Heparin and warfarin are the two main agents in use. Heparin comes in two main formulations – standard unfractionated heparin and low-molecular weight heparin. The former is monitored by the APTT with a therapeutic range of 1.5-2.5 times normal control values.

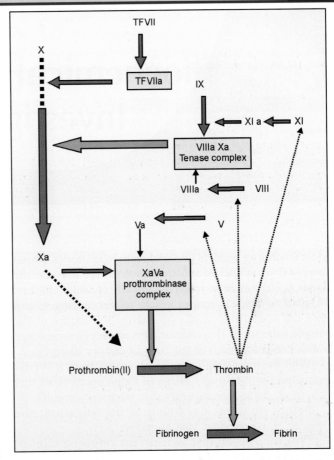

Fig. 28.8: Haematological finding in disseminated intravascular coagulation: A revised coagulation cascade. Thick dashed arrows indicate low efficiency pathways. Thin dashed arrows indicate feedback activation loops. Boxes indicate complexes formed on phospholipid surfaces

Low molecular weight heparin therapy does not prolong the APTT and needs to be monitored by anti-Xa levels. Warfarin therapy prolongs the PT but in order to standardize results between laboratories this level is converted into an international normalized ratio (INR), the target INR varies depending on the indication for anticoagulation.

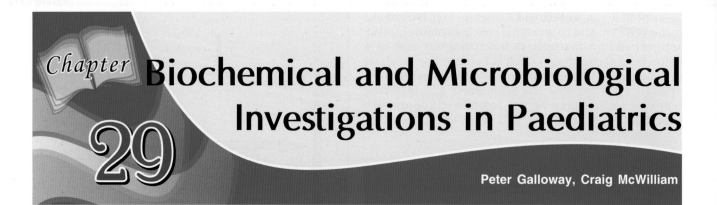

Chapter 29
Biochemical and Microbiological Investigations in Paediatrics

Peter Galloway, Craig McWilliam

Most laboratory work is undertaken in laboratories whose principal workload is adult patients. There are specific issues, which can arise when the unwary consider children as small adults, e.g. inappropriate reference ranges, and how the age of the child may change the nature of the sample submitted. This chapter aims to simply review key issues present in each of the core laboratory disciplines.

With the increasing range of laboratory tests, it is now estimated by the Royal College of Pathologists (UK) that 70% of all diagnoses depend upon laboratory results.

Before undertaking a clinical investigation, the clinician must consider two questions:
1. Will the chosen test confirm (or refute) a clinical suspicion, affecting alteration of management of the patient to obtain a clinical benefit (or avoid a problem), e.g. why identify hypercholesterolaemia in patients over 85? and
2. If the natural evolution of the condition is trivial or self-limiting, what additional information is obtained, e.g. stool culture in acute diarrhoeal illness.

This concept is best summarized in the quote:

"Before ordering a test, decide what you will do if it is either positive or negative, and if both answers are the same, then don't do the test!"

What are the roles of Diagnostic Tests?

There are only four specific reasons for doing a test. These are:

1. Screening

To take a population and pick out those with a disease with few false positive diagnoses. In certain circumstances, we demand 100% sensitivity, i.e. all cases will be diagnosed allowing a few false positives through and using a more specific confirmatory assay, e.g. Neonatal TSH screening using a cut off 30 mU/L on day 6 will identify all congenital hypothyroid cases and a number whose thyroid axis matures over first few weeks. This is necessary to avoid any missed cases.

Down's screening in pregnancy uses markers and maternal age to identify women at high enough risk (1 in 220) to justify amniocentesis with its concomitant 1% pregnancy loss. It fails to identify approximately a third of cases.

2. Diagnosis

While some tests can specifically identify the illness (e.g. abnormal blood film in leukaemia), others may be less specific, e.g. aspartate-amino transferase (AST) commonly used as a marker of liver disease is raised in muscle disease – thus all 1-3 year olds with a raised AST need a Creatine kinase (CK) done concomitantly to exclude Duchenne's muscular dystrophy.

3. Prognosis

This allows estimates of the likely outcome. For example, creatinine in renal impairment can act as a marker of degree of renal damage in an individual, or levels of α-fetoprotein (AFP)/HCG are inversely proportional to outcome in non-seminomatous testicular tumours.

4. Detection of Complications/Monitoring

With increasing laboratory use, there is routine monitoring such as looking for side effects from drugs. Identifying those with marrow suppression on immunosuppressants, e.g. azathioprine.

What Factors are Important in Interpreting Data?

Quality of Information

The laboratory's role is to maximise accuracy and precision of a result. (Accuracy is an indication of how close to the correct value; while precision is how reproducible a result is). To achieve this, laboratories carefully control as many factors as they can. They run quality controls, both internal (allowing regular precision) and intermittent external (to confirm accuracy) (Fig. 29.1).

The expansion of external quality control into rarer analytes has allowed laboratories to improve, particularly, inborn errors of metabolism investigations.

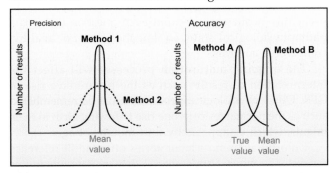

Fig. 29.1: Shows that precision is a measure of reproducibility with Method 1 being more precise than Method 2. From the second figure, both Methods A and B are equally precise but method A is more accurate

Factors Occurring Before the Laboratory

Samples must always be collected under appropriate conditions. If the analyte is unstable, then appropriate preservative or rapid handling is required, e.g. fluoride oxalate tubes for glucose. They must be properly identified especially with multiple births.

More specific factors which can affect the result is to consider the biological diurnal variation in analyte such as cortisol being higher in morning and lower in evening or longer periods, such as gonadotrophin changes post puberty over a month in a female. Without considering the clinical features, interpretation is impossible.

A major effect on many analytes is the acute phase response to any illness. This physiological process identified by simple measures such as elevated C-reactive protein (CRP) is associated with widespread changes. There is vascular leakage of albumin into the extravascular space evident by reduced albumin levels and many micronutrient measurements, such as iron and zinc fall rapidly as the body sequesters them to prevent them being available to bacteria. Prolonged inflammatory responses result in altered endocrine disturbances with, e.g. suppression of thyroid function (Sick Euthyroid syndrome).

Before being able to interpret a result, we need to be able to compare it to the normal homeostatic levels.

What is Normal?

'Normal' is a term that is often used to include only 'healthy' individuals. The term 'normal range' encom-passes a range from two standard deviations greater and less than the median in a 'healthy' population. This assumes the population data is Gaussian distributed (or mathematically transformed into Gaussian distributed) encompasses 95% of these individuals.

Interpretation of laboratory data is then against this healthy group of individuals. But they must be comparable if affected by sex, age, etc. But 2.5% lie above or below that range and are still healthy. The further they lie from the mean the more likely they are to be ill.

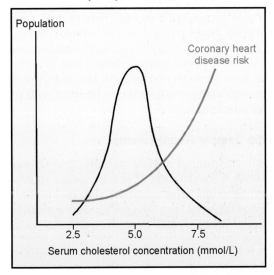

Fig. 29.2: Serum cholesterol concentration (mmol/L)

The second problem is best illustrated by cholesterol (Fig. 29.2). The normal UK range is 3.5-6.7 mmol/L. However, the risk of coronary heart disease increases progressively above 5.2 mmol/L – doubling by 6.7 mmol/L. However, below 5.2 mmol/L the curve is not flat and there remains a shallow gradient of risk. Thus the idea of 'normal' range may be less helpful.

It follows that if 5% of normal results are outside the 'normal' range, the chance of a healthy individual having one abnormal result is $(1-0.95^n)$ where n is number of tests performed. When 20 tests are done 1/3 will have one or more results outwith the 'normal range'. In healthy individuals, chasing perceived abnormalities may not result in any clinical benefit.

What do you Need to know about Biochemical Tests?

Analytical

Major analytical advances occurred during the 70's from manual to automated analysers for common tests. The resulting reduction in sample volume requirements allowed biochemistry to support neonatal care.

Problems still remain, particularly in premature neonates where blood volume is more critical. Specific issues which can occur are excessive evaporation from small samples; concentrating the sample; problems if inadequate volume added to tubes containing liquid anticoagulant where there may be a direct dilution effect. With small sample volumes, it is important to discuss your priorities with the lab to maximise the number of tests which will impact on that child/neonates care.

The Assay Detection Limits

In paediatrics, different normal ranges are expected physiologically. A child with breast development will have an oestrogen level < 100 pmol/L. The normal adult pre-menopausal range being 150-1000 pmol/L (depending upon day of cycle). Truly prepubertal children are < 12 pmol/L. Most routine assay therefore fails to help in the clinical management of children, but highly sensitive radioimmunoassays with detection limits of < 10 pmol/L do offer advantages.

Specific Sample Requirements

An understanding of analyte stability, diurnal variation is required. Consideration of specific issues such as only measuring drugs after adequate pharmokinetic distribution has occurred, e.g. Digoxin remains elevated till six hours post dose, should be addressed prior to sample collection.

Critical Difference

Particularly as more monitoring occurs, it becomes important to be truly certain.

Critical Difference Between Two Results

Particularly as more monitoring occurs, it becomes important to be truly certain that a result has statistically changed. For this, the result must vary by 2.8 times the total variance (i.e. $[(SD\ Biological)^2 + (SD\ Analytical)^2]$ where biological differences are the physiological variability in an analyte during the day and analytical refers to the imprecision in measurement) (Table 29.1).

Analyte	Biological variance (%)	Level (mmol/l)	Critical difference
Na	0.7	140	5
K+	5.1	4.2	0.6
Urea	13.6	5	1.9
Creatinine	4.6	60	14
Calcium	1.7	2.4	0.21
Phosphate	5.1	1.2	0.3
Alkaline phosphatase (iu/l)	6.7	60	20
Albumin (g/l)	3.1	40	4

Table 29.1: Critical difference between two results

With increasing automation of analyses, the analytical imprecision has decreased. At present, typical critical differences for routine analytes are at mid point of adult reference range.

Neonatal Reference Ranges

With modern ethical considerations, collecting blood to perform reference ranges in children is not possible. In premature neonates, one could even question if this is a pathophysiological state, so that there are no 'healthy' comparable controls.

The ongoing maturation processes will affect the interpretation of results such as the progressive rise in GFR. Other physiological processes must be remembered such as the normal testosterone rise following birth in male infants, which disappears by four months of age.

Unfortunately most laboratories offer 'adult reference ranges'. The tables (Appendix A) demonstrate where this can cause particular issues in children. For simplicity, exact data for right age ranges are not given. When interpreting an analyte, the pathophysiological process needs to be considered; particularly inflammation and the acute phase response such that some analytes increase, e.g. α-1-antitrypsin and others decrease, e.g. zinc.

What do you Need to Know about Microbiology Tests?

Urine

There are three major aspects to the microbiological analysis of urine. Microscopy, culture and dipstick testing for leucocyte esterase, a surrogate for the presence of white cells, and nitrite, a bacterial product. Urine can be collected from children at a variety of ages and in a number of ways. The age of the child and the method of collection and storage may effect the interpretation of the results.

Methods of Urine Collection

Type of Sample

Suprapubic aspirate (SPA)
Urine is collected directly via a needle inserted through the skin into the bladder
Clean-catch-urine
Mid-stream specimen of urine
Bag specimen of urine
Catheter specimen of urine

Microscopy of Urine

Microscopy is performed to identify formed elements present within the urine; these include white cells (pyuria), red blood cells (haematuria) bacteria and casts.

Pyuria

The excretion of 400,000 leucocytes per hour which corresponds to > 10 white cells mm^5 correlates with the presence of urinary tract infection. However pyuria in the absence of bacteriuria is not a reliable guide to infection as leucocytes can be found in all types of inflammation and in older females pus cells may come from the vagina. The amount of pyuria also varies with urine flow and pH.

Bacteriuria

The presence of organisms in unspun urine is highly suggestive of significant bacteriuria. Bacteriuria is demonstrable in unspun urine in over 90% of cases with 10^5 bacteria/ml or higher are present. However, a negative result does not rule out infection and has poor sensitivity at lower colony counts.

Dipstick Testing

Dipstick testing can be performed for a number of analytes. In UTI the most useful are leucocyte esterase and nitrite. Overall dipstick testing is less reliable in children under two years of age, in children over two if both leucocyte esterase and nitrite are positive it is suggestive of the presence of a UTI, if both leucocyte esterase and nitrite are negative it is useful to rule out a diagnosis of UTI (Fig. 29.3).

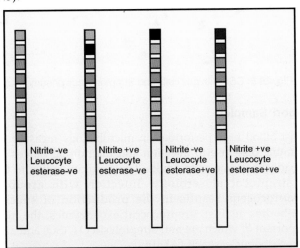

Fig. 29.3: Dipstick testing

Culture of Urine

Most urinary tract infections (UTI) are due to a single organism. Common organisms causing UTI in children include: *Escherichia coli*, which probably causes 75% or more of cases. *Klebsiella spp Proteus spp* and *Staphylococcus saprophyticus*. Less common causative organisms include *Enterobacter spp, Citrobacter spp, Serratia marcescens,* *Acinetobacter* species, *Pseudomonas* spp, and *Staphylococcus aureus*. The number of bacteria taken as significant bacteriuria varies depending upon the type of sample:

- Suprapubic aspiration of the bladder: significant culture if > 10^2 colony-forming units per millilitre (cfu/ml)
- In-out catheterization of the bladder: significant culture if >10^3 cfu/ml
- Clean-voided urine: significant culture if >10^4 cfu/ml
- Carefully collected bag, nappy or pad specimen: significant culture if > 10^5 cfu/ml

A false positive result due to contamination should be suspected when:
- Bacteria but no leucocytes (except in immunocompromised patients)
- Multiple organisms cultured
- Blood, and the specimen is from a menstruating girl
- Prolonged storage greater than 8 hours at room temperature.

A false negative result may be due to:

- Inadequate filling of a specimen bottle containing boric acid (the preservative is bactericidal at high concentrations).
- Antibiotics excreted in the urine.
- Prolonged storage, i.e. greater than 48 hours at fridge temperature.

CSF

CSF is examined microscopically then cultured. Examination for bacterial antigens and polymerase chain reaction (PCR) may also be performed. Meningitis can occur in children with normal CSF microscopy. If it is clinically indicated, children who have a 'normal' CSF should still be treated with IV antibiotics pending cultures.

Microscopy

CSF white cell count is higher at birth than in later infancy and falls fairly rapidly in the first 2 weeks of life. In the first week, 90% of normal neonates have a white cell count less than 18.

The presence of any neutrophils in the CSF is unusual in normal children and should raise concern about bacterial meningitis. Neither a normal Gram stain, nor a lymphocytosis excludes bacterial meningitis; in fact a Gram stain may be negative in up to 60% of cases of bacterial meningitis even without prior antibiotics.

CSF findings in bacterial meningitis may mimic those found in viral meningitis particularly early on and neutrophils may predominate in viral meningitis even after the first 24 hours. Antibiotics are unlikely to significantly affect the CSF cell count in samples taken < 24 hours after antibiotics (Table 29.2).

Table 29.2: Interpretation of CSF findings

	White cell count		Biochemistry	
	Neutrophils (x 10⁶/L)	Lymphocytes (x 10⁶/L)	Protein (g/L)	Glucose (CSF: blood ratio)
Normal (>1 month of age)	0	≤ 5	< 0.4	≥ 0.6 (or 2.5 mmol /L)
Normal term neonate	0	≤ 11	<1.0	≥ 0.6 (or ≥ 2.1 mmol /L)
Bacterial meningitis	100-10,000 (but may be normal)	Usually < 100	> 1.0 (but may be normal)	< 0.4 (but may be normal)
Viral meningitis	Usually <100	10-1000 (but may be normal)	0.4-1 (but may be normal)	Usually normal

Traumatic Tap

In traumatic taps one can allow 1 white blood cell for every 500 to 700 red blood cells however this is not entirely reliable and in order not to miss any patients with meningitis the safest way to interpret a traumatic tap is to **count the total number of white cells, and disregard the red cell count.** If there are more white cells than the normal range for age, then the patient should be treated.

Polymerase Chain Reaction (PCR)

PCR is routinely available for *Neisseria meningitidis*, Herpes Simplex and Enterovirus but results are not usually available in a timescale, which informs immediate management decisions. Meningococcal PCR is particularly useful in patients with a clinical picture consistent with meningococcal meningitis, but who have received prior antibiotics. Enterovirus PCR should be requested on CSF from patients with clinical and/or CSF features of viral meningitis. HSV PCR should be requested for patients with clinical features of encephalitis.

Bacterial Antigens

CSF bacterial antigen tests have low sensitivity and specificity and have little role if any in management.

Culture

The usual organisms causing bacterial meningitis in children over 2 months of age are *Neisseria meningitidis* and *Streptococcus pneumoniae*. *Haemophilus influenzae* type b (Hib) is much less common since the onset of vaccination for Hib.

In infants under 2 months of age Group B streptococcus, *E. coli* and other Gram-negative organisms, and *Listeria*

monocytogenes should also be considered (Figs 29.4 and 29.5).

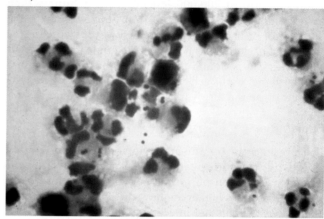

Fig. 29.4: CSF with pus cells and Neisseria meningitides

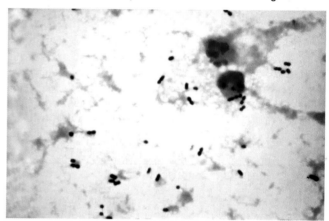

Fig. 29.5: CSF with pus cells and Streptococcus pneumoniae

Blood Samples

Most blood tests performed in microbiology measure the immune response to infection and the normal ranges are broadly the same as in adults. The major exception to this is streptococcal serology. Infection with group A streptococcus results in the production of specific antibodies against streptococcal exoenzymes, the most important of which are anti-streptolysin O (ASO) and anti-deoxyribonuclease - B (ADB).

The ASO response is generally good in pharyngitis and tonsillitis but will not distinguish between infections with groups A, C, and G streptococci, the response is generally poor in impetigo and pyoderma.

The mean ASO normal levels are age dependant:
Pre-school - < 1:200 u/ml
School age - < 1:320 u/ml
Adult - < 1:200 u/ml

The ADB response is good in skin as well as throat infections and may be more specific for Group A Streptococci (GAS) infection. The ADB test shows elevated titres in > 90% of clinically diagnosed cases of pyoderma, acute glomerulonephritis and acute rheumatic fever. ADB titres peak later than ASO levels, and remain elevated for several months. The ADB can therefore be of value if there is a delay in diagnosis.

The mean normal ADB levels are age dependant:

Pre-school - 1:60
School age - 1:170
Adult - 1:85

Examination of Faeces

Pathogens found in the stools of children are broadly the same as those found in adults. However the age of acquisition of such pathogens varies between developed and developing countries. In developing countries, *Campylobacter*, e.g. is the most commonly isolated bacterial pathogen from children less than 2 years old with diarrhoea. The disease does not appear to be important in adults.

In contrast in developed countries infection may occur in adults and children. Poor hygiene and sanitation and the close proximity to animals may all contribute to easy and frequent acquisition of any enteric pathogen. The age of acquisition of campylobacter in a number of countries is illustrated below (Table 29.3).

Table 29.3: Age of acquisition of Campylobacter in different countries	
Countries (ref.)	*Age of infection (months)*
Nigeria	24
Tanzania	18
China	12-24
Thailand	< 12 (18.8%)
	12-23 (12.3%)
	24-59 (10.3%)
Bangladesh	</=12 (38.8%)
	> 12 (15.9%)
Egypt	0-5 (8%)
	6-11 (14%)
	12-23 (4%)

(Adapted from Emerg Infect Dis 8(3), 2002.)

Thus the spectrum of pathogens sought in the microbiology laboratory for children of different ages will need to be determined by a knowledge of local epidemiology.

Antibiotic Monitoring and Interpretation

Antibiotic Monitoring

It is necessary to monitor the levels of antibiotic for two major reasons. Some antibiotics have a narrow theraputic range, that is the ratio between theraputic levels and toxic levels is so antibiotic levels are measured to reduce the potential for toxicity. For other antibiotics it may not always be possible to predict serum levels, in this case antibiotic levels are monitored to ensure efficacy. The antibiotics whose levels are most commonly mesured are the aminoglycosides (gentamicin, tobramycin and amikacin) and the glycopeptide antibiotic vancomycin.

Aminoglycoside Dosing and Monitoring

Gentamicin should preferably be given as an intermittent IV Infusion with the antibiotic diluted with a maximum of 100 ml compatible infusion fluid and administered over 30 minutes. The undiluted solution may however be given as a slow IV Bolus injection administered over 3-5 minutes.

The dosage varies with the age of the child and the indication for gentamicin therapy. For most indications a single daily dose regimen should be employed as it ensures effective peak levels and minimises side effects. In this case the dose should be:

Neonate (< 32 weeks): 4-5 mg/kg every 36 hours
Neonate (> 32 weeks): 4-5 mg/kg every 24 hours
Child 1 month – 18 years: 7 mg/kg every 24 hours

However a single daily dose regimen is not appropriate for all patients, and those with endocarditis, meningitis and cystic fibrosis should be managed with a multiple daily dose regimen. For endocarditis and meningitis the dose is as below:

Neonate (< 29 weeks): 2.5 mg/kg every 24 hours
Neonate (29-35 weeks): 2.5 mg/kg every 18 hours
Neonate (> 35 weeks): 2.5 mg/kg every 12 hours
Child 1 month – 12 years: 2.5 mg/kg every 8 hours
Child 12-18 years: 2 mg/kg every 8 hours

For cystic fibrosis patients with Pseudomonal lung infection the dose should be:

1 month – 18 years: 3 mg/kg every 8 hours

In patients with impaired renal function, the daily dose may need to be reduced and/or the intervals between doses increased to avoid accumulation of the drug.

Gentamicin monitoring single daily dose regimen

Plasma concentrations and renal function should be monitored to ensure efficacy and prevent toxicity. Frequency should be adjusted according to the results obtained.

Measure the first trough concentration immediately before the second dose and peak concentration (if required) 1 hour after second dose.

Neonates: Peak concentration (1 hour post-dose) should measure 8-12 mg/L and trough concentration (pre-dose) should measure less than 2mg/L.

Child 1 month – 18 years: Trough concentration (pre-dose) should measure less than 1mg/L. Peak concentrations are less critical with this dose regimen in this age group.

Multiple Daily Dose Regimen

The first peak concentration should be taken 1 hour after third dose. Measure first trough concentration immediately before the fourth dose.

All age groups: Peak concentration (1 hour post dose) should measure 8-12 mg/L and trough concentration (pre-dose) should measure less than 2 mg/L.

Endocarditis

In endocarditis due to Streptococcus viridans gentamicin is used for its synergistic effects with penicillin and as such lower concentrations are acceptable.

Measure first peak concentration one hour after third dose. The first trough concentration should be taken immediately before the fourth dose.

Peak concentration (1 hour post-dose) should measure 3-5 mg/L and trough concentration (pre-dose should measure less than 1 mg/L.

If there is no change in dosage regimen or renal function, repeat trough levels every 3 days.

Vancomycin Therapy

Vancomycin is a glycopeptide antibiotic, which is active against gram-positive organisms. Critically ill children require higher doses of vancomycin to achieve therapeutic levels.

Trough levels should be taken anytime after 2 hours before the next dose is due prior to the third dose. The target trough level is 8-15 mg/L, however the microbiologist may request higher levels in some infections. Peak levels do not need to be checked routinely.

If trough levels are within accepted range and there is no change in renal function no further monitoring is required.

- If trough levels are low (< 8 mg/L), increase the dosage interval to 6 hrly
- If trough levels are high (> 15 mg/L), reduce dosing interval to 12 hrly
- Re-check levels

If renal function deteriorates (increase in creatinine > 50% from baseline or 50% drop in urine output) during the course of vancomycin therapy recheck trough level as soon as possible. Adjust doses only if necessary, following the guidance above.

Serious Paediatric Problems

Chapter 30

N Doraiswamy

SERIOUS PAEDIATRIC PROBLEMS – MANAGEMENT

	Airway
Anticipate	*Breathing*
Activate	*Circulation*
Act	*Disability*
	Exposure

'problem recognition and treatment have higher priority than definite diagnosis'

Children are not small adults. They are immature in many respects – anatomy, physiology, psychology etc. They do not understand the after-effects, often forget and so would do the same/similar actions repeatedly. The relative incidences of problems vary with seasons, e.g. more children with trauma during summer/school holidays and illnesses in winter/rain/floods/famine. Some congenital conditions may predispose to problems. They can easily acquire infections and rapidly deteriorate. Urgent/emergency problems in childhood and their responses to illnesses or injuries are different from adults as well as at different ages. The initial appropriate and effective management in a structured manner of seriously injured/ill children will have a positive effect on the subsequent management in the wards/ICU/HDU. This finally helps to reduce mortality and morbidity and leading to a better quality of life.

ANTICIPATE

It is of great benefit when a dedicated communication line from and to the Ambulance Service and the Emergency Medicine Department is available. The medical officer or senior nurse should take the call from the ambulance service and record the details, in a specially developed form about name, age, sex, problems (*A, B, C, D*) with duration, drugs given, procedures carried out and expected time of arrival (ETA). Such recorded information can be used later for audit and training of staff and discussion with the Ambulance Service. The information enables the medical and nursing staff to anticipate the possible problems, be prepared and equipped and also to alert the appropriate departments should help would be required soon.

Important charts - formula and weight according to ages, normal range of vital signs – pulse/heart rate, respiratory rate, blood pressure for different ages (Table 30.1), algorithms (cardiac arrest due to asystole, ventricular fibrillation, pulseless electrical activity (Figs 30.1 to 30.3) anaphylactic shock (Fig. 30.4), status epilepticus (Fig. 30.5) and emergency drugs and dosage (Table 30.2), should be displayed in the walls of the emergency room for quick reference with **easily visible large letters**. A clock should be kept on the wall. A folder containing salient features of clinical details, investigations and immediate management of serious illnesses and injuries should be developed according to the requirement of the region and be made available in the room at all times.

Mobile trolley(s) with several drawers, labelled with big letters in the similar order as resuscitation as '*Airway* (e.g. Guedal airway, endotracheal tubes etc.), *Breathing* (e.g. transparent mask with oxygen reservoir bag, Ambu bag, etc.), *Circulation* (e.g. IV/IO needles, crystalloid and

Table 30.1: Normal range of respiratory rate, heart rate/pulse rate and blood pressure according to ages			
Age in years	*Respiratory rate*	*Heart/Pulse rate*	*Systolic BP*
<1	30-40	110-160	70-90
1-2	30-35	100-150	80-95
2-5	30-30	95-140	80-100
5-12	20-30	80-120	90-110
>12	15-20	60-100	100-120

Table 30.2: Emergency drugs and dosage

Useful for resuscitation
Weight in kg = (Age in years + 4) x 2
Initial fluid bolus for shock 20ml/kg
10% Dextrose (if Blood sugar < 3 mmol/l)   5ml/kg in 20 minutes

Name	Dose	Route
Activated charcoal	1g/kg	Oral
Adrenaline - CPR	0.1 ml/kg of 1: 10,000	IV/IO/ETT
Adrenaline - anaphylaxis	0/01 ml/kg of 1:1,000	Deep IM
Adrenaline – croup	1-5 ml of 1:1,000	Nebulised
Aminophylline – acute asthma, anaphylaxis	5 mg/kg	Infusion over 20-30 minutes
Cefotaxime	80 mg/kg	IV/IO
Dexamethasone – brain tumour	500 µg/kg	IV/oral
Diamorphine	0.1 mg/kg	Intranasal
Diazepam – status epilepticus	0.5 mg/kg	Rectal
Dopamine	1-5 µ/kg/min.	Low cardiac output
Glucagon	500 µg if < 30 kg, 1 mg if >30 kg	
Hydrocortisone	4 mg/kg (max. 100 mg)	Severe asthma, shock
Insulin	0.1 unit/kg/hour	Infusion
Mannitol	20% 1.30 – 2.5 ml/kg	Infusion over 30 minutes
Morphine	100 – 200 µg/kg	IV/IO
Naloxone	10 µg/kg	IV/IO
Salbutamol	2.5 – 5 mg	Nebulised
Sodium bicarbonate	1 – 2 mmol/kg	Slow IV/IO

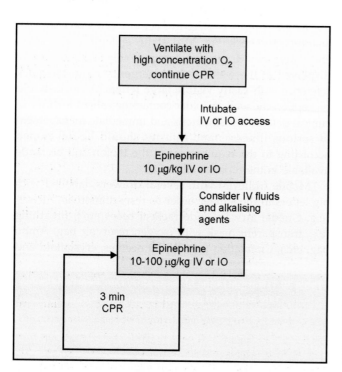

Fig. 30.1: Cardiac arrest – asystole

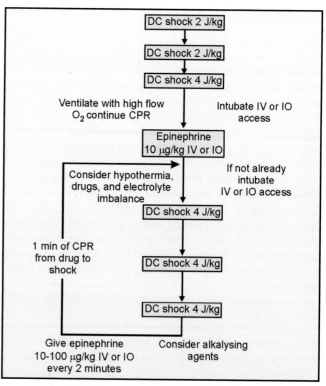

Fig. 30.2: Cardiac arrest – ventricular fibrillation

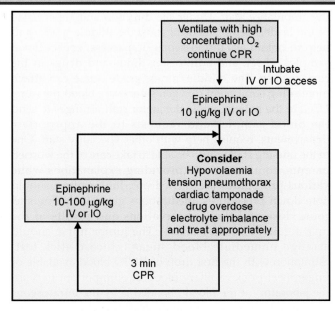

Fig. 30.3: Pulseless electrical activity (PEA) –formerly EMD

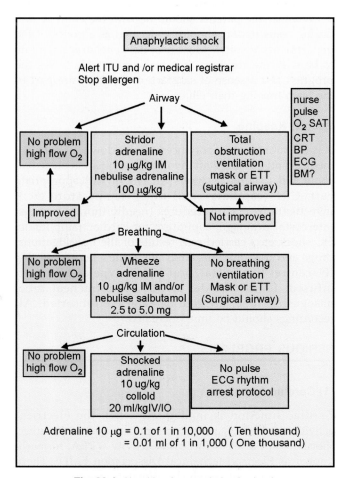

Adpenaline 10 μg = 0.1 of 1 in 10,000   (Ten thousand)
                = 0.01 ml of 1 in 1,000 (One thousand)

Fig. 30.4: Algorithm for anaphylactic shock

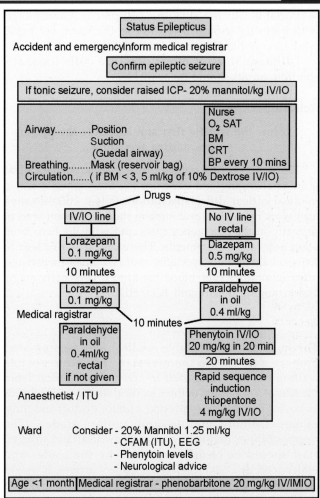

Fig. 30.5: Algorithm for status epilepticus

colloids, etc.) should be kept in the room and a **named nurse** in the department should be made responsible to equip daily and soon after an incident. A lockable cupboard containing the emergency and schedule drugs and a record book should be kept in the emergency room and the key should be with the senior nurse attending the room, at all times.

Cooling equipment (fan, tepid water), heating (heater/ incubator, fluid/blood warming device, aluminium foil, blanket) should be available for use according to the season and the patient.

A board fixed on the wall is useful to calculate and write the requirements for the particular patient by the named medical/nursing staff – name, age, weight (real or calculated), (airway) endotracheal tube size and length, (circulation) fluid required as bolus, dextrose, emergency drugs and dosage (for resuscitation and anaesthesia), DC shocks (ventricular fibrillation).

Portable Glucose stick test equipment (Glucometer) with batteries should be handy in the room for rapid estimation of blood glucose levels (BM).

Different sizes of blood pressure cuffs (neonate, children, adult) should be available.

Activate

'Blow the whistle first and assemble the players before starting the game'

Resuscitation of a patient in the paediatric age can be quite challenging and gone are the days when a single medical officer did resuscitation. It is a collaborative teamwork by medical and nursing staff at different level of seniority in the emergency room and with the help from other relevant departments. Therefore, it is prudent to request help of other speciality staff (viz. anaesthetist) and other laboratory (viz. blood bank) at a very early stage, and arranging theatre and ICU/HDU.

Act

The immediately available medical and nursing staff prepare and initiate the necessary procedures while waiting for the senior staff to arrive. Emergency Team consists of a minimum of three medical staff (a senior doctor as leader, one middle grade and a junior doctor) and three nurses (senior, middle and junior grade). The responsibilities and duties of each medical and nursing staff should be clearly explained by the leader and understood by all even before the patient arrives. If weight is not known or not able to weigh, it can be calculated with the formula:

$$(\text{Age in years} + 4) \times 2 = \dots \text{Kg}$$

For any child over the age of 1 year. In general the birth weight becomes double at 6 months and treble at 12 months of age. If birth weight is not known, full term neonate can be considered to weigh 3-4 Kg and 12-month-old infant as 10 Kg.

A **named** middle grade medical/nursing staff should calculate weight, the dosage of emergency drugs, fluids, dextrose and DC shock and write in the board clearly in large letters in addition to name, age and sex. Arrangement to retrieve the existing record in the hospital should be done soon. A **named** senior nursing staff should arrange the equipment like appropriate needles, syringes, drips, drip stand with pump, ECG, trolleys, cooling/heating equipment, drugs and anaesthetic trolleys with equipments and drugs. Preloaded manufacturers' syringes and correct labelling with doses would eliminate mistakes.

Senior/middle grade medical and nursing staff should receive the patient from the ambulance, transfer to the emergency/resuscitation room and gather the details from the ambulance staff. Under the direction and supervision of the leader (senior medical staff) the middle grade staff help to obtain IV/Intraosseous (IO) access, collect blood samples, check and administer fluids and drugs in the correct dose. The middle/junior grade nurse can attach monitoring equipment (oxygen saturation, blood pressure, ECG) to the patient, while the junior staff arranges to send the blood samples and requests to the appropriate departments, request help with other speciality staff. One of the nursing staff would be able to take care of the worried parents, comforting and providing explanations while various procedures are carried out. Junior nurse should note down procedures, medications given including site, route dose and time, observations and results of the investigations as they arrive. The junior nurse should arrange immediate blood sugar (glucose stick test) estimation with the first drop of IV/IO blood available or finger/heel prick capillary blood. It is important to warn the laboratory if the blood obtained is by the intraosseous route as the white cells are in the blast form (not to mistake as Leukaemia) and minute bony spicules may block the equipment if precautions are not taken.

Whether the parents should be with the child or not, during resuscitation, should be decided as a policy of the department/hospital. Most hospitals encourage parents to be with the child, as they feel comfortable to see the progress and a sense of satisfaction that they are part of the team treating their child.

Record Keeping

It is of paramount importance to write down all details – medical and nursing staff involved, examination on arrival about *A, B, C, D*, observations [RR, HR, BP with appropriate cuff, CRT (capillary refill time), temperature etc.], investigations and procedures (needle thoracocentesis, intercostal drainage, aspiration for cardiac tamponade, DC shock etc.) carried out, results of the investigations, drugs and dose administered, site, route - peripheral IV/IO/central line/rectal/oral - fluid type and amount infused, tubes (Guedal airway, endotracheal tube, nasogastric tube, urethral catheter etc.) inserted. All recordings should be time orientated.

SERIOUS PROBLEMS

(1) Cardiac Arrest

Cardiac function is inadequate when the electrical activities in the ECG are not present (asystole) or disturbed (fibrillation, Pulseless Electrical Activity – PEA, formerly known as Electro Mechanical Dissociation EMD). There are number of causes which ultimately result in *hypoxia (A, B), hypovolaemia (C), hypo/hyperthermia/hypoglycaemia* and lead to deranged cardiac function. Cardiac insufficiency can also be noted in children with congenital or acquired cardiac defect, or cardio-respiratory obstructions.

The ECG monitor should be correctly connected to the body with three electrodes (red to right, amber to left of chest and green below), increased electrical gain to the best, in lead II are used to understand/record the electrical activity of the heart.

Pulse (carotid for child, brachial for baby) should be palpated for the presence or absence and rate according to the age to indicate normal, bradycardia or tachycardia (Table 30.1).

As soon as the patient is brought to the emergency room, *Basic Life Support* and *correction of A, B, C, D* deficits should be carried out starting with high flow oxygen through mask with reservoir bag if spontaneously and adequately breathing or assisted (bag-valve-mask or endotracheal intubation) if spontaneous breathing is not present or inadequate. Vascular access (peripheral or central IV/IO) should be obtained immediately for delivering appropriate sugar, fluid and medication. Asystole, Ventricular fibrillation and Pulseless Electrical Activity (PEA, formerly known as Electro Mechanical Dissociation EMD): In children, precordial thumping is done only when the arrest is **witnessed in the wards** resulting in asystole and should not be attempted if the child is brought from outside the hospital. CPR (Cardio-Pulmonary Resuscitation) should be carried out according to the protocols developed by the Paediatric Life Support Groups[1,2] (Figs 30.1 to 30.3).

(2) Collapsed Patient

Hypoxia (*A, B*) and hypovolaemia (*C*) are the most important common reasons/effects for collapse in the paediatric age. Cardio-respiratory problems, fluid loss (e.g. dehydration – gastroenteritis, burns), blood loss (trauma), septicaemia, serious illness or poisoning are some of the important causes. Due to limited storage of glycogen, hypoglycaemia sets in fast in very ill children due to serious illness.

'Problem recognition and treatment have higher priority than definite diagnosis'

Immediate management in the **first few minutes** is aimed to identify the deficits of *A, B, C, D* and correct each one as recognised rather than spending time to make a diagnosis which can be considered/worked out while/after stabilising the patient.

A, B, C, D, E is carried out in the standard format as in Resuscitation manuals[1,2]. For trauma, assessment and resuscitation are done as a Primary and Secondary survey and adding cervical collar for *A* and control of bleeding for *C*.

If there are enough persons available, several procedures can be done simultaneously. But in the event that only one medical officer is available, it is vital to go through *A, B, C, D, E* in *seriatim* and deficits should be corrected step by step as the problems are recognised (e.g. *A* should be satisfactorily corrected/completed before attempting to improve *B* and so on). Repeated assessments should be done after performing any action to note the desired effect and if no/poor response, further treatment should be considered before proceeding to the next letter – all are recorded *in seriatim* and time orientated.

Airway is corrected with the patient in neutral (infant) or sniffing position (children) with head tilt and chin lift (jaw thrust, without tilting, for trauma), removal of secretions using Yankauer sucker, removing **visible** foreign body in the mouth using Magill or similar forceps, supplemented with oxygen (3 litres/minute for a full-term neonate and increasing amounts to 15 litres/minute to an older child according to the age) through a transparent mask with oxygen reservoir bag. If not improving, respiratory effort can be supported by assisted ventilation (bag-valve-mask – Ambu Bag, endotracheal intubation). In a traumatic situation, appropriate cervical collar and sandbags on either side, taped to chin and forehead (Figure 30.6), should be in place if the patient is symptomatic or unconscious. This can be removed when asymptomatic and satisfactory radiological and neurological examinations.

Breathing should be equal and adequate in both sides. If inadequate on one side, intrathoracic obstruction should be considered and corrected – *tension pneumothorax* (needle thoracocentesis just **under** the midpoint of the clavicle – Fig. 30.6 NT), *haemothorax* [operative intercostal drainage at the (5th intercostal space) in the nipple line in the **midaxillary line** – (Fig. 30.6 ICD) or *haemo-pneumothorax*. These landmarks cannot be missed even in the most obese patient. Sucking effect can be prevented with occlusive dressing on three sides for *open pneumothorax* and at the same time not allowing to develop *tension pneumothorax*. Endotracheal tube ventilation may be required for a *flail segment* when oxygen saturation cannot be improved. Continuous monitoring of oxygen saturation (O_2 Sat.) through the probe in the finger/toe is useful to know the response of the procedure.

Circulation should be improved with fluid (crystalloid 20 ml/Kg or colloid 10 ml/Kg) as a bolus. In a collapsed patient, bolus injection with a 50 ml syringe is of more benefit to the child than dripping through the pump. If the response is not satisfactory second bolus of 20 ml/Kg will be necessary when fluid loss had been considerable. For an inadequate response, the subsequent fluid should be administered as blood to increase the oxygen carrying capacity in addition to filling the vascular compartment. Infusion of colloids and crystalloids can be alternated to take advantage of both types. A blood sample should be

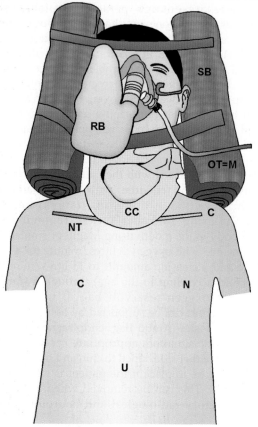

Fig. 30.6: Resuscitation, needle thoracocentesis and intercostal drain

SB – Sand Bag, RB – Reservoir Bag, OT + M – Oxygen Tube and Mask, CC – Cervical Collar, NT – Needle Thoracocentesis, ID – Intercostal Drain, C – Clavicle, N – Nipple, U – Umbilicus

obtained for crossmatching before colloids are administered. The fluid replacement should be aimed to result a urinary out put of about 1ml/Kg/hour.

Blood sugar, full blood count, C reactive protein, urea and electrolytes and blood gases should be done in all patients and other appropriate investigation according to the problem, like poisoning profile tests and metabolic disorders etc. Culture and coagulation profile for patients due to illness, cross match (group or full crossmatch according to the urgency) for trauma problems.

Disability can be assessed using *Glasgow Coma Score* (GCS) and/or AVPU (<u>A</u>lert, response to <u>V</u>oice/<u>P</u>ain or <u>U</u>nresponsive), size, reaction and equality of both pupils and neurological examination including the position of the patient (decorticate or decerebrate). Though many are important, **oxygen and blood sugar are the two *most* vital elements** to sustain some basic cerebral functions. Brain can be insulted by many different ways, but reduced/no oxygen and/or sugar will derange the brain sufficiently worse to disturb all other functions. Sufficient oxygen should be made available to the brain, by effective

oxygenation (through assisted ventilation using oxygen reservoir bag/bag-valve mask/endotracheal intubation). Children have limited storage of glucose and glycogen in the liver, rapidly utilised and depleted in a few hours during any serious illness – leading to symptomatic **hypoglycaemia**. If the finger prick (BM) and/or laboratory blood sugar is below 3 mmol/l, a **bolus injection of glucose.**

5ml/Kg of 10% dextrose, i.e. 0.5 Gm/Kg

in the peripheral IV/IO line or concentrated dextrose (20% - 50%) in the central line (0.5 Gm/Kg) **in addition** to the fluid requirement (as indicated above).

Exposure – The nurse can cut the clothes and remove the footwear so that A, B, C, D can be assessed better. When the patient is lying on the couch, examination is done only for the 50% of the body in the front as there is another 50% on the dorsal aspect, lest open pneumothorax, spinal injuries etc. in an unconscious patient can be missed and resuscitation may not improve the condition of the patient. Coordinated effort to turn the patient as **'log roll'** (3 or 4 persons according to the size of the patient)[1,2] would preserve the existing neurological function even in the presence of vertebral injury.

Trauma and poisoning should also be considered when adequate history is not or could not be obtainable.

Radiological Investigations: Plain X-ray of the shunt system for hydrocephalus is useful to diagnose blocked/disconnected system. Emergency CT scan is useful to understand intracranial problems like oedema, bleeding, vascular malformation, tumour etc.

NON-TRAUMATIC PROBLEMS

(1) Very Ill Child with/without Rash

Children become very ill quickly with onset of septicaemia. Rash in the body may range from one two spots to completely covering the body or even without any rash at all when a child is presenting in the hospital. Rash may be noticeable only after admission in the hospital in some children. Therefore it is vital to suspect septicaemia for vigorous investigation and prompt treatment.

Children are brought because of lethargy ranging to unconsciousness, not responding to parents, refusal of feeds, altered temperature (hyper/hypothermia), vomiting. Parents notice change of behaviour developing very quickly in few hours to 1 or 2 days. In suspected septicaemia, the resuscitation should be carried out in the same sequence as *A, B, C, D* as all of these could be disturbed – details as in the 'collapsed child' section as above.

Maintaining the body temperature (heater, covering the head, limbs and body with blankets/towels, use of aluminium space blanket if hypothermia or removing clothes (cut if necessary), fan, rectal paracetamol if the child is hot), cephalosporin like cefotaxime (100 mg/Kg), use of Fresh Frozen Plasma (FFP) if coagulation screening indicates abnormal results should be considered.

(2) Diabetes

Symptomatic *hypo*glycaemia should be corrected as indicated above when the glucose stick test (finger/heel prick BM) indicates blood sugar < 3 mmol/l.

5 ml/Kg of 10% dextrose, i.e. 0.5 Gm/Kg in peripheral IV/IO lines

In a known diabetic child, *hyper*glycaemia is associated with loss of water and sodium in large amounts and so the initial fluid replacement should be with normal saline, 20 ml/Kg bolus injections till hypovolaemia is corrected.

50 units of soluble insulin added to 50 ml of saline = 1 unit/ml

The infusion is given at a dose of 0.1 unit/Kg/hour, which equals to 0.1 x weight in Kg as ml/hour of the made up fluid (e.g. 20 Kg child requires 2 ml/hour or 35 Kg child requires 3.5 ml/hour of such made up fluid). When the blood sugar is satisfactory, insulin can be reduced to half such dose and fluid changed to 0.45% or 0.18% saline with dextrose. **Rapid correction often leads to cerebral oedema** with high mortality rate and therefore the correction should be at a reasonable slow pace with frequent biochemical monitoring and with the help of a diabetologist.

In diabetic ketoacidosis when the blood pH falls below 7.1 depression of CNS prevents compensation by hyperventilation in the initial period. When blood pH is < 7.1, 8.4% $NaHCO_3$ should be infused over about 2 hours at a dose of 2.5 ml/Kg and the infusion should be stopped when the pH is over 7.1 as the body will correct subsequently.

Potassium loss should be corrected with addition of 20-40 mmol/l of potassium chloride diluted in saline and frequent monitoring of serum and ECG.

(3) Poisoning

Iron, tricyclic antidepressants, opiates, paracetamol, salicylates are some of the commonly ingested medications with high fatality rate. Any unconscious child without any clear history suggestive of illness/injury or choking due to foreign body, ingestions of medications/chemical compounds should be considered. The patient should be stabilised in identifying and correcting the deficits of *A, B, C, D, E* while waiting for the results of poison profile tests in blood, urine and vomitus when the medications are unknown. Specific antidotes should be given in appropriate doses when the substance/medication is known/identified. Gastric lavage or charcoal should be used carefully in certain indications and not as routine.

Accidental ingestion is more common especially in infants and young children although deliberate ingestions are not uncommon in older/teenage children (see chapter 19 on accidental poisoning in childhood).

(4) Child with Seizures

Most of the time, seizure stops by the time the child reaches the hospital though the ambulance message would have been a fitting child, but sometimes continues in status epilepticus on arrival in the hospital. When trained ambulance persons are available, the first dose of rectal diazepam is given at home. At times, parents bring the child with own transport and the child is received fitting. Anticonvulsive medication dose/doses are occasionally missed/vomited and to precipitate fits. Hypoxia and/or hypoglycaemia can precipitate or accentuate fits. Position, falling of tongue, oral secretions, vomiting can obstruct air passage _A_, and should be corrected and oxygen should be administered in an appropriate way. Blood sugar (glucose stick test – finger/heel prick or IV/IO BM) result should be available within a few minutes of arrival. If it is < 3 mmol/l, this should be corrected with a **bolus** dose of 5ml/Kg of 10% dextrose (0.5 Gm/Kg) through peripheral IV/IO or higher concentrated dextrose (20 - 50%) through a central line (0.5 Gm/Kg). It is important to *differentiate* **tonic convulsion** due to **raised intracranial pressure** and in which case mannitol 1.30 ml/Kg should be given IV/IO as a **bolus** soon. Fits should be controlled using the algorithm whether IV line is available or not (Fig. 30.5). Help of Paediatric/ Neurology and Anaesthetic team should be sought if fits could not be controlled. Usual medications and dosages should be verified and ascertained whether they were given at home in time. Parents are helpful to point out the drugs used during previous episodes with success, rather than trying different medications.

Removal of clothes, rectal paracetamol and fan could be used to reduce temperature in cases of high fever. The patient should be warmed, if hypothermic due to drowning, using heaters, electric/space blankets, warm fluids (IV/ intragastric/urinary bladder) using a 'blood warmer' and warm gases.

(5) Acute Respiratory Distress

Reduction in the diameter of the air passage is the common reason for acute respiratory distress in the paediatric age. Larger passages like trachea, bronchi may be narrowed due to infection such as croup (laryngotracheobronchitis), foreign bodies or small passages as in asthma, bronchiolitis. Severe infection like pneumonia affects the parenchymal function.

(a) Epiglottitis: Due to compulsory vaccination against HIB (Haemophilus Influenza B) the incidence of epiglottitis is declining in many countries, but this is a life threatening disease in the unvaccinated childhood population. Acute respiratory distress not settling/getting worse in a few hours, dusky or cyanotic and toxic looking anxious child, unable to speak or whisper and signs of proximal airway obstruction like indrawing intercostal and subcostal muscles and reduced but equal air entry both sides should alert the staff. In such an airway compromised child, no attempt like asking the child to lie down or sight of needles should be done as the upset might precipitate respiratory and followed by cardiac arrest. Immediate explanation and oxygen by mask, held by mother, should be attempted while waiting for the anaesthetist to come and intubate. Should there be a **delay** and child becomes unconscious due to severe hypoxia, **emergency needle cricothyroidotomy** should be carried out and wait for endotracheal intubation by an expert anaesthetist. Cephalosporin like Cefotaxime (100 mg/Kg) and steroids are useful when the airway is controlled.

(b) Croup (laryngotracheobronchitis): Larger and proximal air passages are narrowed due to inflamed and edematous mucosa of the respiratory tract. Well looking child with barking sound, playing well with toys is seen on most of the occasions but can be ill when the diameter of the proximal passage is narrowed enough to result in hypoxia. In ill patients, oxygen by mask with reservoir bag, parenteral cephalosporins and steroids will help to improve the passage within a few hours. In critical patients, endotracheal intubation and ventilation is required and intubation should be attempted by expert anaesthetist, using the tube with considerably less diameter.

(c) Acute exacerbation of asthma: Narrowing of smaller terminal air passages classically produces wheeze due to flow of air in such passage and are usually controlled with inhalers. But when the passage is sufficiently inadequate, resulting hypoxia makes the child very ill. Oxygen saturation and peak flow metre reading give an idea of severity of the problem. In mild to moderate conditions, oxygen through reservoir mask, inhalers and 3 day course of Prednisolone (2 mg/Kg/day single or two divided doses) may be sufficient. But hypoxia is manifest with *GCS* less than 12 or 13 or ranging from 'V' to 'U' in the *AVPU* scale and requiring endotracheal intubation, high concentration and high flow oxygen, adrenaline, hydrocortisone and inhalers are very useful. Antibiotics (like Co-amoxiclav) will be required if precipitating factor is infection. Intravenous fluids/nutrition is mandatory if prolonged ventilation is required.

(d) Bronchiolitis: Hypoxia can be resulted when the small air passages are further narrowed due to inflammation in young babies and infants. Most of the patients can be managed at home but may require hospitalisation if hypoxia and/or feeding is sufficiently interfered. Severely hypoxic patients should be treated with endotracheal tube ventilation and transferred to ICU after stabilising. Moderately hypoxic patients can be treated with oxygen (nasal/mask with reservoir bag) and nasogastric feeding. Antibiotics and steroids are not considered beneficial.

TRAUMA

Radiological investigations: Any child with **trauma** and brought **unconscious**, lateral view of cervical vertebrae, AP chest and pelvis are **mandatory**. Time should not be wasted for X-ray chest, if **tension pneumothorax** is **suspected** and treatment (needle thoracocentesis, at the lower border of the midpoint of clavicle) should be carried out **immediately**.

(a) Head and Neck Injury: Cerebral functions are depressed because of raised intracranial compression due to oedema and/or bleeding. In intracranial injuries with compression of brain, **Cushing's triad** – altered consciousness, **slow pulse rate** and **increased blood pressure** are often noted. Therefore, **increased pulse rate** and/or **low blood pressure** should raise the suspicion of **trauma and bleeding** elsewhere in chest, abdomen, pelvis or major bony injuries and not just concentrating on head injury only. The mechanism of injury, like RTA or fall from a considerable height or hit by heavy solid object, can point to a serious intracranial injury.

When head injury is severe enough to make the person with depressed conscious level (GCS < 13), **injury to cervical vertebra** should be presumed to be present till later neurological and radiological investigations (plain X-rays in two views and oblique if necessary, CT/MRI) prove to be normal. Therefore, it is prudent to immobilise with cervical collar and sandbags on either side of the neck (the Ambulance Service personnel are trained to apply, from the initial scene). Controlled 'log rolling' (with 3 or 4 persons according to age)[1,2] under the orders of the leader who stabilises head and neck, for any examination or procedure at the back, will prevent any iatrogenic cord/nerve injury.

Blood loss can be considerable due to cut injuries of scalp, especially in neonates and infants, as the blood supply to a unit area of scalp is similar to tongue and heart and considerably greater than many parts of the body. Hypovolaemic shock may result especially in babies, even with a haematoma (scalp, fracture femur) with loss of considerable amount of blood.

Blood volume of an infant is 80 ml/Kg (about a can of canned beverages!) and gradually changing to 60 ml/Kg in older children.

Consciousness should be assessed by Glasgow Coma Scale (*GCS*) or quickly with *AVPU* scale. GCS of < 13 indicates a serious problem and head injury should be considered if the mechanism of injury is suspicious.

Pupils are windows of the brain. Size, reaction, equality are under the control of sympathetic (through ophthalmic artery) and parasympathetic fibres (in Oculomotor nerve). Alteration (Hutchinson's pupils) indicates intracranial compression and the side of the problem clinically, though CT scan is required to confirm and for further management.

In an unconscious patient, plain X-ray of skull in AP, Lateral and Towne's view have limited use but CT scan is of more value for management immediately – as this can identify fractures. Tangential view may be required if suspected depressed fracture, but CT scan can also indicate such diagnosis, in addition to other intracranial problems.

Management: Assistance by Neurosurgical colleague should be requested early if the patient was known to be unconscious/unresponsive. BLS should be carried out, even before reaching a definite diagnosis as correction of deficits (hypoxia *A, B,* hypovolaemia *C,* hypo/hyperthermia/hypoglycaemia) may improve conscious status, GCS/AVPU. Assisted ventilation by a mask with an Oxygen reservoir bag or endotracheal intubation is required often in unconscious/unresponsive patients. Provided no other bleeding is known/considered, better to wait for CT scan before giving more parenteral fluids. The first available **blood sample** is used for cross matching **before any colloids are given**. The blood bank should be warned about such parenteral fluid administration in case if the blood sample was collected after colloid administration. Nasogastric tube should be inserted carefully after ruling out basal skull fracture, preferably by anaesthetist under vision, lest the tube may be inserted into the brain! Skills of an expert anaesthetist are required for endotracheal intubation if fracture/dislocation of cervical vertebra(e) is suspected/proven. Mannitol (1.30 ml/Kg) should be used only after agreement with the Neurosurgical team.

Examination findings, actions and repeated observations, should be clearly recorded including pupils' sizes in diagrams and diameter in mm and reaction and equality.

(b) Chest injuries: (1) Pleuro/Pulmonary: The injuries can be life threatening at times and simple emergency procedures could save life. Acute compression of lung(s) results in severe hypoxia, which may **falsely mislead** for a priority diagnosis of head injury.

(i) Pneumo/Haemo-thorax: Acute respiratory distress developing after chest trauma quickly due to air/blood is due to acute compression of the lung(s). The child becomes cyanosed, has fast breathing, hard working intercostal and subcostal muscles, ipsilateral side of chest has reduced/no movement by inspection and palpation, reduced/no air entry or disparity of air entry on both sides. All clinical findings are similar to both conditions except resonant or dull for percussion for air or blood trapped in the pleural cavity respectively. Due to the time taken to arrange for X-ray studies and imminent danger of death, an *emergency needle thoracocentesis* should be done *immediately* when the diagnosis is considered. It is difficult to feel the menubrio-sternal angle or the 2nd rib in children, but even in the most obese child, it is always easy to feel the *lower border of the ipsilateral clavicle* (Figure 30.6– NT) and the needle with cannula should be introduced *below the mid point of the clavicle* till 'hissing noise' of air heard and then attach to an underwater seal drain after removing the needle and properly fixing. The child who was unconscious due to severe hypoxia can respond well when the tension is relieved with improving oxygenation and so the possibility of displacing/removing the needle.

Intercostal drainage should be performed if acute lung compression is due to blood in the pleural cavity (haemothorax). *Nipple line* in children is an easy landmark for incision in the mid-axillary line of the chest (Fig. 30.6, ICD, *5th intercostal space*) and the intercostal drainage tube should be inserted only after enlarging the opening in the intercostal space sufficiently enough and **feeling with a finger** inside. The sharp metal trocar **should not be used** for introducing the drainage tube lest injury may result to underlying structures (like stomach) if there were to be a ruptured diaphragm. It is wise to have two wide bore needle vascular access before inserting the drainage tube as sudden release of accumulated blood could release the tamponade effect and promoting severe bleeding. In acute respiratory distress due to Haemo-Pneumothorax, immediate needle thoracocentesis should be done prior to intercostal drainage if there is only one rescuer is available.

(ii) *Open pneumothorax*: When the pleura from the skin side is cut, the air movement can be bi-directional resulting in hypoxia. Gauze sealed on three sides would allow air to escape from the chest (not allowing to develop tension pneumothorax if all four sides are sealed) and prevents sucking air from the atmosphere till a definite action is planned.

(iii) Lung injuries: Injury to the parenchyma of lung (contusion) should be suspected in a hypoxic child without any acute compression/cut injury as above. Endotracheal intubation and urgent help is sought from the thoracic surgeons, in addition to *A, B, C* and *D* management. Such a diagnosis should be considered only after 'log roll' assessment of the dorsal side of the body.

(2) Rib injuries: Flail Chest: When few ribs are fractured at two sites of the same ribs, 'paradoxical movements' occur due to movement of the segment in the opposite direction of movement of the chest, resulting in hypoxia. Endotracheal intubation may be required if ventilation is inadequate.

(c) Abdominal injuries: Emergency laparotomy is always indicated when hollow viscus like intestine is **perforated/ruptured**. Without disturbing the patient, (Decubitus) lateral view of X-ray abdomen in the supine position is enough to recognise free intraperitoneal gas.

Non-surgical method is mostly satisfactory with careful observation due to intra-abdominal bleeding. Unlike adults, when bleeding due solid viscera like liver/spleen is suspected, peritoneal tapping/lavage is not usually performed in children, as the result and subsequent management may be confused. In general, very few children will require surgical exploration when replacing adequate fluid would not improve and large amounts of fluid/blood is required and not able to stabilise due to continuous bleeding. Emergency splenectomy is a rare procedure in modern trauma care in children. IVP/CT would help to decide further management of renal injuries.

(d) Pelvic injuries: Run-over injuries typically result in pelvic injuries and genito-urinary and other hollow visceral injuries could accompany. Immediate management is on general principles of correction of *A, B, C, D* deficits. Urethral catheterisation should be performed only after discussion with surgical/urological team. Stabilisation with sandbags on either side of pelvis is useful till orthopaedic team takes over the management.

(e) Limb injuries: Blood loss can be considerable for long bone injuries and circulation should be taken care of once *A* and *B* are satisfactory. Emergency action is required for neuro-vascular compromise in conditions like angulated/displaced fractures, compound fractures and compartment syndromes. Immediate manipulation and reduction may restore blood supply, but exploration/adequate incisional release for compartment syndrome should not be delayed if there is no adequate improvement. When delay is anticipated to gain access to operation theatre, incisions deep enough to release acute compression should be done in the emergency room. Immobilisaton and parenteral analgesia and/or nerve blocks (e.g. femoral nerve block for fracture femur) result in the comfort of the child.

THERMAL INJURIES

Mortality rate is high when the airway is compromised in house fires due to smoke inhalation, when mouth and/or nose involved, or inadequate/slow/no fluid replacement when large areas are involved. Oedema of mucosa quickly develops due to inhaled hot air reducing the diameter of the large passages of respiratory tract. Apart from applying cervical collar in an unconscious child, *A, B, C, D, E* deficits should be identified and corrected. Early endotracheal intubation by experienced anaesthetist should be considered when the area involved is around mouth/nose/anterior part of neck and in cases of house fires or large surface. For children, *Rule of nine should **not** be used* and the surface area is calculated using the Paediatric Burn chart. Child's own palm with adducted fingers is about 1% surface area and the area involved can be estimated quickly. IV fluids should be given for burns over 10%. Insertion of intraosseous needle should not be withheld even if the surface of skin at that site is burnt, in extensive burns when IV line could not be obtained in time. Boluses of 20 ml/Kg of crystalloid or 10 ml/Kg of colloids should be injected, as above, aiming for normovolaemia and urinary output of about 1 ml/Kg/hour. Apart from the normal requirement, the *additional* fluid required per day can be calculated using the formula:

$$\text{Percentage of burn} \times \text{weight in Kg} \times 4$$

and *half* this fluid should be given in the *first 8 hours since the time of burn.*

The involved areas should be covered with appropriate dressings.

Apart from inhalation injury to the air passage and lungs, head, bone and visceral injuries should be specifically looked for and managed.

FOREIGN BODIES

Mortality is high when the proximal respiratory passage is obstructed *in toto*. Most of the children brought to the hospital have some or nearly most of the passage in use. Mouth should be inspected with good light and foreign body removed if **visible**, using Magill's or similar forceps. *Blind finger sweeping is contraindicated* in children for fear of traumatising delicate mucosa resulting in bleeding and/or pushing deeper causing total obstruction.

In unconscious patient when witnessed or suspected to have foreign bodies in the respiratory tract, back blows and chest thrust (and abdominal thrust – Heimlich manoeuvre in older children) should be done alternatively till the foreign body comes out by itself or visible enough to remove.

If the foreign body has moved distally, ENT/Thoracic specialists help should be sought early while continuous oxygen from mask with reservoir bag is given.

NAI AND CSA

When the history is not consistent with duration and/or identified injuries or significant delay in presentation, non-accidental injuries should be suspected and investigated. The possibility of child sexual abuse should be thought of when a child is presented with genital and/or anal injuries.

MAJOR INCIDENTS

The hospital should have a well worked out plan to deal with several children presenting at the similar time, due to a disaster, like collapsed school building, drowning in the floods or food poisoning, etc. Resources – manpower, equipments, materials – should be mobilised fast to the scene and all attendants are made aware of their duties and responsibilities while the appropriate senior medical staff as a controlling leader, depending on the problem, i.e. surgeon/orthopaedic surgeon for trauma or paediatrician/anaesthetist for poisoning.

TRANSPORT

Quality rather than speed of transport is beneficial to the child with serious problems. Problems due *A, B, C, D* deficits should be corrected/stabilised (including cervical collar and sand bags if required) and then only the child should be transported to ward/ICU/HDU or from hospital to hospital. Appropriate staff who could manage airway, drips, and monitors should accompany the child. All documentation, laboratory results, blood samples, medication, observation charts, X-rays should be transported with the child and the accompanying person should have the complete knowledge about the child and management since arrival in the department, for handing over. Whether parents should accompany the child, depends upon the policy of the hospital.

REFERENCES

1. Advance Paediatric Life Support – Practical Approach. 4th Edition 2005, BMJ Books, London.
2. European Life Support Course Manual – 1st Edition, 2004, Paediatric Resuscitation Training Office, London.

Disorders of Emotion and Behaviour

Chapter 31

Michael Morton, David James

AN INTRODUCTION TO CHILD AND ADOLESCENT PSYCHIATRY

Knowledge of the emotional processes of child development within a family, social and cultural context is essential in paediatric practice. These factors have a primacy in this chapter that is different in many ways from others in this book. The disturbances discussed are generally not based upon easily defined "organic disease". Although advances in brain scanning and neurochemistry are becoming more relevant, it is only in a minority of these disorders that laboratory investigations yield useful information. While there is a scientific basis to the measurement of symptoms like depression and there are real advances in quantifying parameters of family and social disturbance, these questionnaires or rating scales may appear less objective than most clinical investigations. In organic disease there is usually a primary cause such as an infective agent or a mutant gene. In psychological disorders there is interplay of heredity and environment. Interaction, within a culture, between the patient, the family and the school, contributes to the clinical presentation. When a diagnostic formulation is reached, although there is a good evidence base for some treatments, the management of disorder often varies in the hands of different physicians or psychiatrists and some factors are beyond the reach of medical intervention. The range of knowledge that may contribute to an understanding of emotional and cognitive development is beyond the scope of this chapter. Some discussion of development is given in the context of an overview of the mental health problems and psychiatric disorders that may present in paediatric practice.

There are difficulties in making a diagnosis of a behavioural/emotional disorder using the usual medical model. Diagnosis in medicine depends partly on a collection of symptoms and physical signs fitting into a pattern that is recognised, but the quality of diagnosis improves when the aetiology can be proved. For example

there may be disagreement about a pain of acute onset in the left upper abdomen or lower chest where a patient may be in a state of collapse. One may vote for a myocardial infarct, and another may claim an exacerbation of a peptic ulcer. Once the abdomen is examined and the ECG done, opposing views will be reconciled. With emotional and behavioural difficulties, it is often difficult to get further than the grouping of signs and symptoms to make a diagnosis that does not generally include an assumption of causation.

Some attempt to deal with this complexity is found in classification systems using different axes for different aspects of a presentation, such as the ICD-10 Multi-axial Classification. The first axis in ICD-10 is generally related to the presenting symptoms, e.g. encopresis or hyperkinesis. The second axis offers a range of specific developmental delays, e.g. reading retardation, developmental speech/language disorder. Axis 3 deals with grades of generalized Learning Disability, labelled as 'Mental Retardation'. Axis 4 labels any associated physical disorder in the child, eg asthma or epilepsy. Axis 5 lists categories of psychosocial difficulty including mental disturbances in other family members, discordant intrafamilial relationships, inadequate or inconsistent parental control and familial over-involvement. This axis also includes social transplantation, stresses in school or work environment and other social problems including persecution or discrimination. A sixth axis enables a rating to be made for the degree of disability caused. It is only when all of these axes have been accounted for that a meaningful diagnostic formulation is produced. The skill of the clinician lies in deciding which factors are amenable to change.

While more severe disorders may require the involvement of a child psychiatrist, many can be dealt with by a family doctor or paediatrician. Often problems presenting at clinics in the UK relate to normal stages of child development, which are ill understood by over-anxious or depressed parents. More severe and intractable symptoms may require a more detailed look at why a parent is finding the situation so difficult, and this may involve referral to a specialist service. A parent, who is angry, distressed or of limited ability, may be unable to take in and implement "good advice" until they see that the advisor has understood their difficulties. This process of listening and building up an understanding of a child's problems in the family context requires interpersonal skills more than medical qualification.

The complexity of presentations to specialist child and adolescent mental health service (CAMHS) clinics requires a range of skills to understand them fully. The child and adolescent mental health team usually includes psychiatrically trained nurses, psychiatrists and psychologists and may include occupational therapists, social workers, teachers, child psychotherapists, speech and language therapists and dietitians.

The style of taking the initial history is important in making the shift from the child's presenting symptom to finding out what has actually gone wrong in the family. According to the age of the child they may be seen on their own or with parents/carers, but the adult, who has usually initiated the consultation will require time to express their concern. It is important to begin with clarity about the reasons for consultation and the approach to be taken. Sometimes youngsters have been threatened with the clinic as a response to bad behaviour, they may sit in trepidation awaiting some imagined painful procedure. A child will usually talk readily about his or her interests, friends, school and relationships at home. A more direct discussion of the child's difficulties may be achieved once a shared understanding is established between interviewer and patient.

An attitude of non-judgmental empathy will often enable a child or parent to move from describing the complaint to feelings of despair and anger and then perhaps how unhelpful other members of the family can be. For example, it is not uncommon for a parent of a child with unexplained pain to move on to their own feelings of hopelessness and depression. At the end of half-an-hour or 40 minutes, there may be tears, perhaps about marital difficulties. Although the first part of the initial interview can be time-consuming, it may save hours later on. Having allowed this time, the interviewer may ask a wide range of questions, perhaps including details of the child's eating, problems with elimination, pain, levels of activity, details about temperament and relationships, anti-social behaviour, sexual difficulties, episodic disorders and school progress. The usual run through of systems, cardio-vascular, respiratory, gastro-intestinal, motor and uro-genital are included as appropriate. The personal history pays particular attention to pregnancy, birth and postnatal period, as well as details of personal and social development and the relationship between child and parents during these stages. The family and social history may take more than one interview to complete. It is important to know about the parents or the child's carers, and also to obtain details about grandparents. Information about cultural factors, the parents' childhood experiences, social values and models from families of origin, leads to an understanding of the child's problem within the extended family context. Social inquiry includes details of peer group, education, housing, neighbourhood and finance.

Apart from any physical examination determined by the complaint, it is important to assess the child's emotional state. One notes the child's appearance, communication, mood and self-esteem. The content and nature of the child's free play or creative behaviour during the assessment may be informative. More detailed approaches to observation may be indicated, for example one might make a modified adult style mental state examination or use structured observations, for example looking at behaviours suggestive of hyperactivity in the classroom.

Psychopathology in youngsters is often heightened by family conflict. Adult disharmony leads to inconsistent methods of discipline, which predispose to behavioural difficulty in the children. Children and adolescents can so easily be blamed or blame themselves for one or other parent's unhappiness. This can lead to anxiety and depression, school phobia and other psychogenic symptoms. As there are so often difficulties in family relationships even when there is an obvious physical component to the disorder; some CAMHS clinics begin with a family assessment. In this situation all members of the family living at home are invited to a first appointment. The therapist joins the family, occupying one of a circle of easy chairs. The initial explanation involves an acceptance that the problem with the child or adolescent involves all members of the family. The aim is to help the family discover where the difficulties are so that, with the therapist, they can plan the changes needed to bring about a resolution. While family therapy techniques require special training, it is worth bearing in mind that involving more than just one parent in the interview can often yield here and now information about the style of communication and the degree of mutual support available.

To complete an assessment, consent may be obtained to seek information from third parties such as teachers or social workers. When all this is drawn together a multi-axial classification can be completed and a plan of action made which may involve further assessment that may be medical, neurodevelopmental, psychometric, psycho-therapeutic or more usually of family relationships.

A range of treatment approaches exists. Some are focused upon the child, such as pharmacotherapy and various forms of psychological therapy, of which Cognitive Behavioural Therapy has the strongest evidence base.

Family interventions are common and the therapeutic power of the peer group, especially in adolescence is well recognised. Schools provide an opportunity for environmental management and specific supports for learning. Community projects are often geared to prevention and early intervention in support of parenting. At the other extreme, In-patient care and Intensive Out-reach or Day Services are used in the most severe and complex disorders.

There are social benefits arising from effective mental health interventions in childhood. Not only may cycles of abuse and parental failure be broken down but also there is a prospect of reducing the progression of childhood disturbance into adult disorder. For example, vulnerable children who present with antisocial behaviour may benefit from the collaboration of health and social agencies in a co-coordinated approach to reducing the risk of adult offending.

PROBLEMS IN EARLY CHILDHOOD

Most people readily understand the bodily changes as children grow. The changes involved in intellectual and emotional development are less easily comprehended. The development of speech, with the skills of language amongst the complex tasks of social communication is a crucial factor in further learning and social interaction. A massive amount of learning takes place during the toddler years. By the time a normal child enters school he has a good grasp of language that underpins the development of social and emotional behaviour.

Adverse environmental circumstances can retard physical growth and hold back children to function intellectually below their potential, but the greatest effects of adverse family relationships and social difficulties are generally upon children's feelings and behaviour. The first year of life or infancy is largely to do with the relationship between the caring adult or adults and the child. The infant needs to be kept warm, fed, clean, cuddled and interacted with. The beginning of shaping up vocalisation into speech involves eye-to-eye contact and social communication grows. A child should begin to feel secure in the knowledge of adult care and understanding of his or her needs. Important problems can arise during early development. The initial attachment of infant and caregiver may be adversely affected by maternal depression or illness in the child requiring long hospitalisation.

Pre-school behaviour problems usually start during the next phase of emotional development. During this phase children may appear defiant and demanding. The toddler thinks as if he/she is at the centre of everything and there is little awareness of the needs of others. The toddler's timescale is poorly developed and there is little ability to tolerate frustration, to do it later, or wait until

tomorrow. Temper tantrums are common and may be intolerable for parents who lack awareness of what is normal in this developmental stage.

A baby can be put away in a cot for periods of time but a toddler is mobile. Rapid cognitive development makes for a huge interest in exploring an environment that was previously inaccessible. Under these developmental conditions it is often a full-time job for the mother to keep the toddler safe and involved in learning social skills. Tables are pulled over, taps left running and electrical sockets interfered with. As speech develops there can be constant unanswerable questions, loud singing or protests if visitors or siblings interfere with activities or social discourse with the parent. Where the parent is feeling below par, perhaps living in a high flat where there is no where to go out to play or in an area which is clearly unsafe for youngsters to go out alone, the tension mounts. Where 2 or 3 youngsters are vying for attention in a family, the parent may be reduced to shouting, smacking or ignoring behaviour that requires attention or correction. In such circumstances, social programmes and parent support groups may be effective interventions. Although early childhood problems are often understandable in this way, a significant proportion of children presenting at this age will have temperamental characteristics or developmental disorders contributing to their difficulties.

Discipline should be firm, clear and consistent but also reasonable. It should relate to the child's developmental stage and understanding. A child will learn most easily when they feel secure with their parent or carer. Prompt positive reinforcement with respect, praise and love is the best way to modify behaviour. If punishment is undertaken in any form it should be carefully considered and quickly carried through to emphasise cause and effect. The more frequent the punishment the less its effect and too often threats are postponed until behaviour causes damage or an accident. Most importantly parents must not be split, with one colluding with behaviour, which the other is trying to correct.

A number of problems arise with failures of discipline. These include; feeding problems, temper tantrums, difficulty going to sleep and battles over toilet training. Sometimes a child has particular difficulties that challenge the most competent parent but by the time professional help is sought, parents have usually become quite inconsistent in their management of the problem. Parents will often claim to have "tried everything". Similar themes are found in most discipline problems but each type has particular features (see Case examples).

Case Examples

A child of four who will not go to sleep is told a story. Then he calls out, a reprimand is given and a testing cry tinged with uncertainty follows. Perhaps he will be given a drink and put back to bed. Opportunistically he cries again only to be given a severe telling-off by a mother who is beginning to be irate and exhausted. She says that she will go away if he is not good, so he cries again. Eventually after further loss of temper the mother feels guilty and upset that the child's shrieking will invite criticism. She brings the child back into the living area to watch the television. Another attempt is made to go to bed and the crying starts again. Night after night the situation worsens. Mother confides that she once put a pillow over the child's head momentarily and then became overwhelmed with guilt and took the child to bed with her.

A two year old with food fads raises parental anxiety by refusing to eat and thus manipulates the situation so that their favourite baked beans or biscuits have to be eaten for breakfast, lunch and tea. All kinds of bribes, punishments and ultimata are given while the toddler resolutely refuses to comply with normal meals. There is inconsistency between anxiety that the child may become ill or even not survive, and the adults' temper loss with sometimes-severe smackings and episodes of rejection.

Distraught parents require a sympathetic ear with some exploration of why this stage of development is difficult. Reassurance is important (for example, a parent may fear that the child will grow up delinquent or anorexic). Where possible, the principles of appropriate discipline should be reinforced and some parents need referral on to social services for support and guidance.

WORKING WITH PHYSICALLY ILL CHILDREN

If a child becomes unwell for significant periods of time the task is not only to get them well but also to enable them achieve their developmental potential. Children grow in three ways, they become physically taller, heavier and sexually mature; they increase in cognitive abilities; and they achieve social and emotional development. As children become more mature they are better able to handle extremes of feeling and to give and take in interpersonal relationships. The tasks of adolescence involve issues of separation and dependency as well as coping with adult values and sexual maturation.

The work of CAMHS involves the pathology of inter-personal relationships and any disability, inborn or acquired, will increase the risk of harmful attitudes in other family members, e.g., over-protection and rejection. Sometimes a parent's need to overindulge the child is based on (usually) irrational feelings of guilt about their disorder. It is also important to note that hospitals, like families, sometimes contain 'sick systems' where anxieties, frustrations and interpersonal difficulties of doctors, nurses and other therapists damage the effectiveness of professional networks.

Physical illnesses make children more vulnerable to psychological disorder and this effect is magnified in diseases affecting the brain, such as epilepsy. Technical advances in treatment subject children to stressful situations. Family disruption with frequent hospital attendances, transport problems, the effects of boredom, pain and tiredness take their toll. Such stresses are particularly damaging for vulnerable families. Pre-school children do not always understand why they are being hurt or why their parents sometimes have to leave when they are scared and in pain. The sequence of angry protest followed by despair and then emotional detachment from parents is well recognized in association with hospitalisation of younger children, without their parents. Children's hospitals encourage parents to stay with their children but mothers sometimes have to go home to look after the rest of the family. This kind of separation can have harmful, albeit temporary, effects. Thus a young child perplexed when the mother visited, turned to run towards the mother, halted, then ran to the comfort of the ward sister.

A child can often accept handicaps or painful treatments as long as all is explained honestly and at a level that can be understood. Anxiety increases if the parents do not appear to be at ease with the situation or if the child is told untruths or let down. It is helpful to listen to the child's worries and questions and then discuss with the parents how the questions should be answered in an understandable way. Children think in concrete practical terms and can be confused about illness and the possibility of dying. Death is seen as a reversible phenomenon by the very young. While it may well be unnecessary to trouble a child with details of a poor prognosis it is not helpful to ignore a child's concerns. When distressed children are told not to be silly or "let's see a smile", the anxieties, which are worrying them, are deflected and not dealt with.

Case Example

One young child almost died from a deliberate overdose. A much-loved relative had died and it appeared the only way to visit him was to go to heaven, and the only way to heaven was to become dead. Having been told that medicine cupboard contained poison he drank contents of several bottles and waited for a "sort of aeroplane ride" to get to heaven. When it was explained that there was no way back and he would not see his friends and relatives again, he decided that he had been unwise.

Coping

There are predictable patterns in coping with bad news, for example that mild malaise is actually renal failure and a transplant is required, or that 'anaemia' is really a cancer of the blood. **Denial** is a common mental mechanism, characterised by disbelief. This may be helpful at times but sometimes its effect is that potentially successful treatment regimes are not adhered to, particularly in adolescence. Thus denial becomes unhelpful when insulin injections penetrate the arm of the settee rather than the youngster's subcutaneous tissues. **Reaction formation** occurs where there is opposition to the underlying feeling and there may be pressure on an ill child to achieve more than they are easily able to do. For example, small vulnerable children may need to be big and tough. Others may **regress** to infantile and dependent behaviour. Some youngsters develop rituals before treatment regimes and others dispel their anxiety in fantasy. In children's hospitals there are a lot of bandaged teddies. Adolescents sometimes identify with medical staff by taking an **intellectualised** interest in their disorder.

All these defence mechanisms can be helpful as well as destructive and if these defences fail too rapidly the youngster may be overcome with **anxiety**, become **severely depressed** or on occasion curl up in a fetal position and **withdraw** from treatment or refuse to eat. **Guilt** is anger turned inwards with soul-searching as to how the disease or accident could have been avoided. Sometimes this leads parents to become depressed with an escalation of guilt and sometimes-morbid thoughts with sleep and appetite disturbance. The **marital situation** can deteriorate and where one parent spends a long time in hospital with the child, the other may be marginalised. Exhaustion and disruption of routine causes irritability and sometimes disagreements about the way the child is managed. The **siblings** are also compromised in that the parents do not always meet their basic emotional needs.

Case Example

A young child with a urinary infection was reassured that he would not need dialysis like his sister. In a temper, he slammed out of the room, saying, "Does that mean I am not getting the machine as well then".

The predicament of a sick child affects the whole family and all should benefit from a realistic acceptance of the disorder so that the child is neither over-protected nor expected to do more than he is able. To achieve such adjustment it helps to see both parents together. If the same person sees the parents on a number of occasions it is possible to check out what they took away from previous interviews. However bad the reality, a child's fantasy may be worse. In general a child's questions should be answered directly, honestly and in a way that is understandable. School attainments are important as long-term disorders can interrupt education, which is a major determinant of adult outcome in chronic childhood disease. Sick children need discipline as well as care, which can be difficult for any adult. A team approach ensures that communication is strong enough to avoid anxious parents inadvertently setting one professional up against another. Sometimes anxious parents make staff feel ill at ease but parents

should be given their place. Close relationships may develop with some staff. The work is multidisciplinary and all members of the team should feel appropriately useful and valued. Work will be stressful especially when children do not recover but morale is helped by regular discussion both case centred and more informally so that anxieties are shared and treatment goals sustained.

EMOTIONAL DISORDERS AND MEDICALLY UNEXPLAINED SYMPTOMS

Children express themselves in physical as well as psychological language and it is helpful to understand the different terms used in such presentations. Various terms may be found in the literature and the confusion of language reflects the complexity of the topic.

Neurosis is a term used to describe predominantly psychiatric disorders that nevertheless may cause a number of worrying and apparently "physical" symptoms including abdominal pain, headaches and limb pains, which sometimes can be severe and disabling. Thus, appetite disturbance, nausea and vomiting can be symptoms of anxiety.

The term **Somatoform disorder** covers a range of stress linked physical symptoms that may be the main presentation of emotional disturbance. For example, somatoform abdominal pain can be severe and although there is no real guarding or tenderness, some children appear exquisitely tender or find it difficult to relax to have their abdomens palpated. It is surprising how such pain can become localised to the right iliac fossa or epigastrium when various doctors have made repeated examinations querying acute appendicitis or peptic ulceration.

The term **Psychosomatic disorder** is used in illnesses with a known organic causation, where there are changes in tissue structure or function, but where the disorder or exacerbations of the disorder are partly or mainly induced by stress. A number of illnesses can be included in this category, for example some cases of asthma, skin disorders or bowel problems.

Cyclical vomiting syndrome, where attacks of prostrating vomiting occasionally needing intravenous fluids can last for one or two days, is a complex example, linked to migraine. As the child gets older visual disturbance, photophobia and pulsating headache become more apparent and the vomiting less obvious. In some cases the episodes are triggered by stress. Children with migraine disorders are often normal between episodes and these are best regarded as organic conditions, possibly with a psychosomatic element but they are not neurotic disorders.

Conversion disorders have been thought to involve the psychological mechanism of **dissociation** whereby the patient is not connecting emotions with experience and unaware that the symptom is other than organic.

Conversion symptoms include some disorders of movement, apparent paralysis of limbs and psychological seizures. Children presenting with these disorders may be in some kind of an emotional trap or predicament. Where conversion is suspected one should look at all aspects of the child's life situation and find out what purpose the symptom is serving or how it is protecting the child from whatever happens if the symptom goes away. Episodes of vomiting may keep together parents who are on the verge of separating. A girl's sore tummy may be stopping her highly esteemed father from trying to have sexual intercourse with her. The astute clinician sometimes sees something symbolic in the presenting complaint, as it is not just chance that certain symptoms are unconsciously selected.

The term 'Medically Unexplained Symptom' helps to avoid problems in categorizing such disorders. There are several pitfalls in attempts to distinguish the origin of such symptoms. Some symptoms can be frankly goal directed with conscious awareness of the gain involved, but for a diagnosis of conversion disorder there must be an element of dissociation or unawareness. A diagnosis of conversion requires a satisfactory formulation of the child's difficulty, and is confirmed when attempts to ameliorate that situation bring about a considerable improvement in the disorder. Children and families may resist a conversion diagnosis for many reasons and many find it hard to understand psychosomatic causation. Often there is dual pathology, e.g. psychological seizures are often found in children with epilepsy. Some cases of so-called psychogenic disorder turn out to have an organic basis when followed-up. Unusual presentations of common disorder and sometimes extremely unusual disorders can appear within the course of time. For example peptic ulcers are a more common cause of intermittent abdominal pain than perhaps one would expect and very rarely, peculiar panic attacks are due to cerebral tumours. Where there is doubt, a decision about diagnosis is best made using both paediatric and psychiatric expertise with a capacity for joint review when there is continuing uncertainty. Where there is no organic disease identified it is possible to make progress through psychological interventions geared to the individual presentation without requiring precision on the mechanism of symptom causation.

Emotional Disorders

Emotional disorders occur in at least 2 per cent of the population of late primary school children. The symptoms of **anxiety** and **depression** often co-exist and may be missed when they present in children, especially when expressed through somatic symptoms. More psychological signs of emotional disorder include sleep difficulties with anxious or depressing thoughts keeping the child awake or preventing him/her going to bed, while early wakening, usually regarded as a symptom of endogenous depression can also occur, especially in older children. Poor concentration is frequently present and may have gone unnoticed in school, as children with emotional disorders do not usually present a behavioural problem in the classroom. Tearfulness, over-sensitivity, agitation and irritability are common. Anxious toddlers and young children are unsettled and on the go and may be thought to be hyperkinetic. Where depression predominates the youngster will admit to feeling bad and guilty and sometimes overwhelming feelings of wretchedness can be associated with stealing, tearing up promising work, being unable to accept praise and wanting to die. In pre-school and young primary children the ultimate depressive thought seems to be separation and abandonment from the parents or those looking after them. Feelings of guilt leading to suicidal ideas have to be checked out in the older primary school child and certainly in the adolescent. One might ask, "Do you sometimes feel so bad or unhappy that you would like to run away from home or have a bad accident or die". A reply in the affirmative must be taken seriously and it is a myth that children who talk about harming themselves would not do so.

Self-harming behaviour and attempted suicide are common in adolescent populations although socio-cultural factors lead to varying prevalence across communities. Such presentations require urgent and careful attention to the range of individual and family factors that may have preceded the event. It is important to look for treatable disorders such as depression. Specific interventions may reduce the risk of recurrence and address the underlying difficulties revealed in the crisis.

School phobia and school refusal are terms used for children who develop emotional or unexplained physical symptoms in the morning before school. The symptoms ameliorate either when they have been at school for a while or when the decision is made that they are too ill to attend. Often symptoms are not due to a true phobia of school, but are caused by separation anxiety about leaving home and parents. Some school phobic children are depressed. Such children are often good achievers, and although they may try to go to school, symptoms occur to prevent this happening. Their parent or parents are much in evidence, worrying about the child's pains, vomiting, or else being angry that he/she has failed to leave the home for school. These patterns of behaviour are totally different from truancy.

Truancy

The truant frequently under-achieves, comes from a family who rather than being over-involved with the non-attendance at school are unconcerned or unaware of the situation until the authorities make contact. There are no psychogenic symptoms associated with truants who frequently go off to join friends in conduct disordered activity.

Phobic anxiety presents where there is a specific anxiety in certain situations, e.g. thunderstorms, fear of dogs and being upset by insects. Often these fears are not generalised into other situations and the youngsters may in other ways be quite emotionally robust. Specific psychological intervention with the child can be most helpful. Phobias in children may be learnt from a parent, friend or relative. This is not always volunteered until asked about during a detailed history taking but it is then useful to try and help the affected parent to try and overcome their own difficulties.

Obsessive/compulsive disorder is characterized by feelings of compulsion to carry out some action or repeatedly dwell on an idea that is difficult to resist. This leads to repetitive rituals, e.g. hand washing which has to be performed time and time again, despite the child and the parent wishing this not to happen. Obsessional compulsive disorders are more common in children with neurodevelopmental impairments and there is a genetic contribution to aetiology. In younger children however, rituals can sometimes be a way of reducing anxiety, which may have its roots in disturbed family relationships, schoolwork that is too hard, or pressure from friends. Toddlers and young children love repetitive games and songs. They can exhibit ritualistic behaviour as part of normal development, e.g. needing to go round every lamp-post twice. These pre-occupations are usually short-lived unless re-enforced by an anxious parent.

Genetic factors are important but the **Aetiology** of childhood emotional disorder is often bound up with family relationships. In some cases the mother of the affected child is frankly depressed or very anxious. In the seclusion of a one-to-one interview, mothers will often begin to cry and disclose morbid ideas. Doctors are thought to be missing a fatal disorder in the child and depressive thoughts become unwittingly projected onto the youngster. In school phobia, the parent feels worn out by the daily decision whether to send the child to school after being re-assured he is physically well. Sometimes when asked "Have you ever felt that you could not go any longer?" mothers will disclose feelings of total hopelessness and frustration. If the child is asked if he/she worries that their illness upsets the mother, they may burst into tears. On questioning it emerges that he/she is worried that mother cannot cope. Occasionally the mother has said she can go on no longer and she may leave home or try to "end it all". Separation anxiety is then only too real, the child is scared to allow the depressed parent out of their sight, and the parent requires the child to be around to help her get through the day. Frequently there are associated marital problems and the father may resent the over-closeness of the child and his spouse.

Emotional disorders can be triggered or maintained by stresses affecting the child, especially in school or with friends. Bullying is often a hidden problem in schools and stress may also arise if a child with specific learning difficulties is seen as lazy and ridiculed or punished when trying to do his/her best. Losses and separations can trigger depression. Illness or death of an important family member may cause a bereavement reaction in a parent for many months. The parent is reluctant to discuss this and the child patient feels blamed when his carer is irritable and unresponsive.

Many children are resilient and can adjust well to stress but some are more vulnerable due to constitutional factors and past experience. Stress may trigger a range of problems including **Adjustment Disorders** with conduct and/or emotional symptoms. Extreme stress can lead to **Post Traumatic Stress Disorders** with characteristic avoidance of possible reminders of stress, nightmares and sleep disturbance and some re-experiencing of stress or 'flashback' phenomena.

Classical adult presentations of **Depressive Illness** occur particularly in older children and young people. **Bipolar Affective Disorder** may have onset in adolescence but great care should be taken in the interpretation of symptoms in making this diagnosis.

A small proportion of children have **mixed conduct and emotional disorder.** These children are often brought up in disorganised, delinquent and socially deprived families with patterns of anti-social behaviour. If they become depressed, the symptoms are more likely to be difficult to contain and control. Children exhibit outbursts of self-destructive behaviour and anger with extreme sadness, guilt and feelings of hopelessness. Sometimes such a youngster will have trouble in trusting adults and needs to be contained and controlled because of the disturbed risk-taking aspects of their behaviour. While it may be difficult to understand such emotional symptoms, some children are so frequently undermined and put down by their parents, teachers and potential friends that they can only see themselves as inadequate and hopeless. Anyone trying to be nice to them feels like a phony. Children often exhibit their feelings in the way they behave. A happy child will be spontaneously bright but a child who is feeling bad will sometimes be unable to stop itself from doing bad things.

First line treatment of emotional disorders will generally be psychological and family based for the younger child. In older children and adolescents adult forms of treatment are more likely to be used. There is good evidence for the benefits of individual treatments, particularly cognitive behavioural therapy, which combines behavioural principles with strategies designed to alter thought content. Medication with Specific Serotonin Reuptake Inhibitors may be considered. The risks of heightened arousal and increased suicidality may outweigh the benefits of such antidepressants especially in less severe disorders. Rarely treatment resistance in this group of disorders can lead to complex interventions including in-patient care.

ELIMINATION DISORDERS

Enuresis

Enuresis refers to the persistent involuntary or inappropriate voiding of urine. This can occur while the child is asleep (nocturnal) or during the day (diurnal). The disorder may have been life long (primary) or come on at a later stage (secondary). Nocturnal enuresis is a commonly occurring disorder that affects approximately 10% of UK children at the age of 5 and 5% at the age of 10 with 1 or 2% continuing to wet throughout the teens. There is frequently a family history and it is usually a mono-symptom with emotional factors being secondary. There is an increased incidence of wetting amongst children with child psychiatric problems, but no correlation with any specific emotional disorder. Enuresis more often occurs in children in poor social circumstances where early training has not been established. Some children have had disturbing life events at the time when night-time bladder control should be acquired and the symptom is more frequent in children with other developmental delays and with encopresis. Nocturnal enuresis is not primarily a child psychiatric problem and is generally managed by families with primary care support or in specialist nurse led clinics, with referral to CAMHS clinics restricted to cases where more complex problems are suspected. Associated urinary tract problems and other medical problems are unusual but should be borne in mind and investigated as necessary.

The simple technique of uplifting a child when the parents go to bed sometimes solves the problem at a practical level. The use of star charts should be reserved for those children who wish to fill them in. All too often there is an expectation that the star chart will work and when it does not there is loss of face for the child, the parent and the doctor. Where angry feelings underlie the problem the chart will merely emphasise the extent of the difficulties, which may please the youngster. If the child has regressed the chart will be meaningless. The chart can imply that the child has voluntary control; to be dry is "good" and to have accidents is "bad". Some children who wet are quite depressed and for them it feels appropriate to be smelly, wet and chastised; the chart may reinforce these feelings.

The best behavioural treatment is the enuresis alarm, designed to wake the child when voiding commences. Attention to detail is important as false alarms can be caused. If there is no progress after 3 months, it is better to withdraw the apparatus assuming the child is not developmentally ready to benefit.

Anti-diuretic hormone, in the form of nasal spray or oral preparations, leads to symptomatic improvement. One should be cautious if there is any renal or cardiac problem. Tricyclic anti-depressants are as effective but have side effects and are very dangerous in overdose. Bed-wetting often recurs when drugs are stopped, unless the child has grown out of the problem during the time of the prescription.

Encopresis

Faecal soiling without physical cause is known as encopresis. This may be continuous or discontinuous.

Continuous soiling occurs where the problem has always been present. Such children may come from families with low expectation, poor motivation and inconsistent attempts to start toilet training. Such families have other social difficulties and the carer may have a background with poor models of parenting or be depressed and pre-occupied with other problems in the family.

Discontinuous soilers may have been satisfactorily trained or may have been especially early trained in bowel control. A way of looking at the mechanisms and family attitudes of children with discontinuous soiling is to look for signs of **regressive behaviour** or an **aggressive toileting situation.**

Regressive soilers are usually reacting to stress and anxiety. Stresses arise within the family and may be made worse by the effects of soiling leading to a vicious cycle. Children feel criticized and scapegoated and some have been harshly disciplined when they are soiled. The soiling may not be the only developmental milestone that has slipped back. The child may be clingy, withdrawn and exhibit toddler-like temper tantrums. Such children are often difficult to engage in play and sit dull, poorly motivated and emotionally flat. Discussion about the bowel problem is useless at first as the mental mechanism of regression switches off understanding.

In aggressive soiling the parent may at first describe reasonable attempts to toilet train, but if sufficient interview time is allowed, one becomes aware of considerable tension and anger regarding soiling. All too often a youngster is expected to perform by a harassed mother in a setting where relaxed toilet training cannot occur. The child may respond negatively and, either voluntarily or involuntarily, retains faeces. Megacolon is frequently associated with this situation.

Any child with a history of intermittent, runny stools often with a fusty acrid smell must be suspected of **Megacolon** with overflow incontinence, especially if there is an intermittent history of extremely large bowel evacuations. The condition is frequently chronic with faecal impaction associated with dilatation of the rectum and colon. The bowel becomes flaccid and unable to pass stools in the normal way. As the situation progresses the child completely loses any sensation of needing to go to the toilet. It is often difficult to weight the physical and emotional maintaining factors. Children with lack of continence are not always treated sympathetically, because adults think the cause is behavioural whereas the child has no bowel control. Occasionally an anal fissure results that compounds the problem. Often family psychopathology appears secondary to physical problems and careful medical assessment is required. The details of such assessment and treatment are outwith the scope of this chapter. Dietary advice to increase fibre and fluids may be helpful. Laxatives of various kinds are the mainstay of management but enemata and/or suppositories may be needed and rarely surgical manual evacuation is required.

Case Example

9-year-old boy, sexually abused as an infant, lived with adoptive parents. His discontinuous soiling had become entrenched and he had developed a megacolon. Attempts at paediatric treatment were complicated by his emotional reactions and adoptive parents feelings of failure. The family benefited from an approach that carefully presented the problem of megacolon in a cartoon form that the child could understand. As the child engaged with therapist and adoptive parents in the task of "beating his problem poo" his adherence to a laxative regime and toileting programme led to slow bowel retraining taking around 6 months.

In encopresis where there is no megacolon and where the child passes a normal consistency stool at regular intervals, there seems little value in using laxatives routinely. Excessive use of laxatives impairs function of a healthy bowel. A behavioural approach with the use of a star chart and simple educative advice may be helpful to a child who has not received basic toilet training. If a chart recognises success but not failure this reduces false expectations. Positive reinforcement is always more acceptable than a programme that increases the parents anger or discourages the child especially where there is no voluntary bowel control. If possible, the child and family should be brought together as allies with the therapist in tackling the problem of soiling, which is helpfully thought of as a problem that is external to the child and family and nobody's fault. Where the child is under considerable stress, or where there is too much anger for co-operation with treatment, it may be helpful to review wider issues of family relationships. Psychotherapy often in the form of play therapy for the child can be helpful.

Where ongoing psychological treatment for soiling is needed it may be best to delegate physical treatment to a separate paediatric clinic. Therapy is undermined if the therapist plays the dual role of doctor and psychotherapist. A pre-school toddler, who soiled in anger, attacked a Daddy doll during therapy, buried him in the sand and beat the sand down with a shovel. The Mother doll was also given a hard time for sending the Daddy away. After 30 minutes of this distressing anger it would not feel right for the therapist, let alone the child, for the session to be followed by the therapist giving the child an enema.

BEHAVIOUR DISORDERS

Attention Deficit Hyperkinetic Disorder (ADHD)

Many people believe that ADHD is a straightforward condition manifested by motor restlessness, distractibility, poor concentration, impulsivity and labile mood. The simple explanation that this disorder is caused by brain dysfunction and elegantly responds to Methylphenidate is much too neat and tidy a concept which bears only a limited relationship to the assessment of badly behaved, inappropriately controlled and under-stimulated children who are referred to paediatricians and child psychiatrists. As knowledge of developmental neuro-psychiatry has increased, so the simple story has seen to be flawed. It is important to realise that hyperactivity is not simply a manifestation of brain impairment. It is unlikely that hyperkinesis is a unitary condition and various aetiological theories have been put forward.

Specific learning difficulties not explained by global retardation are common in children with ADHD. Occasionally ADHD may follow brain damage that is identifiable on scanning. This is a recognized outcome of low birth weight and is found in conditions arising from intrauterine adversity, such as foetal alcohol syndrome. The infant's brain is both vulnerable and plastic with an enormous capacity for function to develop in spite of areas of damage. Such damage may be generalised rather than localised, e.g. by anoxia, so that it is reasonable that some years on the effects of damage will be manifest by impulsivity and labile mood. The parents of children with ADHD have increased rates of alcoholism and sociopathy when compared with the relatives of normal children. Theories of disorders of monoamine neurotransmission are well supported and genetic effects have been robustly demonstrated but the constitutional basis for this disorder remains unclear. While specific factors in heredity, pregnancy, delivery or neonatal period may correlate with dysfunction; it can be difficult to confirm such links when dealing with individuals.

Food allergy is considered important by some, but additive-free diets are often expensive and difficult to follow. If there is evidence that certain foods upset the child, a dietitian can devise a trial of diet that is sensible, within the grasp of the parent and unlikely to deprive the child of essential nutrition. Sometimes helpful results are obtained, although it is not always clear what is due to support and what is due to diet. It appears reasonable to keep an open mind and carefully accumulate data. While coeliac disease is considered a respectable paediatric diagnosis, the possibility of wheat allergy is often discounted. There is little doubt that some children are irritable and restless when they are itchy with eczema or frustrated by coryza and nasal stuffiness.

Whatever the underlying constitutional disturbance there always needs to be an emphasis on consistent and positive management. Children with ADHD generally struggle in a classroom, often receiving criticism and negative reinforcements, which alienate them from teachers and sometimes classmates. This leads to over-arousal, making distractibility worse and contributing to the development of poor self-esteem. Depressive feelings may further reduce motivation, and there may be a defensive reaction "that teacher is always bugging me" or "I am not working for him". It can be difficult to sort out cause and effect when parents appear tired, angry or depressed. As the cycle of events winds up, parents become inconsistent being either inappropriately angry or at other times too negative and exhausted to intervene. Follow up of children with ADHD shows a high risk of developing conduct disorder in later childhood and antisocial behaviour and alcoholism in adult life.

Children with ADHD require a treatment plan. This will include advice on their management, often involving the educational psychologist working with the school and sometimes support to the family from a social worker. The neurostimulants, Methylphenidate and Dexamphetamine, are effective with or without a wider treatment programme. Their use can cause appetite impairment (growth should be monitored), anxiety, sleeplessness and very occasionally psychosis. Where there is social deprivation, others may abuse stimulants. Other medications that can help include atomoxetine, clonidine and antipsychotic drugs. All drugs may have a potential for interactions and side-effects, in particular, antipsychotics present the long-term danger of tardive dyskinesia. There is limited evidence that tricyclic antidepressants may be helpful, although they are not widely used because of a poor balance of risk to benefit. Rarely it may be useful to consider an admission to a child psychiatric unit to see how hyperkinesis responds to consistent care before embarking on many years of pharmacotherapy.

Conduct Disorder

Although the management of children with aggressive and destructive behaviour giving rise to social disapproval usually falls to other professionals, doctors are bound to become involved as such problems are common. The incidence of anti-social disorders varies from around 2 to 10% in the mid-childhood years, depending on the kind of population being served.

There are two principal approaches to understanding the learning of social behaviour. First are the well-researched cognitive and behavioural models of social learning where consistent rewards and reprimands and exposure to pro-social attitudes and behaviours are needed to learn appropriate responses. Second, the psycho-dynamic approach concentrates on the quality of relationship between the child and the parent or authority figure. In both models difficulties may arise in the family and/or in other areas of community life, especially in school.

Family norms may not be acceptable to society: many delinquent children have fathers and sometimes mothers with a criminal record. Some families issue no clear guidelines and throw their children into confusion by their response to behaviour, being very punitive on occasion and at another time amused when the youngster does something inappropriate. Some families have unclear roles with perhaps the elder sister taking over when the mother is not coping. The impact of personality disorder or substance misuse in the parent or parents must be taken into account with a range of other social factors.

The community can foster antisocial behaviour. Housing may be allocated so that families with social difficulties are housed together in unpopular housing schemes. Their children are exposed to a peer group with high delinquency rates and neighbours potentiate this downward cycle. The culture of a school can make or break a youngster who is not well supported at home. Children with conduct disorder often fall behind in reading and other school attainments; conversely children with learning difficulties have an increased rate of conduct problems. If the child is encouraged and made to feel an important individual in his own right within school, identification with the school system and certain teachers will exert a positive influence. Conversely if the child does not succeed in school he is much more likely to get recognition from other anti-social youngsters. If specific learning difficulties are missed a child who is of average intelligence is labelled as 'lazy' or 'not trying' in the area of disability. Motivation can fail because of a depressive or angry attitude towards school.

The medical skill lies in identifying conditions within the child that pre-dispose to anti-social difficulties, especially treatable disorders such as ADHD. Children vary in temperament and parents who have successfully reared one or more "easy" children may find that their methods do not succeed with a more challenging child. Children who are hyperkinetic with poor concentration and sometimes poor co-ordination are difficult to discipline. They easily get discouraged with repeated failure or develop negative ways of opposing those putting pressure upon them. Depression can sometimes give rise to stealing and under functioning as the "I am bad" guilt is sometimes acted out or the object stolen may be held for comfort. Lastly some children with long-term illness or handicap who are feeling vulnerable may need to over-react to show friends and teachers that they are a force to be reckoned with.

Conduct disorder may develop out of **Attachment disorders,** where the effects of early emotional deprivation (for example poor quality institutional care or care by a mentally disordered parent) can lead to profound difficulties in relationships, with striking abnormalities in social contact. Classically such children may be inhibited with 'frozen watchfulness' or disinhibited and indiscriminately friendly. There are continuing rages and toddler-like behaviour sometimes for many years even though a child may be in an improved home situation.

Case Example

A 13-year-old boy was brought to the clinic by his social worker and his mother. He had been in trouble with gang related offences of violence, theft and possession of street drugs. His father, an aggressive man, had left home 4 years ago and his mother, was an alcoholic, unable to give consistent care to her children. He was residing in a children's home but not able to relate well to staff, testing their commitment to him. If he began to feel secure he would do something bad. Thus if he were moved on it would be on his terms, which he saw as better than being rejected "for no reason". Nevertheless after an incident he hoped to be allowed to stay. Similar testing behaviour occurred in school. Like his father he had specific learning difficulties as yet unappreciated by teachers who focussed more on his behaviour. Unable to gain satisfaction in lessons, he found it more rewarding to truant and revelled in his role in the gang.

EATING DISORDERS

A range of emotional and behavioral disorders lead to abnormal eating in childhood and unusual eating behaviours are commonplace in adolescence. Although eating disorders may be a focus of considerable parental concern, the insidious development of **Anorexia Nervosa** is still sometimes overlooked. Anorexia nervosa still carries a significant mortality. While approximately one third make a full recovery, many remain vulnerable, psychiatrically disturbed and requiring repeated periods of therapy; some require hospitalisation.

Anorexia nervosa has at its core a morbid fear of fatness and a distorted body image. Weight loss leads to a low body mass index, pubertal development and growth may be retarded. The disorder sometimes develops from dieting with selective rejection of calorific food. Various tactics to lose weight are displayed, the most dangerous of which is vomiting, sometimes done quietly and with remarkable ease. Bursts of frantic exercise may occur openly or in secret while increasing quantities of laxatives and purgatives may be consumed. Girls develop amenorrhea and the disorder is typified by bradycardia, hypotension, a growth of fine hair, and increased pigmentation. Sometimes the parotid glands are swollen and the back teeth decayed because of acid reflux from vomiting. Baggy clothes often disguise weight loss. It is only when one has sight of the protruding ribs, scapulae, clavicles and the scaphoid abdomen with prominent iliac crests that the degree of starvation become apparent. Emotional state is adversely affected often with obsessive or depressive and suicidal thoughts. Some youngsters show attention seeking and confrontational behaviour, which may involve the family and therapists, who become fearful for the fate of the patient and also angry with them.

Aetiology remains a topic for debate. The disorder is more common in girls than boys and often appears during adolescence. Cultural factors may reinforce the fear of fatness and evidence suggests that Anorexia Nervosa is becoming more common in countries where traditional attitudes to weight are replaced by fashionable ideals of thinness. Neurodevelopmental disorders may precede anorexia and, in a small minority, anorexia follows sexual abuse.

In treatment, prescribed food is taken regularly. This may involve the exhausting task of sitting with the patient until food has been finished and after that for at least another hour. Where the patient is very underweight, diet should be built up gradually, with dietetic advice. In very severe cases, re-fed too rapidly, acute gastric dilatation can develop and can be fatal.

Family therapy approaches involve supporting parents in understanding the disorder and taking greater control at mealtimes. Cognitive Behavioural approaches to anorexic beliefs are helpful once a patient has recognised their problem and can engage in individual work. Intensive day-patient programmes that involve group dynamics can enable youngsters to enforce their own dietary control. Sometimes anti-depressants or neuroleptics are used, but dosage should be gradually built-up if the patient is frail.

Those who pursue a relapsing course often develop **Bulimia Nervosa,** where there is intermittent bingeing, often with very large amounts eaten, followed by self-induced vomiting or purging. As with anorexia, treatment plans must be clear, often with contracts drawn up so that therapy is underpinned with behavioural objectives.

PSYCHOTIC DISORDERS

Symptoms suggestive of psychosis require careful assessment in childhood, but true psychoses are very rare in younger children and when they occur an organic cause should be suspected. Careful medical review is required including consideration of a range of disorders such as temporal lobe epilepsy, infectious, inflammatory and degenerative disorder as well as toxic effects of heavy metals and substance misuse. Mental state examination in children requires particular skill. Where children have not established good communication or clear boundaries between fantasy and reality, it is a highly complex task to use diagnostic criteria derived from adult psychiatry. Children with communication disorders and learning disability may present symptoms suggestive of psychosis, but are at particular risk of misdiagnosis, as well as being at increased risk of psychosis. Psychoses such as schizophrenia and hypomania become more prevalent in adolescence.

Treatment approaches need to take account of the young person's stage of development. Family involvement is important and, in particular, neuroleptic drugs have higher rates of side effects in younger people and doses need careful consideration.

Case Example

A 9 years old living with socially isolated parents is seen by an Education officer concerned about non-attendance. He has stopped sleeping at night and plays computer games for hours. He appears distracted by what he describes as 'voices of aliens'. He recovers quickly in a psychiatric unit, where MRI scanning shows cortical dysplasia, consistent with his abnormal pattern of cognitive skills. His psychosis is seen as a consequence of abnormal functioning within an abnormal environment and medication is not required.

COMMUNICATION DISORDER

Normally children are taught language by a two-way process of interaction with an adequately responsive mother or other caring adults. It is a pleasure to watch the intent eye-to-eye contact as the infant sits on the mother's knee while producing baby vocalisations that are praised by the mother as they approximate to some simple well-known word like "Mum". As the noises approximate to the word "Mum" the mother responds, the baby excites and the dialogue slowly and surely proceeds into a basic vocabulary where the child develops some understanding of the meaning of words as well as being able to articulate them. For this process to occur hearing must be intact, the auditory nerve functioning and incoming stimuli from the input side of the brain must work in harmony with memory so that messages can be devised in the output or expressive part of the brain and these coded into impulses going down the motor nerves to the larynx and pharynx. If a child presents with defective speech or language it is worth being satisfied that there is no deafness or even high tone deafness. Some children can imitate the alarm of a fire engine but the frequencies needed to imitate the human voice may not be received in which case incoming language can only be perceived as distorted. If hearing is unimpaired and there are no anatomical or neurological problems of sound producing organs, one can assume that the disorder is in the brain. In practice most language

disorders are not clearly defined, being mixed or central with both receptive and expressive difficulties but it can be helpful to think separately of receptive or expressive language impairments.

Where there is delay in **expressive** communication, the child clearly understands what is being said and will obey verbal instructions but has hesitancy in finding words to express himself. Children with this problem are irritable and demanding, as they live in a frustrating world of adults moving on to the next topic before they have been able to join in. There is frequent gesticulating, pulling parents over to indicate their wishes by body language and general frustration. Providing the child is socially aware and develops an understanding of language the problem may resolve with support and possibly speech and language therapy.

In **receptive** language impairments impulses coming along the auditory nerve cannot be decoded into anything meaningful. Some children appear to repress language in the same way that children with a squint can repress vision, and on occasions it requires an audiogram to be performed with an EEG machine set to give evoked response readings. In this way it can be deduced that the brain receives noises coming into the child's ear. If little meaningful sense can be made of the spoken word the child becomes seriously socially disadvantaged and may begin to withdraw from a world, which increasingly depends on social interaction through language. Children with severe receptive disorders require special education so that a language can be build up with stimuli presented through visual or tactile routes.

The concept of the **Autistic spectrum disorder (ASD)** provides a useful way of thinking about various more severe disorders of communication that in ICD-10 are categorised as **Pervasive developmental disorders**. The core of the difficulties faced in ASD lies in the **autistic triad** of impairments of communication, social development and behavioural rigidity. The recognition of ASDs is the first step towards ensuring that such children achieve their developmental potential. Specific treatments have a limited evidence-base, but early supports for parents, later educational and social interventions, individually tailored, can reduce the impact of a child's impairments.

The signs of **Infantile Autism** usually present within the first 30 months with abnormal responses to both auditory and sometimes visual stimuli. Speech is delayed and if it begins to develop it tends to be echolalic and later lacking in ability to use abstract terms. Autistic children appear detached socially and classically there is impairment of eye-to-eye contact and lack of ability to relate meaningfully to parents or age-mates. Autistic children frequently resist change and may have catastrophic rage reactions for minor causes, e.g. if an item in a room has been moved or if their transport to a school goes by an unusual route. Routines, rituals and obsessional behaviour are commonplace and if the disorder improves patterns of logically concrete thinking emerge with a lack of social empathy.

There are a number of theories of possible aetiology. The disorder is male predominant but not X-linked. Whereas in the past family influences were suspected it now seems clear that genetic factors are highly relevant, with multiple interacting genes and high heritability. Associated medical disorders (e.g. specific disorders of the brain such as tuberous sclerosis) are found in more than 10%. Better prognosis is found where there are not signs of severe generalised learning disability. Many require ongoing family, educational and social support with only a minority achieving more positive adjustment. A few truly gifted individuals achieve great success in areas less dependent upon their areas of difficulty, for example as musicians or scientists.

Asperger's Syndrome has been conceptualized as high functioning autism but this may be misleading as the social deficits of this condition can be as disabling as in infantile autism. The criteria for diagnosis of Asperger's syndrome in ICD 10 are open to debate but the syndrome differs from infantile autism in that the level of speech and language impairment is much less obvious. Such children will still have marked impairments in language in areas such as semantics (the construction of meaning) and pragmatics (the use of language in social interaction). There appears to be increased recognition of this disorder as more subtle social impairments are identified and labeled.

Atypical Autism is a term that is sometimes applied to children with marked autistic features who do not fulfil criteria for another diagnosis, especially where there is Learning disability.

Rett's Syndrome is a rare genetic disorder leading to autistic regression with a characteristic pattern of abnormal hand movements.

DISORDERS WITH MOTOR PRESENTATIONS

Children may present in paediatric clinics with a range of motor disturbances that are best managed with the skills of a child psychiatrist. Repetitive stereotyped movements are common features of Autism and may need to be distinguished from self-stimulating behaviours, which are also common in developmentally impaired children. Tics are rapid repetitive movements that are driven by an internal compulsion that older children may describe as 'like an itch'. Tics may be motor but can also be vocal, involving explosive and sometimes culturally unacceptable utterances, which if sustained are a core feature of **Tourette's syndrome**. Tourette's syndrome often co-exists with obsessional and attentional difficulties. Motor over-activity is a core feature of ADHD but like immobility can more rarely be seen in childhood affective states and psychosis. Awareness of the link between specific

disorders of motor development (**Dyspraxias**) and other developmental and psychiatric disorders should lead to careful global assessment when problems in areas such as co-ordination and visuo- spatial capacity are identified.

PROBLEMS OF LEARNING

Many disorders can directly or indirectly affect learning. Children with emotional disorders are frequently anxious and depressed. They find it difficult to concentrate in class if they are preoccupied by feelings of worthlessness and are worrying that their mother or father may be unwell or in the process of separation. Their distress and falling off of attainments may be missed by the teacher who is more preoccupied by disruptive behaviourally disturbed children. Somatic symptoms including abdominal pains and headache lead to frequent school absence and the continuity of learning is lost.

A child with a chronic or relapsing illness may find learning difficult because of malaise, pain, repeated time consuming or traumatic medical treatments and because of time lost from school. The side effects of medications, e.g. Anti-convulsants are important causes of cognitive impairment.

Attainments are frequently poor in conduct disordered children. The causes are multifactorial. In areas of social deprivation parents' attitude towards education is not always positive, homework is not encouraged, and there is no space to work in overcrowded, noisy, disorganised households. A youngster, behind with his attainments is frequently criticised by teachers. If the child believes that he cannot learn, his motivation will be adversely affected. One mental process guarding against depression and poor self-esteem is to blame the system. It is safer to reject the school and denigrate the teachers than to accept criticism. This attitude can become the group norm and outshining truanting colleagues with anti-social behaviour can preserve self-respect. Under these conditions school attainments fall further and further behind.

In a number of cases constitutional difficulties with attention, concentration or more specific learning skills precede behavioural difficulties. Where such difficulties are not discovered and educational help is not given, a child's self-esteem and motivation worsens and the situation escalates.

Specific learning difficulty is described when children with otherwise normal developmental capacity demonstrate defined problems in one area of learning or development, e.g. dyslexia is specific reading retardation and dyscalculia a similar problem with numbers. There has been enormous pressure from some professionals and parents to get such problems recognized by teachers. Specific learning difficulties may present with depression or conduct disorder. Impressed by a youngster's unhappiness or suicidal ideas, it is all too easy to miss the underlying stress of a child trying his/her hardest and never being able to succeed at school. If a child does not have the innate ability to cope with an aspect of learning it is often wrongly assumed that extensive practise will improve the situation but often the converse is true. It is not surprising that such children may feel despairing and only careful attention to their specific needs will offer a way forward. However the term "dyslexia" can give rise to confusion. Worried parents can be fearful that dyslexia is some frightful illness, others may use this as an explanation for a school failure that is rooted in other factors. The problem about this label is that it does not describe the precise nature of the underlying learning difficulty. Many professionals prefer to describe the nature of the problem in functional terms.

Three cognitive processes are often found to be affected in specific reading retardation. The first is a problem of short-term memory or a sequencing difficulty. This may be associated with difficulty of recall of information obtained through the auditory route, or the problem may be in recalling material, which has recently been read from writing or print (e.g. a person can be told a telephone number and not recall it, whereas they can retain the same number read from a book or vice versa). The second major difficulty is with spatial ability, for example some children have enormous difficulty in learning left from right. The third problem area may be visuo-motor or perceptual difficulties. This is often associated with problems of putting thoughts into legible writing and decoding information from the written page. In some instances a child may acknowledge that his written page is full of mistakes but be unable to correct them.

Severe dyslexic problems may overlap with mild communication disorders and specific learning difficulties can be found in association with hyperkinesis or in children who are clumsy with poor motor control. Three disorders, namely ADHD, Specific Learning Difficulty and Specific Disorder of Motor Development (Dyspraxia) are sometimes grouped together. Aetiological theories are covered above in relation to ADHD.

Severe head trauma, cerebral tumours and other forms of brain injury in childhood may impair learning. Intellectual abilities may appear remarkably intact after marked anatomical damage has occurred, especially if early in the child's life. However, such brain-injured children may become more obviously disabled as the demands of development outstrip their capacity.

A child who has problems affecting all aspects of cognitive development is described in ICD 10 as 'Mentally Retarded' although groups in the UK have campaigned effectively for the term 'Learning disabled' to be used as it is less stigmatising. Stigma is compounded when a child looks dysmorphic or has an associated movement disorder. Learning disability generally does not have an identifiable cause but various aetiologies are recognised.

The commonest single cause is chromosomal disorder, e.g. Down's syndrome. There are a number of genetic disorders where an inborn error of metabolism can be proven; for example, Wilson's disease, which is a defect of copper metabolism, and the mucopolysaccharide disorders, which are progressive. Screening at birth allows for intervention to prevent the insidious mental retardation resulting from phenylketonuria and hypothyroidism. Children born with neurological impairments, such as spastic hemiplegia, frequently have Learning Disability. There are many rare medical causes of deteriorating cognitive capacity or dementia in childhood.

WORKING WITH SOCIAL SERVICES AND POLICE

Professional responsibility in dealing with children includes a responsibility to work within a legal framework governing the acceptable treatment of children as well as attending to the childhood roots of adult criminality. It is important that doctors familiarise themselves with the social arrangements and statutory procedures for liaison with Social Work Departments (or their equivalents) and where necessary with the Police, and the Courts or equivalent legal bodies. In Scotland, the children's hearing system is designed to attend to youth offending as well as child welfare in the under-eighteens.

In certain circumstances a professional opinion is sought in relation to severe **offending behaviour in children.** Adult approaches to forensic examination need to be modified to take account of developmental factors and the influence of family and social factors must be acknowledged. Careful notes should be kept of **forensic** interviews and examinations. Cultures vary in their attitude to antisocial behaviour in childhood but it is generally accepted that the younger the child the more their behaviour must be seen in the context of age. Punishment may then seem less important than attempts to intervene to reduce the risk of further offending.

Physical abuse is often relatively easy to recognise and prove, while **sexual abuse** may be devoid of physical findings. The signs that arouse suspicion of sexual abuse are now legion. Apart from obvious trauma, infections or pregnancy, there is an increased incidence of psychogenic pains, often abdominal, and conversion symptoms that may indicate that a child is under stress which is too difficult to go on tolerating and too difficult to be disclosed. A range of psychiatric symptoms may occur or be made worse as a result of abuse.

The way in which the child behaves should be noted. Abused children may be fearful of adults and appear apprehensive or withdrawn, particularly where circumstances recall the abuse, e.g. a male doctor reminds the child of a male abuser. If a child is taken to a playroom and cowers in the corner when the therapist closes the door this can be very revealing. Children often replicate confusing or worrying incidents in their play. Children's drawings may also indicate fears of sexual objects or sexual knowledge beyond what is age-appropriate. Most of all it is important to listen to what the child has to say. Although children can be regarded as manipulative, it is very unusual (but not unknown) for children to disclose abuse that has not actually occurred. They are more likely to remain mute or ill at ease in order to protect their perpetrators.

If sexual abuse is suspected, it is important that arrangements for paediatric examination give due weight to the emotional needs of the child. Provision of special units with quietness and appropriately comfortable furnishing is helpful. In this setting full explanations can be given and trust built-up between the child and the examining doctor. The skills of being frank and open at a level the child can understand, seeking the child's permission and talking them through the examination go some way to reducing the secondary emotional damage from the fear resulting from disclosure. Attempts to tussle with the child to perform a physical examination must increase the horror of abuse. If a parent or relative has been the perpetrator and then doctors remove the child's clothes and intrude into the child's personal space, it must seem as if no adult can ever be trusted again.

Although dialogue with the child or interpretation of his/her behaviour sometimes leaves little doubt to the clinician that abuse has occurred, the legal system is not always well-equipped to cope so that a number of cases are not proven with resulting further difficulties for those managing the case. Perhaps most difficult of all are the categories of **emotional abuse** and **failure to thrive** where the parents contest the need for intervention. Close co-operation is required across the agencies involved.

Factitious and Induced Illness (FII, formerly known as Munchausen Syndrome by Proxy or Meadow's Syndrome) is described when children are repeatedly brought to hospital with symptoms which tempt the physician or surgeon to subject the child to numerous investigations, sometimes of an increasingly intrusive, traumatic and expensive form. While many anxious parents unwittingly subject their children to the effects of their anxiety and over concern; in FII the problem is that the parent is usually doing something actively to produce the child's symptoms. Mothers have used their own blood to contaminate a child's urine specimen to precipitate investigations for haematuria, and anoxic seizures have been deliberately produced by mothers partially suffocating their children. Such problems may be more likely in medical systems where care is compartmentalised by specialty and consideration of psychosocial mechanisms neglected. Surgical intervention or complex treatment regimes may be set up but the problem fails to resolve. Mothers of children with FII often have personality disorders. They are often co-operative, adapt well to ward routine and are well-acquainted with hospital, where their emotional needs may be met. It is difficult to empathise with their psychopathology and dissociation may be present. The ability to play the competent caring mother and yet behaved destructively in order to gain input from doctors and nurses is hard to comprehend. Confrontation is often not met by an admission of guilt and it is important that appropriate child protection orders are sought. Sometimes after confrontation the parent may decompensate. A needy, distraught mother feels she has failed once again. Adult psychiatric intervention may be necessary as depressive feelings are mobilised when the mechanism of dissociation is broken down.

ACKNOWLEDGEMENTS

The authors wish to acknowledge the published work of RS Illingworth and DW Winnicott , two paediatricians whose influence has shaped medical practice in support of children and young people's mental health.

FURTHER READING

Reference Work:
1. Managing Children with Psychiatric Problems (2002) Garralda E. & Hyde C. BMJ Books.
2. New Toddler Taming: The World's Bestselling Parenting Guide (2005) Green C. Vermilion.
3. Child Psychiatry: Key Facts and Concepts Explained (2005) Goodman R. & Scott S. Blackwell Publishers.
4. Child & Adolescent Psychiatry, a Developmental Approach (2007) Turk, J & Graham, P. Oxford University Press.
5. Child & Adolescent Psychiatry (2005) Rutter, M & Taylor, E. Blackwell Science Ltd.
6. The Normal Child (1991) Tenth Edition, Ronald S. Illingworth, Churchill Livingstone.
   Background Reading:
7. The Spirit Catches You and You Fall Down (1998) Fadiman A. Farrar Straus & Giroux Inc..(The experience of childhood epilepsy amongst the Hmong Chinese in USA).
8. The curious incident of the Dog in the Night-time (2004) Haddon M. Vintage (Growing up with Asperger's Syndrome in England).
9. Nervous Conditions (2004) Dangarembga, T. Ayebia Clarke Publishing Ltd (Developing Eating Disorder symptoms, caught between cultures in Africa).

Chapter

32

Paediatric Radiology

Sanjay V Maroo, Sandra J Butler

GENERAL CONSIDERATIONS IN PAEDIATRIC RADIOLOGY

1. Imaging has assumed an important role in the diagnosis, understanding and in certain cases, treatment of paediatric diseases.
2. The availability of many imaging modalities (plain film, ultrasound, CT, MRI, nuclear medicine, angiography, SPECT scanning,) requires problem-oriented decisions to determine which techniques should be used or omitted in any given clinical situation.
3. The radiologist plays a central role in the diagnostic imaging process and is actively involved in formulating an appropriate pathway of diagnostic evaluation to maximize the benefits from any imaging examination.
4. Adequate clinical information should always be available on the radiology consultation in order to determine, what, if any, imaging modalities are indicated for diagnostic evaluation.
5. Ozpen communication between the referring physician and the radiologist improves quality of patient care.
6. There is no place for routine radiological examinations.

RADIATION EFFECTS ON CHILDREN

1. The biologic effects of radiation result primarily from damage to DNA and the effects are greatest on fastest growing organisms—the foetus, infant and the young child. All ionising radiations are potentially harmful.
2. The consequences of radiation relate to both dose and time of radiation and may appear later in life. There is no existence of a threshold dose in unknown.
3. The ALARA principle states that radiation dose of exposed individuals should be kept as low as is reasonably achievable, with economic and social factors being taken into account.
4. Medical diagnostic X-rays represent the largest source of radiation exposure resulting from human activity. The greatest source of background radiation is radon gas, a decay product in the uranium series.

5. Imaging modalities which deliver ionizing radiation are plain films, fluoroscopy, computed tomography (CT) and isotope studies. The modality which delivers the highest dose is CT and use of this modality is increasing with children (0-15 years) receiving 11.2% of all CT examinations.
6. All effective methodologies to reduce radiation exposure in children should be employed. These include tailoring the examination to the child, adjusting technical factors for plain films, using pulsed fluoroscopy, screening of CT examinations, and utilizing other modalities which don't involve ionising radiation like ultrasound and MRI.
7. Radiology consultation should be obtained to obtain a proper test. Factors utilized in determining the best test include sensitivity in diagnosis, cost, timeliness and safety.
8. Dose may be decreased by performing only examinations that are clinically indicated.

IMAGING MODALITIES USED IN PAEDIATRIC IMAGING

Plain Film Radiography

Conventional radiography is based on the variable attenuation of an X-ray beam as it passes through tissue.

This modality is frequently a starting point for radiological investigations in a number of conditions. The radiology request should provide adequate clinical information and specify the views.

There are standard views for specific anatomic areas and specific conditions.

Head: AP, Towne and lateral

Spine: AP and lateral

Chest: Frontal and lateral

Abdomen: AP

Pelvis: AP

Contrast Media

Contrast media are externally administered agents used to provide positive or negative contrast in certain areas of the body. Areas where contrast media are frequently used include gastrointestinal tract, genitourinary tract, and the vascular system. Barium compounds (Barium sulphate) are used for routine gastrointestinal studies .Water soluble iodinated compounds are used for assessing the gastrointestinal system in emergency cases or where perforation is suspected, for the genitourinary system, the cardiovascular system and CT scanning. Water soluble contrast agents contain iodine. Low osmolar iodinated contrast media should be used as a routine . High osmolar contrast media can have a profound effect on serum osmolality and the haemodynamics status of infants and children .

Fluoroscopy

Indications include gastrointestinal, genitourinary studies, orthopaedic procedures, and diagnostic angiography and during image guided therapeutic procedures. Image intensification is necessary for fluoroscopy of children and most procedures usually involve contrast medium administration. Techniques reducing radiation doses in children without any significant loss in image quality include pulsed fluoroscopy, last image hold and collimation.

Ultrasound

Ultrasound is ideal for imaging children for a number of reasons:
1. Uses no ionising radiation
2. Sedation is almost never required
3. There is no evidence that energy levels of diagnostic ultrasound used in humans are harmful to humans
4. Examination can be performed at the bedside in sick children
5. Paucity of fat in the paediatric abdomen and the smaller size of the patient allow detailed visualisation of the abdominal anatomy.

Indications include intracranial examinations in neonates, urinary tract infections, abdominal pathology, scrotal conditions, anomalies of soft tissues, and certain chest conditions and for interventional procedures.

Computed Tomography (CT)

CT uses a radiation beam that is highly collimated through one cross-sectional slice of tissue from different angles. The data is then computed to record X-ray absorption in a specific volume element which is then converted to an image. CT has high spatial resolution and demonstrates anatomy as a two-dimensional image which helps determine extent of disease. Recent advances in CT and software technology now allow CT imaging in a volume of tissue such as the abdomen in less than 5 seconds and also enable reconstruction of the image in any plane including 3-dimensions.

A major disadvantage in children is the radiation dose.

Magnetic Resonance Imaging

MRI uses a strong magnetic field and radiofrequency energy to generate a synchronised precessional motion of protons in body tissues.

An MRI image reflects the distribution of protons in the section of the body.

Applications of MRI are gradually increasing in paediatrics. Reasons include lack of ionising radiation, multiplanar capabilities, superior contrast resolution and the ability to image blood vessels without using intravenous contrast agents. In addition to illustrating normal and pathologic anatomy MR is also used to assess chemical composition and tissue perfusion.

Disadvantages include need for sedation or anaesthesia in younger children and the examination is contraindicated in children with pace makers and certain implants.

Radio Isotope Studies (Nuclear Medicine)

The imaging energy source for scintigraphy is the isotope attached to a radiopharmaceutical injected into the body. The detection system, a gamma camera, uses a collimator and photo-multiplier tubes to detect the gamma rays emitted from the body to a scintillation crystal. The raw data from the scintillation crystal then yields a raw image after computer reconstruction and signal processing. Most radio isotopes are injected intravenously and the functional information provided by scintigraphy often complements the anatomic information provided by anatomical studies and may provide the only imaging evidence of pathology. Radiopharmaceuticals are given in small doses and are relatively innocuous, i.e. they do not produce significant pharmacologic, haemodynamic, osmotic or toxic effects. Radiation exposures from their use in diagnostic imaging usually fall in the lower range of radiation exposures from common radiological examinations.

The technique has high sensitivity but low specificity.

Common radio isotopes include 99mTc DMSA, 99mTc DTPA, and 99Tcm MDP.

Image Guided Therapeutic (IGT) Procedures

A steady increase in non-vascular and vascular IGT procedures has occurred in the last decade. This increase stems from the growing recognition that many paediatric interventional procedures like their counterparts in the adult world can achieve the same results as surgery without being as invasive and usually with less morbidity and more rapid recovery.

Most of the interventional procedures are performed with ultrasound and fluoroscopic guidance. Use of contrast media is made at every stage, if indicated, as an additional safety margin.

Non-vascular image guided therapeutic procedures include biopsies, drainages, of pleural fluid, abscesses, other fluid collections, balloon dilatation of oesophageal strictures, percutaneous nephrostomy, pyeloplasty, percutaneous gastrostomy/gastrojejunostomy.

Vascular interventional procedures include image guided central and peripheral central venous catheter placement, sclerotherapy of vascular malformations, angioplasty, embolisation and trans-jugular liver biopsy.

RESPIRATORY AND CARDIAC

The Child with Cough and Fever

Common Causes

Acute pneumonias:
1. Viral
2. Bacterial
3. Atypical organism.

Other pneumonias:
1. Tuberculosis
2. Aspiration
3. Cystic fibrosis
4. Opportunistic organisms

Viral Pneumonia

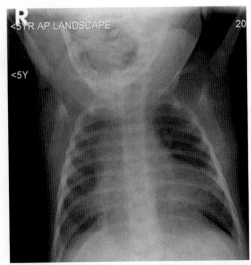

Fig. 32.1: Viral pneumonias are mainly small and large airway disorders and radiological findings are due to partial and complete airway occlusion leading to atelectasis and hyperinflation. Chest radiograph in a month old baby with viral pneumonia showing hyperinflation and atelectasis of the lingua (seen as effacement of the left heart margin) and the middle lobe (seen as effacement of the right heart lobe)

Bronchiolitis

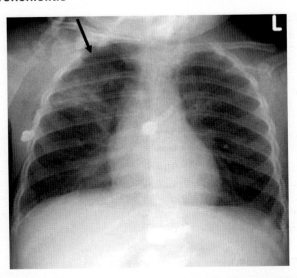

Fig. 32.2: Bronchiolitis is a serious manifestation of a lower respiratory infection occurring in infants in the first 2 years of life. Radiologically air trapping and atelectasis are the common features. The infection is a caused by the respiratory syncytial virus (RSV). Bronchiolitis with air trapping and right apical pneumothorax (arrow). Additional findings include bilateral parahilar infiltrates and atelectases

Bacterial Pneumonia

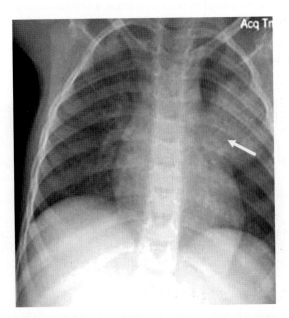

Fig. 32.3: Bacterial infections present as lobar or segmental consolidations or fluffy infiltrates.Even though consolidation may be extensive, volume loss may be minimal .The organisms are commonly *Hemophilus influenzae* in infants less than 2 years and *Streptococcus pneumoniae* in older children. CXR showing segmental consolidation in the left upper lobe with air bronchograms (white arrow)

Round Pneumonia

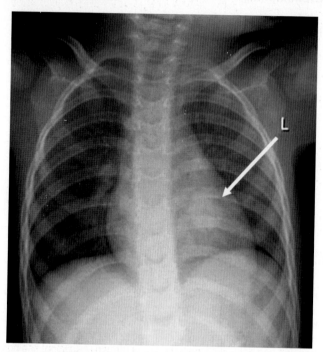

Fig. 32. 4: A round pneumonia (arrow) is seen exclusively in children, usually in the superior segment of the lower lobes. Consolidations in the early phases may appear rounded and one should not be mislead by their appearance which is strictly fortuitous. It can be mistaken for a neoplasm but a history of an acute illness and the extreme rarity of such neoplastic lung nodules in children should confirm the diagnosis. Causative organism is commonly *Streptococcus pneumoniae*

Primary Pulmonary Tuberculosis

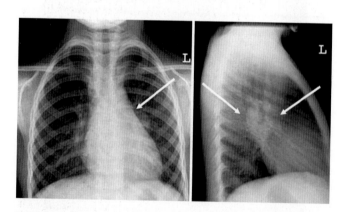

Fig. 32. 5: Primary pulmonary tuberculosis results from inhalation of the organism from an infected individual. The radiologic hall mark is unilateral hilar or paratracheal lymphadenopathy, very often accompanied by atelectasis due to compression of the bronchus by the enlarged nodes. Frontal and lateral CXR showing left hilar adenopathy in a patient with cough and fever (arrows)

Cystic Fibrosis (CF)

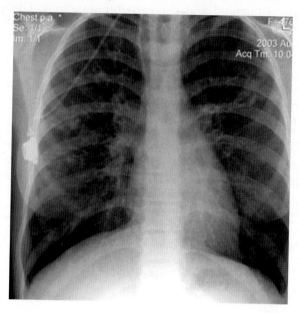

Fig. 32.6: An autosomal recessive error in chloride ion transport results in thick tenacious mucous.Clinical manifestations result from bronchiectasis, lung abscesses, air trapping, airway obstruction and right heart failure. On chest radiograph early CF can be seen as hyper aeration and bronchial wall cuffing. Mucoid impaction is seen as finger like densities radiating from the hilum. Bronchiectasis is seen as tram tracks radiating from the hilum. Chest radiograph showing lung hyperinflation, patchy infiltrates and peribronchial thickening and dilatation in a 11-year old patient with cystic

Bronchiectasis

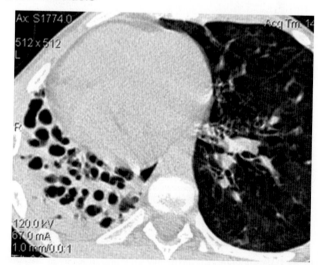

Fig. 32.7: High resolution CT confirms the presence and extent of bronchiectasis. Evaluation of segmental/lobar involvement is important if surgery is contemplated. CT scan showing cystic bronchiectasis in the right lower lobe

Inhaled Foreign Body

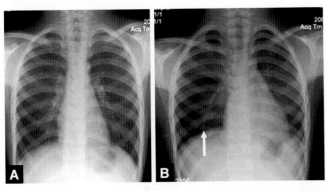

Figs 32.8A and B: Airway obstruction by foreign body (FB) usually affects toddlers and presents with stridor, wheezing, cough or pneumonia. The FB which can be radio or non-radioopaque usually lodges in bronchi (right commoner than left) and can obstruct the airway. Total obstruction can cause collapse. Partial obstruction can cause ball valve effect permitting air to enter but not leave the lungs. The affected side will demonstrate air trapping made prominent on expiration. Inspiratory (A) and expiratory (B) radiographs showing air trapping in the right middle lobe on expiration (arrow)

Complications of Pneumonia

Empyema

The appearance of pleural fluid in the setting of pneumonia suggests an empyema. Ultrasound (US) and Computed Tomography scanning reveal helpful information such as depicting whether the effusion is loculated or free, clear or containing debris. Image guided drainage can be done using ultrasound and fluoroscopy to accurately place the drainage catheter.

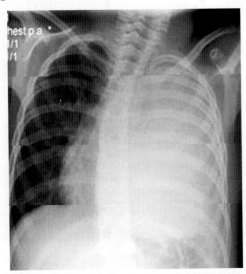

Fig. 32.9: CXR of a 6-year-old girl showing an opaque left haemithorax due to a large empyema. Note the scoliosis concave to the left

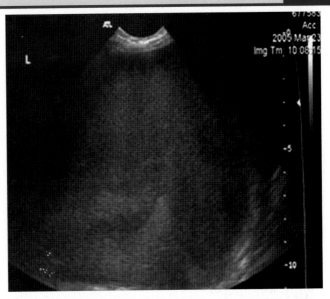

Fig. 32.10: Ultrasound scan in the same patient as above shows debris in the pleural fluid

Lung Abscess

Suppurative parenchymal complications represent a spectrum of abnormalities and include cavitary necrosis, lung abscess, pneumatocele, broncho-pleural fistula and pulmonary gangrene. When lung first becomes necrotic, the necrotic tissue liquefies and forms fluid filled cavities. When portions of this necrotic fluid are expectorated via bronchial communications, the cavities may fill with air. CT is more sensitive to earlier detection of lung abscesses, can assess proximity to pleura and plan drainage.

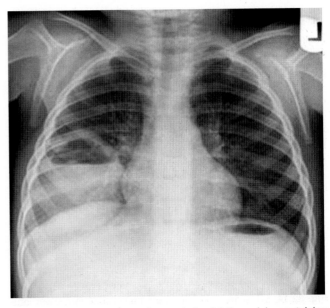

Fig. 32.11: CXR showing an abscess in the right lower lobe containing an air fluid level

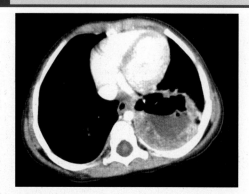

Fig. 32.12: CT scan in another patient showing left basal lung abscess

Pneumatoceles

Pneumatocele is a term given to thin-walled cysts seen at imaging and may represent a later stage of healing necrosis.

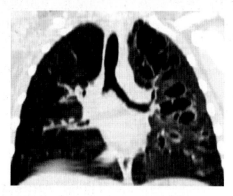

Fig. 32.13: Coronal CT reconstruction shows left upper lobe pneumatoceles as thin-walled cysts containing air

Broncho-pleural Fistula

Broncho-pleural fistula is identified on CT when a direct communication is visualised between the air spaces of the lung and the pleural space. There may be a chronic air leak.

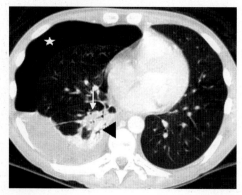

Fig. 32.14: CT scan in a patient with necrotising right lower lobe pneumonia shows right basal consolidation (arrow) and a large right tension pneumothorax (asterisk). The site of the fistula is shown by the arrowhead

The Neonate in Respiratory Distress

Common Causes

1. *Medical:* Respiratory distress syndrome (Surfactant deficiency disorder), Transient tachypnoea of the new born (retained foetal lung fluid), meconium aspiration, neonatal pneumonia
2. *Surgical:* Intrathoracic air leaks, diaphragmatic hernia, Intrathoracic masses of the newborn (Congenital lobar emphysema, Congenital cystic adenomatoid malformation, sequestration, bronchogenic and gut duplication cysts.

Imaging: Chest X-ray, mainly frontal view. Lateral view to localise focal air collections/masses. Ultrasound for solid chest masses. CT/MRI for further assessment of radiologically detected masses.

MEDICAL CAUSES

Respiratory Distress Syndrome (RDS)

RDS results from a deficiency of pulmonary surfactant due to prematurity. Surfactant deficiency leads to instability and collapse of the alveoli producing diffuse micro-atelectasis, stiff lungs and impaired gas exchange with resultant respiratory distress radiologically, the lungs are diffusely involved with a granular pattern of opacification and abnormal air bronchograms.

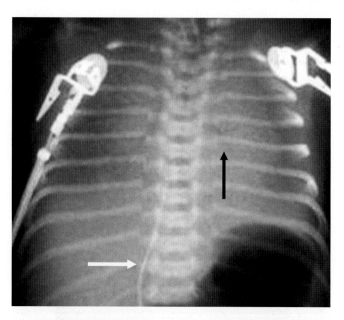

Fig. 32.15: CXR on a premature baby with RDS done on day one shows generalised underaeration of the lungs, reticulogranular densities caused by acinar atelectasis and air bronchograms (arrow). Incidental note is made of the umbilical venous catheter lying at the inferior vena cava and right atrial junction (white arrow)

Surfactant is now administered prophylactically in premature babies and in most infants the lungs clear rapidly. Since the surfactant is unevenly distributed throughout the lungs, the uneven distribution of surfactant leads to a radiographic appearance, which stimulates pneumonia or meconium aspiration syndrome.

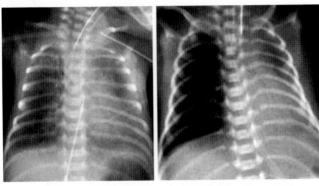

Fig. 32.16: Asymmetric SDD in two patients due to administration of exogenous surfactant. CXRs show asymmetrical opacities in both lungs

Complications of Respiratory Distress Syndrome

Iatrogenic or disease related complications might occur during the course of RDS. These include air leaks (pulmonary interstitial emphysema, pneumomediastinum and pneumothorax), tube malposition (Endotracheal, umbilical catheters), pulmonary haemorrhage and broncho-pulmonary dysplasia.

Pulmonary Interstitial Emphysema (PIE)

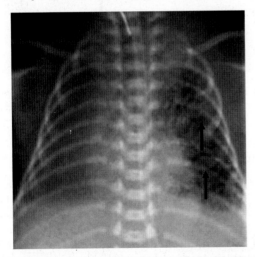

Fig. 32.17: Pulmonary interstitial emphysema in the left lung. This often appears as pseudo-clearing of SDD. Irregular and tubular densities (arrows) extending to the pleural edge are identified as pulmonary interstitial air. Peripheral PIE can produce sub-pleural blebs and can often rupture into the pleural space giving a pneumothorax or extend centrally to produce a pneumomediastinum or pneumo-pericardium

Pneumothorax

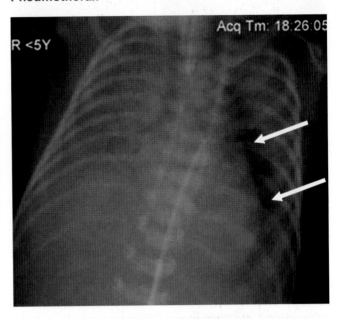

Fig. 32.18: CXR showing an early left medial pneumothorax (arrows) in a 2 days old infant with RDS. When a pneumothorax collects medially, the findings must be differentiated from pneumomediastinum or pneumopericardium. Pneumomediastinal air tends to outline the thymus while pneumopericardium surrounds the heart entirely

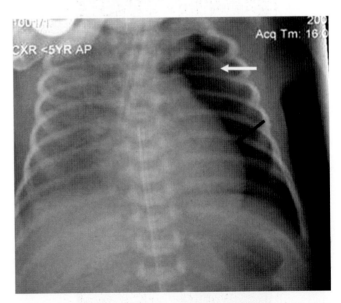

Fig. 32.19: Anterior left pneumothorax in the same infant as above in a CXR taken about 10 hours after the above radiograph. In the supine position air acculmulates over the anterior surface of the lung and produces a hyperlucent large hemithorax, increased sharpness of the ipsilateral mediastinal edge (black arrow) with a visible free edge of the left lung (white arrow). The thymus (T) may be compressed to form a pseudomass. Note the endotracheal tube down the right main bronchus

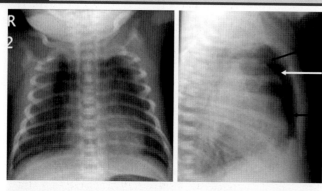

Figs 32.20A and B: Pneumomediastinum: Frontal (A) CXR shows a large lucency overlying the mediastinum. Lateral view (B) shows the air collection in the anterior mediastinum (black arrows) lifting and outlining the thymus (white arrow)

Bronchopulmonary Dysplasia (BPD)

BPD is a distinct pulmonary disease affecting the developing lung after prolonged respirator or oxygen therapy of RDS. Also called chronic lung disease of prematurity, the radiological findings include bubbly appearance to the lungs, hyperaeration and cardiomegaly.

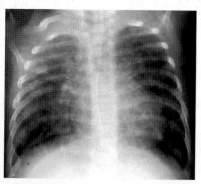

Fig. 32.21: CXR of a month old infant with BPD shows bilateral lung hyperinflation, bubbly appearance of the lungs and cardiomegaly

Endotracheal Tube (ETT) Malposition

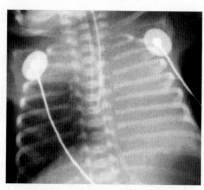

Fig. 32.22: The ideal position of the ETT is 2.0 cm above the carina with the neonates head in a neutral position. CXR showing the ETT down the right mainstem bronchus with total atelectasis of the left lung and right upper lobe

Umbilical Arterial (UAC) and Venous (UVC)

The UAC passes through the umbilicus, umbilical artery, internal iliac artery, common iliac artery and the abdominal aorta. It should ideally be placed away from the vessels to abdominal and pelvic viscera approximately at L3/L4 or T8/T10. The UVC passes through the umbilicus, umbilical vein, medial part of left portal vein, ductus venosus, IVC and right atrium.

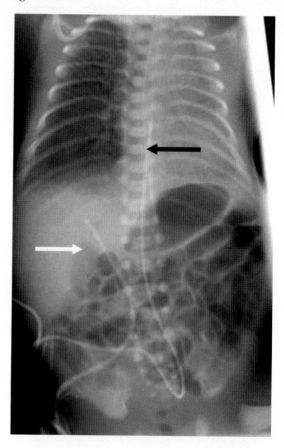

Fig. 32.23: Chest and abdominal film showing UAC (black arrow) in distal thoracic aorta and UVC (white arrow) at the level of left portal vein

Meconium Aspiration Syndrome (MAS)

MAS is caused by the intrauterine or intrapartum aspiration of meconium stained fluid in term or post-term infants. Aspiration of meconium into the tracheobronchial tree causes complete or partial bronchial obstruction leading to patchy areas of subsegmental atelectasis and compensatory areas of hyperinflation. Meconium also causes chemical pneumonitis, which is complicated by bronchopneumonia.

Radiologically, there are patchy, bilateral asymmetric areas of rounded/linear opacities and marked hyperinflation. Air leaks such as pneumomediastinum, pneumothorax is seen in 25% of patients.

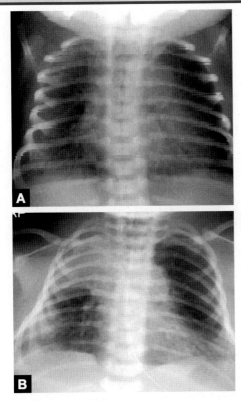

Figs 32.34A and B: Term newborns with MAS. (A) CXR shows assymetrical lung hyperinflation, patchy right basal infiltrates and areas of atelectasis. (B) CXR showing left and right upper lobe atelectasis and right basal infiltrates

Transient Tachypnoea of the Newborn (TTN)

Usually affects full-term infants, often following caesarean section or infants of diabetic mothers and is symptomatic within first 2 to 4 hours of life. It is caused by retained foetal lung fluid and treatment is supportive. CXR reveals normal lung volumes with interstitial oedema, which clears within 1 to 2 days.

SURGICAL CAUSES

Congenital Diaphragmatic Hernia

Left sided hernias, through the foramen of Bochdalek are commoner than right sided ones in the newborn. Variable quantities of intestinal contents, stomach and liver enter the chest during foetal life. The CXR shows an abnormal haemithorax, which is opaque initially but later fills with bubbles representing gas filled bowel and contralateral mediastinal shift. The lungs are hypoplastic. The abdomen is small and narrow. Right-sided hernias are less common in the newborn and usually present later in life.

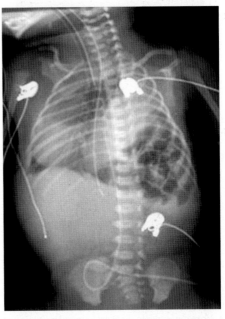

Fig. 32.26: Left diaphragmatic hernia: Many intrathoracic air-filled loops of bowel and absence of normal amounts of gas in the abdomen are seen in this neonate with severe respiratory distress. The prognosis correlates with the degree of underlying lung hypoplasia

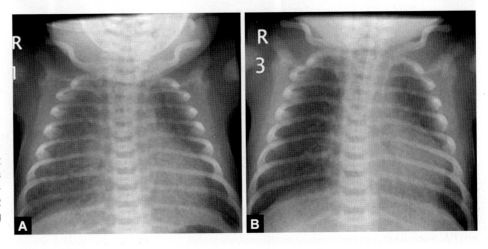

Figs 32.25A and B: CXR in an infant with TTN taken day 1(A) shows cardiomegaly and interstitial pulmonary oedema. Follow-up CXR day 2 (B) shows almost complete clearing of the lungs

Congenital Adenomatoid Malformation (CAM)

A congenital hamartomatous lesion characterised by proliferation of terminal respiratory bronchioles with no alveolar communication and usually presents in the neonate as respiratory distress. The lesion initially appears radio-opaque due to fluid filled cysts. As lungs aerate, these cysts gradually fill with air giving a 'cystic' appearance. The radiological appearance can mimic diaphragmatic hernia. A helpful differentiating feature is the presence of air filled loops of bowel in the abdomen.10 % of CAMs present after first year of life, often with recurrent pneumonias.

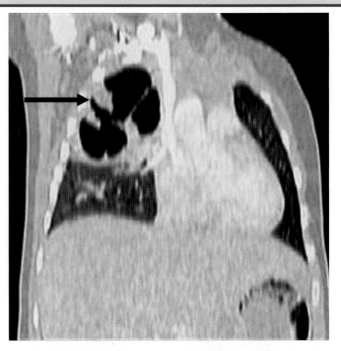

Fig. 32.28: Coronal CT reconstruction shows a CAM in the right upper lobe (arrow)

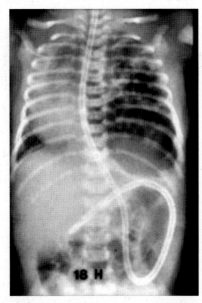

Fig. 32.27: CXR showing multiple cystic lucencies in the left hemithorax. There is mediastinal shift, which can cause progressive pulmonary hypoplasia. Note the multiple air filled loops of bowel in the abdomen and the intra-abdominal nasogastric tube tip

Congenital Lobar Emphysema (CLE)

CLE initially appears as an opacification of one lobe or the whole lung due to partial bronchial obstruction causing retention of fluid. Over a period of few days the fluid is resorbed and replaced by air at which point the diagnosis becomes obvious. Progressive over distension results in air trapping and its consequences, namely mediastinal shift, compression of normal lung or lobes.

Common sites to be affected are left upper and right upper lobes.

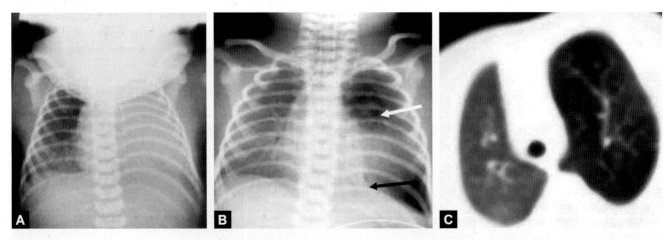

Figs 32.29A to C: CXR (A and B) of a term neonate with respiratory distress. Day 1 (A) shows an opaque left hemithorax. Day 2 (B) shows a hyperinflated left upper lobe (white arrow) and compression collapse of left lower lobe (black arrow). CT scan (C) on day 3 shows an emphysematous left upper lobe and moderate mediastinal shift

Bronchogenic Cyst

Usually arise from an abnormal lung bud from developing foregut. The mediastinal form is usually asymptomatic but can present with respiratory distress if the major airways are compressed due to gradual expansion over time. The cyst is often subcarinal in location and can be mistaken for a duplication cyst.

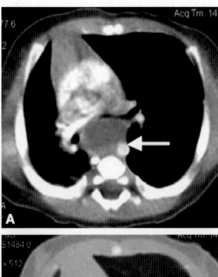

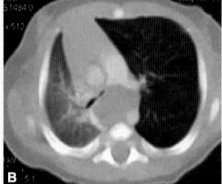

Figs 32.30A and B: CT scans (A) showing a posterior mediastinal cystic lesion (white arrow) causing compression of the left main bronchus (asterisk) and (B) hyperinflation of the left lung. Differential diagnosis includes duplication cyst of the oesophagus

Neurenteric Cyst

Faulty neural tube closure results in abnormal mesenchyme leading to abnormal vertebral body formation and continued neural connection with endoderm. The abnormality is found most commonly in the thoracic spine with a cystic mass in the mediastinum and segmentation anomalies of the spine (butterfly vertebrae or hemivertebrae).

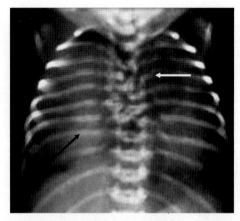

Fig. 32.31: CXR showing a soft tissue mass in the right hemithorax (black arrow) and multiple segmentation anomalies of the thoracic spine (white arrow). Differentials include a large intrathoracic meningocele

A CHILD WITH A MEDIASTINAL MASS

Normal Thymus

The thymus gland is found in the anterior mediastinum and can have a variety of appearances. The 2 lobes of the thymus are often dense enough to obscure the upper and middle mediastinum. A thymus is recognised by its wavy margin from indentation by the ribs, by a sail configuration and by a notch where the thymic shadow intersects the cardiac margin. A normal thymus can be a notorious source of difficulty when interpreting chest films. Sonography can be useful in thymic imaging especially to determine if the anterior mediastinal mass is a normal thymus.

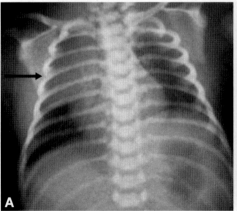

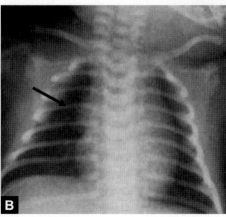

Figs 32.32A and B: Radiographs of neonates showing a prominent normal thymus exhibiting the 'sail sign' (arrow in A) or the wave sign (arrow in B). It is often difficult to ascertain true heart size on the frontal radiograph. Mass effect or mediastinal shift is almost never seen with a normal thymus

Thymic Sonography

Sonographically the thymus has an echotexture similar to liver with punctuate echoes and echogenic lines. Real time sonography demonstrates normal thymic malleability during the respiratory cycle, helping in differentiating from a thymic mass. In the setting of a mass presence of cysts, calcification or heterogeneity of architecture can suggest thymic pathology.

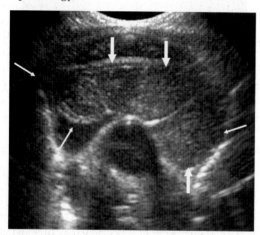

Fig. 32.33: Axial ultrasound of the thymus at the level of ascending aorta (AA) The normal thymus (arrows) can have a bilobed appearance, homogenous texture and some echogenic strands

Lymphoma

Thymic involvement with lymphoma (Hodgkins and non Hodgkins) can be multifocal or diffuse. With lymphoma, the age of the child and presence of other regions of adenopathy can be helpful in prioritising histology. If the lymphoma is confined to the thymus in an older child or adolescent, a Hodgkin's type lymphoma is likely. Non-Hodgkin's lymphoma can occur at any age. On CT, the appearances can be homogenous or heterogenous with areas of fibrosis, necrosis.

Germ Cell Tumours

These tumours include teratomas, seminomas, dysgerminomas and choriocarcinomas. Second to lymphoma as a cause of mediastinal mass, most are located in the superior mediastinum and can be asymptomatic in up to half of the patients. Large tumours can cause tracheal and superior vena caval compression and are malignant in up to 10% of cases. Teratomas are the commonest germ cell tumours and consist of ectodermal, mesenchymal and endodermal derivatives. On CT/MR they contain variable amounts of fat, calcium or soft tissue. Fat or calcium in an anterior mediastinal mass almost always indicates a germ cell tumour.

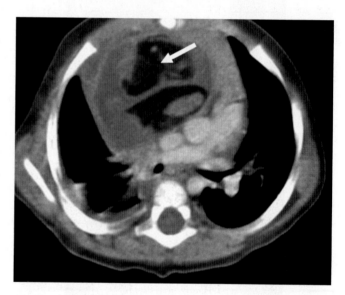

Fig. 32.35: Mixed attenuation mass in the anterior mediastinum containing low attenuation areas representing fat (seen as low attenuation areas, arrow), in a child with chronic stridor from was airway compression

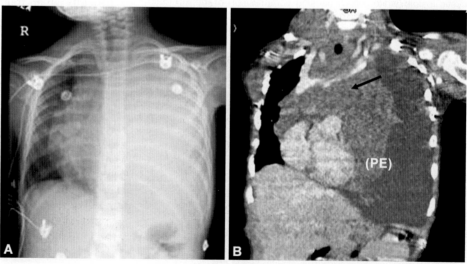

Figs 32.34A and B: CXR (A) and coronal reconstruction of a CT scan (B) of a 5 year old showing a large mediastinal mass (arrow) midline shift and a left pleural effusion (PE). Diagnosis at biopsy was of a T-cell lymphoma

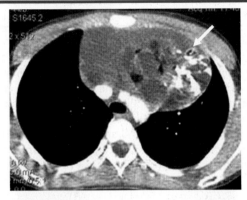

Fig. 32.36: CT scan in another patient with stridor shows a calcified anterior mediastinal mass (white arrow). The low attenuation areas within the mass represent fat

Metastases

Most paediatric malignant tumours are pulmonary metastases, usually found during staging of a known or a new malignancy. Common paediatric tumours associated with lung metastases include Wilms tumour, rhabdomyosarcoma, hepatoblastoma, Ewing's and osteosarcoma. CT is more sensitive than plain films in detecting metastases.

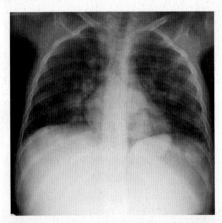

Fig. 32.37: Multiple intrapulmonary metastases from hepatoblastoma

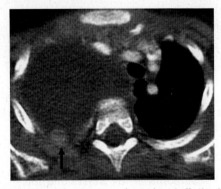

Fig. 32.38: Pleural based metastases (arrow) and effusion in a patient with Wilms tumour

Neuroblastoma

Majority of posterior mediastinal masses in children are of neurogenic origin, namely neuroblastoma, ganglioneurblastoma and ganglioneuroma. Thoracic neuroblastoma has a better prognosis than abdominal neuroblastoma. The plain film suggest the diagnosis with posterior rib erosion and a mass, which may have some calcification. At CT most tumours are well circumscribed fusiform masses in the para-spinal location. Enlargement of the inter vertebral neural foramina and spread into the abdomen via the aortic or oesophageal hiatus may be evident.

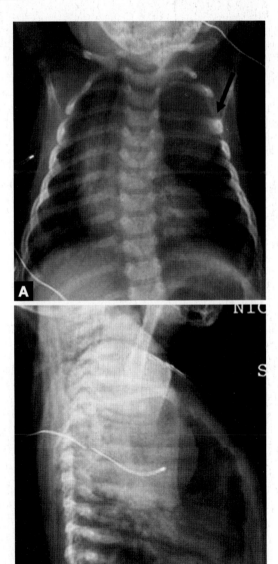

Figs 32.39A and B: AP (A) and lateral (B) CXR in a child showing a well defined left posterior mediastinal mass (arrow) with erosion, splaying and thinning of the posterior ribs

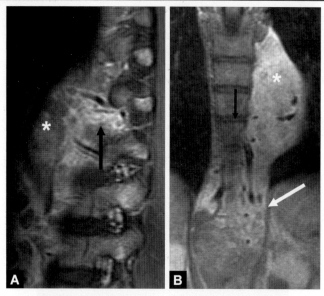

Figs 32.40A and B: Sagittal (A) and coronal (B) MR images show a left paraspinal mass (asterisk) with extension into the intervertebral foramina (black arrows) and into the abdomen via the aortic hiatus (white arrow)

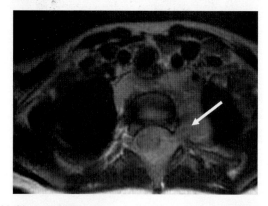

Fig. 32.41: Axial MR in a 6-year-old child showing a well defined left para-vertebral mass with extension into the intervertebral foramen (arrow)

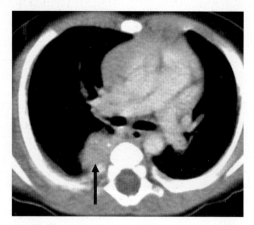

Fig. 32.42: Calcified neuroblastoma in the right para-vertebral area (arrow) in 6 months old infant

CHEST WALL MASSES

Ewing Sarcoma

Ewing sarcoma is a malignant round cell tumour and is the the commonest malignant chest wall mass in children. It usually manifests as a peripheral chest wall mass with or without rib destruction. The CXR will show a mass with intrathoracic growth, rib and chest wall involvement and accompanying pleural effusion. MRI and CT play complimentary roles in staging these tumours.

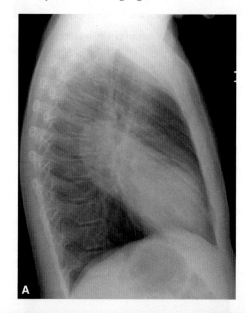

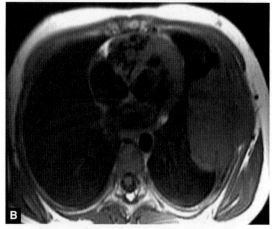

Figs 32.43A and B: Lateral (A) CXR and T1 weighted MR (B) showing a left chest wall mass following the rib contours and extending into the thoracic cavity

Rhabdomyosarcoma

Rhabdomyosarcoma is the most common extrapleural chest wall tumour in children. The radiologic features are difficult to distinguish from Ewing sarcoma.

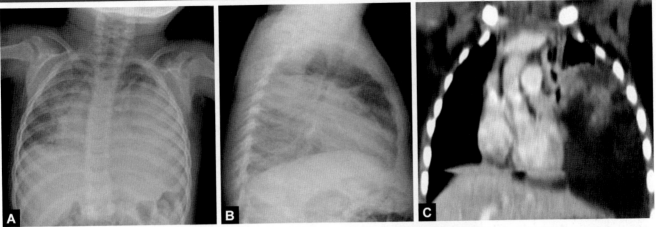

Figs 32.44A to C: AP (A) and lateral (B) CXR showing a left chest soft tissue mass and mediastinal shift. Coronal CT (C) reconstruction shows a mixed density mass with fluid and solid components. These appearances may be confused with empyema

Osteochondroma of the Ribs

Commonest benign tumour of he chest wall, composed of cortical and medullary bone with a cartilaginous cap and usually continuous with the underlying bone.

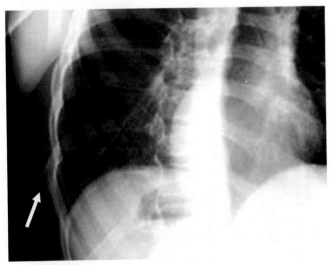

Fig. 32.45: Oblique view of the ribs shows bony lesion attaches to the ribs by a broad base (arrow)

CONGENITAL HEART DISEASE

Imaging approach:
1. Echocardiography
2. Chest radiography
3. Cardiac catheterisation
4. Magnetic resonance imaging (MRI).

Specific Chamber Enlargement on Plain Film

Right Atrium

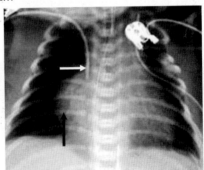

Fig. 32.46: The enlarged right atrium displaces the right heart border to the right and increased curvature of the right heart border. A step like angle (white arrow) between the right atrium and the superior vena cava may be seen.

Right Ventricle

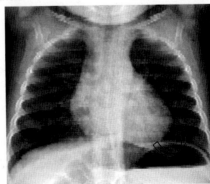

Fig. 32.47: The right ventricle occupies the front of the heart and is non-border forming in the frontal view. Enlargement of the right ventricle results in tilting up and posterior displacement of the left ventricle and a triangular configuration of the heart and elevation of the apex (block arrow)

Left Atrium

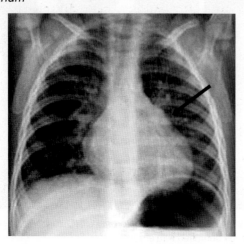

Fig. 32.48: An enlarging left atrium may elevate the left main bronchus, and cause a bulge in the *right* heart border producing a double shadow seen through the right heart border. Particularly in rheumatic heart disease there may be left atrial enlargement seen as a discrete bulge on the left heart border below the pulmonary bay.

Left Ventricle

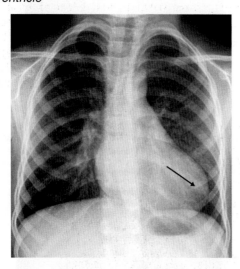

Fig. 32.49: The left ventricle forms the left border and the apex of the cardiac shadow on a frontal CXR. Enlargement leads to rounding of the apex of the heart and elongation of long axis of the left ventricle (arrow)

Acyanotic Child with Congenital Heart Disease

Left to right shunts account for about half of all forms of congenital heart disease.
3 common diagnoses include.

1. Patent ductus arteriosus (PDA)
2. Ventricular septal defect (VSD)
3. Atrial septal defect (ASD).

Ventricular Septal Defect (VSD)

VSD is the commonest congenital cardiac anomaly, usually presenting in infants and toddlers. It may be isolated or associated with other congenital defects. Defects can occur in any part of the inter ventricular septum: Peri membranous, muscular or trabecular, outlet or inlet. The haemodynamics of the VSD are determined by the size of the defect and the pressure difference between the left and right ventricle. In neonates with a high pulmonary vascular resistance significant left to right shunting is uncommon but in large defects congestive heart failure develops at 1-3 months of age due to normal decrease in pulmonary vascular resistance. The CXR in a VSD with a small left to right shunt is normal. In large shunts the main, branch and the intra-pulmonary branches of the pulmonary arteries dilate. There is enlargement of the left atrium and the ventricles.

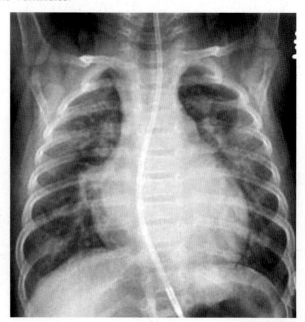

Fig. 32.50: Chest radiograph showing cardiomegaly, biventricular enlargement and increased lung vascularity

Patent Ductus Arteriosus (PDA)

The ductus arteriosus, extends from the origin of the left pulmonary artery to the descending aorta just beyond the origin of the the left subclavian artery and shunts blood from the main pulmonary artery to the aorta. In newborns the PDA is a common cause of congestive heart failure. Small premature infants with a PDA and a left to right shunt may have evidence of left ventricular failure. Patients with small PDA have no radiographic abnormalities. Large PDAs show increased lung vascularity and enlarged left atrium and ventricle.

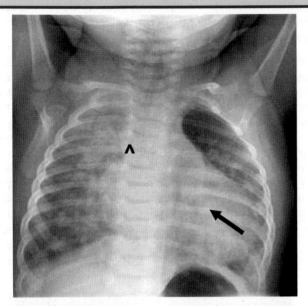

Fig. 32.51: Chest radiograph showing marked cardiomegaly with left ventricular enlargement (downward pointing apex, arrow), left atrial enlargement resulting in carinal splaying (∧) and areas of atelectasis interspersed with hyperinflation, and pulmonary oedema in a patient with a large PDA. Atelectasis is due to a large left atrium compressing the airways

Atrial Septal Defect (ASD)

ASD is commonly an isolated lesion. The shunt is from the left to the right atrium leading to enlargement of the right atrium, ventricle and the pulmonary arteries. Most children are asymptomatic and is usually diagnosed in older children or adults. The condition is usually undetected until a murmur is heard. A moderate sized ASD shows increased lung vascularity, an enlarged heart with prominent right atrium and pulmonary artery. Right ventricular filling may be seen as filling of the retrosternal space on a lateral CXR.

CYANOTIC CHILD WITH CONGENITAL HEART DISEASE

Common causes include Tetralogy of Fallot, Transposition of great vessels and pulmonary atresia with intact ventricular septum.

Tetralogy of Fallot (TOF)

TOF is the commonest cyanotic congenital cardiac disease in children. The four components of TOF are: Right ventricular out flow tract (RVOT) obstruction, subaortic VSD, overriding aorta and right ventricular hypertrophy. The severity of RVOT obstruction determines the amount of left to right shunting across the VSD. The infundibular stenosis progresses with age and left to right shunting increases proportionately. The CXR shows a mild to moderate cardiomegaly, uplifted apex secondary to right ventricular enlargement and concavity in the region of pulmonary artery segment giving a boot shaped heart. A right-sided aortic arch occurs in 25% of patients with TOF.

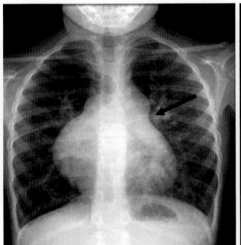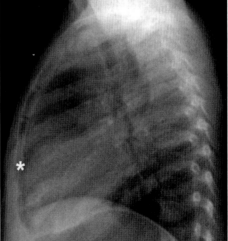

Fig. 32.52: CXR showing enlarged right atrium and right ventricle (shown as filling of the retrosternal space on a lateral CXR, (asterisks) main pulmonary artery (arrow) with increased pulmonary flow

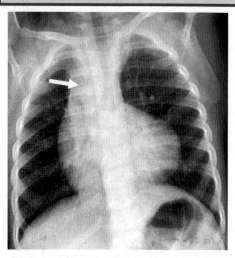

Fig. 32.53: CXR showing a 'boot shaped heart', due to elevation of the apex secondary to right ventricular hypertrophy, right aortic arch (arrow) and pulmonary oligemia

D-Transposition of Great Vessels

TGV is the commonest congenital cardiac disorder causing cyanosis in the first 24 hours of life. The aorta and the pulmonary artery are transposed. The ascending aorta arises from the right ventricle and the pulmonary artery rises from the left ventricle giving two parallel circuits between the pulmonary and systemic circulations. Communications between the two circulations are vital for survival and include PDA, ASD and VSD. The CXR shows a narrow superior mediastinum due to decrease in thymic tissue and abnormal relations of the great vessels and lack of visualisation of the aortic arch which is malpositioned and lack of normal shadow of the main pulmonary artery. The lung vascularity can be increased, decreased or normal.

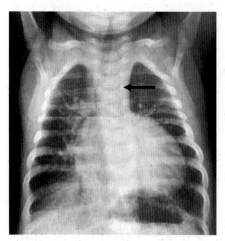

Fig. 32.54: (d-TGV). Newborn with marked cyanosis. The heart is enlarged and there is a narrow superior mediastinum (arrow). The pulmonary vascularity is increased despite an inconspicuous main pulmonary artery segment

Pulmonary Atresia with Ventricular Septal Defect (VSD)

There is severe hypoplasia or atresia of the main pulmonary artery leading to no forward flow from the right ventricle into the lungs. Blood supply to the lungs is usually via collaterals from the aorta. Most infants are hypoxic and cyanotic. Radiologically the heart is enlarged with an upturned apex secondary to right ventricular hypertrophy. There is marked concavity in the region of the main pulmonary artery because of underdevelopment of the infundibulum and the main pulmonary artery. Pulmonary vascular markings have an unusual reticular appearance due to abnormal.

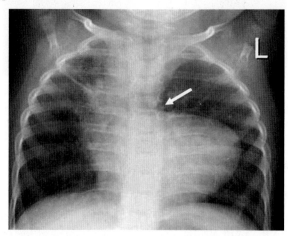

Fig. 32.55: Pulmonary atresia with VSD. Cardiomegaly with a markedly elevated apex, concavity in the region of the main pulmonary artery (arrow) and a right aortic arch with abnormal lung vascularity

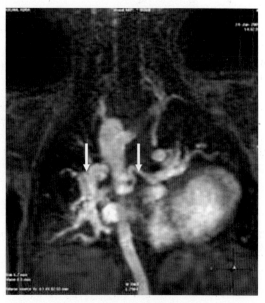

Fig. 32.56: Contrast enhanced MRA shows multiple aorto pulmonary collateral arteries (arrows) supplying the lungs

Truncus Arteriosus

An uncommon anomaly, truncus arteriosus is due to failure of division of the primitive truncus into the aorta and pulmonary artery. One large vessel originates from the heart to supply the systemic, pulmonary and coronary circulations. A large VSD is always present. Several types of truncus are described. Radiologically, cardiomegaly and increased pulmonary flow are seen at birth in a cyanosed infant . There is enlargement of the left atrium, pulmonary oedema and a prominent truncus. The main pulmonary artery segment is concave. The aorta is right sided in one third of patients.

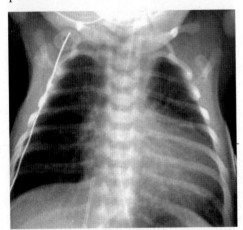

Fig. 32.57: A 2-month-old boy with cyanosis. The heart is enlarged, the main pulmonary artery segment is concave and the pulmonary vascularity is increased

Total Anomalous Pulmonary Venous Drainage (TAPVD)

TAPVD occurs when he common pulmonary vein fails to develop and the branch pulmonary veins connect to other venous structures such as SVC, IVC, right atrium, or portal venous system. TAPVD is divided into 4 types: Supra cardiac, cardiac, infracardiac and mixed. The supracardiac type is the most common. All 4 pulmonary veins converge into a left vertical, which drains into the left innominate vein. Because both systemic and pulmonary veins drain into the right atrium there is increased volume overload of the right heart, which enlarge. Radiologically, the appearance of the mediastinum, is likened to a snow man with the upper half of the 'snowman' consisting of the vertical vein and the dilated SVC.

OTHER CARDIAC AND RELATED CONDITIONS

Coarctation of Aorta (CoA)

CoA results from membranous infolding of the posterolateral wall of the thoracic aorta at the level of ligamentum or ductus arteriosus causing obstruction to forward blood flow. Post-stenotic dilatation of the proximal descending thoracic aorta is present. Significant coarctation impairs blood flow into the descending thoracic aorta necessitating the presence of collaterals to re-establish blood flow. The intercostal arteries are major collaterals resulting in rib notching along the inferior surface of 3-8th ribs in untreated patients usually by 10 years. Other collaterals arise from internal mammary, lateral thoracic and epigastric arteries. On a frontal CXR one can identify a high aortic arch, a reverse '3' indentation at the site of coarctation (reflecting pre-coarctation dilatation, the coarctation and post-coarctation dilatation and rib notching. The coarctation can be well demonstrated by MR angiography.

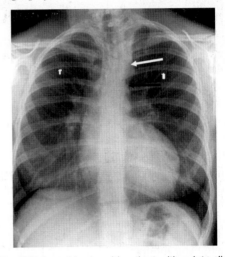

Fig. 32.58: CXR in a 14-year-old patient with a late diagnosis of coarctation shows a high aortic arch (black arrow), a reverse appearance at the coarctation site (white arrow), rib notching (small arrows) and left ventricular hypertrophy

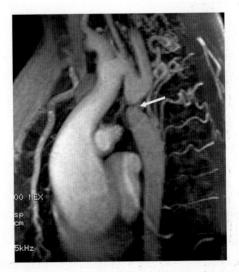

Fig. 32.59: Contrast enhanced MRA of the aorta demonstrates the tight coarctation (arrow) and intercostal, internal mammary and lateral thoracic collaterals

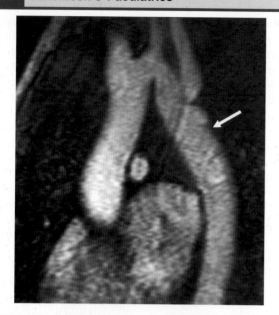

Fig. 32.60: Post-balloon angioplasty of another patient with coarctation shows resolution of the stenosis with a small intimal flap from dissection (arrow).

Epstein Anomaly

An uncommon congenital abnormality in which the septal and posterior leaflets of the tricuspid valve are attached to the wall of the middle of the right ventricular chamber instead of the valve ring. This results in mild to gross tricuspid regurgitation and marked right atrial enlargement. The foramen ovale is patent and the raised right atrial pressure results in right to left shunt and cyanosis. The frontal CXR shows an enlarged globular or square cardiac silhouette and reduced pulmonary vascularity.

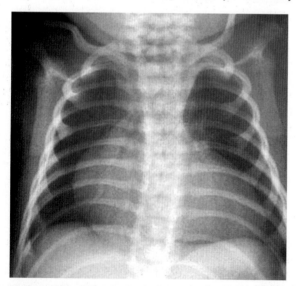

Fig. 32.61: CXR showing a globular cardiomegaly, enlarged right atrium and reduced lung vascularity

Double Aortic Arch

In this type of anomaly the ascending aorta is anterior to the trachea bifurcating into 2 arches that pass to the sides of the trachea before joining posterior to the oesophagus to form the descending aorta. The double aortic arch forms a tight vascular ring that may present with severe stridor and requires surgical intervention.

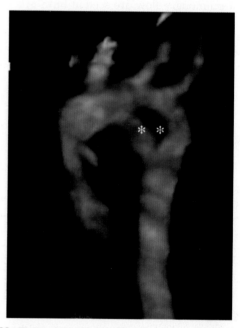

Fig. 32.62: Three dimensional reconstruction of a CT angiogram shows a double aortic arch (asterisks)

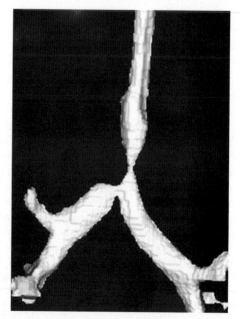

Fig. 32.63: Three-dimensional reconstruction of the airway in a patient with double aortic arch and stridor shows tight narrowing of the distal trachea by the complete vascular ring

ABDOMEN

A NEONATE WITH BILIOUS VOMITING

Common causes:
1. Malrotation with or without small bowel volvulus
2. Duodenal/small bowel atresias and webs
3 Meconium ileus.

Malrotation

Malrotation is a general term for any abnormal variation in intestinal rotation. Any variety of malrotation seen in a child with abdominal symptoms should be assumed to be the cause of the symptoms unless proven otherwise. Malrotation of he intestines is accompanied by malfixation of the mesenteric root, which can have catastrophic consequences. The duodenal junction and the ileocaecal junctions are normal points of fixation of the mesentery, which has a broad base and unlikely to twist. When these points of fixation are not in their usual location the mesentery has a narrow base and there is a tendency for the intestines to twist around it. Abnormal peritoneal bands Ladds bands frequently accompany malrotation and can cause duodenal obstruction. Patients with malrotation can present at any age with bilious vomiting but most patients with symptomatic malrotation present in the first month of life.

Radiological investigations should include a plain film of the abdomen, which may show duodenal obstruction and an upper gastrointestinal studies which demonstrate malfixation of bowel, namely malposition of the duodenojejunal flexure (more accurate indicator of malrotation) and the caecum.

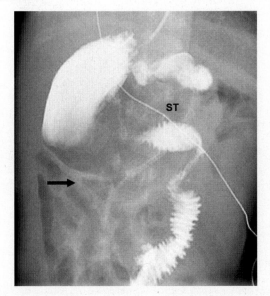

Fig. 32.64: Upper GI contrast exam in a newborn baby with bilious vomiting shows malrotation of the small bowel with the duodenal jejunal flexure and jejunal loops lying to the right of the spine (arrow)

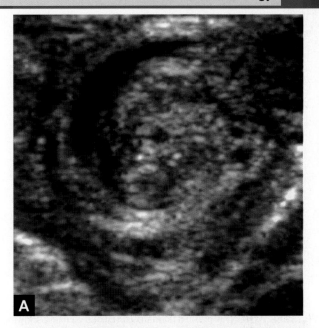

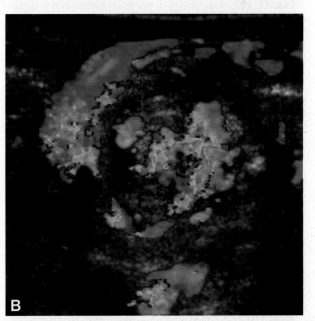

Figs 32.65A and B: Malrotation with volvulus in another patient: Sonography with colour Doppler shows (A) a 'whirlpool' appearance of the volved small bowel and (B) twisting of the superior mesenteric artery and vein

Duodenal Atresia (DA)

Infants with duodenal atresia present with bilious vomiting in the first few hours of life. The obstruction is usually below the ampulla of Vater. Plain abdominal film shows a characteristic double bubble sign. Once this pattern is seen there is no need for further contrast studies. DA is commoner in infants with trisomy 21.

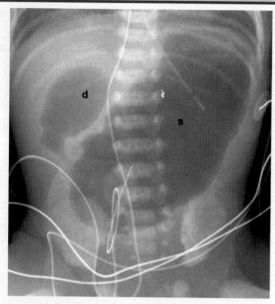

Fig. 32.66: Abdominal film in a neonate with bilious vomiting showing a 'double bubble' appearance in duodenal atresia due to a dilated stomach (s) and first part of duodenum (d). No air is present distal to the stomach

Duodenal Diaphragm

Duodenal diaphragms usually occur in the descending portion of the duodenum and frequently the common bile duct is incorporated in the diaphragm. Vomiting is bile stained and plain abdominal films show obstruction at the level of descending duodenum. Definitive diagnosis is usually made with barium studies.

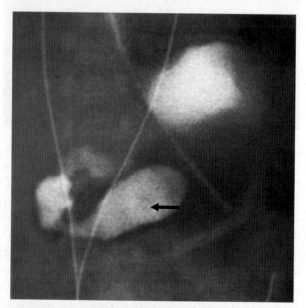

Fig. 32.67: Upper gastrointestinal contrast study in a newborn with bilious vomiting shows the duodenal diaphragm (arrow)

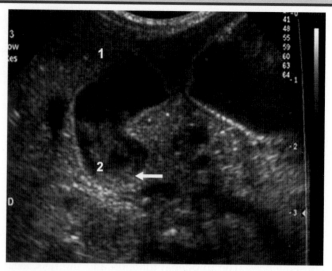

Fig. 32.68: Upper abdominal ultrasound in a neonate showing dilated and fluid filled first (1) and second (2) parts of the duodenum due to a web (arrow)

Small Bowel Atresia

Small bowel atresia presents with abdominal distension and bilious vomiting condition is often not diagnosed until laparotomy. Radiographs show one or two dilated small bowel loops if the obstruction involves jejunum. If distal small bowel is involved multiple dilated loops of small bowel is seen with air fluid levels. A contrast enema is then necessary to assess for colonic obstruction.

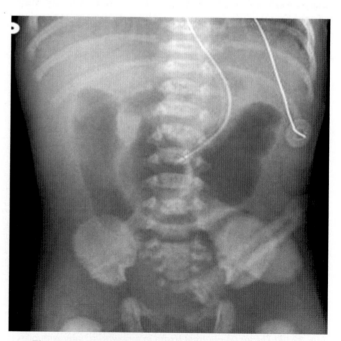

Fig. 32.69: Plain radiograph in an infant with jejunal atresia showing dilatation of proximal bowel loops

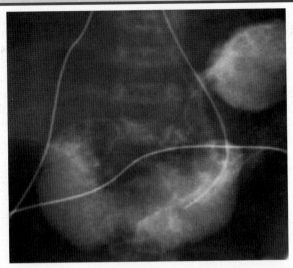

Fig. 32.70: Water-soluble contrast study showing a dilated duodenum and failure of passage of contrast beyond the duodenal jejunal flexure in proximal jejunal atresia

Meconium Ileus

Usually considered a manifestation of cystic fibrosis in neonates. Obstruction results from impaction of thick tenacious meconium in the distal small bowel and complications such as ileal atresia, stenosis, ileal perforation, meconium peritonitis and volvulus with or without pseudocyst formation are common. Infants present with bile stained vomiting, abdominal distension and failure to pass meconium. Plain films show low small bowel obstruction with marked small bowel dilatation. Air fluid levels are generally absent due to tenacious mucous. A contrast enema demonstrates a micro colon. The enema can also be therapeutic.

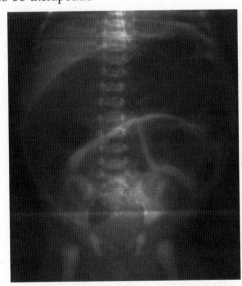

Fig. 32.71: Abdominal film in an infant with meconium ileus shows marked small bowel dilatation

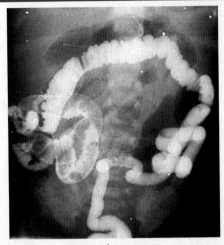

Fig. 32.72: A contrast enema shows a microcolon

OTHER ABDOMINAL CONDITIONS IN CHILDREN

Hypertrophic Pyloric Stenosis (HPS)

HPS is a common condition presenting between 2 to 6 weeks of life in predominantly male infants with non-bilious projectile vomiting . Severe cases also have weight loss and metabolic alkalosis of varying severity with potassium depletion. A small firm mass_the pseudotumor of HPS may be palpable. Sonography is the modality of choice to diagnose HPS. The stomach is emptied prior to exam by inserting a naso-gastric tube and aspirating the contents. Sterile water is then introduced under sonographic guidance. HPS is seen as enlarged hypoechoic pyloric musculature with minimal emptying of the water into the duodenum. A plain film done to assess for other causes of vomiting may show gaseous distension of the stomach with little gas distally.

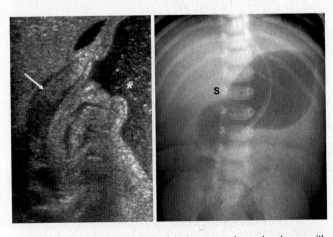

Figs 32.73A and B: (A) US showing an enlarged pylorus with hypoechoic muscle (arrow). Water introduced through a nasogastric tube is seen in the antrum (asterisk). (B) plain abdominal film showing a distended stomach (s)

Acute Appendicitis

Acute appendicitis is the most common indication for emergency abdominal surgery in children. It is caused by obstruction to the appendiceal lumen commonly by a fecalith. The appendix distends with secondary bacterial inflammation, oedema and vascular engorgement. Compromised blood supply may produce necrosis, gangrene and perforation with peritonitis. Complicated peritonitis can lead to a local walled off abscess or multiple intra-abdominal abscesses. Plain abdominal films may be normal or demonstrate a gasless right iliac fossa and a calcified fecalith. Complicated cases may present with small bowel obstruction from the complex appendiceal mass with comprises of the inflamed appendix, adjacent lops of small bowel and inflamed mesentery. Sonography shows the inflamed appendix, abscess and the complex right lower quadrant mass.

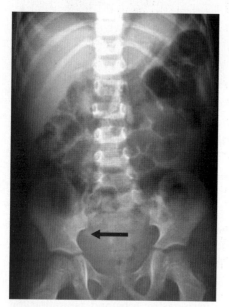

Fig. 32.74: Plain abdominal film shows a calcified fecalith (arrow) in the right iliac fossa and small bowel dilatation in a patient with appendicitis

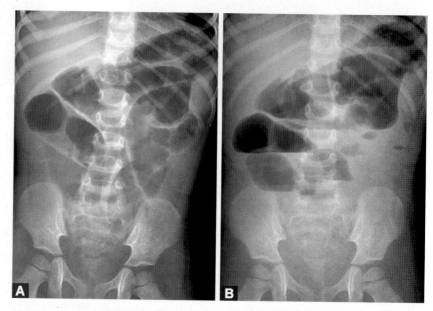

Figs 32.75A and B: Appendicitis with obstruction: (A) Supine view of the abdomen shows small bowel dilatation and a gasless right iliac fossa. (B) Erect view demonstrates air-fluid levels in the small bowel

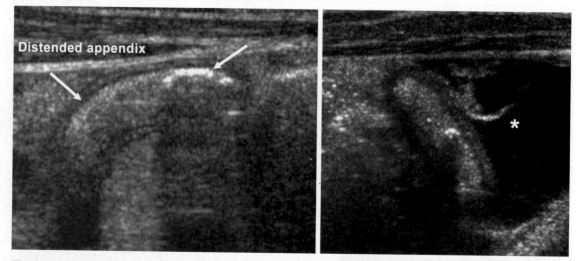

Fig. 32.76: Ultrasound of a patient with complicated appendicitis shows a distended appendix with a phlebolith (arrow). The phlebolith is seen as an echogenic curvilinear structure with posterior acoustic shadowing. There is a focal fluid collection near the appendix (asterisk)

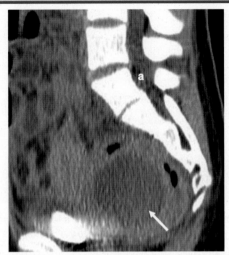

Fig. 32.77: Sagittal reconstruction of a CT scan of the abdomen in a patient with complicated appendicitis shows a thick walled abscess (arrow) which was successfully drained trans rectally

Intussusception

Intussusception is the invagination of the proximal bowel into its distal lumen. Ileocolic intussusceptions are commonest (90%) and may or may not have a lead point. Which include Meckel's diverticulum, polyps, lymphoma or sub-mucosal haemorrhage. Most intussusceptions are idiopathic and the clinical symptoms include intermittent abdominal pain, vomiting, bloody stools and palpable abdominal mass. The plain film is normal in 25% of patients or may show soft tissue mass or small bowel obstruction. Ultra sound helps in the diagnosis and shows a mass with alternating hypo and hyperechoic concentric rings axially and a 'pseudokidney sign' longitudinally. Depending on the sonographic appearances and clinical state of the patient radiological reduction using air is attempted.

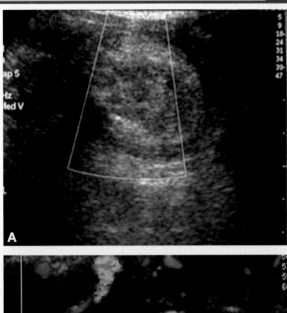

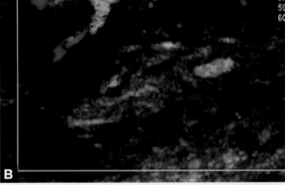

Figs 32.79A and B: Ultrasound shows (A) concentric hypo and hyper- echoic layers in the intussusception and (B) a pseudokidney sign with preserved blood supply on colour Doppler

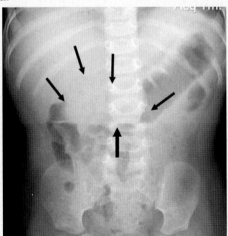

Fig. 32.78: Abdominal radiograph in a patient with typical clinical features of an intussusception shows a soft tissue mass in the right upper quadrant (black arrows)

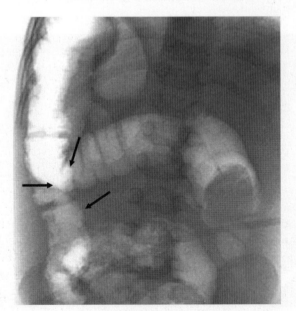

Fig. 32.80: Air enema reduction shows the intussusception reduced to the cecum (arrows)

Abdominal Trauma

Abdominal trauma in children can be penetrating or blunt. Blunt trauma is commoner in children and can cause solid organ or bowel trauma. Various types of solid organ injuries like liver fractures and contusions, splenic fractures, pancreatic and renal injuries can occur. Bowel trauma with contusion and perforation can also occur. The main modality for investigating these surgical emergencies is CT scanning which should be done with intravenous and gut contract enhancement as far as possible. Associated lung trauma like contusions, pneumothoraces and rib fractures may occur. Vertebral injuries like Chance fractures may also occur.

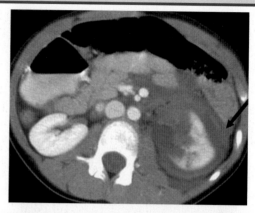

Fig. 32.83: Renal trauma: CT scan shows a left renal fracture and contusion with perirenal fluid (arrow). Note the normal right kidney

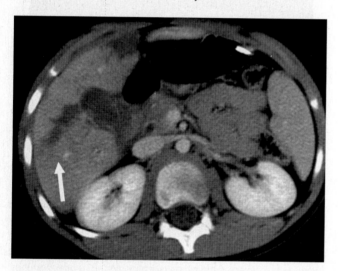

Fig. 32.81: CT scan of a child following a fall from a height shows a fracture of the right lobe of the liver (arrow)

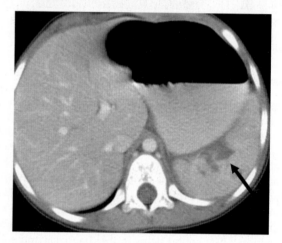

Fig. 32.84: Splenic fracture (arrow) seen in a 7 years old after fall from a horse

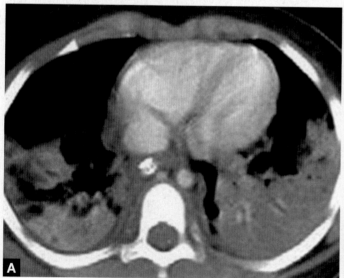

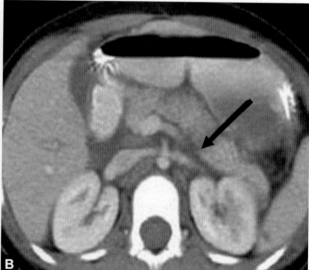

Figs 32.82A and B: CT scan of a child with blunt trauma shows (A) Bilateral lung contusions (B) Pancreatic fracture (arrow)

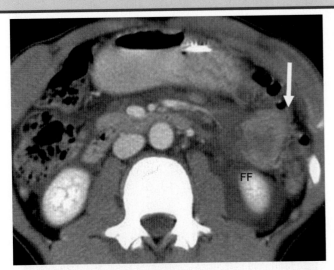

Fig. 32.85: Jejunal contusion (arrow) and free fluid (FF) in the left flank in a patient with blunt trauma to the abdomen from fall from a tree

THE CHILD WITH AN ABDOMINAL MASS

Common masses include:
1. Neuroblastoma
2. Wilms tumour
3. Multicystic dysplastic kidney (MCDK)
4. Hepatoblastoma
5. Pelviureteric junction obstruction (PUJ)
6. Lymphoma

The differential diagnosis varies according to the age. An abdominal mass in the newborn is most commonly benign and of renal origin (neonatal hydronephrosis due to various causes). Renal, neoplasms are unusual in this group but occasionally mesoblastic nephroma may be seen. Other masses include renal enlargement due to renal vein thrombosis, adrenal haemorrhage, bowel related masses and sacro-coccygeal teratoma. In infants and young children the retroperitoneal masses are common. These include neuroblastmas and Wilms tumour. Other masses include hepatoblastomas, lymphomas, teratomas and lymphangiomas.

Abdominal Neuroblastoma

Most common extracranial solid tumour of childhood, and accounts for 10% of all paediatric neoplasms. Presentation is commonly with an abdominal mass. Other modes of presentation include cord compression, constipation, or as a paraneoplastic syndrome. Two of these syndromes are recognised, namely the opsoclonus myoclonus syndrome and the watery diarrhoea, hypokalaemia and achlorhydria syndrome. Radiological evaluation begins with a plain film, which shows a mass with calcification. Sonography shows a tumour, which is

in homogenous, echogenic and a poorly defined extrarenal mass. Hypo-echoic regions may be due to haemorrhage, necrosis or cyst formation. Areas of calcification are echogenic. CT scanning accurately stages the tumour and demonstrates the primary tumour, contiguous spread, vascular encasement retroperitoneal lymphadenopathy and liver metastases. MRI is the imaging modality of choice and is superior in imaging adenopathy, vascular involvement, bone marrow metastases and intraspinal extension.

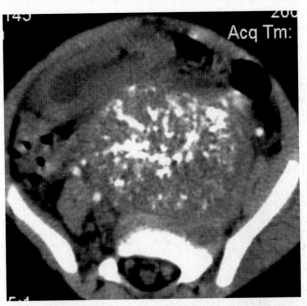

Fig. 32.86: Neuroblastoma: CT scan showing a calcified lower abdominal mass with presacral lymphadenopathy

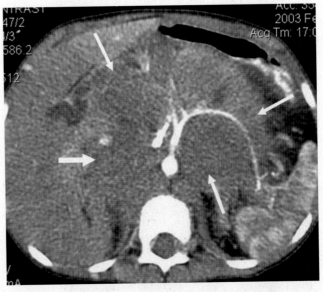

Fig. 32.87: Neuroblastoma: 2 years old with neuroblastoma. An enhanced CT image shows a retroperitoneal mass with vascular encasement (arrows)

Wilms Tumour

Wilms tumour is the commonest renal tumour of childhood and presents mostly as an asymptomatic abdominal mass. Other symptoms include abdominal pain and hematuria. Plain abdominal radiography shows a soft tissue mass with calcification in about 5%. Sonography shows an intra renal mass which is hyper-echoic compared to normal renal parenchyma with areas of necrosis and cysts. Renal vein and inferior caval invasion occurs in 15%. CT scan shows a well defined intra-renal mass distorting the collecting system and with inhomogeneous enhancement postcontrast. MRI is better than CT in the evaluation of the intrarenal mass, assessment of perinephric extension, contra lateral kidney and evaluation of the renal vein and IVC.

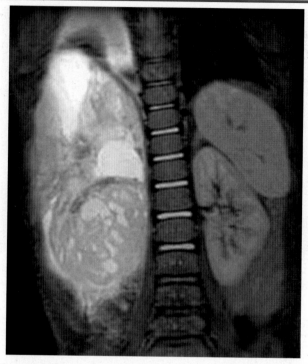

Fig. 32.90: Right sided Wilms tumour: Coronal MRI shows a large right sided mass containing areas of cystic degeneration

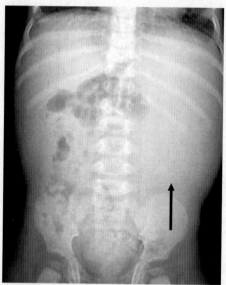

Fig. 32.88: Left sided Wilms tumour. Plain abdominal radiograph shows a left sided soft tissue mass (arrow)

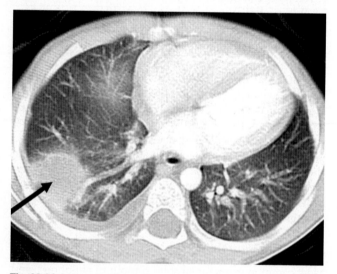

Fig. 32.91: Lung metastases from a Wilms tumour. CT image showing a large right sided lung metastasis (arrow)

Congenital Mesoblastic Nephroma

Most common renal tumour of neonates and the pathologic spectrum ranges from benign congenital mesoblastic nephroma to malignant spindle cell sarcoma. Plain radiographs show a soft tissue mass. Sonographically the mass is well-defined and hypoechoic or hyper-echoic. CT demonstrates the intrarenal location of the mass.

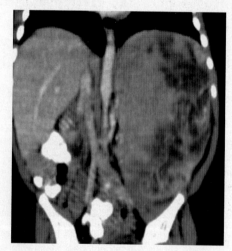

Fig. 32.89: Left sided Wilms tumour (same patient as above). Coronal CT reconstruction shows a mixed density mass containing areas of necrosis and cysts

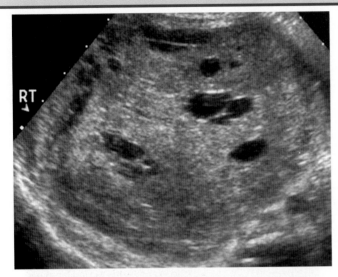

Fig. 32.92: Mesoblastic nephroma: US shows a hyperechoic mass containing cysts in a newborn

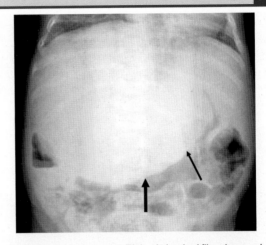

Fig. 32.94: Hepatoblastoma: Plain abdominal film shows a large upper abdominal soft tissue mass in a 3 months old infant (arrows)

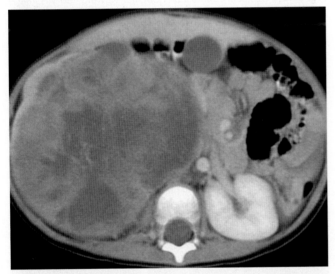

Fig. 32.93: Mesoblastic nephroma (same patient as above). CT image shows a right renal mass of mixed attenuation

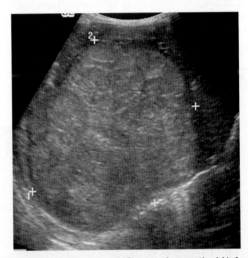

Fig. 32.95: Hepatoblastoma: US scan of a month old infant with an abdominal mass shows a large hyperechoic mass

Hepatoblastoma

Primary liver tumours account for 15% of abdominal neoplasms in children. Most children present with an asymptomatic abdominal mass. Others present with anorexia, weight loss, jaundice and pain. Alpha fetoprotein levels are raised in up to 90% of cases. Plain films reveal a soft tissue mass in the upper abdomen. Sonographically the lesion appears as a large, welldefined intrahepatic hyper echoic mass containing areas of cystic degeneration, necrosis and haemorrhage. Hepatic and portal venous invasion may occur. CT and MRI define the intra hepatic extent, extrahepatic spread and vascular invasion.

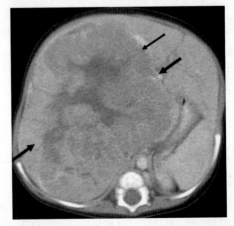

Fig. 32.96: Hepatoblastoma: CT image shows a large well-defined in homogenous lobulated intrahepatic mass (arrows) with slightly lower attenuation and enhancement than the normal liver. Fibrous bands can be seen as un enhancing linear structures

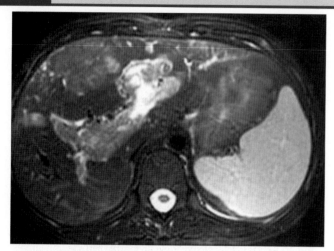

Fig. 32.97: Hepatoblastoma with portal vein invasion: Axial MRI (T2-weighted) shows a distended portal venous confluence (arrows) and multiple tumour thrombi

Burkitt Lymphoma

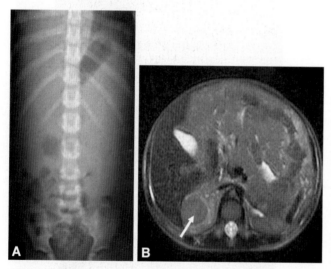

Figs 32.98A and B: Plain abdominal film (A) showing upper abdominal fullness due to masses. (B) MRI showing diffuse bowel wall infiltration and a right renal mass (arrow)

PAEDIATRIC NEURORADIOLOGY

CONGENITAL BRAIN MALFORMATIONS

Cephalocele

A cephalocele is a defect in the skull and dura, through which intracranial structures (cerebrospinal fluid, meninges and brain tissue) can herniate. Magnetic resonance imaging is the study of choice for investigating this condition.

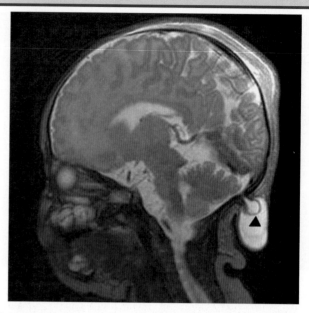

Fig. 32.99: Occipital cephalocele. Sagittal T2-weighted MR image shows a small occipital cephalocele with herniation of CSF and meninges (arrowhead)

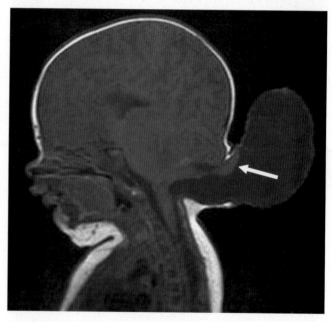

Fig. 32.100: Occipital cephalocele. Sagittal T1-weighted MR image shows a large occipital cephalocele with herniation of cerebellar tissue (arrow) and CSF into the cephalocele

HOLOPROSENCEPHALY

The holoprosencephalies are a group of disorders typified by failure of the embryonic forebrain (prosencephalon) to sufficiently divide into two cerebral hemispheres.

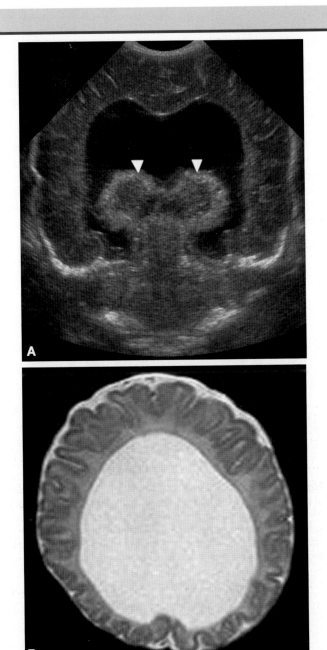

Figs 32.101A and B: Holoprosencephaly. (A) Coronal ultrasound scan shows a holoventricle due to absence of midline structures (septum pellucidum, corpus callosum and falx cerebri). The thalami (arrowheads) are fused in the midline. (B) Axial T2-weighted image shows a holoventricle

Dandy-Walker Malformation

The Dandy-Walker malformation consists of complete or partial agenesis of the cerebellar vermis, an enlarged posterior cranial fossa and cystic dilatation of the fourth ventricle, which almost entirely fills the posterior cranial fossa.

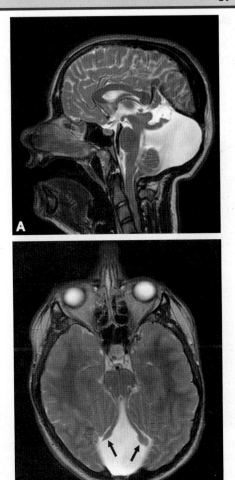

Figs 32.102A and B: Dandy-Walker malformation. (A) Sagittal T2-weighted MR image shows a markedly enlarged posterior fossa and cystic dilatation of the fourth ventricle. (B) Axial T2-weighted MR image shows the markedly hypoplastic cerebellar vermis (arrows)

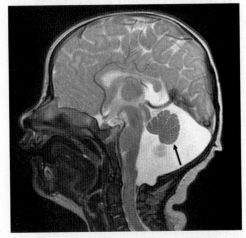

Fig. 32.103: Dandy-Walker malformation. Sagittal T2 MR image shows enlarged posterior cranial fossa with mild hypoplasia of the cerebellar vermis (arrow)

Chiari I Malformation

The Chiari I malformation is defined as caudal (downward) extension of the cerebellar tonsils below the foramen magnum. The cerebellar tonsils are elongated and pointed. There may be mild caudal displacement and flattening or kinking of the medulla. A syrinx is present in the spinal cord in up to 25% of patients.

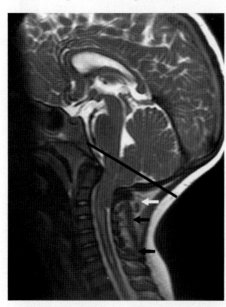

Fig. 32.104: Chiari I malformation on sagittal T2-weighted MR image. The cerebellar tonsil (white arrow) extends well below the foramen magnum (black line). The high signal within the cervical cord (arrowheads) indicates the presence of a syrinx

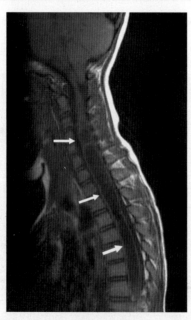

Fig. 32.105: Chiari I malformation. Sagittal T1-weighted MR image shows cerebellar tonsilar descent below the foramen magnum. There is a large syrinx in the cervical and thoracic spinal cord (arrows)

Sturge-Weber's Syndrome

The Sturge-Weber's syndrome is a neurocutaneous disorder with angiomas involving the leptomeninges and the skin of the face (port wine stain). The syndrome can affect one or both cerebral hemispheres.

Contrast-enhanced MRI is the best imaging study for showing the extent of the pial angioma. After IV contrast administration, the angioma is identified as an area of enhancement following the contours of the gyri and sulci. Cortical calcification and cerebral atrophy is seen in long-standing cases. The cortical calcification is best demonstrated on CT scanning.

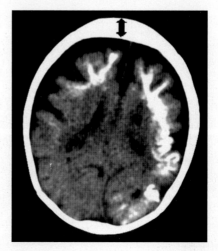

Fig. 32.106: Sturge-Weber's syndrome. Axial unenhanced CT scan of brain shows marked subcortical and cortical calcification in both cerebral hemispheres in a gyriform pattern. The calcification is more extensive in the left cerebral hemisphere. There is evidence of cerebral atrophy with enlargement of the surrounding CSF spaces and thickening of the skull vault anteriorly (black arrow)

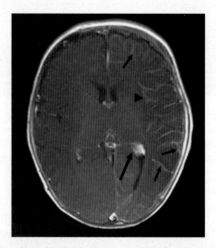

Fig. 32.107: Sturge-Weber's syndrome. Post-contrast axial T1 weighted MR image shows pial enhancement which follows the gyral and sulcal contours of the entire left cerebral hemisphere (arrowheads). The choroid plexus in the left lateral ventricle is enlarged (arrow) - another feature of the syndrome

Tuberous Sclerosis

Tuberous sclerosis is a genetic disorder which results in hamartoma formation in many organs, including the brain. Intracranial manifestations include:

- *Subependymal hamartomas*—small nodules, which protrude into the ventricles (usually the lateral ventricles). These can be calcified.
- *Cerebral hamartomas or cortical "tubers"* - these hamartomas are identified as subcortical areas of abnormal signal intensity associated with adjacent gyral broadening. Cerebral hamartomas can also calcify.

Vein of Galen Malformation

The malformation occurs because of a congenital connection between intracranial arteries and the vein of Galen or other primitive midline vein. On ultrasound, the malformation is usually identified as a round hypoechoic structure posterior to the third ventricle. Colour Doppler studies can show the rapid blood flow within the malformation. On T2-weighted MR sequences, the malformation is identified as a low signal (black) structure posterior to the third ventricle. Intracranial complications include hydrocephalus and brain ischaemia.

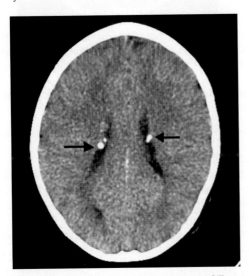

Fig. 32.108: Tuberous sclerosis. Axial unenhanced CT scan of brain shows calcified subependymal nodules within both lateral ventricles (arrows)

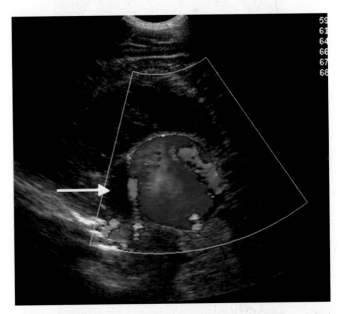

Fig. 32.110: Vein of Galen malformation on ultrasound. Midline sagittal image shows blood flow within the malformation which lies posterior to the third ventricle (arrow)

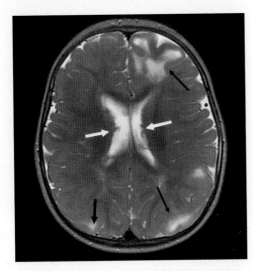

Fig. 32.109: Tuberous sclerosis. Axial T2-weighted MR image shows several subependymal nodules within both lateral ventricles (white arrows). The high signal intensity lesions within the cerebral hemispheres represent cortical tubers (black arrows)

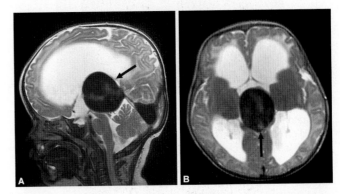

Figs 32.111A and B: Vein of Galen malformation. T2-weighted MR sagittal (A) and axial (B) images demonstrating the malformation (black arrows). There is obstructive hydrocephalus involving the lateral and third ventricles

**TRAUMA, HYPOXIA-ISCHAEMIA
AND HAEMORRHAGE**

Head Injury

As a general rule, CT is the initial study of choice for children who have sustained a head injury. Skull fractures, intracranial haemorrhage and any associated mass effect can be detected with CT.

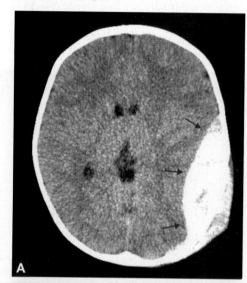

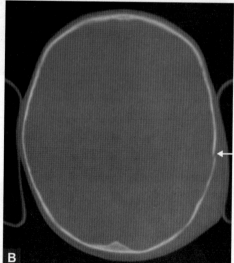

Figs 32.112A and B: Left parietal skull fracture and extradural haematoma. (A) Unenhanced CT brain scan shows a large biconvex collection of blood adjacent to the left cerebral hemisphere (arrows). (B) The left parietal skull fracture is demonstrated (arrow)

On CT, an *extradural haematoma* is a biconvex collection of blood between the brain surface and the skull. The acute haematoma is of increased attenuation (i.e. appears white). A *subdural haematoma* is identified as a crescentic collection of blood between the brain surface and the skull.

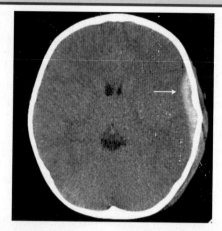

Fig. 32.113: Acute left subdural haematoma. Unenhanced CT scan of brain demonstrates a crescentic collection of blood overlying the left cerebral hemisphere (arrow)

Periventricular and Intra-ventricular Haemorrhage in Premature Infants

Intracranial haemorrhage in the preterm infant has been divided into four grades:
* *Grade 1*—subependymal haemorrhage only
* *Grade 2*—extension of subependymal haemorrhage into non-dilated ventricle
* *Grade 3*—intraventricular haemorrhage associated with ventricular dilatation
* *Grade 4*—periventricular parenchymal haemorrhage associated with intraventricular haemorrhage.

On cranial ultrasound, intraventricular haemorrhage is identified as echogenic material within the ventricle.

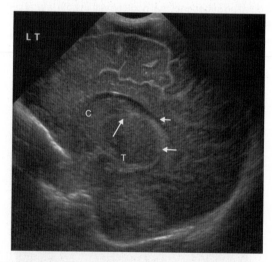

Fig. 32.114: Normal parasagittal view of lateral ventricle (left). The head of the caudate nucleus (C) lies inferior to the body of the ventricle anteriorly. The thalamus (T) is located inferior to the body of the ventricle posteriorly. The echogenic choroid plexus (arrowheads) is seen within the ventricle. The caudothalamic groove is a small echogenic area, which lies between the head of caudate and the thalamus (arrow)

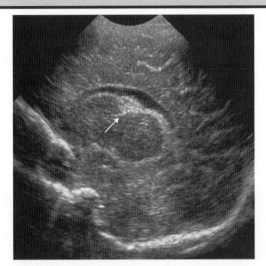

Fig. 32.115: Grade 1 haemorrhage. Left parasagittal ultrasound scan shows a focus of increased echogenicity in the caudothalamic groove in keeping with subependymal haemorrhage (arrow)

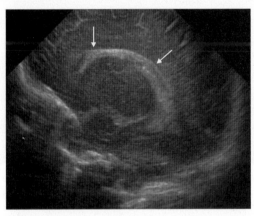

Fig. 32.116: Grade 2 intraventricular haemorrhage. Left parasagittal ultrasound scan shows blood within the left lateral ventricle (arrows). The ventricle is not dilated

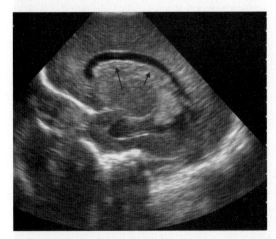

Fig. 32.117: Grade 3 intraventricular haemorrhage. Right parasagittal ultrasound scan shows haemorrhage (arrows) in the right lateral ventricle which is dilated

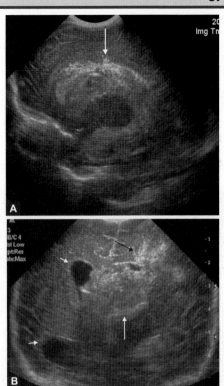

Figs 32.118A and B : Grade 4 haemorrhage. (A) Left parasagittal ultrasound scan shows haemorrhage in the parenchyma adjacent to the left lateral ventricle (arrow). (B) Coronal ultrasound scan shows extensive intraventricular haemorrhage (white arrow) and periventricular parenchymal haemorrhage (black arrow). Note the obstructive hydrocephalus of the right lateral ventricle (small arrows)

Post-haemorrhagic Hydrocephalus

Ventricular dilatation after intraventricular haemorrhage occurs as a result of intraventricular obstruction by clot or septations or because of an obliterative arachnoiditis. The lateral ventricles usually dilate more than the third and fourth ventricles.

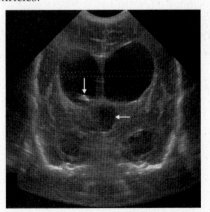

Fig. 32.119: Post-haemorrhagic hydrocephalus. Coronal ultrasound scan shows marked dilatation of both lateral ventricles and the third ventricle (thick arrow). Some residual clot is present in the right lateral ventricle (thin arrow)

Periventricular Leukomalacia

Periventricular leukomalacia (PVL) is an ischaemic brain injury in preterm infants affecting the deep white matter in the immediate periventricular region. The earliest sonographic sign is increased echogenicity in the periventricular white matter. Cystic change becomes evident within the injured periventricular white matter approximately 2-3 weeks following the ischaemic insult.

Infarction

There are a number of causes of hypoxic-ischaemic brain infarction in infants and children. Cardiac causes, thrombotic conditions and metabolic diseases are a few categories of conditions responsible for strokes in the paediatric population.

Cranial ultrasound can be used to investigate neonates and infants in whom cerebral infarction is suspected. It is however less sensitive to CT and MR imaging in the detection of areas of hypoxic-ischaemic brain injury.

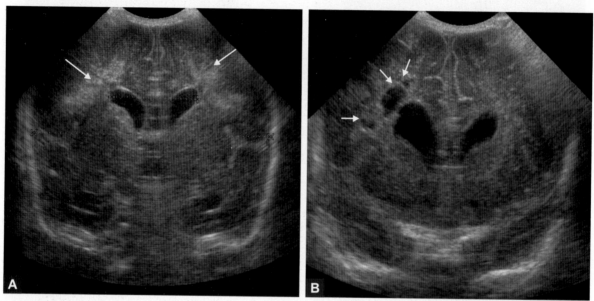

Figs 32.120A and B: Progression of periventricular leukomalacia. (A) Coronal ultrasound scan at approximately one week of age shows increased periventricular echogenicity around the frontal horns of the lateral ventricles (arrows). (B) A follow-up ultrasound scan shows significant cavitation in the right frontal periventricular white matter (small arrows)

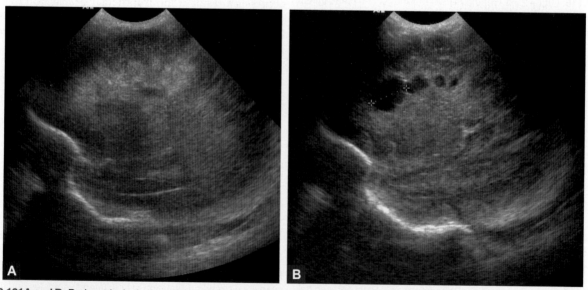

Figs 32.121A and B: Periventricular leukomalacia. (A) Parasagittal ultrasound scan shows increased echogenicity in the white matter adjacent to the right lateral ventricle. (B) Follow-up scan shows cavitation in the same area, consistent with cystic periventricular leukomalacia

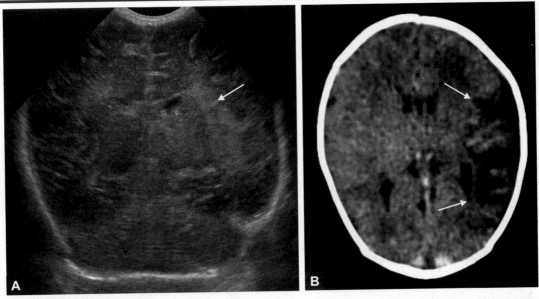

Figs 32.122A and B: Left middle cerebral artery (MCA) territory infarct. (A) Coronal ultrasound scan in a neonate shows subtle increased echogenicity in the left MCA territory (arrow). (B) Unenhanced axial CT scan shows decreased attenuation (dark area) in the left MCA territory, consistent with an infarct (arrows)

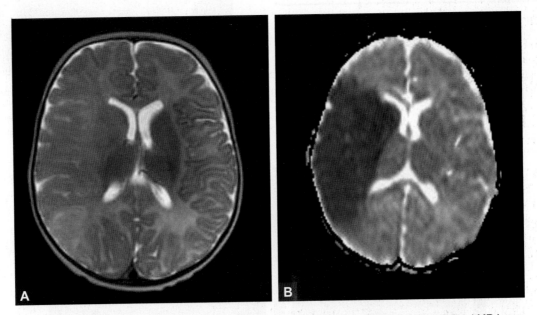

Figs 32.123A and B: Right middle cerebral artery (MCA) territory infarct. (A) Axial T2-weighted MR image shows subtle swelling and loss of grey-white matter differentiation in the right MCA territory, consistent with an acute infarct. (B) The ADC map of the diffusion sequence best demonstrates the acute infarct

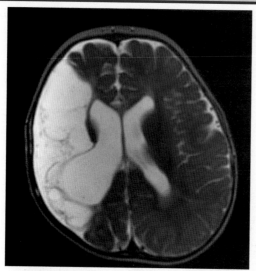

Fig. 32.124: Established right middle cerebral artery (MCA) territory infarct. Axial T2-weighted MR image shows cystic change (encephalomalacia) in the right MCA territory, due to loss of brain tissue. The right lateral ventricle is enlarged due to the adjacent brain loss

INFECTIONS, TUMOURS AND HYDROCEPHALUS

Congenital Brain Infection

Congenital brain infection can be caused by cytomegalovirus, toxoplasmosis, herpes simplex virus, rubella, syphilis and human immunodeficiency virus. Radiological findings generally depend on the timing of the injury and the degree of brain destruction. Brain patterns identified include abnormal brain formation, periventricular white matter injury and intracranial calcification.

Brain Abscess

Pyogenic organisms causing brain infection can reach the brain by haematogenous spread from a distant infection, extension of infection from adjacent sites (sinus or middle ear infection), as a result of congenital heart disease, or as a complication of a penetrating wound or sinus tract. Cerebritis is the earliest stage of purulent brain infection. If undetected or untreated, it can develop into an abscess.

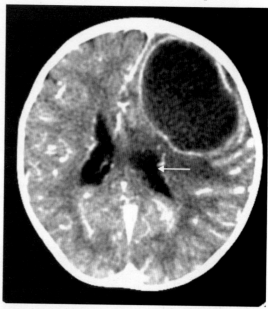

Fig. 32.126: Left frontal lobe cerebral abscess in a child with congenital heart disease. Contrast-enhanced axial CT scan of brain shows a large low density lesion in the left frontal lobe, with an enhancing rim. Note the distortion of the anterior midline brain structures (arrowheads) and the left lateral ventricle (thin arrow).

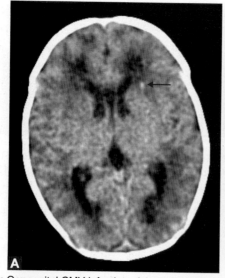
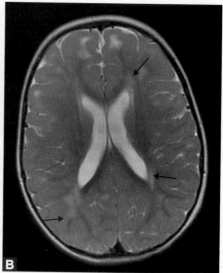

Figs 32.125A and B: Congenital CMV infection of the brain. (A) Unenhanced axial CT scan of brain shows a tiny area of periventricular calcification (arrow) near the frontal horn of the left lateral ventricle. (B) Axial T2-weighted MR image shows abnormal areas of increased signal in the periventricular and deep white matter (arrows)

Tuberculous Meningitis

CNS manifestations of tuberculous (TB) infection include meningitis, tuberculoma, tuberculous abscess or spinal leptomeningitis.

In TB meningitis, a thick exudate fills the basal cisterns. The basal cisterns on contrast-enhanced scans. The thick exudate blocks the subarachnoid spaces, causing hydrocephalus. Another complication is small vessel disease which results in basal ganglia and thalamic infarcts.

Tuberculomas are ring-enhancing lesions within the brain. They can be single or multiple.

Hydrocephalus

Hydrocephalus is a disorder where there is disturbance in the production, flow or absorption of cerebrospinal fluid (CSF). Consequently, there is increased CSF volume within the central nervous system, causing distension of the CSF pathways and increased pressure transmitted to the brain parenchyma.

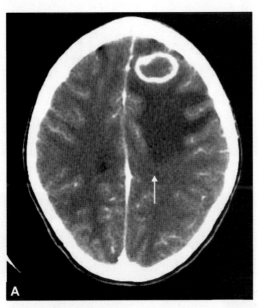

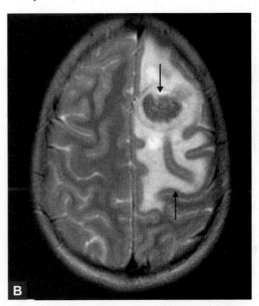

Figs 32.127A and B: Left frontal lobe tuberculoma. (A) Contrast-enhanced axial CT scan shows a ring-enhancing lesion in the left frontal lobe of the brain. There is adjacent white matter oedema (arrow). (B) Axial T2-weighted MR brain image. The tuberculoma (black arrow) is isointense to brain. Note the adjacent white matter oedema (white arrow)

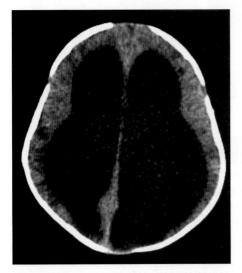

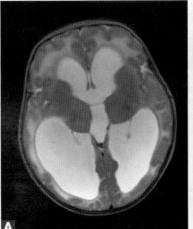

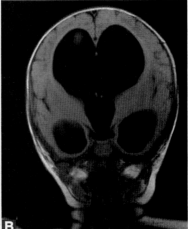

Fig. 32.128: Hydrocephalus. Axial CT scan shows marked dilatation of both lateral ventricles.

Figs 32.129A and B: Examples of hydrocephalus on MR imaging. (A) Axial T2-weighted MR scan demonstrates marked dilatation of both lateral ventricles and the third ventricle (arrow). (B) Coronal MR image from another patient also shows hydrocephalus involving both lateral ventricles and the third ventricle

Tumours

CT is usually the imaging modality employed in the initial diagnosis of intracranial tumours. However, MR is becoming the preferred study because of its multiplanar imaging capability, which is useful for surgical planning. Furthermore, it can image the spine. This is a prerequisite for the staging of intracranial neoplasms which metastasise to the spine.

Craniopharyngioma

On CT scanning, craniopharyngiomas are identified as mass lesions in the suprasellar region, composed of cystic areas and calcification.

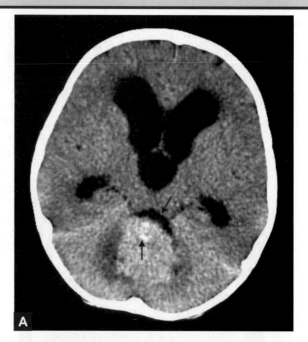

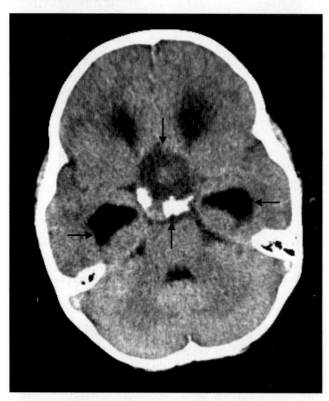

Fig. 32.130: Craniopharyngioma. Unenhanced axial CT brain scan shows a cystic (white arrow) and calcified (black arrow) lesion in the suprasellar region. Note the hydrocephalus affecting the lateral ventricles with marked dilatation of the temporal horns (small arrows)

Medulloblastoma

A medulloblastoma on CT scanning is usually a dense neoplasm arising from the cerebellar vermis. Cystic change can be seen in approximately 50% of tumours and calcification in up to 20%. The tumours enhance with intravenous contrast. Hydrocephalus is usually present at the time of diagnosis.

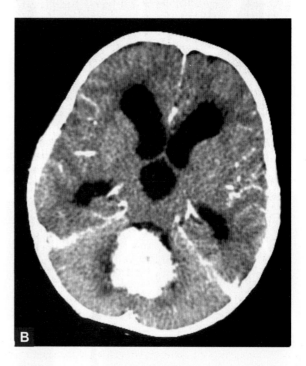

Figs 32.131A and B: Medulloblastoma. (A) Unenhanced axial CT scan shows a dense mass lesion situated within the cerebellar vermis, containing a small area of calcification (black arrow). The tumour is impinging upon the fourth ventricle (white arrow), restricting CSF flow and conse quently there is hydrocephalus of the lateral and third ventricles. (B) After injection of intravenous contrast, there is marked tumour enhancement

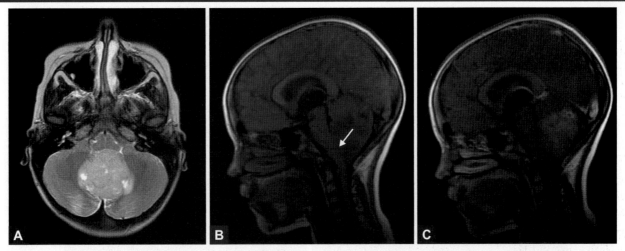

Figs 32.132A to C: Medulloblastoma. (A) Axial T2-weighted MR image shows a midline posterior fossa mass which is of increased signal intensity relative to the cerebellum. (B) Sagittal T1-weighted MR image shows the mass to be hypointense on this sequence. The mass is obstructing the fourth ventricle (arrow). (C) Sagittal T1-weighted MR image following intravenous contrast. The tumour demonstrates enhancement with contrast

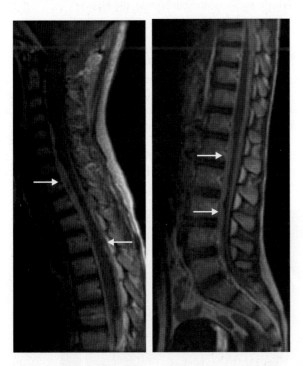

Fig. 32.133: Medulloblastoma spinal metastatic disease. Post-contrast T1-weighted sagittal MR scans of the whole spine show nodular tumour enhancement along the entire cord (arrows) consistent with spinal metastatic disease

Cerebellar Astrocytoma

The cerebellar astrocytoma arises from the vermis or the cerebellar hemisphere. Most tumours are cystic with a tumour nodule located in the cyst wall. The mural nodule enhances with contrast. Hydrocephalus is usually present due to compression of the fourth ventricle.

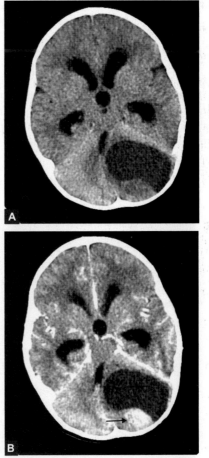

Figs 32.134A and B: Pilocytic astrocytoma. (A) Unenhanced axial CT scan shows a cystic mass centred on the left cerebellar hemisphere. It distorts the fourth ventricle and there is hydrocephalus of the third and lateral ventricles. (B) Following intravenous contrast infusion, there is marked enhancement of a mural nodule in the posterior aspect of the cystic tumour (arrow)

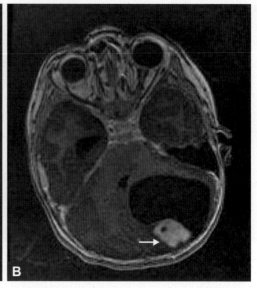

Figs 32.135A and B: Pilocytic astrocytoma. (A) Sagittal T1-weighted MR image shows a hypointense cystic tumour in the cerebellum. The mural nodule is situated posteriorly within the tumour (arrow). (B) Axial T1-weighted MR image shows intense enhancement of the tumour nodule following intravenous contrast administration (arrow)

Ependymoma

Ependymomas arise from the fourth ventricle and frequently grow out of the ventricle into the surrounding cisterns and foramina. Most ependymomas are solid in nature. Calcification is seen in up to 50% of tumours and cystic change in about 20%. Hydrocephalus is usually present at diagnosis.

Brain Stem Glioma

Because of its location, MR is the best imaging modality for assessing the brain stemglioma. It allows multiplanar assessment of the tumour. In contrast to CT scanning, there is no bony artefact from the adjacent skull base.

Most brain stem gliomas arise from the pons. The tumour may be focal or diffuse and typically expands the pons. Tumour enhancement with intravenous contrast agents is variable.

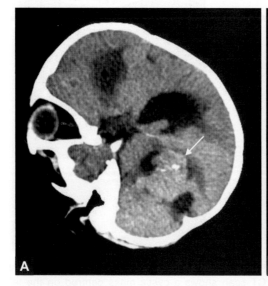
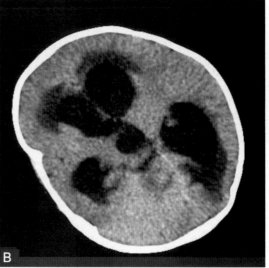

Figs 32.136A and B: Ependymoma. (A) Unenhanced axial CT scan through the posterior cranial fossa shows an isodense mass (arrow) containing punctuate calcification, arising from the fourth ventricle. (B) Axial image from a higher level shows hydrocephalus affecting the lateral ventricles and the third ventricle

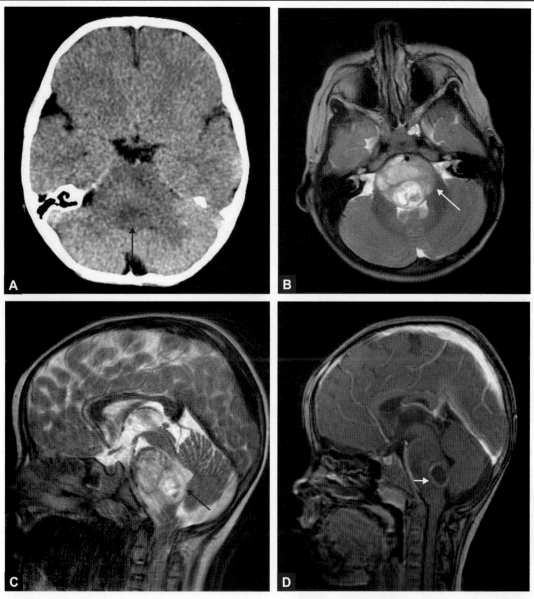

Figs 32.137A to D: Brain stem glioma. (A) Axial unenhanced CT scan shows a poorly defined low density mass in the pons (arrow). (B) Axial and (C) sagittal T2-weighted MR images show a heterogeneous mass of increased signal intensity expanding the pons (arrows). There is minor distortion of the fourth ventricle. (D) T1-weighted sagittal MR scan following intravenous contrast administration. There is peripheral enhancement of a cystic area posteriorly within the tumour (arrow). The remainder of pontine glioma is poorly enhancing

Retinoblastoma

Retinoblastoma is the commonest orbital malignancy and is almost universally a tumour of infancy. The tumour can be unilateral or bilateral. Calcification is present in excess of 90% of tumours.

On CT scanning, the retinoblastoma is identified as a calcified mass within the globe, arising from the retina. It usually enhances with intravenous contrast.

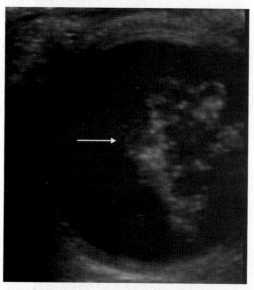

Fig. 32.138: Retinoblastoma. Ultrasound scan of right globe reveals an irregular mass (arrow) containing multiple specks of calcification

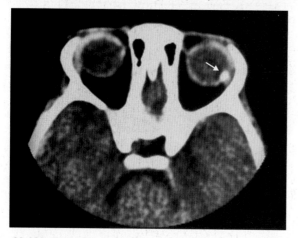

Fig. 32.139: Retinoblastoma left orbit. Unenhanced axial CT scan through the orbits shows a small calcified lesion arising from the retina in the temporal aspect of the left globe (arrow)

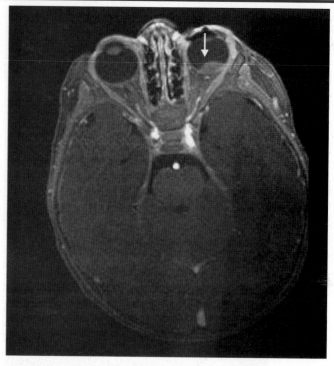

Fig. 32.140: Left-sided retinoblastoma, axial T1-weighted MR image (fat saturated and post-contrast administration) shows an enhancing mass lesion situated posteriorly within the left globe (arrow)

CONGENITAL SPINE LESIONS

Myelomeningocele

Myelomeningocele results from impaired closure of the caudal end of the neural tube. This results in an open lesion or sac containing abnormal spinal cord, nerve roots and meninges which herniate through a posterior defect in the vertebral column.

Closure of the spinal defect is usually performed within 48 hours of delivery and consequently imaging studies of the spine are rarely performed preoperatively.

Myelomeningocele is associated with the Chiari II malformation. The malformation is associated with caudal displacement of the medulla, fourth ventricle and cerebellum into the cervical spinal canal. Consequently there is elongation of the pons and fourth ventricle. In combination, these features impede the flow and absorption of CSF causing hydrocephalus, usually after surgical closure of the spinal defect.

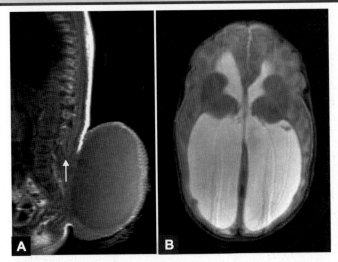

Figs 32.141A and B: Myelomeningocele and hydrocephalus. (A) Sagittal T1-weighted MR image of the lower spine shows a large lumbosacral meningocele. The spinal cord is stretched and can be identified passing through the posterior spinal defect (arrow). (B) Axial T2-weighted MR image of the brain shows marked dilatation of the lateral ventricles due to hydrocephalus

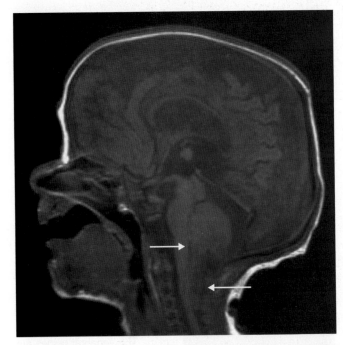

Fig. 32.142: Chiari II malformation. (A) Sagittal T1-weighted MR image shows a small posterior cranial fossa and inferior displacement of the cerebellum through the foramen magnum (white arrow). The fourth ventricle is narrow and displaced caudally (white arrow)

Diastomatomyelia

Diastomatomyelia is the sagittal division of the spinal cord into two hemicords by a bony or cartilaginous spur, or fibrous septum. MRI is the preferred modality for imaging children with suspected diastomatomyelia. The defect is most commonly found in the lumbar region.

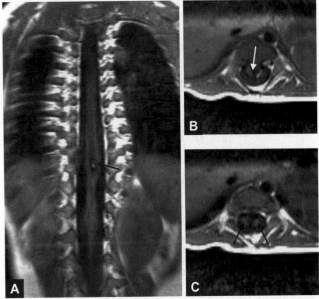

Figs 32.143A to C: Diastomatomyelia. (A) Coronal and (B) Axial T1-weighted MR images show a bony spur (arrow) extending posteriorly from a vertebral body in the lower thoracic spine, splitting the spinal cord into two hemicords. (C) Axial T1-weighted MR image obtained above the level of the bony spur shows the hemicords (arrows)

Sacrococcygeal Teratoma

This is a rare congenital tumour that devel ops in the sacrococcygeal region. The tumour usually presents as an external mass protruding from the gluteal cleft or the per ineum. The tumour is divided into 4 types:

Type I: Tumours are predominantly external, situated posteriorly, and have only a minimal presacral component.
Type II: Tumours have significant pelvic extension but the external portion predominates.
Type III: Tumours have a predominant internal component although the external component is still visible.
Type IV: Tumours are entirely presacral with out any external component.

Plain films will demonstrate a large soft tissue mass associated with the lower sacrum and coccyx. Approximately two-thirds of tumours will contain calcification.

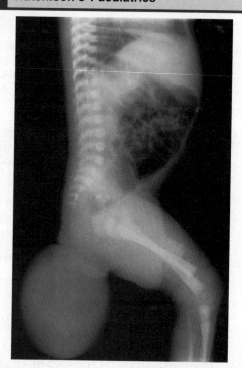

Fig. 32.144: Sacrococcygeal teratoma in a neonate. Lateral radiograph shows a large exophytic soft tissue mass arising from the gluteal region. The lower density area within the lesion represents fat

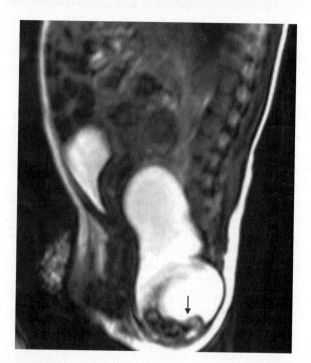

Fig. 32.145: Sacrococcygeal teratoma. Sagittal T2-weighted MR image demonstrates a large cystic structure in the presacral region. Some solid elements are present inferiorly within the lesion (arrow). There is significant anterior displacement of the rectum and bladder by the mass. This is a type III tumour since it has a small external component

PAEDIATRIC SKELETAL RADIOLOGY

SKELETAL DYSPLASIAS

Thanatophoric Dysplasia

Radiographic Findings

- Skull: Proportionately large skull relative to trunk
- Thorax: Long narrow trunk with very short ribs, small abnormal scapulae
- Spine: Small, flat vertebrae with *U* or *H* shaped vertebrae in the AP projection
- Pelvis: Small flared iliac wings, narrow sacrosciatic notches and flat acetabula
- Limbs: Long bone shortening and bowing; *French telephone receiver femurs*
- Hands and feet: Marked shortening and broadening of the tubular bones.

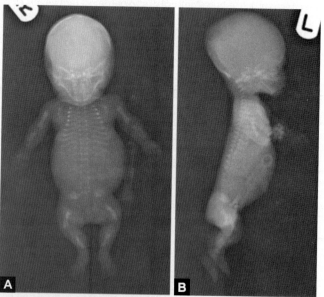

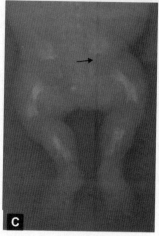

Figs 32.146A to C: Thanatophoric dysplasia. (A) The head is proportionately large and the trunk is long and narrow. There is marked rib shortening and the scapulae are small. There is shortening of the long bones of the limbs (micromelia)- note the *French telephone receiver* femurs. The vertebral bodies are flat and H-shaped. (B) The lateral view shows the flattened vertebrae and the proportionately large skull. (C) Coned view of the pelvis and lower limbs demonstrates small, flared iliac wings, narrowed sacrosciatic notches (black arrow) and horizontal acetabula

ACHONDROPLASIA

Radiographic Findings

- Skull: Large skull with relatively small base and midface hypoplasia
- Thorax: Small short ribs which are splayed anteriorly
- Spine: Short flat vertebral bodies. Short pedicles with decreasing interpedicular distance caudally in lumbar spine. Posterior scalloping of vertebral bodies

- Pelvis: *Champagne glass* appearance of pelvis. Flared iliac wings, narrow sacrosciatic notches and flat acetabular roofs
- Limbs: Short and thick tubular bones, flared metaphyses
- Hands: Shortening and broadening of metacarpal and phalangeal bones.

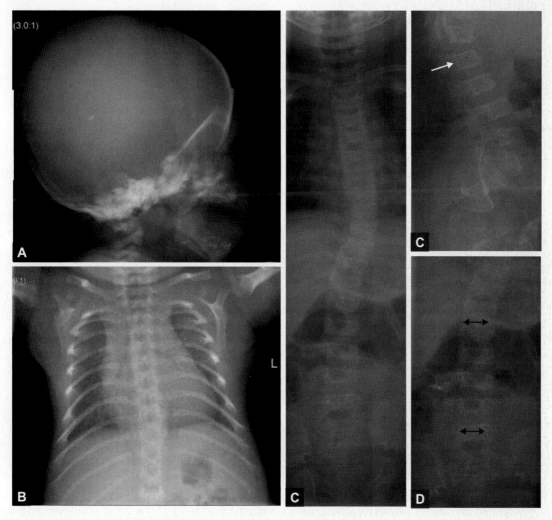

Figs 32.147A to D: Achondroplasia in newborn infant. (A) Large skull with midface hypoplasia. (B) Small thorax with short ribs. (C) AP and lateral views of spine show a thoracolumbar kyphoscoliosis. The lateral view shows posterior vertebral body scalloping (arrow) and a horizontal sacrum. (D) AP view of lumbar spine demonstrates gradual reduction in interpediculate distance caudally (arrows)

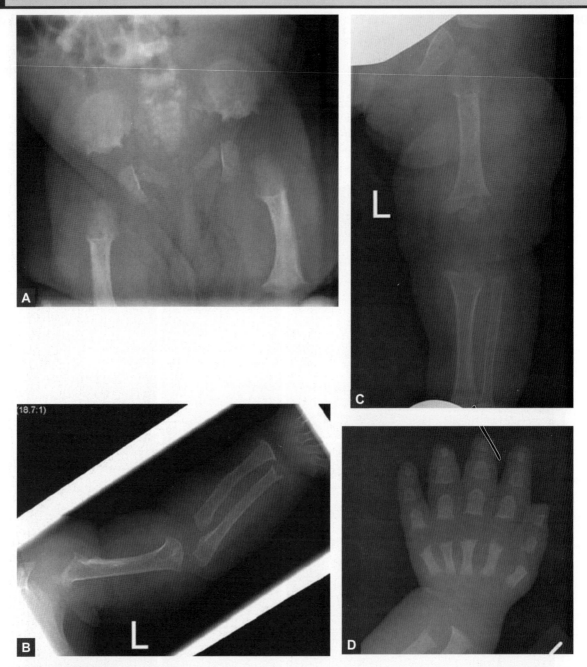

Figs 32.148A to D: Achondroplasia in neonate. (A) The pelvis X-ray shows flared iliac bones, flat acetabular roofs and narrow sacrosciatic notches. (B) and (C) Limb X-rays show shortening of the long bones. (D) Hand: Short and broad metacarpal and phalangeal bones

MUCOPOLYSACCHARIDOSES

Mucopolysaccharidosis 1-H (Hurler Syndrome)

Radiographic findings:
- Skull: Large skull with abnormal J-shaped sella
- Thorax: Short thick clavicles, broad 'oar-shaped' ribs and hypoplastic glenoid

- Spine: Antero-inferior beaking of thoracolumbar vertebral bodies, atlantoaxial subluxation due to hypoplastic dens
- Pelvis: Small, flared iliac wings; steep
- Limbs: Widening of the midshaft of long bones
- Hands: Widening of the diaphyses of the metacarpals and proximal and middle phalanges; phalangeal shortening; small and irregular carpal bones, pointed proximal ends of the metacarpals.

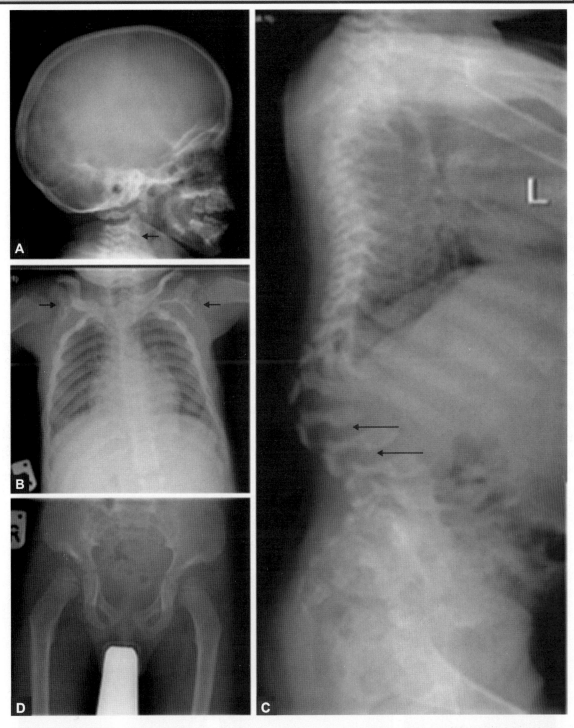

Figs 32.149A to D: Hurler's syndrome. (A) Lateral radiograph demonstrates an enlarged skull. The dens is hypoplastic (arrow). (B) Frontal chest X-ray shows thickened clavicles and broad ribs. The glenoid fossae are poorly formed (arrows). (C) The lateral spine film features a thoracolumbar gibbus, and antero-inferior beaking of the vertebrae at the apex of the gibbus (arrows). (D) The pelvic X-ray demonstrates small, flared iliac wings and steep acetabular roofs

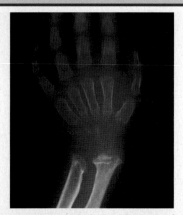

Fig. 32.150: Hurler's syndrome: Hand radiograph. X-ray of right hand reveals widening of the diaphyses of the metacarpals and proximal and middle phalanges. The phalanges are short. The carpal bones are small and irregular. There is proximal tapering of the metacarpals. The distal radius and ulna tilt towards each other

Mucopolysaccharidosis IV (Morquio Syndrome)

Radiographic Findings:
- Thorax: Flaring of ribs
- Spine: Platyspondyly within thoracolumbar spine; central anterior bony beaking; odontoid hypoplasia and atlanto-axial instability
- Pelvis: Steeply oblique acetabular roofs; defective irregular ossification of femoral heads leading to flattening
- Limbs: Widening of the long bone diaphyses; irregular metaphyses

- Hands: Small, irregular carpal bones; proximal tapering of metacarpals.

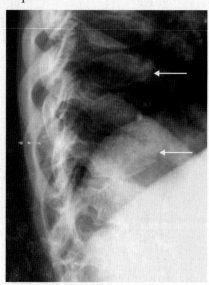

Fig. 32.151: Morquio's syndrome. Lateral radiograph of lower thoracic spine demonstrates decreased height of the vertebral bodies (platyspondyly). Note the central anterior bony protrusion or beaking of the vertebral bodies (arrows).

Osteogenesis Imperfecta

There are a several types of osteogenesis imperfecta. The radiographic findings are variable and depend upon the type and severity of the disease.

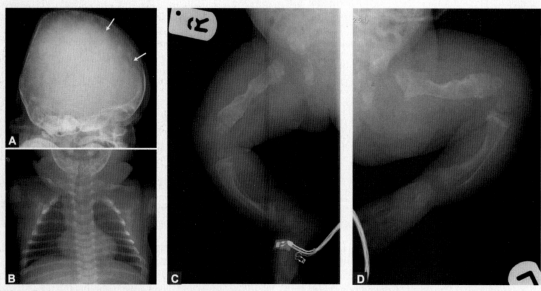

Figs 32.152A to D: Osteogenesis imperfecta in a neonate. (A) Lateral skull film shows multiple intrasutural (Wormian) bones. (B) Chest radiograph demonstrates multiple healing rib fractures giving the ribs a beaded appearance. There is also a healing left clavicular fracture. (C) and (D) There are multiple fractures within both lower limbs. The femurs are short and crumpled due to healing fractures and there is bowing deformity of the tibia and fibula bilaterally. The bones are osteopenic.

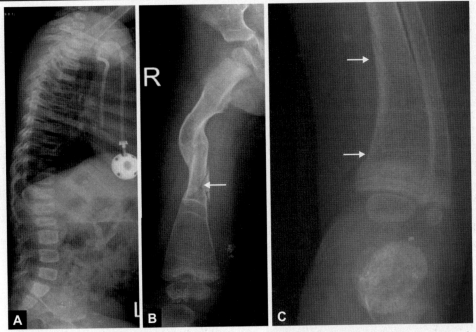

Figs 32.153A to C: Osteogenesis imperfecta in an older child. (A) The lateral spine X-ray shows wedging and collapse of several vertebral bodies. The child has a Portacath device in situ for intravenous biphosphonate treatment. (B) The right leg is in a plaster cast due to a recent midshaft spiral fracture of the right femur (arrow). There is also an older healing fracture in the proximal shaft. (C) There are fractures within the distal left tibia (arrows). Note the osteopenia. There is also lateral bowing of the distal tibia and fibula

Radiographic Findings:
- Skull: Variable decreased ossification, abnormal number of wormian bones (small bones within the cranial sutures)
- Spine: Wedged or collapsed vertebrae, kyphoscoliosis
- Remainder of skeleton: Osteoporosis and fractures.

PAEDIATRIC HIP ABNORMALITIES

Developmental Dysplasia of the Hip

Developmental dysplasia of the hip (DDH) can be diagnosed radiologically using ultrasound or X-ray. Ultrasound is the preferred imaging modality in neonates since the neonatal hip is composed almost entirely of cartilage, thereby making it difficult to establish the relationship of the femoral head to the acetabulum on radiographs.

By 4 to 6 months of age, the femoral head ossifies and radiographs are then used to evaluate infants with suspected DDH. The radiographic findings in DDH are:
- Increased slope of bony acetabulum (acetabular dysplasia)
- Delayed growth of the femoral head ossification centre compared to the normal side

- A pseudoacetabulum, which is a late radiographic sign in DDH.

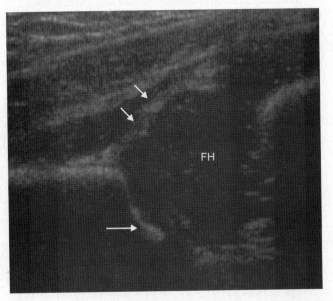

Fig. 32.154: Normal hip ultrasound. Coronal ultrasound scan of hip shows the femoral head (FH) covered by the bony acetabular roof (arrow) and acetabular labrum (arrowheads)

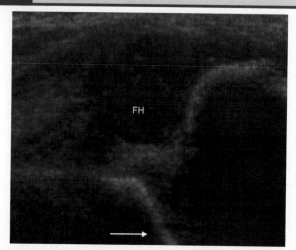

Fig. 32.155: Decentred hip. Coronal ultrasound scan shows the cartilaginous femoral head (FH) lies outwith the bony acetabular roof (arrow)

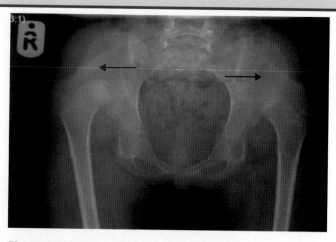

Fig. 32.157: Late diagnosis of bilateral DDH in a four-year-old girl. Both hips are dislocated superiorly and laterally and articulate with pseudoacetabula (arrows)

Legg-Calvé-Perthes Disease

Legg-Calvé-Perthes disease is avascular necrosis of the proximal (capital) femoral epiphysis. The peak incidence is 6-8 years of age. The disease can be bilateral.

The radiographic findings include flattening, sclerosis and fragmentation of the capital femoral epiphysis. Early subchondral fractures can be detected on frog lateral views as a curvilinear lucency within the epiphysis.

With progressive fragmentation and collapse of the femoral head, the femoral neck becomes short and wide. Eventually the epiphysis remineralises and heals. The healed capital femoral epiphysis is flat and wide.

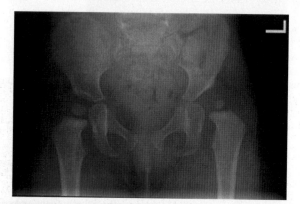

Fig. 32.156: Developmental dysplasia of hip and dislocation. There is increased slope of the left bony acetabulum. The left femoral head ossification centre is hypoplastic. The left femoral head is dislocated superiorly and laterally. The right hip is normal

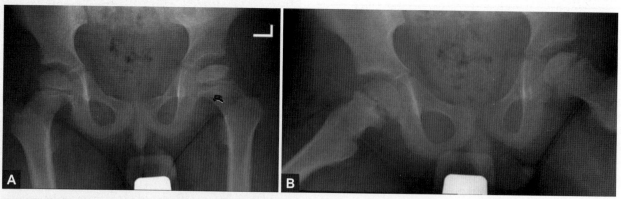

Figs 32.158A and B: Legg-Calvé-Perthes disease left hip. (A and B): Frontal and frog-leg lateral radiographs demonstrate flattening, irregularity, fragmentation and sclerosis of the left capital femoral epiphysis. The right capital femoral epiphysis is normal

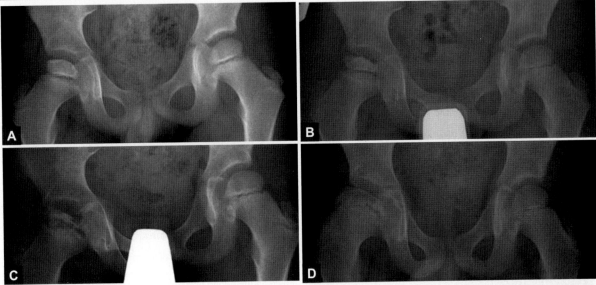

Figs 32.159A to D: Serial radiographic changes of Legg-Calvé-Perthes disease of right hip. (A) Radiograph at presentation demonstrates flattening and sclerosis of the right capital femoral epiphysis. (B) Radiograph five months later reveals further loss of epiphyseal height. (C) Ten months later, there is marked fragmentation and flattening of the right capital femoral epiphysis. (D) Two and a half years after the onset, the capital femoral epiphysis has healed but is flatter and wider to fit the widened femoral neck

Slipped Capital Femoral Epiphysis

Slipped capital femoral epiphysis (SCFE) is a disease of the adolescent hip. The disease can be bilateral.

The radiographic findings of SCFE are:

- Widening of the epiphyseal plate
- Displacement of the femoral head posteriorly and medially.

Medial slippage can be identified on a frontal projection of the pelvis. Mild displacement, which may not be immediately apparent on the frontal projection, is best appreciated on the frog leg lateral view.

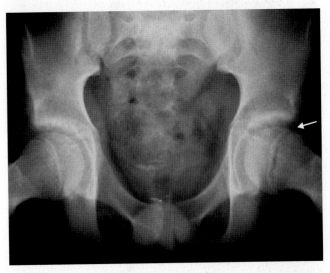

Fig. 32.161: Left slipped capital femoral epiphysis. Frog leg lateral view shows mild slippage of the left capital femoral epiphysis (arrow)

METABOLIC BONE DISORDERS

Rickets

There are a number of clinical conditions which can lead to the development of rickets. The radiographic features of this metabolic disorder is shared, whatever its underlying cause.

Radiographic Findings:
- Demineralisation
- Widening of the growth plate

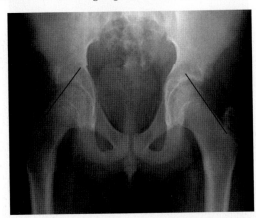

Fig. 32.160: Slipped right capital femoral epiphysis. Frontal radiograph of the pelvis demonstrates medial slippage of the right capital femoral epiphysis. A line drawn along the lateral femoral neck on the normal left side intersects a portion of the femoral epiphysis. However, a similar line drawn along the lateral aspect of the right femoral neck just misses the epiphysis

- Cupping, fraying and splaying of the metaphysis, which is of reduced density
- Thin bony spur extending from the metaphysis to surround the uncalcified growth plate
- Indistinct cortex because of uncalcified subperiosteal osteoid
- Poorly ossified epiphyses with faint, indistinct borders.

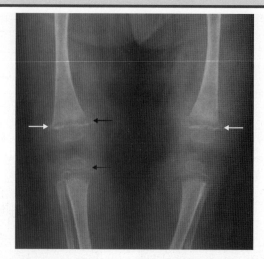

Fig. 32.163: Scurvy. AP radiograph of the knees. Transverse bands of metaphyseal lucency lie adjacent to dense zones of provisional calcification (white arrows). There are metaphyseal corner fractures through the weakened metaphyses (white arrows)

Lead Poisoning

Lead intoxication may occur by ingesting or inhaling the metal. Lead is present in many products including leaded petrol, old water pipes and lead paint. Exposure to lead can lead to anaemia, abdominal symptoms (abdominal pain, vomiting, diarrhoea), a blue line around the gums and encephalopathy. In the skeletal system, lead intoxication causes widening of the cranial sutures (due to increased intracranial pressure) and dense transverse lines in the metaphyses of tubular bones. Opaque lead particles can be seen within bowel on abdominal radiographs.

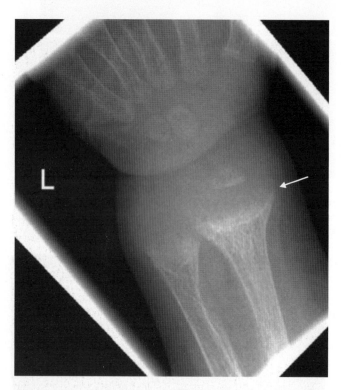

Fig. 32.162: Rickets. Radiograph of the left wrist shows a wide distal radial growth plate. Note the cupping, fraying and splaying of the distal radial and ulnar metaphyses. There is a prominent bony spur extending from the distal radial metaphsysis (arrow). The distal radial epiphysis is poorly ossified and has an indistinct contour. The forearm bones are demineralised with coarsened trabeculae and indistinct cortices

Scurvy

Scurvy is the result of vitamin C deficiency.
Radiographic Findings:
- Generalised osteopenia
- Dense zone of provisional calcification due to excessive calcification of osteoid
- Metaphyseal lucency
- Metaphyseal corner fractures through the weakened lucent metaphyses (Pelkan spurs)
- Periosteal reaction due to subperiosteal haematoma
- Loss of epiphyseal density with a pencil thin cortex

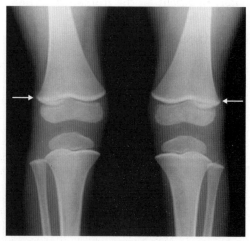

Fig. 32.164: Lead poisoning. AP radiograph of the knees reveals transverse bands of increased density in the metaphyses of the long bones (arrows)

INFLAMMATORY JOINT AND MUSCLE CONDITIONS

Juvenile Idiopathic Arthritis

Plain radiography in the early stages of juvenile idiopathic arthritis (JIA) are usually unhelpful. Soft tissue swelling and periarticular osteopenia may be visible. Late findings include joint space loss (due to cartilage loss), bony erosions and joint subluxation or dislocation. In children, growth disturbance can occur with epiphyseal overgrowth and premature growth plate fusion.

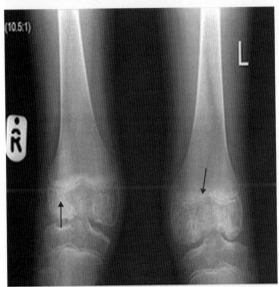

Fig. 32.165: Juvenile idiopathic arthritis of both knees. The bones are osteopenic and there is significant joint space loss at the femoro-tibial joints. Subarticular bony erosions are present (arrow). The epiphyses are enlarged (overgrowth). There is slight lateral subluxation of the tibia in relation to the femur bilaterally

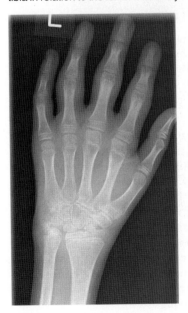

Fig. 32.166: Juvenile idiopathic arthritis of the left hand and wrist. There is osteopenia, especially in a periarticular distribution. There is significant joint space loss at the radio-carpal and carpal joints. Note the irregularity of the carpal bones. Joint space loss is also present at the metacarpo-phalangeal and the inter-phalangeal joints. There is soft tissue swelling of the fingers proximally

Dermatomyositis

Juvenile dermatomyositis is the commonest idiopathic inflammatory condition of muscle in children.

MRI is helpful in establishing the diagnosis of dermatomyositis and is also useful in assessing the response to treatment.

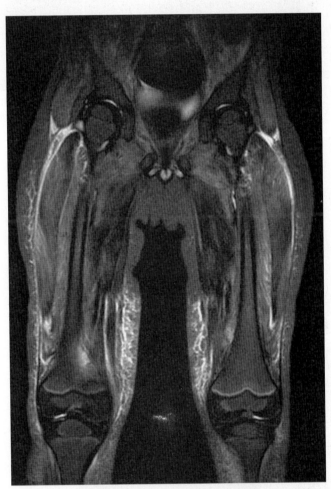

Fig. 32.167: Dermatomyositis. Coronal T2-weighted MR sequence through the thighs with fat saturation shows diffusely abnormal increased signal intensity within the muscles of both thighs and also within the subcutaneous tissues

Soft tissue calcification is best demonstrated on plain films. Calcium deposition in soft tissues usually occurs around pressure-point sites: the buttocks, knees and elbows. Calcium deposition occurs in the cutaneous and subcutaneous tissues, muscles and fascial planes.

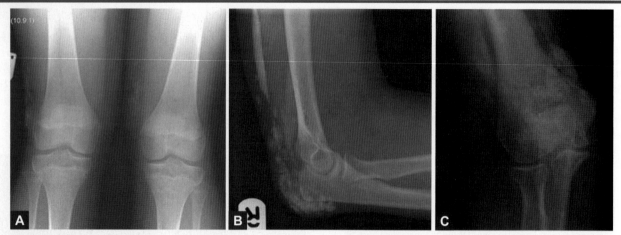

Figs 32.168A to C: Dermatomyositis. (A) AP radiograph of both knees shows amorphous calcification mainly in the cutaneous tissues bilaterally. (B and C) AP and lateral radiographs of right elbow. There is extensive calcification in the cutaneous tissues and in the muscles around the elbow joint

BONE INFECTIONS

Congenital Syphilis

Congenital syphilis is caused by transplacental spread of *Treponema pallidum.*

The radiographic features in infants include:

- Metaphyseal lucent bands
- Metaphyseal serration (sawteeth)
- Metaphyseal bony destruction on the medial aspect of the proximal tibia
- Periosteal reaction
- Diaphyseal destructive lesions.

The radiographic features of congenital syphilis in childhood are:

- Periosteal and cortical thickening
- Focal destructive lesions.

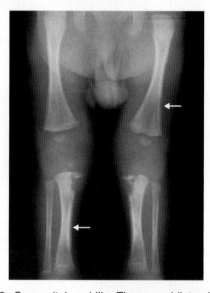

Fig. 32.170: Congenital syphilis. There are bilateral symmetric destructive metaphyseal lesions on the medial aspect of the tibiae. There is also significant periosteal reaction along the diaphyses of the femurs and tibiae (arrows)

Osteomyelitis

Osteomyelitis is an acute or chronic inflammatory condition of bone and its adjacent structures due to pyogenic organisms. Radiographs often show no bony abnormality in the early stages, although soft tissue swelling may be evident. Bony involvement is often not detected on radiographs until the second week of the disease. This is manifest as radiolucent areas, usually in the metaphysis, where bony destruction has occurred. Periosteal reaction is also evident. If treatment is delayed or ineffective, there is an increase in the amount of periosteal reaction to form an involucrum around the fragments of dead bone (sequestrum).

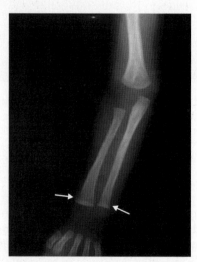

Fig. 32.169: Congenital syphilis. Radiograph of left forearm in a neonate shows metaphyseal lucency within the long bones, best demonstrated in the distal radius and ulna (arrows)

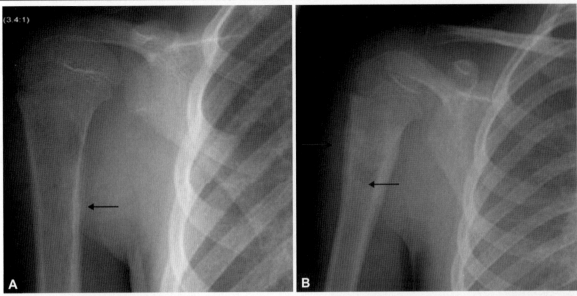

Figs 32.171A and B: Osteomyelitis proximal right humerus. (A) AP radiograph at time of presentation shows patchy radiolucency within the proximal right humeral shaft and faint periosteal reaction (arrow). (B) Follow-up radiograph one month later with treatment. The lucent area within bone is smaller and well-defined. The periosteum has produced new cortical bone (arrows)

HAEMOLYTIC ANAEMIAS

Thalassaemia

Skeletal Findings:

- Skull: Osteoporosis; expansion of the diploic space, especially in the frontal bone; thinning of the outer table of the skull; *hair-on-end* appearance. Hypoplasia of the paranasal sinuses due to expansion of the facial bones; malocclusion of the jaw
- Trunk: Osteoporosis, coarse bony trabeculae and cortical thinning. Accentuation of vertical trabecular pattern in the vertebrae; biconcave vertebral bodies
- Tubular bones: Widened medullary cavity and cortical thinning.

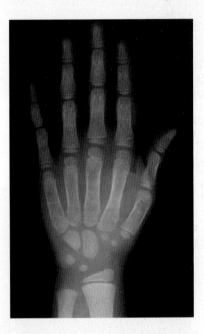

Fig. 32.173: Thalassaemia. Radiograph of the left hand demonstrates widening of the medullary cavity and thinning of the cortex within the tubular bones

Sickle Cell Anaemia

The skeletal findings in sickle cell anaemia are similar to those in thalassaemia. The skull changes are less severe. Compression fractures of the spine can occur due to loss of bony support resulting from marrow hypertrophy. Vertebral fractures however can also be due to infarcts involving the blood vessels supplying the central portions

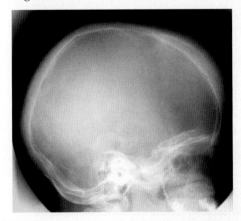

Fig. 32.172: Thalassaemia. There is widening of the diploic space and thinning of the outer table of the skull. Note the *hair-on-end* appearance in the frontal region on this lateral skull radiograph

of the superior and inferior endplates. This latter feature results in a depression of the central portion of the vertebral endplate.

Vascular occlusion due to sickling also results in osteonecrosis in other bones. Diaphyseal or epiphyseal infarcts can occur in the long bones. In young children, the bones of the hands and feet can be affected. This is known as sickle cell dactylitis or hand-foot syndrome. Patients with sickle cell disease are also at risk of osteomyelitis and pyogenic arthritis.

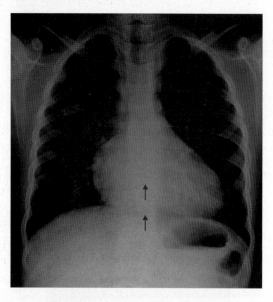

Fig. 32.174: Sickle cell disease. There is central endplate depression within some of the thoracic vertebrae (arrows) due to focal fractures resulting from local vascular occlusion. There is also cardiomegaly due to anaemia

LANGERHANS' CELL HISTIOCYTOSIS

Langerhans' cell histiocytosis (LCH) in the skeleton can be unifocal or multifocal. The commonest affected site is the skull. Other frequent locations include the femur, ribs mandible, pelvis, and spine.

LCH lesions in the skull are usually well-defined lytic lesions with sharp margins. In the spine, the disease causes lytic destruction and collapse of the vertebral body. Elsewhere in the skeleton, LCH lesions are usually well-defined with minimally sclerotic borders.

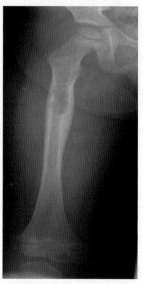

Fig. 32.175: LCH proximal right femur. AP radiograph demonstrates a well-defined, ovoid lytic lesion in the proximal right femur. The margins of the lesion are slightly sclerotic. There is cortical expansion and periosteal reaction

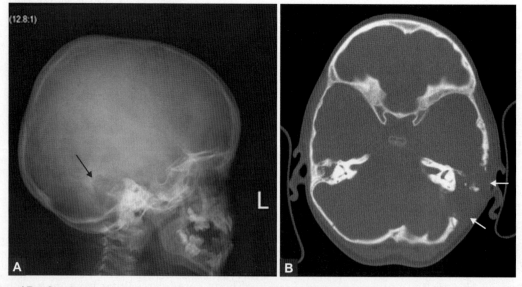

Figs 32.176A and B: LCH of skull. (A) Lateral skull radiograph shows a large, well-defined lytic lesion within the temporal bone region of the skull (arrow). (B) Axial CT scan through the skull on bone window settings. This confirms the presence of an extensive destructive process involving the left petrous temporal bone (arrows)

PAEDIATRIC BONE TUMOURS

Osteoid Osteoma

The osteoid osteoma is a painful lesion, with patients classically complaining of night pain. The commonest sites for osteoid osteoma are the femur and tibia. The typical radiographic appearance is a cortically based sclerotic lesion in a long bone, which has a small lucent area within it known as the nidus.

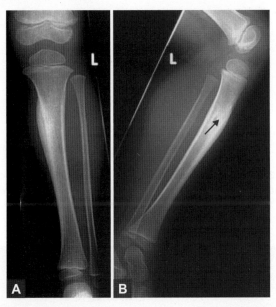

Figs 32.177A and B: Osteoid osteoma of the left tibia. (A) AP radiograph of left lower leg demonstrates dense sclerosis and focal cortical thickening along the medial aspect of the proximal left tibia. (B) The lateral radiograph shows the small radiolucent nidus within the bony lesion (arrow)

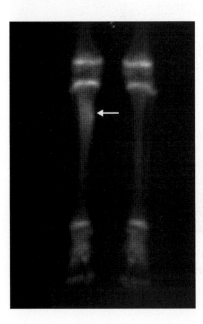

Fig. 32.178: Osteoid osteoma on radionuclide bone scan. Image taken from the front shows increased tracer uptake medially within the proximal right tibia which corresponds to the sclerotic component of the lesion. The smaller more focal area of intense uptake corresponds to the nidus (arrow)

OSTEOSARCOMA

Osteosarcomas can occur anywhere in the skeleton. Frequently encountered sites are the distal femur, proximal tibia, proximal humerus and pelvis. Long bone tumours usually arise from the metaphysis. On X-ray, a typical osteosarcoma is identified as a mixed lytic and sclerotic lesion involving the long bone metaphysis. There is usually cortical erosion and destruction, often with a spiculated 'sunburst' periosteal reaction. Elevated periosteal reaction is also demonstrated at the tumour extremities (Codman's triangle).

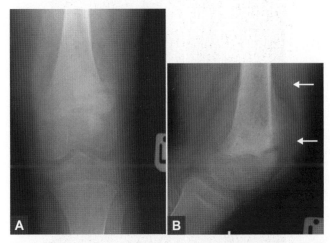

Figs 32.179A and B: Osteosarcoma of distal left femur. (A and B) AP and lateral radiographs of left knee show a sclerotic lesion arising from the distal left femoral diametaphysis. Spiculated periosteal reaction is present (white arrow) and there is also elevated periosteal reaction (Codmans triangle) at the superior margin of the lesion (white arrow)

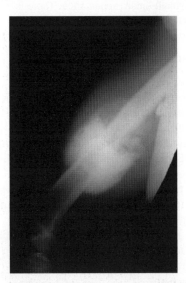

Fig. 32.180: Osteosarcoma of femur. Lateral view of the femur shows marked -sunray- periosteal new bone formation associated with the mid femoral shaft tumour. Osteosarcoma was confirmed pathologically at biopsy

Ewing Sarcoma

The commonest site for Ewing sarcoma is the long bone diaphysis. Flat bones (pelvis and ribs) are also commonly involved.

The typical radiographic appearance of Ewing sarcoma is a *'moth eaten'* lesion (due to multiple small holes) in the diaphysis or, less commonly, the metaphysis of a long bone. There is usually an *'onion skin'* type of periosteal reaction.

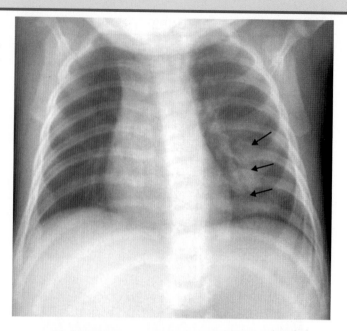

Fig. 32.182: Frontal chest radiograph shows healing posterior rib fractures involving the left seventh, eighth and ninth ribs (arrows)

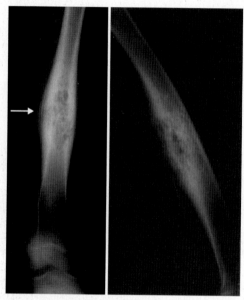

Fig. 32.181: Ewing sarcoma left femur. AP and lateral radiographs show a mixed lytic and sclerotic lesion in the diaphysis of the left femur resulting in a 'moth-eaten' appearance. There is 'onion-skin' type periosteal reaction (arrow)

Non-accidental Injury

Skeletal Findings:
- Multiple fractures in varying stages of healing
- Diaphyseal fractures, especially in the nonambulatory infant/child
- Metaphyseal fractures: The classic metaphyseal fracture is often described as a corner or bucket-handle fracture
- Rib fractures: Posterior rib fractures have a higher specificity for inflicted injury than antero-lateral fractures
- Scapula fracture: Fracture of the acromion is highly specific for abuse
- Spinal fractures
- Skull fractures.

Other types of injury encountered in this situation include intracranial and visceral trauma.

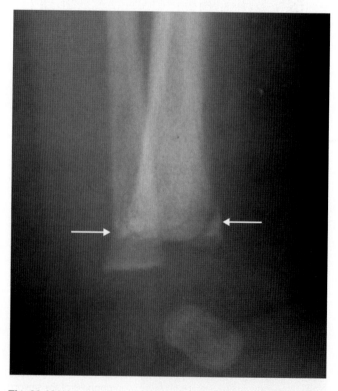

Fig. 32.183: Lateral view of ankle demonstrates metaphyseal corner fractures of the distal tibia (arrows)

PAEDIATRIC RENAL IMAGING

CONGENITAL ANOMALIES

Ureteral Duplication

Ureteral duplication may be partial or complete. In partial duplication, the ureters unite anywhere along their course and then continue inferiorly as a single structure. In completely duplicated systems, the two ureters are separate throughout their entire course. The ureter draining the upper moiety usually inserts into the bladder ectopically, below and more medial to the insertion of the ureter, which drains the lower renal moiety. The ectopic ureter is more likely to become obstructed, sometimes due to an associated ureterocele. The lower-moiety ureter is more prone to reflux. When renal function is adequate, duplication of the pelvocalyceal system and ureter can be visualised on excretion urography. It is sometimes difficult to establish if the ureteric duplication is partial or complete on this study.

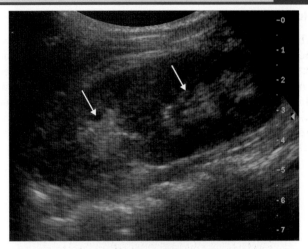

Fig. 32.185: Uncomplicated ureteral duplication. Parasagittal ultrasound scan of left kidney shows two echogenic renal sinuses (arrows). The kidney is also enlarged. These findings are typical for an uncomplicated duplex kidney

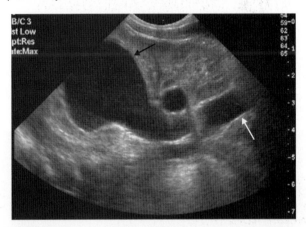

Fig. 32.186: Ureteral duplication with obstructed upper renal moiety. Longitudinal ultrasound scan of left kidney shows a hydronephrotic upper moiety renal pelvis (white arrow) and its associated hydroureter (white arrows)

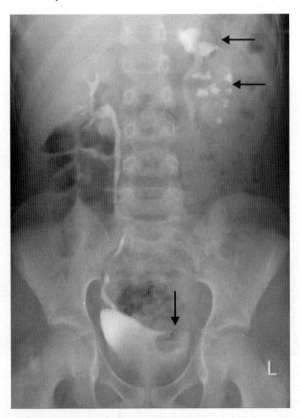

Fig. 32.184: Left-sided upper ureteric duplication. Excretory urogram shows two left-sided pelvocalyceal systems (arrows). The separate proximal ureters are visible. There is a filling defect in the left side of the bladder due to a ureterocele (arrowed). This is causing some obstruction to the upper renal moiety which demonstrates clubbing of its calyces

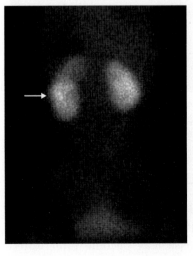

Fig. 32.187: Duplex left kidney. Renal radionuclide study using technetium 99 m dimercaptosuccinic acid (DMSA). This image taken from the back, shows an enlarged left kidney consistent with a duplex kidney (arrow)

Horseshoe Kidney

The horseshoe kidney arises because of fusion of the lower poles of the kidneys across the midline. This fusion produces an abnormal renal axis, which may be detected on ultrasound. The fused portion of the kidney (known as the isthmus) may also be visualised on ultrasound as renal tissue which overlies the spine. The horseshoe kidney is best demonstrated in its entirety on renal scintigraphy (DMSA scan) and abdominal CT or MR scans.

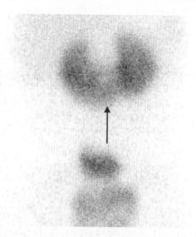

Fig. 32.188: Horseshoe kidney. DMSA scan demonstrates uptake within both kidneys and within the renal isthmus (arrow)

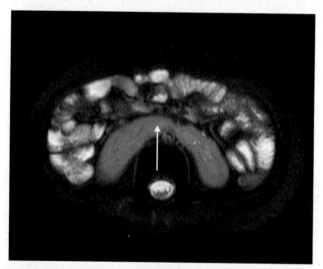

Fig. 32.189: Horseshoe kidney on abdominal MR scan. Axial T2-weighted (fat saturated) image demonstrates fusion of the lower poles of the kidneys anterior to the spine (arrows)

RENAL ECTOPIA

Ipsilateral Renal Ectopia

In the fetus, the normal migration of the kidney from the pelvis to the renal fossa may become interrupted.

Consequently the kidney can be located anywhere along the migrational path. When a kidney cannot be found in its usual position on ultrasound, the pelvis should be closely scrutinised to see if there is an ectopic pelvic kidney. Pelvic kidneys are more prone to vesicoureteric reflux than normal kidneys. They have an abnormal rotation and are also more likely to have ureteropelvic junction obstruction.

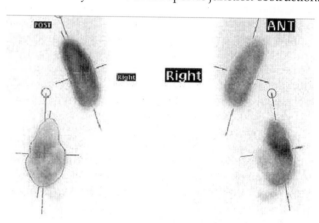

Fig. 32.190: Pelvic kidney on DMSA scan. The right kidney is located in a normal position. The left kidney is ectopic, lying within the pelvis

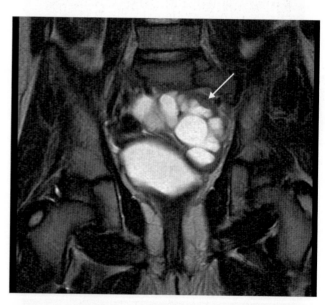

Fig. 32.191: Pelvic kidney. Coronal T2-weighted MR scan shows an ectopic left kidney above the bladder (arrow). The renal pelvis and calyces are dilated

Crossed Fused Renal Ectopia

This is a condition where the bulk of both kidneys is on one side of the spine. Part of the ectopic kidney may extend across the spine. The ectopic kidney is usually smaller than normal and malrotated. It usually lies below the normally-sited kidney. The kidneys are usually fused and surrounded by a common renal fascia, hence the given term *crossed fused renal ectopia*. The ureter from the ectopic lower kidney usually crosses the midline to inert into the bladder in its normal position.

Abdominal ultrasound will reveal an empty renal fossa on one side and an apparently enlarged kidney on the other side, with two renal sinuses. The ectopic kidney is generally positioned medially, extending anteriorly across the spine. Nuclear scintigraphy can also be used to confirm the presence of crossed fused renal ectopia.

Renal Agenesis

Bilateral renal agenesis is a lethal anomaly. If the diagnosis is not made until birth, the infant will have features of Potter's sequence. A renal ultrasound scan in the early neonatal period usually confirms the diagnosis by showing no renal tissue in the renal flanks or in an ectopic location.

Unilateral renal agenesis is sometimes detected antenatally or on postnatal ultrasound because of anomalies elsewhere. It is also associated with anomalies of the genital tract.

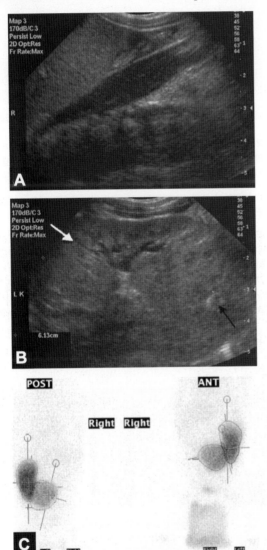

Figs 32.192A to C: Crossed fused renal ectopia. (A) Parasagittal ultrasound scan of right flank shows absent right kidney. (B) Parasagittal scan ultrasound scan of left flank shows a normally positioned left kidney (white arrow) with an apparent –mass of renal tissue at its lower pole (black arrow). This is the ectopic right kidney. (C) DMSA renal scan demonstrates the ectopic right kidney lying medially and horizontally, attached to the lower pole of the left kidney

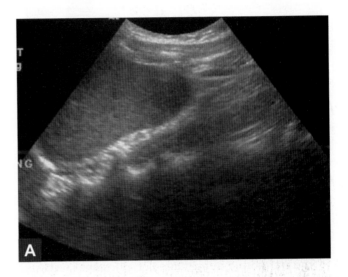

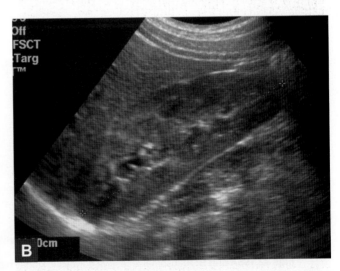

Figs 32.193A and B: Agenesis of left kidney. (A) Left parasagittal ultrasound scan shows no kidney in the left flank (B) Right parasagittal ultrasound scan demonstrates a normal appearing right kidney which is larger than usual due to compensatory hypertrophy

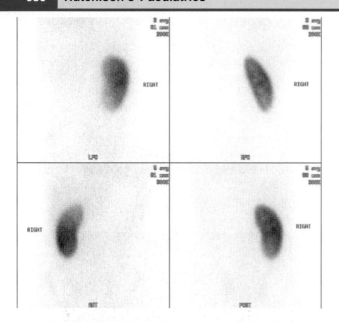

Fig. 32.194: Agenesis of left kidney. Radio-isotope study (DMSA) shows a solitary right kidney. No left kidney or ectopic renal tissue is identified

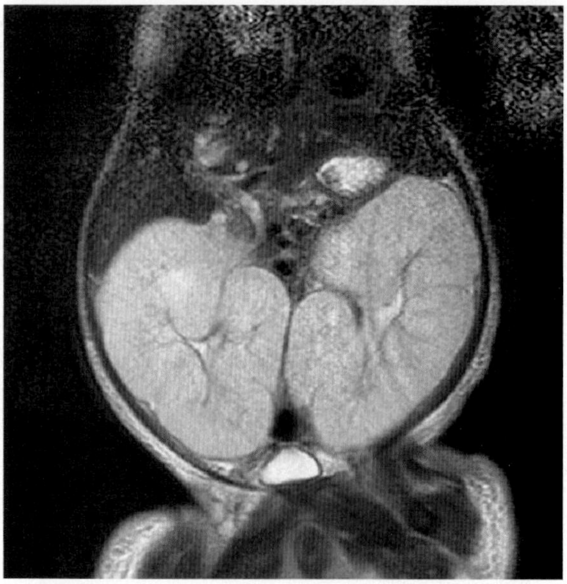

Fig. 32.196: Autosomal recessive polycystic kidney disease on abdominal MR scan. Coronal T2-weighted abdominal MR image from the same patient, shows the extent of the bilateral nephromegaly

Autosomal Recessive Polycystic Kidney Disease

This is a rare disorder involving both kidneys and the liver. The disease causes ectasia of the renal collecting tubules and this is manifest pathologically as numerous tinycysts in the cortex and medulla.

The ultrasound appearances of autosomal recessive polycystic kidney disease in neonates are bilateral enlarged kidneys which are diffusely echogenic. Discrete small cysts may be visible.

Multicystic Dysplastic Kidney

Multicystic dysplastic kidney is a severe form of renal dysplasia which is associated with obstruction of urinary drainage on the affected side, probably occurring in utero. The sonographic features of classic multicystic dysplastic kidney are multiple cysts of variable size which do not communicate with each other. There is absent or dysplastic renal parenchyma and no renal pelvis is identified. There is no function in a multicystic dysplastic kidney.

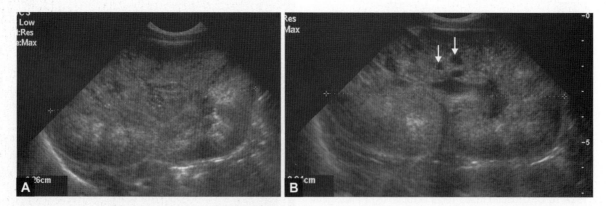

Figs 32.195A and B: Autosomal recessive polycystic kidney disease in a newborn infant. (A) Longitudinal ultrasound scan of right kidney demonstrates a markedly enlarged, echogenic kidney. (B) Longitudinal ultrasound scan of the left kidney also shows an enlarged, echogenic kidney. There are a few small discrete cysts within the renal parenchyma (arrows)

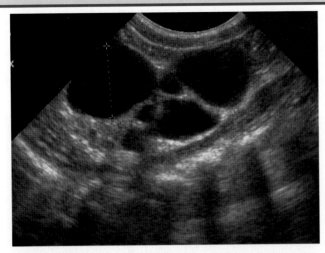

Fig. 32.197: Multicystic dysplastic kidney. Longitudinal ultrasound image of the left kidney reveals several cysts of different size within the kidney. The cysts are non-communicating. No normal renal parenchyma is identified

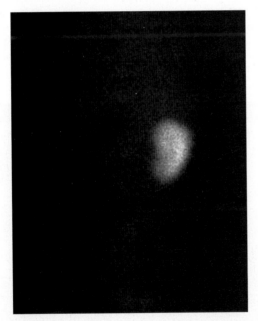

Fig. 32.198: Multicystic dysplastic kidney. DMSA study performed in the same patient. This image, taken from behind, shows tracer uptake only in the normal right kidney. There is no uptake in the dysplastic left kidney

URINARY TRACT STONES AND NEPHROCALCINOSIS

Urinary Tract Stones

Causes of renal tract stones in children include:
- Infection
- Developmental anomalies of the urinary tract

- Immobilisation
- Metabolic disorders such as hypercalcaemia and hypercalciuria
- Idiopathic.

Calcium stones are radiopaque and therefore can be identified on X-ray. Cystine stones are poorly opaque. Uric acid stones are radiolucent.

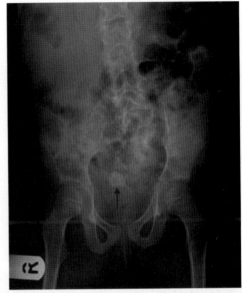

Fig. 32.199: Bladder calculus. AP radiograph shows a large, radiopaque structure projected over the pelvis, consistent with a bladder calculus (arrow)

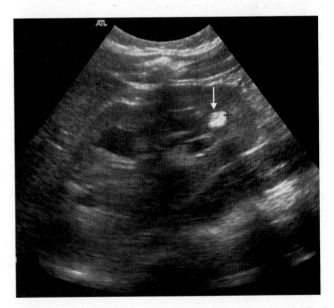

Fig. 32.200: Calculus within lower pole of the left kidney. Longitudinal ultrasound scan of left kidney shows a bright (hyperechoic) structure at the lower pole of the kidney (arrow), consistent with a small renal calculus

Nephrocalcinosis

Nephrocalcinosis is the deposition of calcium in the renal medulla or cortex. Calcium deposition is more common in the medulla than in the cortex.

Causes of medullary nephrocalcinosis include:
- Hyperparathyroidism
- Renal tubular acidosis
- Medullary sponge kidney
- Causes of hypercalcaemia or hypercalciuria
- Hyperoxaluria
- Frusemide.

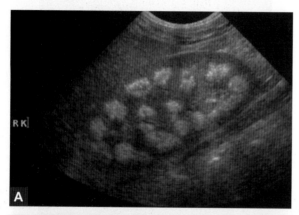

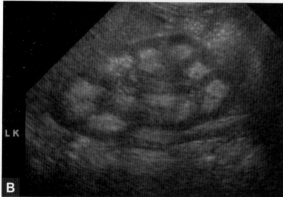

Figs 32.201A and B: Medullar nephrocalcinosis. (A and B) Longitudinal ultrasound images of right and left kidneys respectively. The renal pyramids are markedly hyperechoic due to medullary calcinosis

DILATATION OF URINARY TRACT

Dilatation of the urinary tract can be due to one of three general problems:
- Obstruction
- Vesicoureteric reflux
- A combination of both.

Ureteropelvic Junction Obstruction

Ureteropelvic junction (UPJ) obstruction is the most common cause of upper urinary tract obstruction in infants and children. The characteristic ultrasound findings include dilated calyces with a moderate or large renal pelvis. The renal parenchyma is of varying thickness depending on the degree of pelvocalyceal dilatation. Diuretic renography is commonly performed to assess UPJ obstruction.

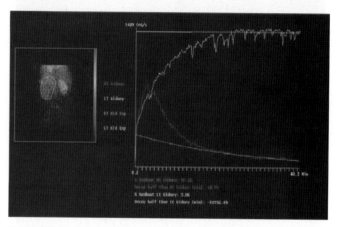

Fig. 32.202: Left-sided ureteropelvic obstruction. On this diuretic renogram study using technetium-99 m mercaptoacetyltriglycine (MAG 3), there is normal excretion of radioisotope from the right kidney. There is no excretion of radioisotope from the left kidney, even after the administration of frusemide at 20 minutes

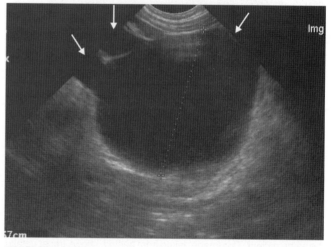

Fig. 32.203: Ureteropelvic junction obstruction. Longitudinal ultrasound scan demonstrates markedly dilated renal pelvis and moderately dilated calyces (arrows)

Posterior Urethral Valves

Posterior urethral valves are the most common cause of urethral obstruction in males and the diagnosis is usually confirmed with a micturating cystourethrogram. The features of posterior urethral valves on this study are:
- Dilated posterior urethra
- Visualisation of valves

- Trabeculated bladder with wide neck
- Usually reflux of contrast into dilated, tortuous ureters.

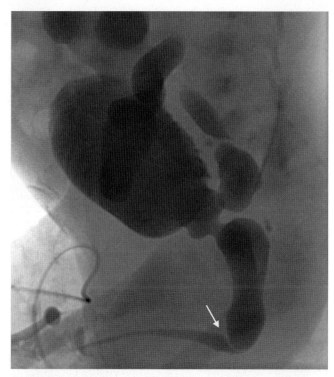

Fig. 32.204: Posterior urethral valves. Micturating cystourethrogram study after urinary catheter removed. There is a filling defect in the posterior urethra due to posterior urethral valves (arrow). The posterior urethra proximal to this is dilated and the bladder neck is wide. There is reflux of contrast into both ureters

Vesicoureteric Reflux

The severity of vesicoureteric reflux is graded according to the degree of upper renal tract dilatation on the micturation cystourethrogram:

- *Grade 1:* Reflux into ureter only
- *Grade 2:* Reflux into ureter, renal pelvis and calyces which are preserved
- *Grade 3:* Reflux into mildly dilated ureter and renal pelvis; the calyces are slightly blunted
- *Grade 4:* Reflux into moderately dilated ureter and renal pelvis; moderately blunted calyces
- *Grade 5:* Reflux into tortuous dilated ureter and markedly dilated renal pelvis; severe calyceal blunting.

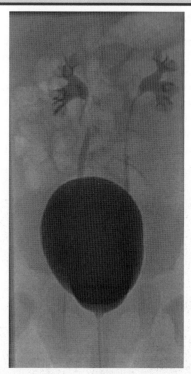

Fig. 32.205: Bilateral grade 2 vesicoureteric reflux. Micturating cystourethrogram study demonstrates reflux of contrast into the pelvocalyceal system and ureter bilaterally. The calyces are preserved

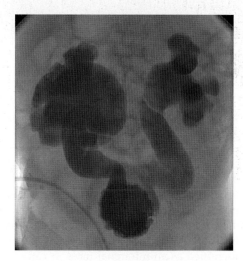

Fig. 32.206: Severe bilateral vesicoureteric reflux. There is grade 5 reflux on the right. The right ureter is dilated and tortuous. There is marked dilatation of the right pelvocalyceal system with severe calyceal blunting. The appearances are slightly less marked on the left side and represent grade 4/5 vesicoureteric reflux

Renal Tract Infection

Urinary tract infection can involve the kidney, bladder or both areas. The role of imaging in the child with a proven urinary tract infection is to diagnose underlying conditions which predispose to infection such as hydronephrosis and reflux, and to detect renal scarring.

The ultrasound scan often appears normal in uncomplicated cases of pyelonephritis. Renal cortical scarring is usually detected using renal scintigraphy.

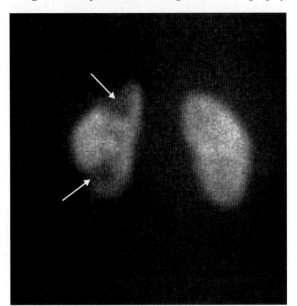

Fig. 32.207: Cortical scarring left kidney. This DMSA study reveals photopenic areas (arrows) in the upper and lower poles of the left kidney, consistent with renal cortical scarring. The right kidney is normal

NEOPLASTIC DISEASES

Wilms' Tumour

Wilms' tumour is the commonest abdominal malignancy of childhood. Radiologic examinations help to stage the disease in order to assist surgical planning and treatment, and to evaluate response to treatment. The tumour is usually identified as an intrarenal mass. It can extend via the renal vein into the inferior vena cava and right atrium and it can metastasise to the lungs. Bilateral Wilms' tumours can occur.

Where possible, an MR scan of the abdomen should be used to stage Wilms' tumour since this avoids ionising radiation. CT scanning however is required to image the chest.

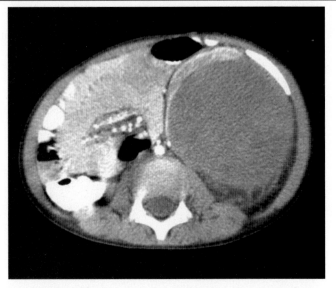

Fig. 32.208: Wilms' tumour of the left kidney. Contrast-enhanced axial CT scan through the abdomen demonstrates a large mass arising from the left kidney. There is a thin rim of normal renal parenchyma around the tumour anteriorly (arrow)

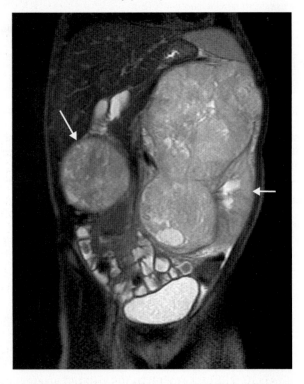

Fig. 32.209: Bilateral Wilms' tumour (stage V). Coronal T2-weighted scan (fat saturated) shows a bilobed mass within the left kidney. There is normal left renal tissue laterally (arrow). There is a smaller mass within the right kidney (arrow)

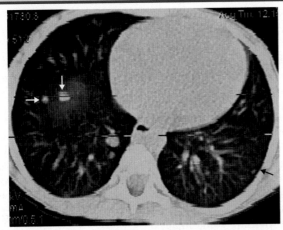

Fig. 32.210: Lung metastases from Wilms' tumour. Axial CT scan through the chest on lung window settings. There are a number of intrapulmonary nodules within both lungs on this image (some of which are arrowed), consistent with intrapulmonary metastases

Neuroblastoma

Among paediatric abdominal neoplasms, neuroblastoma is the second most common after Wilms' tumour. Neuroblastomas which arise within the abdomen, are staged with an abdominal MR scan (where possible) and a CT scan of the chest. Neuroblastomas arising from the adrenal gland can invade the adjacent kidney. The tumour spreads

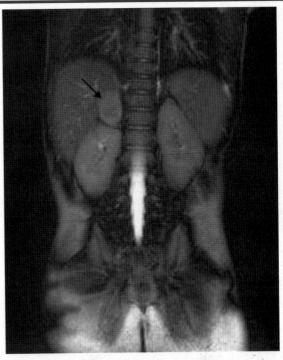

Fig. 32.211: Right adrenal neuroblastoma. Coronal T2-weighted (fat saturated) MR scan of abdomen demonstrates an ovoid mass situated above the upper pole of the right kidney in the right adrenal gland (arrow)

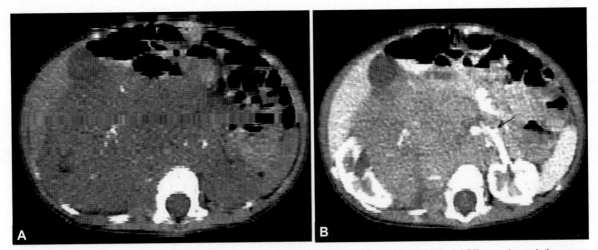

Figs 32.212A and B: Right adrenal neuroblastoma with nodal metastases. (A) Unenhanced axial CT scan through the upper abdomen demonstrates a large low density mass in the right flank which crosses the midline. The mass contains small areas of increased density, which are flecks of calcium. This is a feature in up to 90% of tumours on CT scanning. (B) Contrastenhanced axial CT scan through the same region shows the conglomerate mass of tumour and retroperitoneal lymphadenopathy. The lymphadenopathy is displacing the aorta and left renal artery anteriorly (arrow)

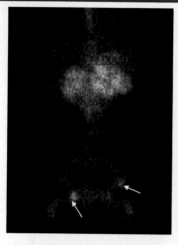

Fig. 32.213: Abdominal neuroblastoma with metastases on MIBG scan. There is increased tracer uptake in the upper abdomen at the site of the tumour and nodal disease. There are also other areas of increased uptake in the pelvis, consistent with skeletal metastases

to lymph nodes, bone, bone marrow, liver and skin. Bone metastases are best identified with radionuclide bone studies.

I-131-metaiodobenzylguanidine (MIBG) scintigraphy assesses functional uptake by the tumour and metastases.

ACKNOWLEDGEMENTS

The authors are grateful to Dr Ruth Allen, Consultant Paediatric Radiologist, Dr Greg J Irwin, Consultant Paediatric Radiologist, Dr Andrew J Watt, Consultant Paediatric Radiologist, Mr Rod Duncan, Consultant Orthopaedic Surgeon and Mrs Morag Attaie, Lead Sonographer at Royal Hospital for Sick Children, Glasgow for providing some images.

Prescribing for Children

James Wallace

THE CHALLENGE

Prescribing for children presents a number of challenges. Children are not "little adults" and should not be treated as such. Their bodies handle medicines differently to adults and the response of young children differs from older ones. Detailed care and attention is needed when making prescribing decisions for children, taking into account their developmental stage. Yet they experience the same range of illnesses that can affect adults. Children can require both specialised care for serious conditions such as cancer or transplantation and general care for more common complaints like asthma and diarrhoea. The paediatric prescriber requires a sound knowledge of the concepts of care within the whole age range of paediatrics. Neonatology can probably be regarded as a specialty in its own right with different clinical situations and huge differences in pharmacokinetics and dynamics.

The Table 33.1 below defines the descriptors commonly used for the different age groups, and the key stages, which define the development of a child.

Table 33.1: Descriptors used for different age groups		
Descriptor	*The age of the child*	*Key stages*
Neonate	Birth to one-month	Normal initial period of human development and growth
Infant	One month to one-year	High growth rates and rapid changes
Child	One to 12 years	Slower growth and development
Adolescent	12-18 years	Final period growth and puberty, stretching into adulthood

Lack of evidence on the use of medicines in children leads to uncertainty in dosing and increases the risk of medication errors. Even the most appropriate dose may lead to differences in effectiveness and adverse effects to those seen in adults. The evidence suggests that medication safety needs to be improved, particularly in babies and young children. Medication errors occur in children in hospital at similar rates to adults but have three times the potential to cause harm.

It is worth remembering that medicines are an important part of treatment strategies but a holistic approach to care of the child is required. Consideration also needs to be given to other approaches where possible including, for example, psychological management and nutrition.

Many changes occur in the way infants and children handle drugs in the period from birth to adulthood. They are important to take into consideration terms of understanding how doses are derived.

PHARMACOKINETICS

Absorption

Absorption of both orally and parenterally administered drugs is similar in children and adults. The exceptions to this are:

- Increased oral absorption of penicillin antibiotics
- Reduced oral absorptions of phenobarbitone, phenytoin and rifampicin in infants.

This is mainly due to decreased gastric acid secretion and an increased gastric emptying time at birth. Normal emptying times and pH are reached at about the age of three years.

Absorption from intramuscular (IM) administration is erratic, just as it is in adults, and the same types of drugs should be avoided with this route, i.e. phenytoin, digoxin and diazepam.

Percutaneous absorption is enhanced in infants and children. Their skin is much thinner and better hydrated than adults' and this can lead to problems with topical steroids. This is particularly the case if the skin is broken or burnt. Potent topical steroids should be avoided as systemic adverse effects have been reported in infants.

Rectal administration is particularly useful in infants and children who are vomiting or are reluctant to take oral medication. However, as in adults, there is considerable variation in individuals' blood supply to the rectum, causing variation in the rate and extent of absorption of rectally administered drugs. Diazepam can be given rectally and this is often the most convenient route in a child who is fitting. Paracetamol is also given rectally to treat pyrexia usually in children who are too ill to take their medication orally.

Distribution

The two main factors influencing drug distribution are body composition and plasma protein binding.

Body Composition

Extracellular fluid volume is much higher in newborn infants (50%). It decreases gradually with increasing age, 25% at one year of age and 20-25% by adulthood. More importantly, total body water is much higher in premature infants (85%) than term infants (75%) and adults (60-50%). In addition, the body fat content changes dramatically with age, from 3% in a premature newborn to 12% in full term infants, 30% at one year and 18% in adulthood.

This tends to mean greater doses of water-soluble drugs, e.g. penicillin and aminoglycosides on a weight-for-weight basis. For example, the normal dose of IV flucloxacillin for a premature neonate is 25 mg/kg. If you were to give this to a 70 kg adult the dose would be 1.75 gm.

Protein Binding

In premature babies, plasma protein binding is reduced resulting in higher concentrations of free (active) drug. This is due to reduced levels of circulating proteins and a reduced ability to bind. Thus these patients have a higher apparent volume of distribution than adults.

Elimination

The neonatal liver and kidneys are immature in their capacity to eliminate drugs. Both hepatic metabolism and kidney function are reduced in premature babies resulting in increased plasma half-lives of both hepatically and renally cleared drugs.

This leads to longer plasma half-lives and increased plasma concentrations. The more premature the infant, the more depressed the hepatic metabolism.

Hepatic Metabolism

Enzyme systems in the liver are immature in newborn and pre-terms infants, particularly oxidation and glucuroni-

dation. In the past this led to the "grey baby" syndrome when large doses of chloramphenicol were administered to infants with meningitis.

In older children, hepatic function is greater than in adults. Most anti-epileptics and theophylline require a larger dose per kilogram than in adults to achieve therapeutic plasma concentrations. This is thought to be due to the fact that, relative to body size, the liver is larger than in adults.

Renal Excretion

Renal excretion is the most important parameter, which affects dosing of children of any age. Renal function is immature in premature infants, leading to extended half-lives of drugs such as aminoglycosides or penicillins. Dosing changes are made in the same way as adults with poor renal function, i.e. increasing the dosing interval or decreasing the dose.

Conversely, patients with cystic fibrosis are able to clear aminoglycoside at a much higher rate than normal children of the same age. The reasons for this have never been fully explained but theories include enhanced tubular secretion, increased extra-renal clearance and increased volume of distribution.

These patients nearly always require much higher doses of aminoglycosides to achieve therapeutic plasma concentrations.

COMPLIANCE AND CONCORDANCE

Medicines should only be prescribed for children when absolutely necessary and always after careful consideration of the benefits of administering the medicine versus the risk involved from side effects and adverse drug reactions. It is important to discuss treatment options carefully with the child and the child's carer.

Compliance

Factors that contribute to poor compliance with prescribed medicines include:
- Difficulty in taking the medicine, (e.g. inability to swallow tablets)
- Unpalatable formulation (e.g. unpleasant taste or unwillingness to administer medicines rectally)
- Purpose of medicine not clear
- Perceived lack of effectiveness
- Real or perceived side effects
- Difference between the carer's or child's perception of risk and severity of side effects from that of the prescriber
- Unclear instructions for administration.

Concordance

The concept of compliance (the extent to which the prescriber's instructions are followed) is now giving way to that of concordance, where the patient is an active participant in decisions about treatment. Concordance is paramount between the health care professional, the child and the family. Time, effort and understanding are needed to achieve effective use of medicines in children. Children and parents need to be empowered to become active partners in discussions about the risks and benefits of their medicines. Their values and beliefs need to be taken into account as well as the effects of the proposed treatment on daily living.

THE ISSUES IN PRACTICE

Dosage Dilemmas

Choosing the most appropriate dose for children is no easy task. Their weight can range from around 0.5 kg for the very young to 120kg for adolescents. However, adults' weight can also vary from 40 kg-120 kg and no prescriber would think twice about giving any adult a 150 mg dose of ranitidine, for example, even though the plasma concentrations obtained will vary enormously. The difference is that we know this dose is safe and effective for most adults – there is less certainty in prescribing for children.

Most paediatric formularies will state that the ranitidine dose in children is 2 mg/kg, making a 26.4 mg dose for a 13.2 kg child. Ranitidine suspension comes as 15 mg/ml requiring the carer to draw up 1.76 ml. We know that decimal points are a major area of risk so would it be appropriate to give 2 ml (30 mg) to this same child?

The answer in this case is "yes" as ranitidine has a wide therapeutic range in children just as it does in adults. Good practice would be to round the dose and avoid decimal points. The skill is to know when this is appropriate with individual drugs and how far rounding can be taken.

Although few drugs are licensed for children, we need to look at what the license really tells us. Let us take the example of aciclovir, which has a licensed dose for children of 10 mg/kg tds for under three months; 500 mg/m² tds for three months up to 12 years and 10 mg/kg tds for 12 years and over. (Note here that this particular license has different units of measurement for these age groups, depending on how trials were carried out). There is good evidence that these doses are safe and effective for these age groups. But should an 11-year-old be treated differently than a 12-year-old? How rigidly should these age-related criteria be applied? In practice an 11-year-old is often given a higher dose than a 12-year-old. It is important to ensure that whatever dose, and whatever source of information is being used, that treatment meets the needs of the individual child.

Information Sources

Prescribers should always use reliable sources of paediatric dose information where these are available. However, the lack of paediatric data means that prescribers are occasionally left to extrapolate information from adult doses. Although this is plausible, it can also be dangerous. The metabolism and dynamics of babies, for instance, may be totally different to those in adults and may have unpredictable and serious adverse effects.

Dose Calculation

Many methods have developed over the years for calculating doses in paediatrics. The percentage method and the mg/kg method are the only two that should be used.

Percentage method (surface area method)

The percentage method for estimating doses is calculated as follows:

$$\frac{\text{Surface area of child (m}^2)}{1.76 \text{ m}^2} \times 100 = \text{percent of adult dose}$$

(1.76 m² being the average adult surface area).

Weight, height and body surface area.

The Table 33.2 shows the mean values for weight, height and body surface area by age; these values may be used to calculate doses in the absence of actual measurements. However, the child's actual weight and height might vary considerably from the values in the table and it is important to see the child to ensure that the value chosen is appropriate. In most cases the child's actual measurement should be obtained as soon as possible and the dose re-calculated.

Table 33.2: Mean values for weight, height and body surface area by age			
Age	Weight kg	Height cm	Body surface m²
Full-term neonate	3.5	50	0.23
1 month	4.2	55	0.26
2 months	4.5	57	0.27
3 months	5.6	59	0.32
4 months	6.5	62	0.34
6 months	7.7	67	0.40
1 year	10	76	0.47
3 years	15	94	0.62
5 years	18	108	0.73
7 years	23	120	0.88
10 years	30	132	1.05
12 years	39	148	1.25
14 years	50	163	1.50
Adult male	68	173	1.80
Adult female	56	163	1.60

(Reproduced by the kind permission of: Paediatric Formulary Committee. BNF for Children (edition 2006) London: BMJ Publishing Group, RPS Publishing, and RCPCH Publishing Ltd; 2006).

Children are often said to tolerate or require larger doses of drugs than adults based on a mg/kg basis. The percentage method helps explain this phenomenon.

Body water (total and extracellular) is known to equate better with surface area than body weight. It therefore seems appropriate to prescribe drugs by surface area if they are distributed in the extracellular water.

Example

Iain is a three-month-old baby. He weights 5.23 kg. His body surface area is 0.31 m². Calculate the dose of aciclovir required for him using the percentage method (the adult dose is 800 mg).

$$\frac{0.31}{1.76} \times 100 = 17.6\%$$

Dose is $0.176 \times 800 = 140.8$ mg

Use 140 mg = 3.5 ml of 200 mg/5 ml aciclovir suspension.

Mg/kg method

$$\frac{\text{Adult dose (mg)}}{70 \text{ kg}} = \text{mg/kg dose}$$

(70 kg being the average adult weight).

This method will give lower doses than the percentage method using surface areas. It is far less accurate in clinical terms but much easier to use since weights are usually more accessible than surface areas. Within limited age bands it is appropriate to state doses on a mg/kg basis. This form of extrapolation from adults is usually inappropriate for accurate therapeutic dosing, although it is unlikely to lead to toxic dosing.

Example

Iain is a three-month-old baby. He weights 5.23 kg. His body surface area 0.31 m². Calculate the dose of aciclovir required for him using the mg/kg method (the adult dose is 800 mg).

$$\frac{800}{70} = 11.4 \text{ mg/kg}$$

Dose is $11.4 \times 5.23 = 59.6$ mg

Use 60 mg = 1.5 ml of 200 mg/5 ml aciclovir suspension.

Using body surface area to calculate drug dose is the most accurate method, because it reflects cardiac output, fluid requirements and renal function better than weight-based dosing. In practice, however, it is impractical and necessary for only a limited number of drugs, e.g. cytotoxic agents. Weight-based doses are mainly used. Doses based on age bands may be used for some drugs with a wide therapeutic index.

PRESCRIBING IN PAEDIATRICS

General

Good prescribing is essential in all patients. However there are key points of good practice in prescribing for children. They can be summarised as follows:

- Always prescribe so that anybody can read it
- Never prescribe or administer without knowing the allergy status of the child
- Always be as clear as you can with units: **mg, micrograms, nanograms, units** are acceptable: **mcg, ng, ug, iu are not acceptable**
- Decimal points must always have a number in front of them even it is a "0"
- Try to be logical with doses. There are a few drugs that need precise prescribing on a mg/kg basis. Most drugs however can be rounded up or down with no clinical consequences (this reduces the use of decimal points and aids administration)
- Only medication with no strength (e.g. lactulose) or with multiple components (e.g. Abidec) can be prescribed in ml. All others must be in **mg, micrograms or mmol** for all electrolytes.

Practical Issues

The lack of licensed drugs for children causes practical problems every day for the paediatric pharmacist, doctor, nurse, family and patient. These include a lack of dose information. Prescribing too small doses may result in suboptimal therapy, or over-dosing may lead to adverse drug reactions. Many paediatric dose reference sources are available but, in some cases, they provide conflicting advice. They tend to be based on local practice and experience rather than hard evidence. A reputable paediatric dose reference source should be used.

Lack of Suitable Formulations

Children are often unable to swallow tablets or capsules and may be in danger of aspiration if they are pushed to do so. Palatable liquid formulations are needed to facilitate administration and accurate measurement of paediatric doses. Often these are not commercially available.

Suitable products such as oral liquid, powders or capsules may therefore have to be prepared extemporaneously. Little information may be available on the bio-availability of the drug or the physical, chemical and microbial stability of the preparation. The result is often unpleasant to take and the preparation will have a short shelf life.

Extemporaneous Dispensing

Extemporaneous dispensing should be seen as a last resort. Standards of extemporaneous dispensing are extremely variable and mistakes have happened with devastating consequences. Currently there are no common regulations or guidelines to regulate extemporaneous dispensing. It may be performed in a highly equipped laboratory, in a licensed "specials" manufacturing unit or in a hospital. In such areas, good manufacturing practice guidelines must be met and are enforced by regulatory authorities. This will involve trained personnel who are using strict checking and documentation procedures, suitable equipment and ingredients of a high standard, and are supported by appropriate quality assurance facilities. The whole production process is auditable in terms of ingredients used and personnel involved.

By contrast, extemporaneous dispensing can also be carried out on the dispensary bench in a community pharmacy, often with little equipment and documentation available. There are many variations between these extremes. Although some countries are developing, or have introduced, guidelines and standards, adherence is usually not a requirement. There needs to be a professional, ethical and legal obligation on practitioners to observe uniformed consistent standards in all areas where extemporaneous dispensing is performed.

Extemporaneous preparation also carries a health risk to pharmacy personnel. An extreme example is infertility and miscarriage in relation to cytotoxic drug handling. Measures are usually taken to ensure the safety of hospital and community pharmacy staff but much better facilities and standards of preparation are required in industry. It would be preferable for all such products to be prepared in a high quality environment to protect the staff involved, the product and the patient.

Alternatives to Extemporaneous Dispensing

A range of options to extemporaneous dispensing is available including:
- Choosing an alternative drug that is commercially available in a more suitable form for administration
- Obtaining a paediatric formulation for a "specials" manufacturer
- Using solutions prepared for injections by the oral route. This must be done with care as different formulations may include different salts and therefore have different bioavailability and stability. The pH of some injection solutions can cause problems and other excipients must be checked to be safe. The taste of many injections is problematic and the cost of using an expensive injectable form orally must be considered.
- Cutting tablets to half or quarter size with a tablet cutter. This may help though it is inaccurate and dose equivalence is unlikely to be achieved.
- Dissolving or dispersing tablets in water to make doses of less than a full tablet. Doses can be made up by dissolving a whole tablet in a specified volume and administering an aliquot of the resulting liquid with an oral syringe. Some tablets are soluble or dispersible even if they are not marketed as such. Having a list of such tablets can be helpful. There is a lack of research however to confirm the drug contents of aliquots of liquids when doses are measured in this way.
- Importing licensed formulations from other countries may be a preferable alternative. However, difficulties around importation of free movement of medicines between countries can make this a complicated process. It is also expensive and gaining access to information on such product availability is not always easy.

Excipients

It is important to be aware of inappropriate excipients in some medicine formulations (including some licensed products). The existence of colourings and preservatives has been highlighted in the press. Other examples include:
- A commercial formulation of Phenobarbital elixir containing 38% alcohol, which is clearly undesirable for children. It has been estimated that if a 5 ml (15 mg) dose was given to a 3 kg baby, this would be equal to an adult swallowing a couple of glasses of wine.
- Phenobarbital injection (200 mg in 1ml) contains 80-90% propylene glycol that can cause hyperosmolality if the injection is not diluted appropriately. The potential for toxicity is increased with babies and infants.
- Some excipients are undesirable in children with specific disorders. Children with phenylketonuria must avoid aspartame, for instance.

An EC Directive issued in 1997 stated that "benzyl alcohol is contraindicated in infants/young children". This has implications for formulation of medicines used in children. Summary of Product Characteristics (SPCs) for amiodarone and lorazepam injections now both state that they contain benzyl alcohol and are contraindicated in infants or young children up to three years old. This poses a dilemma given the lack of more appropriate alternatives for these patients.

The sugar content of medicines must also be considered, particularly with long-term treatment. However, it is unlikely to be a major issue in short-term medication.

OTHER ISSUES

Medication Errors

The lack of suitable, licensed formulations for children increases the risk of medication errors by complicating administration. Frequently, a small proportion of the content of an injection vial is required to administer a calculated dose. Miscalculation can lead to a ten-fold or even a 100-fold overdose for a small baby from one vial.

Dilution of adult strength injections is also often needed which can involve complex calculations. Fatal errors have indeed occurred.

Other complications are that displacement values must be taken into account and syringes have to be used carefully to avoid administration of the contents of the 'dead space' and overdosing with a concentrated drug.

Different reference sources quote doses in different ways. Some provide dose information as the total daily dose per kg bodyweight, which should then be divided into the appropriate number of doses per day. Others give the individual dose per kg bodyweight and the number of time daily this should be administered. Errors are common due to confusion between these systems. It is therefore essential that prescribers are familiar with the way the reference works to minimise the risk of prescribing errors.

Advanced Formulation

More advanced formulations are becoming increasingly available for adult patients, such as transcutaneous delivery system, fast dissolving drug formulations and multiple unit dose systems, which all offer potential major improvements. Generally, however, this new technology is not benefiting children as their needs are not being addressed in the development of these innovate products. This is unacceptable and must also be addressed at government and regulatory levels.

ACKNOWLEDGEMENTS

Thanks are due to NES (Pharmacy), the Scottish Neonatal Paediatric Pharmacists Group, and particularly to Steve Tomlin and Sharon Conroy for permission to use and adapt their material for this Chapter.

BIBLIOGRAPHY

1. An Introduction to Paediatric Pharmaceutical Care. NHS Education Scotland (Pharmacy) 2005.
2. The British National Formulary for Children. BMJ Publishing Group Ltd/RPS Publishing/RCPCH Publications Ltd 2006.

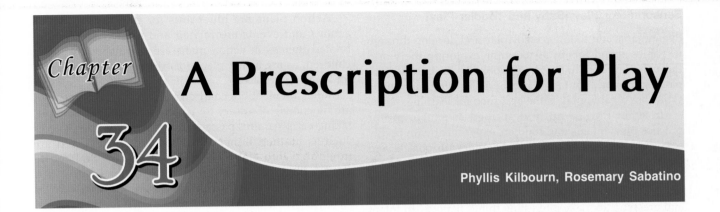

A Prescription for Play

Chapter 34

Phyllis Kilbourn, Rosemary Sabatino

INTRODUCTION

Play! What a wonderful word—the very essence of childhood! For those whose family saw the importance of play, it calls up memories of our own childhood years when playing was the main focus of our waking hours. "Will you play with me?" is one of the most expressive, expectant questions asked. The query carries with it hope and anticipation about a time of fun and make-believe, a world of adventure and exploration, the world of the child. Play becomes an activity in which the child takes control, is motivated from within and uses his or her imagination. The absence of play is viewed as an obstacle to the development of healthy and creative individuals. For this reason, play is important for health care providers to consider and prescribe play as a vital intervention that facilitates healthy childhood development and learning.

DEFINING PLAY

Play for children has been likened to work for an adult. It is what they do. Through play children learn about their world and the things in it.

Play also has been likened to a child's rehearsal or practice for life since through play a child finds the root of future successes. During play children can switch roles, control situations and experiment with a variety of scenes where they can be the authors, stars and directors of their world. Research has shown that if children can play well, they will adjust well as adults.

The dynamic process of play develops and changes, becoming increasingly more varied and complex. Considered a key facilitator for learning and development across domains, play reflects the social and cultural contexts in which children live.

Play is a window to the child's world and the adult who knows the value of play is committed to learning about children while they play. Play tells us much about children's lives, health and level of development. From observing their play we learn how children think, feel and believe. Play also can tell us of a child's pain, conflict and insecurity. Those who value the personhood of children should also value the play of children.

IMPORTANCE OF PLAY

Play allows children the chance to explore their environment, to learn how it works and how they relate to it. A child can express feelings and emotions through various types of play activities (games, art, stories, etc.) far earlier than they can express them in words. For older children, play may be the outlet through which they convey emotions that they are either unwilling to share verbally or do not have the sufficient vocabulary to express. Through play children can be anyone, at anyplace, at anytime.

Play is how children reconstruct their world in order to understand and master it. To be a child is to be little and powerless; someone big always has charge, telling you what to do.

In play children are autonomous; they're independent. They make the decisions, solve the problems and deal with the consequences. As Piaget[1] has said, autonomy should be the aim of education and to understand is to invent. In play, children are autonomous inventors.

DESCRIPTION OF FORMS OF PLAY

Play takes many forms. Children play when they sing, dig in the mud, build a block tower, or dress up. Play can be purely physical (running, climbing, ball throwing) or highly intellectual (solving an intricate puzzle, remembering the words to a song). Play also can be creative using crayons, clay and finger-paint. Play's emotional form is expressed when children pretend to be mummies, daddies or babies. Skipping rope with a friend or sharing a book are examples of the social side of play.

Sensorimotor Play (Baby and Toddler Play)

Even infants and toddlers enjoy play and develop through it. Babies spend lots of awake time exploring the world through play. To adults, it might look like the baby is "just playing around." In fact, the baby is learning many new skills. For a baby, play is the best time for learning.

In what Piaget[2] aptly described as sensorimotor practice play, infants and toddlers experiment with bodily sensation and motor movements, and with objects and people. By six months of age, infants have developed simple but consistent action schemes through trial and error and much practice. Infants use action schemes, such as pushing and grasping, to make interesting things happen. an infant will push a ball and make it roll to experience the sensation and pleasure of movement.

As children master new motor abilities, simple schemes are coordinated to create more complex play sequences. Older infants will push a ball, crawl after it and retrieve it. When infants of nine months are given an array of objects, they apply the same limited actions to all objects and see how they react. By pushing various objects, an infant learns that a ball rolls away, mobile spins around and a rattle makes noise. At about twelve months, objects bring forth more specific and differentiated actions.

A toddler's second year, brings a growing awareness of the functions of objects in the social world. The toddler puts a cup on a saucer and a spoon in her mouth. During the last half of this year, toddlers begin to represent their world symbolically as they transform and invent objects and roles. They may stir an imaginary drink and offer it to someone. Adults initiate and support such play. They may push a baby on a swing or cheer its first awkward steps. Children's responses regulate the adult's actions. If the swing is pushed too high, a child's cries will guide the adult toward a gentler approach. In interactions with adults such as peek-a-boo, children learn to take turns, act with others and engage others in play.

Toddlers play well on their own (*solitary play*) or with adults. They begin solitary pretend play around one year of age. During the toddler years, as they become more aware of one another, they begin to play side by side, without interacting (*parallel play*). They are aware of and pleased about other persons, but are not directly involved with them. During this second year toddlers begin some form of *coordinated play*, doing something with another child. This form is similar to the preschooler's *associative play*.[3]

Early Childhood (Pretend Play)

As children develop the ability to represent experience symbolically, pretend play becomes a prominent activity. In this complex type of play, children carry out action plans, take on roles and transform objects as they express their ideas and feelings about the social world.

Action plans are blueprints for the ways in which actions and events are related and sequenced. Family-related themes in action plans are popular with young children, as are action plans for treating and healing and for averting threats.

Roles are identities children assume in play. Some roles are functional, necessary for a certain theme. For example, taking a trip requires passengers and a driver. Family roles such as mother, father and baby are popular and are integrated into elaborate play with themes related to familiar home activities. Children also assume stereotyped character roles drawn from the larger culture, such as nurse, and fictional character roles drawn from books and television, such as Spider Man. Play related to these roles tends to be more predictable and restricted than play related to direct experiences such as family life.

By the age of four or five, children's ideas about the social world initiate most pretend play. While some pretend play is solitary or shared with adults, preschoolers' pretend play is often shared with peers in the school or neighborhood. To implement and maintain pretend play episodes, a great deal of shared meaning must be negotiated among children. Play procedures may be talked about explicitly, or signalled subtly in role-appropriate action or dialogue. Players often make rule-like statements to guide behaviour ("You have to finish your dinner, baby"). Potential conflicts are negotiated. Though meanings in play often reflect real world behaviour, they also incorporate children's interpretations and wishes.

Preschoolers learn differently from school-age children. Play is essential to their early learning and is the main way children learn and develop ideas about the world. It helps them build the skills necessary for critical thinking and leadership. It's how they learn to solve problems and to feel good about their ability to learn.

Children learn the most from play when they have skilled teachers who are well trained in understanding how play contributes to learning. Most child development experts agree that play is an essential part of a high-quality early learning program. Play is not a break from learning—it's the way young children learn.

The preschool years bring many changes for children in relation to social development. Children have more quality relationships outside the home and have a growing ability to play with other children. When children verbalize, plan and carry out play, cooperative play is established. This is the most common type of peer interaction during a child's pre-school years.[4]

Construction play with symbolic themes is also popular with preschoolers, who use blocks and miniature cars and people to create model situations related to their experiences. Rough and tumble play with a lot of motion is popular with preschoolers. In this play groups of children run, jump and wrestle. Action patterns call for these behaviours to be performed at a high activity level. Adults may worry that such play will become aggressive and they should probably monitor it. Children, who participate in this play become skilled in their movements, distinguish between real and pretend aggression and learn to regulate each other's activity.

School-age Play: Structured or Spontaneous

School-age children's playful activities can occur in two forms: structured and creative. Structured play tends to focus on a child's physical skill, natural talent or mental abilities to successfully engage in or with the game. Therefore structured play is extremely beneficial to the physical, mental and social development of a child and should be encouraged and practiced. Such a plan enables a child to gain skills, knowledge and self-confidence.

Structured play includes sports, board games and simple fun events such as jump rope or marbles. Regardless of the game's complexity or intensity, set rules govern the proper way to play. A child's unique personality is confined within the boundary of the rules.

Most play is unstructred and happens naturally when opportunity for play arises. Such spontaneous play is the unplanned, self-selected activity in which children freely participate. Children's natural inclinations are toward play materials and experiences that are developmentally appropriate. Therefore, when children are allowed to make choices in a free play situation, children will choose activities that express their individual interests, needs and readiness levels.

Dramatic play—or imaginative play—is a common form of spontaneous play. Here children assume the roles of different characters, both animate and inanimate. Children identify themselves with another person or thing, playing out situations that interest or frighten them. Dramatic play reveals children's attitudes and concepts toward people and things in their environment. Much play of this sort addresses a child's sense of helplessness and inferiority. Through dramatic play, they are the big superhero, capable of any feat!

Creative play engages the imagination. Creative play is the natural childlike ability to express one's personality, feeling and attitudes with imaginative words and actions. This play focusses on having fun and sharing in a relationship by using the imagination. A child's ability to make-believe adventures, activities or events—not game rules—sets the limits of the game. Participants win by playing with imagination rather than by competing successfully against each other. A child's skill, strength, intelligence or age is of no consequence.

PLAY: AN ESSENTIAL ELEMENT IN CHILD DEVELOPMENT

Practices and paradigms of what would be considered good child rearing and teaching have been debated, shifted, embraced and discarded over the years—yet basic concepts still remain. One of them is the child's intrinsic desire and tendency to play, which transcends age, time, culture, ethnicity, geography, socioeconomic circumstances, and abilities.[5] Acknowledging the child's inherent need to play, and that it effectively fulfils his desire to explore, learn, and discover, is key to understanding that play is a building block as essential to healthy child development as are food and rest.

According to early childhood specialist, Eric Strickland "Play involves the whole child. Play builds physical skills (such as balance, agility, strength, and coordination), cognitive skills (including language, problem solving, strategizing, and concept development), social skills (sharing, turn-taking, cooperation, and leadership), and the components for emotional well-being (joy, creativity, self-confidence, and so on). It is the fundamental process underlying most of the learning children do before they come to school."[6]

Physical Development

Because play often involves physical activity it aids in the development and refinement of both gross and fine motor skills for children of all ages. This process can be observed as infants playfully begin to explore their world and are given room to roll, scoot and eventually crawl. Babies enjoy reaching for small objects like mobiles, streamers, rattles and small toys and as a consequence even begin to develop some of the finer motor skills like hand-eye co-ordination.

Throughout childhood, as children vigorously and joyfully use their bodies in physical exercise-running, jumping, skipping, climbing, or throwing a ball, etc.—they are simultaneously releasing energy and developing muscles, balance, and skills that will help them feel confident, secure, and self-assured. As they gain increasing control over their bodies, and develop awareness of the space around them they learn to move safely and confidently in their environment.

In addition, during play children gradually become more adept at actions that involve different parts of the body. As they increase their skill at manipulating malleable materials and small items of equipment, they are also aiding the development of their small muscles. Fine motor control and hand-eye co-ordination are needed, for example, to build a tower of blocks, complete a jigsaw puzzle, draw a picture, manipulate play dough or interact with small toy figures. Large construction toys can help children's muscular development through any lifting, carrying, stretching or balancing they may do, and throwing and catching a ball will develop fine gross motor skills.[7]

No one is more convinced of the effects of play on learning and a child's physical development than education officials in Wales who introduced a play based curriculum for 3-7 year-olds in 40 schools throughout the country with Physical Activity as the foundational phase. According to Wales' officials, who see play as a vehicle for learning, the Physical Activity Phase is of prime importance because it impacts all other areas of learning. For example, they consider activities like legos, painting and pegboard as pre-writing experiences, since fine motor control is pre-requisite to holding a pencil properly in order to make marks on a paper and later produce precise writing patterns, letters and number.[8]

Recent findings from research on the brain and learning have bolstered the importance of play as having a physical impact on children. It is well known that active brains make permanent neurological connections that are critical to learning, and inactive brains do not make the necessary permanent neurological connections. Research on the brain demonstrates that play is a scaffold for development, a vehicle for increasing neural structures, and ameans by which children practice skills they will need later in life. These findings raise the importance of play to a more serious exercise that has a powerful impact on physical as well as cognitive development.

Cognitive Development

Have you ever watched children at play? If the answer is no, then try it some time. You will notice how totally absorbed they become in what they are doing, and their vivid imaginations and clever ideas will amaze you. They approach play with intense focus and inquiring minds.

No wonder then that practically all forms of play engage and enhance the development of cognitive related skills including imagination, creativity, problem solving, sorting and using information and negotiation skills with peers. For example, block building and sand and water play lay the foundation for logical matchematical thinking, scientific reasoning and cognitive problem solving.

Play fosters creativity and flexibility in thinking. Play has no right or wrong way to do things; a chair can be a car or a boat, a house or a bed. Pretend play fosters communication, developing conversational skills, turn-taking, perspective taking and the skills of social problem solving/persuading, negotiating, compromising and cooperating. Pretend play requires complex communication skills: children must be able to communicate and understand the message, "this is play." As they develop skill in pretend play, they begin to converse on many levels at once, becoming actors, directors, narrators, and audience, slipping in and out of multiple roles.[9]

We can see that play can have a beneficial effect on a child's development in the area of language. Through play children learn to ask questions or to develop an understanding of a new set of rules in a game. For example, in the case of construction play when children are building something with others, they need to be able to form an understanding of instruction. The same can be said of board games, where the explanation and understanding of the rules or instructions can aid the development of language skills.

Finally, research indicates a strong relationship between play and cognitive development. In her extensive study on the effects of pretend play and cognitive development, Doris Bergen of Miami University concluded, "There is a growing body of evidence supporting the many connections between cognitive competence and high-quality pretend play. If children lack opportunities to experience such play, their long-term capacities related to metacognition, problem solving, and social cognition, as well as to academic areas such as literacy, mathematics, and science, may be diminished. These complex and multidimensional skills involving many areas of the brain are most likely to thrive in an atmosphere rich in high-quality pretend play.[10,11]

Social and Emotional Development

The American Medical Association believes that the majority of a child' social skills come as a result of play since play enables children to interact and respond to others from an early age.[12] Children, like all human beings, have a basic need to belong to and feel part of a group and to learn to live and work in groups with different compositions and for different purposes. Play serves as a wonderful avenue for children to satisfy these needs and to develop social and emotional life skills. Children of all ages need to be socialized as contributing members of their respective cultures, and playing with others gives children the opportunity to match their behaviour with others and to take into account viewpoints that differ from their own.

Through play children can develop social skills, such as sharing with others, waiting their turn to do something, learning how to cooperate and how to lead and follow.

Children learn about themselves and others through play. By pretending, daydreaming, imitating others and having a good time, children learn to recognize their feelings and how to deal with them. In pretend play, children can be disobedient or uncooperative without getting in trouble. They can confront and overcome fears and, when under stress, play helps them forget their worries and gives them a chance to feel more in control of their world. At all levels of development, play enables children to feel comfortable and in control of their feelings by: (i) allowing the expression of unacceptable feelings in acceptable ways and (ii) providing the opportunity to work through conflicting feelings. In fact, children who play more seem to be happier and healthier.[13]

More than a respite from structured learning experiences, play is the cornerstone of learning and an integral link in the chain of healthy child development. As Dana Johnson, leading child play therapist puts it, "Play fosters the growth of healthy children in every aspect of development—physically, cognitively, socially and emotionally. It really is food for children's bodies, minds and spirits."

THE DANGERS OF PLAY DEPRIVATION

Sadly, in many parts of the World children are losing, and many have lost, the opportunity to engage in the crucial activity of play. Child soldiering, trafficking, exploitation, abuse, and abandonment are just some of the reasons that children, even at an early age, are being stripped of the fundamental rights and necessities of a meaningful childhood. In the United States, and many other countries, the emphasis on academic achievement and testing, the predominance of computer and electronic games, and the increased incidence of highly scheduled children in extra-curricular activities have diminished the importance of, and time allotted for, adequate and purposeful play experiences both in the classroom and at home. The effects of this loos could be far reaching.

No Time for Play

According to a study published by Dr Kenneth R Ginsberg and the American Academy of Pediatrics in 2006, a survey conducted by the National Association of Elementary School Principals in 1989 found that 96 percent of surveyed schools had at least 1 recess period. A decade later it was found that only 70 percent of even kindergarten classrooms had a recess period. In addition, since the introduction of the No Child Left Behind Act of 2001, the amount of time committed to recess, the creative arts and even physical education has been reduced considerably.

"This change may have implications on children's ability to store new information," stated Ginsberg, "because children's cognitive capacity is enhanced by a clear cut and significant change in activity." In addition, the reduced time for physical activity may also account for the present discordant academic abilities between girls and boys, since boys find it more difficult to navigate in that environment.

The Academy recognizes that play is important for optimal child development. It further endorses the position that every child deserves the opportunity to develop their unique potential and urges all child advocates to press for circumstances that allow each child to reap the advantages of play.[14]

The American Academy of Pediatrics has the following advice that can be applied worldwide:

- Promote free play as an essential part of childhood.
- Emphasize the advantages of active play and discourage parents from the overuse of passive entertainment.
- Emphasize that active child-centered play is a time-tested way of producing healthy, fit young bodies.

- Emphasize the benefits of "true" toys such as blocks and dolls, with which children use their imagination fully, over passive toys that require limited imagination.
- Educate families regarding the protective assets and increased resiliency developed through free play and some unscheduled time.
- Reinforce that parents who share unscheduled spontaneous time with their children and who play with their children are being wonderfully supportive, nurturing, and productive.
- Support parents to organize playgroups beginning at an early preschool age.
- Support children having an academic schedule that is appropriately challenging and extracurricular exposures that offer appropriate balance.

ADVICE FOR PARENTS (OR CAREGIVERS)

- *Allow for exploration:* Children play using their entire bodies and all of their senses. Let them see, hear, touch, smell and feel things to try them out. This means lots of supervision and regular checks to make sure they are exploring safely.
- *Watch your child play:* Be prepared for surprises! While watching your child play, you learn a lot about their interests, attention span and skills. Your observations tell you how to play with your children and when to offer new playthings as they grow. You'll also find the best time to join in.
- *Accept invitations to play:* Young children usually spend most of their time with parents and caregivers. Children may include you in their play naturally. Be ready to join in, but avoid taking over. Remember that children learn and enjoy more when they stay in charge of their own play. When adults respect children as they play with them, children play longer. This increases their attention span. Children learn more and show more advanced play when they have chances to play with adults.
- *Provide play space:* Small children need room to play. If your home or yard is unsafe or twoo small, find a park to play in several times a week. At home, teach your child the house rules and allow him to play in spaces where he can jump, climb, crawl and creep safely.
- *Provide playtime:* Young children play all the time. Routines like bathing, eating and dressing can be just as much fun and adventurous as trips to the park. Allowing a little extra time for everyone to have fun during these routines helps children develop a sense of time management and responsibility. This can help them now with their play skills and later in school and at work.

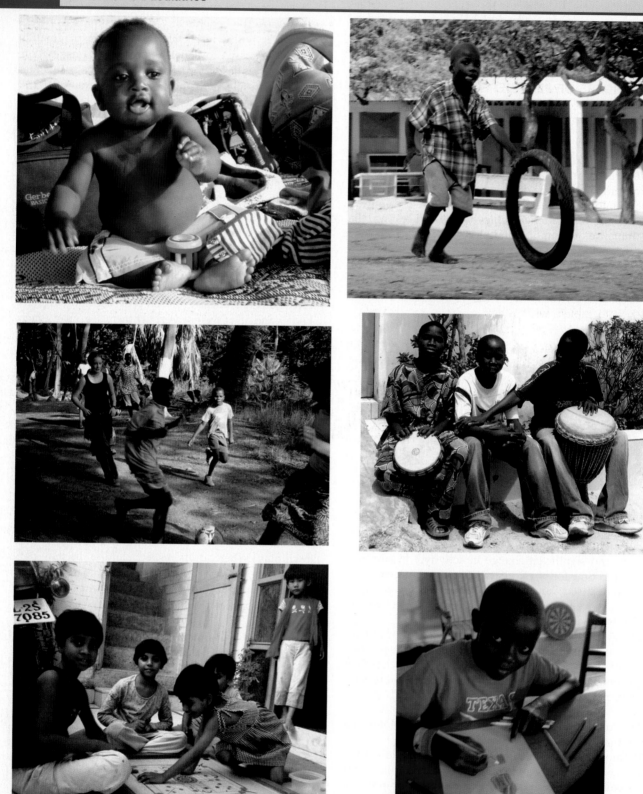

Figs 34.1 to 34.6: Figure games children play for fun and enjoyment

- *Provide play materials:* Children can create their own fun with crumpled paper, pots and pans, large cardboard boxes, play dough, paper, crayons and bubbles. Arrange a place for playthings where children can select them. A shelf is better than a clothes basket so children don't have to search for playthings. It also makes it easier for them to learn clean-up skills. When children lose interest in certain toys and other play materials, put those objects out of sight. Bring them back out a few weeks or months later. You may notice the children now use the toys differently because they have learned new skills.

- *Encourage different types of play:* Young children learn from many kinds of play. Encourage both quiet and active play. Encourage your children to play outdoors as well as indoors. Find ways to let them use their big muscles (legs, arms) and small muscles (fingers, toes). Let your children practice and repeat activities. Use words to explain what is happening when they play.

Through creative play, health providers and parents are given the unique opportunity to speak to a child in the language he or she understands and loves. And speaking in their language results in strong bonding and building of relationships (Figs 34.1 to 34.6 show Games children play for fun and enjoyment).

REFERENCES

1. Gordon, Ann Miles, Kathryn, Williams Browne; Beginning and Beyond: Foundations in Early Childhood Education (Delmar Publishers, NY& Canada, 1989), p.32.
2. Piaget, J. Play, Dreams and Imitation in Childhood, New York: Norton.
3. www.Kidsource.com/nature of child's play.
4. Gordon, Ann Miles and Browne, Kathryn Williams, Beginnings and Beyond: Foundations in Early Childhood Education (Delmar Publishers, California, 1989), pp. 324.
5. Playing for keeps, 2005, playingforkeeps.org.
6. Strickland, Eric, Ph.D.; Power olf Play; March 2000; Early Childhood Today.
7. Rise, Gabriel; Play and Child Development; 2006; Ezine @articles.
8. Teacher's TV; Learning Through Play; www.teachers.
9. Lessons in Learning; November 8, 2006; Canadian Counsel on Learning early Childhood Research and Practice.
10. Bergen, Doris: The Role of Pretend Play in Children's Cognitive Development; 2002, vol.4: Early Childhood Research and Practice.
11. American Medical Association; www.medem.com
12. Children at Play; The Creativity Institute; www.creativity institute.com
13. Johnson, Dana; When is Play Not Playing; 2007; Natural Family Online.
14. Ginsberg, Kenneth R: The importance of play in promoting healthy child development and maintaining strong parent-child bonds; 2006; American Academy of Pediatrics.

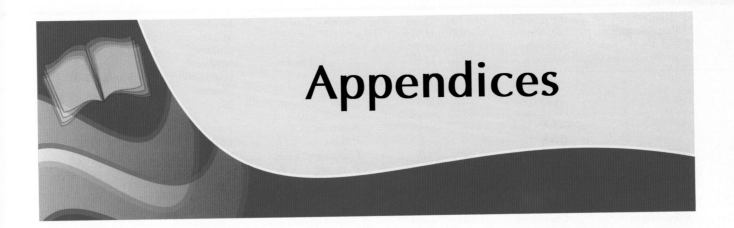

Appendices

Notes on International System of Units (SI Units)

Examples of Basic SI Units

Length	metre (m)
Mass	kilogram (kg)
Amount of substance	mole (mol)
Energy	joule (J)
Pressure	pascal (Pa)

Units of Volume and Concentration

Volume. The base SI unit of volume is the cubic metre (1,000 litre). Because of its convenience the litre is used as the unit of volume in laboratory work.

Amount of Substance ('Molar') Concentration (e.g., mol/l, μmol/l) is used for substances of defined chemical composition. It replaces equivalent concentration (mEq/l) which is not part of the SI system – for reporting measurements of sodium, potassium, chloride and bicarbonate (the numerical value of these four measurements is unchanged because the ions are univalent).

Mass Concentration (e.g., g/l, μg/l) is used for all protein measurements, for substances which do not have a sufficiently well-defined composition and for plasma vitamin B_{12} and folate measurements. The numerical value in SI units will change by a factor of 10 in those instances previously expressed in terms of 100 ml.

Haemoglobin is an exception. It is agreed internationally that meantime haemoglobin should continue to be expressed in terms of g/dl (g/100 ml).

APPENDIX A

A Guide to Biochemical Values

Those where large differences occur when compared to adult reference ranges are highlighted.

Blood

Acid-base [H^+]	38-45 nmol/l	pH 7.35-7.42
	(Neonates especially premature pH 7.2 - 7.5)	
pCO_2	4.5-6.0 kPa	(32-45 mmHg)
pO_2	11-14 kPa	(78-105 mmHg)
Bicarbonate [HCO_3^-]	22-27 mmol/l	
	(Preterm/< 1 month 17-25 mmol/l)	
Base excess	– 4 to +3 mmol/l	

Plasma: Electrolytes and Minerals

Sodium		135-145	mmol/l
Potassium	Newborns	4.3-7.0	mmol/l
	Older children	3.5-5.0	mmol/l
Chloride		95-105	mmol/l
Calcium	Preterm	1.5-2.5	mmol/l
	First year	2.25-2.75	mmol/l
	Children	2.25-2.70	mmol/l
Phosphate (lower in breast fed)	Preterm	1.4-3.0	mmol/l
	First year	1.2-2.5	mmol/l
	Children	0.9-1.8	mmol/l
Magnesium	Children	0.7-1.0	mmol/l
Copper	Birth to 4 weeks	5.0-12.0	μmol/l
	17-24 weeks	5.0-17.0	μmol/l
	25-52 weeks	8.0-21.0	μmol/l
	>1 year	12.0-24.0	μmol/l
Zinc		9.0-18.0	μmol/l
Iron	< 3 years	5.0-30.0	μmol/l
	>3 years	15.0-45.0	μmol/l
Ceruloplasmin	Newborn	0.05-0.26	gm/l
	Children	0.25-0.45	gm/l
Ferritin	**Infant**	**20-200**	**ng/ml**
	Children	**10-100**	**ng/ml**

Plasma: Other Analytes

Acetoacetate (incl. acetone)	<30	mg/l
AFP	< 6 months	

(Very high levels especially if premature – rapid fall over a week expected)

Alkaline phosphatase	> 6 months	< 10	U/ml
	Newborn	<800	U/l
	Children	100-500	U/l
Alanine aminotransferase (ALT)	Infants	10-60	U/l
	Children	10-40	U/l
Ammonia	Preterm	<200	µmol/l
	Newborn	50-80	µmol/l
	Infants and children	10-35	µmol/l
Amylase		<200	U/l
Ascorbic acid		15-90	µmol/l
Aspartate aminotransferase (AST)	<4 weeks	40-120	U/l
	>4 weeks	10-50	U/l
Bilirubin total (preterm greater)	Cord blood	<50	µmol/l
	Term day 1	<100	µmol/l
	Term days 2-5	<200	µmol/l
	>1 month	<20	µmol/l
Cholesterol	Cord blood	1.03-3.0	mmol/l
	Newborn	2.0-4.8	mmol/l
	Infants and children	2.8-5.7	mmol/l
Cortisol	Neonates use synacthen test		
	Diurnal variation after 10 weeks post-term		
Creatine kinase (CK)	Newborn	<600	U/l
	Infants	<300	U/l
	Children	<200	U/l
Creatinine	Newborn	20-100	µmol/l

Reflects Maternal level and declines over first month

	Infants and children	20-80	µmol/l
Creatinine clearance	0-3 months	30-70	ml/min/m²
	12-24 months	50-100	ml/min/m²
	Older children	90-120	ml/min/m²
C-reactive protein (CRP)		<7	mg/l
Folic Acid		10-30	nmol/l
Follicle-stimulating hormone (FSH)		<3	U/l
Gammaglutamyltransferase (γGT)	Newborn	<200	U/l
	1-6 months	<120	U/l
	>6 months	<40	U/l
Glucose	Newborn (<48h)	2.2-5.0	mmol/l
	Infants and children	3.0-5.0	mmol/l
Glycosated haemoglobin		4:1-6.1	%
	(DCCT aligned)		
17 OH Progesterone		>4 days	<13 nmol/l
		>60 confirms CAH	
Insulin	Fasting	<13	mU/l
	(Always measure glucose)		
Lactate (blood)	Newborn	<3.0	mmol/l
	Infants and children	1.0-1.8	mmol/l
		?0.7-2.1	
Lactate dehydrogenase (LDH)	<1 month	550-2100	U/L
	1-12 months	400-1200	U/l
	1-6 years	470-920	U/l
	6-9 years	420-750	U/l
	>9 years	300-500	U/l
Lipids – Triglycerides	Fasting	0.3-1.5	mmol/l
Luteinising hormone (LH)		<1.9	U/l
Osmolality		275-295	mmol/kg

Protein – Total	Newborn	45-70	gm/l	
	Infants	50-70	gm/l	
	Children	60-80	gm/l	
- Albumin	Newborn	25-35	gm/l	
	Infants and Children	35-50	gm/l	
- Immunoglobulins (g/l)	IgG		IgA	IgM
Newborn	2.8-6.8		0-0.5	0-0.7
Infants	3.0-10.0		0.2-1.3	0.3-1.5
Children >3 years	5.0-15.0		0.4-2.5	0.4-1.8
Pyruvate (blood)		50-80	µmol/l	

(Ratio Lactate/Pyruvate > 20 abnormal)

Free Thyroxine (T₄)	<1 month	6-30	pmol/l
	>1 month	9-26	pmol/l
Thyroid-stimulating hormone (TSH)	1-30 days	0.5-16	mU/l
	1 month-5 years	0.5-8	mU/l
	5 years -	0.4-6	mU/l
Tri-iodthyronine (T₃)	Newborn	0.5-6.0	nmol/l
	Infants and children	0.9-2.8	nmol/l
Urea		2.5-6.0	mmol/l

(Neonates often 1.0-5.0 mmol/l)

Uric acid	<9 years	0.11-0.3	mmol/l
Vitamin A	Preterm	0.09.1.7	µmol/l
	<1year	0.5-1.5	µmol/l
	1 year-6 years	0.7-1.7	µmol/l
	Older	0.9-2.5	µmol/l
25 Hydroxyvitamin D		>15	nmol/l
	Ideally > 25 + <100 nmol/l		
Vitamin E (α-tocopherol)	< 2 months	2-8	µmol/l
	1-6 months	5-14	µmol/l
	2 years	13-24	µmol/l

Urine

The kidney develops rapidly over the first year of life. Its handling of many filtered compounds is substantially different, e.g.

Urine calcium	Birth – 6 months	< 2.4 mmol/mmol Creatinine
	6-12 months	0.09-2.2 mmol/mmol Creatinine,
	1-3 years	0.06-1.4 mmol/mmol Creatinine,
	3-5 years	0.05-1.1 mmol/mmol Creatinine,
	7 years to adult	0.04-0.07 mmol/mmol Creatinine
Urine phosphate	7-12 months	1.2-19 mmol/mmol Creatinine
	1-3 years	1.2-12 mmol/mmol Creatinine
	3-6 years	1.2-8 mmol/mmol Creatinine
	Adult	0.8-2.7 mmol/mmol Creatinine

CSF

Protein	<1 month	0.26-1.2 gm/l
	1-3 months	0.1-0.8 gm/l
	>3months	0.1-0.5 gm/l

APPENDIX B

Age	Haemoglobin (g/dl)	Hct	MCV (fl)	WBC (× 10⁹/l)	Neutrophils (× 10⁹/l)	Lymphocytes (× 10⁹/l)	Monocytes (× 10⁹/l)	Eosinophils (× 10⁹/l)	Basophils (× 10⁹/l)	Platelets (× 10⁹/l)
Birth (term)	14.9-23.7	0.47-075	100-125	10-26	2.7-14.4	2.0-7.3	0-1.9	0-0.85	0-0.1	150-450
2 weeks	13.4-19.8	0.41-0.65	88-110	6-21	1.5-5.4	2.8-9.1	0.1-1.7	0-0.85	0-0.1	170-500
2 months	9.4-13.0	0.28-0.42	84-98	5-15	0.7-4.8	3.3-10.3	0.4-1.2	0.05-0.9	0.02-0.13	210-650
6 months	10.0-13.0	0.3-0.38	73-84	6-17	1-6	3.3-11.5	0.2-1.3	0.1-1.1	0.02-0.2	210-560
1 year	10.1-13.0	0.3-0.38	70-82	6-16	1-8	3.4-10.5	0.2-0.9	0.05-0.9	0.02-0.13	200-550
2-6 years	11.0-13.8	0.32-0.4	72-87	6-17	1.5-8.5	1.8-8.4	0.15-1.3	0.05-1.1	0.02-0.12	210-490
6-12 years	11.1-14.7	0.32-0.43	76-90	4.5-14.5	1.5-8.0	1.5-5.0	0.15-1.3	0.05-1.0	0.02-0.12	170-450
12-18 years female	12.1-15.1	0.35-0.44	77-94	4.5-13	1.5-6	1.5-4.5	0.15-1.3	0.05-0.8	0.02-0.12	180-430
Male	12.1-16.6	0.35-0.49	77-92							

Table B1: A guide to normal ranges for the FBC in infancy and childhood

Reproduced with permission from P. Simpson and R. Hinchcliffe/R. Arceci, I.Hann and O. Smith; Table of normal ranges and blood counts from birth – 18 years; Paediatric Haematology, Blackwell Publishing, 2006.

APPENDIX C

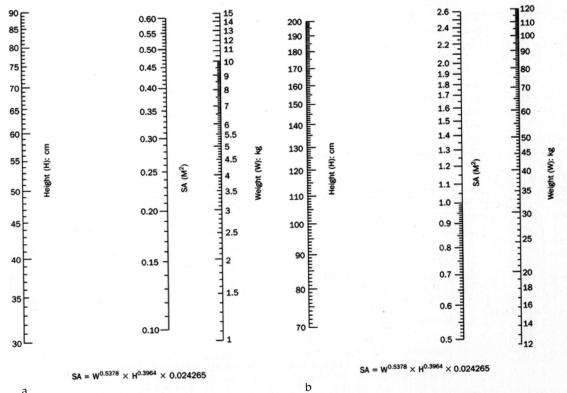

$$SA = W^{0.5378} \times H^{0.3964} \times 0.024265$$

a

$$SA = W^{0.5378} \times H^{0.3964} \times 0.024265$$

b

a. Nomogram representing the relationship between height, weight and body surface area in infants. (After Haycock et al. (1978) Geometric method for measuring body surface area: A height-weight formula validated in infants, children and adults. J Pediatrics 93,64-65).

b. Nomogram representing the relationship between height, weight and body surface area in children and adults. (After Haycock et al. (1978) Geometric method for measuring body surface area: A height-weight formula validated in infants, children and adults, J pediatrics 93, 64-65 (The editors and publisher gratefully acknowledge to reproduce the nomograms in this book).

APPENDIX D: PERCENTILES OF AGE SPECIFIC BLOOD PRESSURE MEASUREMENTS IN BOYS AND GIRLS
(Figures D1 to D4: Reproduced with permission from pediatrics: 79; 1-25, 1987. Copyright © AAP)

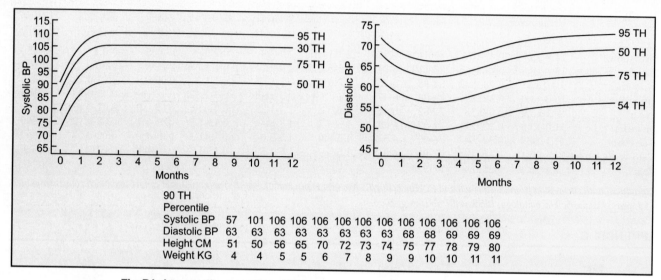

90 TH Percentile													
Systolic BP	57	101	106	106	106	106	106	106	106	106	106	106	106
Diastolic BP	63	63	63	63	63	63	63	63	68	68	69	69	69
Height CM	51	50	56	65	70	72	73	74	75	77	78	79	80
Weight KG	4	4	5	5	6	7	8	9	9	10	10	11	11

Fig. D1: Age-specific percentiles of BP measurements in boys—birth to 12 months of age.
Korotkoff phase IV (K4) used for diastolic BP

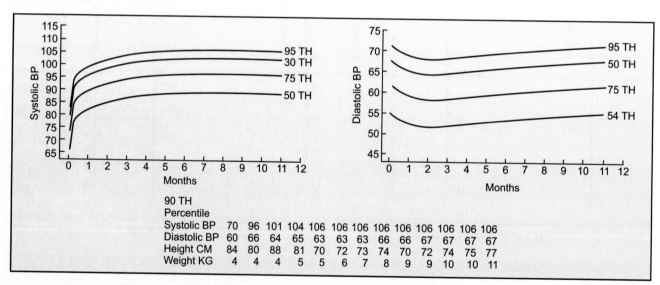

90 TH Percentile													
Systolic BP	70	96	101	104	106	106	106	106	106	106	106	106	106
Diastolic BP	60	66	64	65	63	63	63	66	66	67	67	67	67
Height CM	84	80	88	81	70	72	73	74	70	72	74	75	77
Weight KG	4	4	4	5	5	6	7	8	9	9	10	10	11

Fig. D2: Age-specific percentiles of BP measurements in girls—birth to 12 months of age;
Korotkoff phase IV (K4) used for diastolic BP

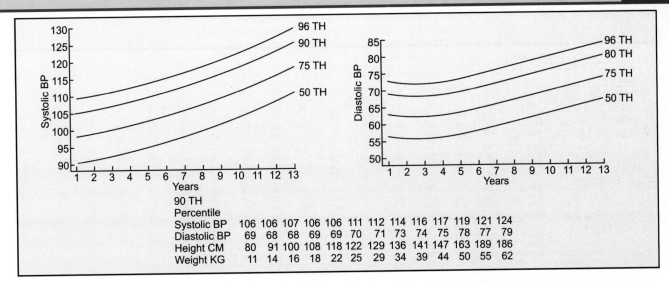

Fig. D3: Age-specific percentiles of BP measurements in boys—1 to 13 years of age;
Korotkoff phase IV (K4) used for diastolic BP

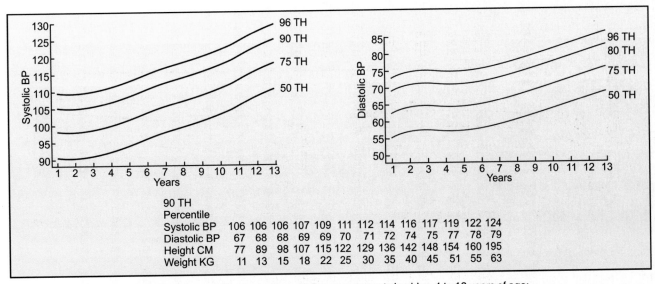

Fig. D4: Age-specific percentiles of BP measurements in girls—1 to 13 years of age;
Korotkoff phase IV (K4) used for diastolic BP

Table D1: BP levels for boys by age and height (Table D1 and D2 reproduce with permission from pediatrics 114:556-576, 2004. Copyright © AAP

Age, y	BP Percentile	SBP, mmHg Percentile of Height							DBP, mmHg Percentile of Height						
		5th	10th	25th	50th	75th	90th	95th	5th	10th	25th	50th	75th	90th	95th
1	50th	80	81	83	85	87	88	89	34	35	36	37	38	39	39
	90th	94	95	97	99	100	102	103	49	50	51	52	53	53	54
	95th	98	99	101	103	104	106	106	54	54	55	55	57	58	58
	99th	105	106	108	110	112	113	114	61	62	63	64	65	66	66
2	50th	84	85	87	88	90	92	92	39	40	41	42	43	44	44
	90th	97	99	100	102	104	105	106	54	55	56	57	58	58	59
	95th	101	102	104	106	108	109	110	59	59	60	61	62	63	63
	99th	109	110	111	113	115	117	117	66	67	68	69	70	71	71
3	50th	86	87	89	91	93	94	95	44	44	45	46	47	48	48
	90th	100	101	103	105	107	108	109	59	59	60	61	62	63	63
	95th	104	105	107	109	110	112	113	63	63	64	65	66	67	67
	99th	111	112	114	116	118	119	120	71	71	72	73	74	75	75
4	50th	88	89	91	93	95	96	97	47	48	49	50	51	51	52
	90th	102	103	105	107	109	110	111	62	63	64	65	66	66	67
	95th	106	107	109	111	112	114	115	66	67	68	69	70	71	71
	99th	113	114	116	118	120	121	122	74	75	76	77	78	78	79
5	50th	90	91	93	95	96	98	98	50	51	52	53	54	55	55
	90th	104	105	106	108	110	111	112	65	66	67	68	69	69	70
	95th	108	109	110	112	114	115	116	69	70	71	72	73	74	74
	99th	115	116	118	120	121	123	123	77	78	79	80	81	81	82
6	50th	91	92	94	96	98	99	100	53	53	54	55	56	57	57
	90th	105	106	108	110	111	113	113	68	68	69	70	71	72	72
	95th	109	110	112	114	115	117	117	72	72	73	74	75	76	76
	99th	116	117	119	121	123	124	125	80	80	81	82	83	84	84
7	50th	92	94	95	97	99	100	101	55	55	56	57	58	59	59
	90th	106	107	109	111	113	114	115	70	70	71	72	73	74	74
	95th	110	111	113	115	117	118	119	74	74	75	76	77	78	78
	99th	117	118	120	122	124	125	126	82	82	83	84	85	86	86
8	50th	94	95	97	99	100	102	102	56	57	58	59	60	60	61
	90th	107	109	110	112	114	115	116	71	72	72	73	74	75	76
	95th	111	112	114	116	118	119	120	75	76	77	78	79	79	80
	99th	119	120	122	123	125	127	127	83	84	85	86	87	87	88
9	50th	95	96	98	100	102	103	104	57	58	59	60	61	61	62
	90th	109	110	112	114	115	117	118	72	73	74	75	76	76	77
	95th	113	114	116	118	119	121	121	76	77	78	79	80	81	81
	99th	120	121	123	125	127	128	129	84	85	86	87	88	88	89
10	50th	97	98	100	102	103	105	106	58	59	60	61	61	62	63
	90th	111	112	114	115	117	119	119	73	73	74	75	76	77	78
	95th	115	116	117	119	121	122	123	77	78	79	80	81	81	82
	99th	122	123	125	127	128	130	130	85	86	86	88	88	89	90
11	50th	99	100	102	104	105	107	107	59	59	60	61	62	63	63
	90th	113	114	115	117	119	120	121	74	74	75	76	77	78	78
	95th	117	118	119	121	123	124	125	78	78	79	80	81	82	82
	99th	124	125	127	129	130	132	132	86	86	87	88	89	90	90
12	50th	101	102	104	106	108	109	110	59	60	61	62	63	63	64
	90th	115	116	118	120	121	123	123	74	75	75	76	77	78	79
	95th	119	120	122	123	125	127	127	78	79	80	81	82	82	83
	99th	126	127	129	131	133	134	135	86	87	88	89	90	90	91
13	50th	104	105	106	108	110	111	112	60	60	61	62	63	64	64
	90th	117	118	120	122	124	125	126	75	75	76	77	78	79	79
	95th	121	122	124	126	128	129	130	79	79	80	81	82	83	83
	99th	128	130	131	133	135	136	137	87	87	88	89	90	91	91
14	50th	106	107	109	111	113	114	115	60	61	62	63	64	65	65
	90th	120	121	123	125	126	128	128	75	76	77	78	79	79	80
	95th	124	125	127	128	130	132	132	80	80	81	82	83	84	84
	99th	131	132	134	136	138	139	140	87	88	89	90	91	92	92
15	50th	109	110	112	113	115	117	117	61	62	63	64	65	66	66
	90th	122	124	125	127	129	130	131	76	77	78	79	80	80	81
	95th	126	127	129	131	133	134	135	81	81	82	83	84	85	85
	99th	134	135	136	138	140	142	142	88	89	90	91	92	93	93
16	50th	111	112	114	116	118	119	120	63	63	64	65	66	67	67
	90th	125	126	128	130	131	133	134	78	78	79	80	81	82	82
	95th	129	130	132	134	135	137	137	82	83	83	84	85	86	87
	99th	136	137	139	141	143	144	145	90	90	91	92	93	94	94
17	50th	114	115	116	118	120	121	122	65	66	66	67	68	69	70
	90th	127	128	130	132	134	135	136	80	80	81	82	83	84	84
	95th	131	132	134	136	138	139	140	84	85	86	87	87	88	89
	99th	139	140	141	143	145	146	147	92	93	93	94	95	96	97

The 90th percentile is 1.28 SD, the 95th percentile is 1.645 SD, and the 99th percentile is 2.326 SD over the mean. For research purposes, the SDs in Table B1 allow one to compute BP Zscores and percentiles for boys with height percentiles given in Table 3 (ie, the 5th, 10th, 25th, 50th, 75th, 90th, and 95th percentiles). These height percentiles must be converted to height Zscores given by: 5% = −1.645; 10% = −1.28; 25% = − 0.68; 50% = 0; 75% 0.68; 90% = 1.28; and 95% = 1.645, and then computed according to the methodology in steps 2 through 4 described in Appendix B. For children with height percentiles other than these, follow steps 1 through 4 as described in Appendix B.

Table D2: BP levels for girls by age and height percentile

Age, y	BP Percentile	SBP, mmHg Percentile of Height							DBP, mmHg Percentile of Height						
		5th	10th	25th	50th	75th	90th	95th	5th	10th	25th	50th	75th	90th	95th
1	50th	83	84	85	86	88	89	90	38	39	39	40	41	41	42
	90th	97	97	98	100	101	102	103	52	53	53	54	55	55	56
	95th	100	101	102	104	105	106	107	56	57	57	58	59	59	60
	99th	108	108	109	111	112	113	114	64	64	65	65	66	67	67
2	50th	85	85	87	88	89	91	91	43	44	44	45	46	46	47
	90th	98	99	100	101	103	104	105	57	58	58	59	60	61	61
	95th	102	103	104	105	107	108	109	61	62	62	63	64	65	65
	99th	109	110	111	112	114	115	116	69	69	70	70	71	72	72
3	50th	86	87	88	89	91	92	93	47	48	48	49	50	50	51
	90th	100	100	102	103	104	106	106	61	62	62	63	64	64	65
	95th	104	104	105	107	108	109	110	65	66	66	67	68	68	69
	99th	111	111	113	114	115	116	117	73	73	74	74	75	76	76
4	50th	88	88	90	91	92	94	94	50	50	51	52	52	53	54
	90th	101	102	103	104	106	107	108	64	64	65	66	67	67	68
	95th	105	106	107	108	110	111	112	68	68	69	70	71	71	72
	99th	112	113	114	115	117	118	119	76	76	76	77	78	79	79
5	50th	89	90	91	93	94	95	96	52	53	53	54	55	55	56
	90th	103	103	105	106	107	109	109	66	67	67	68	69	69	70
	95th	107	107	108	110	111	112	113	70	71	71	72	73	73	74
	99th	114	114	116	117	118	120	120	78	78	79	79	80	81	81
6	50th	91	92	93	94	96	97	98	54	54	55	56	56	57	58
	90th	104	105	106	108	109	110	111	68	68	69	70	70	71	72
	95th	108	109	110	111	113	114	115	72	72	73	74	74	75	76
	99th	115	116	117	119	120	121	122	80	80	80	81	82	83	83
7	50th	93	93	95	96	97	99	99	55	56	56	57	58	58	59
	90th	106	107	108	109	111	112	113	69	70	70	71	72	72	73
	95th	110	111	112	113	115	116	116	73	74	74	75	76	76	77
	99th	117	118	119	120	122	123	124	81	81	82	82	83	84	84
8	50th	95	95	96	98	99	100	101	57	57	57	58	59	60	60
	90th	108	109	110	111	113	114	114	71	71	71	72	73	74	74
	95th	112	112	114	115	116	118	118	75	75	75	76	77	78	78
	99th	119	120	121	122	123	125	125	82	82	83	83	84	85	86
9	50th	96	97	98	100	101	102	103	58	58	58	59	60	61	61
	90th	110	110	112	113	114	116	116	72	72	72	73	74	75	75
	95th	114	114	115	117	118	119	120	76	76	76	77	78	79	79
	99th	121	121	123	124	125	127	127	83	83	84	84	85	86	87
10	50th	98	99	100	102	103	104	105	59	59	59	60	61	62	62
	90th	112	112	114	115	116	118	118	73	73	73	74	75	·76	76
	95th	116	116	117	119	120	121	122	77	77	77	78	79	80	80
	99th	123	123	125	126	127	129	129	84	84	85	86	86	87	88
11	50th	100	101	102	103	105	106	107	60	60	60	61	62	63	63
	90th	114	114	116	117	118	119	120	74	74	74	75	76	77	77
	95th	118	118	119	121	122	123	124	78	78	78	79	80	81	81
	99th	125	125	126	128	129	130	131	85	85	86	87	87	88	89
12	50th	102	103	104	105	107	108	109	61	61	61	62	63	64	64
	90th	116	116	117	119	120	121	122	75	75	75	76	77	78	78
	95th	119	120	121	123	124	125	126	79	79	79	80	81	82	82
	99th	127	127	128	130	131	132	133	86	86	87	88	88	89	90
13	50th	104	105	106	107	109	110	110	62	62	62	63	64	65	65
	90th	117	118	119	121	122	123	124	76	76	76	77	78	79	79
	95th	121	122	123	124	126	127	128	80	80	80	81	82	83	83
	99th	128	129	130	132	133	134	135	87	87	88	89	89	90	91
14	50th	106	106	107	109	110	111	112	63	63	63	64	65	66	66
	90th	119	120	121	122	124	125	125	77	77	77	78	79	80	80
	95th	123	123	125	126	127	129	129	81	81	81	82	83	84	84
	99th	130	131	132	133	135	136	136	88	88	89	90	90	91	92
15	50th	107	108	109	110	111	113	113	64	64	64	65	66	67	67
	90th	120	121	122	123	125	126	127	78	78	78	79	80	81	81
	95th	124	125	126	127	129	130	131	82	82	82	83	84	85	85
	99th	131	132	133	134	136	137	138	89	89	90	91	91	92	93
16	50th	108	108	110	111	112	114	114	64	64	65	66	66	67	68
	90th	121	122	123	124	126	127	128	78	78	79	80	81	81	82
	95th	125	126	127	128	130	131	132	82	82	83	84	85	85	86
	99th	132	133	134	135	137	138	139	90	90	90	91	92	93	93
17	50th	108	109	110	111	113	114	115	64	65	65	66	67	67	68
	90th	122	122	123	125	126	127	128	78	79	79	80	81·	81	82
	95th	125	126	127	129	130	131	132	82	83	83	84	85	85	86

* The 90th percentile is 1.28 SD, the 95th percentile is 1.645 SD, and the 99th percentile is 2.326 SD over the mean.
For research purposes, the SDs in Table B1 allow one to compute BP Z scores and percentiles for girls with height percentiles given in Table 4 (ie, the 5th, 10th, 25th, 50th, 75th, 90th, and 95th percentiles). These height percentiles must be converted to height Z scores given by: 5% = −1.645; 10% = −1.28; 25% = −0.68; 50% = 0; 75% = 0.68; 90% = 1.28; and 95% = 1.645 and then computed according to the methodology in steps 2 through 4 described in Appendix B. For children with height percentiles other than these, follow steps 1 through 4 as described in Appendix B.

Index